Emergency Care
in the Streets

EMERGENCY CARE IN THE STREETS

FIFTH EDITION

Nancy L. Caroline, M.D.

Adjunct Professor of Anesthesiology/Critical Care Medicine,
University of Pittsburgh School of Medicine,
Pittsburgh, Pennsylvania

Little, Brown and Company
Boston   New York   Toronto   London

Library of Congress Cataloging-in-Publication Data

Caroline, Nancy L.
    Emergency care in the streets / Nancy L. Caroline.—5th ed.
        p.   cm.
    Includes bibliographical references and index.
    ISBN 0-316-12891-0
    1. Medical emergencies.   2. Emergency medical technicians.
I. Title.
    [DNLM: 1. Emergency Medical Services.   2. Emergency Medical
Technicians.   3. Emergency Medicine.   WB 105 C292e 1995]
RC86.7.C38   1995
616.02'5—dc20
DNLM/DLC
for Library of Congress   94-30822
                                                     CIP

Printed in the United States of America

SEM

Editorial: Evan R. Schnittman
Production Editor: Marie A. Salter
Copyeditor: Debra Corman
Production Supervisor: Cate Rickard
Cover Designer: Cate Rickard

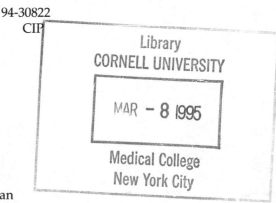
The publisher acknowledges photographers Jay K. Bradish, Brian
Clark, and Michael S. Kowal, NREMT-P. Special thanks to all
emergency medical personnel shown in this book; in particular, Bob
Anthony, Kurt Augustine, Jeff Dowling, Pamela Foster, Michael Gant,
Steve Knott, Alan Moore, Jaydee Prohosky, Daniel Tate, Mark Terry,
and Randy Wilkening.

To Peter Safar

Contents

Preface

In the late autumn of 1974, when Dr. Peter Safar talked me into leaving my relatively calm and secure enclave in the intensive care unit for the world of emergency care outside the hospital, I didn't know I was getting myself mixed up in a revolution. The revolution was in the immediate care of the critically ill and injured, and unwittingly I was being shipped off to the front lines, to marshal a new type of medical shock troops that went by the name of *paramedics*. My job presumably was to teach those troops the sophisticated techniques of advanced life support, but I had a great deal to learn from them as well. The first time I climbed into a sewer to do a resuscitation, I realized there were lots of things they never told me in medical school.

Nonetheless, I was in good hands. My teachers were veteran emergency medical technicians of the Freedom House Ambulance Service and were also very special human beings. They had been recruited by Dr. Safar in 1967 from among the "unemployables" of Pittsburgh's black ghetto and had been among the first ambulance personnel in the country to receive training in advanced life support. They were tough, skilled, compassionate, and professional.

For many months, I rode the ambulances with them. While they learned more emergency medicine, I learned the special stresses and constraints of rendering care outside the controlled conditions of a hospital: CPR in a crowded restaurant, childbirth in the lingerie section of a department store, splinting at the bottom of an elevator shaft, intravenous infusions inside a wrecked automobile. It was an education for all concerned—for the EMTs, for me, and also for the public, who were in those days unaccustomed to the idea that the emergency room had sprouted wheels and definitive care could now begin at the scene.

Out of that experience, the first edition of *Emergency Care in the Streets* was born, together with the first United States Department of Transportation (USDOT) curriculum for paramedics. Now this book is going into its fifth edition, the USDOT curriculum has been completely revised, and the revolution in immediate care of the ill and injured has become commonplace on the streets and byways of the United States and many other countries. The paramedic is no longer a strange new creature on the public scene, but rather has become an accepted and respected member of the medical community.

Nonetheless, the revolution isn't over yet. Many things are still changing out on the streets. Paramedics are better trained today and are deploying a variety of skills that were not part of the original curriculum. Thus, in this fifth edition of *Emergency Care in the Streets*, along with the updating of *all* previous material, there are entirely new sections on

- Critical incident stress debriefing
- Pulse oximetry
- End-tidal carbon dioxide monitoring
- New devices for maintaining an open airway
- Metered-dose inhalers and nebulizers
- 12-Lead electrocardiograms
- Active compression-decompression CPR
- Use of adenosine in cardiac dysrhythmias

There is only one certainty in the field of medicine, and that is that things change. At any time, new research and new data may overthrow some of our most cherished and firmly held concepts. That is another reason why this book—like other books in the medical field—must undergo periodic revision. It is likely, therefore, that also during the lifetime of *this* edition, there will be changes in the theory and practice relating to emergency medical care. Even as I write, debate continues over the use of anti-shock trousers, optimal techniques for cardiopulmonary resuscitation, early pharmacotherapy of spinal cord injury, and so forth. For that reason, this text (or any other text, for that matter) should not be regarded as the "last word" on every subject. It is, rather, an attempt to give the paramedic a firm grounding in the fundamental concepts—a basis on which to build through a professional lifetime of learning. The treatment recommendations presented here reflect, as much as possible, the current medical consensus. But that consensus may change, and local practice may differ. The paramedic, therefore, should keep abreast of new developments in prehospital emergency care through the professional journals in the field and should be guided in his or her practice by the policies of the local EMS system.

A note about the illustrations in this textbook: Throughout the text, for reasons of clarity, most procedures are shown carried out with ungloved hands.

It is taken for granted that in actual practice, the paramedic will wear surgical gloves for activities involving contact with blood or bodily secretions. Here too, things have changed.

Looking back now on the days I spent riding ambulances full time, I realize they were the best days I have known in medicine. They were days of adventure and challenge and the shared pride in having done a tough job well. I learned a lot from the paramedics, and this book belongs to them.

N.L.C.

A Word to Paramedic Instructors

In 1974, I wrote the first version of this book. A lot has changed since then. Paramedics today are a lot more sophisticated, a lot more professional, and have to do a job that has become a lot tougher.

Already by the 1980s it had become clear that the basic body of knowledge to be taught to an EMT-paramedic needed to be expanded; in 1982, the United States Department of Transportation (USDOT) created a support committee to ensure that the changes occurring in prehospital care were reflected in paramedic training curricula. The committee surveyed paramedic training programs in all 50 states and recommended updating the National Standard Training Curriculum for the EMT-paramedic to expand the knowledge base of the paramedic and include topics such as geriatrics, crisis intervention, the biomechanics of injury, and so forth. Accordingly, in 1985 USDOT issued a revised National Standard Training Curriculum reflecting the expanded knowledge objectives defined by the support committee.

The new curriculum clearly required a new textbook, and in 1991 *Emergency Care in the Streets* was entirely rewritten in accord with the revised USDOT curriculum and covers *all* of the objectives of that curriculum. In one or two places, I have introduced material in a sequence somewhat different from that of USDOT, when it seemed to me that the sequence of the current USDOT course was not optimal from a teaching standpoint. But all of the knowledge objectives of the USDOT course are fully covered in this textbook.

There is a great deal of new material in this edition of *Emergency Care in the Streets*, much of it added in response to requests from paramedic instructors. Thus the current edition now has **wholly new sections on**

- Critical incident stress debriefing
- Pulse oximetry
- End-tidal carbon dioxide monitoring

- New devices for maintaining an open airway
- Metered-dose inhalers and nebulizers
- 12-Lead electrocardiograms
- Active compression-decompression CPR
- Use of adenosine in dysrhythmias

as well as fully updated material in all subject areas.

Emergency Care in the Streets is intended, first and foremost, as a *learning* tool, and toward that objective it employs various didactic devices built into the format of the book. Each chapter begins with a list of **knowledge objectives** to enable the student to define precisely what is expected of him or her. Each of those knowledge objectives is systematically tested in the *Study Guide for Emergency Care in the Streets, Fifth Edition,* which was written to accompany this edition. Important points are highlighted in **boxed summaries** throughout the text, to permit quick reference during review. Logical processes are summarized in **flowcharts,** to help the student identify key decision points in evaluating and managing various emergencies. New vocabulary is highlighted in boldface type when it is first introduced, and summarized in **glossaries** both at the end of each chapter and at the end of the book. **Skill evaluation checklists** have been provided as an aid to practicing manual skills. At the end of each chapter, there is a list of **further reading** for those instructors or students who wish to pursue any particular subject in greater depth. Throughout the text, **illustrations** and **tables** help clarify and summarize important concepts.

The information on specific medications has again been collected in the **Drug Handbook** at the back of the textbook, for easier reference both during and after the course. The Drug Handbook contains detailed information on all of the field medications mentioned by USDOT, along with some others that are in common use in American EMS systems. A second section of the Drug Handbook contains an **Index to Commonly Prescribed Drugs,** organized alphabetically by trade name, to enable the paramedic to quickly identify the medications taken by a patient at home and the indications for which those medications are prescribed.

As I mentioned, a great many of the changes and additions made to this book were the result of suggestions from paramedic instructors throughout the United States, who were more than generous in sharing their teaching experiences with me. I hope that, thanks to their help, this fifth edition of *Emergency Care in the Streets* will prove a more effective aid to the very able teachers who are preparing the current generation of paramedics to do the best job possible.

N.L.C.

Acknowledgments

Not long ago, a medical colleague of mine congratulated me on the fact that I'd written one of the last remaining single-authored medical textbooks in the United States (or perhaps in the whole world). His tone was similar to the inflection one adopts on congratulating someone who has reached her 105th birthday, and there was also a small note of doubt lurking behind the compliment: How could any one person in this day and age be smart enough—that was the implication—to encompass medical disciplines as various as trauma, pediatrics, obstetrics, psychiatry, cardiology, and so forth? The fact is, I am *not* smart enough to do so. But what my colleague did not realize is that *Emergency Care in the Streets* is not, in any meaningful sense, a single-authored textbook. True, it is my name only that appears on the cover. But in fact I've had a lot of help, since the very first edition of this book, from some *really* smart and well-informed people in a variety of medical and other disciplines. For this fifth edition, I need particularly to acknowledge the help of:

Dr. Gerry Baum, wise physician and pulmonary specialist par excellence, who took time from his own formidable textbook of pulmonary medicine to review my chapters on respiratory emergencies, and whose unshakable optimism has carried me through many nonrespiratory emergencies

Dr. Eric Cassell, whose enthusiasm for this book kept me at it when my own enthusiasm had flagged, while his own wonderful books about the practice of medicine (and his practice of medicine itself) have helped me keep the faith

Ms. Debra Corman, veteran copy editor of all five editions of this book, who has kept me on the grammatical straight-and-narrow path for more than 16 years and who should, by now, be able to pass a paramedic certifying exam

Dr. Yoel Donchin, EMS cabbellero, who has been more than generous in sharing his wide knowledge of traumatology, both in person and via 20-page messages that come spilling off my fax machine in the small hours of the night

Dr. Mickey Eisenberg, classmate, penpal, writer of textbooks, chronicler of CPR, and innovator in EMS research, who still somehow finds time to keep me up to date on new developments in prehospital resuscitation

Mr. David Ladd, EMS leader, who has helped nurture this book in innumerable ways and who exemplifies the very best that a paramedic can be

Dr. Eugene Nagel, "father of the paramedics," treasured friend, and genie of the magic lamp, for whom my merest wish (for 50 ECGs, for a book I needed yesterday) is his command

Dr. Peter Safar, pioneer of resuscitation research, who got me into this business in the first place and who never forgets my birthday

Dr. Yakov Schweitzer, who reviewed the chapter on psychiatric emergencies, and whose "doing" and "being" have been equally impressive to the writer of that chapter

Ms. Mikki Senkarik, whose drawings were a highlight of the previous edition of this book and who came through at short notice with fine new illustrations for this edition

Dr. Alexander Waller, who reviewed the geriatrics chapter and whose day-to-day work as a hospice physician has been a continuing reminder to me, when reminders are often scarce, of all that is best in the practice of medicine

Dr. Gary Zentner, who once again went over the chapters on pediatric emergencies and neonatal care and provided genuine talmudic (even if sometimes irreverent) commentary thereon

Dr. Rodney Zenter, who examined the obstetrics and gynecology chapters line by line and found all the inaccuracies I had missed, and who has taught me, over the last two editions, more about obstetrics and gynecology than I ever hoped (or wanted) to know

The editorial and production team at Little, Brown—Evan Schnittman, my editor; Amy Mastrodomenico, Editorial Assistant; Priscilla Hurdle, Managing Editor; and Sue Michener, Production Manager—who called cheery messages to me through a Microsoft Window and saw this book safely through its various stages of production; and Marie Salter, Production Editor, who served as midwife through the book's difficult labor and delivery

The ICU nurses of Winter Haven Hospital in Winter Haven, Florida—particularly Mary-Jo Schreiber, Clinical Specialist, and Dorothy Ruggieri, Supervisor, Neurosurgical/Surgical ICU—who unfailingly managed to come up with precisely the electrocardiograms I needed, once again in the shortest time ever recorded

The paramedics of Boston, Pittsburgh, and Kiryat Shmona, Israel, with whom I continue to share adventures now and then and who set a standard of professionalism that any paramedic anywhere could be proud to match

My students, wherever they may be, whose relentless questions keep life interesting

I

THE PREHOSPITAL WORLD

1
Roles and Responsibilities of the Paramedic

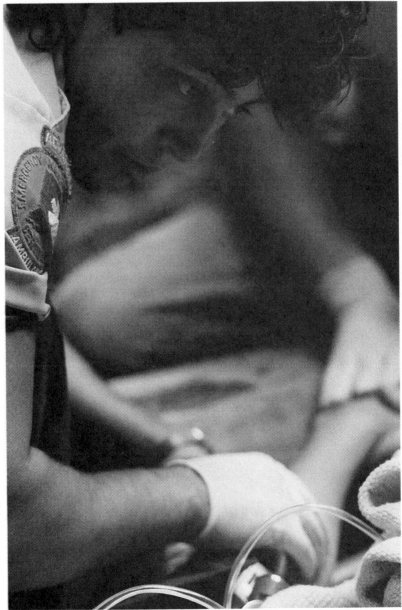

Parke County Emergency Medical Services, Rockville, Indiana. Photo by Michael S. Kowal.

OBJECTIVES

In real life, paramedics try to comfort little old ladies with broken hips, and they sometimes help derelicts who are dirty and smell bad. Other times, they take abuse from people who are under the influence of drugs or alcohol. Occasionally, they get called to exciting and dangerous emergencies that would make a good TV show, but that doesn't happen every day.

Good paramedics understand that the routine and *un*glamorous parts of their job are important too. Their occupation may not be as exciting or glamorous as the TV version, but what could be more important than having the right and the responsibility to protect and care for the life and health of other people?

Jim Page, Editor-in-Chief of *JEMS**

In this chapter, we shall examine how paramedics came to be, what paramedics do, and what gives paramedics the authority to function. By the end of this chapter, the student should be able to:

1. Describe the attributes desirable in a paramedic
2. List at least five responsibilities of a paramedic
3. List at least five skills performed by paramedics that may not be performed by the emergency medical technician–ambulance (EMT-A)
4. Explain why medical control is necessary for paramedic services
5. Give an example of
   - Prospective medical control
   - Immediate medical control
   - Retrospective medical control
6. Identify the correct definition of
   - Certification
   - Licensure
7. List at least three ways of preventing skills and knowledge from getting "rusty"

HOW DID PARAMEDICS COME TO BE?

Thirty-five years ago, there was no such thing as an emergency medical technician–paramedic (EMT-paramedic, EMT-P). Today, there are more than 75,000 EMT-paramedics in the United States and another several thousand in various other countries, including Australia, Canada, the United Kingdom, and Germany.

The story begins, in fact, in Belfast, Northern Ireland, as well as in Germany and several countries of Eastern Europe, where mobile intensive care units

(MICUs) were introduced in the 1950s and 1960s to enable early care of the critically ill and injured. The idea was very simple: Bring the emergency room *to* the patient before bringing the patient to the emergency room and thereby save precious minutes that could mean the difference between life and death. It soon became clear that the idea worked, and MICUs—staffed with specialist physicians—began to proliferate in various European countries.

In the United States, however, it proved unfeasible to staff a sufficient number of ambulances around the clock with physicians specially trained in emergency care. To begin with, at that time—in the early 1960s—there *were* no physicians specially trained in emergency care. The early MICUs in the United States—such as Dr. William Grace's mobile heart unit in New York City or Dr. James Warren's Heartmobile in Columbus, Ohio—were staffed principally by cardiologists. But very few American physicians, specially trained or not, were interested in riding around in ambulances; most preferred working in the more controlled setting of a hospital, clinic, or medical office. So it became necessary to look for alternatives to physician staffing of MICUs, and various doctors in the United States began asking the question: Can a *nonphysician* be taught the sophisticated skills of advanced life support?

The first doctor to provide an affirmative answer to that question was Dr. Eugene Nagel, then of Miami, Florida. Dr. Nagel, considered to be "the father of the paramedics," trained Miami firemen in advanced emergency skills to supplement the basic first aid that they had learned as part of their fire training. In addition, Dr. Nagel developed a telemetry system that enabled the firemen to transmit a patient's electrocardiogram to doctors at Jackson Memorial Hospital and to receive radio instructions from the doctors regarding what measures to take. With the introduction of that radio/telemetry communication, the rescuer working in the street became an extension of the doctor working in the emergency room.

The idea of paramedic-staffed MICUs operating under radio command by physicians spread quickly. And by 1970, the question—can a nonphysician be taught the sophisticated skills of advanced life support?—had been answered with a resounding affirmative. Pioneering programs in Miami, Seattle, Pittsburgh, and several other cities demonstrated that highly trained paramedics under radio command from a physician could indeed do the job, and the paramedic came into his (and her!) own. By 1976, the United States Department of Transportation (US-DOT) issued the first set of national standards and guidelines for paramedic training. And by the end of the 1980s, more than 50,000 paramedics were certified in the United States (Table 1-1).

*Quoted from *JEMS* 11(8):S–8, 1989.

TABLE 1-1. EMTs IN THE UNITED STATES AND CANADA, 1993

STATE/PROVINCE	EMT-As	EMT-Is	EMT-Ps
Alabama	6,552	1,675	2,202
Alaska	2,000	900	180
Arkansas	4,200	217	644
California	40,000	300	7,000
Colorado	10,600	500	1,200
Connecticut	16,387	1,345	938
Delaware	1,238		132
District of Columbia	1,400	10	220
Florida	18,547	0	7,860
Georgia	6,500	350	2,300
Hawaii	350	0	249
Idaho	3,877	637	115
Illinois	19,934	1,434	5,924
Indiana	12,439	1,474	1,228
Iowa	2,503	4,874	960
Kansas	6,378	784	
Kentucky	9,750		750
Louisiana	3,472	364	681
Maine	2,670	573	417
Maryland	11,000	1,300	600
Massachusetts	13,959	375	900
Michigan	12,007	1,601	2,928
Minnesota	13,185	254	1,167
Mississippi	2,025	175	404
Missouri	6,077		2,054
Montana	2,300	180	90
Nebraska	6,800	31	127
Nevada	4,500	530	144
New Hampshire	4,000	616	269
New Jersey	16,000		1,030
New Mexico	3,550	645	455
New York	30,580	2,361	2,728
North Carolina	16,523	1,872	1,900
North Dakota	2,174	192	134
Ohio	21,914	3,336	6,285
Oklahoma	4,007	545	630
Oregon	3,493	1,717	1,392
Pennsylvania	26,132		4,488
Rhode Island	2,000	577	65
South Carolina	3,619	832	1,430
South Dakota	3,237	85	81
Tennessee	6,000		1,450
Texas	24,959	3,172	8,121

TABLE 1-1   (continued)

STATE/PROVINCE	EMT-As	EMT-Is	EMT-Ps
Utah	4,785	100	265
Vermont	1,012	288	34
Virginia	22,267		1,103
Washington	10,491		1,542
West Virginia	8,435	6	691
Wisconsin	6,450	878	906
Wyoming	1,500	800	19
TOTALS	463,778	37,905	76,432
Alberta	1,350	—	500
British Columbia	No information	—	No information
Manitoba	No information	—	No information
New Brunswick	No information	—	No information
Newfoundland	700	—	—
Ontario	4,917	—	No information
Prince Edward Island	71	—	—
Quebec	—	3,100	—
Saskatchewan	1,800	—	—
TOTALS	8,838	3,100	500

EMT-A = EMT-ambulance (basic EMT); EMT-I = EMT-intermediate; EMT-P = EMT-paramedic.
Source: Data from the state and province survey published in *Emergency Medical Services* 22(12):188, 1993.

WHAT IS A PARAMEDIC?

What, then, *is* a paramedic, and what does he or she do? The EMT-P provides prehospital emergency care, under the command of a physician, to acutely ill or injured patients. The precise role of a paramedic is, in fact, defined by a specific body of knowledge and skills. It is with that particular collection of knowledge and skills that this book is concerned. But in more general terms, a paramedic is a *health care professional,* and the paramedic's role is defined by that phrase:

Health is the state of being sound in body, especially freedom from disease or pain.
Care is painstaking or watchful attention, caring management, and solicitude.
A *professional* is a person having certain special skills and knowledge in a specific area and con-

forming to the standards of conduct and performance in that area.

Putting it all together, the paramedic is a person who has special, well-defined skills and knowledge in prehospital emergency care; who is concerned for the well-being of others; and who exercises in his or her daily work painstaking attention to all assigned tasks in order to promote the well-being of others.

The special status of the paramedic as a professional entails many special responsibilities. As a paramedic, you will be responsible for the care of the vehicle and its gear; you must know how to troubleshoot every piece of equipment in the vehicle and must be certain that the vehicle is fully stocked before every emergency run. As a paramedic, you must be capable of a prompt and efficient response to the scene of an emergency, with due regard for traffic safety and local laws pertaining to the operation of an emergency vehicle. You must be able to gain control of a scene rapidly, managing bystanders and removing patients from possible hazard. As a paramedic, you are the representative of the patient's best interests, and you must not permit the actions of others, including police, to compromise the patient's care. You must know how to stabilize a patient prior to transport and must ensure the continuing care of the patient while en route to the hospital. At the hospital, you must be able to supply a thorough and accurate report of the patient's history, physical findings, and treatment. You should know when to seek help from the medical director or from supporting services such as fire and police. You must be conversant with the regulations governing communications over the radio. And you must know the essentials of good record-keeping.

In your personal conduct as a paramedic, you must remain in complete self-control in emergency situations, staying calm under stress and dealing sympathetically with those whose behavior may be altered by illness or anxiety. You must demonstrate interest in the patient's feelings and respect for his or her privacy, making an effort to shield the patient from the stares of curious bystanders. Your personal appearance, as a paramedic, should also reflect the standards of a professional—hair combed, uniform clean and pressed, shoes shined. For if you are sloppy about your appearance, the patient may legitimately wonder whether you are also sloppy about carrying out your job. Professionalism means taking pride in who you are and what you do.

WHAT DOES A PARAMEDIC DO?

The paramedic must master a variety of complex skills that are not practiced by the basic-level emergency medical technician (EMT-A). The skills that define a paramedic are summarized in Table 1-2. Many of those procedures can be very hazardous if performed by persons poorly trained in their use; thus the paramedic must take responsibility for maintaining competence in the skills necessary to sustain life and prevent injury.

In addition to being a health care *provider*, the paramedic—like any other health professional—must also be a health *educator*. In some regions, for example, paramedics participate as CPR instructors for the American Heart Association and the American Red Cross. Paramedics serve as teachers in many other situations as well: advising patients on sound health practices; training other emergency medical technicians; and even teaching other health professionals,

such as nurses and medical students, the fundamentals of prehospital emergency care. Teaching helps the paramedic keep his or her own skills sharp; at the same time, teaching identifies the paramedic as a resource person in the community.

Perhaps the most special aspect of the paramedic's job, however, derives from his or her unique relationship with the doctor in charge of the service. For the paramedic is no more nor less than the eyes, ears, and hands of the medical director. Through the paramedic's observations and report, the doctor in charge must be able to make an accurate assessment of a patient that the doctor can neither see nor touch; through the paramedic's hands, the doctor must render skilled, appropriate treatment. In their management of the critically ill and injured, paramedic and doctor are linked only by a radio, and the success of their endeavor depends on earned mutual trust and respect.

MEDICAL CONTROL

What principally distinguishes the paramedic (EMT-P) from the basic-level emergency medical technician (EMT-A) is that the paramedic carries out a variety of invasive procedures—procedures that otherwise are permitted only to doctors. The law, however, does not give the paramedic any independent authority to act. In carrying out invasive procedures in the field, the paramedic functions solely as an extension of a licensed physician. Ultimately, responsibility for the patient belongs to the physician, so the physician must exercise control and supervision of paramedics acting on his or her behalf. **Medical control** is what provides the legal framework for paramedics to act in behalf of doctors.

Probably the most conspicuous part of medical control is the direct radio communication between paramedics in the field and a doctor at a base station, usually in a hospital. In fact, that dialogue between paramedic and doctor—however important—is only a small part of what goes into effective medical control of prehospital emergency medical services (EMS). To begin with, long before the paramedics take their first call, qualified physicians have to participate in various planning activities to establish training standards, medical protocols, and operational guidelines for the system. All of those activities can be regarded as *prospective* medical control, that is, medical control activities that are carried out before the EMS system goes into operation.

The next phase of medical control is *immediate* medical control, which is the control exercised by the

TABLE 1-2.   PARAMEDIC SKILLS

Airway management	Endotracheal intubation
	Cricothyrotomy*
	Transtracheal jet ventilation*
	Pharyngeal and endotracheal suctioning
Ventilatory support	Mouth-to-mouth ventilation
	Pocket mask ventilation
	Bag-valve-mask ventilation
	Demand valve ventilation
	Oxygen administration
	Pneumothorax decompression*
Circulation/shock	Intravenous cannulation
	Vagal stimulation techniques
	Cardiac monitor lead placement
	Cardiac rhythm interpretation
	Cardioversion/defibrillation
	Transthoracic pacemaker*
Clinical assessment	Rapid, thorough patient history and physical examination
	Prioritization of care
	Triage multiple casualties
Fractures and dislocations	Spinal immobilization
	Use of extrication devices
	Traction and splinting
Administration of medications	Intravenous, intramuscular, subcutaneous
	Oral, topical
	Inhaled, nebulized, endotracheal
	Correct drug, dosage
Obstetric techniques	Emergency childbirth
	Neonatal resuscitation
	Fundal massage
Communication	Accurate, appropriate patient information
	Accurate, appropriate response to verbal and standing orders
	Accurate written reports
	Emergency scene management
	Crisis intervention and other communication skills

*Not required in all paramedic programs

medical director or his designee over the care being delivered to individual patients. There remains some controversy over how much immediate medical control is necessary. In some EMS systems, direct voice communication between physician and paramedics ("on-line medical control") is required for every advanced life support procedure; that is, the paramedic must obtain a voice order from a physician to start an intravenous (IV) infusion, intubate the trachea, give medications, and so forth. In other EMS systems, paramedics function entirely by protocol and standing orders: For any given medical emergency, they have a list of instructions as to what steps to take, and they need not radio for orders until after they have

carried out the protocol. Most EMS systems employ some combination of those two approaches. For cases of cardiac arrest, for example, paramedics might have standing orders to initiate CPR, attempt defibrillation, and start an IV before calling in by radio for further instructions.

Finally, there is a third aspect of medical control, *retrospective* medical control, which is, in fact, a form of continuing education for all concerned. Retrospective medical control involves reviewing cases with all those who took part—the paramedics, emergency department personnel, the medical director—to see how the care of the patient could have been improved. Was the patient accurately assessed in the field? Was he given appropriate care? Were there unwarranted delays at any stage of the response? Retrospective medical control also involves statistical analyses of ambulance calls: How many calls come in per month? What kind of calls? What is the average response time? What percentage of patients with cardiac arrest outside the hospital survive to hospital discharge?

Asking those questions and going over individual cases help us to identify shortcomings in the system—in training, in paramedic performance, in medical command itself—and thereby to find ways to improve the system. The object of the exercise, of course, is to improve the care given to patients.

Ultimately, that is what medical control is really all about—ensuring the best possible care for the patient, an objective shared by the whole EMS team. Some paramedics, especially those who are insecure about their own capabilities, tend to resent the "interference" of an EMS medical director in individual calls; such paramedics feel that any intervention by a doctor indicates lack of confidence in the paramedic. It is useful to remember, however, that the physician asking you questions over the radio is trying, as you are, to do the best for the patient. It is also very reassuring to know, when you are out there on the streets, that there is expert advice just a radio call away.

CERTIFICATION AND LICENSURE

Not just anyone can walk into the local ambulance service and call himself a paramedic. Just as there are agencies and procedures for credentialing doctors and nurses, so too there are agencies and procedures for granting credentials to paramedics. Whether for doctors, nurses, or paramedics, the objectives of credentialing are the same: to protect the public from incompetence and to provide for professional identification.

In general, there are two forms of credentialing. The first is **certification,** or **registration.** Certification is the process by which an agency, such as a specialty board in medicine, grants recognition to an individual who has met predetermined qualifications specified by that agency. For example, the National Registry of Emergency Medical Technicians (NREMT) gives a written and practical examination for certification as a paramedic. Many states will accept NREMT certification in lieu of taking the state examination.

Most states also require periodic **recertification,** usually every 2 or 3 years. Recertification requirements may include accumulating a certain number of hours of continuing medical education along with passing a state recertification examination.

The second form of credentialing, **licensure,** is a process by which a governmental agency, on verifying that an applicant has attained the minimal degree of competency necessary, grants permission to the individual to engage in a given occupation. In the United States, licensing of medical professionals is a state function, although a state may opt to use a national examination as the basis for granting state licensure. The state of Ohio, for example, requires that a person seeking a license as a paramedic must have taken a state-accredited paramedic training program and passed the NREMT paramedic examination. In Pennsylvania, on the other hand, the licensure requirement is the attainment of a score of 75 percent on the state licensure examination. Since such licensing prerequisites vary from state to state, it is essential for each paramedic to be familiar with the licensing requirements of the state in which he or she is working and to maintain certification and licensure as required under state law.

CONTINUING MEDICAL EDUCATION

As noted, nearly every state in the United States requires a certain number of hours of continuing medical education as a prerequisite for paramedic recertification. For example, in California, a paramedic must complete 48 hours of continuing education, including CPR and field care audits, in addition to passing a recertification examination every 2 years. The reason for a continuing education requirement is simple: Facts get forgotten. Skills get rusty. And a patient's life may depend on one of those facts that you've forgotten or one of those skills that you can no longer perform competently. So it is absolutely crucial to take time periodically to review what you learned and to practice your skills. In medicine, furthermore, new facts and new equipment, often requiring new skills, are appearing all the time. Continuing education is a way of keeping up-to-date.

Continuing medical education need not be a tedious chore. There are a lot of ways of staying sharp, for example:

- Reading some of the **professional journals** that are published specifically for EMTs. (See Additional Reading at the end of this book for some suggestions.)
- Attending **workshops,** conferences, or other medical meetings.

- Organizing weekly **debriefing** sessions with the medical director to discuss interesting or difficult cases.
- **Teaching** others what you have learned.

No matter what requirements are mandated by the state licensing agency, responsibility for continuing medical education ultimately rests with each individual paramedic. You are the only person who knows which subjects have become alarmingly foggy in memory, which procedures leave you feeling as if you have ten thumbs. And you are the person who will have to live with the questions and doubts that inevitably arise after something goes wrong in the field. Continuing medical education is a way to help make sure that things *don't* go wrong.

CONCLUSION

The role of paramedic entails new prestige, but it also imposes new responsibilities. Paramedics are entrusted with the lives of other human beings, and there is no more awesome or sacred responsibility than that. Your education as a paramedic must not stop with this text. You must continue to read and study and ask questions, to refine your knowledge and skills, so that you may give to each patient the best of which you are capable. You must learn to conduct yourself with humility, to accept criticism, to learn from mistakes as well as from triumphs, and to demand of yourself and your colleagues nothing less than the best. For only then will the title of paramedic signify what it is meant to signify: a commitment to other human beings.

GLOSSARY

certification   The process by which a professional association grants recognition to an individual who has met predetermined qualifications specified by that association.

licensure   The process by which a governmental agency grants permission to an individual to engage in a given occupation.

medical control   The supervision of paramedics by physicians that provides the legal framework for paramedics to function.

MICU   Abbreviation for *mobile intensive care unit*, an ambulance staffed and equipped to give advanced life support.

FURTHER READING

ROLE OF THE PARAMEDIC

Allison EJ et al. Specific occupational satisfaction and stresses that differentiate paid and volunteer EMTs. *Ann Emerg Med* 16:676, 1987.

Benson K. The drive to license: What lies ahead on the road to EMS as a profession? *Emergency* 26(1):32, 1994.

Caroline NL. Will the real paramedic please stand up? *Emerg Med Serv* 6:16, 1977.

Dunn JJ et al. Patient and house officer attitudes on physician attire and etiquette. *JAMA* 257:65, 1987.

Frey R, Nagel E, Safar P (eds.). *Mobile Intensive Care Units*. New York: Springer-Verlag, 1976.

Jacobs LM et al. Congruency in physician-EMT assessment. *Ann Emerg Med* 10:205, 1981.

Latman N, Wooley K. Knowledge and skill retention of emergency care attendants, EMT-As and EMT-Ps. *Ann Emerg Med* 9:183, 1980.

McManus WF, Darin JC. Can the well-trained EMT-paramedic maintain skills and knowledge? *JACEP* 5:984, 1976.

Page JO. Paramedic services—a true extension of emergency medicine. *Ann Emerg Med* 14:994, 1985.

Page JO. Making a difference in an angry world. *JEMS* 17(10):5, 1992.

Pelta K. *What Does a Paramedic Do?* New York: Dodd, Mead, 1978.

Safar P, Esposito G, Benson D. Emergency medical technicians as allied health professionals. *Anesth Analg* (Cleve.) 51:27, 1972.

Smith JP, Bodai BI. The urban paramedic's scope of practice. *JAMA* 253:544, 1985.

MEDICAL CONTROL

American College of Emergency Physicians. Medical control of prehospital emergency medical services. *Ann Emerg Med* 11:387, 1982.

American College of Emergency Physicians. Control of advanced life support at the scene of medical emergencies. *Ann Emerg Med* 13:547, 1984.

Amey BD, Straub EJ, Harrison EE. Medical control of paramedic services. *Emerg Med Serv* 7(4):20, 1978.

Bourn S. Mother, may I? *JEMS* 19(1):43, 1994.

Boyd DR et al. Medical control and accountability of emergency medical services (EMS) systems. *Vehicular Tech* 28:249, 1979.

Burney RR. Is the flight physician needed for helicopter emergency medical services? *Ann Emerg Med* 15:174, 1986.

Caroline NL. Medical care in the streets. *JAMA* 237:43, 1977.

Caroline NL. Quo vadis, Rampart One? *JACEP* 3:376, 1977.

Dickinson ET. Who's in charge? *Emergency* 25(5):28, 1991.

Erder MH, Davidson SJ, Cheney RA. On-line medical command in theory and practice. *Ann Emerg Med* 18:261, 1989.

Hoffman JR et al. Does paramedic-base hospital contact result in beneficial deviations from standard prehospital protocols? *West Med J* 153:283, 1990.

Holliman CJ et al. Medical command errors in an urban advanced life support system. *Ann Emerg Med* 21:347, 1992.

Holroyd BR, Knopp R, Kallsen G. Medical control: Quality assurance in prehospital care. *JAMA* 256:1027, 1986.

Hunt RC et al. Standing orders vs. voice control. *JEMS* 4:26, 1982.

McSwain NE. Medical control—what is it? *JACEP* 7:114, 1978.

Pepe PE, Stewart RD. Role of the physician in the prehospital setting. *Ann Emerg Med* 15:1480, 1986.

Pepe PE et al. Effect of full-time, specialized physician supervision on the success of a large, urban emergency medical services system. *Crit Care Med* 21:1279, 1993.

Pointer JE. The advanced life support base hospital audit for medical control in an emergency medical services system. *Ann Emerg Med* 16:557, 1987.

Polsky S et al. Guidelines for medical direction of prehospital EMS. *Ann Emerg Med* 22:742, 1993.

Pons P. Medical control of prehospital care. *J Emerg Med* 1:449, 1984.

Pozen MW et al. Effectiveness of a prehospital medical control system: An analysis of the interaction between emergency room physician and paramedic. *Circulation* 63:442, 1981.

Shanaberger CJ. The license you lose may not be your own. *JEMS* 11(6):66, 1989.

Smith M. "Hello . . . I'm a doctor." *JEMS* 17(5):37, 1992.

Swor RA, Krome RL. Administrative support of emergency medical services medical directors: A profile. *Prehosp Disaster Med* 5(1):25, 1990.

Wasserberger J et al. Base station prehospital care: Judgment errors and deviations from protocol. *Ann Emerg Med* 16:867, 1987.

2
EMS Systems

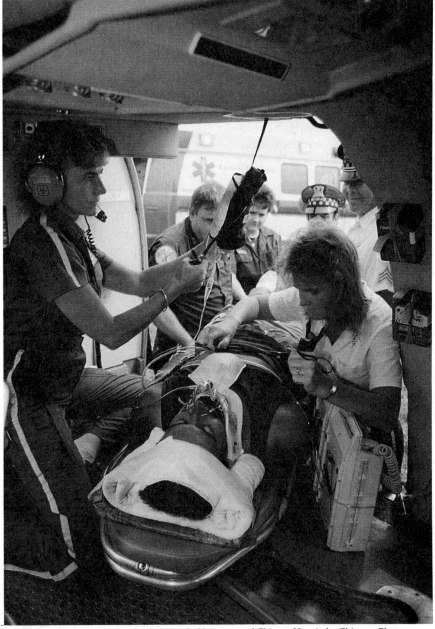

University of Chicago Aeromedical Network, University of Chicago Hospitals, Chicago. Photo by Michael S. Kowal.

Objectives
Links in the EMS Chain: Overview
Public Education
Activating the System
Treatment at the Scene
Transport
Hospital Treatment

Communication
Training
Organization and Planning
Evaluation and Research
Conclusion
Further Reading

OBJECTIVES

Emergency medical care is not a single entity but rather a *chain* of services involving a whole array of personnel and equipment. Each link in the chain is vital for the effective provision of emergency care. If even one link is weak, the whole chain of emergency medical services (EMS) can fail. In this chapter, we shall examine the links in the EMS chain in some detail. By the end of the chapter, the student should be able to

1. List the links in the EMS chain
2. Describe what an educated public needs to know in order to make optimal use of an EMS system
3. List the requirements for activating an EMS system
4. Explain the rationale for starting treatment at the scene and indicate under what circumstances it is not feasible to stabilize a patient fully before transport
5. List two ways in which ambulance transport today differs from ambulance transport 40 years ago
6. Identify the most appropriate hospital to which to transport a patient, given a description of the patient's condition and the capabilities of several different hospitals
7. List the components of an EMS communications system, that is, indicate who should be able to communicate with whom
8. List at least five questions that need to be answered in the planning phase of an EMS system
9. Propose a research project that could improve the quality of EMS in his or her region

LINKS IN THE EMS CHAIN: OVERVIEW

Prehospital emergency care by paramedics is only one facet of a properly organized EMS system. A fully developed EMS system must have the following components:

EMS SYSTEM

- RECOGNITION of the emergency and FIRST AID by bystanders (public education and awareness)
- INITIATION of the EMS RESPONSE system (e.g., 911, CB radios)
- TREATMENT AT THE SCENE by members of the system (firefighters, other first responders, ambulance crews)
- TRANSPORTATION WITH ADVANCED LIFE SUPPORT by members of the system (paramedics, nurses, medical command)
- TREATMENT IN THE HOSPITAL (emergency department, operating room, intensive care unit)
- COMMUNICATIONS (patient-to-system, dispatch-to-ambulance, paramedic-to-doctor)
- EDUCATION and TRAINING (lay public, EMTs, nurses, physicians)
- PLANNING and ORGANIZATION
- EVALUATION and RESEARCH

Those are the links in the EMS chain, and the EMS system as a whole is only as strong as its weakest link. A given city may, for example, have a world-class hospital and a paramedic service worthy of a television series. But that won't help John Q. Citizen if he doesn't realize he is having a heart attack, if he doesn't know what number to call for help, or if the people around him don't know what to do if he collapses. Let us take a closer look, then, at each link in the EMS chain and what is required to make each link sturdy.

PUBLIC EDUCATION

The very first link in the EMS chain involves the public, and the whole system can break down right from the beginning if the public doesn't know how to use the system. In essence, John Q. Citizen needs to know three things:

- HOW TO RECOGNIZE AN EMERGENCY when it happens. Recognizing an emergency generally is not a major problem in the case of trauma, such as a road accident. But recognition of serious *medical* emergencies is often delayed by the patient's ignorance of basic symptoms. The average heart attack victim, for example, waits 3 hours after the onset of his symptoms before seeking help, a delay that may be—and often is—fatal. The public must be educated, therefore, in how to recognize the symptoms of heart attack, major allergic reactions, poisoning, and other potentially life-threatening medical emergencies, so that they will seek help before it is too late.
- HOW TO CALL FOR HELP. Having reached the conclusion that an emergency exists, John Q. Cit-

izen must then know how to get help. We shall look at that problem in more detail when we discuss the second link in the EMS chain: activating the system.

- WHAT TO DO UNTIL HELP ARRIVES. Let us assume that John Q. Citizen has collapsed at home. He doesn't seem to be breathing. His wife has telephoned for an ambulance. What should she do during the 5 to 10 minutes it may take until the ambulance arrives? If she has taken a course in cardiopulmonary resuscitation (CPR), she will know what to do. If she is fortunate enough to live in a city in which the EMS dispatchers are trained to give *CPR instruction by telephone*, she may be able to learn what to do on the spot. Otherwise, John Q. Citizen's chances of survival are quite small. Public education for EMS should therefore include basic first aid training—how to perform CPR, how to treat choking, how to stop bleeding, how to manage a person in shock—to enable that vital member of the public, the bystander, to provide assistance until professional help arrives.

ACTIVATING THE SYSTEM

As noted, it is critically important to the effectiveness of an EMS system that every member of the public knows how to activate the system. Activating the system requires

- KNOWING WHAT TELEPHONE NUMBER TO CALL. In much of the United States, that problem has been vastly simplified by the introduction of a universal emergency telephone number, **911**. But implementation of the 911 phone system is not complete nationwide, and in many areas John Q. Citizen must still call either the police or one of several dozen private ambulance services listed in the telephone book. If your ambulance service operates in one of those regions, it is worthwhile having telephone stickers printed up that list the telephone numbers of the police, fire department, and ambulance service and then going door-to-door to distribute the stickers. (You can also take advantage of your door-to-door trek to offer other EMS education services, such as a poison control inspection.)
- KNOWING WHAT TO TELL THE EMS DISPATCHER. Here again there is a need for public education. Generally when a person telephones 911, he is immediately asked for his name, address, and phone number. A person who is ill or who is panicky over someone else's illness may

not understand the reason for such questions and may become angry. The caller who has not been taught how to make use of the EMS system may complain, "Why are you wasting time collecting all that bureaucratic information?" (And then the dispatcher *will* have to waste time—explaining the need for the information.)

So far in our discussion of the second link in the EMS chain, we have dealt with the responsibilities of the person seeking help—to know what number to call and to know what information to provide. For the optimal means of activating the EMS system, however, we also need professional personnel and a good deal of sophisticated hardware. Specifically, this link of the EMS chain also requires

- TRAINED DISPATCHERS who are skilled in gathering information from panicky callers, in giving instruction by telephone for what to do until help arrives, and in making quick decisions regarding the most appropriate unit to dispatch to the call (EMT-As only? paramedics? police backup?).
- 911 TECHNOLOGY.
- Highway telephones and other PUBLIC PHONES THAT DO NOT REQUIRE A COIN to dial 911.
- INTERFACE WITH OTHER RADIO SYSTEMS. If, for example, a CB radio enthusiast is driving along a lonely country road and comes across the victims of a vehicular accident, he should have a reliable means of contacting the EMS dispatcher by CB radio. The same applies to taxi drivers and others who carry mobile radio equipment.
- DISPATCHER-TO-EMS COMMUNICATIONS. Having received the call for help, the dispatcher must, as noted, mobilize the most appropriate members of the EMS team, which may include police or fire fighters as first responders or hazard control personnel, a basic life support ambulance, a mobile intensive care unit, or any combination thereof. To mobilize the appropriate people, the dispatcher needs to be able to contact them immediately—by telephone if they are at their base, by beeper or radio if they are elsewhere.

TREATMENT AT THE SCENE

This link in the EMS chain—treatment at the scene— is one of the features that distinguishes a modern EMS system from the ambulance services of the past. It is not so many years ago that the function of an ambulance was solely to race to the scene, snatch the patient, and career off to the hospital; and the sole qualification required of an ambulance attendant was a driver's license. In those days of "swoop and scoop," ambulances were sometimes sarcastically referred to as "meat wagons," and not without some justification. Simply tossing a critically ill or injured person in the back of a vehicle and then subjecting that person to the further trauma of a wild ride to the hospital was not, it turned out, a very effective method for saving lives. So the concept evolved of bringing the emergency room *to* the patient, to initiate treatment at the scene, before bringing the patient to the hospital. This was the concept of prehospital *care*—a way of extending hospital care out into the community.

Clearly, to bring the emergency room to the patient, one needs to bring along

- TRAINED MEDICAL PERSONNEL. In most of Europe, "trained medical personnel" has meant doctors, and in some European EMS systems, such as that of Bruges, Belgium, only the most highly qualified medical specialists ride ambulances. In the United States, on the other hand, it was found that nonphysicians with varying degrees of physician guidance could do the job in the field. Today treatment at the scene may therefore involve
  1. FIRST RESPONDERS: police officers, fire fighters, lifeguards, and a variety of others who have received basic first aid training and who are situated such that they are most likely to reach the average call first.
  2. EMT-A (EMT-ambulance): an individual who has passed a nationally standardized course that includes CPR, airway management, artificial ventilation, basic trauma life support, emergency childbirth, rescue and extrication, and other noninvasive skills.
  3. EMT-I (EMT-intermediate): an individual who has passed a nationally standardized course including all the material in an EMT-A course plus use of the esophageal obturator airway, intravenous infusions, and in some cases endotracheal intubation and defibrillation.
  4. EMT-P (EMT-paramedic): an individual who has passed a nationally standardized course that includes all of the material in the EMT-A and EMT-I courses plus additional invasive techniques, administration of medications, and advanced trauma life support.
  5. NURSES, particularly those specializing in emergency nursing, coronary care nursing, neonatal intensive care, and so forth.
  6. DOCTORS. While still rarely seen in American ambulances, doctors maintain radio contact with paramedics at the scene and are occasionally summoned for backup support, especially in multicasualty incidents.
- LIFE SUPPORT EQUIPMENT. An emergency room consists not only of skilled personnel. It also contains the equipment and supplies necessary to save lives, such as oxygen, devices to provide artifical ventilation, and so forth. Bringing the emergency room to the patient means bringing the most critical gear that the emergency room contains.

The concept of treatment at the scene is sometimes misunderstood, both by the public and by some of the medical community. The objective of the prehospital phase of emergency care is to START DEFINITIVE TREATMENT OF THE PATIENT AT THE SCENE. For many patients with medical problems, it will be possible to stabilize the patient's condition fully in the field before moving on to the hospital. When, however, the patient needs definitive control of bleeding and replacement of lost blood—which is often the case in a seriously injured person—full stabilization of the patient will not be possible until he reaches the operating room. For such patients, resuscitation measures must be started expeditiously in the field or in transport, and the patient must be moved rapidly to the appropriate hospital. Among paramedics, the "pros" are the ones who can distinguish between the two situations just described, that is, between those patients who can be stabilized in the field and those who require urgent transport.

TRANSPORT

The next link in the EMS chain is transportation with advanced life support by members of the system. Gone are the old meat wagons and the untrained attendants who drove them. Today, emergency medical transport requires the following:

- AMBULANCES must meet minimum design specifications (in the United States, those specifications are detailed in document KKK-A-1822B of the U.S. Department of Transportation). Previously just about any vehicle in which it was possible to stuff a stretcher could qualify as an ambulance, and as recently as around 20 years ago, station wagons, hearses, and a motley variety of vans constituted nearly half of the ambulances in the United States.
- MEDICAL EQUIPMENT carried on ambulances must also meet minimum standards (in the United States, the minimum equipment stan-

dards for ambulances are set out in the document "Essential Equipment for Ambulances," furnished by the American College of Surgeons). Additional equipment and supplies, over and above the minimum standards, are required for MICUs—usually including a portable monitor/defibrillator, a whole variety of drugs, equipment for giving intravenous fluids, and so forth.

- As in the stage of treatment in the field, the stage of transport with advanced life support also requires that there be PARAMEDICS UNDER MEDICAL CONTROL. As we learned in the previous chapter, immediate medical control may be exercised through standing orders, voice orders by radio, or some combination thereof.

HOSPITAL TREATMENT

In the days of "swoop and scoop," there was one simple rule that governed where the ambulance took the patient: to the *closest* hospital. There was a certain logic in that rule, for at least, on arriving at the closest hospital, the patient might begin to receive some sort of care; almost certainly he had not been given any treatment up to that point. With the advent of prehospital emergency care, however, and the possibility of initiating stabilizing measures in the field, it became necessary to take another look at the old "Nearest-Hospital Rule."

Hospitals vary enormously in their capabilities and in their preparedness to deal with different types of emergencies. In the United States, only approximately 5 percent of admissions to hospital emergency departments constitute life-threatening emergencies. The remainder are noncritical emergencies (about 25%) and nonemergencies (i.e., primary care, about 70%). Thus a hospital's preparedness to deal with life-threatening emergencies may be less than optimal, especially in emergency departments seeing a small volume of patients.

Recognizing that not all hospitals have equal capabilities, those responsible for EMS planning have devised a system of *hospital categorization* to assess the emergency services in any given region. The criteria for hospital categorization include the following:

CRITERIA FOR HOSPITAL CATEGORIZATION

- The number of physicians on staff and their availability
- The medical specialties of staff physicians
- The medical specialties of staff nurses
- Availability of life support equipment and supplies
- 24-hour physician coverage in the emergency room
- 24-hour coverage of x-ray and laboratory facilities
- Availability and adequacy of special-care facilities (e.g., coronary care unit, trauma center, poison center, burn unit, spinal cord injury unit)

In consultation with medical command, the paramedic must evaluate the patient's condition and then decide, based on the capabilities of the medical facilities in the area, which facility is best staffed and equipped to care for that particular patient. A patient with a serious head injury, for example, needs to be taken to a facility in which a neurosurgeon is immediately available. A patient with critical burns should, ideally, be treated at a burn center. The ability of the paramedic to provide life support in transit is what makes it possible today to take the patient directly to the neurosurgical unit or the burn center rather than having to stop first at the nearest hospital.

COMMUNICATION

One of the most critical links in the EMS chain—the one that helps keep all of the other links together—is the communication network that enables transfer of information from one part of the system to another. We shall deal with the logistics and the hardware of EMS communications in Chapter 39. For our purposes here, it is sufficient to note that EMS communications must include at least the following elements:

- CITIZEN TO EMS SYSTEM: the means by which a person who needs help activates the EMS system (e.g., 911)
- DISPATCHER TO EMS TEAM: the means by which the dispatcher contacts those needed to respond to the call (dedicated telephone line to the EMTs' base station, radio, beeper)
- DISPATCHER TO OTHER SERVICES: the means by which the dispatcher can request assistance from the police, fire department, public utilities company, and so forth
- PARAMEDIC TO DOCTOR: the means by which paramedics in the field can consult their medical

director for advice or verbal orders (radio, telephone patch, or cellular phone)
- AMBULANCE TO RECEIVING HOSPITAL: the means by which the EMT-A or paramedic can notify a hospital of an incoming patient

In large metropolitan areas, it is very useful if the communications system also includes

- HOSPITAL-TO-HOSPITAL connections, through dedicated telephone lines or radio or both, to facilitate interhospital transfers of critically ill or injured patients
- EMS COMMUNICATIONS CENTER–TO-HOSPITAL connections, again by telephone or radio or both, to enable coordination in the event of a mass casualty incident

TRAINING

As mentioned earlier, it is not very long ago that the sole qualification required for a person to become an ambulance attendant was a driver's license. With the advent of modern EMS systems, all that has changed. In most states, the minimum acceptable standard for ambulance personnel is EMT-A, which requires anywhere from 80 to 120 hours of course work. Paramedic training takes anywhere from 500 to 1500 hours. And for all members of the EMS team, training is not something that ends with graduation and a diploma; training is a lifelong commitment to continuing education.

ORGANIZATION AND PLANNING

The links in the EMS chain we have described so far do not just magically come together. As anyone who has participated in setting up such a system can testify, an enormous amount of planning (which may include an enormous amount of political wrangling) goes into the establishment of even the most rudimentary EMS system. Ideally, the widest possible cross section of the community should be involved in the planning process—representatives of the medical profession, hospital administration, local government, the business community, and private individuals. Together, those representatives will form a local or regional EMS council, to address the many questions that arise in the course of planning and implementing a community-wide emergency care system: Where should the ambulances be stationed? How many levels of response are necessary? Who will pay

the bill? Who will give medical command? Until those and many similar questions are answered in any given community, EMS will remain on the drawing boards.

EVALUATION AND RESEARCH

The last link in the EMS chain—evaluation and research—does not at first seem like a link at all. Research, indeed, sounds suspiciously like what scientists in ivory towers do for a living, not like something that has any relevance to the day-to-day work of a paramedic out in the real world. In fact, however, evaluation and research are as critical to the EMS chain as any other link, for it is by evaluating the job we do that we learn how to do it better. In Seattle, Washington, for example, Dr. Mickey Eisenberg and his colleagues evaluated the success rate of EMS providers in resuscitating patients found in cardiac arrest. Their studies showed that the most critical single factor in determining whether a patient would be successfully resuscitated was the time elapsed between the moment his heart stopped beating and the delivery of a defibrillating shock. The sooner defibrillation was carried out, the better the patient's chances of surviving.

Dr. Eisenberg's findings suggested that one way to improve the performance of the EMS system was to find a means to get a defibrillator to a cardiac arrest victim more quickly. So the Seattle group then undertook another study. They trained and equipped EMT-As in one district around Seattle to perform defibrillation. Then they compared the "save rate" in cardiac arrest cases occurring in two districts around Seattle: one where EMT-As *were* trained and equipped to defibrillate, the other where EMT-As did *not* have defibrillation capability. What they found was that giving defibrillation capability to EMT-As, who generally reached a cardiac arrest victim several minutes earlier than did the paramedics, doubled the overall salvage rate in out-of-hospital cardiac arrest. As a consequence of that research, many thousands of EMT-As all over the United States have now received training in defibrillation, and many thousands of lives have been saved. Evaluation and research saved those lives.

CONCLUSION

We have seen, then, that EMS is not a single entity. It is a chain of many interconnected links. But what does all this have to do with *me*? the aspiring paramedic may well ask. The answer is that it has *everything* to do with you and your chances of working effectively in your chosen career. As a paramedic, you need to be concerned not only with your own limited phase of emergency care, but also with the total system in which the ambulance service operates—for very practical reasons: You may have a gold star in CPR performance, but those resuscitation skills aren't going to do anyone any good if bystanders are not educated to call for help in time and to take appropriate measures until you can reach the victim. Similarly, the best prehospital emergency care in the world is doomed to failure if the receiving facilities are not equipped to carry on a high standard of care after you have transferred responsibility for the patient to the emergency department. Thus the paramedic needs to be interested in all phases of emergency care in the community and should seek to remedy deficiencies found at every level. Paramedics are, for example, particularly well suited to assist in the education of lay persons. Paramedics can also take political action to press for whatever improvements are needed in the system. The problem is not to identify the deficiencies in the system. Ask any working paramedic what's wrong with the EMS system in which he is employed, and he will spend the rest of the day giving you a list of everything that's wrong. Then the rest of his crew will give you *their* lists. Compiling those lists, however, is only a first step. The next step is *doing* something about it.

FURTHER READING

EMS SYSTEMS, GENERAL
Becker LB, Pepe PE. Ensuring effectiveness of community-wide emergency cardiac care. *Ann Emerg Med* 22:354, 1993.

Cady G, Scott T. EMS in the United States: 1994 survey of providers in the 200 most populous cities. *JEMS* 19(1):88, 1994.

Committee of Emergency Medical Services, National Academy of Sciences. *Emergency Medical Services at Midpassage.* Washington, D.C.: National Academy of Sciences, 1978.

Johnson JC. Prehospital care: The future of emergency medical services. *Ann Emerg Med* 20:426, 1991.

PUBLIC EDUCATION
Eisenberg M et al. Emergency CPR via telephone. *Am J Public Health* 75:47, 1985.

Guzy PM, Pearce ML, Greenfield S. The survival benefit of bystander cardiopulmonary resuscitation in a paramedic-served metropolitan area. *Am J Public Health* 73:766, 1983.

Haas JC. A public education and prevention program. *Emerg Med Serv* 5:38, 1976.

Ritter G et al. The effect of bystander CPR on survival of out-of-hospital cardiac arrest victims. *Am Heart J* 110:932, 1985.

Sampsel RE. Telephone-directed CPR: Does it work? *Emerg Med Serv* 18(4):49, 1989.

Spaite DW et al. Prehospital cardiac arrest: The impact of witnessed collapse and bystander CPR in a metropolitan EMS system with short response times. *Ann Emerg Med* 19:1264, 1990.

Steuven H et al. Bystander/first responder CPR: Ten years experience in a paramedic system. *Ann Emerg Med* 15:707, 1986.

Troiano P et al. The effect of bystander CPR on neurologic outcome in survivors of prehospital cardiac arrests. *Resuscitation* 17:91, 1989.

ACTIVATING THE SYSTEM
Clawson JJ. Quality assurance: A priority for medical dispatch. *Emerg Med Serv* 18(7):53, 1989.

Curka PA. Emergency medical services priority dispatch. *Ann Emerg Med* 22:1688, 1993.

Dreifuss R. 911 misuse. *Emerg Med Serv* 18(7):43, 1989.

Slovis CM et al. A priority dispatch system for emergency medical services. *Ann Emerg Med* 14:1055, 1985.

Yandell DC. 911 update. *Emerg Med Serv* 18(7):36, 1989.

TREATMENT AT THE SCENE
Cummings RO, Eisenberg M. Prehospital cardiopulmonary resuscitation: Is it effective? *JAMA* 16:2408, 1985.

Dean NC, Haug PJ, Hawker PJ. Effect of mobile paramedic units on outcome in patients with myocardial infarction. *Ann Emerg Med* 17:1034, 1988.

Eisenberg M, Bergner R, Hallstrom A. Cardiac resuscitation in the community. *JAMA* 241:1905, 1979.

Jakobsson J et al. Effects of early defibrillation of out-of-hospital cardiac arrest patients by ambulance personnel. *Eur Heart J* 8:1189, 1987.

TRANSPORT
Committee on Trauma, American College of Surgeons. Essential equipment for ambulances. *Bull Am Coll Surgeons*, 1977.

Safar P, Esposito G, Benson D. Ambulance design and equipment for mobile intensive care. *Arch Surg* 102:163, 1971.

United States Department of Transportation/General Services Administration. *Emergency Medical Care Surface Vehicle: Federal Specification-Ambulance KKK-A-1822B.* Washington, D.C.: Government Printing Office, 1985.

United States Department of Transportion/National Highway Traffic Safety Administration. *Ambulance Design Criteria* (pamphlet). Washington, D.C.: Government Printing Office, 1973.

COMMUNICATION
Henke S, Orcutt L. Portable radio communications for emergency medical services. *Emerg Med Serv* 12(4):32, 1983.

Howell JE. Amateur radio: An alternative means of emergency communication. *Emerg Med Serv* 14(4):28, 1985.

McCorkle JE et al. *Basic Telecommunications for Emergency Medical Services.* Cambridge, Mass.: Ballinger, 1978.

U.S. Department of Health, Education, and Welfare. *Emergency Medical Services Communications System.* DHEW Publication No. (HSM)732003. Washington, D.C.: Government Printing Office, 1972.

TRAINING

Benson D et al. Mobile intensive care by "unemployable" blacks trained as emergency medical technicians (EMTs). *J Trauma* 12:408, 1971.

Benson K. An EMT by any other name. *Emergency* 25(6):28, 1993.

Curry L, Gass D. Effects of training in cardiopulmonary resuscitation on competence and patient outcome. *Can Med Assoc J* 137:491, 1987.

Lightfoot S. Getting your training programs on the right track. *Emergency* 25(1):39, 1993.

Rowley JM et al. Advanced training for ambulance crews: Implications from 403 consecutive patients with cardiac arrest managed by crews with simple training. *Br Med J* 295:1387, 1987.

ORGANIZATION AND PLANNING

Safar P (ed.). *Public Health Aspects of Critical Care Medicine and Anesthesiology.* Philadelphia: Davis, 1974. See especially Chapter 4, by P. Safar et al, Emergency and Critical Care Medicine: Local Implementation of National Recommendations.

Urban N et al. Costs of a suburban paramedic program in reducing deaths due to cardiac arrest. *Med Care* 19:379, 1981.

EVALUATION AND RESEARCH

Alexander RH et al. The effect of advanced life support and sophisticated hospital systems on motor vehicle mortality. *J Trauma* 24:486, 1984.

American College of Emergency Physicians. *Continuous Quality Improvement in EMS.* Dallas: ACEP, 1992.

Eisenberg M et al. Management of out-of-hospital cardiac arrest: Failure of basic emergency medical technician services. *JAMA* 243:1049, 1980.

Eisenberg M et al. Out-of-hospital cardiac arrest: Improved survival with paramedic services. *Lancet* 1:812, 1980.

Eisenberg M et al. Treatment of ventricular fibrillation: Emergency medical technician defibrillation and paramedic services. *JAMA* 251:1723, 1984.

Gibson G. Measures of emergency ambulance effectiveness: Unmet need and inappropriate use. *JACEP* 6:389, 1977.

Lombardi G, Gallagher J, Gennis P. Outcome of out-of-hospital cardiac arrest in New York City. *JAMA* 271:678, 1994.

Luterman A et al. Evaluation of prehospital emergency medical service (EMS): Defining areas for improvement. *J Trauma* 23:702, 1983.

Nagel EL. Improving emergency medical care. *N Engl J Med* 302:1416, 1980.

Pergner L et al. Health status of survivors of out-of-hospital cardiac arrest six months later. *Am J Public Health* 74:508, 1984.

Pressley JC et al. A comparison of paramedic versus basic emergency medical care of patients at high and low risk during acute myocardial infarction. *J Am Coll Cardiol* 12:1555, 1988.

Rademaker AW, Powell DG, Read JD. Inappropriate use and unmet need in paramedic and nonparamedic ambulance systems. *Ann Emerg Med* 16:553, 1987.

Sidel VW, Acton J, Lown B. Models for the evaluation of prehospital coronary care. *Am J Cardiol* 24:674, 1969.

Solomon NA et al. What are representative survival rates for out-of-hospital cardiac arrest? *Arch Intern Med* 153:1218, 1993.

Spaite DW. Outcome analysis in EMS systems (editorial). *Ann Emerg Med* 22:1310, 1993.

Steuven HA et al. Prehospital cardiac arrest: A critical analysis of factors affecting survival. *Resuscitation* 17:251, 1989.

Swor RA (ed.). *Quality Management in Prehospital Care.* St. Louis: Mosby Lifeline, 1993.

Vertesi L, Wilson L, Glick N. Cardiac arrest: Comparison of paramedic and conventional ambulance services. *Can Med Assoc J* 128:809, 1983.

3
Medicolegal and Ethical Issues

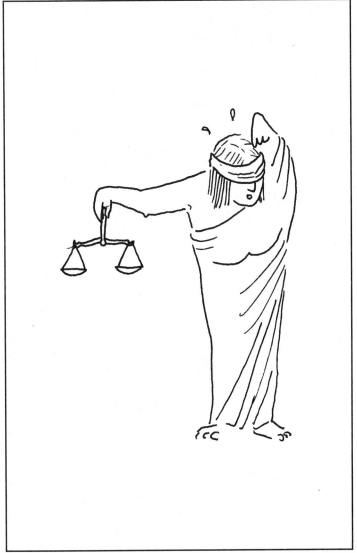

Peter Caroline

OBJECTIVES

Being a paramedic imposes both legal and moral obligations. In a democratic society, all of us must function within the framework of laws—laws that define our obligations and that protect our rights and the rights of others. A paramedic responding to an emergency works within a framework of several types of laws: laws regarding the operation of an emergency vehicle, medical licensing regulations, and civil and criminal statutes relating to touching, transporting, and possibly injuring another person. It is essential, therefore, that the paramedic have a basic understanding of laws applicable to prehospital emergency care. In this chapter, we shall review the more important legal concepts affecting the paramedic. We shall also examine the ethical obligations that being a paramedic entails. By the end of this chapter, the student should be able to

1. Identify, given a list of definitions, the correct definition of
   • Liability
   • Tort
   • Assault
   • Battery
   • False imprisonment
   • Negligence
   • Informed consent
   • Implied consent
   • Abandonment
   • Duty to act
   • Protocol
2. List the provisions of the Good Samaritan Act in his or her state, specifically:
   • Who is protected under the act?
   • Under what circumstances is that protection given?
   • What actions are *excluded* from protection under the act?
3. List the four elements required to prove negligence
4. Specify the requirements for obtaining consent to treat
   • A conscious, mentally competent adult
   • A child
5. Identify situations in which a paramedic may treat a patient without obtaining expressed consent, given a description of different situations
6. List three criteria for establishing mental competence
7. List the actions to be taken when a mentally competent adult refuses medical treatment
8. List six components of a complete trip sheet
9. List four categories of cases that you are required by state law to report to the appropriate authorities
10. List four categories of cases that are generally considered to be coroner's cases
11. Summarize in one or two sentences the basic principle of medical ethics

SOME BASIC CONCEPTS

A substantial part of the law is concerned with establishing **liability**, or responsibility. When a person suffers an injury and seeks redress for that injury, the judicial process must determine who was responsible. Sometimes, for example, a patient or (if the patient died) the survivor of a patient may be unsatisfied with the medical care the patient received; the patient or survivor may feel that inadequate care led to a bad outcome. That person has a constitutional right to take legal action against the doctor, nurse, EMT, or anyone else he feels was responsible for the bad outcome. A legal action of that sort is called a **civil suit**—that is, an action instituted by a private individual (the plaintiff) against another private individual (the defendant)—and the wrongful act that gives rise to a civil suit is called a **tort.** The objective of a civil suit is usually some sort of compensation (**damages**) for the injury the plaintiff sustained. In medical liability cases, the plaintiff usually seeks monetary compensation for physical suffering, mental anguish, hospital and medical bills, and sometimes loss of earnings or earning capacity. To succeed in a civil suit, the plaintiff need only show that the balance of believable evidence favors his position.

Sometimes the same allegedly wrongful act (tort) that gave rise to a civil suit may also elicit criminal prosecution. A **criminal suit** is an action taken by the government when a person has violated criminal laws. In a criminal case, the government must prove guilt beyond all reasonable doubt; if it does so, the defendant can be fined or imprisoned or both. The criminal laws most likely to be applicable to prehospital emergency care are those relating to assault, battery, and false imprisonment.*

Assault is said to occur when a person instills the fear of immediate bodily harm or breach of bodily security—whether or not the threat of harm is actually carried out. **Battery** occurs when the defendant touches another person without his consent. Thus,

---
*Assault, battery, and false imprisonment may also be grounds for a *civil* suit.

declaring to someone, "I'm going to kick your teeth in," is assault. Actually kicking his teeth in is battery. Clearly just about any act of medical treatment performed without consent may be considered assault or battery or both, for such acts constitute a threat to the patient's bodily security ("Now I'm going to stick you with this needle . . .") and an unsanctioned contact with the patient's body.

False imprisonment occurs when a person is intentionally and unjustifiably detained against his will. In prehospital care, charges of false imprisonment are most likely to arise if an EMT transports a patient without the patient's consent or uses restraints in a wrongful manner.

As we shall see later in this chapter, a paramedic's best protection against charges of the sort just described is to obtain informed consent wherever applicable.

LAWS GOVERNING THE PARAMEDIC

A variety of laws and ordinances, many of which differ considerably from state to state, regulate the actions of the paramedic. Probably the most important law affecting paramedics is one that doesn't appear in any of the statute books; it is the LAW OF DOING WHAT IS BEST FOR THE PATIENT. Paramedics are trained in emergency medical care, not jurisprudence. Every decision regarding patient care that a paramedic makes, therefore, should be based on the standards of good medical care—*not* on the possible legal consequences.

Medical Practice Act

As to those statutes that *are* on the books, in most regions emergency medical technicians and paramedics are enabled to function through the provisions of a **Medical Practice Act.** That act usually defines the minimum qualifications of those who may perform various health services, defines the skills that each type of practitioner is legally permitted to use, and establishes a means of certification for different categories of health professionals. The paramedic should become familiar with the terms of the Medical Practice Act in his or her region and should stay within the limits of that law. A paramedic carrying out procedures for which he or she is not authorized under the Medical Practice Act is practicing medicine without a license, which is a criminal offense.

As we noted in our discussion of medical control in Chapter 1, the actions of the paramedic in the field are considered the **delegated practice** of a physician.

It is worth reiterating the implications of that proviso. Delegated practice means that the physician has delegated the paramedic to carry out certain actions on his or her behalf. In the eyes of the law, however, the delegated actions are *still* those of the physician, and the physician bears legal responsibility for them. For that reason, many of the paramedic's activities require an order from a licensed physician. Orders may be given by radio or may be defined by **protocols** (standing orders), but in any case, the paramedic is not at liberty to disregard or countermand a physician's order. That fact may give rise to difficult situations, such as instances where paramedics find themselves at the scene of an emergency together with a physician who may not be knowledgeable in prehospital emergency care. Under those circumstances, the paramedics may feel that the orders of the physician on the scene are inappropriate. However, paramedics are on shaky legal ground if they choose to disregard a physician's orders. To avoid such situations, it is best to develop policies ahead of time defining the paramedic's relationship with the medical director of the service and with other physicians in the community. When conflicts do arise between paramedics and physician bystanders in the field, the medical director, not the paramedic, should resolve them.

Good Samaritan Legislation

Most states have, in addition to the Medical Practice Act, some form of **Good Samaritan law** designed to provide freedom from liability to individuals who stop and help at the scene of an emergency. The Florida Good Samaritan legislation of 1965 is fairly representative of such acts:

> Any person, including those licensed to practice medicine, who gratuitously and in good faith renders emergency care or treatment at the scene of an emergency outside of a hospital, doctor's office or other place having proper medical equipment, without objection of the injured victim or victims thereof, shall not be held liable for any civil damages as a result of any act or failure to act in providing or arranging further medical treatment where the person acts as an ordinary reasonable prudent man would have acted under the same circumstances. [Florida Stat. Ann. 768.13.]

Note that there is a "hooker" in the Florida Good Samaritan legislation (and in that of most other states) that limits the legal protection provided: The emergency care must be given free of charge (gratuitously). An EMT or paramedic giving emergency care while on the job is probably not, therefore, protected under Good Samaritan laws. Note also the last clause of the Florida statute. It requires that the person responding to an emergency do all that he can, *within his knowledge,* to support and sustain life and to prevent further injury. The paramedic is not expected to function as a physician would; but the paramedic *is* expected to deploy those skills that any other person with similar training would use under the same circumstances.

The Maryland code of 1964 makes specific reference to ambulance and rescue personnel:

> The members of volunteer ambulance and rescue squads shall not be liable for damages . . . except for gross negligence, and shall have the defense provided therein, except for gross negligence. In order to be eligible for the exemption from liability provided in this section, a person must have completed a basic and an advanced Red Cross or equivalent course of instruction in first aid, and must be on active duty as a member of a volunteer ambulance and rescue squad which (1) is a bona fide and permanent organization and (2) is organized and operated as a nonprofit group. [Maryland Ann. Code, art. 43, 149a.]

Negligence

The Maryland statute illustrates that even Good Samaritan legislation does not ordinarily protect an individual from liability for **negligence**. Negligence occurs when

- An INJURY happened.
- The person accused of negligence had a DUTY TO ACT. In the case of an EMT, a duty to act is established as soon as he or she reports to work.
- There was a BREACH OF DUTY; that is, the person accused of negligence failed to act as another prudent person with similar training would have acted under the same circumstances. Breach of duty may involve doing *less* than one is trained to do (e.g., an EMT who fails to splint an injured extremity) or doing *more* than one was trained to do (e.g., an EMT who stitches up a laceration).
- That failure to act appropriately was the proximate cause of the plaintiff's injury.

The lesson in all of this is that paramedics are protected from liability so long as they perform according to the standards expected of paramedics. Thus the paramedic's best protection is to behave in all circumstances according to established procedures. Furthermore, many codes have been formulated, by groups such as the National Research Council and the National Highway Traffic Safety Administration, regarding ambulance design and equipment. While those codes do not have the force of law, they may be introduced as evidence in litigation and may affect the outcome of a suit. For that reason, it is also in the paramedic's best interests to make sure that his or her vehicle is maintained in optimal condition and equipped according to prevailing standards.

Most of the other laws or legal concepts pertaining to emergency medical care have evolved in terms of the physician's relationship to the patient. However, since the paramedic functions as a direct extension of the physician, those laws are also of concern to emergency medical technicians.

Duty to Act

The **duty to act** requires that a public or municipal ambulance operator respond to the aid of an injured person in his jurisdiction. That requirement does not, in most instances, apply to private ambulance providers, who are generally permitted to select patients and answer calls at their own discretion. However, ambulance providers who do not accept remuneration for their work, such as public, municipal, and volunteer services, are obliged to respond to *every* call for help.

Consent

Giving emergency medical care requires the **consent** of the patient, for any touching of a patient's body without his or her consent may give rise to charges of technical assault and battery. There are several important aspects of consent:

- Consent must be *informed;* that is, the patient must be told, in a manner he or she can understand, the nature and extent of the procedure to be performed and the possible risks involved.
- Consent must be obtained from every conscious, mentally competent adult.
- In the unconscious adult, consent for emergency, lifesaving treatment is said to be *implied*. (This is known as the **emergency doctrine.**)
- In the case of *children* or of adults who are *mentally incompetent,* consent must be obtained from a parent or legal guardian of the patient. If the parent or guardian is not available, emergency treatment to sustain life may be undertaken without consent.
- If a conscious and mentally competent adult refuses to consent to treatment, that person may not be treated without a court order. In such in-

stances, the paramedic should consult the local medical director for instructions. Generally the most prudent approach is to inform the person in a calm and sympathetic manner of the possible consequences of refusing treatment. Bear in mind that many people who refuse medical treatment do so out of fear and emotional distress, and the patient's distress needs to be recognized and dealt with in an understanding way. It is *not* appropriate to consider the person who refuses treatment as a "bad patient" and to behave in a hostile or aggressive manner toward him. Remember, the object of the exercise is to help the patient. So try to find out what is bothering him and why he is rejecting help. Bear in mind that some patients refuse treatment as a way of denying that they have a problem—such as the middle-aged macho man with chest pain who refuses treatment in order to deny the possibility that he might be suffering a heart attack. A sympathetic ear and a little reassurance will often convert the "problem patient" into someone you can help. Sometimes having the patient talk by radio or telephone with your medical director may also be helpful. If, however, after your best efforts to talk with the patient about his situation and to explain the possible consequences of refusing treatment, the patient still declines your care, there is little more that you can do. Even at that point, though, do not close any doors. Let the patient know that, should he change his mind, you will be willing and ready to help him, because that is your job.

WHEN A COMPETENT ADULT REFUSES TREATMENT

- Maintain a courteous, sympathetic attitude. Let the patient know that your chief concern is his well-being.
- Let the patient know that it is all right to change his mind.
- Urge the patient to seek further medical evaluation by the doctor of his choice. Help him make concrete plans for follow-up.
- Try to make sure that someone will be with the patient after you leave, to call for help if he needs it.
- Document *everything!*
  1. The patient's history
  2. All findings of your physical examination and mental status examination

3. The patient's stated reasons for refusing care
4. All advice given to the patient, including explanations of the risks of refusing care
5. The trip sheet should be signed by the patient and, preferably, by an impartial observer (e.g., a police officer, if present).

A problem sometimes arises in determining whether a person who refuses transport to hospital is indeed mentally competent. Suppose, for example, you are called for a patient who has had a seizure in a downtown store. By the time you arrive, the seizure is over, and the patient is conscious. He says he is all right, and he refuses to go to the hospital. You smell alcohol on his breath. Is that patient mentally competent to refuse treatment?

To make that determination, you need to spend a little time evaluating the patient. You should explain to him, "I can't let you go until I've checked you over and until you talk to me enough to convince me that you're OK and that you understand your problem." In general, any patient with altered mental status or unstable vital signs probably cannot be considered competent to refuse transport to the hospital. The criteria for determining mental competence should be spelled out in detail in the protocols of every ambulance service. As a rule, such criteria will include the following:

CRITERIA FOR ESTABLISHING MENTAL COMPETENCE

- The patient is oriented to person, place, and time.
- There is no significant mental impairment from alcohol, drugs, head injury, or other organic illness. (Ask family members, if present, whether the patient is behaving the way he normally does.)
- The patient understands the nature of his condition and the risks of not going to the hospital for immediate care.
- The patient can describe a reasonable plan for follow-up care.

When the patient has a potentially life-threatening illness or injury and there is any doubt as to his mental competence, it is preferable to transport him to hospital, even against his will. The decision to allow a potentially impaired patient to refuse treatment is a *medical* decision, requiring judgment and experience. That decision is best made by a doctor in the hospital, not by a paramedic on the street. Furthermore, the potential legal consequences of using reasonable force to bring a patient to hospital (false imprisonment) are far less serious than the consequences—legal and medical—of a bad outcome (wrongful death or malpractice) if a patient in need of care is released at the scene. So it is preferable to err on the side of transporting a patient, but in all cases confer first with your medical director.

Psychiatric emergencies present particularly vexing problems of consent. When a person's life is not in danger, a police officer is generally the only individual given the authority to restrain and transport that person against his or her will. An ambulance service should not do so except at the express request of the police. Notably, neither a physician nor the patient's family may, in most regions, authorize such transport; they may authorize involuntary *commitment*, but their authority does not extend to the forcible transport of a patient against his or her will. Therefore, it is essential for every ambulance service to establish procedures, based on local laws, for dealing with the mentally disturbed patient who refuses transport. In many instances, the participation of the police will be required, and the role of each agency involved should be clearly defined beforehand.

Abandonment

Abandonment is the termination by a physician of the doctor-patient relationship without consent of the patient and without allowing the patient sufficient time to find another physician. The term also implies that the patient had a continuing need for medical treatment and that the abrupt termination of treatment was the cause of subsequent injury or death. While the definition of abandonment is framed in terms of the physician, clearly it applies as well to those who serve as agents of a physician. Therefore, once you have responded to an emergency, you may not leave a patient in need of medical treatment until another competent health professional has taken responsibility for that patient's care. While that would seem obvious, on more than one occasion a critically ill or injured patient was left in a busy emergency department by an ambulance service and died before emergency room personnel took note of his presence. It is the responsibility of the paramedic to stay with the patient until proper transfer of care has taken place. "Proper transfer of care" means transfer of care

to another health professional, not to a gurney! Thus, if you arrive at a busy emergency room with a seriously ill patient, you may have to remain with that patient in the waiting area until emergency department personnel are free to attend to him.

Medical Records

Even the most skilled and conscientious health professional may eventually have to go to court as a witness or defendant in a civil or criminal action. The paramedic's best protection in court is a THOROUGH AND ACCURATE MEDICAL RECORD. This cannot be overstressed. Whenever a paramedic cares for a patient in the field, a careful, detailed record should be made of at least the following information:

MEDICAL RECORD

- DATE and TIMES (time call was received, time of arrival at the scene, time of departure from the scene, time of arrival at hospital).
- Information elicited from the patient and bystanders (HISTORY).
- Observations of the scene.
- Findings of PHYSICAL EXAMINATION.
- Any TREATMENT rendered. Be precise! Do not write, for example, "IV therapy was given," but rather "An IV was initiated under orders from Dr. Smith with an 18-gauge Angiocath and D5/W to a keep-open rate."
- Any CHANGES in the patient's status while under your care.

Complete your records as soon as possible after the call. Even a few hours later, the details may become vague in your memory. Write legibly in ink. Be as precise and detailed as possible. Document everything you did. Remember, **if you don't document it, you can't prove you did it.** Your trip sheet becomes a permanent part of the patient's record. It is also a legal document and reflects on its author. A sloppy, incomplete record suggests to the reader (and to the court!) that the care of the patient may also have been sloppy and incomplete. So take time to make your records accurate and thorough. Needless to say, the medical record is not the place for flippant or derogatory remarks about a patient; at the very least, such remarks could cause the author considerable embarrassment should they later be read aloud in a court of law.

Reportable Cases

Each state in the United States has its own requirements regarding certain categories of cases that must be reported to the appropriate authorities. All 50 states, for example, have passed laws to protect abused children, and many of those laws impose a reporting obligation on various individuals, which may include EMTs and paramedics. Thus it is essential for the paramedic to be familiar with the reporting requirements of his or her own state.

The obligation to report is most frequently applied to the following categories of cases:

- Neglect or abuse of children
- Neglect or abuse of the elderly
- Injury sustained during the commission of a felony, or specific injuries considered to be of suspicious origin (e.g., gunshot wounds, stab wounds)
- Drug-related injuries
- Childbirth occurring outside a licensed medical facility
- Rape
- Animal bites
- Certain communicable diseases

As noted, reporting requirements vary widely from state to state. Learn the laws of your state and observe the reporting obligations that apply to you.

Coroner's Cases

Every ambulance service, finally, should have a list of procedures for CORONER'S CASES. While the Coroner's Law varies somewhat from state to state, the following guidelines are generally applicable:

**GUIDELINES FOR
CORONER'S CASES**

- Notify the police of all coroner's cases, including
  1. Obvious or suspected homicide.
  2. Obvious or suspected suicide.
  3. Any other violent or sudden, unexpected death.
  4. Death of a prison inmate.
- Try not to disturb the incident scene.

- Stay with the body until the police arrive.
- In most jurisdictions, a paramedic is not legally authorized to pronounce a patient dead.
- When in doubt about the possibility of saving the patient, start CPR and transport to the hospital.

MEDICAL ETHICS

Ethics is the science of right and wrong, of moral duties, and of ideal behavior. Medical ethics is simply that part of ethics having to do with the health care of human beings. Thus medical ethics must inevitably form a part of, and be consistent with, a health professional's ethical code in general.

Throughout the ages, there have been many published codes of ethics for health professionals. The Oath of Geneva, drafted by the World Medical Association in 1948, provides a good example; it is the oath taken by many medical students on completion of their studies, at the time of being admitted to the medical profession:

> I solemnly pledge myself to consecrate my life to the service of humanity; I will give to my teachers the respect and gratitude which is their due; I will practice my profession with conscience and dignity; the health of my patient will be my first consideration; I will respect the secrets which are confided in me; I will maintain by all the means in my power the honor and noble traditions of the medical profession; my colleagues will be my brothers; I will not permit considerations of religion, nationality, race, party politics, or social standing to intervene between my duty and my patient; I will maintain the utmost respect for human life from the time of conception; even under threat, I will not make use of my medical knowledge contrary to the laws of humanity. I make these promises solemnly, freely and upon my honor.

Very similar principles underlie the more detailed *Code of Ethics for Emergency Medical Technicians* issued by the National Association of Emergency Medical Technicians in 1978:

> Professional status as an Emergency Medical Technician is maintained and enriched by the willingness of the individual practitioner to accept and fulfill obligations to society, other medical professionals, and the profession of Emergency Medical Technician. As an Emergency Medical Technician, I solemnly pledge myself to the following code of ethics:
> - The fundamental responsibility of the Emergency Medical Technician is to conserve life, to alleviate suffering, and to promote health.
> - The Emergency Medical Technician provides services based on human need, with respect for hu-

man dignity, unrestricted by considerations of nationality, race, creed, color, or status.

- The Emergency Medical Technician does not use professional knowledge and skill in any enterprise detrimental to the public good.
- The Emergency Medical Technician respects and holds in confidence all information of a confidential nature obtained in the course of professional work unless required by law to divulge such information.
- The Emergency Medical Technician as a citizen understands and upholds the laws and performs the duties of citizenship; as a professional person, the Emergency Medical Technician has a particular responsiblity to work with other citizens and health professionals in promoting efforts to meet the health needs of the public.
- The Emergency Medical Technician maintains professional competence and demonstrates concern for the competence of other members of the medical profession.
- The Emergency Medical Technician assumes responsibility in defining and upholding standards of professional practice and education. The Emergency Medical Technician assumes responsibility for individual professional actions and judgment, both in dependent and independent emergency functions and knows and upholds the laws which affect the practice of the Emergency Medical Technician.
- The Emergency Medical Technician has the responsibility to participate in the study of and action on matters of legislation affecting Emergency Medical Technicians and emergency service to the public.
- The Emergency Medical Technician adheres to standards of personal ethics which reflect credit upon the profession.
- The Emergency Medical Technician may contribute to research in relation to a commercial product or service, but does not lend professional status to advertising, promotion, or sales.
- The Emergency Medical Technician, or groups of Emergency Medical Technicians, who advertise professional services, do so in conformity with the dignity of the profession.
- The Emergency Medical Technician has an obligation to protect the public by not delegating to a person less qualified any service which requires the professional competence of an Emergency Medical Technician.
- The Emergency Medical Technician works harmoniously with, and sustains confidence in, Emergency Medical Technician associates, the nurse, the physician, and other members of the health team.
- The Emergency Medical Technician refuses to participate in unethical procedures and assumes the responsibility to expose incompetence or unethical conduct in others to the appropriate authority.

These oaths, and others like them, are simply an amplification of a very basic concept: concern for the welfare of others. All of the various codes of right and wrong must ultimately arise from that concern, and it is a safe generalization that **if you place the welfare of the patient ahead of all other considerations, you will rarely if ever commit an unethical act in medical care.** It would be impossible to enumerate here all the

ethical dilemmas with which you may at one time or another be faced in your work as a paramedic. However, if each time you are confronted with a dilemma of right and wrong you ask youself, "What is in the best interest of the _patient?_" you will be on firm footing.

GLOSSARY

abandonment   Abrupt termination of contact with the patient without giving the patient sufficient opportunity to find another suitable health professional to take over his medical treatment.

assault   To create in another person a fear of immediate bodily harm or invasion of bodily security.

battery   Any act of touching another person without that person's consent.

civil suit   An action instituted by a private individual against another private individual.

consent   Agreement by the patient to accept a medical intervention.

  implied consent   Assumption on behalf of a person unable to give consent that he would have done so (see _emergency doctrine_).

  informed consent   A patient's voluntary agreement to be treated after being told about the nature of the disease, the risks and benefits of the proposed treatment, alternative treatments, or the choice of no treatment at all.

criminal suit   An action instituted by the government against a private individual for violation of criminal law.

damages   Compensation for injury awarded by a court.

duty to act   Legal obligation of public and certain other ambulance services to respond to a call for help in their jurisdiction.

emergency doctrine   A form of implied consent to medical treatment. When a person's life or limb is in imminent danger and the person is unable to consent to treatment, the law implies consent to emergency treatment and assumes that the person would consent if otherwise able.

false imprisonment   The intentional and unjustified detention of a person against his will.

Good Samaritan Act   Statute providing limited immunity from liability to persons responding voluntarily and in good faith to the aid of an injured person outside the hospital.

liability   A finding in civil cases that the preponderance of the evidence shows the defendant was responsible for the plaintiff's injuries.

negligence   Professional action or inaction on the part of the health worker that does not meet the standard of ordinary care expected of similarly trained and prudent health practitioners and that results in injury to the patient.

protocols Written procedures, established by the medical director and forming part of the official policy of the system, for diagnosis, triage, treatment, transport, or transfer of specified emergency medical cases.

tort Wrongful act that gives rise to a civil suit.

FURTHER READING

LAWS GOVERNING THE PARAMEDIC

Berne M. Prehospital emergency treatment of people who say, "No, thank you." *Emerg Med Serv* 15:62, 1986.

Chayet NL. *Legal Implications of Emergency Care.* New York: Appleton-Century-Crofts, 1969.

Clark LA. Documentation: A lingering impact. *Emergency* 20(4):42, 1988.

Cohn BM, Cohn E. Limiting liability in prehospital care. *Emergency* 26(1):54, 1994.

Curran WJ. Economic and legal considerations in emergency care. *N Engl J Med* 312:374, 1985.

Donvito MT. State legislative requirements: CPR certification of EMS personnel. *Emerg Med Serv* 14(2):89, 1985.

Drane JF. Competency to give informed consent. *JAMA* 252:925, 1984.

Frew SA. *Street Law: Rights and Responsibilities of the EMT.* Reston, Va.: Reston, 1983.

George J. *Law and Emergency Care.* St. Louis: Mosby, 1980.

Goldberg RJ et al. A review of prehospital care litigation in a large metropolitan EMS system. *Ann Emerg Med* 19:557, 1990.

Goldstein AS. *EMS and the Law.* Bowie, Md: Brady, 1983.

Griglak MJ, Bucci RL. Medicolegal management of the organically impaired patient in the emergency department. *Ann Emerg Med* 14:685, 1985.

Heck LL. Emergency care and Good Samaritan legislation. *J Kans Med Soc.* 68(1):15, 1967.

Henry GL. Legal Rounds. Problem: What constitutes negligence? *Emerg Med* 17(13):67, 1985.

Henry GL. Legal Rounds. Problem: Preventing malpractice suits. *Emerg Med* 18(13):53, 1986.

Henry GL. Legal rounds: About the medical record. *Emerg Med* 22(2):47, 1990.

Hirsch H. Legal implications of patient records. *South Med J* 72:726, 1979.

Holder AR. Minors' rights to consent to medical care. *JAMA* 257:3400, 1987.

Holroyd B et al. Prehospital patients refusing care. *Ann Emerg Med* 17:957, 1988.

Lavoie FW. Consent, involuntary treatment, and the use of force in an urban emergency department. *Ann Emerg Med* 21:25, 1992.

Mosher CB. The EMT and the law. *Emerg Med Serv* 6(5):44, 1977.

Neely K. "No way!" Handling patients who refuse care. *Emerg Med Serv* 21(11):29, 1992.

Owens BA. Suits happen. *Emerg Med Serv* 22(8):51, 1993.

Penven DS. EMTs at the crime scene. *Emerg Med Serv* 13(5):28, 1984.

Shanaberger CJ. Escaping the charge of false imprisonment. *JEMS* 15(3):58, 1990.

Shanaberger CJ. Protect yourself: Avoiding the claim of abandonment. *JEMS* 15(1):143, 1990.

Shanaberger CJ. Vehicle maintenance: Who's responsible? *JEMS* 15(10):70, 1990.

Shanaberger CJ. Defining a sense of duty. *JEMS* 16(6):91, 1991.

Shanaberger CJ. The trials of no-transport. *JEMS* 17(2):75, 1992.

MEDICAL ETHICS

Adams JR et al. Ethical conflicts in the prehospital setting. *Ann Emerg Med* 21:1259, 1992.

Ethics Committee, National Association of Emergency Medical Services Physicians. Ethical challenges in emergency medical services. *Prehosp Disaster Med* 8(2):179, 1993.

Gillon R. Philosophical medical ethics: Consent. *Br Med J* 291:1700, 1985.

4
Stress Management

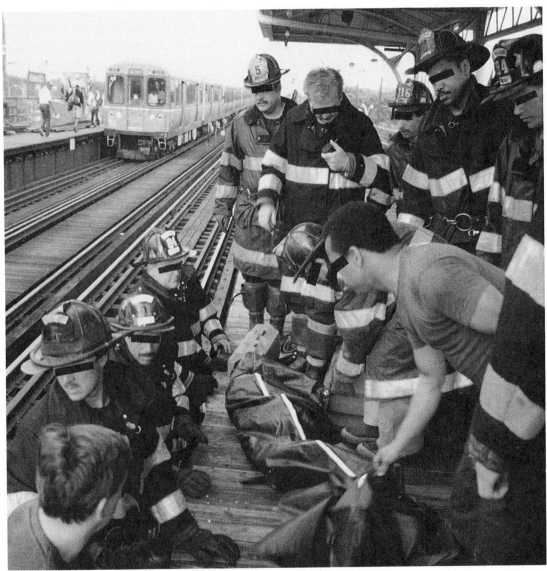

Chicago Fire Department, Chicago. Photo by Michael S. Kowal.

OBJECTIVES

Stress is a word everybody uses these days, but not everyone has a clear idea of what stress really is and how it affects us. There is no doubt, however, that stress is very much a part of the paramedic's working environment—the stress experienced by other people in the context of illness and injury; the stress experienced by the paramedic in dealing with emergencies and also nonemergencies. And because stress plays a big part in the paramedic's job, we need to understand as much as we can about stress. In this chapter, therefore, we shall take a closer look at stress—what stress is (and isn't), how it affects different people, and how the paramedic can learn to cope with stress effectively. By the end of this chapter, the student should be able to

1. Identify, given a list of definitions, the correct definition of
   • Stress
   • Alarm reaction
   • Alerting response
   • Denial
   • Regression
   • Projection
   • Displacement
   • Conversion hysteria
   • Burnout
2. List five situations or events that he or she personally finds stressful
3. List four symptoms or physical signs of an acute stress response (alarm reaction)
4. List four ways a person may respond to being injured or becoming ill
5. Identify the psychologic mechanism of defense being deployed, given a description of specific behavior
6. Identify various bystander reactions to a mass casualty situation, given a description of the behavior of several bystanders
7. List the stages in the grieving process
8. List guidelines for dealing with
   • A dying patient
   • A grieving family
9. List eight symptoms or signs of impending burnout
10. Describe his or her personal strategy for preventing burnout

WHAT STRESS IS ALL ABOUT

All of us have experienced what is commonly regarded as stress at one time or another. In fact, vir-

tually every human activity involves some degree of stress—sometimes pleasant, sometimes unpleasant, sometimes mild, sometimes intense; and virtually all living creatures are equipped with some sort of inborn stress reaction that enables them to deal effectively with their environment. Hans Selye, considered to be the "father of stress theory," has *defined* biologic **stress** as the "nonspecific response of the body to any demand made upon it." Stress, that is to say, is a stereotyped *reaction* of the body to any agent or situation (**stressor**) that requires the individual to adapt. Adaptation of one sort or another is necessary all the time, for growth, for development, or just for meeting the demands of everyday life. By itself, then, stress is neither a good thing nor a bad thing, nor should all stress be avoided. After all, self-preservation, one of the most basic requirements of life, would be impossible without a stress-alarm mechanism. That mechanism also serves us in a variety of other endeavors, such as motivating us to study for examinations! Therefore it is important to distinguish between injurious and noninjurious stress responses. Selye, for that reason, has classified stress into two categories: *eu*stress (positive stress), the kind of stress that motivates an individual to achieve; and *di*stress (negative or injurious stress), the stress that a person finds overwhelming and debilitating. In the rest of this chapter, when we speak about "stress," we shall in fact be talking about *di*stress, the negative kind of stress.

WHAT TRIGGERS STRESS

The stress response is usually associated with events that are perceived as threatening or demanding, but the specific events that fall into that category vary enormously from individual to individual. One person may, for example, go into a cold sweat even at the *thought* of air travel, while another isn't happy unless he is up among the clouds piloting an airplane. Learned attitudes, that is, strongly affect the situations people find stressful. Nonetheless, it is possible to list certain categories of experience that serve as stress triggers in the vast majority of people:

STRESS TRIGGERS

• LOSS of a loved person or thing
  Examples: death of a spouse or family member; divorce
• Personal INJURY or ILLNESS

- MAJOR LIFE EVENTS
  Examples: starting or finishing school; marriage; pregnancy; children leaving home; retirement
- JOB STRESS
  Examples: conflicts with the boss or co-workers; excessive responsibility; change in responsibilities; unclear job description; work overload or underload; time pressure; being fired; changing jobs

To deal effectively with stress, each individual needs to make a personal appraisal of the stress triggers in his or her life, for by recognizing the specific stressors in our lives, we can take steps to minimize their effects.

THE PHYSIOLOGY OF ACUTE STRESS

One of the fundamental models for stress evolved from studies of how man and many other animals respond to a threatening situation. It was observed that when a person or a laboratory animal is confronted with a situation that he *perceives* as threatening, a standard series of physiologic reactions is triggered, irrespective of the nature of the threat (that is why Selye referred to stress as a *nonspecific* response). Typically those physiologic reactions are initially such to prepare the animal for "fight or flight," through activation of the **sympathetic nervous system.** We shall learn about the sympathetic nervous system in considerably more detail later, in Chapter 23. For our purposes here, suffice it to say that the sympathetic nervous system is the part of the autonomic, or involuntary, nervous system whose function is to prepare the body to meet an emergency.

Generally, the first stage of the stress response is an **alarm reaction,** which occurs within a fraction of a second after being confronted with a strong stimulus—for instance, a sudden loud noise. The alarm reaction begins with a quick **alerting response,** in which one immediately stops whatever one was doing and orients toward the source of stimulation. Anyone who has ever startled a grazing deer will have seen a very good example of the alerting response: The deer will suddenly stop grazing, look toward the sound that startled it, and stand absolutely still. Together with the alerting response there is a sudden stimulation of the sympathetic nervous system, producing constriction of the blood vessels, in-crease in the heart rate, dilatation of the pupils, erection of the hair follicles on the skin, increased secretion of sweat, and a variety of other physiologic effects. Indeed, we often describe our reactions to a stressful experience in terms of the sympathetic nervous system effects: "My heart was pounding in my chest." "I broke out in a cold sweat." "I had goose bumps all over." "My mouth went dry." Those are all part of the body's "fight-or-flight" response to a perceived threat.

For most animals, the fight-or-flight response is a very useful and adaptive mechanism, mobilizing them either to defend themselves (fight) or run away (flight) in the face of possible danger. Taking either of those steps dissipates the stress, and the animal then goes through a stage of relaxation ("I breathed a sigh of relief when it was over.") and finally returns to its original internal balance. For modern man, however, the automatic fight-or-flight response to stressful circumstances is probably not as useful as it was in an earlier stage of his evolution; for most of the stressors that humans face in the modern world are not, as we saw in the previous section, of a type that can be effectively handled either by fighting or running away. When a loved one dies, for example, or when one loses one's job, there is no outlet for the stress either in fighting or running away. Under such circumstances, stress becomes chronic, placing our bodies in a continuous, unrelieved state of alert leading eventually to exhaustion and ill health.

It is important to point out that the stress response, even if it is not perhaps as useful to us as it once was, is nonetheless perfectly normal. Yet very many people misunderstand the normal physiologic reactions to stressors and interpret the body's preparations for fight or flight as signs of disease, which only serves to increase the level of anxiety. In commenting on that tendency to misread the stress signals of our bodies, one stress researcher has written:

> [Modern man] speaks of indigestion when apprehensiveness kills his appetite, and insomnia when fright keeps him awake at night. . . . The increased heartbeat becomes palpitation, the sudden elimination of waste matter he calls diarrhea, the clenching of his back muscles he calls lumbago.*

As we shall discuss in a later section when we deal with the prevention of "burnout," it is essential that the paramedic learn to recognize the symptoms of the stress response for what they are. Chronic stress can exact a high toll when it goes unrecognized and unrelieved.

---

*Simeons ATW. *Man's Presumptuous Brain: An Evolutionary Interpretation of Psychosomatic Disease.* New York: Dutton, 1961.

HOW PEOPLE REACT TO STRESSFUL SITUATIONS

Anyone who is involved in the situation of critical illness or injury—the patient, the family, bystanders, health professionals—responds in some way to the stresses of an emergency. It is important that paramedics understand the range of normal responses to an emergency, both in others and in themselves, in order to deal with those responses effectively.

Responses of the Patient to Illness and Injury

The reactions of a given patient to critical illness or injury will be largely determined by the mechanisms that individual has developed over the years for dealing with stressful situations. Among those mechanisms are certain common patterns. If the emergency is a medical illness, there is usually a transition period from health to illness, during which most people first become aware of some painful or unpleasant sensations and perhaps a decrease in energy and strength as well. The common response to that awareness is ANXIETY. Some patients will attempt to deny or minimize their symptoms at that point, while others become irritable and angry. Once the patient comes to view himself as ill or once he has been injured, any of several common reactions may occur:

- REALISTIC FEARS, such as fear of pain, disability, death, or economic difficulties resulting from disability.
- DIFFUSE ANXIETY, often stemming from a feeling of HELPLESSNESS. Nearly every person who finds himself transformed into a patient feels that he has lost a degree of control over his own existence; furthermore, he must place himself in the hands of someone, often a stranger, on whom he must depend completely and whose competence he cannot really evaluate. People whose self-esteem depends on being active, independent, and aggressive are particularly prone to anxiety when they become ill or injured; but nearly all individuals will experience some degree of diffuse anxiety at the prospect of losing control over their lives.
- DEPRESSION is a natural response to *loss*. In the case of the patient with critical illness or injury, what he has lost is some bodily function as well as some degree of control over his own destiny. The patient who has suffered a stroke, for example, may have lost the ability to move the arm or leg on one side of his body and even the ability

to speak. It is only natural to feel depressed under such circumstances.
- ANGER. The angry patient poses one of the most difficult problems for many health professionals to deal with. Suppose, for example, a paramedic arrives at the scene of an accident and starts tending immediately to one of the injured, and the patient becomes hostile and abusive. The paramedic's natural tendency, under the circumstances, is to think, "Here I am trying to save this guy's life, and he's dumping all over me. Well, he can just go straight to blazes." It is crucial, therefore, to understand that often people respond to discomfort or limitation of function by becoming resentful and suspicious of those around them. A patient who feels angry may vent his anger on the rescuer, by becoming impatient and irritable or excessively demanding, simply because the rescuer is the most convenient target. What a health *professional* will realize in such circumstances is that the patient's anger stems from fear and discomfort and is not really directed at the rescue team.
- CONFUSION is especially common among the elderly, in whom illness or injury may precipitate disorientation. Such confusion is furthered by the presence of unfamiliar people and equipment, which may overwhelm the patient. When a patient appears confused, therefore, it is very important to explain carefully at the outset who you are and what your mission is; thereafter, you should keep up a running commentary on what you are doing, to help orient the patient to your role.

In addition to experiencing the reactions just described, most people suffering sudden illness or injury will mobilize one or another psychologic **mechanism of defense.** All of us use psychologic defense mechanisms all the time. We deploy those defense mechanisms mostly automatically and without even being aware of them (i.e., unconsciously) as a way of obtaining relief from stressful situations. The defense mechanisms most commonly encountered in the practice of prehospital emergency care include the following:

- DENIAL. Many patients attempt to ignore their problem, especially in the case of medical illness, because of the anxiety it causes. Denial is often evident in a tendency to dismiss all symptoms with words such as *only* or *a little* (e.g., the middle-aged man with chest pain who says, "I'm fine, I'm fine. It's only a little indigestion."). When a patient tries to minimize his or her symptoms in that way, it may be necessary to find a reliable informant among the patient's family or friends from whom to obtain more details.

- REGRESSION is a return to an earlier mode of behavior or level of emotional adjustment. Regression is often evident in children under stress; for instance, a 10-year-old who sailed through his toilet training years earlier may suddenly start wetting the bed at night after a stressful experience. Adults too often revert to more childish behavior under stress. Indeed, when a person is injured or becomes ill, his role as a patient *forces* him back into a state of dependency on others that has much in common with the situation of a child.

- PROJECTION involves attributing to others one's own unacceptable feelings, motives, or desires. The patient who expresses vehement indignation or anger at the behavior of others may in fact be unconsciously "aware" that his own behavior is not exemplary.

- DISPLACEMENT occurs when a person redirects an emotion from the original object to a more acceptable substitute object. Displacement is often the operative mechanism when a patient expresses anger at the paramedic. In reality, the patient is angry at someone else—himself, a family member, fate, God—but he unconsciously redirects his anger toward the stranger who comes to provide medical care.

As noted, most of the psychologic mechanisms that a person deploys to deal with stress are not under conscious control. The injured patient who responds with anger toward the paramedic usually "can't help" behaving the way he does. It is his automatic way of dealing with stress. For you, seeing a person with a heart attack, a stroke, or a broken leg will become a routine part of the job. For the person who has suffered that heart attack or stroke or broken leg, it is a major personal calamity. Try to keep that in mind and to understand the enormous distress that lies behind difficult behavior.

Responses of Family, Friends, and Bystanders

Those at the scene may show many of the responses just described. Family members, for example, may be anxious, panicky, or angry—the last reaction often stemming from their FEELINGS OF GUILT. Suppose, for example, you are called to care for a 4-year-old child who has been struck by a car. The parents of the child are at the scene. Consciously or unconsciously, they feel guilty for what has happened; they may believe, deep down, that if they had kept a

closer eye on the child, he would not have run out into the street. But, using the mechanisms of *projection* and *displacement*, the parents express their guilt feelings in aggressive behavior toward the rescue team. To cope with their own anxieties, they may demand immediate action or put pressure on you to move immediately on to the hospital. Especially galling may be inferences that you are not competent to handle the situation (e.g., "Hurry up and get him to the hospital so that he can be seen by a *doctor!*"). The paramedic needs to recognize that the patient's family and friends have concerns too and that their behavior, however irritating, arises from distress. Step back emotionally from the situation for a moment. Keep your cool. Reassure the patient's family or friends that there is radio contact with the physician at all times and that you are working under the physician's guidance for the best interests of the patient.

In summary, whether dealing with the behavior of the patient or of those around him, the paramedic must constantly remain aware of the distress that lies behind the behavior. When you are summoned to an emergency, you are not being invited to a tea party. You are entering a situation in which *everyone is under stress*, so people are not going to behave the way they do on social occasions. People who are ordinarily calm and polite in everyday life may not be calm and polite in the circumstances in which you find them. But if *you* can stay calm and polite, irrespective of what is going on around you, it will go a long way to improve the behavior of everyone else at the scene.

> **REMEMBER: IN EMERGENCY SITUATIONS, EVERYONE IS UNDER STRESS.**

Responses in Multicasualty Incidents

In a situation involving multiple casualties, such as a train derailment, building collapse, or natural disaster (tornado, flood, earthquake), both victims and bystanders may react by becoming dazed, disorganized, or overwhelmed. The American Psychiatric Association has identified five categories of reactions in such circumstances:

- The NORMAL REACTION to such incidents consists of symptoms of extreme *anxiety*, including sweating, tremulousness, weakness, nausea, and sometimes vomiting. Individuals experiencing this response may recover fully within a few minutes and provide useful assistance if properly directed. EMS personnel are not immune to this type of reaction, and if you see one of your crew looking a little shaky, the best remedy is to give him or her a specific task (e.g., "Get this IV started.").

- A more worrisome reaction is BLIND PANIC, in which the individual's judgment seems to disappear entirely. Blind panic is particularly dangerous because it is "catchy," and it may precipitate mass panic among others present. For that reason, a panicky bystander needs to be separated quickly from others and, if at all possible, placed under the supervision of a calmer person.
- DEPRESSION is seen in the individual who sits or stands in a numbed, dazed state. The depressed bystander needs to be brought back to reality and given something constructive to do.
- OVERREACTION is typified by the person who talks compulsively, jokes inappropriately, becomes overly active, and races from one task to another without accomplishing anything useful. The person who is overreacting needs to be removed from the area where casualties are being treated.
- In CONVERSION HYSTERIA, the patient subconsciously converts his anxiety into a bodily dysfunction; he may be unable to see or hear or may become paralyzed in an extremity.

We shall deal in more detail with how to cope with bystanders at mass casualties when we discuss multicasualty incidents in Chapter 21.

Responses of the Paramedic

Health professionals are not immune to the stresses of emergency situations, and it is to be expected that those dealing with the critically ill and injured will experience a multitude of feelings, not all of them pleasant. The paramedic may feel ANGRY at the demands of the family or the patient; ANXIOUS in the face of life-threatening injuries; DEFENSIVE at inferences he or she is not competent to handle a situation; SAD in response to the death of a patient. Those feelings are all perfectly natural, but it is preferable to keep such feelings to yourself during the emergency situation. An attitude of outward calm and confidence on your part will do much to relieve the anxieties of others at the scene—and that too is part of the paramedic's therapeutic role.

One reaction that is common among health professionals is a feeling of *irritation at the patient who does not appear to be particularly ill.* That reaction is especially prevalent among emergency personnel, who are psychologically geared to deal with life-threatening and catastrophic cases and who therefore tend to regard an apparently minor complaint as a burdensome annoyance. Recall, however, that when a person calls for help, he does so because something is worrying him. It may be an injury, a pain, a disturbing feeling, or a bodily function that the patient perceives as somehow disordered. IT IS NOT THE PARAMEDIC'S FUNCTION TO PASS JUDGMENT ON THE VALIDITY OF THE PATIENT'S COMPLAINT. While it is much more dramatic to rescue the victim of multiple trauma than to reassure the patient with a minor cold, both patients have, by virtue of a stated or implicit request for help, indicated that they are in some way distressed and are looking to the rescuer for assistance. The paramedic's role is to be supportive and nonjudgmental, rendering whatever care is needed under the circumstances. The paramedic who uses derogatory terminology (such as "turkey" or "crock") to refer to a patient is simply betraying immaturity and lack of compassion for others.

COPING WITH DEATH AND DYING

Sooner or later, just about every emergency care provider is going to have to deal with death because a certain proportion of patients requiring urgent care are going to die. When that happens, what do you do? What do you say to a dying patient? What do you say to a parent when there's nothing else you can do for his or her child? How do you deal with your own feelings when a patient has died while under your care? Each of us ultimately has to answer those questions for ourself, after taking a close look at our own attitudes toward death and taking care of the "unfinished business" connected with our attitudes. But there *are* some general guidelines and techniques for dealing with the dying patient, the grieving family, and your own stress.

Stages of the Grieving Process

In her classic study, *On Death and Dying*, Dr. Elisabeth Kubler-Ross defined five stages through which grieving people—such as the dying patient himself or the surviving family—often proceed when dealing with loss. Each of those stages in some way helps the grieving person to adapt to the reality he or she must confront. It is useful to be aware of those stages and to consider the behavior of dying patients or their families in the context of the grieving process.

- STAGE 1: DENIAL

  We have already mentioned denial as a mechanism by which a person attempts to ignore a problem or pretend it does not exist. Denial is a way of buffering bad news until one can mobilize the resources to deal with that news more effectively.

- STAGE 2: ANGER

  When a person can no longer deny the reality of his situation, anger over the loss replaces denial. The patient or the family ask, "Why me?" and displace their anger randomly to those around them. As we mentioned earlier, such anger may be very difficult for health care personnel to deal with, and it is necessary again and again to remind oneself, "This patient (or this family member) is not really angry at me. He is angry at the unfair hand life has just dealt him."

- STAGE 3: BARGAINING

  When anger does not change the painful reality, the grieving person will often turn to bargaining, that is, trying to make some sort of deal in hopes of postponing the inevitable: "If I can just live long enough to see my daughter's wedding, then I'll die in peace."

- STAGE 4: DEPRESSION

  When bargaining fails to change the reality and the individual must come to terms with dying, there is suddenly an enormous sense of loss. The patient may become very quiet, and many people make the mistake of trying to "cheer the patient up" at this point. The patient does not *want* to be cheered up. He wants permission to express his sorrow—in words, in tears, or in what Kubler-Ross has called "the silence that goes beyond words."

- STAGE 5: ACCEPTANCE

  In the final stage, the patient prepares to disengage from the world around him. He sheds his fears and most of his other feelings as well and begins to loosen the ties that bind him to other people. When the dying patient enters the stage of acceptance, it is often the family that is in need of the most help.

Dealing with the Dying Patient

The patient who is dying generally knows, at the very least, that his situation is serious; he may, in fact, be well aware that he is dying, and he may want to talk about it. Many health professionals are reluctant to discuss death with a patient, mostly because of their own anxiety about the subject. So they try to maintain an attitude of cheery reassurance ("Everything is going to be all right . . ."), when both they and the patient know that everything will *not* be all right. The message the patient gets is that the subject of dying is taboo and that he'd better keep his feelings about dying to himself. In fact, perhaps the most important thing one can do for a dying patient is to let him know that it *is* OK to talk about it. There are many ways of doing so. One needn't come right out and ask, "Do you want to talk about dying?" It's enough to say, "If there's anything worrying you, I'd be glad to listen."

Having made the offer to listen, be prepared to do so. Let the patient talk as much as he wishes to. And make some physical contact with him: Hold his hand, put a hand on his shoulder, or make some other gesture of human warmth.

What if the patient comes straight out and asks you, "Am I going to die?" There is no simple answer as to how to reply to that question, but the answer should acknowledge the seriousness of the patient's condition without taking away all hope. For example, one might say, "Sir, you seem to have had a quite severe heart attack. We're going to give you the best care available, and there's every chance you'll come out of this OK. But the situation *is* serious." For a patient who knows that he is dying, it may be a great relief to have someone else acknowledge the fact and thereby give him permission to talk about it.

The dying patient also needs to feel that he still has some control over his life; for when a person loses all control over his life, he loses a large measure of his dignity and self-respect. To the degree possible, explain to the patient what you are doing and allow him to participate in the treatment. Ask him if there is anyone he would like you to contact or if he has any special instructions he wants conveyed to someone. If the patient *does* ask you to convey a message, *write it down* word-for-word as he states it to you.

Dealing with a Grieving Family

Suppose you are called to the scene of an accident where a child has been run over by a truck. You can see at a glance that the child is dead and beyond hope of resuscitation—his skull has been smashed open and his brains are all over the street. Two police officers are restraining the child's mother, who is crying hysterically.

The fact that there is nothing you can do for the child does *not* mean that the call is over. There is another "patient" at the scene, the child's mother, and the call is not over until you have done all you can for her.

What kind of things *can* you do for a grieving family? How can you help them begin the process of dealing with their loss? Here are a few guidelines:

- Do *not* try to hide the body of the deceased from the family, even if the body has been badly mutilated. People who are prevented from seeing the body of a loved one may later have enormous difficulty in working through their grief, for they may not be able to get beyond the stage of denial.
- For similar reasons, do not use euphemisms for death, such as *expired* or *passed away*. The family needs to hear the word *dead*.
- Do not be in a hurry to clear away all your resuscitation equipment. Let the family see the equipment before you start tidying up and packing away your gear, so that they will know that everything possible was done to try to save the patient.
- Give the family some time with the body, especially when the victim is a child. If the death occurred in a public place—as in the hypothetical road accident described—move the body into the ambulance and let the family be alone with it there. Give them a chance to say good-bye in their own way.
- Try to arrange for further support. Recruit a neighbor to come over, or offer to call the family's clergy.
- Accept the family's right to experience a variety of feelings—guilt, shock, denial, anger. And when family members do respond with anger, remind yourself yet again, "They aren't really angry at *me*."

After the Call Is Over

It can be a shattering experience to have a patient die while under your care, especially if the patient is a young person or if you and your crew invested a lot of time and effort trying to save the patient. In such cases, everyone involved in the call is likely to experience some heavy-duty feelings. If those feelings stay bottled up, there may be all sorts of problems later on down the line. Every ambulance service, therefore, needs to develop routine procedures for debriefing after any call that involved the death of a patient. All those who participated in the call need a chance to sit down together, in an atmosphere of confidentiality, and air their feelings about what happened.

Increasingly, EMS systems throughout the United States and abroad are deploying specially trained teams to conduct **critical incident stress debriefings** (CISD) with emergency personnel who

have been involved in particularly traumatic calls or other painful incidents. By definition, a critical incident is one that overwhelms the ability of an EMS worker to cope, either at the scene or some time later. The sorts of incidents that are apt to require a CISD include

- Serious injury or death of a fellow worker in the line of duty
- Suicide of a fellow worker
- Multicasualty incidents, such as an airliner crash or train wreck
- Serious injury or death of a child
- Intense media attention to an incident

It is impossible, however, to predict how any given person will react to a particular incident. A call that may be very disturbing to one paramedic may not bother his or her partner at all. So when a potentially critical incident occurs, what is important is to be on the lookout for signs and symptoms that suggest a need for psychologic intervention.

CRITICAL INCIDENT STRESS DEBRIEFING MAY BE NEEDED WHEN

- You have trouble putting the incident out of your thoughts
- You keep having "flashbacks" of the incident
- You have nightmares or other sleep disturbances after the incident
- You find yourself withdrawing from co-workers and family members after an incident

---

The purpose of the CISD is to accelerate the normal recovery process and to help EMS personnel realize that they are normal people having a normal reaction to *ab*normal events. As mentioned, many EMS systems now have critical incident stress management *teams* to provide support after a traumatic call—and sometimes even during the incident itself. The intervention may take the form of a brief (30-minute) **defusing** session right after the call, in which all of those who were involved in the incident are given a chance to express their feelings about what happened. As the name implies, a defusing session is intended to remove the explosive potential from a situation and thereby prevent more serious psychologic consequences later on.

A formal **debriefing** is usually conducted 24 to 72 hours after an incident when it becomes clear that the incident has had a serious impact and is causing persisting symptoms among the crew. A debriefing usually takes about 3 hours. It ideally includes all the personnel who were involved in the incident. It is conducted away from the workplace and in an atmosphere of confidentiality, so that each participant can feel secure to speak freely.

HOW TO KEEP FROM BURNING OUT

What's all this? We've scarcely started the paramedic course, and already we're talking about burnout! Why should we start worrying now about something that may (or may not) happen 10 years down the line?

We need to consider burnout now—at the earliest stage of paramedic training—because now is the time to start developing attitudes and habits that will help prevent burnout, whether 1 year or 20 years down the line.

The dictionary defines *burnout* as the exhaustion of physical or emotional strength. Burnout is, in fact, a consequence of chronic, unrelieved stress. The paramedic's job, by its very nature, is full of potential stresses. There are the obvious stresses imposed by having to deal, day after day, with mutilating trauma or catastrophic illness. There are, as well, more subtle stresses associated with interpersonal relations, pay, prestige, fringe benefits, and so forth. Consider, for example, this list of grievances from one apparently burned-out EMT:

1. I'm tired of nurses who complain about medics "stealing their jobs" and turn around and want to run calls and tell us what to do without experience.
2. I'm tired of the public's misconception of what we do, and I'm tired of our complacent attitude toward correcting this misconception.
3. I'm tired of not having equipment work (including vehicles) when we need [it].
4. I'm tired of system abuse: those who use an ambulance as a taxi. . . .
5. I'm tired of supervisors and administrators not listening to those of us who are in the field every day and have good, common-sense ideas that would make the job easier and keep morale up.
6. I'm tired of making less money than most of the people who work in the hospital, ranking right up there with unit clerks and LPNs.*

All of the complaints and stresses listed by the EMT are, no doubt, legitimate. But burnout does not occur

*McQueen I. Sick and tired. *Emergency* 21(7):40, 1989.

solely because of stress. Burnout develops because of the way a person *reacts* to stress. During the past decade, considerable scientific study has been devoted to the ways different people respond to stress and the implications for health and disease.

We mentioned earlier that one person's eustress may be another's distress. The reason is that distress is a *learned* reaction, based on the way an individual perceives and interprets the world around him. In other words, distress is nearly always the result of what a person *believes*.

Some beliefs are more likely than others to produce stress. Here are some beliefs that are common among EMS personnel:

- I have to be perfect all the time.
- My safety depends on being able to anticipate every possible danger.
- I am totally responsible for what happens to the patient; if he dies, it is wholly my fault.
- If there's something I don't know, people will think less of me.
- A good paramedic never makes mistakes.

Those beliefs are very likely to produce stress. They are also false beliefs. Prevention and relief of stress among EMS personnel begin with the recognition that such beliefs are unrealistic and invalid.

Like many of the conditions we shall study in this textbook, burnout is also a sort of illness. And like any other illness, it has signs and symptoms. Learn to look for the symptoms of burnout in yourself and in your co-workers. Those symptoms are warning signals, telling you to stop and reexamine your beliefs and your ways of responding to stress.

SYMPTOMS OF IMPENDING BURNOUT

- Chronic fatigue and irritability
- Cynical, negative attitudes
- Lack of desire to report to work
- Emotional lability (crying easily, flying off the handle without provocation, laughing inappropriately)
- Changes in sleep patterns (insomnia or sleeping more than usual), and waking without feeling refreshed
- Feelings of being overwhelmed, being helpless, hopeless
- Loss of interest in hobbies
- Decreased ability to concentrate

- Declining health—a lot of colds, stomach upsets; muscle aches and pains (especially headaches, backaches)
- A feeling of constant tightness in your muscles
- Overeating; smoking; abusing drugs, alcohol

It is preferable, of course, not to wait until symptoms of burnout develop. There are paramedics who have been in the field for 20 years and show no signs whatsoever of burnout, who still report to work every day with the same enthusiasm they had as rookies.

What is their secret? In general, the paramedics who do not suffer burnout are those who have learned to respect and value *themselves*. That is not as easy as it sounds. The type of person who chooses to become a paramedic is usually altruistic—someone who puts the needs of others ahead of his or her own needs. In theory, that is very laudable. But in fact, no one can give his best to others for very long if he ignores his own personal needs.

Guidelines for Preventing Burnout

Practically speaking, what does it mean to respect and value yourself? How can you translate that attitude into concrete action? Some of the steps you can take to protect yourself from burnout are summarized in the following guidelines:

- Paramedic heal thyself! TAKE CARE OF YOUR OWN HEALTH.
  1. Get enough REST. Fatigue reduces a person's ability to cope with stress. People who are tired, furthermore, experience increased irritability, anxiety, and dissatisfaction as well as impairments in thinking and judgment.
  2. Eat a balanced DIET (see Further Reading at the end of this chapter). Avoid sugar and highly processed food. Go easy on the caffeine. Eating a diet low in fat and sugar and high in complex carbohydrates (starches) before and during a shift can elevate your energy level. On the other hand, junk food diets, which are often the mainstay of firehouse cuisine, produce fatigue, nervousness, and irritability.
  3. Get regular physical EXERCISE—*at least* 30 minutes of aerobic activity (e.g., walking, running, swimming) 3 to 4 times per week. Physical activity, besides keeping you fit, helps relieve tension and stress.

  4. DON'T ABUSE YOUR BODY. Smoking, overindulgence in alcohol, taking recreational drugs, or self-prescribing any other drugs—all of these are forms of self-abuse. If you value yourself, you will value your body.
- GIVE YOURSELF SOME "ME" TIME EVERY DAY. Some of the most stress-resistant paramedics are those who have learned the techniques of meditation and can thereby escape now and then to a quiet place within themselves. Try out different methods of meditation or relaxation (see Further Reading at the end of this chapter), and see what works best for you.
- LEARN HOW TO RELAX.
  1. Take time for hobbies.
  2. Engage in social activities with people *not* involved in EMS.
  3. Leave your job behind when your shift is over.
- DO NOT MAKE UNREASONABLE DEMANDS ON YOURSELF.
  1. Forget the idea that you have to be perfect. No one is perfect. If you do the best job you can, that is good enough.
  2. You don't have to be right all the time. Accept the fact that now and then you will make a mistake—and that the world will not come to an end on account of it.
- DO NOT MAKE UNREASONABLE DEMANDS ON OTHERS.
- STAY IN TOUCH WITH YOUR FEELINGS.
  1. Find someone you can talk to. Share the stress.
  2. Cry when you need to. There's no shame in being sad sometimes.
- LEARN TECHNIQUES FOR SHEDDING STRESS WHILE ON DUTY. Don't let stress accumulate. Kate Dernocoeur, an experienced paramedic and teacher, has described three techniques for dealing with the emotions and frustrations of a tough shift:
  1. CLEAN-SLATING. Picture a blackboard in your mind. Every time you go on a call, new data are written on the mental blackboard. When the call is finished, wipe the slate clean. By doing so, you provide yourself with a fresh framework for the next call, and you don't muddle up the feelings that are generated by different calls.
  2. ROLL-OFF-THE-BACK. If you find yourself taking a lot of verbal abuse on a call, treat that abuse by letting it roll past you, just as a wave rolls over your back at the seashore. Let it roll on and be gone. "Holding onto it," as Ms. Dernocoeur points out, "means you have to do something else with it!"
  3. COMPARTMENTALIZATION. "Knowing how to focus on just one task at a time can also help minimize the sense of being overwhelmed and

pressured, either on an emergency call or in daily life. Imagine a place in your mind where there are slots like those for mail in a mail room; assign only one task per 'box.' Below these slots is your 'work space.' The goal is to strive to have only one task pulled from its slot and spread out on the work space at once."*

- DEBRIEF AFTER TOUGH CALLS. If your ambulance service does not have a program for critical incident stress debriefing, insist that such a program be started. As mentioned earlier, your health and your career as a paramedic depend on having a means of ventilating your feelings after tough calls; it is the responsibility of your employer to make sure you have those means.

GLOSSARY

alarm reaction   The first stage of the acute stress response.

alerting response   The beginning of an alarm reaction, in which the animal suddenly stops all activity and orients toward the source of stimulation.

burnout   The exhaustion of physical or emotional strength as a result of chronic stress.

CISD   Critical incident stress debriefing.

conversion hysteria   A condition in which a person unconsciously translates an emotional conflict into a physical symptom, such as paralysis.

critical incident   An incident that overwhelms the ability of an EMS worker to adjust emotionally.

debriefing   Formal session, usually conducted 24 to 72 hours after a critical incident, to deal with the feelings and reactions of the personnel involved.

defusing   Brief meeting shortly after a potentially critical incident to vent feelings and prevent serious psychologic sequelae.

denial   The psychologic defense mechanism of dealing with unwanted feelings or information by ignoring them.

displacement   The redirection of an emotion from the original object to a substitute object more acceptable to the patient.

fight-or-flight reaction   Instinctive response to acute stress, mediated by the sympathetic nervous system.

projection   Attributing to others one's own unacknowledged feelings.

regression   Return to an earlier mode of behavior or level of emotional adjustment.

stress   The nonspecific response of the body to any demand made upon it.

sympathetic nervous system   A subdivision of the autonomic nervous system that prepares the body to meet emergencies.

FURTHER READING

DEATH AND DYING

Cooke MW et al. Management of sudden bereavement in the accident and emergency department. *Br Med J* 304:1207, 1992.

Costello L. Death and dying. *Emerg Med Serv* 18(8):17, 1989.

Floren T. Impact of death and dying on emergency care personnel. *Emerg Med Serv* 13(2):43, 1984.

Gassaway B. Death and the EMT. *Emerg Med Serv* 5:66, 1976.

Kubler-Ross E. *On Death and Dying.* New York: Macmillan, 1969.

Meoli M. Supporting the bereaved: Field notification of death. *JEMS* 18(12):39, 1993.

O'Keefe K. Death and dying. *JACEP* 8:275, 1979.

Osterweis M et al (eds.). *Bereavement: Reactions, Consequences, and Care.* Washington, D.C.: National Academy Press, 1984.

Schmidt TA, Tolle SW. Emergency physicians' responses to families following patient death. *Ann Emerg Med* 19:125, 1990.

STRESS MANAGEMENT: PREVENTION OF BURNOUT

Applebaum SH. *Stress Management for Health Care Professionals.* Rockville, Md: Aspen, 1981.

Benson H. *The Relaxation Response.* New York: Morrow, 1975.

Benson H. *Your Maximum Mind: Changing Your Life by Changing the Way You Think.* New York: Random House, 1987.

Brody J. *Jane Brody's Nutrition Book.* New York: Norton, 1981.

Dernocoeur K. Total self-care: Basic stress management—and more. *Emerg Med Serv* 18(2):29, 1989.

Feiner B, Helin K. Beating burnout. *Emerg Med Serv* 19(2):24, 1990.

Hinds C. The heat of burnout: How to reduce stress. *Emerg Med Serv* 17(10):52, 1988.

Kabat-Zinn J. *Full Catastrophic Living.* New York: Delacorte, 1990.

Kallop S. Finding the ability to cope. *Emergency* 22(7):48, 1990.

Light J. How to steer clear of burnout. *Emergency* 26(1):40, 1994.

LeShan L. *How to Meditate.* Boston: Little, Brown, 1974.

McQueen I. Sick and tired. *Emergency* 21(7):40, 1989.

Metz DL. *Running Hot: Structure and Stress in Ambulance Work.* Cambridge, Mass: ABT, 1982.

O'Rear J. Post-traumatic stress disorder: When the rescuer become the victim. *JEMS* 17(11):30, 1992.

Richards T. Emotional fortresses. *JEMS* 19(1):17, 1994.

Selye H. *The Stress of Life.* New York: McGraw-Hill, 1956.

Simeons ATW. *Man's Presumptuous Brain: An Evolutionary Interpretation of Psychosomatic Disease.* New York: Dutton, 1961.

Wirth SR. Job satisfaction in EMS: A different approach. *Prehosp Disaster Med* 5(1):9, 1990.

---

*Dernocoeur K. Total self-care: Basic stress management—and more. *Emerg Med Serv* 18(2):29, 1989.

II

THE BASICS

5
Medical Terminology

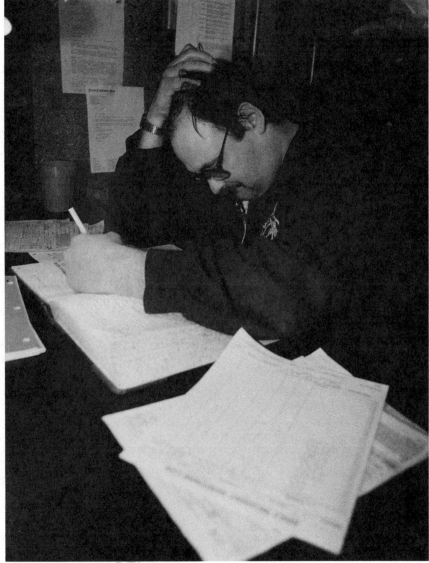

Chicago Fire Department, Chicago. Photo by Michael S. Kowal.

OBJECTIVES

Every specialized field has its own vocabulary to communicate its special concepts and concerns, and medicine is no exception. Over the centuries, medicine has acquired tens of thousands of words to express various ideas clearly. As a paramedic, you will need to know a considerable number of those technical words. You will need that vocabulary, first of all, simply to understand what is being said in class and what is written in the textbooks you are studying. As you continue learning, an understanding of medical terminology will enable you to think with more precision about medical problems. And, equally important, a knowledge of the terminology will also help you communicate effectively with other health professionals—doctors, nurses, other paramedics—for in order to communicate, people have to speak the same language.

Learning "thousands" of new words sounds like a daunting task, but in fact the task is not that difficult at all—there is a trick to it! In this chapter, we shall learn the trick of mastering medical terminology, and by the end of this chapter the student should be familiar with approximately 100 medical root words and be able to

1. Explain the meaning of a medical term, given a term composed of two or more of the root words learned in this chapter
2. Form the technical term for a medical condition, using root words learned in this chapter, given a definition of the condition
3. Describe the topographic relationship of various parts of the body to one another, using the correct terminology of position and location
4. Identify the meaning of common medical abbreviations
5. Locate terms in a medical dictionary

THE BUILDING BLOCKS OF MEDICAL WORDS

Medicine has an enormous vocabulary. But there is, as mentioned, a trick to mastering that vocabulary. That trick is based on the fact that medical terms are put together from a limited number of *root words*. The root words come mostly from the Greek and Latin and can be assembled in many different ways, like the pieces of a Lego set. So by learning only a relatively small number of root words, you will be able to figure out the meanings of many medical terms. For example, *nephro-* is a root that means "kidney"; *pyelo-* is a root meaning "the central part of the kidney," called the "pelvis" of the kidney; *-itis* is a root that means "inflammation of"; and *-ectomy* is the root

that means "surgical removal of." So we have now learned four root words:

nephro-	kidney
pyelo-	pelvis
-itis	inflammation of
-ectomy	surgical removal of

Let's put them together in a few different ways and see what comes out. (*Note*: When root words are combined, some of the vowels may drop out to make the resulting word easier to pronounce.)

nephro- + -itis	*nephritis* (an inflammation of the kidney)
pyelo- + nephro- + -itis	*pyelonephritis* (an inflammation of the pelvis of the kidney)
nephro- + -ectomy	*nephrectomy* (surgical removal of the kidney)

Let's learn a couple more roots:

chole-	bile
cyst-	sac; bladder

Now we have learned six root words, and our medical vocabulary is multiplying exponentially:

cysto- + -itis	*cystitis* (inflammation of the bladder)
chole- + cysto- + -itis	*cholecystitis* (inflammation of the gallbladder)
chole- + cysto- + -ectomy	*cholecystecomy* (surgical removal of the gallbladder)

Medical root words in fact come in three basic forms: prefixes, combining words, and suffixes.

Prefixes

The first group of medical root words we shall examine are those that tell us *in what direction, how,* or *how much*. The vast majority of these root words are *prefixes*, that is, words that appear at the beginning of a medical term (*pre-* means "before" or "in front of," so a "prefix" is a root affixed to the *front* of another word).

COMMON PREFIXES (HOW, IN WHAT DIRECTION, HOW MUCH)

a-, an-	absence of
ab-	away from
ad-	toward, near

ante-	before
anti-	against
bi-	two, double
brady-	slow
circum-	around
contra-	against
dys-	disordered, painful, difficult
ecto-	outside
endo-	within
epi-	upon
extra-	outside of
hemi-	half
hyper-	above, excess
hypo-	below, deficient
in-, intra-	inside
inter-	between
mal-	bad, disordered
olig-	few, little
ortho-	straight
para-	beside
per-	through
peri-	around
poly-	many, much
post-	after
pre-	before
quadr-	four
retro-	behind
sub-	below
super-, supra-	above
tachy-	rapid
trans-	across
tri-	three

Note that many of these prefixes are already familiar to you from their use in nonmedical words. Consider the following:

A ship that goes *below* the water is a _____ -marine.

The distance *around* a circle is its _____ -ference.

Activities *outside* regular schoolwork are _____curricular.

A sports program *within* a school is _____ -mural.

A man who has *many* wives is _____ -gamous.

Combining Words

A second class of root words include those that tell us *what organ or substance* we're talking about, such as *nephro-*, meaning "kidney." Roots in this class often appear at the beginning of a word, as in "nephri-

tis," but they may also appear in the middle of a word ("pyelo*nephr*itis") or even at the end ("peri*nephr*ic").

**COMBINING WORDS
(WHAT ORGAN OR SUBSTANCE)**

adeno-	gland
angio-	blood vessel
arthro-	joint
cardio-	heart
cephalo-	head
cerebro-	brain
chole-	bile
cyst-	sac, bladder
cyt-	cell
derm(at)o-	skin
entero-	gut
erythro-	red
gastro-	stomach
glyco-	sugar
hem(ato)-	blood
hepato-	liver
hystero-	uterus
leuko-	white
meningo-	meninges
myo-	muscle
nephro-	kidney
neuro-	nerve
orchi-	testicle
osteo-	bone
oto-	ear
pharyngo-	throat
phlebo-	vein
pneumo-	air
pulmo-	lung
pyo-	pus
rhino-	nose
sclero-	hardness
thoraco-	chest
uro-	urine, urinary
vaso-	vessel

Some of those roots are shown in Figure 5-1.

Here again, as in the case of the prefixes, there are several roots you have been using in your day-to-day speech. So you doubtless already know the meaning of words such as

arthritis (arthro- + -itis)
epigastric distress (epi- + -gastro)
hysterectomy (hystero- + -ectomy)

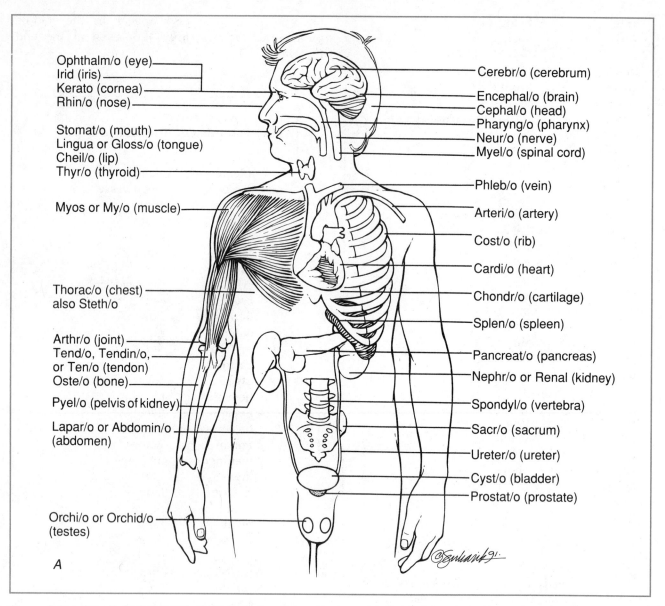

Ophthalm/o (eye)
Irid (iris)
Kerato (cornea)
Rhin/o (nose)

Stomat/o (mouth)
Lingua or Gloss/o (tongue)
Cheil/o (lip)
Thyr/o (thyroid)

Myos or My/o (muscle)

Thorac/o (chest)
also Steth/o

Arthr/o (joint)
Tend/o, Tendin/o,
or Ten/o (tendon)
Oste/o (bone)
Pyel/o (pelvis of kidney)

Lapar/o or Abdomin/o
(abdomen)

Orchi/o or Orchid/o
(testes)

Cerebr/o (cerebrum)
Encephal/o (brain)
Cephal/o (head)
Pharyng/o (pharynx)
Neur/o (nerve)
Myel/o (spinal cord)

Phleb/o (vein)
Arteri/o (artery)
Cost/o (rib)
Cardi/o (heart)
Chondr/o (cartilage)
Splen/o (spleen)
Pancreat/o (pancreas)
Nephr/o or Renal (kidney)
Spondyl/o (vertebra)
Sacr/o (sacrum)
Ureter/o (ureter)
Cyst/o (bladder)
Prostat/o (prostate)

A

FIGURE 5-1.   MEDICAL ROOT WORDS.

To form words like *arthritis* and *hysterectomy,* we need to consider one last category of root words—those that go at the *end* of the word: suffixes.

Suffixes

The third class of roots are those that tell us *what is going on* with the organ involved, for instance -*pathy* (there is disease in the organ), -*megaly* (the organ is abnormally enlarged), or -*ectomy* (the organ was surgically removed). Roots in this category are nearly always *suffixes;* that is, they appear at the *end* of the word.

**COMMON SUFFIXES
(WHAT IS GOING ON)**

-algia	pain in
-asthenia	weakness in
-centesis	puncture of
-ectomy	surgical removal of
-emia	(in the) blood
-esthesia	sensation
-genic	causing
-graph(y)	visualization of
-itis	inflammation of

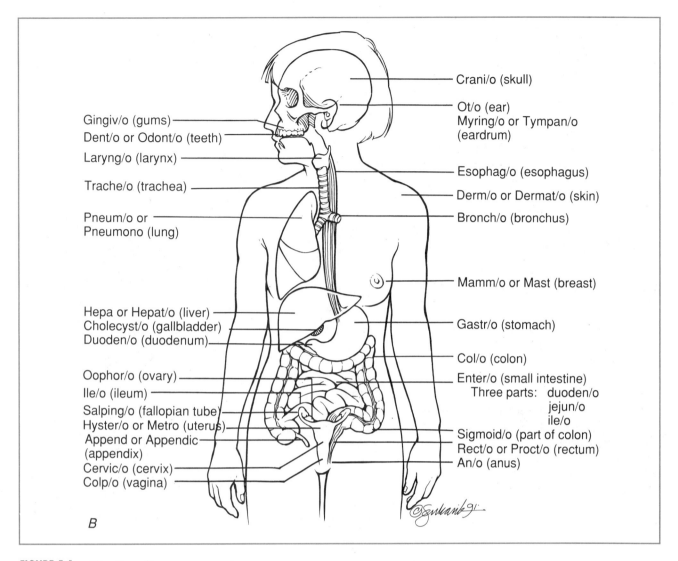

Crani/o (skull)

Ot/o (ear)
Myring/o or Tympan/o
(eardrum)

Gingiv/o (gums)
Dent/o or Odont/o (teeth)
Laryng/o (larynx)
Trache/o (trachea)

Esophag/o (esophagus)
Derm/o or Dermat/o (skin)

Pneum/o or
Pneumono (lung)

Bronch/o (bronchus)

Mamm/o or Mast (breast)

Hepa or Hepat/o (liver)
Cholecyst/o (gallbladder)
Duoden/o (duodenum)

Gastr/o (stomach)

Col/o (colon)

Enter/o (small intestine)
Three parts: duoden/o
jejun/o
ile/o

Oophor/o (ovary)
Ile/o (ileum)
Salping/o (fallopian tube)
Hyster/o or Metro (uterus)
Append or Appendic
(appendix)
Cervic/o (cervix)
Colp/o (vagina)

Sigmoid/o (part of colon)
Rect/o or Proct/o (rectum)
An/o (anus)

B

FIGURE 5-1.   (Continued)

-megaly	enlargement of
-oma	tumor of
-osis	disease of
-ostomy	opening into
-otomy	incision into
-paresis	weakness
-pathy	disease of
-penia	deficiency of
-plegia	paralysis
-pnea	breathing
-rrhagia	bursting forth
-rrhea	profuse flow
-scopy	to examine, see
-uria	urine

We have now learned somewhat fewer than 100 root words (many of which were already familiar from everyday speech), but we should already be able to figure out a very large number of medical terms. For example, what do you think is the meaning of the following?

myasthenia (myo- + -asthenia)
hepatitis (hepato- + -itis)
erythrocyte (erythro- + -cyte)
hematuria (hemato- + -uria)
hyperglycemia (hyper- + glyco- + -emia)
pericarditis (peri- + cardio- + -itis)

In the chapters that follow, you will encounter several hundred new vocabulary words (new words will be printed in **boldface type** the first time they appear). The majority will already be at least partially familiar to you if you know the roots from which they were derived. Learn the root words listed in this chapter, for those are the roots that appear most frequently. A more comprehensive list of medical root words is presented in the first glossary at the end of the book; there is also a glossary of common medical terms. Use the glossaries to refresh your memory on words you have forgotten, and use a medical dictionary to look up words you cannot decipher from their roots (see the section, Using a Medical Dictionary).

THE TERMINOLOGY OF LOCATION AND POSITION

In all of our medical work, the object of our scrutiny is ultimately the human body, and a great deal of the new terminology we shall learn relates to the human body and its structure (anatomy). Specific anatomic terms will be introduced as we deal with illness and injury involving different organ systems. We shall, for example, learn the names of the bones when we study musculoskeletal injuries. But we still need some more general terminology to help us describe where things are on the body or in what position the body and its parts are found.

Words Describing Location

On a map, we refer to north, south, east, and west. For the human body, we have other terms to indicate direction and location. The point of reference is always the *patient's* body, not the examiner's. Thus if we say that the liver is on the right side of the abdomen, we mean the *patient's* right side. Right and left are defined by drawing an imaginary line from top to bottom down the middle of the patient's body. We call that line the **midline** of the body (Fig. 5-2). When the patient is facing the examiner, everything to the "east" of the midline is on the patient's **left** side, and everything to the "west" of the midline is on the patient's **right** side.

Next we need to know which is the *front* of the body and which is the *back!* When the patient is facing the examiner, the front is called the **anterior** surface, and the back is called the **posterior** surface. Those terms may also be used in a relative sense, for example, "The toes are anterior to the heel" (the toes are more toward the front of the body than the heel is).

The next distinction we need to make is between

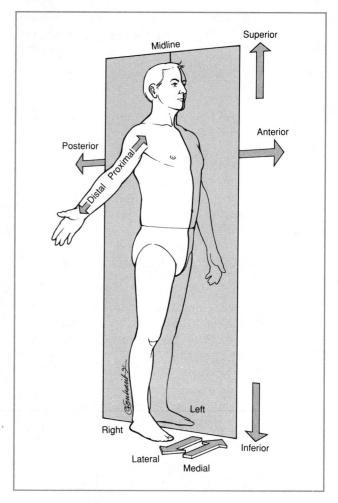

FIGURE 5-2. LOCATIONS AND DIRECTION ON THE HUMAN BODY.

things that are *up* and things that are *down*. Things that are more toward the patient's head we call **superior,** and things that are more toward his feet we call **inferior.** Those are relative terms. Thus we say, "The neck is inferior to the chin" (the neck is more toward the feet than the chin is), or "The Adam's apple is superior to the belly button" (the Adam's apple is more toward the head than the belly button is).

It is also important to be able to indicate whether the thing we are referring to—say, a particular injury—is *near the center* of the body or *near the side*. Things that are *nearer* to the center, that is, nearer to the *midline* of the body, are said to be **medial,** while locations *farther* from the midline are called **lateral,** irrespective of whether they are on the right or the left side of the body. For instance, one would say that the eye is medial to the ear (the eye is closer to the midline of the body than the ear is); conversely, the breast is lateral to the sternum (the breast is farther from the midline of the body than the sternum, or breast bone, is). [If a gunshot wound is 2 inches superior to and 2 inches lateral to the umbilicus on the right side, what organ is likely to have been hit?]

Finally, when we are talking about the extremities, we want to be able to indicate whether the part we are talking about is *near* to or *far* from the point where the extremity attaches to the body. A part of the extremity that is *nearer* to the point of attachment to the body is called **proximal**, while a part that is *farther* from the point of attachment to the body is called **distal**. Thus one may say that the elbow is proximal to the wrist (the elbow is nearer to the point of attachment to the body than the wrist is), but the ankle is distal to the knee (the ankle is farther than the knee from the point where the leg attaches to the body). [Is a burn on the distal thigh closer to the hip or closer to the knee?]

So far, we have been referring to locations on the surface of the body (**external**). We may also want to indicate that a process, like bleeding, is going on *inside* the body, that is, an **internal** process. Things affecting the inside of the body, like gunshot wounds, for example, may be near the surface (**superficial**) or remote from the surface (**deep**).

To summarize:

WORDS DESCRIBING LOCATION

midline	imaginary vertical line down the middle of the front surface of the body
anterior	toward the front
posterior	toward the back
superior	above; toward the head
inferior	below; toward the feet
medial	nearer the midline of the body
lateral	farther from the midline of the body
proximal	nearer the point of attachment to the body (or to the heart)
distal	farther from the point of attachment to the body (or from the heart)
internal	inside
external	outside
superficial	near the surface
deep	remote from the surface

Words Describing Position

We also need some vocabulary to describe the position in which we find the patient. Commonly used words, such as *sitting, standing,* and *lying down,* are perfectly acceptable. But in talking with medical professionals, you are apt to hear some more technical terminology to describe the patient's position.

A person who is standing upright is said to be **erect,** while someone who is lying down is **recumbent.** If he is lying on his back, faceup, he is **supine;** if he is lying facedown, he is **prone.** And if he should be lying on his side, he is said to be in the **lateral recumbent** position ("left lateral recumbent" if he is lying on his left side, and "right lateral recumbent" if he is on his right side).

WORDS DESCRIBING THE PATIENT'S POSITION

erect	standing upright
recumbent	lying down
supine	lying faceup
prone	lying facedown
lateral recumbent	lying on a side (left or right)

Finally, we need some terminology to describe the position or motion of extremities—whether they are straight or bent at a joint, whether they are displaced toward or away from the body. The act of bending a part of the body, or the state of being bent, is called **flexion.** When a body-builder *flexes* his biceps, for instance, what he is actually doing is bending his forearm so that it forms an angle with the upper arm. The act of straightening the arm out again, on the other hand, is called **extension.** When the chin is bent forward so that it touches the chest, the head is in flexion. When the head is tilted back to normal position, it is in extension. If you tilt the head back even farther, it is in *hyper*extension.

We can also move our extremities toward or away from the midline of the body. Any movement *away* from the midline of the body is called **abduction** (*ab-* is a prefix meaning "away"). If you hold your arms straight out to the sides, your arms are *ab*ducted. A movement of an extremity *toward* the midline of the body, on the other hand, is called **adduction** (*ad-* is a prefix meaning "toward"). [In anterior dislocation of the hip, the hip is flexed, abducted, and externally rotated. Can you picture the position of the dislocated hip?]

Finally, when the arm is *externally* rotated so that the palm faces forward, we call that **supination;** when the arm is *internally* rotated so that the back

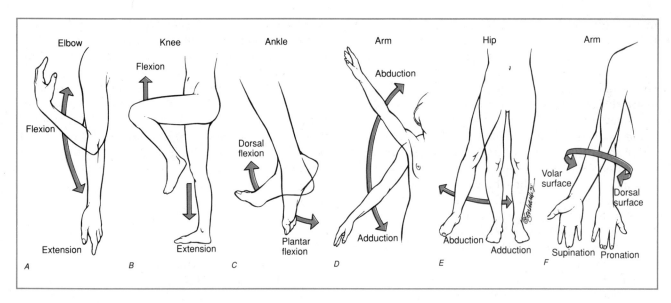

FIGURE 5-3.   **MOVEMENT AT JOINTS.**   A. Flexion and extension at the hinge
joint of the arm. B. Flexion and extension at the knee and hip. C. Flexion
(dorsiflexion) and extension (plantar flexion) at the ankle. D. Abduction and
adduction of the arm. E. Abduction and adduction of the hip. F. Supination
(external rotation) and pronation (internal rotation) of the arm.

(dorsum) of the hand faces forward, the arm is said to be in **pronation.**

Some of the positions of the extremities we have described are shown in Figure 5-3.

**WORDS DESCRIBING MOTION
AT A JOINT**

flexion	the act of bending a part, or the condition of being bent
extension	the movement that brings the parts of a limb toward a straight condition
abduction	movement away from the midline
adduction	movement toward the midline
supination	external rotation of the arm so that the palm faces forward
pronation	internal rotation of the arm so that the dorsum of the hand is forward

---

COMMON MEDICAL ABBREVIATIONS

Abbreviations are for people in a hurry, and doctors seem to be in more of a hurry than most other people.

Probably for that reason, medical language is filled with abbreviations, to the point that often a patient's medical record will be completely incomprehensible to the average layperson. For example, a typical emergency room chart might read, "The pt is a 50 yo WM c/o DOE," which translates to "The patient is a 50-year-old white male complaining of dyspnea on exertion." There is no doubt that such abbreviations save time and ballpoint pen mileage. And it would certainly be cumbersome to do without abbreviations altogether (imagine if you had to say, "We are performing cardiopulmonary resuscitation," every time you wanted to report that you were doing CPR!). Nonetheless, probably the best advice regarding the use of medical abbreviations is: AVOID THEM!!

The problem with abbreviations is that they don't always mean the same thing to different people. To an emergency room doctor, *MS* usually means "morphine sulfate," but to a neurologist it means "multiple sclerosis." Not much chance of confusion there, you say? The meaning will be clear from the context? Let's take another example. If you announce over your two-way radio, "The patient is S.O.B.," the doctor at the other end of the radio may know that what you mean is "The patient is short of breath." But the patient and his family, right there beside you, may make a different interpretation altogether, and they may not like what they hear! So try to avoid using abbreviations, especially when there is any possibility of their being misinterpreted.

Even if you are virtuously stingy with abbreviations, however, the doctors and nurses with whom you work will continue using abbreviations with happy abandon. It is therefore useful to become familiar with some of the more common medical abbreviations, which are summarized in Glossary B at the end of the book. Don't try to memorize all the abbreviations listed in the glossary! Those that you need to know will become familiar through frequent usage, both in this textbook and in your daily work. The others can lie quietly in Glossary B and needn't clutter up your head.

USING A MEDICAL DICTIONARY

Even after you have mastered the lists of basic medical root words, sooner or later you will come upon a technical term that you cannot decipher. When that moment arrives, you are going to need a medical dictionary. Check out the dictionaries at the local medical bookstore, and find one that is suited to you. The biggest, most comprehensive dictionary may not be the best. Look at the definitions in the dictionary and make sure they are written in a way that you can easily understand them. See what other features the dictionary has, such as diagrams, color plates, various tables, and lists.

Once you have purchased a medical dictionary, spend a little time getting to know what's inside. Most medical dictionaries contain, in addition to words, various illustrations and a large variety of tables (e.g., weights and measures; laboratory tests; lists of arteries, veins, muscles, and nerves).

When you are looking up a specific word, the dictionary will give you several types of information about the word. Let us consider, for example, the word *cardiomyopathy*. We already know a lot about that word, having learned the basic medical roots listed in this chapter. So we know that the word *cardiomyopathy* was put together from *cardio-* (heart), *myo-* (muscle), and *-pathy* (disease of); thus *cardiomy-*

opathy must have something to do with disease of the heart muscle. The citation in *Dorland's Illustrated Medical Dictionary* reads as follows:

> **cardiomyopathy** (kar'de-o-mi-op'ah-the) [Gr. *kardia* heart + *mys* muscle + *pathos* disease]. A subacute or chronic disorder of heart muscle of unknown or obscure etiology, often with associated endocardial, and sometimes with pericardial involvement, but not atherosclerotic in origin.

Immediately following the word *cardiomyopathy* in the above citation the somewhat strange-looking letters in parentheses indicate how to pronounce the word (one learns, thus, that the accent is on the syllable *op*). Immediately after the pronunciation, there is information in brackets about the root of the word, indicating that it comes from the Greek [Gr.] words *kardia*, meaning "heart"; *mys*, meaning "muscle"; and *pathos*, meaning "disease." Then comes the definition of the word as it is used today in medicine.

Remember:

WHEN YOU LOOK IT UP, WRITE IT DOWN!

Keep a notebook of new medical terms as you encounter them, unless you want to keep looking up the same words over and over again.

FURTHER READING

Dorland's Illustrated Medical Dictionary (27th ed.). Philadelphia: Saunders, 1988.
Frenay AC. *Understanding Medical Terminology* (6th ed.). St. Louis: Catholic Health Association, 1971.
Rothenberg RE. *Medical Dictionary and Health Manual.* (5th rev. ed.) New York: Signet Classics, 1992.
Smith GL, Davis PE. *Medical Terminology: A Programmed Text* (5th ed.). New York: Delmar, 1988.
Stedman's Medical Dictionary (25th ed.). Baltimore: Williams & Wilkins, 1990.
Steen EB. *Abbreviations in Medicine.* New York: Macmillan, 1978.
Taber's Cyclopedic Medical Dictionary (17th ed.). Philadelphia: Davis, 1993.

6
The Primary Survey: Overview

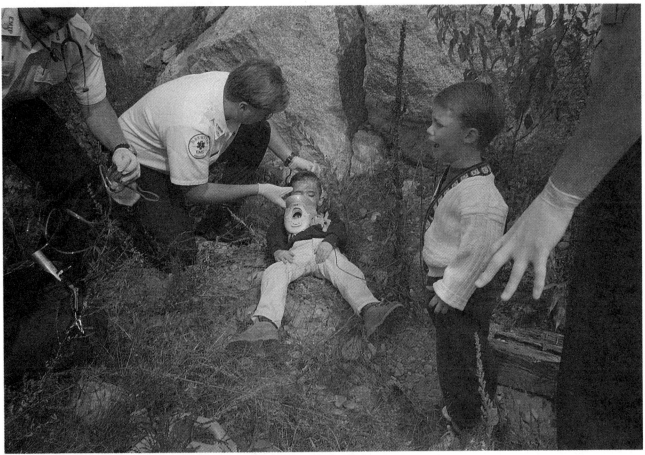

Brewster Ambulance Service, Brewster, Massachusetts. Photo by Nancy L. Caroline.

OBJECTIVES

The next few chapters will take us on a tour of emergencies that pose an immediate threat to life and that, therefore, must be dealt with urgently. In this chapter, we shall examine the priorities governing emergency care outside the hospital—what steps need to be taken first and what steps follow. We shall then review the major way stations along the pathway from life to death and identify the points at which a patient travelling down that pathway can be intercepted and brought back to safety—through a process we call the "primary survey." The three chapters that follow this one will then examine each step of the primary survey in detail.

By the end of *this* chapter, the student should be able to

1. State the reason why it is important to establish priorities in evaluating and treating a patient in the prehospital setting
2. Arrange the steps of prehospital care in the correct order, given a case description and a list of actions in random order
3. List the questions about the incident scene that need to be answered before approaching the patient, given a description of the incident, and describe the measures that need to be taken to deal with each question
4. List the way stations on the pathway from life to death, and indicate at which points along the pathway it is possible to intervene and reverse the process
5. Given a list of definitions, identify the correct definitions of
   • Respiratory arrest
   • Cardiac arrest
   • Clinical death
   • Biologic death
6. Arrange the steps of the primary survey in the correct sequence, given a list of steps in random order

INTRODUCTION: THE PRIORITIES OF PREHOSPITAL CARE

In the day-to-day practice of medicine, a patient comes to see a doctor for help in solving a problem, usually a problem relating to dysfunction of some part of the body. The doctor asks a lot of questions (takes a history), examines the patient, perhaps orders some laboratory tests, and *then* decides what is wrong and what needs to be done about it. If the doctor is a good doctor, the whole process is carried out in a systematic, unhurried manner. In prehospital emergency medicine, however, the job is a little more complicated.

It would be very nice indeed if the paramedic could, like the doctor sitting in an office or clinic, take a detailed history, then carry out a thorough physical examination, then ponder the findings, and only after all those steps go back and treat whatever abnormalities were found. That, however, is impossible by the very nature of a paramedic's work. To begin with, the paramedic does not work in an office or clinic. The paramedic works in an *uncontrolled environment*—by the side of the road at a traffic accident, amidst the rubble of a collapsed building, at a football stadium or a movie theater or a bar full of disorderly patrons. Those are not situations that foster leisurely history-taking and physical examination. In the second place, the paramedic in many instances deals with *critically ill or injured patients,* from whom there isn't time to obtain a complete history before taking action. Some problems, such as an obstructed airway or profuse bleeding, must be managed as soon as they are detected; they cannot wait until you have inquired about the patient's family history or examined his reflexes.

What the paramedic needs, then, is a strategy for evaluating and caring for the patient under the special conditions imposed by the prehospital setting. That is to say, the paramedic needs to have a set of **priorities** that specifies what to do first, what to do second, and so on. Those priorities will, of necessity, be based on the degree to which any given situation or condition presents a threat to life (the patient's life *or* the paramedic's!). We therefore turn our attention first to those things that represent the greatest threat to life; next we address problems that are a less immediate threat to life; and only afterward do we take up the problems that are not life-threatening but that might be aggravated if not treated. The most important skill for a paramedic to acquire—and it takes a lot of experience to do so—is to be able to distinguish among those situations and to act accordingly.

As a general rule, *every* ambulance call should proceed according to the following sequence:

**THE STAGES OF
PREHOSPITAL CARE**

1. **Survey of the scene**:
   • Check for **hazards** to the rescuers or patient, and eliminate any hazards detected.
   • Initial determination of whether **backup** is needed.

- Is special equipment needed to gain **access** to the patient?
2. **Primary survey**: rapid assessment to identify and treat conditions that involve an immediate threat to life:
   - Initiate **airway** management.
   - Make certain the patient is **breathing**.
   - Check the adequacy of the **circulation**.
     a. Start CPR for cardiac arrest.
     b. Control hemorrhage and start treatment of shock.
   - Continuing reassessment and management of ABCs.
3. **Secondary survey**:
   - Closer look at the **scene** (mechanisms of injury).
   - More detailed **history**.
   - Head-to-toe **physical assessment**.
4. **Definitive field management**, conditions permitting:
   - Wound care.
   - Stabilization of **fractures**.
   - **Packaging** for transport.
5. Ongoing **reevaluation** of the patient's condition.

SURVEY OF THE SCENE

The very first step on reaching the scene of *any* emergency is to TAKE A LOOK AROUND. If the call is for a "possible heart attack" in a quiet suburban neighborhood, taking a look around may require no more than a quick glance for oncoming traffic before you leap out of the driver's seat onto the road. If, on the other hand, the call is for a road accident in which a semitrailer hit a school bus, you are going to have to give the scene more than a cursory glance before you jump out of the ambulance and start tearing over to the disabled vehicles. Your preliminary survey of *that* scene will have to establish at least the following:

- Are the vehicles positioned on the road in such a way that other vehicles are likely to pile into them?
- Is either of the vehicles on fire? Is there spilled gasoline on the road?
- Is the semitrailer carrying a hazardous cargo?
- Is either of the vehicles in an unstable position and likely to tip over?
- Are there downed electrical wires at the scene?

- Will you need special equipment to gain access to the victims?
- Will you need backup (more ambulances, fire department, police)?

If you do not take a few moments to survey the scene and answer those questions, you are very likely to become one of the casualties yourself. And a paramedic who is injured, because he or she rocketed out of the ambulance without taking a good look around, will be of no benefit to the patient(s). Indeed, an injured paramedic just increases the number of victims that the remaining rescue personnel have to care for, and that will very likely detract from the care given to the other patients. The moral is:

> **DEAD HEROES CAN'T SAVE LIVES. INJURED HEROES ARE A NUISANCE. SO CHECK THE SCENE FOR HAZARDS BEFORE YOU LURCH IN.**

The survey of the scene, like the primary and secondary surveys, needs to be *systematic*. For any given type of incident (e.g., road accident, structural fire, hostile situation), you need to have a mental checklist of what needs to be established before you approach the incident scene. In general, the checklist will be something like the following:

1. IS IT SAFE FOR *ME* TO APPROACH THE VICTIM(S)?
   - *At a road accident*:
     a. Is there a fire or imminent danger of fire or explosion?
     b. Are any of the vehicles carrying hazardous materials?
     c. Are the disabled vehicles out of the flow of traffic?
     d. Are there downed electrical wires on or near the disabled vehicles?
   - *At a hostile situation* (e.g., shooting, crowd violence):
     a. How many perpetrators were there? Have they been captured? If not, what is their precise location?
     b. What is the mood of bystanders? Hostile? Supportive?

If there is a significant hazard to the rescue team, that hazard must be neutralized before proceeding further. Once it is relatively safe to approach the victims, the next question to ask is:

2. IS THERE ANY HAZARD TO THE PATIENT?
   - *Environmental hazards*:
     a. Fire.
     b. Rain, snow, heat, cold.
   - *Structural hazards*:
     a. Unstable disabled vehicle.
     b. Unstable structure (e.g., cave-in).
   - *Hostile situation*:
     a. Perpetrator.
     b. Bystanders.

If there is an immediate danger to the patient at the scene, the patient must be removed from danger *even if it means disregarding the usual treatment priorities.* Consider for example a vehicular accident in which the driver may have sustained spinal injury. Ordinarily the rule is to extricate the victim carefully from the damaged vehicle using a long and short backboard, cervical collar, and so forth. But suppose the vehicle is on fire and you don't have the means to control the fire quickly. The fire constitutes an immediate danger to the patient's life, so he must be removed from the vehicle as fast as possible, even at the risk of aggravating the injury to his spine—for the first priority is to save the patient's *life.*

THE SALVAGE OF LIFE TAKES PRECEDENCE OVER THE SALVAGE OF LIMB.

That is, in fact, one of the fundamental principles of *triage* (sorting of patients), about which we shall learn in more detail in Chapter 21.

When you have seen to your own safety and that of the patient, the next question to ask is:

3. AM I GOING TO NEED HELP IN DEALING WITH THIS EMERGENCY?
   - Will one ambulance be enough to deal with the number of victims immediately apparent? (If you have any doubts, call for help.)
   - Are any other services needed?
     a. Police, for traffic or crowd control, or to secure a hostile situation.
     b. Fire personnel.
     c. Hazardous materials specialists.
     d. Power company technicians for downed wires.

Radio for help early, so that backup personnel can set out for the scene while you get started with the primary survey.

4. DO I NEED ANY SPECIAL EQUIPMENT TO REACH THE VICTIM(S)?
   - Self-contained breathing apparatus.
   - Access equipment (for an entrapped patient).
   - Protective clothing (e.g., for a radiation accident).
   - Equipment to protect the patient during access (e.g., a blanket to shield the patient from shattered glass if access must be obtained by breaking through a window).

Clearly, each emergency situation will have its own peculiar hazards, and it is impossible to specify here every question that needs to be asked in making the initial survey of the incident scene. What is important is to remember the four basic questions:

SUMMARY: SURVEY OF THE SCENE

1. Is it safe for *me* to approach the victims?
2. Is there any hazard to the patient?
3. Am I going to need any help?
4. Do I need any special equipment to reach the patient?

Once you have answered those questions and taken care of any life-threatening hazards, you may proceed to the primary survey.

THE PRIMARY SURVEY

We have stated that the primary survey is the initial, rapid assessment of the patient to identify and treat those conditions that present an immediate threat to life. To understand the rationale behind the primary survey, we need first to look a little more closely at the path that a person travels on the journey from life to death.

The Pathway from Life to Death

In fact, there is more than one pathway a person can take on the journey toward death, depending on the events that precipitated the journey. Thus the sequence of events will be slightly different if the primary insult was, for example, cardiac arrest due to electrocution as opposed to primary respiratory arrest due to choking. Nonetheless, it is possible to describe in general terms the usual sequence of events when a person dies a "natural death."

The first way station along the pathway from life to death is **loss of meaningful communication**. The dying person becomes less and less aware of his surroundings and stops making any attempt to communicate. After a variable period, **loss of consciousness** occurs. The patient becomes totally unresponsive to external stimuli. His muscles become slack, among them the muscles of the jaw, thus permitting the back of the tongue to sag against the posterior part of the throat. That in turn leads very quickly to **airway obstruction**. Air can no longer enter the lungs, and within a few minutes the patient stops breathing altogether; that is, he suffers **respiratory arrest**. The heart cannot continue to function very long without the oxygen normally furnished by respiration, so shortly after the patient stops breathing, the heart stops beating as well; that is, **cardiac arrest**, or **clinical death**, occurs. Now there is no longer blood flow to *any* organ in the body, and lacking the oxygen that the circulation ordinarily brings, body cells begin to suffocate and die. The cells most vulnerable to even short periods of oxygen deprivation (hypoxia) are those in the brain. Within a very few minutes of clinical death, the number of brain cells that have been irreversibly damaged is so great that meaningful human existence can no longer be restored. At that point, the patient has suffered **biologic death**—death of the organism. In general, we estimate that irreversible brain damage begins within about 4 to 6 minutes after cardiac arrest, but the time may vary depending on the previous condition of the patient and the circumstances in which cardiac arrest occurred. Irreversible brain damage may be significantly delayed, for example, sometimes even for hours, when cardiac arrest takes place in a very cold environment. On the other hand, irreversible brain damage may occur within only 1 or 2 minutes of cardiac arrest in circumstances where the patient collapsed in an environment lacking in oxygen (e.g., in a house fire). In any case, if circulation cannot be restored within a very few minutes of clinical death, biologic death will inevitably follow.

3. Airway obstruction
4. Respiratory arrest
5. Cardiac arrest (clinical death)
6. Irreversible brain damage (biologic death)

The journey down the pathway from life to death may be gradual, as in the case of an elderly person dying after a long illness. Or it may be sudden and unexpected, as when a young person chokes on a piece of food and collapses. It is with that second kind of death—the sudden and unexpected death of a person who might otherwise live many more years—that emergency care of the critically ill and injured is chiefly concerned. The job of those who provide emergency care is to try to intervene in the pathway from life to death before the last stop on the pathway—irreversible brain damage—and to turn the process around so that the patient may continue to live (Fig. 6-1).

Only a few conditions can cause sudden death: airway obstruction, respiratory arrest, cardiac arrest, and severe bleeding. Often those conditions are reversible, but to reverse them, one has to be able to recognize them quickly and take immediate steps to correct them. That is what the primary survey is all about.

CONDITIONS THAT POSE AN IMMEDIATE THREAT TO LIFE

- Airway obstruction
- Respiratory arrest
- Cardiac arrest
- Profuse bleeding

Components of the Primary Survey

The first step in the primary survey of *every* patient is to DETERMINE WHETHER THE PATIENT IS CONSCIOUS. If not, the primary survey proceeds through three steps, *always in the same sequence*—**ABC**—to answer the following questions:

1. Does the patient have an open AIRWAY (**A**)?
2. Is the patient BREATHING (**B**)?

PATHWAY FROM LIFE TO DEATH

1. Loss of meaningful communication
2. Loss of consciousness

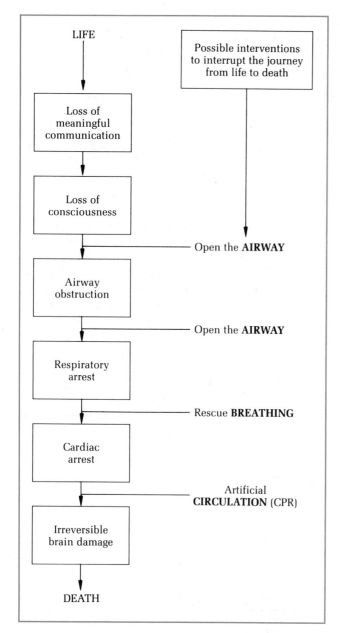

FIGURE 6-1.   THE PATHWAY FROM LIFE TO DEATH.

3. Does the patient have an adequate CIRCULATION (**C**)?
   a. Is there a *pulse*?
   b. Is there profuse *bleeding*?

In some cases, the primary survey can be performed at a glance. If the patient is alert and talking, for example, it is clear that his airway is open, he is breathing, and he has a pulse; patients in respiratory or cardiac arrest don't talk! If, on the other hand, the patient is unconscious, it will be necessary to proceed step-by-step through the ABCs and correct any problems as they are detected. If the airway is obstructed, the obstruction must be relieved. If the patient isn't

breathing, you will have to breathe for him (artificial ventilation); if he has no pulse, you will need to provide an artificial circulation by performing external chest compressions. If he is bleeding, you will have to try to stop the bleeding.

There are two important rules relating to the primary survey:

**RULES OF THE
PRIMARY SURVEY**

- The primary survey is the FIRST assessment made of EVERY patient.
- The primary survey of an unconscious patient is ALWAYS performed in the same sequence: ABC.

Why are those rules important? Suppose, for example, that you are called to the scene of an accident in which a 20-year-old motorcyclist has been struck by a car and hurled from his bike onto the road. You find him lying unconscious with a pool of blood around his leg. Because the blood is the most obvious and dramatic thing that meets your gaze, you forget about the ABCs and start searching for the source of bleeding. You become so engrossed in that task that you fail to notice that the victim has an obstructed airway; and while you are carefully cutting away the patient's trouser leg, he stops breathing on account of the airway obstruction and goes quietly into cardiac arrest. You finally find the laceration on the patient's leg, but meanwhile he has died—died of causes you could have easily prevented if you had performed the primary survey systematically, in the correct sequence. THE MOST DRAMATIC INJURY IS NOT ALWAYS THE MOST SERIOUS. The ABCs provide a list of *priorities* and thus help rescuers carry out their jobs in a logical and systematic way. That is particularly important when a patient has multiple injuries and treatment may at first seem overwhelmingly complicated. The ABCs tell us where to start and where to go from there.

In this chapter, we have presented only an overview of the primary survey, summarized in Figure 6-2. In the three chapters that follow, we shall look at each step of the primary survey—airway, breathing, and circulation—in considerable detail and learn how to manage those conditions that present an immediate threat to life.

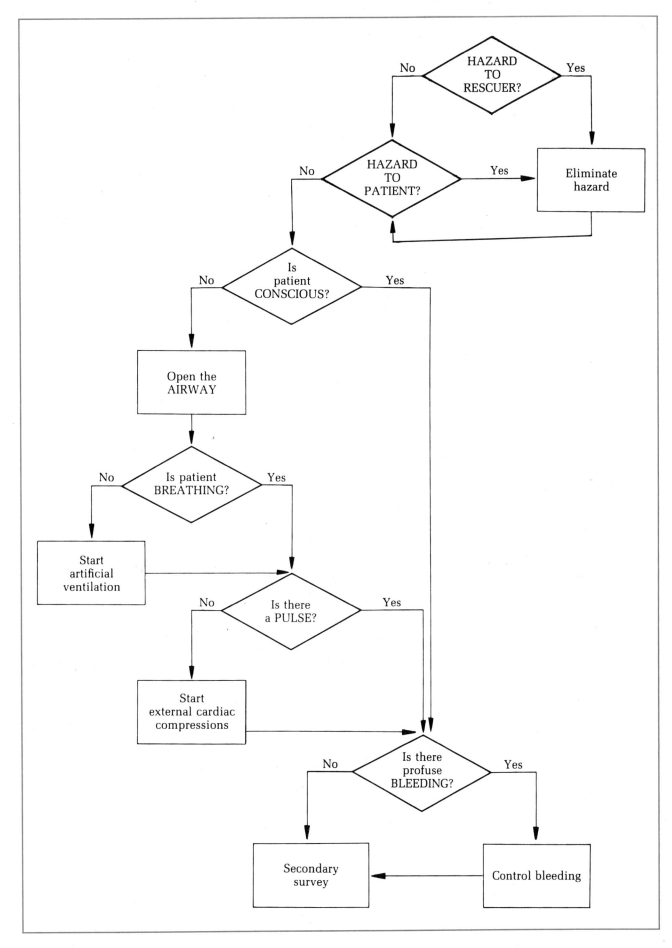

FIGURE 6-2. **THE PRIMARY SURVEY.**

GLOSSARY

ABC Airway, breathing, and circulation—the steps of the primary survey.

biologic death Death of the organism, when irreversible brain damage has occurred; also called *brain death.*

cardiac arrest The cessation of effective cardiac action, detected clinically by absence of a pulse.

clinical death The moment when the heart stops beating, as determined by the absence of a pulse.

primary survey The rapid, orderly initial assessment of a patient to detect and correct conditions that pose an immediate threat to life.

respiratory arrest The cessation of breathing.

7
The Airway

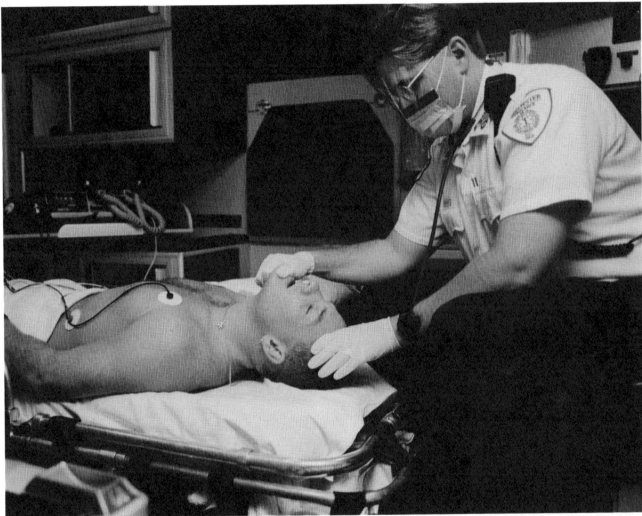

Brewster Ambulance Service, Brewster, Massachusetts. Photo by Brian Clark.

OBJECTIVES

Every course in saving lives—from the most basic first aid instruction of lay persons to postgraduate training of doctors in intensive care—starts with the ABCs: **A**irway, **B**reathing, and **C**irculation. There is nothing more important or fundamental in the training of emergency medical personnel than the ABCs, which is why we go over them again and again.

Establishing an airway is the first step of the ABCs. The airway comes first because it is the body's lifeline to the outside world. If the airway is blocked, that lifeline is cut, and death will occur within a few minutes. In this chapter, we shall examine the airway in detail. We shall look first at its structure (anatomy) to understand the ways in which the airway can be jeopardized. We shall then consider the various causes of airway obstruction and how to manage a patient with an obstructed airway. Finally, we shall discuss various airway adjuncts—equipment that can help secure and maintain an open airway in an ill or injured patient. By the end of this chapter, the student should be able to

1. Identify the major structures in the airway, given a model or a diagram of the airway
2. Identify the most common cause of upper airway obstruction, given a list of several causes, and describe the methods of relieving airway obstruction from that cause
3. Choose the most appropriate method for opening the airway of an unconscious patient, given a description of the patient's condition
4. Recognize a person who is choking, given a description of several patients with different signs and symptoms, and select the most appropriate method for treating the choking victim
5. Recognize a person suffering from allergic laryngeal edema, given a description of several patients with different signs and symptoms, and select the most appropriate treatment for that patient
6. List the indications and contraindications for
   • An oropharyngeal airway
   • A nasopharyngeal airway
7. List the equipment needed for suctioning and the steps in carrying out
   • Suctioning of the mouth and pharynx
   • Suctioning through an endotracheal tube
8. Identify the principal hazard associated with suctioning through an endotracheal tube, and describe what actions can be taken to minimize that hazard
9. List three indications for orotracheal intubation
10. List at least four advantages of endotracheal intubation over other methods of airway control

11. List the two principal potential complications of endotracheal intubation and describe
    • How each can be prevented
    • How each can be detected if it does occur
12. Describe the steps in preparing for orotracheal intubation, and list the equipment that is needed for the procedure
13. Describe, or demonstrate on a manikin or fellow student, the correct position of a patient for orotracheal intubation
14. State the maximum permissible time for an intubation attempt
15. Identify a patient for whom cricoid pressure may be helpful in bringing the vocal cords into view, given a description of several patients
16. List two ways of confirming that an endotracheal tube has been inserted into the right place
17. Describe the method for performing orotracheal intubation without a laryngoscope
18. State the principal danger in using neuromuscular blockers before carrying out endotracheal intubation
19. List four anatomic features that forewarn of a difficult intubation
20. List four indications and four contraindications for blind nasotracheal intubation
21. List the equipment required for blind nasotracheal intubation, and describe the steps of the procedure
22. Identify the phase of the respiratory cycle during which a nasotracheal tube should be advanced through the vocal cords
23. List the indications and contraindications for the esophageal obturator airway (EOA)
24. List in the correct sequence the steps in inserting the EOA
25. Identify errors in the use of an EOA, given a description of incorrect uses, and indicate what complications may result from the errors described
26. Indicate under what circumstances the EOA may be removed, and describe the steps in removing it
27. List the indications for cricothyrotomy, and describe the steps in performing the procedure*

ANATOMY OF THE AIRWAY

One way to describe the anatomy of the airway is to follow the path taken by a breath of air as it is inhaled from the atmosphere into the lungs.

---

*Not required by United States Department of Transportation standards for certification as a paramedic.

On inhalation, air normally enters the body through the NOSTRILS, or **nares**, and passes into the NASAL CAVITY (Fig. 7-1), where it is warmed and humidified and where particles are trapped by nasal hairs and mucus. The nasal cavity, in fact, is divided into *two* passages by a rigid partition composed of bone and cartilage, called the **nasal septum**. Normally, the nasal septum is in the midline of the nose, but in some people the septum may be deviated to one side or the other—a fact that becomes important when contemplating nasotracheal intubation. Another fact about the nasal cavity that becomes relevant in performing nasotracheal intubation is that the mucous membrane lining the nasal passages has a rich blood supply. Therefore, any trauma to the nasal passages, which may occur during hurried nasotracheal intubation, may result in profuse bleeding.

From the nasal cavity, air passes into the NASOPHARYNX, which becomes continuous with the back of the throat, or OROPHARYNX, at the level of the soft palate. The oropharynx, in turn, forms the posterior portion of the oral cavity, which is bordered superiorly by the hard and soft palates, laterally by the cheeks, and inferiorly by the tongue. Probably the most important anatomic fact about the *tongue*, from the standpoint of the airway, is that it is attached to the lower jaw (mandible). Thus when the jaw goes slack, the tongue can flop back against the posterior wall of the pharynx and close off the airway. We shall consider the significance of that fact in our discussion of airway obstruction.

Continuing down the airway from the oropharynx, air then enters the LARYNX, a boxlike structure that lies in front of the esophagus (the conduit for food), and perches on top of the trachea, opposite the fourth, fifth, and sixth cervical vertebrae. Protecting the entrance to the larynx is a structure called the EPIGLOTTIS, which flops over the laryngeal opening during swallowing, thus preventing aspiration.

The larynx (Fig. 7-2) is actually just a sort of valve that helps protect the airway from aspiration, regulates pressure within the lung, generates the force needed for coughing, and vibrates air passing through it to control the pitch of speech. The larynx is made up of nine cartilages connected by ligaments and moved by muscles. The THYROID CARTILAGE is the main cartilage of the larynx, its two plates joining in a V shape anteriorly to form the prominence known as the *Adam's apple*. Below the thyroid cartilage lies the CRICOID CARTILAGE, or cricoid ring, which forms the lowest portion of the larynx. Between the thyroid and cricoid cartilages is the CRICOTHYROID MEMBRANE, which can be punctured to provide an emergency airway (cricothyrotomy—see later section in this chapter). Above and behind the cricoid cartilage lie the ARYTENOID CARTILAGES, which are attached to the vocal cords and can be seen when the cords are visualized for intubation.

The VOCAL CORDS are, in fact, composed of the upper, free edge of the cricothyroid membrane (Fig. 7-2C). The anterior two-thirds of that membrane is true membrane, but the posterior third is cartilage. For that reason, it is very difficult to try to slip an endotracheal tube through closed vocal cords; the cartilaginous portion of the cords will resist passage of the tube, and any attempt to force the tube through may dislocate an arytenoid cartilage and lead to permanent hoarseness.

Because the vocal cords are anchored to the cricoid ring, pressing down on the cricoid during an intubation attempt can help bring the vocal cords into view when they are obscured by the tongue. Posteriorly, the vocal cords are attached to the arytenoid cartilages (Fig. 7-3). As the arytenoid cartilages pivot, the vocal cords open and close, which regulates the passage of air through the larynx and controls the production of sound (hence the larynx is sometimes called the "voice box"). The vocal cords and the opening between them are together termed the **glottis**. At rest, the vocal cords are partially separated (i.e., the glottis is partially open). During forceful inhalation, the cords open widely to produce an opening that provides minimum resistance to air flow.

FIGURE 7-1. THE UPPER AIRWAY.

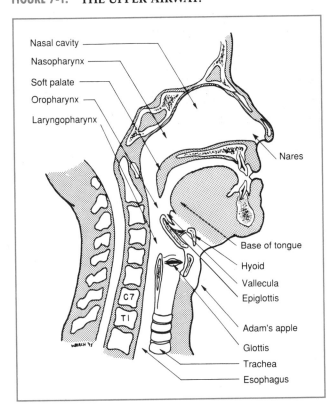

Nasal cavity
Nasopharynx
Soft palate
Oropharynx
Laryngopharynx

Nares

Base of tongue
Hyoid
Vallecula
Epiglottis

Adam's apple

Glottis
Trachea
Esophagus

C7
T1

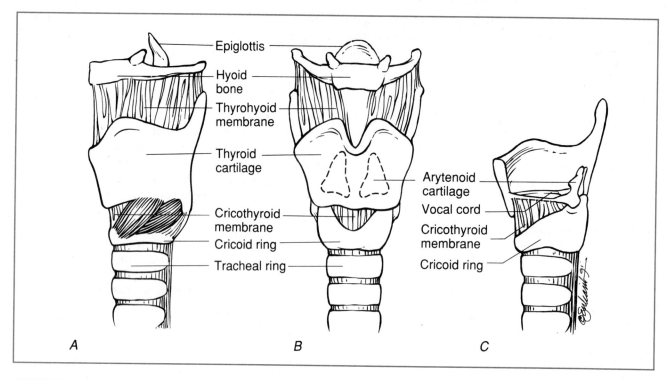

FIGURE 7-2.   ANATOMY OF THE LARYNX.   Lateral view (A) and anterior view
(B) show the basic cartilaginous and membranous structures of the larynx.
Lateral view of the cricoarytenoids (C) shows the relationship among the ary-
tenoid cartilages, cricothyroid membrane, and vocal cords.

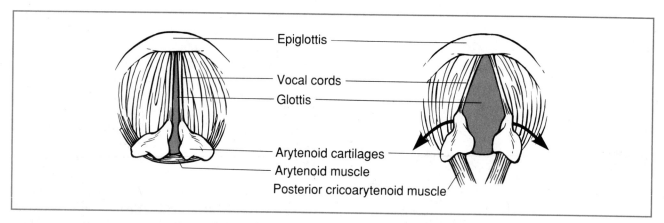

FIGURE 7-3.   VOCAL CORD FUNCTION.   As the arytenoids pivot, the vocal
cords are tensed, and the glottis opens.

The whole larynx descends on inhalation and
rises on exhalation; it also rises during coughing or
swallowing. (To confirm this, watch your Adam's apple in the mirrow as you swallow.) Elevating the larynx opens the airway, while lowering it facilitates closure of the airway by the epiglottis and base of the
tongue.

When the airway is stimulated, for example by
the aspiration of foreign material, defensive reflexes
cause the vocal cords to close spasmodically (**laryn-**

gospasm), which in turn seals off the airway and, in
its most severe form, prevents ventilation altogether.

From the larynx, air passes into the TRACHEA,
or windpipe, a tubular structure composed of a series
of C-shaped cartilaginous rings. The trachea begins
in the neck, where it is continuous with the cricoid
cartilage of the larynx (Fig. 7-4). From there, it descends anteriorly down the midline of the neck and
chest to the level of the fifth or sixth thoracic vertebra;
at that point, the trachea divides into the right and

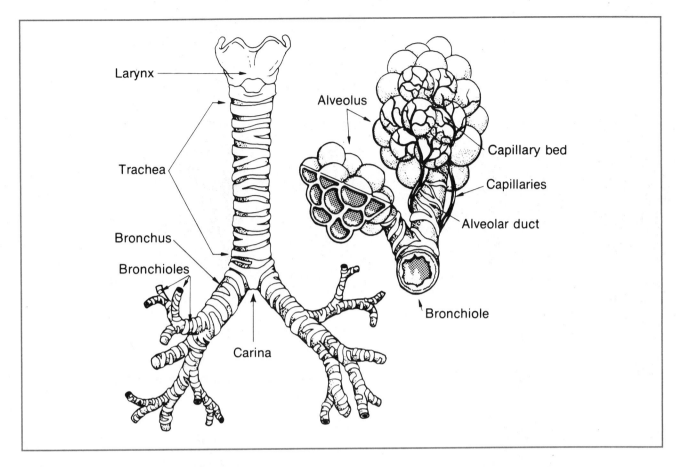

FIGURE 7-4. THE LOWER AIRWAY.

left main BRONCHI (the point of bifurcation is called the **carina**). The right bronchus is somewhat shorter and straighter than the left; thus an endotracheal tube inserted too far will often come to lie in the right main bronchus.

On entering the lungs, each bronchus divides into smaller and smaller bronchi, which in turn subdivide into BRONCHIOLES, finally connecting with the air spaces, or ALVEOLI, which conduct the business of gas exchange. Each alveolus is surrounded by tiny capillaries carrying blood to and from the air spaces. We shall learn in the next chapter how gas exchange occurs in the pulmonary alveolus.

**SUMMARY: THE ROUTE AIR
TAKES THROUGH THE AIRWAY**

- Nasal cavity
- Nasopharynx
- Oropharynx
- Hypopharynx (or laryngopharynx)
- Larynx
- Trachea
- Bronchi
- Bronchioles
- Alveoli

AIRWAY OBSTRUCTION

As noted earlier, the airway is what connects the body to the life-giving oxygen in the atmosphere. If the airway becomes obstructed, the lifeline is cut and the organism dies—dies within minutes. Thus the greatest urgency attends the detection and correction of an obstructed airway.

Obstruction by the Tongue

By far the most common source of upper airway obstruction is the *tongue*. In the stuporous or comatose patient, the jaw becomes slack and the tongue as a consequence tends to fall back against the posterior wall of the pharynx, thereby closing off the airway

(Fig. 7-5). A patient with *partial* obstruction from the tongue will have snoring respirations; a patient whose airway is *completely* obstructed will have no respirations at all—a very unhealthy situation! Fortunately, obstruction of the airway by the tongue is simple to correct using one of several maneuvers that elevate the base of the tongue away from the back of the throat. Perhaps the simplest of those maneuvers is the HEAD TILT, in which the rescuer places one hand on the victim's forehead and applies firm pressure backward with the palm to tip the victim's head maximally back. Head tilt is usually augmented by using the other hand either to support the victim's chin (head tilt–chin lift) or to lift the victim's neck (head tilt–neck lift).

HEAD TILT–CHIN LIFT (Fig. 7-6) is the method for opening the airway now favored by the American Heart Association. To perform this maneuver, use one hand to press backward on the victim's forehead (head tilt); at the same time, place the fingers of your other hand under the bony part of the victim's chin and pull the chin forward (chin lift), so that the victim's upper and lower teeth are nearly brought together. Avoid closing the victim's mouth completely, however, unless you are performing mouth-to-nose ventilation. If the victim has loose dentures, use your thumb to hold them in position. The head tilt–chin lift maneuver supports the jaw and helps keep the head held back. Be careful, though, to keep your fingers on the *bony* part of the chin and not to compress the soft tissues under the chin, for pressing on those soft tissues may itself cause airway obstruction.

An alternative maneuver for opening the airway, and one that some rescuers find more comfortable, is

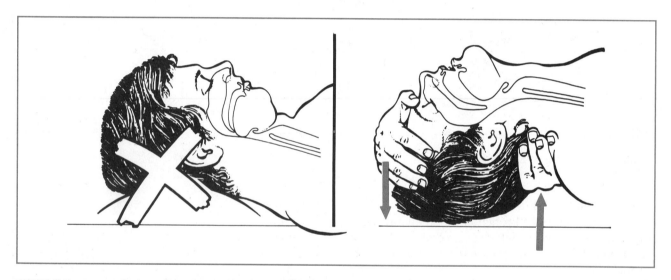

FIGURE 7-5.   OBSTRUCTION OF THE UPPER AIRWAY BY THE TONGUE can be relieved by tilting the head back. Reproduced courtesy of Asmund Laerdal, Stavanger, Norway.

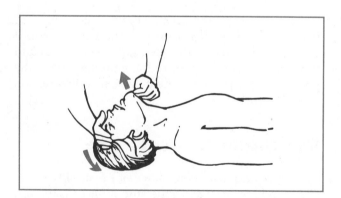

FIGURE 7-6.   HEAD TILT–CHIN LIFT MANEUVER. Reproduced courtesy of the American Heart Association.

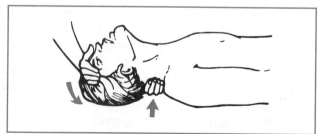

FIGURE 7-7.   HEAD TILT–NECK LIFT MANEUVER. Reproduced courtesy of the American Heart Association.

the HEAD TILT–NECK LIFT (Fig. 7-7). To perform the head tilt–neck lift, place one hand on the victim's forehead and press backward, as described; at the same time, slip your other hand beneath the victim's neck and lift gently upward. The aim is to extend the head backward at its junction with the neck, not to hyperextend the cervical vertebrae, so the hand lifting the neck should be positioned at the top of the cervical spine, close to the back of the head.

Another useful technique for opening the airway, which often works when head tilt maneuvers have failed, is the TRIPLE AIRWAY MANEUVER (Fig. 7-8), so named because it has three components. The rescuer places his or her fingers behind the angles of the patient's jaw and

- Forcefully displaces the mandible forward
- Tilts the head backward
- Retracts the patient's lower lip (with the rescuer's thumbs)

The triple airway maneuver is particularly useful when using a pocket mask to provide artificial ventilation.

All of the maneuvers described so far require some extension of the neck and thus could be dangerous when there is injury to the cervical spine. In such cases, any motion of the head and neck—whether backward, forward, to the left, or to the right—*must* be avoided. If it is necessary to open the airway of a patient in whom you suspect a cervical spine injury, you must therefore use a modified technique. One useful approach is the JAW THRUST, performed by pushing upward on the angles of the patient's jaw *with the head in neutral position*. Alternatively, you may place a thumb inside the patient's mouth and pull upward on the lower jaw and tongue, again avoiding any movement of his head and neck.

In the comatose patient, an oropharyngeal or nasopharyngeal airway may be useful in helping to keep the airway open, especially during ventilation with a bag-valve-mask. Conscious patients seldom tolerate such devices (and seldom need them).

If an unconscious patient must be left unattended temporarily—as in a situation where there are many casualties and few rescuers—the patient's airway can be somewhat protected by placing the patient in the RECOVERY POSITION (also known as the *stable side position*). The patient is placed onto one side—preferably the left side—with the lower knee and thigh flexed beneath him to stabilize him. The head is extended and rests, facing down, on the flexed arm (the right arm if the patient is lying on his left side). That position permits saliva, blood, and vomitus to drain out of the patient's mouth rather than down into his

FIGURE 7-8. TRIPLE AIRWAY MANEUVER. Reproduced courtesy of Asmund Laerdal, Stavanger, Norway.

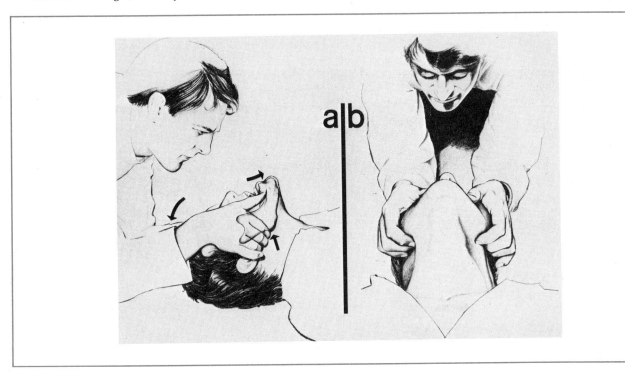

lower respiratory tract. Extension of the head is still required to keep the base of the tongue off the back of the throat. Since placing the patient in the recovery position requires rolling the patient onto his side and extending his head, the recovery position should *not* be used when there is any possibility that the patient has sustained an injury to the spine.

To place a patient in the recovery position, kneel at his left side and flex his left leg at a sharp angle (Fig. 7-9A), so that the foot is near the buttocks. Extend his left arm and put his left hand beneath his hip (Fig. 7-9B). Then pull the right arm toward you, gently rolling the patient onto his left side (Fig. 7-9C). Guide the movement with your hand on his left knee. When the patient is on his side, tilt his head backward and put his right hand under his cheek to maintain his face in position. Then pull his left hand away from his back (Fig. 7-9D).

Obstruction by a Foreign Body (Choking)

According to the National Safety Council, each year an estimated 4,000 people die suddenly while eating;

in a significant proportion of those cases, the cause of death is choking on a piece of food. The typical victim of the so-called café coronary is middle-aged or elderly and often a denture wearer. He has usually had a few drinks, which both depress his protective reflexes and adversely affect his judgment as to how large a piece of food can be prudently placed in the mouth. (The largest piece of meat extracted from the throat of a choking victim at autopsy was over 8 inches long! Since the offending piece of food very often *is* a chunk of meat, choking has also sometimes been called the "sirloin strangle.") When a piece of solid food of any type lodges in the airway, the victim becomes completely **aphonic,** that is, unable to talk, groan, or cry out; he may try to get up and walk from the table or may pitch forward—all in complete silence. Sometimes the victim will signal his distress by the universal distress sign for choking (Fig. 7-10).

FIGURE 7-9. RECOVERY POSITION. Also called the stable side position. Adapted with permission from Asmund Laerdal, Stavanger, Norway.

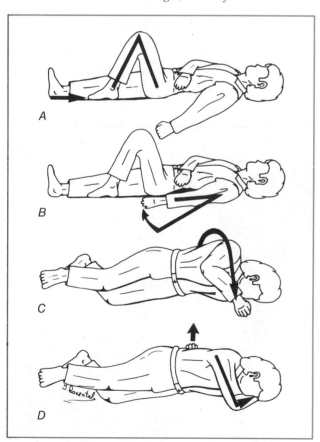

SIGNS OF CHOKING
• Victim cannot speak or make any sound. • Universal distress signal for choking: Victim clutches his neck between his thumb and index finger. • Dusky or cyanotic skin. • Exaggerated but ineffective breathing movements. • Collapse.

FIGURE 7-10. UNIVERSAL DISTRESS SIGNAL FOR CHOKING. Reproduced courtesy of the American Heart Association.

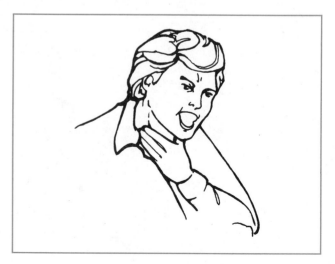

The most definitive *treatment* for the patient with a chunk of food lodged in the upper airway is to visualize the larynx directly with a laryngoscope and remove the offending piece of food, under direct vision, with a Magill forceps, Kelly forceps, finger, or strong suction (see section Direct Laryngoscopy later in this chapter). For that reason, the paramedic team should make it standard procedure to carry an intubation kit with them whenever they respond to an emergency in a restaurant.

> **CARRY YOUR INTUBATION KIT WITH YOU WHENEVER YOU RESPOND TO A CALL IN A RESTAURANT.**

There will, however, be circumstances when you do not have a laryngoscope and forceps handy when someone starts to choke, and you must take alternative actions.

The treatment of choking involves the application of various techniques in different sequences, with the aim of dislodging the obstructing material from the airway. We shall look first at the techniques themselves and then see how they are applied in different specific situations.

The first "technique" is a normal physiologic mechanism, and that is a COUGH. If a person's airway is only *partially* obstructed by a foreign object and there is still good air exchange, *a forceful cough is the most effective means of dislodging the obstruction.* A choking victim with "good air exchange" is one who remains conscious and can cough forcefully. He may wheeze between coughs but does not become cyanotic (blue). So long as the choking victim has good air exchange, do not interfere with his own attempts to expel the foreign body by coughing.

If the choking victim develops poor air exchange or if the airway is *completely* obstructed, you must apply other methods. A patient with "poor air exchange" has a weak, ineffective cough and is in marked respiratory distress. He may make a high-pitched, barking noise (**stridor**) on inhalation, and his lips may take on a bluish tinge. *Complete* airway obstruction is signalled by the total absence of air exchange. The patient cannot speak, breathe, or cough at all.

The technique now favored to relieve choking is the delivery of MANUAL THRUSTS—quick thrusts to the victim's upper abdomen (abdominal thrust) or lower chest (chest thrust). The purpose of manual thrusts is to try to create an *artificial cough* by forcing air out of the victim's lungs and thereby to blow the foreign body out of the airway.

The ABDOMINAL THRUST, or Heimlich maneuver, is the technique now recommended by the American Heart Association. It can be performed with the victim sitting, standing, or supine. *When the victim is sitting or standing* (conscious), stand behind him and wrap your arms around his waist, grasping your fist (thumb side against the victim's abdomen) with your other hand (Fig. 7-11). Be sure that your fist is in the midline slightly above the victim's navel and *below* his xiphoid, to avoid damage to the liver and other internal organs. Then press your fist into the victim's abdomen with a quick inward, upward thrust. Each thrust should be a separate movement. Repeat until the object is expelled from the airway or the patient becomes unconscious.

If the victim is lying down (unconscious), he should be positioned supine. Straddle the victim's hips and

FIGURE 7-11. HAND PLACEMENT FOR ABDOMINAL THRUST. Reproduced courtesy of the American Heart Association.

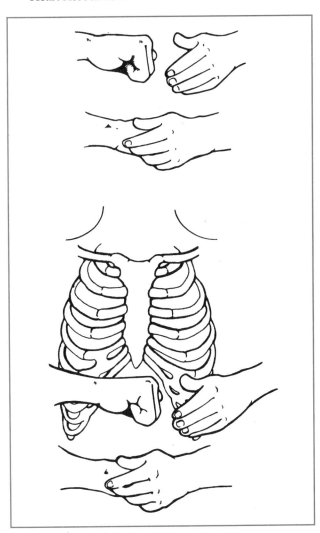

place the heel of one hand in the victim's midabdomen, slightly above the navel and well below the xiphoid. Place your other hand directly on top of the first. Then lock your elbows, and thrust inward and upward. Repeat until the object is expelled.

The CHEST THRUST is now recommended only for choking victims who are very obese or in the late stages of pregnancy. This technique may also be applied with the victim sitting, standing, or supine. *If the victim is sitting or standing* (conscious), you should stand directly behind him with your arms encircling his chest, just beneath the armpits (Fig. 7-12). Place the thumb side of your fist (palm down) over the *middle* of the victim's sternum—taking care to stay off the xiphoid and the ribs. Then grasp your fist with your other hand, and thrust directly backward (toward you). Repeat until the foreign body is expelled or the patient loses consciousness. If you are tall enough, it is best to have the victim leaning forward during the maneuver, so that gravity will work to your advantage.

If the victim is lying down (unconscious), position him on his back. Kneel beside him, with your knees close to his body, and position your hands just as you would for external cardiac compressions; that is, place the heel of one hand over the lower half of the sternum and your other hand on top of the first, fingers off the chest. Line your shoulders up so that they are directly over your hands, and then give a quick downward thrust. Repeat as needed until the foreign body is expelled. Deliver each thrust slowly and separately.

In addition to manual thrusts, there is a second technique used to treat the choking victim, and that is the FINGER SWEEP. That maneuver is an attempt to clear the airway manually of the obstructing object. Don protective gloves. With the (unconscious) victim supine, grasp his tongue and lower jaw between your thumb and index finger, to pull the tongue away from the back of the throat (tongue-jaw lift). Holding the jaw in that position, insert the index finger of your other hand down along the inside of the victim's cheek and into his throat at the base of the tongue. Then try to hook the foreign body to dislodge it and maneuver it into the mouth. Take care not to force the foreign body deeper into the airway. Do *not* place any object other than your fingertip into the victim's mouth to remove a foreign body.

> **BLIND INSERTION OF ANY INSTRUMENT, WHETHER IMPROVISED OR SPECIALLY DESIGNED, INTO A PATIENT'S PHARYNX IS EXTREMELY DANGEROUS. DON'T DO IT!!**

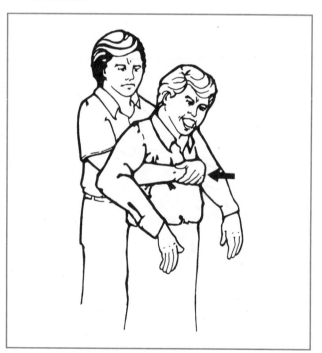

FIGURE 7-12. CHEST THRUST WITH VICTIM STANDING. Reproduced courtesy of the American Heart Association.

An instrument jammed blindly into the throat when the rescuer cannot see what he is doing can tear apart delicate structures of the pharynx and compound the obstruction with hemorrhage.

We have described three maneuvers for the treatment of choking: cough, manual thrusts, and finger sweeps. Which maneuver do we use when? There are basically three scenarios of airway obstruction that paramedic may encounter: (1) the conscious choking victim; (2) the choking victim who becomes unconscious in the paramedic's presence; and (3) the victim who is found unconscious and the cause is unknown. Let us take those situations one at a time.

If the victim is conscious (Fig. 7-13), first determine whether the obstruction is complete. (Can he talk? Can he move any air past the obstruction?) If the obstruction is not complete, encourage the victim to cough. If, however, the obstruction *is* complete, apply **manual thrusts**. Keep repeating the thrusts until successful or until the victim loses consciousness.

If the victim becomes unconscious in your presence (Fig. 7-14), place him on his back, open his mouth (tongue-jaw lift), and perform a quick **finger sweep** to remove any accessible obstructing material. Then

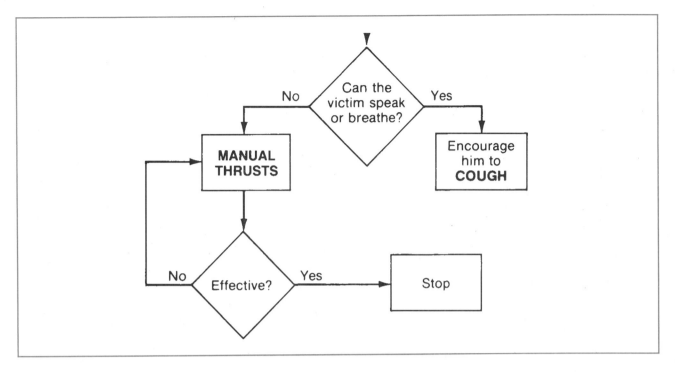

FIGURE 7-13. Treatment sequence for the **CONSCIOUS CHOKING VICTIM.**

open the airway (head tilt–chin lift) and **attempt** mouth-to-mouth **ventilation**. (The technique of mouth-to-mouth ventilation is described in detail in Chap. 8.) If you cannot force any air past the obstruction, apply **up to five manual thrusts** followed by a **finger sweep**. Reposition the victim's head, and again attempt to ventilate. Repeat the sequence as needed.

If the victim is found unconscious and the cause is unknown (Fig. 7-15), proceed through the usual ABCs of cardiopulmonary resuscitation (CPR), as described in Chapter 9. In brief, determine whether the victim is truly unresponsive (shake and shout). If not, open the **airway** (head tilt–chin lift). Determine whether the patient is **breathing**. If not, **attempt to ventilate**. If the attempt is unsuccessful, **reposition the** victim's **head** and try again. Should you still be unable to ventilate, then proceed through the series of manual thrusts and finger sweeps described previously.

> **THERE ISN'T A SECOND TO SPARE IN TREATING A VICTIM OF CHOKING.**

Whatever technique you use to relieve the obstruction, TIME IS OF THE ESSENCE! Death from asphyxia occurs within about 5 minutes, and you can-

not waste time hunting for equipment or trying to decide what to do. Don't wait for anything. Let someone else run back to the vehicle for the intubation kit, oxygen, or whatever. You must act *immediately*.

What happens if you arrive at the scene of a café coronary when the patient's muscles have already become rigid from asphyxiation and his jaws are therefore clenched tightly shut? While the muscle spasms will probably subside after the patient has progressed to cardiac arrest, it is not particularly desirable to stand there and wait for cardiac arrest to occur. In such instances, as well as when other maneuvers have failed and equipment for direct laryngoscopy is not available, **cricothyrotomy** (making an opening into the cricothyroid membrane) may be required as a last resort. We shall describe the technique of cricothyrotomy later in this chapter.

In the case of the CHOKING INFANT or SMALL CHILD, there is still considerable merit to the time honored technique of holding the baby upside down while sharply slapping its back, and the AHA still recommends back blows for the treatment of choking infants (Fig. 7-16). Chest thrusts may be combined with back blows as needed. *Abdominal* compression techniques should *not* be used in infants and small children because of the vulnerability of the liver and other abdominal organs to serious injury. (For a more detailed discussion of pediatric resuscitation and AHA performance checklists pertaining to infants and children, see Chap. 30).

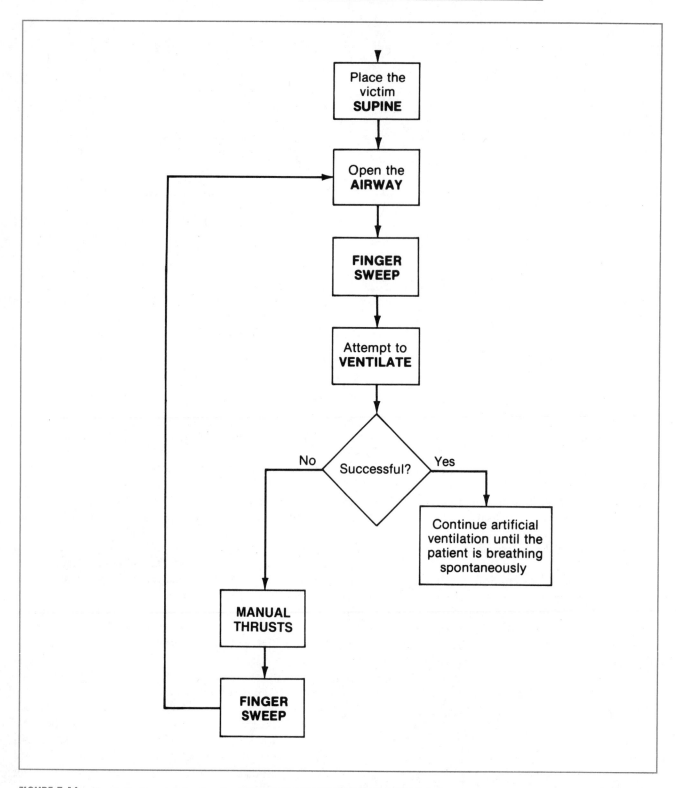

FIGURE 7-14. Treatment sequence for the **CHOKING VICTIM WHO BECOMES UNCONSCIOUS.**

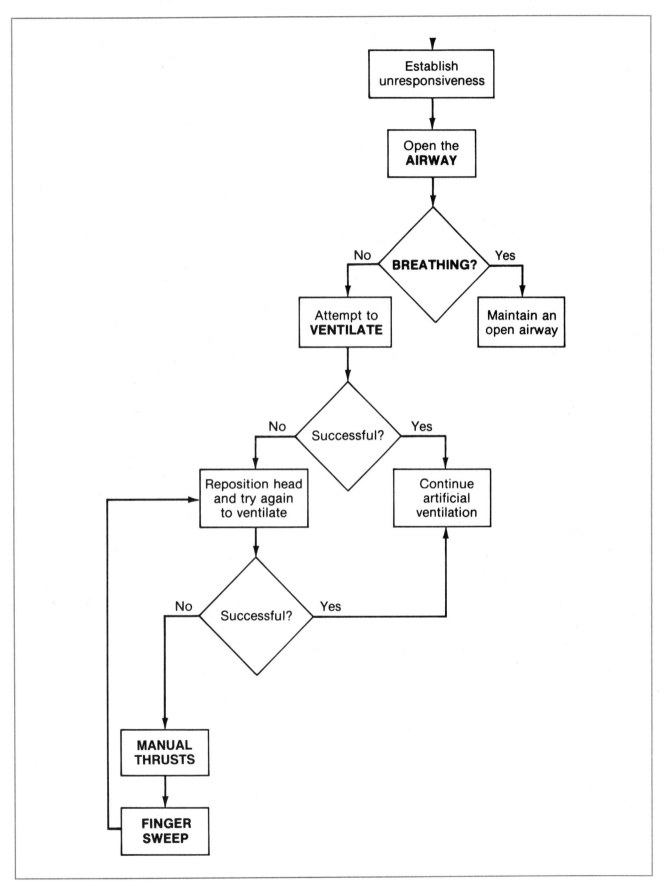

FIGURE 7-15. Treatment sequence for the **PERSON WHO IS FOUND UNCONSCIOUS AND THE CAUSE IS UNKNOWN.**

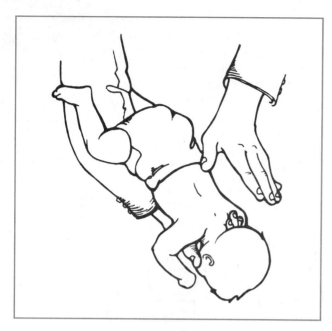

FIGURE 7-16. BACK BLOWS FOR THE CHOKING INFANT. Reproduced courtesy of the American Heart Association.

Obstruction from Swelling and Trauma

The upper airway may become obstructed not only by the tongue or foreign bodies, but also by SWELLING of its component tissues. In CROUP, for example, there is edema of the loose tissue immediately below the vocal cords, and the child has a "brassy" cough, with stridulous respirations. EPIGLOTTITIS in children leads to marked swelling of the epiglottis, with pain on swallowing, and may result in complete airway obstruction (see Chap. 30). In the adult, laryngeal edema can occur from BURNS TO THE AIRWAY and from allergic reactions. The most severe form of allergic reaction, called ANAPHYLAXIS, may occur in sensitive individuals on exposure to a food, medication, or inhalant to which they are allergic. We will deal with anaphylaxis in detail in Chapter 26. For our purposes here, we are primarily interested in the effects of anaphylaxis on the airway.

Typically, the patient has been stung by a bee or has recently ingested a food to which he or she is sensitive (often shellfish) and begins to notice *itching* of the palate and a sensation of a "lump in the throat." That sensation is produced by **laryngeal edema,** that is, swelling of the larynx. There may also be swelling of the posterior pharynx, uvula, and vocal cords. The net effect is to produce progressive upper airway obstruction. The patient's voice grows *hoarse* and then very quickly, as his airway narrows

further, develops a harsh, barking sound called **stridor.** Finally, the airway may close off altogether. That entire sequence of events—from the first vague feeling of an itchy palate to complete airway obstruction—can occur within minutes, so speed in recognizing the problem and initiating treatment is crucial.

MANAGEMENT OF ACUTE LARYNGEAL EDEMA DUE TO AN ALLERGIC REACTION

- Establish an AIRWAY.
- Administer OXYGEN.
- Give EPINEPHRINE 1:1,000, 0.3 to 0.5 ml subcutaneously. The dose may be repeated in 10 to 20 minutes as necessary. If you carry an aerosol form of epinephrine (e.g., Medihaler-Epi), give the patient 2 to 3 deep inhalations of the aerosolized drug as well.
- Give diphenhydramine (Benadryl), 25 mg intramuscularly.
- Patients with severe airway obstruction who do not respond promptly to epinephrine and antihistamines may require an emergency airway. If trained and authorized to do so, perform CRICOTHYROTOMY, as described later in this chapter; otherwise, move with all possible speed to the hospital, where emergency access to the airway can be obtained.
- As with all patients having acute, life-threatening emergencies, the patient with acute laryngeal edema merits an IV LIFELINE. Start the IV en route to the hospital if the patient's airway is in jeopardy.

Finally, upper airway obstruction may occur secondary to TRAUMA TO THE FACE AND NECK. Facial trauma can cause airway obstruction from collapse of the mandible; hemorrhage; tongue injury; aspiration of tissue, teeth, or dentures; and associated coma. The strategy of management will depend on the site of the trauma and the extent of related injuries. In general, the patient's head should be turned to the side (if there is injury or suspected injury to the neck, the patient's whole body should be logrolled to the side, with the head and neck kept in alignment), so that blood will drain out of the patient's mouth rather than down his throat. Suction the mouth to remove blood and small particles from the upper airway. If the trauma involves primarily the mandible, a nasopharyngeal airway (see next section) may be useful. Trauma to the neck can result in laryngeal fracture or contusion and may require urgent cricothyrotomy. The details of management of facial and neck injuries are discussed further in Chapter 16.

SUMMARY: AIRWAY OBSTRUCTION

Cause	*Response*
Tongue	Head tilt–chin lift, or Triple airway maneuver, or Jaw thrust (trauma victim), or Recovery position
Foreign body	Cough Finger sweep Direct laryngoscopy Cricothyrotomy (last resort)
Allergic laryngeal edema	Administration of oxygen Administration of drugs (epinephrine, diphenhydramine) If above unsuccessful, cricothyrotomy
Trauma to the airway	Bite-block or naso-pharyngeal airway Patient turned as a unit to the side

---

AIRWAY ADJUNCTS

The first step in the primary survey of an unconscious patient is to open the airway, initially by manual methods (e.g., head tilt–chin lift). If the patient is not deeply unconscious and is capable of breathing spontaneously, a manual maneuver to open the airway is usually all that is necessary. In the deeply unconscious patient, however, an artificial airway may be needed to help maintain an open air passage. It should be emphasized, however, that AN ARTIFICIAL AIRWAY IS NOT A SUBSTITUTE FOR PROPER HEAD POSITION. Even after an airway has been inserted, backward tilt of the head should be maintained.

Artificial Airways

The OROPHARYNGEAL AIRWAY (also called an oral airway) is a device made of plastic, rubber, or metal and curved in such a way that it fits over the back of the tongue with one end in the posterior hypopharynx. (Where is the hypopharynx? Do you remember?!) The oral airway is designed to hold the tongue away from the posterior pharyngeal wall, and its use makes it much easier to ventilate patients with a bag-valve-mask. The oral airway can also serve as an effective bite-block in an intubated patient, preventing the patient from chomping down on the endotracheal tube.

Because its distal end sits in the back of the throat, the oral airway is a powerful stimulant to gagging and retching in a patient who is conscious or semiconscious. For that reason, the oropharyngeal airway should be used only in deeply unconscious, unresponsive patients. (If you're not sure whether a patient is unconscious enough to tolerate an oropharyngeal airway, try—gently—to insert one. If the patient gags, his protective reflexes are intact, and he will not tolerate the airway; probably he doesn't need it either!)

USE THE OROPHARYNGEAL AIRWAY ONLY IN DEEPLY UNCONSCIOUS PATIENTS.

Oropharyngeal airways come in a range of sizes to fit infants, children, and adults. To choose the right size airway for a particular patient, hold the airway alongside the patient's face; if it is the right size, it will extend from the mouth to the angle of the jaw.

To insert the oropharyngeal airway, first turn it so the convex part of its curve faces toward the top of the patient's head (Fig. 7-17A) and its tip is pointed toward the roof of his mouth. Then open the patient's mouth, and gently advance the tip of the airway along the roof of the mouth (Fig. 7-17B). When the tip reaches the soft palate, rotate the airway 180 degrees (Fig. 7-17C) and advance it into the hypopharynx until its flange is flush against the patient's mouth (Fig. 7-17D).

The reason for rotating the airway is to avoid pushing the tongue backward into the throat during airway insertion, which would only aggravate the problem of airway obstruction. Another method of inserting the oropharyngeal airway is to hold it with its tip pointing downward (toward the patient's feet)

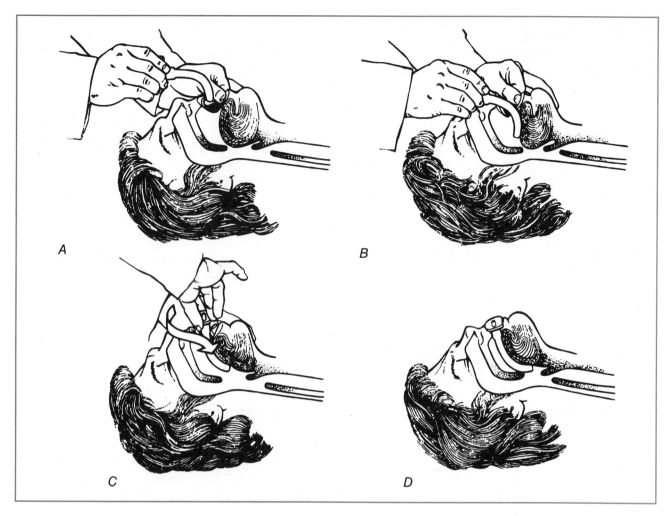

FIGURE 7-17.   STEPS IN INSERTION OF AN OROPHARYNGEAL AIRWAY.
(A) Orient airway with tip upward. (B) Advance tip. (C) Rotate airway 180
degrees. (D) Airway correctly seated in oropharynx. Reproduced courtesy of
Asmund Laerdal, Stavanger, Norway.

and use a tongue depressor to push the tongue forward and downward; then slip the airway along the
tongue into the hypopharynx.

The NASOPHARYNGEAL AIRWAY is a soft,
rubber tube about 6 inches long that is inserted
through the nose into the posterior pharynx behind
the tongue, thereby allowing passage of air from the
nose to the lower airway. (The hard, plastic varieties
of nasopharyngeal airway are unnecessarily traumatic and should not be used.) The nasopharyngeal
airway is much better tolerated than an oral airway
in awake or semiconscious patients who still have an
intact gag reflex. It should not, however, be used
when there is trauma to the nose or reason to suspect
a basilar skull fracture (e.g., when there is blood or
clear fluid coming from the nose).

The nasopharyngeal airway must be inserted

gently to avoid precipitating epistaxis (nosebleed).
Lubricate the airway generously with a water-soluble
jelly, preferably one that contains local anesthetic,
and slide it gently, tip downward, into one nostril
(Fig. 7-18). Do *not* try to force it. If you meet resistance, try to pass it down the other nostril.

Suctioning

When the patient's mouth or throat becomes filled
with vomitus, blood, or secretions, a suction apparatus enables you to remove the liquid material
quickly and efficiently. Ambulances should carry
both a fixed suction, which operates off the engine
manifold, and a portable suction that can be carried
from the vehicle to the patient.

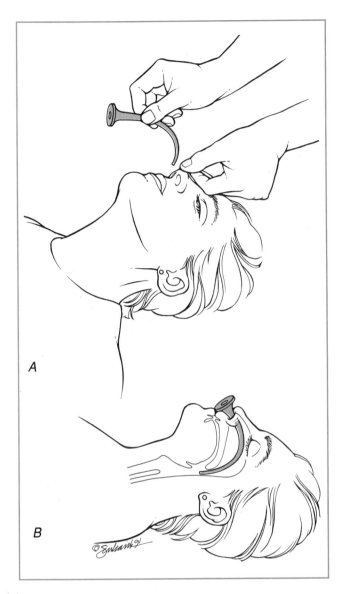

FIGURE 7-18. **INSERTION OF A NASOPHARYNGEAL AIRWAY.** (A) Hold the airway so that its curvature follows that of the floor of the nose. (B) Slide the airway into the nostril until its flange is flush against the opening of the nostril; at that point, its distal end will be in the oropharynx.

Equipment for Suctioning

A FIXED SUCTION unit is one that is permanently installed in the ambulance and is usually powered by vacuum from the engine manifold or by an electric pump. Whatever the power source, the suction unit should be capable of generating a *vacuum* of 300 mm Hg within 4 seconds of clamping off the collection tube, and it should be able to provide a constant air flow of at least 30 liters per minute. Check the vacuum on the fixed suction apparatus at the beginning of every shift by switching on the suction, clamping the tubing, and making sure the pressure gauge registers 300 mm Hg.

In addition to a strong vacuum, a fixed suction unit should be equipped with a nonbreakable **collection bottle;** a stiff, transparent **collection tube** long enough to reach easily to the patient's head; and a variety of sterile, disposable **suction catheters.** Catheters come in two forms. The *flexible rubber catheter* is used for suctioning the nose and pharynx as well as for suctioning through an endotracheal tube. The rigid *tonsil-tip suction catheter*, or Yankauer suction catheter, is a plastic or metal catheter that is very useful for suctioning the mouth and pharynx of an unconscious patient, for its rigid tip is easier to direct where you want it to go.

Whichever type of suction catheter you use, you will need a supply of **water** for rinsing the system after suctioning. You will also need a means of periodically interrupting the suction without having to turn the whole system off and on each time. One way of controlling the suction is to insert a small piece of plastic shaped like a Y between the collection tubing and the catheter. Two arms of the Y are thus connected into the system, while the third arm is left open. So long as that third arm remains open, air will be pulled in through it, and the suction at the end of the catheter will be minimal. But when you need to activate the suction, all you have to do is cover the open end of the Y with your fingertip, and air will then be pulled in through the suction catheter. (*Note:* Some suction catheters have a built-in side hole that serves the same function as the open arm of the Y connector.)

PORTABLE SUCTION UNITS come in several types, depending on the power source used to create the required vacuum. *Electrically-powered units* operate off either a rechargeable battery or a 110-volt outlet and are, on the whole, the most satisfactory portable units for everyday use in the field. Electrically-powered suction kits are compact, relatively lightweight, and capable of generating a vacuum well above the 300 mm Hg standard.

The *oxygen-powered suction unit* operates off an oxygen-powered resuscitator (see Chap. 8). It does not generate as strong a vacuum as an electrically-powered suction unit, and it very quickly uses up the oxygen in a cylinder. Oxygen is too valuable to waste on suctioning! *Air-powered suction units*, which operate off tanks of compressed air, do not have the disadvantage of wasting oxygen, and they tend to be more effective than oxygen-powered units besides. However, in comparison to electrically-powered suction units, those powered by compressed air are generally heavier and more cumbersome to carry around.

Suction units may also be powered by compressed *freon* in disposable cans. Those units generate powerful suction, but occasional freezing of the valves and the necessity to maintain an inventory of freon cans limit their usefulness for daily work; they are, however, a good device to stock in disaster kits.

Finally, there are suction units powered by the rescuer. The suction in *manually-powered units* is generated by squeezing a rubber bulb or stepping rhythmically on a foot pump. Most manually-powered suction units are ineffective and unsatisfactory for emergency work.

Suctioning the Mouth and Throat

Suctioning removes not only liquids from the airway; it removes air as well. For that reason, any patient who is to be suctioned should first be *preoxygenated* by inhaling a high concentration of oxygen for at least 3 minutes. That will give him a small reserve of oxygen in his tissues that he can draw upon while you are suctioning. The oxygen reserve *is* very small, however, so each suctioning attempt must be kept brief (less than 15 seconds), with a period of oxygenation—and, if necessary, artificial ventilation—in between.

Use a RIGID, TONSIL-TIP CATHETER to suction the mouth and throat of an unconscious patient, for the rigid catheter is easier to direct than a flexible catheter, and it can remove large volumes of fluids quickly, along with small food particles. Thus the tonsil tip catheter is ideally suited for dealing with a mouth filled with vomitus or for clearing secretions that obstruct your vision during an intubation attempt. The steps in suctioning the mouth and throat are as follows:

1. **Inspect the suction unit** to make sure all the parts are correctly assembled and the unit is functioning properly. Switch on the suction, clamp the tubing, and verify that the pressure reaches 300 mm Hg.
2. If the unit is working properly, **attach the** tonsil-tip **catheter** to the tubing and recheck the suction by placing the catheter tip in rinse water with the thumb hole or Y tube closed; water should flow rapidly into the collection bottle.
3. **Position yourself** at the patient's head, and **turn his head to the side.**
4. **Open the patient's mouth** using the **crossed-finger maneuver** (Fig. 7-19), by inserting the thumb and middle finger of your right hand as far as possible into the right corner of the patient's mouth; cross your thumb in front of your index finger and use it to push down against the patient's *lower* molars while your index finger pushes upward against the *upper* molars. When

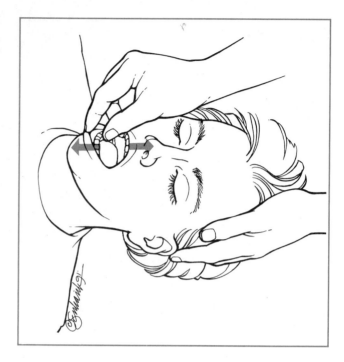

FIGURE 7-19.   CROSSED FINGER MANEUVER.   Use your right hand to open the patient's mouth, with your thumb on the lower jaw and your middle finger crossed behind it to press on the upper jaw.

the patient's mouth is open, use the fingers of your other hand to clear the mouth of any solid debris or large collections of fluid.
5. **Insert the suction catheter** into the patient's mouth so that the convex side goes along the roof of his pharynx. **Keep the vacuum** *off* until the suction tip is in place. *Then* occlude the side hole or Y tube and move the catheter tip around the pharynx to "vacuum clean" it out.

USE A TONSIL-TIP SUCTION CATHETER ONLY UNDER DIRECT VISION. NEVER JAM IT BLINDLY INTO THE PATIENT'S MOUTH OR THROAT.

Bear in mind also that a semiconscious patient may gag or vomit if a hard object touches the back of his throat.
6. DO NOT SUCTION FOR MORE THAN 15 SECONDS AT A TIME. Count out loud ("One-one thousand, two-one thousand . . .") if that will help you keep track of the time elapsed. Then remove your finger from the thumb hole to release the vacuum, draw the catheter back from

the pharynx, and quickly suction the patient's mouth. Remove the catheter, and RINSE the system through with water while you REOXYGENATE THE PATIENT.

7. **Reoxygenate** at least 3 minutes before suctioning again.

Suctioning Through the Nose

If the patient's mouth is clamped shut and you cannot open it by the crossed finger maneuver, you may use a FLEXIBLE RUBBER CATHETER to suction the back of the throat through the nose. To do so, proceed as follows:

1. **Moisten the catheter** in rinse water, while you are preoxygenating the patient.
2. **Insert the catheter** *gently* through one nostril, with the SUCTION OFF. Advance it smoothly about 10 inches, or as far as it will go before meeting resistance.
3. Slowly **withdraw the catheter,** applying **intermittent suction** as you do so. Once again, do *not* suction for more than 15 seconds at a time.
4. **Reoxygenate the patient** for at least 3 minutes while you **rinse the catheter** with water.

If you need to suction the patient during CPR, make it quick! Do not interrupt artificial ventilations for more than about 5 seconds for suctioning, and resume ventilations—preferably with oxygen—*immediately* upon completing the suctioning procedure.

**SUCTIONING THE MOUTH
AND THROAT:
POINTS TO REMEMBER**

- PREOXYGENATE the patient for at least 3 minutes before each time you suction.
- CHECK YOUR EQUIPMENT *before* you insert a suction catheter into the patient's mouth or nose.
- Do not use a rigid (tonsil-tip) suction catheter to suction the throat of a conscious or semiconscious patient.
- Keep the SUCTION OFF as you are inserting the catheter.
- Do not suction for more than 15 SECONDS at a time. REOXYGENATE the patient immediately after suctioning.
- Do not interrupt artificial ventilation for more than 5 seconds for suctioning.

Suctioning Through an Endotracheal Tube

The first rule to remember about suctioning through an endotracheal tube in the intubated patient is: DON'T DO IT IF YOU DON'T HAVE TO. Endotracheal suctioning, first of all, requires strict attention to sterile technique, which is very nearly impossible to maintain when you're in a ditch by the side of the road or in any of the other interesting locations where paramedics have to function. In the second place, suctioning the trachea is a powerful stimulus to cardiac dysrhythmias; cardiac arrest has been reported during endotracheal suctioning. So it is best to avoid suctioning through an endotracheal tube *unless secretions are so massive that they interfere with ventilation.* In that case, endotracheal suctioning must be carried out with full sterile technique and under cardiac monitoring. The procedure is as follows:

1. If the patient is not already being monitored for cardiac rhythm, **hook the patient to a cardiac monitor,** and turn on the audible beep tone so that you will hear any changes in cardiac rhythm.
2. **Preoxygenate** the patient with 100% oxygen for at least 3 minutes before each time you suction. If the patient is not breathing spontaneously, that will mean bagging him for at least 3 minutes with 100% oxygen (bag-valve device with an oxygen reservoir and 12 liter per minute oxygen flow; see Chap. 8).
3. **Assemble the necessary equipment**:
   a. **Suction** apparatus.
   b. Two to three sterile suction **catheters.** The catheters should be of flexible rubber or plastic with a thumb hole or Y tube to permit intermittent suction. Their external diameter should be no greater than one-third the internal diameter of the endotracheal tube, for a suction catheter that nearly fills the endotracheal tube will pull out too much gas (hence oxygen) from the airway. A 14- or 16-gauge French catheter is adequate for most adult patients.
   c. Sterile **gloves.**
   d. **Sterile water.**
   e. Sterile **container** for the water.
   f. A **sterile cloth** on which to lay out the equipment.
4. **Test the suction apparatus.** Make sure all the connections are tight. Turn the suction on, clamp the tubing, and make sure the pressure reaches 300 mm Hg (if not, check for a leak in the system). If you can regulate the vacuum on your suction machine, set it to between 80 and 120 mm Hg.

5. Unfold and **spread out the sterile cloth,** taking care not to touch the upper surface, on which you will be laying out your sterile equipment.

6. **Lay the sterile equipment out on the sterile cloth.** To do so, handle only the *outside* of the sterile packages as you open them, and let their contents drop onto the sterile cloth.

7. Open a bottle of sterile water, and pour it into the sterile container.

8. Touching only the proximal end of the suction catheter, **connect** that end of **the catheter** to the collection tubing of the suction unit.

9. **Don sterile gloves.** Once you have put on the sterile gloves, take care not to touch *anything* that is not sterile.

10. Dip the distal end of the suction catheter in sterile water to lubricate the catheter, and occlude the side vent or Y tube with your thumb to test the suction; water should move rapidly up through the catheter.

11. Have your partner **disconnect the** ventilating **bag** from the endotracheal tube (don't *you* touch the bag or the tube; they are not sterile!).

12. **Insert the catheter** gently into the endotracheal tube **with the suction off,** taking care not to let the catheter touch the outside of the endotracheal tube. Advance the catheter until it will not advance farther.

13. **Apply intermittent suction while slowly withdrawing the catheter,** rotating it as you withdraw it.

14. **Do not apply suction for more than 10 seconds.** Remember, prolonged suctioning can cause **hypoxemia** (inadequate levels of oxygen in the blood) and cardiac arrest! Keep an eye on the monitor; discontinue suctioning and ventilate the patient with 100% oxygen at the first sign of a dysrhythmia.

15. If there are still secretions that need to be removed after your first 10 seconds of suctioning, have your partner **reoxygenate** the patient—by ventilating him with 100% oxygen for 3 minutes—before you try again. Meanwhile **flush the catheter** with sterile water. Take care not to let the catheter touch anything that is unsterile.

16. When you have finished suctioning through the endotracheal tube, you may suction the patient's nasopharynx and mouth with the same catheter. But once the catheter has been used in the nose, mouth, or throat, do not use it again in the endotracheal tube. The human mouth is full of nasty germs; it is preferable not to introduce those germs into the patient's lungs!

17. If at any point during suctioning, cardiac dysrhythmias, bronchospasm, or other problems arise,

STOP SUCTIONING *IMMEDIATELY,* withdraw the catheter, and ventilate the patient with 100% oxygen.

SUCTIONING THROUGH AN ENDOTRACHEAL TUBE: POINTS TO REMEMBER

- DON'T carry out endotracheal suctioning in the prehospital setting unless absolutely necessary.
- Always PREOXYGENATE the patient for 3 minutes with 100% oxygen before *every* suctioning attempt.
- Observe STRICT STERILE TECHNIQUE.
- Never suction the trachea for more than 10 SECONDS at a time.
- REOXYGENATE the patient the moment you finish suctioning.
- Do not put the suction catheter back into the endotracheal tube after it has been in the patient's mouth or in contact with any other unsterile object.

Direct Laryngoscopy

Earlier in this chapter, we learned several techniques, such as the abdominal thrust, that are applied to treat a choking patient in circumstances where the rescuer does not have any ancillary equipment. In many instances, those techniques will be effective in relieving the airway obstruction. The *most* efficient way to remove a foreign body that is obstructing someone's upper airway, however, is to look into the patient's larynx, reach inside with some sort of a snare, and pull out the foreign body under direct vision. Direct laryngoscopy enables you to do just that. Direct laryngoscopy is the visualization of the larynx and associated structures with a laryngoscope and is usually performed to locate and remove a foreign body that is obstructing the airway. Direct laryngoscopy is also part of the procedure for endotracheal intubation.

Equipment for Direct Laryngoscopy

To perform direct laryngoscopy, it is first necessary to become familiar with the *equipment* required for the procedure. The **laryngoscope** (Fig. 7-20) consists of a battery-containing *handle* and a removable *blade.* Blades come in two types: curved (MacIntosh) and straight (Miller, Guedel). The *curved blade* is designed

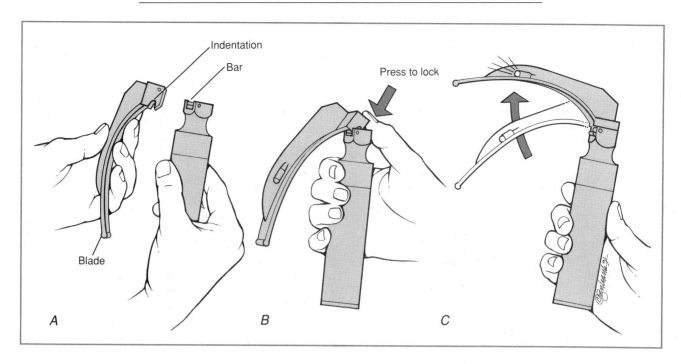

FIGURE 7-20. THE LARYNGOSCOPE. (A) Attaching a blade to the laryngoscope handle. (B) Aligning the indentation on the blade with the bar on the handle and pressing forward to lock. (C) Elevating the blade to a right angle to activate the light.

to slip between the epiglottis and the base of the tongue, while the *straight blade* exposes the vocal cords by lifting the epiglottis itself.

The blade is attached to the handle by inserting the blade's U-shaped indentation onto the small bar at the end of the handle (Fig. 7-20A). After you have lined up the indentation with the bar, press the blade forward to lock it into place (Fig. 7-20B); then lift the blade until it clicks into position at a right angle to the handle (Fig. 7-20C). At that point, the light on the blade should go on.

The laryngoscope must be checked before each use and periodically between use to ensure that the batteries and bulb are functioning optimally. *The light should be bright white and steady;* a flickering yellow light is worse than useless, for it distorts the image of the anatomy. Make it a daily practice, therefore, to assemble the laryngoscope in your intubation kit and check the light on each blade. Replace aging batteries or bulbs promptly, and keep a set of spare, fresh batteries in the intubation kit.

Another piece of equipment you will need is a **Magill forceps,** a long, curved forceps designed to reach into the posterior pharynx. The Magill forceps are ideally suited for grasping and extracting a foreign body visualized during direct laryngoscopy. As we shall see later, the Magill forceps can also help in guiding an endotracheal tube into place during nasotracheal intubation.

A tonsil-tip suction catheter attached to a strong suction can also be used to help remove a foreign body from the airway if Magill forceps are not readily available.

Carrying Out Direct Laryngoscopy

In the usual case of choking, you will not have time to make elaborate preparations; you will have to assemble the laryngoscope and blade rapidly, grab the Magill forceps, and get to work. Remember:

> **EVERY SECOND COUNTS WHEN A PERSON IS CHOKING.**

1. Quickly **flex the patient's neck** forward and **extend his head** backward to enable optimal visualization of the upper airway. Meanwhile, send your partner back to the vehicle for an oxygen cylinder (and a pocket mask, if you don't have one in your pocket).

2. **Grasp the laryngoscope** in your left hand **and the Magill forceps** in your right. Insert the laryngoscope blade into the *right* side of the patient's mouth, and use the blade to push the patient's tongue gently toward the left.

3. Slowly **advance the laryngoscope blade** toward the epiglottis, exerting gentle traction upward at a 45-degree angle until you can *see* the foreign body (Fig. 7-21A).

> **YOU MUST SEE THE FOREIGN BODY BEFORE YOU TRY TO SNARE IT. NEVER POKE ANY INSTRUMENT BLINDLY INTO THE PHARYNX!**

4. Use the Magill forceps to **grasp the foreign body** securely (Fig. 7-21B) and pull it free.

5. As soon as you have removed the obstructing material from the airway, immediately **withdraw the laryngoscope blade,** and **attempt to ventilate** the patient. If you cannot blow air into the patient's lungs when his head is properly posi-

tioned, part of the obstructing material may still be in the airway. Take another look. Time is critical.

6. Once you have removed the obstructing object and have successfully ventilated the patient, **connect your pocket mask to an oxygen source** so that artificial ventilation can continue, as needed, with supplemental oxygen.

Orotracheal Intubation

Endotracheal intubation consists of passing a tube directly into the trachea. When the tube is passed into the trachea through the *mouth*, we call the procedure *oro*tracheal intubation, and when the tube is passed into the trachea through the *nose*, we call the procedure *naso*tracheal intubation. The endotracheal tube itself is open at both ends. At the proximal end, it contains a standard 15-mm adapter for attachment of a bag-valve or other ventilating device; near the distal end there is an inflatable cuff, which effectively seals off the airway. Intubation of the trachea is the most definitive means to achieve complete control of the airway, offering the following *advantages* over other techniques of airway management:

FIGURE 7-21.   DIRECT LARYNGOSCOPY TO REMOVE A FOREIGN BODY.
(A) Elevate the tongue and jaw until you can see the foreign body. (B) Use the Magill forceps to snare the foreign body under direct vision.

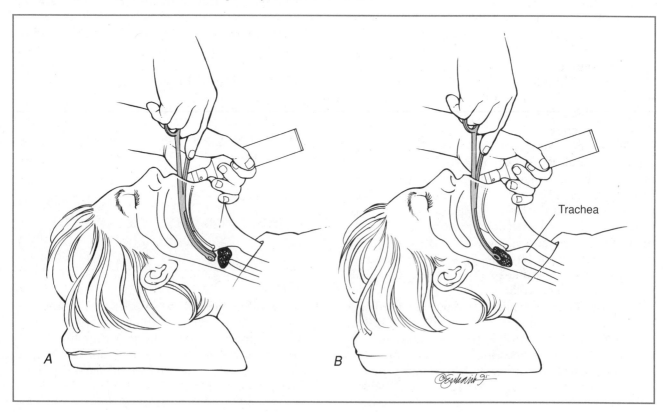

- The cuffed endotracheal tube PROTECTS THE AIRWAY from aspiration.
- Endotracheal intubation permits intermittent positive pressure ventilation (IPPV) with 100% oxygen.
- The endotracheal tube provides ACCESS to the tracheobronchial tree FOR SUCTIONING of secretions when those secretions are seriously interfering with the patient's breathing.
- Ventilation through an endotracheal tube DOES NOT CAUSE GASTRIC DISTENTION and the associated danger of regurgitation that are apt to occur with mouth-to-mouth or bag-valve-mask ventilation.
- An endotracheal tube MAINTAINS A PATENT AIRWAY in patients who develop obstruction despite the use of an oropharyngeal or nasopharyngeal airway.
- An endotracheal tube enables DELIVERY OF AEROSOLIZED MEDICATION, such as epinephrine, directly to the lungs, where it can be absorbed quickly into the bloodstream.

For all of these reasons, endotracheal intubation remains the gold standard among all the methods for controlling the airway.

Endotracheal intubation *does*, however, have some hazards. In the acute situation, the principal potential *hazards* of the procedure are

- Accidental intubation of the esophagus instead of the trachea
- Passage of the endotracheal tube past the carina into the right main bronchus

Both those hazards can be minimized by proper technique and by careful auscultation after intubation to be certain that breath sounds are equally audible on both sides of the chest. Additional immediate complications of attempted intubation may include injury to the teeth, lips, mouth, pharynx, or larynx; bronchospasm; and aspiration of blood or vomitus while being intubated.

One of the most common *mistakes* in the situation of cardiac arrest is to attempt endotracheal intubation too early, wasting precious time in the initiation of treatment in an already hypoxemic patient.

DO NOT ATTEMPT ENDOTRACHEAL INTUBATION UNTIL THE PATIENT HAS BEEN ADEQUATELY OXYGENATED BY SOME OTHER MEANS.

Use mouth-to-mouth ventilation, mouth-to-pocket mask ventilation, or bag-valve-mask ventilation—with supplemental oxygen as soon as possible—to initiate CPR, and carry on for at least 3 minutes after oxygen therapy has been started. The patient needs that period of oxygenation to tolerate the 15 to 20 seconds without ventilation that will occur during insertion of the endotracheal tube. Furthermore, the rescuer needs the time to check his or her equipment properly.

Who Needs an Endotracheal Tube?

Endotracheal intubation in the prehospital setting is indicated for any patient whose airway is in jeopardy, specifically:

- Any patient in CARDIAC ARREST
- Any patient in DEEP COMA who cannot protect his airway (that is, whose GAG REFLEX IS ABSENT)
- Any patient in IMMINENT DANGER OF UPPER AIRWAY OBSTRUCTION, for example, a person who has suffered burns to the airway

Endotracheal intubation in the prehospital setting should be *avoided*, on the other hand, in

- Patients with an *intact gag reflex* (it will be very difficult to intubate such patients without a struggle!)
- Patients likely to react with laryngospasm to an intubation attempt (for example, children with epiglottitis)

Preparing the Equipment for Endotracheal Intubation

While another rescuer manages the patient's airway and performs artificial ventilation as needed, assemble the equipment for endotracheal intubation (Fig. 7-22):

- **Choose an ENDOTRACHEAL TUBE of the appropriate size.** Tubes are sized on the basis of their internal diameter. Normally an adult male will require an 8.0- to 8.5-mm tube, while an adult female will require a 7.5- to 8.0-mm tube. The appropriate size tube for infants and children can be roughly determined from standard tables (Table 7-1); one practical guideline is to select an endotracheal tube approximately the diameter of the patient's little finger. Bear in mind, though, that all attempts to predict the tube size required for a given patient are estimates—so have *three* endotracheal tubes ready: one tube of the size

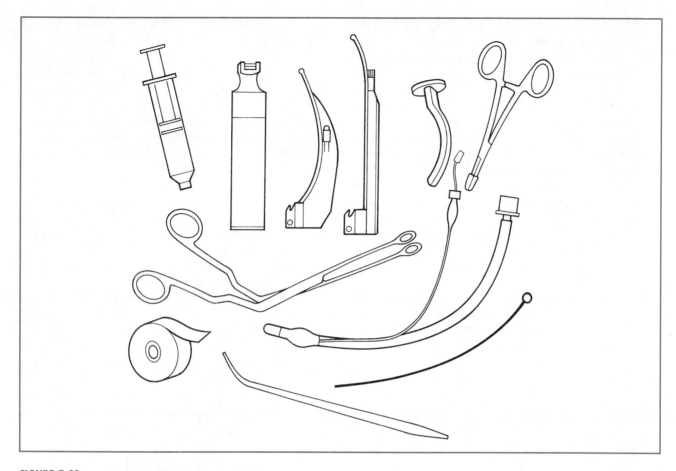

FIGURE 7-22.   EQUIPMENT FOR OROTRACHEAL INTUBATION.   Assemble and check all your equipment before you start the intubation.

TABLE 7-1.   DIMENSIONS OF ENDOTRACHEAL TUBES

AGE	WEIGHT (KG)	INTERNAL DIAMETER (MM)	OPTIMAL LENGTH (CM)
Newborn	To 4	2.5	10
1–6 months	4–6	3.5	11.5
7–12 months	6–9	4.0	12
1 year	9	4.5	13
2 years	11	5.0	14
3–4 years	14–16	5.5	15
5–6 years	18–21	6.0	15
7–8 years	22–27	6.5	17
9–11 years	28–36	7.0	18–19
12–13 years	37–46	7.5	20
14 years–adult	46+	8.0	20–24
Adult female	46+	7.5–8.0	20–24
Adult male	46+	8.0–8.5	20–24

you *think* will be appropriate, one a size bigger, and one a size smaller.

Adjust the length of the endotracheal tube if necessary. Endotracheal tubes are usually longer than necessary when received from the manufacturer, and a tube that is too long easily passes beyond the trachea into a main bronchus. So the tube should be cut to a more manageable size before it is inserted. Table 7-1 shows approximately what length a tube should be for a patient of a given age, but you can make a good estimate of the desired length by placing the tube alongside the patient's face and neck; the tube should be long enough to reach from the patient's teeth to the angle of Louis (the prominence on the sternum at the level of the second intercostal space).

Once you have adjusted the length of the endotracheal tube, **insert a connector** (a standard 15-mm/22-mm adapter) of the appropriate size. The connector should fit very snugly into the endotracheal tube, distending the end of the tube as it is pushed into place. A connector that slips easily into the tube will also slip *out* very easily, inevitably at some very inconvenient moment.

Next, inflate the cuff of each of the tubes you've chosen to **check for leaks,** then deflate them again, and keep the 20-ml SYRINGE attached to the tube you plan to try first. Have a HEMOSTAT ready to clamp off the inflation line of the endotracheal tube after the cuff has been inflated.

Many people find an endotracheal tube easier to direct through the vocal cords if a STYLET has been placed inside the tube to stiffen its curve. If used, the **stylet should be lubricated** to facilitate its removal, and its end should be bent to form a gentle "hockey stick" curve (Fig. 7-23). The end of the stylet should rest at least ½ inch back from the end of the endotracheal tube; if the stylet protrudes beyond the end of the endotracheal tube, it may damage the vocal cords and surrounding structures. Bend the other end of the stylet over the tube connector, so that the stylet cannot slip farther into the tube.

Lubricate the end of the endotracheal tube with a WATER-SOLUBLE JELLY.

- **Assemble and test the LARYNGOSCOPE.** Choose an appropriate laryngoscope BLADE. As noted earlier, there are basically two types of blades: straight blades and curved blades. The *straight* blade is designed so that its tip will extend beneath the epiglottis and lift it up. That feature is particularly useful in infants and small children, because they often have a long, floppy epiglottis that is difficult to elevate out of the way with a curved blade. In the *adult*, use of a straight blade requires great care, for if used improperly, levered across the upper jaw, the straight blade is more apt to damage the patient's teeth. The

FIGURE 7-23. USE OF A MALLEABLE STYLET. Insert the stylet into the endotracheal tube so that the tip of the stylet comes to rest ½ inch back from the tip of the tube. Bend the proximal end of the stylet over the tube adapter, and bend the distal end into a "hockey stick" angle.

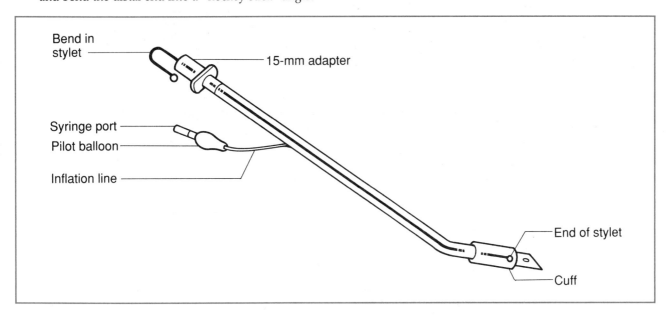

curved blade is less likely to be levered against the teeth by an inexperienced rescuer and is usually preferred by beginners. The direction of the curve conforms to that of the tongue and pharynx, so the blade will follow the outline of the pharynx with relative ease. The tip of the curved blade is placed in the **vallecula** (the space between the epiglottis and the base of the tongue) rather than beneath the epiglottis. It is best to have *both* curved and straight blades available, along with spare bulbs and batteries. **Check the light** on each of the blades you think you may use. *The light should be bright white and steady.* If it isn't, you need a new set of batteries or a new bulb. Keep one blade—the one you plan to use—snapped onto the laryngoscope handle, but folded down in the "off" position until you are ready to intubate.

- **Check the SUCTION apparatus,** as described earlier. Attach a TONSIL-TIP SUCTION CATHETER to the tubing, and put the suction where you will be able to reach it easily with your right hand.
- Prepare a BITE-BLOCK (an oropharyngeal airway will do very nicely) to insert after intubation. As the name of the device implies, the bite-block is used to prevent the patient from biting down on the endotracheal tube.
- Prepare strips of ADHESIVE TAPE 6 to 8 inches long for securing the endotracheal tube in place. Alternatively, umbilical tape cut into 30-inch lengths can be used to *tie* the tube in place, which is often preferable under field conditions (adhesive tape can peel off!).
- Keep a MAGILL FORCEPS handy in the event you have to remove a foreign body obstructing the airway.
- Secure a FOLDED TOWEL OR SMALL PILLOW to place beneath the patient's head.

The equipment required for endotracheal intubation is summarized in Table 7-2. It is a good idea to make a copy of that table and tack it to your intubation kit, so that you can check the kit systematically at the beginning of every shift. The time to discover that the laryngoscope batteries are dead or that you don't have any lubricating jelly is *before* the big cardiac arrest case, not during it.

Carrying Out the Intubation

While you are preparing the equipment, your partner should be hyperventilating the patient with 100% oxygen. He should also remove the patient's dentures or partial plates, if present, before you start the intubation procedure.

TABLE 7-2.   EQUIPMENT FOR ENDOTRACHEAL INTUBATION

AMOUNT	EQUIPMENT
1–2	Laryngoscope handles with fresh batteries
4	New batteries
2	Curved laryngoscope blades (MacIntosh)—medium and large
1	Straight laryngoscope blade (Miller or Guedel)
1	Spare bulb for laryngoscope blades
3	Plastic or rubber endotracheal tubes with intact cuffs (sizes 7.5, 8.0, and 8.5 for adults*)
3	15-mm/22-mm connectors, one for each endotracheal tube
1	Bandage scissors (to cut tube to correct length)
1	20-ml syringe
1	Hemostat for clamping off the inflation tube
1	Flexible metal stylet
3–4	Packets of water-soluble lubricant
1	Suction apparatus
1	Tonsil-tip suction catheter
1	Magill forceps
2–3	Flexible suction catheters (sterile)
1	Bite-block or oropharyngeal airway
1	Roll of 1-inch adhesive tape, or
2–3	Strips of umbilical tape cut in 30-inch lengths
1	Folded towel to place beneath patient's head

*It is preferable to keep equipment for pediatric intubation in a separate kit.

Having checked all your equipment, move to the patient's vertex (top of his head) to intubate, and place your equipment where it will be within easy reach of your right hand (your left hand will be occupied, holding the laryngoscope). From here on, your actions must be *unhurried but swift:*

1. **Position the patient** to bring his upper airway into alignment with his trachea: Flex his NECK FORWARD and his HEAD BACKWARD so that he is in the "sniffing position" (Fig. 7-24). If the patient is on an elevated surface, such as a bed, it may be helpful to put a folded towel or small pillow under his head. If, as is more often the case, the patient is on the floor or outside on the

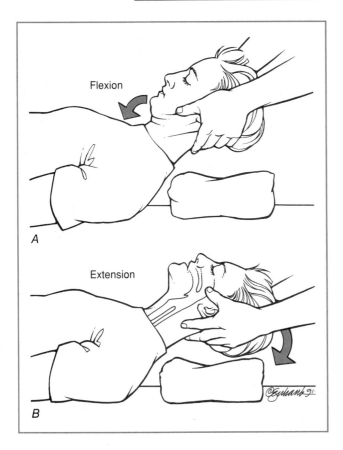

FIGURE 7-24. SNIFFING POSITION. To facilitate endotracheal intubation, the pharynx needs to be aligned with the trachea by (A) flexing the patient's neck and then (B) extending the patient's head.

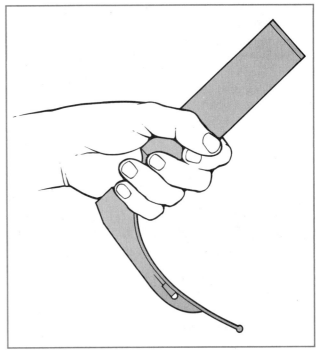

FIGURE 7-25. HOLDING THE LARYNGOSCOPE. Grasp the laryngoscope low on the handle with your wrist held rigid.

ground, you may find it easier to sit and straddle the patient's head with your thighs. If you intubate from this position, you'll have to lean back slightly to visualize the larynx. Alternatively, in cramped quarters, you may lie down supine beside the patient (on the patient's right), with your left arm encircling his head.

2. **Recheck the patient's mouth** for dentures, and remove them if present. Also use this opportunity to **suction the mouth** of vomitus or secretions. Then let your partner ventilate the patient again for a minute or so.

3. **Grasp the laryngoscope** in your left hand. Hold the laryngoscope as low down on the handle as possible (Fig. 7-25), and keep your left wrist rigid (that will help prevent you from using the patient's upper teeth as a fulcrum).

4. With your right hand, **open the patient's mouth** using the crossed-finger technique. **Insert the blade** into the *right* side of the patient's mouth, and use the blade to push the patient's tongue gently to the left (Fig. 7-26). Take care not to catch the patient's lips between the laryngoscope blade and his teeth.

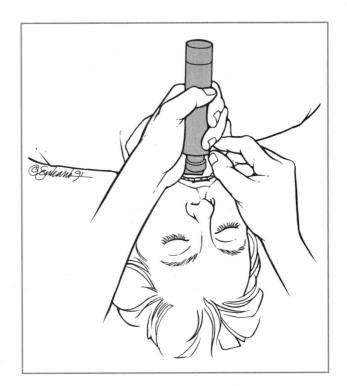

FIGURE 7-26. INSERTING THE LARYNGOSCOPE. Insert the laryngoscope from the right side of the patient's mouth and use the blade to move the patient's tongue to the left.

5. Slowly **advance the blade**—the curved blade into the vallecula, the straight blade beneath the epiglottis, at the same time sweeping the tongue to the left. Exert *gentle* traction at a 45-degree angle to the floor (Fig. 7-27). Keeping your back and your left arm straight as you pull upward allows you to use the strength of your shoulders to lift the patient's head and decreases the likelihood of levering the laryngoscope blade against the patient's teeth.

> ## DO NOT USE THE UPPER TEETH AS A FULCRUM!!

6. **Continue** lifting as described **until the vocal cords come into sight** (Fig. 7-28). Suction any secretions that obscure your view. In some patients, especially those who have a *short, thick neck*, you may catch a glimpse of the vocal cords floating up near the top of your line of vision, behind the epiglottis, but it may be difficult to bring them clearly into view. If that is the case, ask your partner to *push the cricoid downward* by placing his thumb on one side of the cricoid ring and his index finger on the other side (Fig. 7-29) and then pushing downward (toward the patient's spine). That maneuver also squeezes the esophagus shut, and for that reason the American Heart Association recommends applying cricoid pressure for every intubation during CPR.

7. Pick up the preselected endotracheal tube in your right hand, holding it near the connector as you would hold a pencil. *Under direct vision,* **insert the tube** from the right corner of the patient's mouth through the vocal cords.

> ## YOU MUST SEE THE TIP OF THE ENDOTRACHEAL TUBE PASS THROUGH THE VOCAL CORDS. IF YOU CANNOT SEE THE CORDS, DO NOT TRY TO INSERT THE TUBE.

An endotracheal tube shoved blindly down the throat will more often than not come to rest in the esophagus, not in the trachea; the only way to be certain that the tube has passed through the vocal cords is to *see* it pass through the vocal cords.

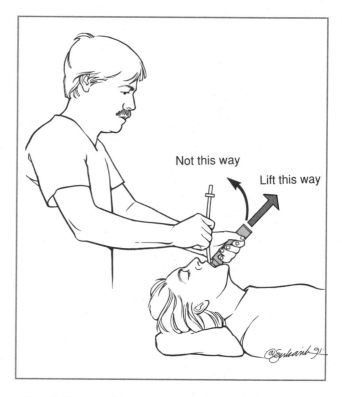

FIGURE 7-27.   LIFTING THE HEAD.   Keeping your back and your left arm straight, lift the laryngoscope away from you at a 45-degree angle.

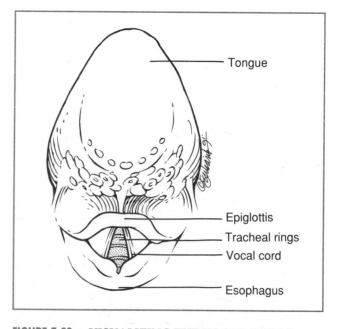

FIGURE 7-28.   VISUALIZING THE VOCAL CORDS. The rings of the trachea may be visible through the glottis.

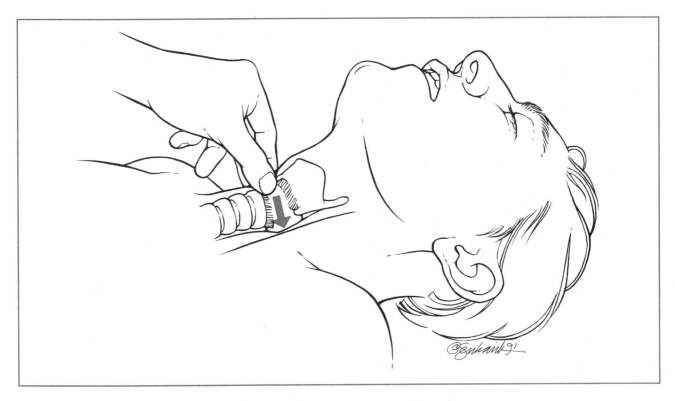

FIGURE 7-29. CRICOID PRESSURE (Sellick maneuver). Firm downward pressure on the cricoid ring pushes the vocal cords downward toward the field of vision while at the same time sealing the esophagus against the vertebral column.

8. When you have seen the cuff of the endotracheal tube pass about 1 inch (not more—Fig. 7-30) beyond the vocal cords, hold the tube securely in place with your left hand and **remove the stylet** from the tube with your right hand.

9. **Check the position of the tube.** Hold the tube securely in place with your left hand, and attach a bag-valve to the tube connector with your right hand. (The bag-valve should in turn be connected to an oxygen cylinder with a flow rate of at least 8 liters/min.) While you ventilate through the tube, *look* at the patient's chest to see whether it rises or falls with each ventilation. At the same time, have your partner *listen* with a stethoscope to both sides of the patient's chest to make sure that breath sounds are audible and are equal on both sides. Your partner should listen over the right and left sides of the *upper* chest, over the right and left *midaxillary lines* (just below the armpits), over the *sternal notch*; and over the *epigastrium.*

   a. **If breath sounds are absent bilaterally** when you ventilate through the tube, or if you hear gurgling over the epigastrium during inflation, chances are that you have intubated the esophagus rather than the trachea. In that case, you must **immediately remove the endotracheal tube,** and ventilate the patient with 100% oxygen for at least 3 minutes before you make another attempt at intubation.

   b. **If breath sounds are audible on only one side of the chest** (usually the right side) or are much louder on one side of the chest, the tube has probably been inserted too far and has entered a main bronchus (Fig. 7-31). In that case, pull back the tube *very slowly* while you continue to ventilate—until your partner reports that he can hear breath sounds equally on both sides of the chest.

We shall look at a *technical* means for assessing tube position—end-tidal carbon dioxide monitoring—in Chapter 8.

10. When the tube is in the correct position, ask your partner to **inflate the cuff.** Continue ventilating the patient while he does so. Before the cuff is inflated, you will hear leakage of air around the tube. The cuff should be inflated only until that leakage ceases. At that point, the inflation line should be clamped off beyond the small pilot balloon.

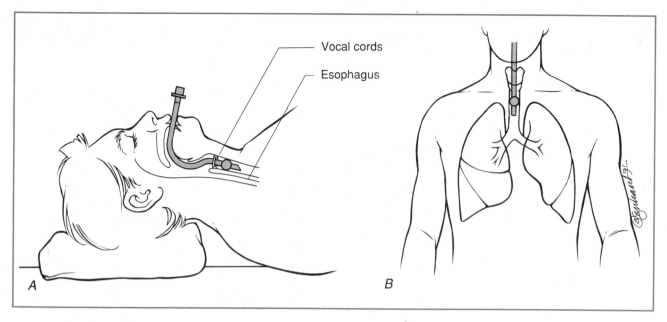

Vocal cords

Esophagus

A

B

FIGURE 7-30.   CORRECT PLACEMENT OF THE ENDOTRACHEAL TUBE.
When properly positioned, the cuff of the endotracheal tube should be just
below the vocal cords (A), and the distal tip of the tube should be above the
carina (B).

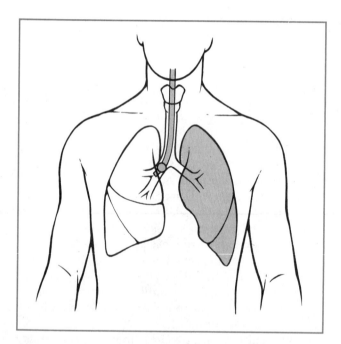

FIGURE 7-31.   ENDOBRONCHIAL INTUBATION.   An
endotracheal tube inserted too far will often come to
lie in the *right* main bronchus. If that occurs, the left
lung will not be ventilated.

11.   While continuing to hold the tube firmly in place,
insert an oropharyngeal airway to serve as a bite-
block, alongside the tube. Continue ventilation.

12.   **Secure the endotracheal tube in place**. In the
field, probably the best way to do so is to *tie* it in

place with umbilical tape. Loop the tape around
the endotracheal tube and around the oropharyngeal airway; bring one end of the tape around
the back of the patient's neck, and then tie the
two ends of the tape at the side of the patient's
neck.

> **NEVER TAKE YOUR HAND OFF THE ENDOTRACHEAL
> TUBE BEFORE IT HAS BEEN SECURED WITH
> TAPE OR TIES.**

Even after the tube has been secured, it is still a
good idea to support the tube manually while
you ventilate the patient, lest a sudden jolt from
the bag-valve device yank the tube from its place.
There are few things more discouraging than to
accomplish a difficult intubation only to have the
tube slip out of the trachea. You may be certain
that reintubation will be even more difficult.

13.   **Mark the endotracheal tube** with an ink line or
piece of tape at the point where it emerges from
the patient's mouth to enable medical personnel
caring for the patient later to determine whether
the tube has slipped in or out.

14.   If bronchial secretions are interfering with ventilation (and *only* if secretions are interfering with

ventilation), you may at this point suction through the endotracheal tube, as described in an earlier section.

15. Once the endotracheal tube has been secured in place, with its cuff inflated, you may pass a nasogastric tube, if necessary, to decompress the stomach. (See Chap. 27 for the technique of passing a nasogastric tube.)

A word of caution:

AN INTUBATION ATTEMPT SHOULD NOT TAKE MORE THAN 15 OR 20 SECONDS.

If you are unable to accomplish intubation in that period, withdraw the laryngoscope, and ventilate the patient for a few minutes with 100% oxygen before trying again. One way to keep track of the time elapsed during an intubation attempt is to HOLD YOUR OWN BREATH; when *you* become uncomfortable from lack of oxygen and accumulation of carbon dioxide, you may be certain that the patient's tissues are at least as uncomfortable. So breathe again, and do the same for the patient.

The steps of orotracheal intubation are summarized in a performance checklist at the end of this chapter.

Orotracheal Intubation Without a Laryngoscope

Suppose you are in the midst of attempting to intubate the patient and suddenly the light on your laryngoscope sputters out. Of course, things like that are not *supposed* to happen, and when they do happen, malpractice lawyers are apt to have a boost in business. But the fact is that such things occasionally do happen, and it's a good idea to have a contingency plan for unexpected occurrences of that nature.

Fortunately in the case of the defunct laryngoscope, there *is* a way to intubate the trachea without a laryngoscope, a technique sometimes referred to as "blind" or "tactile" orotracheal intubation. Tactile intubation in fact provides a quick method of airway control in circumstances other than that of the nonfunctional laryngoscope; the procedure can also be quite useful for patients in whom direct laryngoscopy may be hazardous or ineffective, such as

- Patients with extensive trauma
- Patients immobilized in cervical collars

- Patients with a short neck
- Very fat patients
- Patients whose airway is completely obscured by bleeding or secretions

Thus it is useful to know how to intubate without a laryngoscope even if you are the type who will never be caught short with a dead laryngoscope and no set of fresh batteries.

The procedure for intubating without a laryngoscope is as follows:

1. **Assemble your equipment** as for standard endotracheal intubation. Insert a stylet in the endotracheal tube, and curve the distal end of the tube into a J shape.
2. Don **gloves**.
3. **Position yourself.** Stand or kneel at the patient's right shoulder, facing his head.
4. **Position the patient.** Once again, extend his head backward.
5. Insert the index and middle fingers of your left hand into the right side of the patient's mouth; press down against the tongue as you slide your fingers along the midline of the tongue until you can feel the epiglottis. Then **pull the epiglottis forward** (Fig. 7-32) with your finger. (If the pa-

FIGURE 7-32. TACTILE INTUBATION. Hyperextend the neck, pull the epiglottis toward you with your left index finger, and advance the tube slowly along the outer surface of your finger.

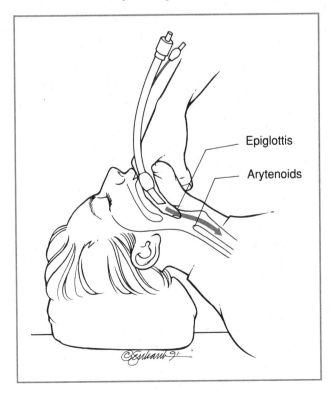

Epiglottis

Arytenoids

tient is not deeply comatose, protect your finger from being bitten by inserting a bite-block between the patient's upper and lower molars before you insert your finger!)

6. Hold the endotracheal tube in your right hand, as you would hold a pencil, and insert it into the left side of the patient's mouth; **advance the tube along the outer surface of your left index finger** or between your middle and index fingers, and guide its tip toward the glottis. Once you feel the cuff of the tube pass about 2 inches beyond the tip of your finger, stabilize the tube in place with your right hand while you gently withdraw your two left fingers from the patient's pharynx.

7. **Check the location of the tube** by ventilating through it and (a) watching the chest to see whether it rises and falls with each ventilation, and (b) listening with a stethoscope for breath sounds on both sides of the chest. If the tube has been properly positioned, secure it in place as described earlier. If not, withdraw it, and ventilate the patient with oxygen before trying again.

OROTRACHEAL INTUBATION: POINTS TO REMEMBER

- Never attempt endotracheal intubation before the patient has been thoroughly OXYGENATED.
- Assemble and CHECK ALL YOUR EQUIPMENT before you start.
- POSITION IS EVERYTHING IN LIFE! *Flex* the patient's neck forward, and *extend* his head backward.
- DON'T RUSH. Work with *deliberate* speed.
- HOLD YOUR BREATH during each intubation attempt. When *you* become uncomfortable, reoxygenate the patient.
- GET IT RIGHT THE FIRST TIME. The second try will be much harder.
- CONFIRM THAT THE TUBE IS IN THE RIGHT PLACE. Take nothing for granted.
- SECURE THE ENDOTRACHEAL TUBE WELL. Otherwise you'll soon be trying to put it back in again.
- Even when the tube is tied in place, STABILIZE IT WITH YOUR HAND as you ventilate the patient.

Paralyzing the Patient for Intubation

In some EMS systems, paramedics are trained and authorized to use neuromuscular blocking agents— drugs that induce temporary paralysis—to facilitate endotracheal intubation of conscious or semiconscious patients. The proponents of the technique argue that endotracheal intubation in the prehospital setting is sometimes hampered by spasm of the patient's jaw muscles or vocal cords or by combativeness of the patient; therefore it is sometimes necessary to paralyze the patient to get the endotracheal tube in.

The prehospital use of neuromuscular blocking drugs is still quite controversial, largely because the experience with those drugs in the prehospital setting is still small and the potential hazards of the drugs are considerable. Within about a minute of receiving an intravenous dose of a blocking agent such as *succinylcholine* (Anectine), a patient will become *totally* paralyzed. That means, first of all, that the patient will stop breathing. It also means that his jaw muscles will go slack, and the base of his tongue will flop back against his throat to obstruct his airway. What administration of succinylcholine does, in other words, is to convert a breathing patient with a marginal airway into a nonbreathing (apneic) patient without any airway. Before you bring about such a metamorphosis, you need to be *absolutely* sure that you will be able to whip a tube into the patient's trachea within the next 20 seconds; for if you cannot do so, the only hope left for the patient is a surgical procedure (within the next few seconds!) to open an airway through the neck. Thus the first thing to remember about using neuromuscular blocking agents in the field is

---

NEVER ADMINISTER A NEUROMUSCULAR BLOCKER TO A PATIENT UNLESS YOU ARE ABSOLUTELY CERTAIN YOU WILL BE ABLE TO INTUBATE HIM WITHIN 20 SECONDS AFTER THE BLOCKER TAKES EFFECT.

That means having all your equipment assembled, checked, and double-checked. It means having a careful look at the patient's anatomy for **features that could make intubation difficult** (e.g., "bull" neck, receding chin, overbite, large or swollen tongue, severe facial trauma). If you have any doubts as to whether you will be able to intubate the patient on the first try, *don't* use neuromuscular blockers!

The patient most likely to benefit from skilled use of a neuromuscular blocker during endotracheal intubation is one who

- *Needs* to be intubated (cannot protect his own airway)
- Has a decreased level of consciousness, but is still

conscious enough that he is combative (therefore won't lie still for an intubation attempt without blocking agents)

The patient who most often fits that description is one with closed head injury and airway complications in whom a struggle during intubation would be doubly dangerous: It could aggravate any associated cervical spine injury as well as increase intracranial pressure (pressure inside the skull).

Procedure for Intubation Under Neuromuscular Blockade

1. Have the patient breathe **100% oxygen** by mask while you get set up for the intubation.
2. **Assemble and double-check all the required equipment:**
   a. All equipment listed in Table 7-2
   b. Cricothyrotomy kit (in case intubation fails)
   c. Medications (each drawn up in a separate, labelled syringe):
      (1) Atropine, 1 mg
      (2) Succinylcholine, 1.5 mg per kilogram
      (3) Diazepam, 5 mg
      (4) Lidocaine, 100 mg
3. Make sure the patient has a secure, **functioning intravenous line.**
4. Hook the patient up to a **cardiac monitor,** and assign one team member to watch the monitor throughout the intubation. (A slowing of the heart—bradycardia—is one possible side effect of succinylcholine; see detailed discussion of succinylcholine in the Drug Handbook at the end of the book.)
5. **Premedicate** the patient as needed:
   a. For *awake* patients, sedate with *diazepam*, 3 to 5 mg by IV push.
   b. For *children and adolescents*, give *atropine*, 0.01 mg per kilogram, to inhibit the bradycardic response to succinylcholine.
   c. For patients with *head injury, intracranial bleeding*, or risk of *ventricular dysrhythmias*, give *lidocaine*, 1 mg per kilogram by IV push.
6. **Administer succinylcholine** 1 mg per kilogram by IV push.
7. Have an assistant **apply cricoid pressure** (Sellick maneuver) to block the esophagus until the endotracheal tube is in place (and thereby decrease the risk of regurgitation).
8. The patient's muscles will usually twitch (*fasciculate*) for a few minutes. When fasciculations stop, **check muscle relaxation** by ventilating the patient for a minute with a bag-valve-mask.
9. **Intubate the trachea** as described earlier. If you cannot accomplish the intubation within 15 to 20 seconds (hold your breath!), stop and ventilate the patient for at least 2 minutes with 100% oxygen before trying again. If the muscles are inadequately relaxed, you may give a second dose of succinylcholine.
10. Once intubation is completed, **verify the correct position of the endotracheal tube** (listen with a stethoscope just below each armpit), and **inflate the cuff.**
11. Release the pressure on the cricoid, and **secure the tube in place.**
12. **Ventilate** the patient with a bag-valve until he resumes spontaneous breathing.

Troubleshooting

There are several potential complications that can arise during an intubation attempt under neuromuscular blockade. The best way to deal with them is to be *ready* for them:

- *If the patient develops bradycardia* (i.e., if his heart starts beating very slowly—less than 60/min), give *atropine*, 0.01 mg per kilogram by IV push (you should have the right dose already drawn up and ready in a syringe—remember?). Stop the intubation attempt, and hyperventilate the patient with 100% oxygen until his heart rate comes back up to normal.
- *If the patient develops ventricular dysrhythmias* (we shall learn to recognize ventricular dysrhythmias in Chap. 23), give *lidocaine*, 1 mg per kilogram by IV push.
- *If several intubation attempts fail*, ventilate the patient with a bag-valve-mask and oxygen until the effects of succinylcholine wear off and spontaneous respirations return (usually in around 6–10 minutes). If you are unable to ventilate the patient because of persisting airway obstruction, urgent cricothyrotomy will be required (see later section).

Nasotracheal Intubation

As the name implies, nasotracheal intubation is the insertion of a tube into the trachea through the nose; it can be performed either without visualizing the vocal cords ("blind") or with the help of a laryngoscope to bring the cords into view.

Blind nasotracheal intubation is an excellent technique for establishing control over the airway in situations where it is either difficult or hazardous to perform laryngoscopy. And since it can (indeed, *must*) be carried out while the patient is breathing spontaneously, blind nasotracheal intubation is less likely to result in hypoxemia. Furthermore, the procedure itself is much better tolerated by a conscious or semiconscious patient than is orotracheal intubation, and the nasotracheal tube is more comfortable for the patient than an orotracheal tube.

Nonetheless, blind nasotracheal intubation isn't for every patient. The success of the procedure depends a great deal on proper patient selection. Patients most likely to benefit from blind nasotracheal intubation are those with *spontaneous respirations* who require intubation to stabilize their condition:

INDICATIONS FOR BLIND NASOTRACHEAL INTUBATION

- Suspected trauma to the CERVICAL SPINE
- Trauma to the MOUTH or MANDIBLE
- Mouth clamped shut (TRISMUS) or wired shut
- RESPIRATORY DEPRESSION from drugs, alcohol, stroke, and so on
- Severe CONGESTIVE HEART FAILURE
- COMA from any cause, if protective reflexes are depressed

There are, on the other hand, patients in whom blind nasotracheal intubation should *not* be attempted. Chief among those are patients in *respiratory or cardiac arrest*. To begin with, in performing the "blind" procedure, one needs the patient's audible breath sounds to guide the tube into the trachea. Furthermore, the fine maneuvering required to pass the tube through the nares, nasopharynx, oropharynx, and larynx takes *time*; often the first attempt is unsuccessful, which means even more time. And time is something you don't have to spare when dealing with a patient who is not breathing. So for patients in cardiac arrest, stick to standard orotracheal intubation.

CONTRAINDICATIONS TO BLIND NASOTRACHEAL INTUBATION

- APNEA
- Known DEFECT IN BLOOD CLOTTING mechanism (e.g., patient taking anticoagulant drugs)
- Possible BASILAR SKULL FRACTURE (as evidenced by blood or clear fluid draining from the nose or ears, black-and-blue mark behind the ear)

- Severe NASAL POLYPS or other obvious abnormalities of the nose

---

Preparing the Equipment

As in performing orotracheal intubation, to carry out blind nasotracheal intubation it is first necessary to gather and check all the equipment needed for the procedure. While you are doing so, have the patient breathe 100% oxygen by mask so that he will be well-oxygenated by the time you start the intubation.

- Select an **endotracheal tube.** The SIZE of the tube should be 0.5 to 1.0 mm smaller than that you would use to intubate the patient through the mouth, and the tip of the tube should be slightly smaller than the nostril into which it will be inserted. TEST THE CUFF of the tube for leaks with a **10-ml syringe** in the usual manner, and LUBRICATE THE TIP generously with **water-soluble jelly.** (Some sources recommend using lidocaine jelly, to anesthetize the nares and back of the throat. Lidocaine jelly, however, does not lubricate as well, and it can cause considerable irritation to the vocal cords.) Do *not* insert a stylet!
- Keep a **laryngoscope** and **Magill forceps** within easy reach, in case you are unable to thread the tip of the tube through the glottis blindly and need to finish the procedure under direct vision. TEST THE LIGHT on the laryngoscope blade; it should be bright white and steady.
- Tear off several long strips of **adhesive tape** or cut a piece of umbilical tape around 30 inches long, for securing the tube once it has been correctly placed.
- Draw up the **medications** that may be needed, and label the syringes or containers:
  1. PHENYLEPHRINE HYDROCHLORIDE (Neo-Synephrine) NASAL SPRAY 0.5%, to produce vasoconstriction of the nasal mucosa and thereby decrease the likelihood of severe nosebleed.
  2. A TOPICAL ANESTHETIC SPRAY, such as Cetacaine, for numbing the mucous membranes of the nose if the patient is awake.
  3. ATROPINE, 0.01 mg per kilogram, for intravenous injection if the patient should develop bradycardia (a slow heart rate) during the procedure.

Preparing the Patient

Once you have all your equipment ready, you may prepare the patient for the procedure.

- If the patient is *awake*, **explain** the procedure and **obtain consent.** Explain that the nose will be made numb and that a small breathing tube will be slipped through the nose to make breathing easier and safer. Explain also that the patient will not be able to speak when the tube is in place.
- If the patient is *not fully awake*, use roller gauze or leather restraints to **secure his hands,** so that he won't reach up and yank out the tube the moment you have succeeded in inserting it.
- Hook the patient up to a **cardiac monitor** and turn on the audible beep tone so that you will immediately be able to *hear* if the heart rate slows down.
- **Inspect the patient's nose** to determine whether there is any deviation of the septum or other abnormality that will make it more difficult to insert the tube into one side or the other. Use your penlight to illuminate both nostrils. Choose the nostril that looks clearer and straighter.
- **Spray phenylephrine into both nares** (you may have to use the second nostril if the one you've chosen turns out to be obstructed—so prepare both nostrils).
- If the patient is *awake,* **spray a topical anesthetic** into both nostrils as well. Also anesthetize the back of the tongue, the soft palate, and the back of the throat.
- **Position the patient.** The optimal position for nasotracheal intubation is the same as that for orotracheal intubation: the "sniffing position" (see Fig. 7-24), which is best achieved by placing a folded towel beneath the patient's head. If there is a possibility of injury to the cervical spine, however, the *head and neck must be kept in neutral position* throughout the intubation attempt.

Intubating the Trachea Through the Nose

Once the patient is positioned, intubation can proceed:

1. **Lubricate the nares and the endotracheal tube copiously** with water-soluble jelly, so that passage of the tube will be as smooth as possible. Grasp the tube as you would hold a pencil, with its distal tip pointing down (i.e., the convex curve of the tube pointing toward the top of the patient's head).
2. **Introduce the tip of the tube gently** into the nostril you have selected. The tube should be held nearly perpendicular to the patient's face, so that the **tube is advanced straight back** along the floor of the nasopharynx and *not* pointed upward toward the top of the head. There is often some resistance to passage of the tube within the first

1 or 2 cm of its entry into the nostril, as the tip becomes hung up in the nasal turbinates. To overcome that resistance, it may be necessary to use a slight back-and-forth rotary motion. If the tube still will not advance, remove it and try the other nostril.

> **NEVER TRY TO FORCE A NASOTRACHEAL TUBE PAST A POINT OF RESISTANCE.**

Once the tube has gone about 3 or 4 cm into the nostril, its tip will have entered the nasopharynx and it should become much easier to advance the tube farther.

3. **Continue advancing the tube** toward the larynx, to a depth of about 12 to 18 cm (5–7 inches).
4. As the tip of the tube approaches the larynx, position yourself behind the patient's head and **place your ear over the proximal end of the tube** (Fig. 7-33). At the same time, place your nondominant hand gently over the larynx.
5. Continue advancing the tube slowly as you **listen for breath sounds** and **look for misting in the**

FIGURE 7-33. BLIND NASOTRACHEAL INTUBATION. Listen over the tube for breath sounds as you advance it toward the glottis.

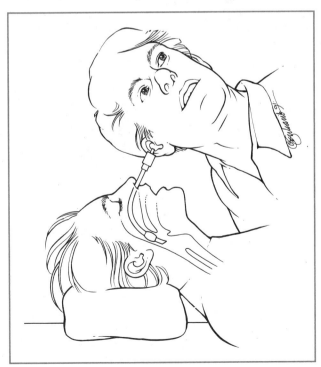

tube; both are signs that the tip of the tube is moving toward the trachea rather than the esophagus. Meanwhile, the hand that is palpating the larynx can detect whether the tube has drifted off course—a bulge will be felt in the neck over the tip of the tube. (For those who find it difficult to listen for breath sounds, an endotracheal tube whistle is now being marketed. The device, about the size of a thimble, fits onto the 15-mm connector of the endotracheal tube and emits a whistling sound with inhalation and exhalation. The whistle may be especially useful when rescuers have to perform blind nasotracheal intubation in a noisy environment, where it would be otherwise difficult to hear the patient's breath sounds.)

Some anesthetists recommend inflating the cuff of the endotracheal tube when the tip of the tube reaches the oropharynx. The idea is that the inflated cuff centers the tube and directs it more anteriorly, so it is more likely to head toward the larynx. From the oropharynx, the tube is advanced until you feel resistance, indicating contact between the cuff and the vocal cords. At that point, the cuff is deflated and the tube is passed through the vocal cords into the trachea.

6. *If at any point breath sounds start to become faint* or disappear altogether while you are advancing the tube, the tip of the tube has probably entered the esophagus. In that case, pull back gently on the tube until you can hear breath sounds again, and (assuming the patient is not suspected to have injury to the cervical spine) extend the neck before attempting to advance the tube once more.

7. When the breath sounds become loudest, the tip of the tube has reached the vocal cords. Recall from our discussion of airway anatomy that

---

THE OPENING BETWEEN THE VOCAL CORDS IS WIDEST DURING INHALATION.

That means that your best chance of whipping the tube through the cords is when the patient is starting to inhale. If, therefore, the patient is awake, ask him to take a deep breath, and **give the tube a final push at the beginning of inhalation.** If the patient is comatose, watch the rise and fall of his chest, and give the tube a push just after the chest completes a descent.

8. Usually SUCCESSFUL PASSAGE OF THE TUBE INTO THE TRACHEA IS SIGNALLED BY A POWERFUL COUGH, as the airway responds to the presence of a foreign body. But whether or not the patient coughs, you need to **check the position of the tube.** LISTEN AND FEEL for air moving in and out of the tube, and LOOK for misting of the tube with respiration. **Inflate the cuff and check again.** Attach a bag-valve to the tube and ventilate a few times while you listen with a stethoscope to both sides of the chest, just beneath the armpits.

9. When you have confirmed that the tube is in the right place, **secure the tube in place** with tape or ties.

DON'T RELEASE YOUR GRIP ON THE TUBE UNTIL IT IS SECURELY TAPED OR TIED IN PLACE.

Nasotracheal Intubation with the Aid of a Laryngoscope

Sometimes the tip of the endotracheal tube simply will not enter the larynx despite repeated attempts to direct it there. In such instances, you will need to use a laryngoscope and Magill forceps to finish the job. We take up the procedure at the point where the tip of the endotracheal tube is in the posterior oropharynx:

1. If the patient is suspected to have a cervical spine injury, **have an assistant hold the patient's head steady in neutral position.**

2. Position yourself at the patient's vertex. Grasp the laryngoscope in your left hand and a Magill forceps in your right hand. **Insert the laryngoscope** as for orotracheal intubation, as described earlier, and gently lift the tongue and jaw forward.

3. When the vocal cords come into view, **grasp the end of the endotracheal tube** with the Magill forceps (Fig. 7-34), and use the forceps to **advance the tube through the glottis** under direct vision. Keep advancing the tube until you have seen the cuff pass beyond the vocal cords.

4. Remove the laryngoscope and Magill forceps from the patient's mouth, and **check the position of the tube** as usual.

5. **Inflate the cuff** on the tube, and **recheck the position.**

6. When you have confirmed that the tube is in the right place, **secure the tube in place** with adhesive tape or ties.

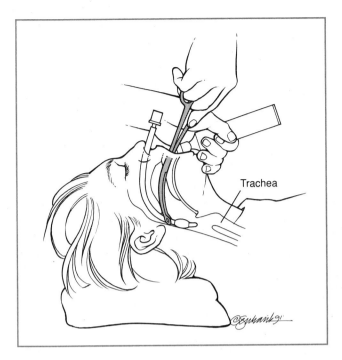

FIGURE 7-34. NASOTRACHEAL INTUBATION WITH MAGILL FORCEPS. Use the forceps to direct the end of the tube through the vocal cords.

Esophageal Obturator Airway

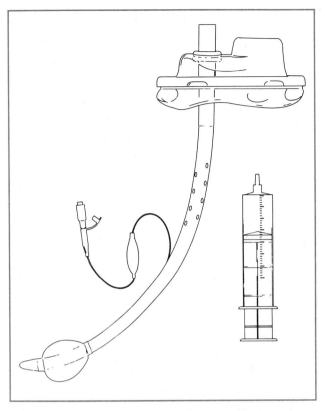

FIGURE 7-35. ESOPHAGEAL OBTURATOR AIRWAY. Reproduced courtesy Cavitron, Anaheim, California.

The esophageal obturator airway (EOA) is a flexible tube approximately 15 inches long that opens into a mask adapter at the proximal end and is sealed off at the distal end (Fig. 7-35). The upper third of the tube has numerous side holes, to permit air flow into the hypopharynx. A mask fits over the tube at its proximal end, and an inflatable cuff surrounds the tube near the distal end. When the EOA is properly placed into the esophagus and the mask is seated firmly on the patient's face, air blown in by mouth or bag-valve device enters the patient's pharynx through the side holes in the tube (Fig. 7-36). Since the inflated cuff obstructs the esophagus and the mask seals off the mouth and nose, the only path that air can take is into the larynx and down the trachea. The EOA thus minimizes progressive gastric distention during assisted ventilation and therefore also lessens the likelihood of regurgitation of stomach contents.

The name "esophageal obturator *airway*" is somewhat misleading. The EOA is *not* really an airway. It does *not* eliminate the need to maintain proper backward tilt of the head. It does *not* provide better ventilation than any other properly used bag-valve-mask device. Furthermore, use of the EOA has several *hazards*: Rough handling during insertion may damage structures in the pharynx, and excessive inflation of the cuff can rupture the esophagus. In addition, in-

advertent intubation of the trachea occurs in 5 to 10 percent of insertion attempts. (What would be the consequence of accidently inserting the EOA in the trachea? Study Figure 7-36, and picture what would happen if the obturator was placed in the trachea rather than the esophagus.)

The *advantage* of the EOA is said to be its relative ease of insertion. The device does not, however, provide definitive control of the airway. It can be used for only short periods (up to 2 hours), and it must be removed—after intubating the trachea—as the patient's level of consciousness starts to improve; its use in prehospital care is associated with three times the complication rate of endotracheal intubation. It is the opinion of this author, therefore, that endotracheal intubation is the method of choice for securing the airway of an unconscious person. The EOA and similar devices are most appropriately used as an interim form of airway control in patients who prove difficult to intubate endotracheally.

The main *indication* for the EOA is full CARDIO-PULMONARY ARREST, for the EOA can be used only in deeply unconscious patients. A conscious or semiconscious patient will not tolerate having a rigid tube jammed down the esophagus. The EOA also should not be used in very short or very tall patients,

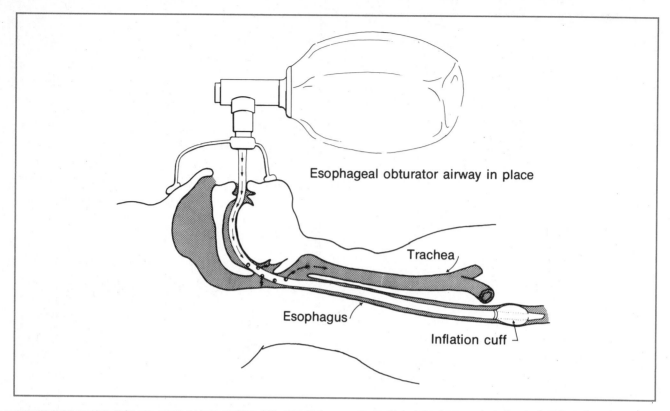

FIGURE 7-36. EOA IN POSITION IN THE ESOPHAGUS. Air blown into the pharynx can enter only the trachea, since the esophagus is obstructed by the cuffed obturator.

in children under 16, in patients with known esophageal or liver disease, or in those who have swallowed a corrosive substance.

A variant of the EOA called the esophageal gastric tube airway (EGTA) is now commercially available. The EGTA has no side holes on the tube, and the tip of the obturator is open, rather than closed in the fashion of the EOA. When the tube of the EGTA is inserted into the esophagus, a No. 16 gastric tube may be inserted through the tube into the stomach to remove gastric contents. Ventilation is meanwhile performed through a *second* hole in the mask (labelled "ventilate here"). The technique for passing the EGTA is the same as that for passing the EOA. The only advantage of the EGTA over the EOA is that it permits passage of a gastric tube to decompress the stomach; its disadvantages and contraindications are the same as for the EOA. Another variation of this device is the tracheoesophageal airway (TEA), whose design is similar to that of the EGTA; but the TEA permits you to ventilate through the tube if you have accidently placed the tube into the trachea!

Insertion of the EOA

Insertion of the EOA requires at least two rescuers—one (or more) to initiate and continue CPR while an-

other prepares the EOA for insertion. CPR should be started with mouth-to-mouth methods and continued with a pocket mask and oxygen or bag-valve-mask and oxygen (see Chap. 8) while one rescuer is getting set up to insert the EOA, as follows:

1. **Assemble the EOA**
   a. Make sure all the components are present—the OBTURATOR tube, the MASK, a 35-ml SYRINGE, and a tube of WATER-SOLUBLE LUBRICANT.
   b. If the **mask** has an inflatable rim, prepare it for use by injecting air through the one-way valve until the mask cushion is firm enough to provide a good seal against the patient's face (don't inflate it *too* hard!).
   c. **Test the cuff** on the obturator for leaks (Fig. 7-37) by injecting 35 ml of air through the valve on the pilot tube. When you have verified that there are no leaks, deflate the cuff and leave the syringe attached to the pilot tube.
   d. **Snap the obturator into the mask** so that they form a single unit.
   e. If the patient's mouth is dry, **lubricate the distal end of the obturator** with a water-soluble jelly.

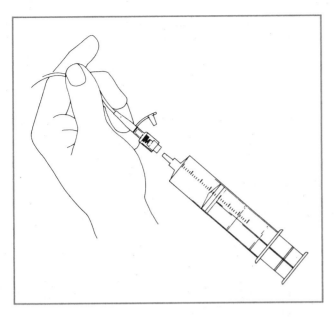

FIGURE 7-37. **CHECKING THE CUFF FOR LEAKS.** Reproduced courtesy Cavitron, Anaheim, California.

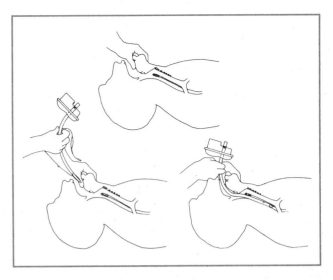

FIGURE 7-38. **STEPS IN INSERTING THE EOA.** Lift the patient's tongue and jaw forward and gently advance the EOA into the esophagus. Reproduced courtesy Cavitron, Anaheim, California.

2. **Position yourself.** Grasp the tube in one hand, just below the face mask, and position yourself at the patient's **vertex** (the top of his head). The tip of the tube should be pointing toward the patient's feet. Notify your partner (who has been doing CPR all this time) that you are ready.
3. **Position the patient.** As soon as your partner completes two ventilations and moves to the patient's chest, *flex* the patient's head slightly, and pull his jaw forward by hooking your thumb beneath his lower teeth and your fingers beneath his chin (Fig. 7-38). Lift straight up without hyperextending the patient's neck, and insert the tip of the obturator into his mouth.
4. While holding the jaw upward, *gently* and **slowly advance the tube** down the patient's throat and into the esophagus until the mask is firmly seated on the patient's face.

NEVER TRY TO FORCE THE EOA INTO THE ESOPHAGUS.

Forcing the tube down may tear the esophagus. If you meet resistance, pull back and gently try to advance the tube again. In most instances, the tube will follow the natural curvature of the throat and move easily into the esophagus. However, because there is always a possibility of ac-

cidentally intubating the trachea with this device, you must:

5. **Check the location of the tube!** Tilt the patient's head back, hold the mask in place as you would hold a pocket mask (see Chap. 8), and blow into the obturator tube. WATCH THE PATIENT'S CHEST as you blow to see whether it rises and falls with each ventilation. To double-check, have your partner listen with a stethoscope over both sides of the chest, just below the collar bones, as you ventilate through the opening in the mask. If the obturator is in the right place, you should see the chest rise and fall with each ventilation, and your partner should be able to hear air entering the patient's lungs each time you blow into the tube. If the chest does *not* move with each ventilation or if your partner does *not* hear breath sounds over the chest (and he *does* hear bubbling noises over the epigastrium), the obturator is probably in the trachea and must be removed *immediately.* Withdraw the obturator smoothly, and have your partner resume CPR for at least 2 to 3 minutes before you try again to insert the EOA.
6. When you have confirmed that the obturator is in the right place, **inflate the cuff** of the EOA to close off any leaks between the tube and the walls of the esophagus; that usually requires about 20 to 30 ml of air. Then detach the syringe from the one-way valve.
7. **Recheck the position of the tube.** Attach a bag-valve device to the port on the mask or put your lips around the port (Fig. 7-39), and ventilate through the mask while your partner listens again to the chest for breath sounds. If the chest

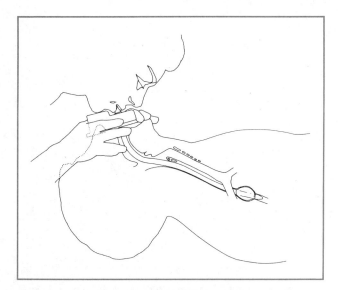

FIGURE 7-39. **VENTILATING THROUGH THE EOA.**
Reproduced courtesy Cavitron, Anaheim, California.

does not expand as you ventilate or if breath sounds are not heard, deflate the cuff and remove the obturator *at once*.

Removal of the EOA

The first rule to remember about removing an EOA is DON'T! Under most circumstances, an EOA should not be removed until the airway has been secured with an endotracheal tube to protect the patient from aspiration. The reason is that removal of an EOA is almost invariably accompanied by massive regurgitation. If the patient is still unconscious and lacking a gag reflex when he regurgitates, and if his trachea is not isolated by an endotracheal tube, a significant proportion of what was in his stomach is going to end up in his lungs, and that is *not* a Good Thing! So the general rule about removing an EOA is

> **NEVER REMOVE THE EOA FROM AN UNCONSCIOUS PATIENT UNTIL HIS AIRWAY HAS BEEN SECURED WITH AN ENDOTRACHEAL TUBE.**

There are times, however, when the patient resumes spontaneous breathing and seems to be waking up before you've had a chance to intubate his trachea. A patient with intact reflexes will not tolerate having a big, thick tube down his throat, and if you don't take it out, he will! So you will have to act with dispatch to get the EOA out safely:

1. Have a good, strong **suction apparatus** with a rigid, tonsil-tip catheter close at hand. As always, check the suction unit to make certain it is working properly, and place the catheter where you can grab it in a hurry.
2. **Turn the patient onto his side.**
3. **Snap off the mask** from the EOA. To do so, pinch the obturator tube where it extends through the mask (i.e., where it emerges from the patient's mouth), and lift the face mask off the obturator. Insert the 35-ml syringe back into the one-way valve of the pilot tube and **deflate the cuff** of the obturator.
4. Hold the suction catheter ready in one hand while you smoothly withdraw the EOA with the other hand. If the contents of the stomach follow the obturator, as they very likely will, **suction the mouth and pharynx** thoroughly. Leave the patient in the stable side position, so that any further vomitus will drain out from his mouth and not down his throat.

Endotracheal Intubation with the EOA in Place

As noted above, the airway of an unconscious patient should ordinarily be protected with an endotracheal tube before the EOA is removed. To intubate the trachea of a patient who has an EOA in place, follow these steps:

1. Have your partner hyperventilate the patient for several minutes with 100% oxygen while you **assemble the equipment for intubation**—suction, laryngoscope and blade, endotracheal tube, syringe, clamp, bite-block, and tie. Once the mask is removed from the EOA, there will be no way to ventilate the patient until the endotracheal tube is in place—so speedy intubation is essential.
2. When the intubation equipment is checked and ready by your right side, **remove the mask from the obturator.**
3. Push the obturator tube over to the *left* side of the patient's mouth, **insert the laryngoscope blade** into the *right* side of the patient's mouth, **and intubate in the usual manner** (see previous section, Carrying Out the Intubation).
4. As in any other endotracheal intubation, YOU MUST SEE THE VOCAL CORDS BEFORE YOU PASS THE ENDOTRACHEAL TUBE. *The presence of an obturator in the esophagus is no guarantee against accidental intubation of the esophagus with an endotracheal tube.* There is plenty of room in the distensible esophagus for both tubes. So take nothing for granted. **Look for the vocal cords,** which will lie *above* the esophageal obturator.
5. When you have seen the tip of the endotracheal

tube pass through the vocal cords, **inflate the cuff of the endotracheal tube.**

6. **Check the position of the endotracheal tube** by ventilating through it. Watch the chest to see if it rises and falls with each ventilation. Meanwhile have your partner listen to both sides of the chest for breath sounds.

7. Once you have confirmed the correct location of the endotracheal tube, **secure the endotracheal tube in place.** Use umbilical tape to tie it snugly.

8. While your partner continues to ventilate through the endotracheal tube, **suction the back of the patient's throat** with a rigid (tonsil-tip) catheter.

9. Instruct your partner to **hold the endotracheal tube firmly in place.** No matter how securely it has been taped or tied in, the endotracheal tube should be held manually in place while the EOA is being withdrawn, lest it be pulled out together with the obturator.

10. Hold the suction catheter in your left hand, in anticipation of massive regurgitation, deflate the EOA cuff, and **gently remove the obturator** with your left hand.

GUIDELINES FOR USE OF THE EOA: SUMMARY

- Use the EOA ONLY IN DEEPLY UNCONSCIOUS PATIENTS. It will cause gagging and vomiting in conscious or semiconscious patients.
- Do *not* use the EOA in
  1. Children under 16 years old.
  2. Patients known to have esophageal or liver disease.
  3. Patients known to have swallowed corrosives.
- DO NOT INTERRUPT CPR FOR MORE THAN 20 SECONDS to insert the EOA.
- PREOXYGENATE the patient before attempting to insert the EOA.
- NEVER USE FORCE to try to insert the EOA.
- MAINTAIN PROPER HEAD TILT to ventilate through an EOA.
- DO NOT REMOVE THE EOA from an unconscious patient until the airway has been secured with an endotracheal tube.

Pharyngeotracheal Lumen Airway

As noted previously, there are at least two potentially serious difficulties with the esophageal obturator airway. First, the EOA may be inadvertently placed in the trachea instead of the esophagus. And, second, even when the EOA is properly inserted, adequate ventilation depends on maintaining a very good seal with the mask.

To overcome those drawbacks, another type of airway device—called the pharyngeotracheal lumen (PTL) airway—was developed. The PTL has two tubes: a short, large-bore tube and a longer tube resembling an endotracheal tube. There is a large, proximal balloon designed to seal the airway by filling the oropharynx and a smaller distal balloon that acts like the cuff on an endotracheal tube (Fig. 7-40). The PTL is inserted blindly, and it may come to rest in *either* the trachea *or* the esophagus. Once the tube is inserted, its location—tracheal or esophageal —is assessed, and the patient is ventilated through the port that will provide lung inflation. The *advantages* of the PTL over an EOA are as follows:

- The problem of inadvertent tracheal intubation is no longer significant, for if the trachea is intubated, one simply uses the PTL as a standard endotracheal tube.
- If the long tube is placed in the esophagus, on the other hand, a face-mask seal is not required to deliver adequate tidal volumes to the lungs, because the proximal balloon seals off the airway (Fig. 7-41).

FIGURE 7-40. PHARYNGEOTRACHEAL LUMEN (PTL) AIRWAY. Reprinted with permission from JJ Niemann et al., *Ann Emerg Med* 13:591, 1984.

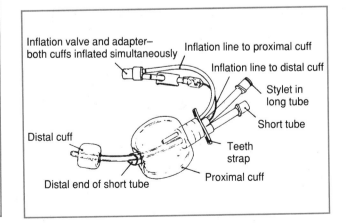

Inflation valve and adapter– both cuffs inflated simultaneously

Inflation line to proximal cuff

Inflation line to distal cuff

Stylet in long tube

Short tube

Distal cuff

Teeth strap

Proximal cuff

Distal end of short tube

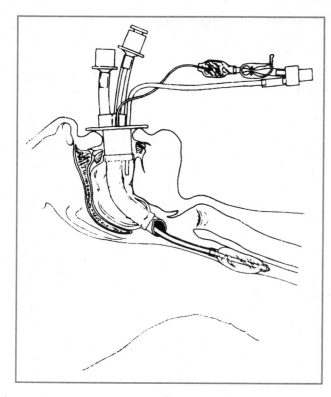

FIGURE 7-41.   PTL IN PLACE. The long tube sits in the esophagus, with its cuff blocking the esophagus to prevent regurgitation. The short tube sits above the vocal cords. The proximal cuff occludes the upper airway. Reprinted with permission from JJ Niemann et al., *Ann Emerg Med* 13:591, 1984

Studies so far seem to indicate that the PTL can provide adequate oxygenation and ventilation without significant complications. Some researchers have reported an inadequate seal with the pharyngeal balloon, and the design of the PTL may make replacement with a standard endotracheal tube difficult. Further studies are thus needed before organizations like the American Heart Association can give this device an unqualified endorsement. The PTL, in any event, is *not* an adjunct to be used by untrained operators. Insertion of the PTL, like any other skill, requires training and practice.

Steps in Inserting the PTL

- **Position the patient** as you would for endotracheal intubation, that is, in the "sniffing position," with the neck flexed and the head extended.
- Stand at the patient's vertex.
- With your left hand, **lift the patient's lower jaw** to bring the base of the tongue forward.
- With your right hand, **insert the PTL** and advance it until the teeth strap touches the patient's teeth.

- **Inflate both cuffs** simultaneously by blowing into the main inflation valve.
- **Determine the location of the long tube**:
  1. Ventilate through the **short (green) tube**. *If the chest rises*, continue ventilating through that tube (the long tube is in the esophagus).
  2. *If the chest does not rise*, **remove the stylet** from the **long, clear tube,** and ventilate through it.
  3. To double-check the location of the tube, **listen with a stethoscope** over both sides of the chest and over the epigastrium as you ventilate through the port you have selected.

Esophageal-Tracheal Double-Lumen Airway (Combitube or ETC)

A device similar in design to the PTL is the esophageal-tracheal double-lumen airway, also known as the Combitube or ETC (esophageal-tracheal Combitube). Like the PTL, it is a double-lumen tube that is inserted blindly, without visualization of the vocal cords; as with the PTL, the location of the tube is assessed after insertion, and then the patient is ventilated through the appropriate port. The principal theoretic advantage of the Combitube over the PTL in a resuscitation situation is that the Combitube has a self-adjusting, self-positioning balloon for occluding the posterior pharynx. There is limited prehospital experience with this device, so it has not yet been endorsed for widespread use. Studies so far suggest that the Combitube provides good ventilation and oxygenation with a low rate of complications. Like any invasive airway procedure, insertion of a Combitube requires training and practice.

Steps in Inserting the Combitube

- **Position the patient** as you would for endotracheal intubation.
- Standing at the patient's vertex, use your left hand to **lift the patient's tongue and lower jaw upward**.
- With the other hand, hold the Combitube as you would an endotracheal tube (Fig. 7-42A). **Insert the tip into the patient's mouth and advance gently** until the printed ring on the tube is aligned with the teeth (Fig. 7-42B). DO NOT TRY TO JAM THE TUBE AGAINST RESISTANCE. If it does not slide in easily, withdraw it slightly, redirect it, and try again.
- **Inflate line 1** (blue pilot balloon leading to the pharyngeal cuff) **with 100 ml of air.** (The Combitube may move slightly in the patient's mouth as you do so.)

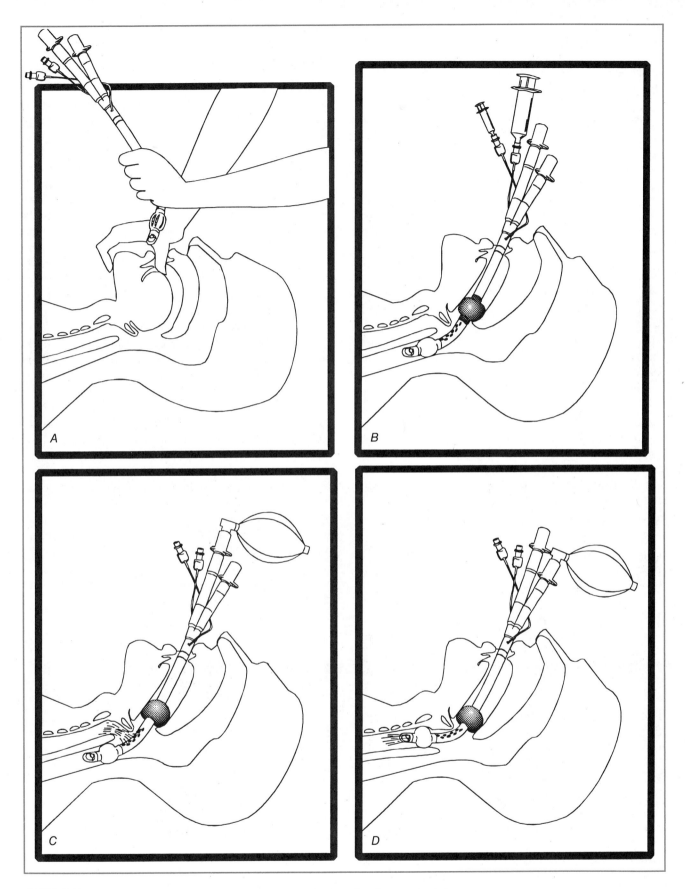

FIGURE 7-42. COMBITUBE INSERTION. (A) Hold the Combitube in your left hand. (B) Advance the tube into the patient's mouth until the printed ring is aligned with the teeth. (C) Ventilate through the longer (blue) tube. (D) If the chest does not rise, switch the bag-valve to the shorter tube. Reproduced courtesy of Sheridan Catheter Corporation, Argyle, New York.

- **Inflate line 2** (white pilot balloon leading to the distal cuff) **with about 15 ml of air.**
- **Determine the location of the tube:**
  1. Ventilate through the *longer* (blue) connecting tube (Fig. 7-42C). *If the chest rises*, continue ventilating through that tube; a suction catheter may be passed through the *other* tube to remove gastric contents.
  2. *If the chest does not rise*, disconnect the bag-valve-mask from the longer tube and ventilate instead through the *shorter* (clear) tube (Fig. 7-42D).
  3. **Double-check the location** of the tube by **listening with a stethoscope** over both sides of the chest and over the epigastrium as you ventilate through the port you have selected.

Since both the PTL airway and the Combitube may enter the esophagus during proper use, both have the same *contraindications* as the esophageal obturator airway:

- Patients under age 16
- Patients under 5 feet tall
- Patients with known esophageal disease
- Patients who have ingested caustic substances
- Patients with an intact gag reflex

Cricothyrotomy*

Cricothyrotomy—the establishment of an opening in the cricothyroid membrane—is indicated for relief of life-threatening upper airway obstruction when

- Manual measures (head tilt methods, triple airway maneuver) and attempts at ventilation have failed, and
- Endotracheal intubation is for some reason not feasible.

Such circumstances might arise, for example, in a patient with severe laryngeal edema or with trauma to the face and upper larynx. Cricothyrotomy may also be useful in a patient whose upper airway is obstructed by a foreign body that cannot be extracted by direct laryngoscopy.

The cricothyroid membrane is the site chosen for making a surgical opening because there are no important structures lying between the skin and the airway that can be damaged by an incision at that site. The airway at this level lies relatively close to the skin

and is easy to enter through the thin cricothyroid membrane. At the same time, the posterior wall of the airway at this level is formed by the tough cricoid cartilage, which helps prevent accidental perforation through the back of the airway into the esophagus.

Nonetheless, cricothyrotomy does have several potential *hazards*. Possible complications include bleeding into the airway and faulty placement of the cannula into the subcutaneous tissue rather than the trachea, resulting in the leakage of air into subcutaneous tissues (**subcutaneous emphysema**) or into the space between the lungs (**mediastinal emphysema**). Cricothyrotomy should not be attempted in infants or children, in whom the hazards are greater. In all patients, endotracheal intubation is the method of first choice when it can be accomplished.

Cricothyrotomy does not require a great deal of EQUIPMENT—a fortunate thing because usually in the circumstances that demand cricothyrotomy, there isn't a lot of time to get set up. One commercially available cricothyrotomy kit consists of a knife blade and cannula (Fig. 7-43). The knife blade is mounted in a rubber holder, such that the blade is long enough to puncture the cricothyroid membrane but not long enough to damage the posterior laryngeal wall. The emergency airway is a metal cannula with a smoothly rounded 90-degree angle; on the outside end, it has a standard 15-mm adapter to enable its attachment to ventilation devices such as a bag-valve. If a cricothyrotomy kit is not available, any sterile scalpel blade and a standard 90-degree tracheostomy tube may be used instead.

Cricothyrotomy is performed by the "cut and poke" technique:

FIGURE 7-43. CRICOTHYROTOMY KIT. A scalpel blade mounted in a rubber stopper and a metal tracheostomy tube are the essentials of a cricothyrotomy kit.

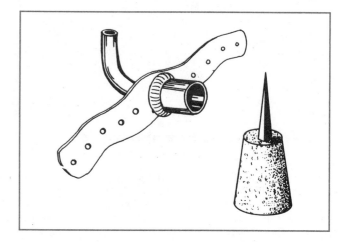

---

*Not required by the United States Department of Transportation standards for certification as a paramedic.

1. **Position the patient.** Place a rolled towel under his shoulders and hyperextend his neck to give optimal exposure to the anatomic features you need to identify.
2. If there is time and the materials are immediately available, **wash the neck with antiseptic solution.**
3. **Identify the cricothyroid membrane** (Fig. 7-44) by palpating for the V notch of the thyroid cartilage (Adam's apple), which feels like a high, sharp bump. Stabilize the larynx between your thumb and middle fingers while you palpate with your index finger. When you have located the V notch, slide your index finger down into the depression between the thyroid and cricoid cartilages; that is the cricothyroid membrane.
4. **Puncture the cricothyroid membrane** by guiding the knife blade along your fingernail and inserting it transversely through the soft tissues of the neck in the midline. Make the puncture cleanly to avoid later complications.
5. Keep your left hand on the larynx to stabilize it. Pick up the cannula in your right hand, and **poke the cannula through the puncture hole** with the cannula tip pointing toward the patient's feet. Use controlled force to insert the cannula, and advance it until the flange is flush with the skin.
6. **Check that the cannula is in the right place.** Listen and feel for air flow through it. Then ventilate through it. The chest should rise and fall with each ventilation, and breath sounds should be audible and equal on both sides of the chest.
7. When the cannula is correctly positioned, **secure the cannula in place** with the tapes provided.

Because of its potential hazards, cricothyrotomy should be performed ONLY by personnel who have been thoroughly trained in the method in the animal laboratory and who have been approved by their medical director to carry out the procedure in the field.

FIGURE 7-44. ANATOMIC LANDMARKS FOR CRICOTHYROTOMY. Slide your finger down from the V notch of the thyroid cartilage into the depression between the thyroid and cricoid cartilages.

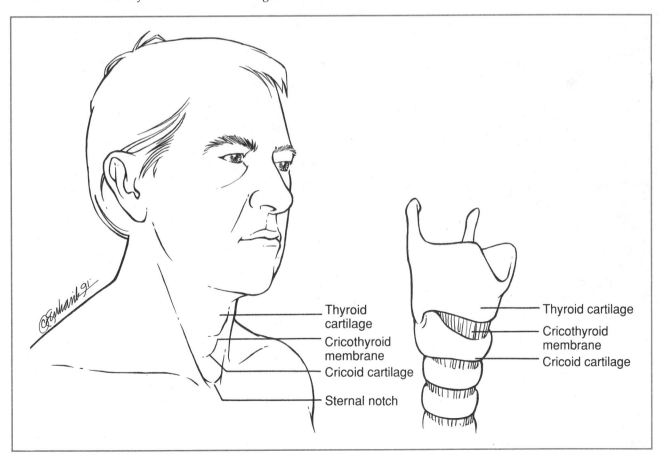

Thyroid cartilage
Cricothyroid membrane
Cricoid cartilage
Sternal notch

Thyroid cartilage
Cricothyroid membrane
Cricoid cartilage

GLOSSARY

alveolus   Saccular unit at the end of a terminal *bronchiole* where gas exchange takes place in the lung (plural = alveoli).

anaphylaxis   An exaggerated allergic reaction that often involves laryngeal edema, severe bronchospasm, and vascular collapse and that may be fatal within minutes.

angle of Louis   Prominence on the sternum that lies opposite the second intercostal space.

aphonia   Loss of voice.

apnea   Absence of breathing.

arytenoid cartilage   One of the paired, pitcher-shaped cartilages at the back of the larynx, at the upper border of the *cricoid cartilage.*

aspiration   Inhalation of foreign material into the lungs.

bronchiole   A small subdivision of a *bronchus.*

bronchus   One of the main branches of the *trachea* carrying air into various parts of the lung (plural = bronchi).

café coronary   Choking incident, so named because its suddenness may lead observers to mistake it for a heart attack.

carina   The point at which the *trachea* bifurcates into the right and left main *bronchi.*

cricoid cartilage   A ringlike cartilage forming the lower and back part of the *larynx.*

cricothyroid membrane   The membrane between the *cricoid* and *thyroid* cartilages of the *larynx.*

cricothyrotomy   Puncture of the *cricothyroid membrane* for the purpose of establishing an emergency airway in cases of upper airway obstruction.

croup   A common disease of childhood characterized by spasm of the *larynx* and resulting upper airway obstruction.

epiglottis   A thin structure, located behind the root of the tongue, that shields the entrance to the *larynx* during swallowing, thus preventing the *aspiration* of food into the *trachea.*

epiglottitis   A common illness of childhood, characterized by swelling of the *epiglottis,* high fever, and pain on swallowing. Complete airway obstruction may result with alarming rapidity.

gag reflex   Automatic spasm of the airway in response to irritation of the throat.

glottis   The opening between the *vocal cords.*

hypoxemia   Inadequate oxygen in the blood.

laryngeal edema   Swelling of the larynx.

laryngospasm   Severe constriction of the *larynx,* often in response to allergy or noxious stimuli.

larynx   The organ of voice production.

lumen   The channel within a tube.

mediastinal emphysema   Air in the space between the two lungs.

naris   One of the openings of the nasal cavity (plural = nares).

nasal septum   The partition separating the two nasal cavities in the midline, composed of cartilage, membrane, and bone.

pharynx   The portion of the airway between the nasal cavity and the larynx, consisting of the nasopharynx, oropharynx, and laryngopharynx.

regurgitation   A passive, retrograde flow of gastric contents from the stomach into the *pharynx* and mouth (to be distinguished from the active process of vomiting).

Sellick maneuver   Pressure applied over the cricoid to seal off the esophagus and prevent reflux of gastric contents.

sniffing position   The position of a patient for endotracheal intubation, with the neck flexed and the head extended.

stable side position   Position in which the patient is lying on his left side with his left thigh and leg flexed and his head resting on his extended left arm.

stridor   A harsh, high-pitched respiratory sound associated with severe upper airway obstruction, such as *laryngeal edema.*

subcutaneous emphysema   The presence of air or gas in the subcutaneous tissues of the body.

thyroid cartilage   The largest cartilage of the *larynx* whose two plates join anteriorly in a V shape to form the Adam's apple.

trachea   The cartilaginous tube extending from the *larynx* superiorly down to the *carina,* where it divides into the main *bronchi;* the windpipe.

vallecula   The groove between the base of the tongue and the *epiglottis.*

vertex   The top of the head.

vocal cords   Paired structures in the *larynx* whose vibrations produce sound.

FURTHER READING

AIRWAY MANAGEMENT: GENERAL

Baughman RP et al. Stridor: Differentiation from asthma or upper airway noise. *Am Rev Respir Dis* 139:1407, 1989.

Boidin MP. Airway patency in the unconscious patient. *Br J Anaesth* 57:306, 1985.

Cooper R, Bourn S. Clearing the way to airway control. *JEMS* 15(6):40, 1990.

Fogues M. Airway: Step one. *Emergency* 22(2):23, 1990.

Garret RC, Timberlake GA. Problem: Management of the difficult upper airway. *Emerg Med* 19(21):91, 1986.

Guildner CW. Resuscitation: Opening the airway. A comparative study of techniques for opening an airway obstructed by the tongue. *JACEP* 5:588, 1976.

Iserson KV. Strangulation: A review of ligature, manual, and postural neck compression injuries. *Ann Emerg Med* 13:179, 1984.

Martin SW. The basics in review. *Emergency* 22(2):42, 1990.

McSwain N. Airway compromise by hematoma. *Emerg Med* 22(11):48, 1990.

Rund DA. Airway management. *Emerg Med Serv* 19(1):19, 1990.

Safar P. Recognition and management of airway obstruction. *JAMA* 208:1008, 1969.

Wertz EM. Airway control. *Emergency* 24(6):29, 1992.

Whitten CE. Management of the airway. *Emerg Med* 22 (5):113, 1990.

Williams EG, Dymock M. Acute airway obstruction after aspiration of boiling tea from teapot spout. *Br Med J* 307:923, 1993.

CHOKING

Addy DP. The choking child: Back bangers against front pushers. *Br Med J* 286:536, 1983.

Agia GA, Hurst DJ. Pneumomediastinum following the Heimlich maneuver. *JACEP* 8:473, 1979.

Banerjee A et al. Laryngo-tracheo-bronchial foreign bodies in children. *Laryngol Otol* 102:1029, 1988.

Chapman JH, Menapace FJ, Howell RR. Ruptured aortic valve cusp: A complication of the Heimlich maneuver. *Ann Emerg Med* 12:446, 1983.

Day RL. Differing opinions on the emergency treatment of choking. *Pediatrics* 71:976, 1983.

Day RL et al. Choking: The Heimlich abdominal thrust vs back blows: An approach to measurement of inertial and aerodynamic forces. *Pediatrics* 70:113, 1982.

Dupre MW, Silva E, Brotman S. Traumatic rupture of the stomach secondary to Heimlich maneuver. *Am J Emerg Med* 11:611, 1993.

Eller WC, Haugen RK. Food asphyxiation—restaurant rescue. *N Engl J Med* 289:81, 1973.

Emergency Cardiac Care Committee and Subcommittees, American Heart Association. Guidelines for cardiopulmonary resuscitation and emergency cardiac care. *JAMA* 268:2171, 1992.

Gann DS. Emergency management of the obstructed airway. *JAMA* 243:1141, 1980.

Guildner CW, Williams D, Subitch T. Airway obstruction by foreign material: The Heimlich maneuver. *JACEP* 5:675, 1976.

Harris CS et al. Childhood asphyxiation by food: A national analysis and overview. *JAMA* 251:2232, 1984.

Haugen RK. The cafe coronary: Sudden deaths in restaurants. *JAMA* 186:142, 1963.

Heimlich HJ, Uhley MH. The Heimlich maneuver. *Clin Symp* 31:3, 1979.

Hoeve LJ et al. Foreign body aspiration in children: The diagnostic value of signs, symptoms and pre-operative evaluation. *Clin Otolaryngol* 18:55, 1993.

Hoffman JR. Treatment of foreign body obstruction of the upper airway. *West J Med* 136:11, 1982.

Meredith MJ. Rupture of the esophagus caused by the Heimlich maneuver (letter). *Ann Emerg Med* 15:106, 1986.

Mittleman RE, Wetli CV. The fatal cafe coronary. *JAMA* 247:1285, 1982.

Orlowski JP. Vomiting as a complication of the Heimlich maneuver. *JAMA* 258:512, 1987.

Redding JS. The choking controversy: Critique of evidence on the Heimlich maneuver. *Crit Care Med* 7:475, 1979.

Robison P et al. Heimlich maneuver in children. *Tex Med* 81(6):60, 1985.

Ruben H, MacNaughton FI. The treatment of food choking. *Practitioner* 221:725, 1978.

Sladen A. Relief of airway obstruction (editorial). *JACEP* 5:710, 1976.

Sofer S et al. Pulmonary edema following relief of upper airway obstruction. *Chest* 86:401, 1984.

Tami TA et al. Pulmonary edema and acute upper airway obstruction. *Laryngoscope* 96:506, 1986.

Torrey SB. The choking child—a life-threatening emergency: Evaluation of current recommendations. *Clin Pediatr* 22:751, 1983.

Trott A. Recurrent upper airway obstruction. *JACEP* 8:407, 1979.

Valero V. Mesenteric laceration complicating a Heimlich maneuver (letter). *Ann Emerg Med* 15:105, 1986.

Visintine RE, Baick CH. Ruptured stomach after Heimlich maneuver. *JAMA* 234:415, 1975.

Wiseman NE. The diagnosis of foreign body aspiration in children. *J Pediatr Surg* 19:521, 1984.

SUCTIONING

Dahlgren BE et al. Appropriate suction device in rescue medicine. *Ann Emerg Med* 16:1362, 1987.

Marx GF et al. Endotracheal suctioning and death. *NY J Med* 68:565, 1968.

Shim C et al. Cardiac arrhythmias resulting from tracheal suctioning. *Ann Intern Med* 71:1149, 1969.

Smith SJ. Suctioning the airway. *Emergency* 25(3):41, 1993.

White PF et al. A randomized study of drugs for preventing increases in intracranial pressure during endotracheal suctioning. *Anesthesiology* 57:242, 1982.

Winston SJ, Gravelyn TR, Sitrin RG. Prevention of bradycardic responses to endotracheal suctioning by prior administration of nebulized atropine. *Crit Care Med* 15:1009, 1987.

OROTRACHEAL INTUBATION: GENERAL

Abarbanell NR. Esophageal placement of an endotracheal tube by paramedics. *Am J Emerg Med* 6:178, 1988.

Aijian P et al. Endotracheal intubation of pediatric patients by paramedics. *Ann Emerg Med* 18:489, 1989.

Applebaum AL, Bruce DW. *Tracheal Intubation*. Philadelphia: Saunders, 1976.

Bissinger U, Lenz G, Kuhn W. Unrecognized endobronchial intubation of emergency patients. *Ann Emerg Med* 18:853, 1989.

Bivins HG et al. The effect of axial traction during orotracheal intubation of the trauma victim with an unstable cervical spine. *Ann Emerg Med* 17:25, 1988.

Chander S et al. Correct placement of endotracheal tubes. *NY State J Med* 79:1843, 1979.

DeLeo BC. Endotracheal intubation by rescue squad personnel. *Heart Lung* 6:851, 1977.

Dick T. Tubular tricks: Fool-proofing your field intubations. *JEMS* 14(5):26, 1989.

Fassoulaki A et al. Does atropine premedication affect the cardiovascular response to laryngoscopy and intubation? *Br J Anaesth* 54:1065, 1982.

Forgues M. Airway: Step two. *Emergency* 22(3):26, 1990.

Guss DA, Posluszny M. Paramedic orotracheal intubation: A feasibility study. *Am J Emerg Med* 2:399, 1984.

Hardwick WC et al. Digital intubation. *J Emerg Med* 1:317, 1984.

Jacobs LM et al. Endotracheal intubation in the prehospital

phase of emergency medical care. *JAMA* 250:2175, 1983.

Kalpokas M, Russell WJ. A simple technique for diagnosing oesophageal intubation. *Anaesth Intensive Care* 17:39, 1989.

Knopp RK. The safety of orotracheal intubation in patients with suspected cervical-spine injury (editorial). *Ann Emerg Med* 19:603, 1990.

Krill RL. Difficult laryngoscopy made easy with a "burp." *Can J Anaesth* 40:279, 1993.

Majernick TG et al. Cervical spine movement during orotracheal intubation. *Ann Emerg Med* 15:417, 1986.

Natanson C, Shelhamer J, Perrillo J. Intubation of the trachea in the critical care setting. *JAMA* 253:1160, 1985.

Owen RL, Cheney FW. Endobronchial intubation: A preventable complication. *Anesthesiology* 67:255, 1987.

Paturas JL. Endotracheal intubation. *Emergency* 24(4):50, 1992.

Pepe PE, Copass MK, Joyce TH. Prehospital endotracheal intubation: Rationale for training emergency medical personnel. *Ann Emerg Med* 14:1085, 1985.

Pointer JE. Clinical characteristics of paramedics' performance of pediatric endotracheal intubation. *Am J Emerg Med* 7:364, 1989.

Rhee KJ et al. Oral intubation in the multiply injured patient: The risk of exacerbating spinal cord damage. *Ann Emerg Med* 19:511, 1990.

Salem MR, Mathrubhutham J, Bennet EJ. Difficult intubation. *N Engl J Med* 295:879, 1976.

Scannell G et al. Orotracheal intubation in trauma patients with cervical fractures. *Arch Surg* 128:903, 1993.

Sellik BA. Cricoid pressure to control regurgitation of stomach contents during induction of anesthesia. *Lancet* 2:404, 1961.

Shapiro BA. Airway access in the struggling patient. *Emerg Med* 16(7):102, 1984.

Smith M. Backward tubes. *JEMS* 18(2):23, 1993.

Stanford TM. ET: A different approach. *Emergency* 20(12):34, 1988.

Stein JM. Endotracheal intubation in a hurry. *Emerg Med* 14(15):129, 1982.

Stein JM. Difficult adult intubation. *Emerg Med* 17(3):121, 1985.

Stemp LI, Singleton M. Intubating the awake patient. *Emerg Med* 23(17):113, 1991.

Stewart RD. Tactile orotracheal intubation. *Ann Emerg Med* 13:175, 1984.

Stewart RD, Paris PM. Signs of endotracheal intubation in the field setting (letter). *Ann Emerg Med* 14:276, 1985.

Stewart RD et al. Effect of varied training techniques on field endotracheal intubation success rates. *Ann Emerg Med* 13:1032, 1984.

Stewart RD et al. Field endotracheal intubation by paramedical personnel: Success rates and complications. *Chest* 85:341, 1984.

Stratton SJ, Gunter CS. Teaching intubation. *JEMS* 17(11):54, 1992.

Stratton SJ et al. Prospective study of manikin-only versus manikin and human subject endotracheal intubation training of paramedics. *Ann Emerg Med* 20:1314, 1991.

Vollmer TP et al. Use of a lighted stylet for guided orotracheal intubation in the prehospital setting. *Ann Emerg Med* 14:324, 1985.

White RD, Billes BP. Endotracheal vs. esophageal intubation. *Emergency* 10(9):49, 1978.

Whitten CE. Intubation for the primary physician (series):

Common errors and how to avoid them. *Emerg Med* 21(15):91, 1989.

Complications. *Emerg Med* 22(7):89, 1990.

Difficult intubations: Tricks to remember. *Emerg Med* 22(1):85, 1990.

Endotracheal anatomy. *Emerg Med* 21(8):171, 1989.

Equipment for airway management. *Emerg Med* 21(12):91, 1989.

Oral intubation in adults. *Emerg Med* 21(14):81, 1989.

Preintubation evaluation: Predicting the difficult airway. *Emerg Med* 21(10):107, 1989.

Tests for tube placement. *Emerg Med* 21(17):93, 1989.

USE OF NEUROMUSCULAR BLOCKERS FOR INTUBATION

Berve MO. Easing intubation with succinylcholine. *JEMS* 15(11):60, 1990.

Dronen SC et al. A comparison of blind nasotracheal and succinylcholine-assisted intubation in the poisoned patient. *Ann Emerg Med* 16:650, 1987.

Hedges JR et al. Succinylcholine-assisted intubations in prehospital care. *Ann Emerg Med* 17:469, 1988.

Koenig KL. Rapid-sequence intubation of head trauma patients: Prevention of fasciculations with pancuronium versus minidose succinylcholine. *Ann Emerg Med* 21:929, 1992.

Kuchinski J et al. Emergency intubation for paralysis of the uncooperative trauma patient. *J Emerg Med* 9:9, 1991.

Ligier B et al. The role of anesthetic induction agents and neuromuscular blockade in the endotracheal intubation of trauma victims. *Surg Gynecol Obstet* 173:477, 1991.

Miller K. Paralysis for intubation. *Emergency* 21(5):19, 1989.

Murphy-Macobabby M et al. Neuromuscular blockade in aeromedical airway management. *Ann Emerg Med* 21:664, 1992.

Rhee KJ, O'Malley RJ. Neuromuscular blockade-assisted oral intubation versus nasotracheal intubation in the prehospital care of injured patients. *Ann Emerg Med* 23:37, 1994.

Roberts DJ, Clinton JE, Ruiz E. Neuromuscular blockade for critical patients in the emergency department. *Ann Emerg Med* 15:152, 1986.

Rotondo MF et al. Urgent paralysis and intubation of trauma patients: Is it safe? *J Trauma* 34:242, 1993.

Severud SA et al. Prehospital use of neuromuscular blocking agents in a helicopter ambulance program. *Ann Emerg Med* 17:236, 1988.

Thompson JD, Fish S, Ruiz E. Succinylcholine for endotracheal intubation. *Ann Emerg Med* 11:526, 1982.

Tressa J. Neuromuscular blocking agents. *Emergency* 24(7):57, 1992.

NASOTRACHEAL INTUBATION

Adams AL, Cane RD, Shapiro BA. Tongue extrusion as an aid to blind nasal intubation. *Crit Care Med* 10:335, 1982.

Berry FA. The use of a stylet in blind nasotracheal intubation. *Anesthesiology* 61:469, 1984.

Danzl DF, Thomas DM. Nasotracheal intubations in the emergency department. *Crit Care Med* 8:677, 1980.

Greiff SJ. Blind nasotracheal intubation. *Emergency* 23(11):53, 1991.

Hartigan ML et al. A comparison of pretreatment regimens for minimizing the hemodynamic response to blind nasotracheal intubation. *Can Anaesth Soc J* 31:497, 1984.

Holdgaard HO et al. Complications and late sequelae following nasotracheal intubation. *Acta Anaesth Scand* 37:475, 1993.

Iserson KV. Blind nasotracheal intubation. *Ann Emerg Med* 10:468, 1981.

Iserson KV. Blind nasotracheal intubation: A model for instruction. *Ann Emerg Med* 13:601, 1984.

Krishel S, Jackimczyk K, Balazs K. Endotracheal tube whistle: An adjunct to blind nasotracheal intubation. *Ann Emerg Med* 21:33, 1992.

O'Brien DJ et al. Prehospital blind nasotracheal intubation by paramedics. *Ann Emerg Med* 18:612, 1989.

Rhee KJ et al. Does nasotracheal intubation increase complications in patients with skull base fractures? *Ann Emerg Med* 22:1145, 1993.

Sessler CN et al. Comparison of 4% lidocaine/0.5% phenylephrine with 5% cocaine: Which dilates the nasal passage better? *Anesthesiology* 64:274, 1986.

Stein JM. Nasotracheal intubation. *Emerg Med* 16(13):183, 1984.

Tintinalli JE, Claffey J. Complications of nasotracheal intubation. *Ann Emerg Med* 10:142, 1981.

Van Elstraete AC et al. Tracheal tube cuff inflation as an aid to blind nasotracheal intubation. *Br J Anaesth* 70:691, 1993.

Verdile VP et al. Nasotracheal intubation using a flexible lighted stylet. *Ann Emerg Med* 19:506, 1990.

Veron KA. NT intubation review. *Emergency* 21(9):19, 1989.

Whitten CE. Intubation for the primary care physician: Nasal techniques. *Emerg Med* 22(3):137, 1990.

ESOPHAGEAL OBTURATOR AIRWAY AND
RELATED DEVICES

Auerbach PS, Geehr EC. Inadequate oxygenation and ventilation using the esophageal obturator gastric tube airway in the prehospital setting. *JAMA* 250:3067, 1983.

Bass R, Allison E, Hunt R. The esophageal obturator airway: A reassessment of use by paramedics. *Ann Emerg Med* 11:358, 1982.

Benumof JL. Laryngeal mask airway: Indications and contraindications. *Anesthesiology* 77:843, 1992.

Brain A. The laryngeal mask: A new concept in airway management. *Br J Anaesth* 55:801, 1983.

Carlson WJ, Hunter SW, Bonnabeau RC. Esophageal perforation with obturator airway. *Emerg Med Serv* 9(5):74, 1980.

Don Michael T. Mouth-to-lung airway for cardiac resuscitation. *Lancet* 2:1329, 1968.

Donen N et al. The esophageal obturator airway: An appraisal. *Can Anaesth Soc J* 30:194, 1983.

Garvin JM. The esophageal obturator airway—an improved model. *Emerg Med Serv* 8(4):48, 1979.

Geehr EC, Bogetz MS, Auerbach PS. Prehospital tracheal intubation versus esophageal gastric tube airway use: A prospective study. *Am J Emerg Med* 3:381, 1985.

Gertler JP et al. Esophageal obturator airway: Obturator or obtundator? *J Trauma* 25:424, 1985.

Goldenburg IF et al. Morbidity and mortality of patients receiving the esophageal obturator airway and the endotracheal tube in prehospital cardiopulmonary arrest. *Minn Med* 69:707, 1986.

Gordon AS. The tongue-jaw lift for EOA and EGTA. *Emergency* 13(6):40, 1981.

Greenbaum DM, Poggi J, Grace WM. Esophageal obstruction during oxygen administration: A new method for use in resuscitation. *Chest* 65:188, 1974.

Grigsby JW, Rottman SJ. Prehospital airway management: Esophageal obturator airway or endotracheal intubation? *Top Emerg Med* 1:25, 1981.

Hammargren Y, Clinton JE, Ruiz E. A standard comparison of esophageal obturator airway and endotracheal tube in cardiac arrest. *Ann Emerg Med* 14:953, 1985.

Hankins DG et al. Complication rates for the esophageal obturator airway and endotracheal tube in the prehospital setting. *Prehosp Disaster Med* 8(2):117, 1993.

Harrison E et al. Esophageal perforation following use of the esophageal obturator airway. *Ann Emerg Med* 9:21, 1980.

Hunt RC, Sheets CA, Whitley TW. Pharyngeal tracheal lumen airway training: Failure to discriminate between esophageal and endotracheal modes and failure to confirm ventilation. *Ann Emerg Med* 18:947, 1989.

Johnson KR, Genovesi MG, Lassar KH. Esophageal obturator airway: Use and complications. *JACEP* 5:36, 1976.

Kassels SJ, Robinson WA, O'Bara KJ. Esophageal perforation associated with the esophageal obturator airway. *Crit Care Med* 8:386, 1980.

Meislin HW. The esophageal obturator airway: A study of respiratory effectiveness. *Ann Emerg Med* 9:54, 1980.

Michael TAD. Comparison of the esophageal obturator airway and endotracheal intubation in prehospital ventilation during CPR. *Chest* 87:814, 1985.

Miller AC, Bickler P. The laryngeal mask airway: An unusual complication. *Anaesthesia* 46:659, 1991.

Schofferman J, Oill P, Lewis AJ. The esophageal obturator airway: A clinical evaluation. *Chest* 69:67, 1976.

Shea SR et al. Prehospital endotracheal tube airway or esophageal gastric tube airway: A critical comparison. *Ann Emerg Med* 14:102, 1985.

Smith JP et al. The esophageal obturator airway. *JAMA* 250:1081, 1982.

Smith JP et al. A field evaluation of the esophageal obturator airway. *J Trauma* 23:317, 1983.

Strate RG, Fischer RP. Midesophageal perforations by esophageal obturator airways. *J Trauma* 16:503, 1976.

PHARYNGEOTRACHEAL LUMEN AIRWAY
AND COMBITUBE

Atherton GL, Johnson JC. Ability of paramedics to use the Combitube in prehospital cardiac arrest. *Ann Emerg Med* 22:1263, 1993.

Frass M et al. Ventilation with the esophageal tracheal Combitube in cardiopulmonary resuscitation: Promptness and effectiveness. *Chest* 93:781, 1988.

Hunt RC, Sheets CA, Whitley TW. Pharyngeal tracheal lumen airway training: Failure to discriminate between esophageal and endotracheal modes and failure to confirm ventilation. *Ann Emerg Med* 18:947, 1989.

Johnson JC, Atherton GL. The esophageal tracheal Combitube: An alternate route to airway management. *JEMS* 16(5):29, 1991.

McMahon S et al. Multi-agency, prehospital evaluation of the pharyngeo-tracheal lumen (PTL) airway. *Prehosp Disaster Med* 7(1):13, 1992.

Niemann JT et al. The pharyngeo-tracheal lumen airway: Preliminary investigation of a new adjunct. *Ann Emerg Med* 13:591, 1984.

Pepe PE, Zachariah BS, Chandra NC. Invasive airway techniques in resuscitation. *Ann Emerg Med* 22:393, 1993.

Schwartz BL. Airway alternatives: The PTL and the Combitube. *JEMS* 19(2):29, 1994.

Staudinger T et al. Emergency intubation with the Combi-tube®: Comparison with the endotracheal airway. *Ann Emerg Med* 22:1573, 1993.

CRICOTHYROTOMY

Brantigan CO, Grant JB. Cricothyroidotomy: Elective use in respiratory problems requiring tracheotomy. *J Thorac Cardiovasc Surg* 71:72, 1976.

Carlton DM et al. An easily constructed cricothyroidotomy device for emergency airway management. *J Oral Surg* 38:623, 1980.

Dobbinson TL et al. Needle tracheostomy: A laboratory study. *Anaesth Intensive Care* 8:72, 1980.

Esses BA et al. Cricothyroidotomy: A decade of experience in Denver. *Ann Otol Rhinol Laryngol* 95:519, 1987.

Grace TL. The crico-ventilating device: A method for ventilation of the needle cricothyroidotomy. *Emerg Med Serv* 12(4):45, 1983.

Kress TD, Balasubramanjam S. Cricothyroidotomy. *Ann Emerg Med* 11:197, 1982.

McGill J, Clinton JE, Ruiz E. Cricothyrotomy in the emergency department. *Ann Emerg Med* 11:361, 1982.

Nugent WL, Rhee KJ, Wisner DH. Can nurses perform surgical cricothyrotomy with acceptable success and complication rates? *Ann Emerg Med* 20:367, 1991.

Safar P, Penninckz J. Cricothyroid membrane puncture with special cannula. *Anesthesiology* 28:943, 1967.

Simon RR, Brenner BE. Emergency cricothyroidotomy in the patient with massive neck swelling. Part 1: Anatomical aspects. Part 2: Clinical aspects. *Crit Care Med* 11:114, 119, 1983.

Spaite DW, Joseph M. Prehospital cricothyrotomy: An investigation of indications, technique, complications, and patient outcome. *Ann Emerg Med* 19:279, 1990.

Werdman MJ. Emergency cricothyroidotomy. *Emergency* 27(7):49, 1993.

PERFORMANCE CHECKLISTS

The following pages contain checklists for correct performance of some of the skills described in this chapter. The checklists can be used as a review and as a guide for practicing the respective skills.

Performance Test
Obstructed Airway: Conscious Adult

Student _____ Date _____

Instructor: Place an "X" in the Fail column beside any element that is done incorrectly, out of sequence, or omitted.

Step	Activity	Critical Performance	Fail
Assessment	Determine airway obstruction	Asks, "Are you choking?"	
		Determines if victim can cough or speak	
Heimlich maneuver	Perform abdominal thrusts	Stands behind victim	
		Wraps arms around victim's waist	
		Makes a fist with one hand and places the thumb side against the victim's abdomen	
		In the midline	
		Slightly above navel and well below tip of the xiphoid	
		Grasps fist with other hand	
		Presses into victim's abdomen with quick upward thrusts	
		Each thrust distinct	
		Repeats thrusts until foreign body is expelled or victim loses consciousness	

Victim with obstructed airway becomes unconscious (manikin):

Step	Activity	Critical Performance	Fail
Additional assessment	Position the victim	Turns victim on back as a unit	
		Places faceup, arms by side	
Foreign body check	Perform finger sweep	Keeps victim's face up	
		Uses tongue-jaw lift to open mouth	
		Sweeps deeply into mouth to remove foreign body	
Breathing attempt	Attempt ventilation (airway is obstructed)	Opens airway with head tilt–chin lift	
		Seals mouth and nose properly	
		Attempts to ventilate	
Heimlich maneuver	Perform abdominal thrusts	Kneels astride victim's thighs	
		Places heel of one hand against victim's abdomen	
		In the midline	
		Slightly above navel and well below tip of xiphoid	
		Places second hand directly on top of first	
		Presses into abdomen with quick upward thrusts	
		Performs up to 5 manual thrusts	

Foreign body check	Perform finger sweep	Keeps victim's face up	
		Uses tongue-jaw lift to open mouth	
		Sweeps deeply into mouth to remove foreign body	
Breathing attempt	Reattempt ventilation	Opens airway with head tilt–chin lift	
		Seals mouth and nose properly	
		Attempts to ventilate	
Sequencing	Repeat sequence	Repeats Heimlich maneuver, foreign body check, and breathing attempts until successful	

Instructor _____

Based on the recommendations in Emergency Cardiac Care Committee and Subcommittees, American Heart Association. Guidelines for cardiopulmonary resuscitation and emergency cardiac care. *JAMA* 268:2172, 1992.

Performance Test
Obstructed Airway: Unconscious Adult

Student _____ Date _____

Instructor: Place an "X" in the Fail column beside any element that is done incorrectly, out of sequence, or omitted.

Step	Activity	Critical Performance	Fail
Assessment	Determine unresponsiveness	Taps or gently shakes shoulder	
		Shouts, "Are you O.K.?"	
Airway	Position the victim	Turns victim on back as unit, supporting head and neck (4–10 sec)	
	Open the airway	Uses head tilt–chin lift maneuver	
	Determine breathlessness	Ear over mouth	
		Observes chest	
		Looks, listens, feels for breathing (3–5 sec)	
Breathing attempt	Attempt ventilation (airway is obstructed)	Maintains open airway	
		Seals mouth and nose properly	
		Attempts to ventilate	
	Reattempt ventilation (airway remains blocked)	Seals mouth and nose properly	
		Again attempts to ventilate	
Heimlich maneuver	Perform abdominal thrusts	Kneels astride victim's thighs	
		Places heel of one hand against victim's abdomen:	
		In the midline	
		Slightly above navel and well below tip of xiphoid	
		Places second hand directly on top of first	
		Presses into abdomen with quick upward thrusts	
		Each thrust distinct	
		Applies up to 5 manual thrusts	

Performance Test
Suctioning the Mouth and Pharynx

Student _____   Date _____

Instructor: Place an "X" in the Fail column beside any element that is done incorrectly, out of sequence, or omitted.

Maximum Time (sec)	Activity	Critical Performance*	Fail
	Preoxygenation	Patient given oxygen while student prepares equipment	
		Oxygen administered for at least 3 min before suction	
	Equipment assembly	Checks that collection bottle is screwed tight	
		Connects collection tubing to suction	
		Connects catheter or suction tip to collection tubing	
		Turns on suction unit	
	Equipment check	Kinks collection tubing to block flow	
		Checks that pressure gauge reaches 300 mm Hg	
		Unkinks tubing	
		Places catheter tip in rinse water and flushes through	
	Catheter measurement	Measures off catheter from patient's mouth to ear lobe	
	Opening victim's mouth	Removes oxygen mask from patient's face	
		Turns patient's head to side	
		Crossed-finger maneuver to open mouth	
		Uses fingers of other hand to sweep mouth of debris	
	Catheter insertion	Suction OFF (Y tube open) during insertion	
		Inserts catheter correct distance	
		If tonsil suction, inserts convex side up	
15	Suction	Occludes Y tube	
		Moves catheter tip around	
		Pulls catheter tip back into mouth	
		Suctions mouth	
	Catheter removal	Suction OFF (Y tube open)	
		Replaces oxygen mask on patient's face	
		Flushes system with water	

*Assume spontaneously breathing, unconscious patient.

Instructor _____

Performance Test
Endotracheal Intubation

Student _____ Date _____

Instructor: Place an "X" in the Fail column beside each item that is performed incorrectly, out of sequence, or omitted.

Maximum Time (sec)	Activity	Critical Performance*	Fail
	Preparation of equipment	Chooses endotracheal tube	
		Measures length against patient	
		Cuts tube to correct length	
		Inserts tight-fitting connector	
		Tests cuff; leaves syringe attached	
		Lubricates stylet	
		Inserts stylet into endotracheal tube	
		Stylet distal end not protruding	
		Bends proximal stylet over connector	
		Bends endotracheal tube to hockey-stick shape	
		Lubricates endotracheal tube	
		Assembles laryngoscope	
		Checks light for brightness, constancy	
		Leaves laryngoscope in "off" position	
		Turns on suction	
		Tests vacuum	
		Attaches tonsil-tip catheter to suction	
		Places within easy reach: Bite-block (or oropharyngeal airway)	
		Magill forceps	
		Umbilical tape	
		Hemostat	
20	Positioning the patient	Neck flexed on pillow	
		Head extended	
	Intubation	All equipment accessible at right hand	
		Grasps laryngoscope in left hand	
		Snaps blade into "on" position	
		Opens patient's jaws with right hand	
		Patient's lips spread apart	

Maximum Time (sec)	Activity	Critical Performance*	Fail
		Inserts blade into right corner of mouth	
		Suctions mouth/pharynx as needed	
		Advances blade to vallecula	
		Lifts mandible/head with laryngoscope	
		Blade not touching teeth	
		Visualizes vocal cords	
		Passes tip of endotracheal tube through cords under direct vision	
		Removes laryngoscope from patient's mouth	
		Removes stylet from endotracheal tube	
		One hand stabilizing tube at all times	
		Attaches bag-valve to endotracheal tube	
		Ventilating, inflates cuff until no leak	
	Testing position	Instructs assistant to listen to six areas on chest during ventilations	
		Watches for rise and fall of chest	
		Palpates sternal notch for cuff	
	Securing tube	Asks assistant to ventilate and hold tube	
		Inserts bite-block (or oropharyngeal airway)	
		Marks endotracheal tube where it emerges from mouth	
		Ties tube/bite-block securely in place	
		Resumes ventilations, holding tube with one hand to stabilize it	

*It is assumed that someone else is ventilating the patient (or manikin) while the student prepares for intubation.

Instructor _____

Performance Test
Esophageal Obturator Airway

Student _____   Date _____

Instructor: Place an "X" in the Fail column beside any element that is performed incorrectly, out of sequence, or omitted.

Maximum Time (sec)	Activity	Critical Performance*	Fail
	Preparation of equipment	Checks to see there is a mask, obturator, and syringe	
		Inflates cuff of mask until firm	
		Inflates cuff of obturator to check for leaks	
		Deflates cuff of obturator and leaves syringe attached	
		Snaps obturator into mask	
		Lubricates obturator	
12	Obturator insertion	Moves to patient's head	
		Tells rescuer doing CPR, "Ready."	
		Tilts patient's head slightly forward	
		Uses thumb and forefinger to pull jaw forward	
		Does not hyperextend neck	
		Slowly advances obturator until mask is flush with face	
10	Testing position	Performs triple airway maneuver from vertex; mask tight	
		Takes deep breath	
		Exhales into mask	
		Observes to see if chest rises	
		Records volume of at least 1,000 ml for each breath	
5	Cuff inflation	Inflates cuff with 20–30 ml of air	
		Detaches syringe	
		Resumes ventilations	
	Interposition of ventilations	Interposes ventilation between every 5 compressions	
		No pause for ventilation	
		Adequate volumes (at least 1,000 ml)	
	Use of adjunct	Attaches bag-valve with O_2 to EOA	
		Interposes ventilation between every 5 compressions	
		No pause for ventilations	
	EOA removal	Instructor says, "The patient is breathing spontaneously." Assembles and tests suction (tonsil tip)	
		Turns patient's head to side	
		Snaps mask off obturator	
		Deflates cuff	
		Smoothly withdraws obturator, with suction in other hand	
		Suctions pharynx and mouth	
		Places oxygen mask or cannula on patient	

*CPR is in progress; second student doing compressions.

Instructor _____

8
Breathing

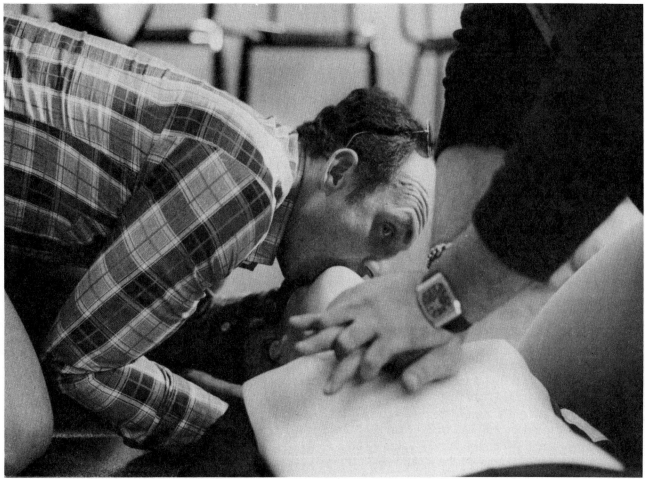

Photo by Nancy L. Caroline.

OBJECTIVES

Recall the primary survey: ABC. The first step, after a check for hazards, is to ensure the patient's *airway*, as described in the previous chapter. Having done so, we come to the next letter of the rescue alphabet: **B** for **breathing;** so our next task is to make certain that the patient is breathing adequately. That is what this chapter is about—how we breathe; what breathing does for us; what happens when breathing is disrupted; and how to help someone who is not breathing adequately or who stops breathing altogether. By the end of this chapter, the student should be able to

1. Identify, given a list of definitions, the correct definition of
   - Respiration
   - Ventilation
   - Tidal volume
   - Minute volume
   - Dead space
   - Shunt
   - Hypoventilation
   - Hyperventilation
   - Atelectasis
2. Describe the optimal position for an unconscious patient, and explain the anatomic reason why that position is preferred
3. State the correct anatomic names of the airways and of the membranes that surround the lung
4. Explain how air flow in and out of the lung is produced
5. Calculate a patient's minute volume, given the patient's respiratory rate and tidal volume
6. List two ways in which the minute volume could fall below normal, and describe what would happen to a person's arterial blood gases as a consequence
7. Explain the physiologic function of
   - Coughing
   - Sighing
8. Describe the difference between venous and arterial blood in terms of their
   - Oxygen (O_2) content
   - Carbon dioxide (CO_2) content
9. List four conditions that can result in an elevated level of carbon dioxide in the blood (hypercarbia), and explain how the blood CO_2 level can be normalized
10. List six conditions that can cause hypoxemia, and state the treatment for hypoxemia
11. Identify, given a description of several mechanisms, the mechanism that
    - Stimulates a healthy person to breathe
    - Stimulates some patients who suffer from chronic obstructive pulmonary disease to breathe
12. List at least six indications for oxygen therapy
13. Identify a person with respiratory insufficiency, given a description of several people with different clinical symptoms and signs
14. Calculate how long the oxygen supply in a cylinder will last, given the reading on the pressure gauge, the size of the cylinder, and the flow rate being used
15. Identify unsafe practices in handling oxygen equipment, given a description of various practices
16. Choose the most appropriate device for administering oxygen to a patient, given a description of the patient's clinical condition
17. List six potential causes of respiratory arrest, and indicate which of them is the most common cause
18. State how one can diagnose respiratory arrest with certainty
19. Describe the purposes of artificial ventilation, and explain the difference between controlled and assisted ventilation
20. List three ways to tell if one is providing adequate volumes of air during mouth-to-mouth or mouth-to-nose ventilation
21. List two ways of minimizing gastric distention during artificial ventilation, and describe what to do if gastric distention does occur
22. List four advantages of a pocket mask over other methods of giving artificial ventilation in the prehospital setting
23. State the main indication for using a demand valve, and list three situations in which the demand valve is not desirable
24. List at least two advantages of automatic transport ventilators over bag-valve or demand valve devices for ventilating a person who isn't breathing
25. List the maximum oxygen concentrations that can be delivered via
    - Mouth-to-mouth ventilation
    - Pocket mask ventilation (with and without supplemental O_2)
    - Bag-valve-mask ventilation (with and without supplemental O_2)
    - Demand valve ventilation
26. State the primary indication for percutaneous translaryngeal ventilation, and describe how the procedure is carried out*
27. List at least three indications for pulse oximetry

---

*Not required by the United States Department of Transportation for certification as a paramedic.

28. List four potential sources of erroneous readings from a pulse oximeter
29. Identify patients who have respiratory compromise, given the pulse oximetry readings and relevant clinical data about the patients
30. Identify the location of an endotracheal tube—within the trachea or within the esophagus—given the reading from an end-tidal carbon dioxide monitor

THE MECHANICS OF BREATHING

Broadly speaking, **respiration** is the exchange of gases between a living organism and its environment. In the simplest, single-cell organisms, that exchange takes place by diffusion of gases across the cell membrane. When we speak of respiration in a complex organism like man, however, we are referring to the exchange of *oxygen* and *carbon dioxide* among the body tissues, the lungs, and the atmosphere.

Oxygen is vital to life. Every living cell in the body requires an uninterrupted supply of oxygen to carry out its metabolic processes. No living cell can survive very long without oxygen. Some cells are more sensitive than others to oxygen deprivation. The cells of the *brain* and *heart*, for example, can tolerate only very short periods of oxygen deprivation—usually less than about 5 minutes—after which they will die. And once brain cells or myocardial (heart muscle) cells have died, they can never be replaced. It is critical, therefore, that the body have a mechanism to ensure a constant oxygen supply.

The same metabolic processes that consume oxygen produce carbon dioxide as a waste product. Like the wastes of any factory, carbon dioxide must be carried away from the cell and disposed of, lest it accumulate to toxic levels. So the body also needs a mechanism for flushing away the carbon dioxide produced by metabolism.

As it happens, the body very economically uses the same mechanism to accomplish both tasks, that is, to ensure a constant oxygen supply and to remove the carbon dioxide generated by metabolism. That mechanism is what we call *breathing*.

Anatomy of the Respiratory System

To understand how breathing is accomplished, we need first to take a look at the anatomy of the respiratory system (Fig. 8-1). That system includes all the structures of the body that contribute to respiration: the AIRWAYS, through which air passes from the atmosphere into the body; a PULMONARY CIRCULATION, which brings blood to and from the terminal airways; the LUNGS, where gas exchange occurs; and the RESPIRATORY MUSCLES, the diaphragm and the muscles between the ribs, which cause the expansion and contraction of the lung that produce air flow.

We have already learned quite a bit about the anatomy of the *airway*. Recall that air normally enters the body through the **nares** to be warmed, filtered, and humidified in the **nasal cavity.** From there, air proceeds down the **nasopharynx, oropharynx,** and **laryngopharynx** to pass through the **vocal cords** in the **larynx.** All of the structures above the vocal cord are referred to as the UPPER AIRWAY.

As air passes through the vocal cords, it enters the LOWER AIRWAY, starting with the **trachea,** a semirigid tube about 5 inches long. The trachea is composed of a stack of cartilaginous rings, which give the trachea its stiffness and keep it from collapsing under the negative pressure generated during inhalation. At about the level of the fourth or fifth thoracic vertebra (T4 or T5), the trachea branches into two main **bronchi,** the right bronchus and the left bronchus. The point at which the trachea divides into the two bronchi is called the **carina.** [If an endotracheal tube is inserted too far, which bronchus is it more apt to enter? Why?]

The right main bronchus is wider and shorter than the left, and its direction is almost identical with that of the trachea. That is why an endotracheal tube inserted too far is more likely to enter the right main bronchus than the left main bronchus. That is also why most aspirated material enters the right lung. For that reason, unconscious patients should always be placed in the lateral recumbent position with the *right side up*, assuming they do not have injuries that preclude that position.

> **PLACE UNCONSCIOUS PATIENTS IN THE LATERAL RECUMBENT POSITION—RIGHT SIDE UP.**

Each main bronchus immediately branches within the lung into smaller and smaller airways—first bronchi to the main pulmonary lobes (three lobes on the right and two on the left) and from there segmental bronchi to the 18 anatomic segments of the lung. As the bronchi pass more and more distally, they divide

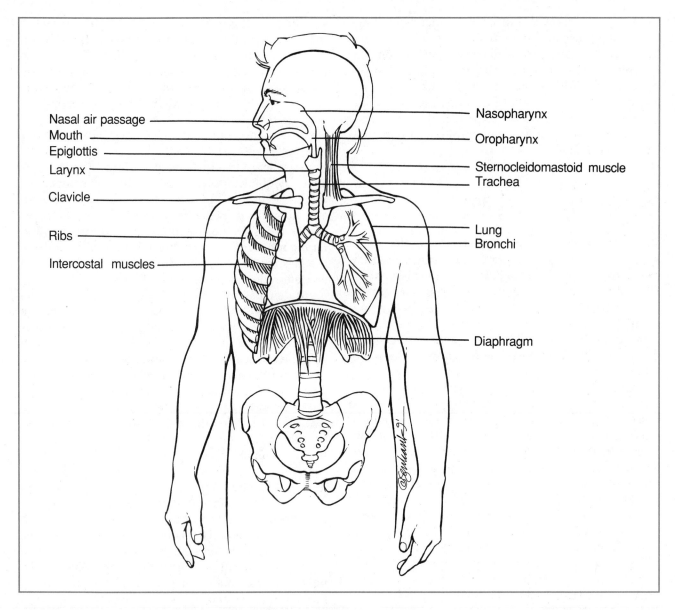

FIGURE 8-1. ANATOMY OF THE RESPIRATORY SYSTEM.

approximately 20 times until they become **bronchioles** and then respiratory bronchioles. The respiratory bronchioles lose their cartilaginous support and divide into alveolar ducts, which in turn pouch out into alveolar sacs. The **alveolus** is the terminal air space of the lung, where the business of gas exchange actually takes place.

Alveoli (Fig. 8-2) are very thin air sacs closely surrounded by tiny blood vessels (capillaries). The proximity of the capillaries to the alveolar wall is what makes gas exchange possible between the alveolar air and the blood. There are approximately 500 million alveoli in the lung, so their combined surface area is enormous, permitting a large volume of blood to participate in gas exchange at any given moment.

For gas exchange to occur, there has to be a way for "stale" blood to enter the lungs and for "refreshed" blood to leave. That is accomplished by the PULMONARY CIRCULATION (Fig. 8-3). Venous blood (blood low in oxygen) from the tissues reaches the lungs via the right heart (right atrium and right ventricle) and **pulmonary arteries.** The pulmonary arteries subdivide into many smaller arterioles. The arterioles in turn divide into **capillaries** surrounding the alveoli, where the blood gives up its excess carbon dioxide and takes up a fresh load of oxygen. The oxygen-enriched blood then passes from the alveolar capillaries into a system of **pulmonary veins,** which eventually join to form the two principal pulmonary veins that empty into the left atrium of the heart. The

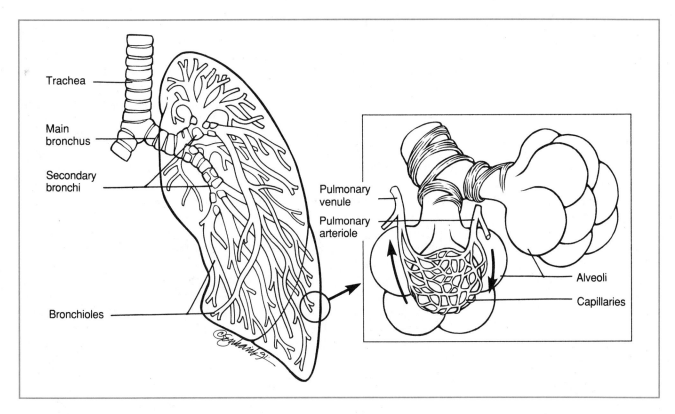

FIGURE 8-2. **THE ALVEOLUS** (*inset*) is the terminal air space in the lung, where gas exchange with the capillary blood takes place.

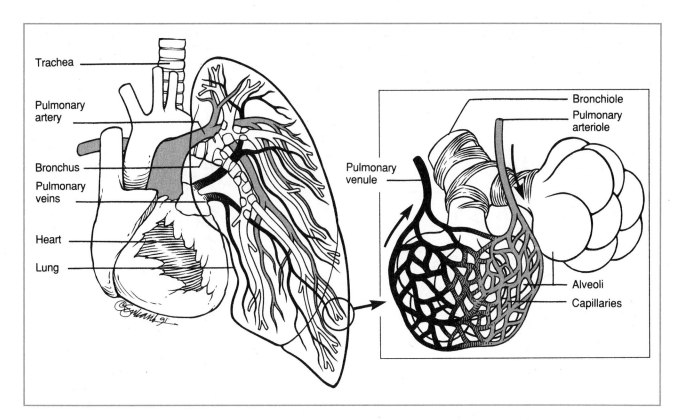

FIGURE 8-3. **THE PULMONARY CIRCULATION.** Pulmonary arteries bring oxygen-poor blood to the lungs from the right heart. Gas exchange takes place across capillary walls (*inset*). Pulmonary veins return oxygen-enriched blood from the lungs to the left heart.

freshly oxygenated blood is then pumped into the left ventricle of the heart and out into the systemic circulation.

The LUNGS, then, actually consist of airways and blood vessels. The lungs are suspended within the thoracic cavity (the chest cavity) by the trachea, arteries and veins, and pulmonary ligaments. Grossly, the lungs look like two cone-shaped structures with their bases resting on the diaphragm. The lungs are covered by a very thin, smooth layer of connective tissue called the **visceral pleura.** Another layer of pleura, the **parietal pleura,** lines the inside wall of the thoracic cavity. The space between the two pleural membranes, called the **pleural space,** is in fact not an actual space but only a potential space, since the visceral and parietal layers of the pleura are applied closely to one another, virtually sealed together by a thin layer of fluid that lubricates the lining membranes and permits free movement of the lungs within the chest. If air is introduced between the two layers of the pleura, however, as happens in some cases of trauma to the chest, the potential pleural space can become an actual one, a condition known as **pneumothorax.** Ordinarily, the pleural "space" has a negative (subatmospheric) pressure. Pneumotho-

rax decreases or abolishes that negative pressure, thereby permitting the lung to collapse.

Since the lungs do not have any muscular tissue, they cannot move by themselves, so their expansion and contraction to create air flow must be produced by other mechanisms. The moving force that activates the whole respiratory system is supplied by the RESPIRATORY MUSCLES. The principal muscle of respiration is the **diaphragm,** a powerful, dome-shaped muscle that forms the floor of the pleural cavity. Assisting the diaphragm are the muscles between the ribs, called the **intercostal muscles.**

The Mechanics of Breathing

Breathing is accomplished through pressure changes in the lungs, which in turn are brought about by contraction and relaxation of the respiratory muscles. INHALATION (Fig. 8-4A) is initiated by contraction of the respiratory muscles. As the *diaphragm* contracts, it descends and flattens out, thus increasing the vertical dimensions of the thorax. At the same time, the *intercostal muscles* contract, causing the ribs and sternum to move upward and outward and thereby in-

FIGURE 8-4. THE MECHANICS OF BREATHING.   (A) On *inhalation* the diaphragm descends, the ribs move up and outward, and the chest expands; pressure in the chest and lungs decreases, and air flows into the lungs. (B) On *exhalation,* the chest contracts passively, and air flows out of the lungs.

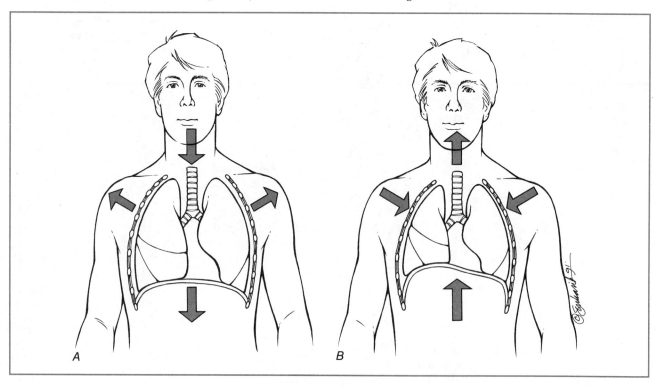

A   B

creasing the horizontal dimensions of the chest cavity. The net effect is to *increase the volume of the chest.* The lungs, being highly elastic and "glued" via the visceral pleura to the chest wall, undergo a comparable increase in volume. The air in the lungs now suddenly occupies a larger space, so the *pressure* within the lungs drops rapidly. Any gas will move from an area of higher pressure to an area of lower pressure. So as the air pressure inside the chest falls lower than that in the outside atmosphere, air begins to flow from the region of higher pressure (outside the body) to the region of lower pressure (the lungs). Air flow continues until the pressures inside and outside the lungs are equalized, at which point inhalation stops.

In contrast to inhalation, which is an active process requiring muscular contraction, EXHALATION (Fig. 8-4B) is a passive process. At the end of inhalation, the respiratory muscles relax, and the chest wall recoils; intrathoracic pressure rises, and air is expelled from the lungs.

A patient in respiratory *distress* may also deploy **accessory muscles,** such as muscles of the neck, to aid in breathing, and the contractions of those accessory muscles may be quite prominent during inhalation.

Measures of Respiratory Function

The RESPIRATORY RATE in the normal adult during quiet breathing is 14 to 18 per minute, with inhalation occupying approximately one-third of the respiratory cycle. In infants, the normal respiratory rate may be 40 to 60 per minute, while in children it is about 24 per minute. Many factors can influence the rate of breathing. Fever, anxiety, and insufficient oxygen *increase* the respiratory rate, while depressant drugs and sleep *decrease* the respiratory rate.

The TOTAL LUNG CAPACITY (the volume of gas contained in the lung at the end of a maximal inhalation) is about 6 liters (6,000 ml) in the adult. However, we breathe only a small portion of that total capacity. The normal TIDAL VOLUME, or volume of gas inhaled or exhaled during each respiratory cycle, is only about 500 ml for the adult man. Of that amount, about 150 ml remains in the upper air passages, where it is unavailable for gas exchange; that volume is called **dead space air,** because it is not available for gas exchange (it is in an inaccessible, or "dead" space). The remaining 350 ml of air, which *does* reach the alveoli and therefore does participate in gas exchange with the capillary blood, is called **alveolar air.**

A useful concept in evaluating the adequacy of a person's respirations is that of MINUTE VOLUME, the amount of gas that moves in and out of the lungs and air passages per minute. The minute volume is determined by the volume of each breath (tidal volume) and the number of breaths per minute (respiratory rate).

$$\text{MINUTE VOLUME} = \text{TIDAL VOLUME} \times \text{RESPIRATORY RATE}$$

Thus,

> Normal minute volume
> = normal tidal volume × normal respiratory rate
> = 500 ml/breath × 14 breaths/min
> = 7,000 ml/min [= 7 liters/min]

It is apparent from the equation that the minute volume will increase if *either* the tidal volume *or* the respiratory rate (or both) increases; similarly, the minute volume will decrease if either the tidal volume *or* the respiratory rate (or both) decreases. [Question: What will happen to the minute volume in a patient who has taken a heroin overdose and who is breathing only 6 times/min? What will happen to the minute volume in a patient with a cervical spine injury who is breathing at a normal rate but with a tidal volume of 300 ml/breath?]

Modified Forms of Respiration

COUGHING is a forceful exhalation produced with a greater than normal volume of breath. The abdominal muscles contract forcefully against a closed glottis, with a resulting increase in intrathoracic pressure. Then, as the vocal cords open, a gust of air is propelled past them with gale force, dislodging any foreign particles from the air passages and expelling them from the body. Coughing thus serves a crucial protective function, and it is the most effective means of expelling a foreign body that is partially obstructing the upper airway. The patient whose cough mechanism is suppressed—whether by drugs, by pain, by trauma, or by any other cause—is at serious risk of aspirating foreign material.

SNEEZING is also a sudden, forceful exhalation, but in this instance air is expelled through the nose rather than through the mouth. Sneezing is usually elicited by irritation of the nose.

HICCUPING (**singultus**) is a sudden *inhalation*, due to spasmodic contraction of the diaphragm, cut short by closure of the glottis. Hiccuping serves no useful physiologic purpose; it is usually harmless and self-limited, but sometimes it may signal the presence of serious illness.

SIGHING is a slow, deep inhalation followed by a prolonged and sometimes quite audible exhalation. In addition to expressing sorrow and unrequited love, sighing serves a valuable physiologic function by periodically hyperinflating the lungs, thereby reexpanding areas that might have become collapsed (**atelectatic**). Studies have shown that women sigh more often than men, but the significance of that finding is not clear.

EXCHANGE OF GASES IN THE LUNGS

The business of the alveoli is to supply oxygen to and remove carbon dioxide from the blood flowing past them. The blood coming from the tissues *to* the alveoli is relatively poor in oxygen, since oxygen has been consumed by the tissues in their metabolism. At the same time, the blood reaching the alveoli has an elevated level of carbon dioxide, for it is carrying away carbon dioxide that has been produced during tissue metabolism. By contrast, the air in the alveoli, drawn directly from the outside atmosphere, is much higher in oxygen and has scarcely any carbon dioxide. So essentially the task of the alveoli is to enable the blood to trade its "stale" air for a fresh supply. That process is shown in Figure 8-5.

The number of molecules of oxygen and carbon dioxide in the alveoli and capillaries is usually expressed in terms of their **partial pressures.** At sea level, the *total* gas pressure is equal to atmospheric pressure, or 760 mm Hg (760 *torr*). The *partial pressure* of any particular gas reflects its fractional concentration in the total gas mixture; and if you add up the partial pressures of all the gases present in a mixture, the sum must equal the total gas pressure (i.e., 760 torr at sea level).

In a person breathing room air—which contains 21% oxygen and 0.03% carbon dioxide—the partial pressure of oxygen (PO_2) in the alveoli will be about 140 to 150 torr, while the partial pressure of carbon dioxide (PCO_2) will be close to zero. The *venous* blood coming from the tissues through the right heart has a PO_2 of approximately 40 torr and a PCO_2 of about 46 torr. Gas diffuses from areas of higher partial pressure to areas of lower partial pressure. Therefore, oxygen will diffuse from the alveolar air into the pulmonary capillaries, while carbon dioxide will diffuse in the opposite direction—from the pulmonary capillaries into the alveoli. After exchange with the alveolar gases, the blood returning to the left heart (i.e., *arterial* blood) normally has a PO_2 of 80 to 100 torr and a PCO_2 of 35 to 40 torr (Fig. 8-6). The partial pressures of oxygen and carbon dioxide in the blood can be measured with an apparatus available in most hospitals, and those measurements are often referred to as "blood gases."

The alert reader will have noticed that the normal partial pressures of oxygen and of carbon dioxide do not add up to atmospheric pressure. Something is missing! What accounts for the rest of the partial

FIGURE 8-5. GAS EXCHANGE IN THE ALVEOLUS. Oxygen is taken up from the alveolus while carbon dioxide is released into the alveolus.

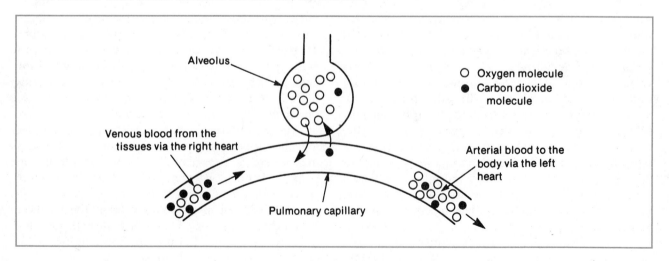

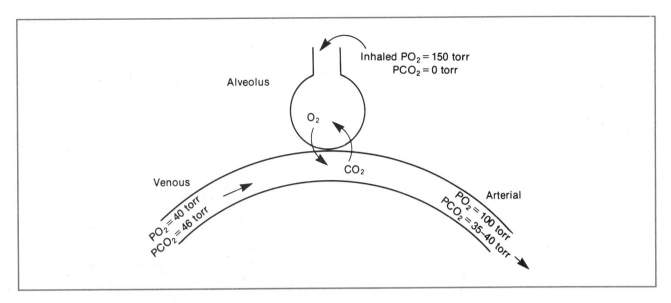

FIGURE 8-6.   PARTIAL PRESSURE OF GASES IN THE ALVEOLI AND CAPILLARIES.   Venous blood (PO_2 = 40 torr) is oxygenated as it passes the alveolus, yielding arterial blood (PO_2 = 100 torr).

pressure, in fact, is NITROGEN, which constitutes about 79 percent of the air we breathe. Nitrogen has no metabolic function, but it helps maintain the inflation of those body cavities that are filled with gas.

In summary, then, oxygen continuously diffuses from the alveoli into the pulmonary capillary blood, while carbon dioxide diffuses from the pulmonary capillary blood into the alveoli. During inhalation, the oxygen that has been absorbed from the alveoli is replenished, and during exhalation, the carbon dioxide that has accumulated in the alveoli is blown out.

Factors Influencing Carbon Dioxide in the Blood

The PCO_2 measured in the arterial blood represents a balance between the CARBON DIOXIDE PRODUCED in metabolism and the CARBON DIOXIDE ELIMINATED in ventilation. The amount of CO_2 *produced* is normally relatively constant and is determined by the rate and type of metabolism. As the metabolic *rate* goes up, as in fever, more CO_2 is produced; as the metabolic rate falls, as in a hibernating bear in winter, the production of CO_2 falls as well. The *type* of metabolism also influences CO_2 production. Any metabolic process that results in the formation of acids will increase the amount of CO_2 in the blood. Thus, the presence of excess *lactic acid* in the blood (which results from metabolism in the absence of sufficient oxygen) or excess *ketoacids* in the blood (which result from metabolism in the absence

of sufficient insulin) will increase the circulating levels of carbon dioxide. That is because acids liberate hydrogen ions and, as we shall learn in Chapter 9, thereby drive the bicarbonate buffer equation to the left in order to rebalance the system:

$$H_2O + CO_2 \leftarrow H_2CO_3 \leftarrow HCO_3^- + \boxed{H^+}$$

Thus, whenever we add acid to the body, we increase the amount of carbon dioxide that dissociates from carbonic acid (H_2CO_3). Paradoxically, the same is true, at least transiently, if we add the buffer bicarbonate (HCO_3^-) to the body:

$$H_2O + CO_2 \leftarrow H_2CO_3 \leftarrow \boxed{HCO_3^-} + H^+$$

What that means, practically speaking, is that whenever you administer sodium bicarbonate to a nonbreathing patient—as, for example, in some cases of prolonged cardiopulmonary resuscitation—it is necessary to increase the patient's ventilations in order to blow off the excess carbon dioxide thereby produced.

So far, we have looked at the CO_2 production side of the equation and have seen that CO_2 will increase whenever the metabolic rate or the level of acid in the blood increases. The other side of the picture is CO_2 *elimination*. Clearly, if the body simply kept producing CO_2 and had no way to get rid of it, the levels of CO_2 in the blood would keep rising indefinitely. Fortunately, the body *does* have a way to get rid of CO_2—

by blowing it out through the lungs. The larger the volume of air that moves in and out of the lungs, the more CO_2 that is eliminated. That is to say, *carbon dioxide elimination is directly proportional to minute volume*. Recall that

$$\text{MINUTE VOLUME} = \text{TIDAL VOLUME} \times \text{RESPIRATORY RATE}$$

Thus there are two ways one can increase the elimination of carbon dioxide from the body:

- One can take *deeper breaths* (increase the tidal volume)
- One can *breathe faster* (increase the respiratory rate)—or both

That is precisely what the normal body does when the level of CO_2 in the blood rises. If you run to catch a bus, for instance, the increased muscle metabolism required by that exertion dumps more CO_2 into the blood. As the level of CO_2 in your blood rises, you will feel "out of breath," because your normal minute volume is no longer sufficient to get rid of that increased amount of CO_2. So you will automatically start breathing more deeply and faster, to blow off the excess CO_2 from your blood.

The two factors determining arterial PCO_2, then, are CO_2 production and CO_2 elimination. When those two are in balance, the arterial PCO_2 is about 40 torr, as shown schematically in Figure 8-7.

If CO_2 production exceeds the body's ability to eliminate CO_2 in breathing, the PCO_2 rises. That condition, by definition, is **hypoventilation.** Theoretically, hypoventilation can occur in two ways: CO_2 production can increase beyond the body's ability to

blow it off; or CO_2 elimination can be depressed to the extent that it no longer keeps up with normal metabolism. In fact, hypoventilation is nearly always due to *decreased CO_2 elimination*, which means decreased minute volume. Looking once again at our equation:

$$\text{MINUTE VOLUME} = \text{TIDAL VOLUME} \times \text{RESPIRATORY RATE}$$

we see that anything that decreases either the depth of breathing or the rate of breathing will decrease the minute volume and thus decrease the elimination of CO_2. What kinds of problems are we talking about? Let us consider, for instance, an injury to the cervical spine that results in paralysis of the intercostal muscles. A person with that type of injury cannot expand his chest fully, so the *volume* of each breath (tidal volume) is reduced. That leads to reduction of the minute volume, which in turns means that less CO_2 is eliminated from the body. The net effect is an increase in arterial CO_2 (**hypercarbia**). Now let us consider the second element in the equation, the respiratory *rate*. A person who has taken an overdose of narcotics may have a very slow respiratory rate—sometimes as low as 4 breaths per minute instead of the normal 14 to 18 per minute. Looking at our equation, it is clear that a decrease in respiratory rate will also lead to a decrease in minute volume, and once again the net effect is the accumulation of CO_2 in the blood. The mechanism of hypoventilation is shown schematically in Figure 8-8.

At the other extreme is a state called **hyperventilation,** which occurs when elimination of CO_2 *exceeds* CO_2 production. If, for example, while you are sitting quietly, reading a book, you start breathing very deeply and very fast (i.e., you increase your

FIGURE 8-7.   CARBON DIOXIDE EQUILIBRIUM. Under normal circumstances, CO_2 production and elimination are in balance.

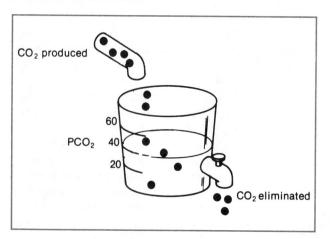

FIGURE 8-8.   HYPOVENTILATION. When carbon dioxide elimination is reduced, CO_2 accumulates in the blood.

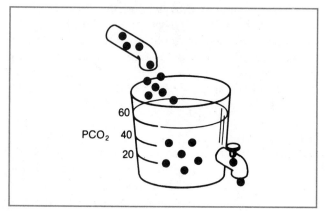

minute volume), you will blow off CO_2 at a rate faster than your body is producing it. The level of CO_2 in your blood will thus fall below normal, and you will start to feel rather dizzy and develop other symptoms besides (see Chap. 22). The mechanism of hyperventilation is shown schematically in Figure 8-9.

To sum up, the level of CO_2 in the blood is determined by the balance between CO_2 production (metabolism) and CO_2 elimination (breathing). Given a steady rate of CO_2 production:

> **CARBON DIOXIDE ELIMINATION IS DIRECTLY PROPORTIONAL TO MINUTE VOLUME.**

FIGURE 8-9. HYPERVENTILATION. When carbon dioxide elimination is increased, the level of CO_2 in the blood falls.

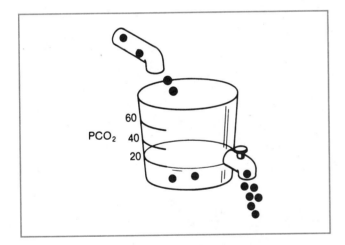

Decrease the minute volume, and you decrease CO_2 elimination, so CO_2 builds up in the blood (hypercarbia). Increase the minute volume, and you increase carbon dioxide elimination, so the level of CO_2 in the blood falls. Those concepts are summarized in Table 8-1.

Factors Influencing Oxygen in the Blood

In the normal alveolus/capillary unit, blood is fully oxygenated in the course of its transit past the alveolus (Fig. 8-10). However, there are several situations in which the blood may *not* become adequately oxygenated during its passage through the lungs.

For example, FLUID may occupy the alveoli (Fig. 8-11) and prevent air exchange. That situation is called **pulmonary edema**, and it may come about as a consequence of heart failure, drowning, or toxic inhalations. Fluid in the alveoli increases the distance that O_2 must diffuse to get from the alveolar space to the pulmonary capillary, so the amount of O_2 reaching the capillary blood is decreased.

Alveoli may also COLLAPSE (**atelectasis;** Fig. 8-12), either from external forces, such as the pressure from a pneumothorax, or internal causes, such as secretions plugging the airways or depressed coughing and sighing mechanisms. Blood that passes by collapsed alveoli will not pick up any oxygen, so the arterial blood as a whole will be less than fully oxygenated.

When alveoli are either filled with fluid or collapsed, we call the resulting situation **shunt** because a portion of the blood from the right heart never picks up oxygen and thus behaves as if it had been shunted past the lungs altogether. When doctors say that a patient "has a big shunt," therefore, what they

TABLE 8-1. CARBON DIOXIDE BALANCE

	HYPOVENTILATION	HYPERVENTILATION
Minute volume	↓	↑
CO_2 elimination	↓	↑
Arterial PCO_2	↑ (*hyper*carbia)	↓ (*hypo*carbia)
Resulting condition	Respiratory acidosis	Respiratory alkalosis
Treatment	Increase the patient's rate and depth of respirations (assisted or controlled ventilation with bag-valve-mask)	Coach the patient to slow his breathing; reassurance and explanation

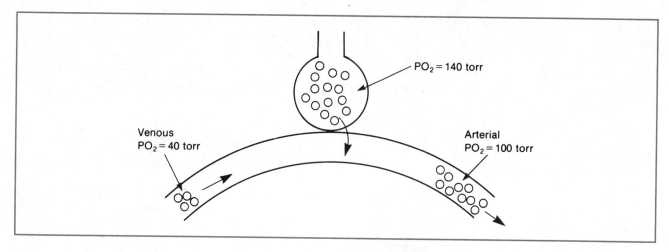

FIGURE 8-10.   OXYGENATION OF BLOOD IN THE LUNGS.   In the normal alveolus/
capillary unit, blood is fully oxygenated in its transit past the alveolus.

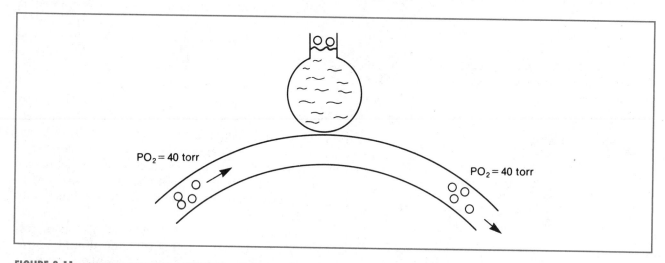

FIGURE 8-11.   FLUID IN THE ALVEOLI.   When fluid occupies an alveolus,
blood passing by it cannot be oxygenated.

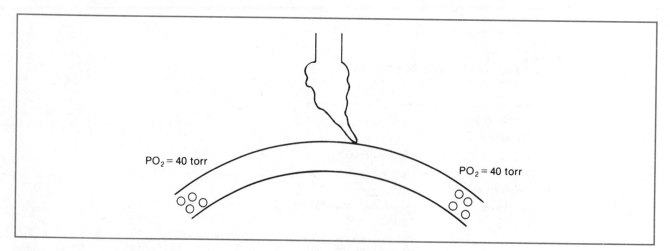

FIGURE 8-12.   COLLAPSED ALVEOLI.   When an alveolus is collapsed, blood
passing by it cannot be oxygenated.

mean is that a substantial proportion of the patient's blood passed through the lungs without becoming oxygenated. Shunt, then, is invariably associated with a decreased PO_2. When the arterial PO_2 falls below about 60 torr, we say that the patient has **hypoxemia** (*hypo-* + *oxy-* + *-emia*).

We attempt to overcome a patient's shunt, at least in part, by supplying a higher oxygen concentration to those alveoli that *are* still functioning, that is, by giving the patient supplemental oxygen to breathe (Fig. 8-13). Intermittent positive pressure ventilation, or IPPV for short (e.g., with a demand valve), may also be useful in such circumstances. In pulmonary edema, for instance, IPPV creates a driving pressure to force fluid out of the alveolar spaces; in atelectasis, IPPV may pop open collapsed alveoli.

It is clear, then, that

> **THE AMOUNT OF OXYGEN IN THE BLOOD IS DIRECTLY PROPORTIONAL TO THE AMOUNT OF OXYGEN DELIVERED TO THE ALVEOLI.**

If we want to increase the amount of oxygen in the blood, we have to increase the concentration of oxygen in the alveoli, and the only way to do that is to give the patient a higher concentration of oxygen than that normally present in ambient air.

REGULATION OF VENTILATION

While we are able to exert considerable voluntary control over breathing—for example in talking, sighing, and breath-holding—respiratory movements are primarily *involuntary*. (Imagine what life would be like if you had to think about each breath!) The rate and depth of breathing are controlled mainly by a RESPIRATORY CENTER located in the brainstem. The object of the respiratory control mechanisms is to regulate arterial PO_2, PCO_2, and pH within very narrow limits.

Any *rise* in arterial PCO_2 above about 40 torr or *fall* in the pH (i.e., increase in acidity of the blood) stimulates chemoreceptors in the respiratory center of the brain. The respiratory center responds by sending messages to the respiratory muscles to increase the rate and depth of respiration (i.e., increase

FIGURE 8-13.   EFFECT OF INHALING ENRICHED OXYGEN MIXTURES. By increasing the concentration of oxygen in those alveoli that *are* functioning, one can increase the net concentration of oxygen in the blood returning to the left heart.

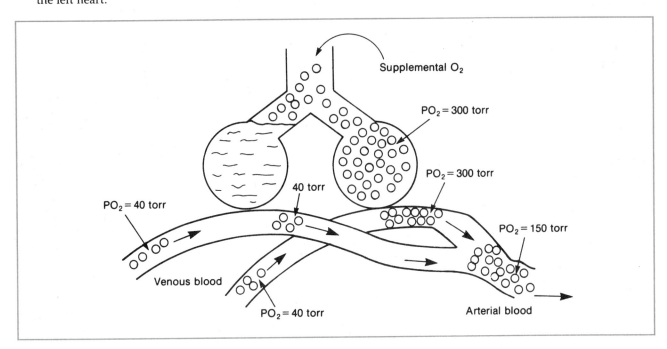

the minute volume); in that way, the excess CO_2 is blown off.

Under normal circumstances, those fluctuations in PCO_2 and pH are the dominant influence on respiration, and the RESPIRATORY DRIVE derives from the body's attempt to regulate the PCO_2 around normal levels. However, as we shall discuss in greater detail in Chapter 22, there are some patients with chronic respiratory diseases who are unable to eliminate CO_2 normally and whose respiratory centers have gradually accommodated to high PCO_2 levels. What, then, stimulates those individuals to breathe?

We used to assume that in patients with hypercarbia another control center became ascendant. Receptors located in the aorta and carotid arteries are sensitive to *decreases in PO_2*. When the arterial oxygen tension falls below 60 torr, those centers are activated and in turn activate the respiratory muscles to increase their activity, so the minute volume is increased. It was assumed that patients with chronic hypercarbia operated on that **hypoxic drive**; that is, that their primary stimulus to breathe came about from a fall in PO_2 rather than a rise in PCO_2. For that reason, there was reluctance to administer oxygen to such patients, lest it suppress the drive to breathe. Recent studies, however, have called the whole matter into question, as we shall discuss in more detail in Chapter 22.

HYPOXEMIA: PATIENTS WHO NEED OXYGEN

Oxygen is a colorless, odorless gas present in the atmosphere in a concentration of approximately 21%. For healthy individuals, that concentration of inhaled oxygen is more than adequate to supply the oxygen needs of all the cells in the body. Patients who are ill or injured, however, may require higher concentrations of inhaled oxygen to maintain their blood levels of oxygen in a range compatible with life.

Probably the most obvious candidates for oxygen therapy are patients whose lungs, for one reason or another, are not performing their task of gas exchange efficiently. We saw earlier, for example, that if a person's alveoli become filled with *fluid*, red blood cells circulating past those alveoli will not find any oxygen there; those red blood cells will leave the lungs empty-handed, so to speak. That is the situation in PULMONARY EDEMA (plasma in the alveoli), PNEUMONIA (pus in the alveoli), and some cases of CHEST TRAUMA (blood in the alveoli). Red blood cells circulating past the nonfunctional alveoli will not find any oxygen to carry back to the tissues. Basically the same thing will happen to red blood

cells passing by *collapsed* alveoli; they too will leave the lung empty-handed. Alveoli are likely to collapse (i.e., *atelectasis* is likely to occur) any time there is partial or complete AIRWAY OBSTRUCTION. Atelectasis is also likely under any circumstances in which a patient fails to take deep enough breaths to keep his alveoli open—for example, because of PAIN (as in rib fractures); PARALYSIS of the respiratory muscles (as in spinal cord injury); or DEPRESSION OF THE RESPIRATORY CENTER (as in head injury or drug overdose). Needless to say, if the whole lung collapses, as in PNEUMOTHORAX, alveolar collapse will be particularly widespread.

All of the conditions mentioned so far are examples of *shunt*—blood leaving the lungs without being oxygenated. Shunt can also occur if OTHER GASES OCCUPY THE ALVEOLI, as in inhalation of smoke or toxic fumes.

The most extreme form of shunt, of course, is RESPIRATORY ARREST. The moment a person stops breathing, the oxygen remaining in his alveoli is rapidly depleted. Even if circulation continues, the blood flowing past the alveoli finds nothing there to take home to the tissues. So tissue oxygen is also rapidly depleted. If at that point a rescuer arrives on the scene and starts artificial ventilation with ambient air, the oxygen-starved tissues will consume whatever oxygen the rescuer can provide.

As we saw in Figure 8-13, the only way to compensate for a significant shunt is to furnish a high concentration of oxygen to those alveoli that *are* functional, which means providing the patient as a whole with oxygen in higher concentrations than are found in the ambient air.

Another class of patients who need oxygen very urgently are those undergoing cardiopulmonary resuscitation (CPR) for CARDIAC ARREST. As we shall see in the next chapter, even perfectly performed CPR produces a blood flow only 25 to 30 percent of normal; that is, red blood cells are plodding through the pulmonary circulation at only one-third to one-fourth their usual rate. At the same time, the peripheral tissues still have the same (if not increased) need for oxygen, so the peripheral tissues are not at all happy about the slowdown in the circulation. If, however, a given volume of blood could carry *more* oxygen on each trip out to the periphery (which it could, if it had access to a higher concentration in the alveoli), the net supply of oxygen per minute would increase even though blood flow remained severely compromised. That is why patients undergoing CPR for cardiac arrest need oxygen.

Cardiac arrest is one example—indeed, the most extreme example—of a larger category of disorders known as SHOCK. Shock occurs whenever there is a failure of tissue perfusion. And, for the same reasons mentioned in connection with cardiac arrest, patients with shock need oxygen.

In many cases, the patient himself will tell us—either in words or in clinical signs and symptoms—that he needs oxygen. When, for whatever reason, not enough oxygen is reaching a person's tissues, his body responds with characteristic signs and symptoms of acute respiratory insufficiency:

SIGNS AND SYMPTOMS OF RESPIRATORY INSUFFICIENCY

- A *feeling* of shortness of breath (**dyspnea**)
- Rapid breathing (**tachypnea**)
- Very deep breathing (**hyperpnea**)
- Use of accessory muscles in the neck and abdomen to assist respirations
- Flaring of the nostrils on inhalation
- Bluish tinge to the lips and nail beds (**cyanosis**)
- If the respiratory center is depressed, SLOW, SHALLOW RESPIRATIONS

A patient showing any of those symptoms or signs is telling us that he NEEDS OXYGEN, so the very *first* thing to do in such circumstances is to *give* him oxygen—and ask questions afterward.

Up to now, we've considered patients whose total body supply of oxygen is compromised—patients with impaired or even absent pulmonary function, patients whose circulatory systems are not moving blood effectively around the body, patients showing clear signs of respiratory distress. But what about patients with perfectly normal lungs who do not show any signs of respiratory distress whatsoever? Are there circumstances in which patients in that category might need oxygen?

The answer is yes.

There are some conditions in which a *part* of the patient's body is not getting enough oxygen, even though the oxygen supply to the body as a whole is entirely adequate. That is the case, for example, in a patient suffering a HEART ATTACK (**acute myocardial infarction**). The basic pathologic process in acute myocardial infarction is narrowing of the coronary arteries. At a certain point, the lumen of a coronary artery may become so narrow that the blood flow through it is reduced to a trickle. At that point, the segment of heart muscle (myocardium) supplied by the blocked artery will experience a lack of oxygen (hypoxia), *even though the rest of the body is well oxygenated*. The only way to try to relieve that localized hy-poxia is to increase the oxygen supply to the whole body, so that those red blood cells that do squeeze through the narrowed coronary artery will be able to deliver a larger oxygen load to the beleaguered segment of myocardium.

Very much the same mechanism is at work in STROKE, except that in stroke it is a part of the *brain* rather than a part of the heart that has become relatively deprived of oxygen. Once again, the only way to improve oxygenation of the threatened section of the brain is to increase oxygenation of the whole body.

We shall learn about these conditions in much more detail as we progress through this textbook. What is important to remember here is that a very considerable proportion of seriously ill and injured patients need oxygen (Table 8-2)—*even when they appear to be breathing normally.* Oxygen is one of the most powerful drugs for saving lives that you will carry in your ambulance. Don't be afraid to use it!

TABLE 8-2. PATIENTS WHO NEED OXYGEN

- Any patients likely to have significant SHUNT from
  1. FLUID IN THE ALVEOLI
     a. Pulmonary edema
     b. Pneumonia
     c. Near drowning
     d. Chest trauma
  2. COLLAPSED ALVEOLI (atelectasis)
     a. Airway obstruction
        (1) Any unconscious patient
        (2) Choking
     b. Failure to take deep breaths
        (1) Pain (rib fracture)
        (2) Paralysis of the respiratory muscles (spine injury)
        (3) Depression of the respiratory center (head injury, drug overdose)
     c. Collapse of an entire lung (pneumothorax)
  3. OTHER GASES IN THE ALVEOLI
     a. Smoke inhalation
     b. Toxic inhalations
     c. Carbon monoxide poisoning
  4. RESPIRATORY ARREST
- Any patient in CARDIAC ARREST
- Any patient in SHOCK
- Any patient complaining of SHORTNESS OF BREATH
- Any patient with SIGNS OF RESPIRATORY INSUFFICIENCY
- Any patient BREATHING FEWER THAN 10 TIMES PER MINUTE
- Any patient complaining of CHEST PAIN
- Any patient suspected to be suffering a STROKE

WHEN IN DOUBT, GIVE OXYGEN.

IMPROVING A PATIENT'S OXYGENATION

When a patient needs oxygen, the paramedic's first priority is to provide that oxygen quickly. To do so, you need to be completely familiar with all of the equipment and procedures of oxygen administration.

Oxygen Cylinders

Pure or 100% oxygen is obtained commercially by fractional distillation, in which air is liquefied and the gases other than oxygen (mostly nitrogen) are boiled off. Liquid oxygen is then converted under high pressure to a gaseous state and stored in steel cylinders (Fig. 8-14) under pressure of about 2,000 pounds per square inch (**psi**). Clearly 2,000 psi is far too much pressure to deliver directly into a patient's airway, unless the objective is to blow the patient away altogether. Therefore gas flow from an oxygen cylinder is controlled by a pressure regulator (**reducing valve**) that—as the name implies—reduces the high pressure of gas in the cylinder to a safe range (about 50 psi). A second regulator, the **flow meter,** is attached in series after the reducing valve and controls the flow of oxygen across a range of about 1 to 15 liters per minute. Both the reducing valve and the flow me-

ter attach to the oxygen cylinder by a **yoke.** Each yoke is designed so that its pins or threading will fit only the cylinders for one type of gas (e.g., oxygen or helium). In addition, all gas cylinders are color-coded according to their contents. Oxygen cylinders are color-coded *green* in the United States (which is why anesthesiologists sometimes refer to oxygen as the "green gas" even though oxygen is, in fact, colorless). Both the color coding of cylinders and the specificity of the yokes are safety precautions, to prevent accidental administration of the wrong gas to a patient.

Some regulator valve units are also fitted with a **humidifier** jar—basically a small bottle of water through which the oxygen leaving the cylinder is bubbled before it reaches the patient. The rationale behind the device is sound enough: Oxygen stored in cylinders has zero humidity. It is not a good idea to deliver dry gases to a patient's airway, for gases entirely devoid of moisture will rapidly dry up the patient's mucous membranes—an undesirable effect. So it is logical to try to humidify the oxygen before it reaches the patient. The problem is that bubble humidifiers of the type shown in Figure 8-14 add scarcely any moisture to the inhaled oxygen, but meanwhile they often become sources of bacterial contamination. Bubble humidifiers are also a bit of a nuisance in emergency work, since they have to be kept upright; so they are practical only for the fixed oxygen unit in the ambulance, not for the portable cylinders you carry to the patient. No harm would be done, therefore, if bubble humidifiers were eliminated altogether from prehospital emergency care.

FIGURE 8-14.   OXYGEN DELIVERY SYSTEM.

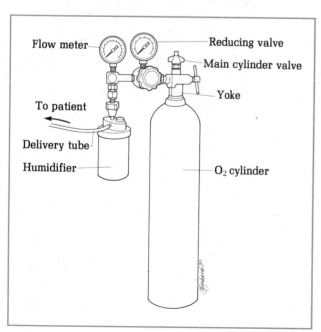

Flow meter — Reducing valve — Main cylinder valve — Yoke — To patient — Delivery tube — Humidifier — O₂ cylinder

Calculating How Long an Oxygen Cylinder Will Last

Oxygen cylinders are given letter designations according to their size; for example, an E cylinder is 4.5 inches in diameter by 30 inches high, a G cylinder is 8.5 inches by 55 inches, and so forth. If you know the size of your cylinder and the reading on the pressure gauge, you can calculate how much longer the supply of oxygen in your cylinder is going to last—a critical bit of information, since it is very poor form to run out of oxygen in the middle of a call.

Since it's not desirable to wait until a cylinder is completely empty, which would invariably happen at the most inconvenient moment, it is customary to replace an oxygen cylinder with a fresh one when the pressure falls to **200 psi.** That level is called the **safe residual,** and the term implies that it is therefore *un*safe to continue using an oxygen cylinder whose pressure is less than 200 psi. The question is, how can you tell how much oxygen you have left in the cylinder when the pressure reading is *above* the safe residual of 200 psi. The calculation is made as follows:

CALCULATING HOW LONG THE OXYGEN WILL LAST

$$\text{Duration of flow} = \frac{(\text{gauge pressure} - 200 \text{ psi}) \times C}{\text{flow rate (L/min)}}$$

where C = the cylinder constant

Cylinder Constants:
D cylinder = 0.16 L/psi
E cylinder = 0.28 L/psi
G cylinder = 2.41 L/psi
M cylinder = 1.56 L/psi

A glance at the above equation confirms what is already intuitively obvious: The higher the pressure inside the cylinder, the more oxygen is left; and the faster we run that oxygen (the higher the flow rate), the quicker it will be depleted. Let us take an example: You are doing CPR by the side of the road. You are ventilating the patient with a pocket mask, into which you are running 10 liters per minute of oxygen from a portable E cylinder. The pressure gauge on the E cylinder reads 1,200 psi. How long can you continue before the pressure reaches the safe residual and you have to go back to the ambulance for a fresh oxygen cylinder? To find out, you need to plug the numbers into the equation we just learned:

$$\text{Duration of flow} = \frac{(\text{gauge pressure} - 200 \text{ psi}) \times C}{\text{flow rate (L/min)}}$$

$$= \frac{(1{,}200 \text{ psi} - 200 \text{ psi}) \times 0.28 \text{ L/psi}}{10 \text{ L/min}}$$

$$= \frac{280 \text{ L}}{10 \text{ L/min}}$$

$$= 28 \text{ minutes}$$

Thus even though the reading on your pressure gauge looks pretty good, the cylinder isn't going to last very long because it isn't very large and it is being emptied at a rapid rate. [For practice, calculate how much longer your oxygen supply would last if you were using the M cylinder in the ambulance instead of a portable E cylinder, at the same flow rate and pressure gauge reading.]

It should be routine procedure at the beginning of every shift to open the main cylinder valve on the vehicle's oxygen supply and check the pressure remaining in the cylinder. The pressure gauges on all portable cylinders should be checked after every call in which oxygen was used. It is extraordinarily discouraging, not to mention negligent, to arrive with lights and sirens and other fanfare at the scene of a gasping patient only to discover that your oxygen cylinder is empty. So check your cylinders often and replace them when the pressure is at 200 psi or below. Always carry a backup cylinder in the vehicle; you may not have a chance to return to base for a fresh cylinder after that big cardiac arrest call.

Safety Precautions in Handling Oxygen Cylinders

Any cylinder containing compressed gas under high pressure has a potential, under the right conditions (actually, the *wrong* conditions!), to assume the properties of a rocket. A cylinder containing compressed *oxygen*, furthermore, presents the additional hazard of fire, for oxygen supports combustion. Therefore a variety of safety precautions are necessary in handling oxygen cylinders:

- KEEP COMBUSTIBLE MATERIALS, such as oil or grease, AWAY from contact with the cylinder itself, the regulators, fittings, valves, or tubing.
- DO NOT PERMIT SMOKING in any area where oxygen cylinders are in use or on standby.
- Store oxygen cylinders in a COOL, WELL-VENTILATED AREA. Do not subject the cylinders to temperatures above 125°F (approximately 50°C).
- USE an oyxgen cylinder ONLY WITH A SAFE, PROPERLY FITTING REGULATOR VALVE. Regulator valves for one gas should never be modified for use with another gas.
- CLOSE ALL VALVES when the cylinder is not in use, even if the tank is empty.
- SECURE CYLINDERS SO THEY WILL NOT TOPPLE OVER. In transit, they should be in a proper carrier or rack, or strapped onto the stretcher with the patient.
- When working with an oxygen cylinder, always position yourself to its side. NEVER PLACE ANY PART OF YOUR BODY OVER THE CYLINDER VALVE! A loosely fitting regulator can be blown off the cylinder with sufficient force to amputate a head or demolish any object in its path.
- HAVE THE CYLINDER TESTED EVERY 10 YEARS, to make sure it can still sustain the high pressures required. The original test date is stamped onto the cylinder together with its serial number.

Operating the Oxygen Cylinder

With the preceding precautions in mind, the procedure for initiating oxygen administration is as follows:

- Place the **cylinder** securely **upright,** and position yourself to the side.
- **"Crack" the tank** with the wrench supplied; that is, slowly open and rapidly close the main cylinder valve to clean it of dust.
- **Inspect the regulator valve** (reducing valve) to be certain it is the right type for an oxygen cylinder and that it has an intact washer.
- **Apply the regulator valve,** and tighten it securely to the yoke.
- **Open the main cylinder valve** slowly to about one-half turn beyond the point where the regulator valve becomes pressurized.
- **Open the flow control valve** to the desired liter flow.
- When you are ready **to stop** giving oxygen (e.g., when the patient has been transferred to the oxygen supply in the emergency room), **shut off the flow control** valve until the liter flow is at zero.
- **Shut off the main cylinder valve.**
- **Bleed the valves** by opening the flow control valve and leaving it open until the needle or ball indicator returns to zero flow.
- **Shut the flow control valve.**

Devices for Giving Oxygen to Patients Who Are Breathing Spontaneously

There are a variety of cannulas and masks available to provide supplemental oxygen to patients who are breathing on their own, and the paramedic needs to be familiar with the general characteristics of those devices (Table 8-3).

Nasal Catheter

The nasal catheter (Fig. 8-15A) is a soft rubber or plastic tube with many holes at the end—somewhat resembling a flexible suction catheter. At a flow rate of 6 to 8 liters per minute, the nasal catheter can deliver concentrations of oxygen of 30 to 50%; higher flows will cause irritation of the nasal and pharyngeal mucosa without delivering a higher concentration of oxygen to the alveoli. The nasal catheter should *not* be used in comatose, debilitated, or elderly patients, for such patients are apt to have impaired reflexes and therefore may not be able to prevent large amounts of gas from flowing into the stomach; the consequence in such patients can be severe gastric distention and regurgitation.

The nasal catheter is inserted as follows:

- **Explain** the procedure to the patient.
- **Measure** the distance from the tip of the patient's nose to his ear lobe, and mark that distance off on the catheter.

TABLE 8-3.   OXYGEN DELIVERY SYSTEMS

DEVICE	FLOW RATE USED (L/MIN)	% O$_2$ DELIVERED	COMMENT
Nasal catheter	6–8	30–50	Do not use in comatose patient
Nasal cannula	4–6	25–40	Usually well tolerated
Plastic face mask	8–12	50–60	
Venturi mask			Useful in long-term treatment of patients with COPD; limited value in the field
24%	4	24	
28%	4	28	
35%	8	35	
40%	8	40	
Partial rebreathing mask	6–10	35–60	
Nonrebreathing mask	10–12	90	Permits administration of high oxygen concentration

COPD = chronic obstructive pulmonary disease.

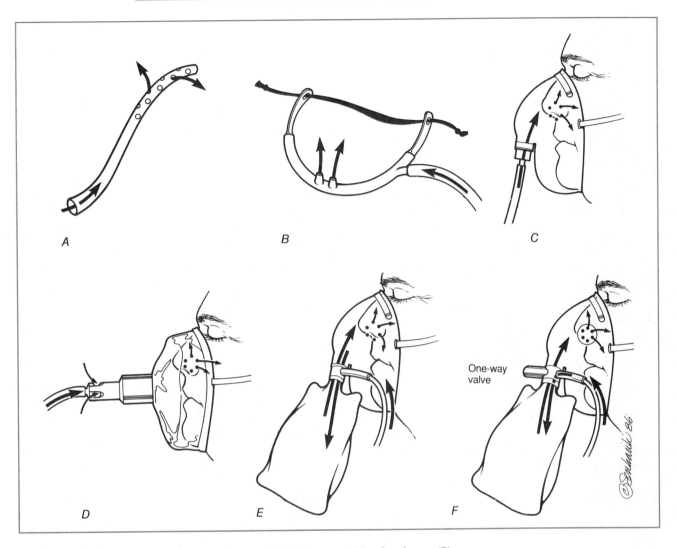

FIGURE 8-15.   OXYGEN ADMINISTRATION DEVICES.   (A) Nasal catheter. (B) Two-pronged nasal cannula. (C) Simple face mask. (D) Venturi mask. (E) Partial rebreathing mask. (F) Nonrebreathing mask.

- **Lubricate** the end of **the catheter** with a water-soluble jelly.
- Gently **insert the catheter** into one nostril until the tip is visible in the oropharynx, just behind the uvula. If you encounter resistance, try the other nostril.
- **Withdraw the catheter slightly** just until the tip is no longer visible in the back of the throat.
- **Tape the catheter** securely to the patient's nose and cheek, so that it cannot slip farther down the throat.
- **Open the oxygen flow** control valve, and adjust the flow to the desired setting (around 6 liters/min).

Do not advance the catheter beyond the point you marked on it. If it is advanced too far, the catheter may enter the esophagus and literally inflate the stomach.

Because of its potential to produce gastric distention, the nasal catheter is of limited usefulness in the field. There is, however, one quite effective—even though rather unusual—use for the nasal catheter that justifies stashing a couple in your jump kit: to provide the patient with supplementary oxygen during mouth-to-mouth ventilation. What makes use of the catheter unusual in those circumstances is the fact that the rescuer inserts the catheter into his *own* nose, not the patient's! By doing so, the rescuer can fill his own airway with a moderately high oxygen concentration; then, when the rescuer exhales into the patient's lungs, he can deliver up to about 40% oxygen rather than the 16 to 18% normally present in exhaled air.

Two-Pronged Nasal Cannula

The two-pronged nasal cannula (Fig. 8-15B) is much to be preferred over the nasal catheter when only moderate concentrations of oxygen are required. The nasal cannula is devised from a semicircle of plastic tubing with two plastic tips that insert into the nostrils. It will deliver an oxygen concentration of 25 to 40% with a 4- to 6-liter flow. Higher flow rates will only irritate the nasal mucosa without increasing the delivered oxygen concentration.

The nasal cannula is usually well tolerated, but it can cause some soreness around the nostrils, and the maximum oxygen concentration it will deliver is limited. For that reason,

> **THE TWO-PRONGED NASAL CANNULA IS THE PREFERRED MEANS OF DELIVERING OXYGEN TO A SPONTANEOUSLY BREATHING PATIENT WHEN ONLY MODERATE CONCENTRATIONS OF OXYGEN ARE REQUIRED.**

Uncomplicated myocardial infarction, for example, is an ideal situation in which to use the nasal cannula.

Simple Plastic Face Mask

The simple plastic face mask (Fig. 8-15C) can deliver up to 60% oxygen, depending on the oxygen flow rate and the patient's tidal volume. Exhaled air is vented through holes on each side of the mask. At low oxygen flow rates and high tidal volumes, the patient may also draw *in* room air through the side holes, which will dilute the concentration of oxygen that reaches his airway. Therefore the simple plastic face mask should be used with a flow rate of 8 to 12 liters per minute, to ensure adequate oxygen delivery. Even so, the simple face mask can deliver oxygen concentrations only slightly higher than those delivered by the nasal cannula. And many patients tend to feel "suffocated" when a plastic mask is clamped over their nose and mouth. So on the whole, the simple face mask offers no advantages over the nasal cannula.

Venturi Mask

The Venturi mask (Fig. 8-15D) is designed to drag specific volumes of room air into the mask along with the oxygen flow; the mixture of precisely known proportions of air and oxygen permits delivery of accu-

rate, *low* oxygen concentrations. Venturi masks are available to deliver 24%, 28%, 35%, and 40% oxygen. Such masks are especially useful in the hospital management of patients with chronic obstructive pulmonary disease and CO_2 retention; they offer no advantage in prehospital care, except in the long-range transport of such patients.

Partial Rebreathing Mask

The partial rebreathing mask (Fig. 8-15E) resembles a simple plastic face mask but has a reservoir bag that permits the patient to rebreathe about one-third of his exhaled air. Since that air is principally from his dead space—that is, the area of the respiratory tract where gas exchange does not take place (like the trachea and bronchi)—it contains mostly oxygen inspired during the previous inhalation. At flow rates of 6 to 10 liters per minute, a partial rebreathing mask can provide an oxygen concentration of 35 to 60%.

Nonrebreathing Mask

The nonrebreathing mask (Fig. 8-15F) looks a lot like the partial rebreathing mask, in that both have an oxygen reservoir, but it is equipped in addition with a *one-way valve* that permits the patient to inhale from the reservoir bag but not to exhale back into it. The only gas that can enter the reservoir, therefore, is 100% oxygen piped in from the oxygen cylinder. The oxygen flow rate is adjusted to prevent collapse of the bag during inhalation; usually that requires about 10 to 12 liters per minute. If the nonrebreathing mask is fitted tightly to the face, it can deliver oxygen concentrations approaching 100%. Therefore:

> **THE NONREBREATHING MASK IS THE PREFERRED MEANS OF DELIVERING HIGH OXYGEN CONCENTRATIONS TO A SPONTANEOUSLY BREATHING PATIENT.**

The nonrebreathing mask, then, is ideally suited to patients with severe hypoxemia, for example those with chest trauma or pulmonary embolism. Some patients, however, tolerate a mask poorly no matter how badly they need the oxygen and complain of feelings of suffocation when the mask is placed over the nose and mouth. In such situations, the two-pronged nasal cannula is a better alternative than no oxygen at all. Whatever device is used, it is important to explain to the patient what it is and why it is necessary. Forewarning the patient that a mask may feel confining but is nonetheless providing "more air" than breathing without it may enable the patient to tolerate the mask with less anxiety.

HYPERCARBIA: PATIENTS WHO NEED VENTILATION

Up to this point, we have discussed ways of improving the oxygenation of a patient who is breathing spontaneously. When a patient is *not* breathing, however, we have an additional problem: Not only do we need a way of providing such a patient with oxygen, but we also have to move air in and out of his lungs in order to wash out the carbon dioxide that is constantly being dumped into the alveoli. Thus, while we can manage problems of shunt and hypoxemia simply by giving oxygen, the problem of hypoventilation and hypercarbia requires artificial ventilation. The most extreme case of hypoventilation is respiratory arrest, in which there is no ventilation at all.

Respiratory Arrest

As the term implies, to suffer a respiratory *arrest* is to stop breathing, which is not a healthy thing to do. Respiratory arrest can occur for several reasons. The most common cause is a condition we have already studied—AIRWAY OBSTRUCTION in an unconscious person. Recall the pathway from life to death: When a person loses consciousness, his muscles become slack, and the base of his tongue tends to fall back against the posterior pharynx, thereby closing off the airway. Respiratory arrest will follow within seconds to minutes if steps are not taken to reopen the airway. The moral of the story is clear:

> **MOST CASES OF RESPIRATORY ARREST COULD BE PREVENTED BY ENSURING AN OPEN AIRWAY.**

Less commonly, respiratory arrest occurs because of *depression of the respiratory center* in the brainstem. OVERDOSE OF certain DRUGS, such as narcotics for example, may depress the respiratory center to the point that the patient stops breathing altogether. HEAD INJURY can do the same, especially if there is

swelling (edema) of brain tissue that causes the brainstem to be compressed against the skull. A similar mechanism may be operative in certain cases of STROKE, while a powerful ELECTRIC SHOCK can produce respiratory arrest by temporarily stunning the respiratory center. Finally, respiratory arrest may come about as a consequence of PRIMARY CARDIAC ARREST; for if the heart stops beating for any reason, as may occur in a massive heart attack, the respiratory center in the brain will, along with every other organ in the body, be cut off from its blood supply and literally suffocate. It will no longer be able to send signals to the respiratory system. For that reason, a person whose heart stops beating will stop breathing by about a minute later.

CAUSES OF RESPIRATORY ARREST

- AIRWAY OBSTRUCTION
  Tongue (in the unconscious patient)
  Foreign body (choking)
  Swelling (laryngeal edema) or laryngospasm
  Trauma to the airway
- DEPRESSION OR DAMAGE TO THE RESPIRATORY CENTER
  Drugs (narcotics, barbiturates)
  Head injury
  Stroke
  Electric shock
- PRIMARY CARDIAC ARREST

Recognition of Respiratory Arrest

To treat respiratory arrest promptly, one has to be able to recognize it promptly. Fortunately, it is not very difficult to do so.

When a healthy person is breathing normally, his chest rises and falls with each breath, and air flow can be felt and heard at his nose and mouth. In a person who is not breathing, those signs are absent. Therefore,

> **TO DIAGNOSE RESPIRATORY ARREST, *LOOK, LISTEN,* AND *FEEL* FOR BREATHING.**

We are, however, getting ahead of our story. First things first:

FIRST, OPEN THE *AIRWAY!*

Why is it necessary to open the airway *before* checking whether the patient is breathing? The reason is that even a person with a perfectly intact breathing mechanism will be unable to move air in and out of his lungs if his airway is obstructed. Furthermore, opening the airway is sometimes the only maneuver required to restore breathing in an apneic (nonbreathing) patient. So the first step in diagnosing respiratory arrest is to relieve any obstruction that might be hindering air flow, by tilting the person's head back (head tilt–chin lift or a similar maneuver). *Then* (Fig. 8-16):

- LOOK at the patient's chest for breathing movements, and
- Bring your face close to the patient's face and LISTEN and FEEL for air being exhaled against your cheek.

[Question: Why not simply observe the chest to see if it is moving? Why bother to listen and feel as well?]

FIGURE 8-16.   DIAGNOSING RESPIRATORY ARREST. Look, listen, and feel for breathing.

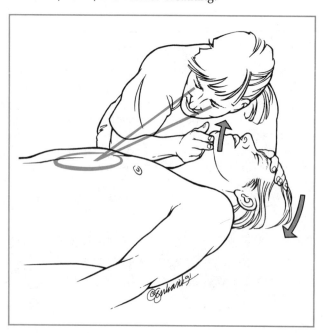

If breathing movements are absent and you do not detect any air flow, the diagnosis is respiratory arrest, and you're going to have to do something about it fast. Since the patient has stopped breathing, what you are going to have to do, in fact, is to *breathe for him,* that is, provide *artificial ventilation.*

IMPROVING A PATIENT'S VENTILATION

There are a number of ways of providing artificial ventilation to a patient who is not breathing (or not breathing adequately). All of them are based on the same principle: blowing air into the patient's lungs. The techniques differ only in the power source used to generate the pressures and air flows required for inflating a patient's lungs.

The most readily available power source for that job are the *rescuer's lungs,* which may be used to blow air into the patient's mouth directly (mouth-to-mouth ventilation) or into the patient's mouth through an interposed pocket mask (mouth-to-mask ventilation). In either case, the rescuer's exhaled air will effectively "wash out" the carbon dioxide that is accumulating in the patient's alveoli and thereby correct the patient's hypercarbia.

In a person who has suffered respiratory arrest, however, hypercarbia is only half the problem. The other half is *hypoxemia.* Because he isn't breathing, the apneic patient is not bringing any oxygen from the outside world into his alveoli. And while it is clear that a rescuer blowing into the patient's lungs will be able to flush out excess carbon dioxide, it is legitimate to ask whether the "second-hand" air exhaled by the rescuer contains enough oxygen to sustain a person who is in respiratory arrest.

The answer is yes.

We have already mentioned that room air contains 21% oxygen. Not all of that oxygen, when taken into the body, is consumed by body tissues; some of it gets exhaled again. As a consequence, our exhaled air contains anywhere from 16 to 18% oxygen, which—although not an optimal concentration—is enough to sustain life when blown into another person's lungs.

Mouth-to-Mouth Ventilation

Consider the following scenario. You are relaxing by the side of a local swimming pool when you see a teenager being fished out of the water, apparently unconscious. You race over to him and tilt his head back to open his airway; then you look, listen, and feel for breathing. The boy isn't breathing. What do you do next? Since you don't ordinarily bring resuscitation equipment with you to the pool (although perhaps you will hereafter!), you will have to start artificial ventilation with the only equipment immediately available to you—your own lungs, airway, and mouth:

- Keeping the patient's head tilted back, use the thumb and index finger of the hand that is on his forehead to **pinch his nostrils closed** (Fig. 8-17A) so that air will not escape through the nose when you blow into the mouth.
- **Take a deep breath.**
- Open your mouth wide, and **seal your mouth over the patient's mouth** (Fig. 8-17B).
- **Exhale forcefully** into the patient's mouth while watching out of the corner of your eye to see if his chest is rising.
- **Remove your mouth** from the patient's mouth, and allow him to exhale passively while you take another breath.

If your ventilation is adequate, you should be able to

- *See* the patient's chest rise and fall
- *Feel* the compliance of the patient's lungs in your own airway (just as you feel the "give" when you inflate a balloon)
- *Hear and feel* air escape through the patient's mouth during his passive exhalation

When you are *starting* artificial ventilation, give TWO FULL, SLOW BREATHS, one after the other, allowing for complete exhalation between the two breaths. Deliver each lung inflation over 1½ to 2 seconds. Each breath you give should be of a sufficient volume to make the patient's chest rise—usually around 800 to 1200 ml. Take a breath each time you complete a lung inflation. Thereafter, if you are dealing with respiratory arrest only, give A BREATH EVERY 5 SECONDS (i.e., 12 breaths/min). After each ventilation, turn your head to the side to watch the

FIGURE 8-17. MOUTH-TO-MOUTH VENTILATION. (A) Tilt the patient's head back and seal his nose shut. (B) Encircle the patient's open mouth with your mouth and exhale.

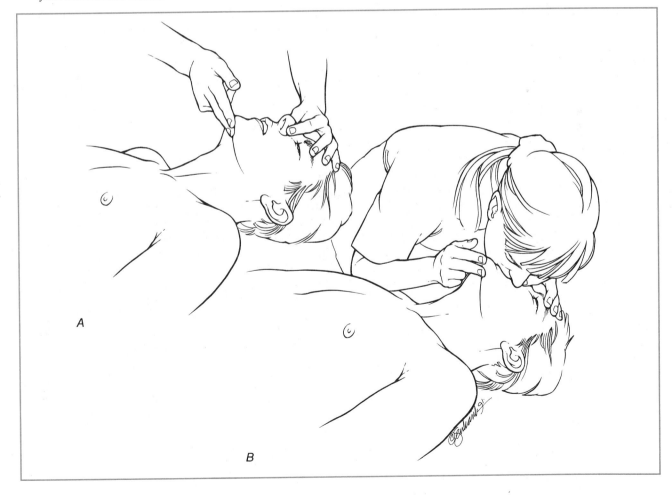

fall of the patient's chest as *you* take another breath. If at any point the patient resumes spontaneous breathing, simply keep his airway open (head tilt–chin lift) and monitor his respirations.

If Air Won't Enter . . .

What if you have opened the airway, taken a deep breath, sealed your mouth over the victim's mouth, and then—nothing! You cannot force any air into the victim's lungs; something seems to be obstructing the airway. As discussed in Chapter 7, the most likely source of that airway obstruction is the victim's tongue, so you should in most cases be able to relieve the obstruction by improving the position of the patient's head and jaw. Switch to the head tilt–neck lift and try again to ventilate, or use the triple airway maneuver. If you still cannot get any air in, there may be a foreign body obstructing the victim's airway. In that case you will need to proceed through the steps described in Chapter 7 for the unconscious choking victim (review Fig. 7-15).

Gastric Distention

Any form of artificial ventilation that blows air into the patient's mouth—as opposed to blowing air directly into the trachea, via an endotracheal tube—may lead to distention of the victim's stomach. Gastric distention is especially likely to occur when excessive pressure is used to inflate the lungs or when the airway is partially obstructed during inflation attempts. In both instances, the pressure in the airway forces open the esophagus, and air flows into the stomach.

Gastric distention occurs most often in children undergoing CPR, but it is common in adults as well. A distended stomach is harmful to the patient for at least two reasons. First of all, gastric distention *promotes regurgitation* of stomach contents, and vomitus creeping up the back of the throat rapidly finds its way into the victim's lungs (aspiration). Vomitus is not good for lungs, nor is its presence in the victim's mouth very pleasant for the rescuer doing mouth-to-mouth ventilation. In the second place, a distended stomach *pushes the diaphragm upward into the chest,* thereby reducing the amount of space in which the lungs can expand. So ventilation volumes are reduced.

You can minimize gastric distention during artificial ventilation by

- Keeping the patient's airway fully open
- Delivering each breath slowly, over 1½ to 2 seconds
- Allowing complete exhalation between breaths

- Limiting the volume of each ventilation you give to just that amount necessary to cause the chest to rise

If despite those measures the victim's stomach still becomes distended, CONTINUE RESCUE BREATHING WITHOUT ATTEMPTING TO EXPEL THE AIR FROM HIS STOMACH. Routinely putting pressure over the victim's abdomen in an attempt to relieve gastric distention has been shown to cause regurgitation and is thus extremely dangerous. So if you see the victim's stomach becoming distended, just recheck the airway and moderate your ventilations.

Only if severe gastric distention prevents adequate lung inflations should you attempt to decompress the stomach. To do so, roll the victim quickly to his side (so that he is facing *away* from you), and press firmly over his epigastrium. Be prepared to wipe (or, ideally, suction) his mouth free of vomitus before rolling him back to a supine position.

Can AIDS or Other Diseases Be Contracted from Doing Mouth-to-Mouth Ventilation?

As we shall learn in Chapter 28, a certain percentage of patients suffering from acquired immunodeficiency syndrome (AIDS) carry the human immunodeficiency virus (HIV) in their saliva. There is, therefore, a *theoretical* possibility of becoming infected with HIV as a result of performing mouth-to-mouth ventilation. The emphasis is on the word *theoretical,* because as of this writing, there has never been a single documented case of HIV transmission in this fashion, despite the fact that there *are* documented instances of rescuers giving mouth-to-mouth ventilation to patients suffering from AIDS. For that reason, it is the current opinion of most experts that the risk of becoming infected with HIV as a result of performing mouth-to-mouth ventilation is extremely small. Similarly, there are no documented cases of hepatitis transmission via mouth-to-mouth ventilation.

A more serious risk to rescue workers performing mouth-to-mouth ventilation is the transmission of tuberculosis from an infected patient to a rescuer (especially if the rescuer's immune system is in any way impaired). The risk is probably quite low, since in general, transmission of tuberculosis requires prolonged close exposure, such as among people living in the same household. Nonetheless, any rescuer who performs mouth-to-mouth ventilation on a patient suspected of having tuberculosis should have a follow-up skin test 12 weeks later to see whether infection occurred. If the skin test is positive, preventive drug therapy should be started.

The best way to avoid potential exposure to communicable diseases while performing artificial ventilation is to make sure you keep a pocket mask—one equipped with a one-way valve—on your person at all times.

Mouth-to-Nose Ventilation

In some cases, mouth-to-nose ventilation may be more effective or more acceptable to the rescuer than mouth-to-mouth ventilation. Mouth-to-nose ventilation is favored, for example, when it is impossible to open the victim's mouth, when there is extensive trauma around the victim's mouth, or when you cannot achieve an effective seal around the victim's mouth (often the case if the patient has no teeth!). To perform mouth-to-nose ventilation:

- Keep the patient's **head tilted back** by pressing one hand on his forehead.
- Use your other hand to **lift the patient's lower jaw and close his mouth.**
- **Take a deep breath.**
- **Seal your mouth around the patient's nose** (Fig. 8-18).

- **Exhale** until you see the chest rise and feel the lungs expand.
- **Remove your mouth** from the patient's nose.
- **Open the patient's mouth to permit passive exhalation.** (The soft palate commonly causes nasopharyngeal obstruction, which may interfere with passive exhalation through the nose. Thus, if the patient's mouth is not opened to permit exhalation between ventilations, progressive gastric distention is likely to occur.)

Mouth-to-Stoma Ventilation

On rare occasions, the paramedic may have to give artificial ventilation to a person who has had a **laryngectomy**, a surgical procedure in which the larynx is removed (*laryngo-* + *-ectomy*) and part of the trachea is brought out through a hole (called a **stoma**) on the front or side of the neck (Fig. 8-19). A person who has had this operation is called a **laryngectomee**, or "neck breather"; that is, he breathes through the hole in his neck. The stoma may be simply a large round opening in the skin, or the patient may wear a breathing tube in the stoma. Since the larynx has been cut out, there is no longer any connection between the patient's pharynx and lower airway. What that means, practically speaking, is that you cannot ventilate such a patient by the mouth-to-mouth or mouth-to-nose technique, for air blown into the mouth or nose will not reach the lower airway but can only go down the esophagus into the stomach.

To make matters more complicated, there is also another kind of surgery in which only *part* of the larynx is removed. People who have had that operation are called *partial neck breathers* because they breathe

FIGURE 8-18. MOUTH-TO-NOSE VENTILATION. With the patient's mouth held shut, seal your mouth over his nose and exhale.

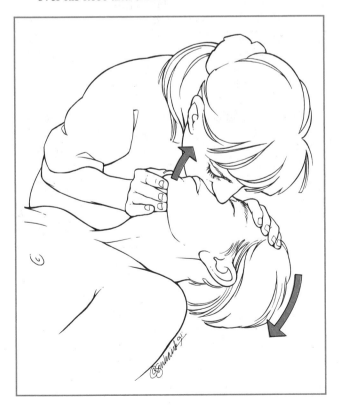

FIGURE 8-19. LARYNGECTOMEE. In this patient, there is no longer any connection between the pharynx and the lower airway.

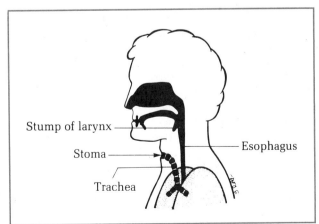

Stump of larynx

Stoma

Trachea

Esophagus

through both the stoma and the nose or mouth. A special tube—a so-called speaking tube—is grafted from just within the stoma to the base of the tongue. In practice, it may be impossible to tell initially if an apneic laryngectomee is a neck breather or only a partial neck breather until you attempt artificial ventilation.

Mouth-to-stoma ventilation is actually easier to perform than mouth-to-mouth ventilation, since you do not need any special maneuvers to open the airway. You exhale directly into the patient's trachea. Furthermore, because there is no contact between the airway and the throat, you do not have to deal with regurgitated stomach contents that sometimes make mouth-to-mouth ventilation a bit unsavory.

To perform mouth-to-stoma ventilation, first remove all coverings (e.g., scarf, tie, necklace) from the stoma area. Then clear the stoma of any foreign material that may have accumulated there. If the patient is wearing a breathing tube, make sure it is not clogged. If the tube is clear, it can be left in place; otherwise it should be removed. Take a deep breath, and make a seal with your mouth over the stoma. Blow into the stoma until you see the victim's chest rise. In general, it will not be necessary to close off the mouth and nose of a laryngectomee, since there is no direct connection between the trachea and the upper airway. However, if the chest does not rise when you ventilate, the patient may be a *partial* neck breather, and you will have to close off the nose and mouth. To do so, pinch the nose closed between your third and fourth fingers while you seal the lips with the palm of your hand; then press upward and backward on the jaw with your thumb under the chin.

After you see the chest rise, remove your mouth from the stoma and allow the victim to exhale passively. Use the usual sequence of two slow, full breaths to start mouth-to-stoma ventilation, and continue, as usual, at a rate of one inflation every 5 seconds.

Ventilation with a Pocket Mask

For those who are a bit squeamish about mouth-to-mouth or mouth-to-nose ventilation, the pocket mask employs the same readily available power source (the rescuer's lungs) but eliminates direct contact with the patient's mouth or nose. Use of a one-way valve over the mask's mouthpiece also virtually eliminates any possibility of contact with the patient's secretions and diverts the patient's exhaled air away from the rescuer's mouth. Furthermore, when its inlet valve is connected to an oxygen source at a flow rate of about

10 liters per minute, the pocket mask can deliver up to 50% oxygen. The pocket mask is used as follows:

- Perform a **triple airway maneuver** from the patient's vertex (Fig. 8-20A).
- **Apply the rim of the pocket mask** between the patient's lower lip and chin to retract the lip down and hold the mouth open (Fig. 8-20B).
- Use both thumbs along the sides of the mask to **clamp the remainder of the mask to the patient's face** (Fig. 8-20C). At the same time, use your fingers to grasp the jaw just beneath the angles and pull upward, maintaining backward tilt of the head and jaw thrust.
- **Exhale into the mask** until you see the chest rise (Fig. 8-20D).

If the pocket mask is connected to an oxygen cylinder and the oxygen flow rate is high enough (flow control valve wide open), the rescuer can simply occlude the opening of the mask periodically with his tongue and allow the oxygen flow to ventilate the patient—which will yield an inhaled oxygen concentration approaching 90 to 100%.

The pocket mask has several important *advantages* over other methods of delivering artificial ventilation in the field:

- The pocket mask is readily available, since the paramedic can, as the name of the device implies, carry the mask in a pocket. Thus there is no need to race back to the vehicle for other equipment.
- There is no need to switch to another device once oxygen becomes available. Simply attach the oxygen line to the inlet valve on the mask and continue ventilating.
- Similarly, there is no need to switch to another device if the patient resumes spontaneous breathing, for the pocket mask can then be strapped to the patient's face and used as a simple face mask to deliver 40 to 60% oxygen.
- It is much easier to maintain a good seal around the patient's mouth with a pocket mask than with a bag-valve-mask, because you can use *both* hands to hold the mask in place. The triple airway maneuver used in conjunction with the pocket mask meanwhile ensures an optimal airway. The net result is that you can deliver larger ventilation volumes to the lungs (and less to the stomach!) through a pocket mask than via a bag-valve-mask.
- Using a pocket mask, you can, as in direct mouth-to-mouth ventilation, feel the resistance of the patient's lungs in your own lungs and can adjust the volume of ventilations accordingly.

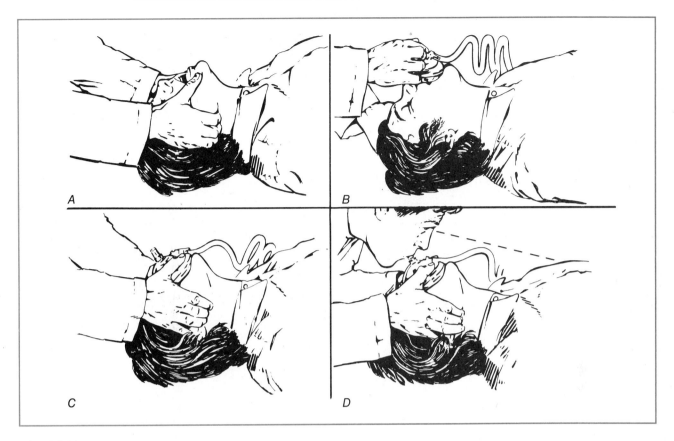

FIGURE 8-20. **APPLICATION OF A POCKET MASK.** (A) Perform triple airway maneuver from the vertex. (B) Fit the mask over the patient's nose and mouth. (C) Clamp mask to face, maintaining head tilt. (D) Exhale into mask until the chest rises. Reproduced courtesy of Asmund Laerdal, Stavanger, Norway.

For the reasons mentioned,

> **THE POCKET MASK IS THE PREFERRED DEVICE FOR GIVING ARTIFICIAL VENTILATION IN THE PREHOSPITAL SETTING.**

Ventilation with a Bag-Valve-Mask

As noted earlier, both mouth-to-mouth ventilation and mouth-to-mask ventilation utilize the rescuer's lungs as a power source. A second potential power source for artificial ventilation is the rescuer's *hand*, used to squeeze the contents of a bag containing air or oxygen into the patient's lungs. That is the principle behind the bag-valve-mask.

The *bag* component of a bag-valve-mask is self-inflating and, when used without supplemental ox-

ygen, delivers room air (21% oxygen) to the patient. If a source of oxygen at a flow rate of 12 liters per minute is attached to the bag, the delivered oxygen concentration can be increased to 40%. The addition of an oxygen reservoir to the bag (Fig. 8-21) can further increase the inspired oxygen concentration to the range of 90%.

The *mask* used with the bag-valve device should be transparent to enable the rescuer to see vomitus or secretions around the patient's mouth. Applying the mask properly is half the battle, for the frequent failure to provide an adequate ventilatory volume with a bag-valve-mask is nearly always due to the difficulty in maintaining a leakproof seal between the mask and the patient's face. To use a bag-valve-mask device, then,

- **Select a mask of the correct size** for the patient you are treating; a mask that is either too small or too large will make it difficult to get a good seal. The mask should just cover the area between the bridge of the nose and the indentation beneath the lower lip. (That usually means using a small

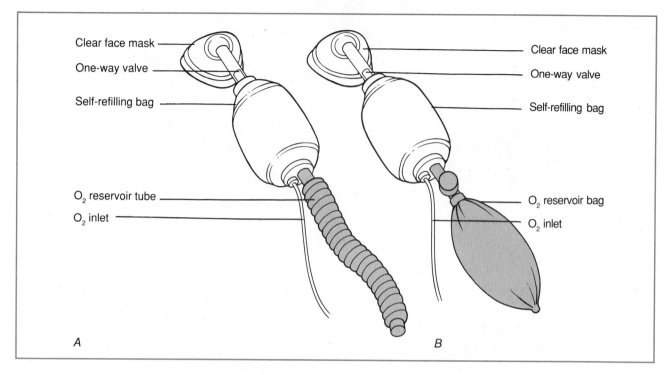

FIGURE 8-21. BAG-VALVE-MASK UNIT WITH OXYGEN. (A) With reservoir
tube. (B) With reservoir bag.

mask for the average woman and a medium mask
for the average man.)

- **Position yourself at the patient's vertex.**
- Use the crossed finger maneuver to **open the patient's mouth, and insert an oropharyngeal airway.**
- **Tilt the patient's head back** (Fig. 8-22A).
- Depending on the design of the mask and the
  grip you find most comfortable, use either the "C
  clamp" grip (Fig. 8-22B) or the palm grip (Fig. 8-
  22C) to hold the mask securely to the patient's
  face. With either grip, use your fingers to grasp
  the patient's mandible (lower jaw) and hold a
  tight seal, while pulling toward you to maintain
  backward tilt of the head.
- Use your other hand to **squeeze the bag.** Watch
  to see whether the chest rises and falls each time
  you squeeze the bag. Pay attention as well to the
  resistance in the bag as you ventilate. If it's very
  hard to squeeze the bag, the airway is probably
  obstructed, and you need to adjust the patient's
  head position. If squeezing the bag is very *easy,*
  there's probably a leak somewhere in the system!

If all that sounds difficult, it is—so difficult, in fact,
that in one study more than half of 320 experienced
EMTs tested were unable to provide adequate ventilation volumes to a manikin with a bag-valve-mask

(the majority *were* able to provide adequate ventilation volumes with a pocket mask, even though three-
quarters of them had never used a pocket mask before).

The principal advantage of the bag-valve-mask
device, then, is an aesthetic one: It distances the rescuer from the patient's oral secretions, a feature that
has considerable appeal when the patient's breakfast
is oozing from his mouth. Effective use of the bag-
valve-mask, however, takes a lot of skill and practice;
and even under optimal conditions, ventilation with
a bag-valve-mask is going to produce gastric distention. For that reason, it is usually preferable to *start*
artificial ventilation with a pocket mask (oxygen
added as soon as possible) and then intubate the trachea at the earliest possible opportunity.

It should be mentioned that bag-valve-mask devices with oxygen supplementation may also be used
to *assist* the ventilations of a spontaneously breathing
patient. Assisted ventilation may be required, for example, in a patient whose tidal volume is very shallow, perhaps because of drug overdose or spinal cord
injury. To assist ventilations in such a patient, apply
the mask to the patient's face in the fashion described
earlier, and squeeze the bag *gently* each time the patient takes a breath. The object of the exercise is to
boost the tidal volume of each breath, thereby improving the elimination of carbon dioxide from the
lungs.

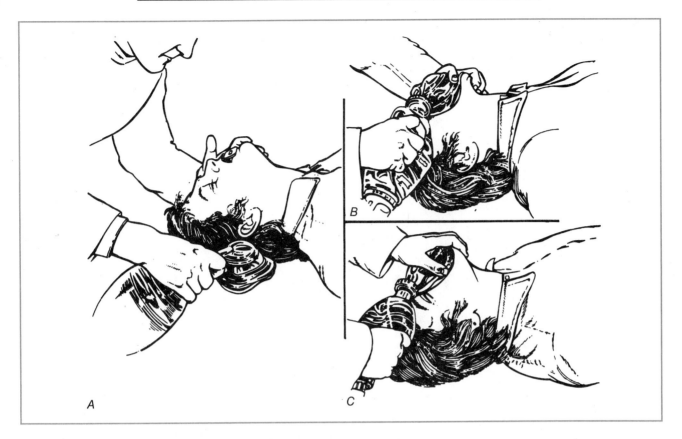

FIGURE 8-22. **USE OF BAG-VALVE-MASK.** (A) Patient's head tilted back, oropharyngeal airway in place. (B) "C clamp" grip to hold mask to face. (C) Use
of palm to hold mask to face. Reproduced courtesy of Asmund Laerdal, Stavanger, Norway.

Ventilation with a Demand Valve

A third potential power source for artificial ventilation—besides the rescuer's lungs and the rescuer's
hand—is the flow from an *oxygen cylinder*, and one
device that makes use of that power source is called
a demand valve.

A demand valve assembly (Fig. 8-23A)—also
known as a manually-triggered oxygen-powered resuscitator—consists of the valve itself; a reinforced
rubber tube by which it is connected to the reducing
valve of the oxygen cylinder; and an adapter that fits
into a standard mask, into an esophageal obturator
airway, or onto an endotracheal tube. On top of the
valve unit, there is a push button that controls oxygen flow: When the button is depressed, 100% oxygen streams out at flow rates anywhere from 50 to 150
liters per minute; oxygen flow continues either until
the operator takes his finger off the button or until a
preset pressure (40–60 mm Hg) is reached, at which
point oxygen flow abruptly stops. (That pressure
limit is a safety measure to prevent blowing a hole in
the patient's lung!) As the lungs are inflated, therefore, and the pressure within them rises to the valve's
preset maximum, oxygen flow automatically shuts
off.

If the demand valve is used with a mask for artificial ventilation of a nonbreathing patient, the mask
should be held as you would hold a pocket mask—
clamped to the patient's face with both hands, with a
triple airway maneuver. Since that position makes it
awkward to reach the push button on top of the
valve, it is advisable to fit the valve with an extension
lever (Fig. 8-23B), positioned so that it is possible to
trigger the valve without taking either hand off the
mask. When the valve is triggered periodically to
provide ventilation to a nonbreathing patient in that
fashion, we call the process **controlled ventilation,**
because the rescuer has control over the patient's
breathing.

The demand valve, however, has another mode
of operation, from which the valve gets its name: It
can give breaths "on demand" of the patient. That is,
the demand valve can augment the ventilations of a
patient who is breathing spontaneously. When the
mask is sealed against the patient's face, the negative
pressure created by the patient's inhalation will trigger the valve automatically, without the rescuer de-

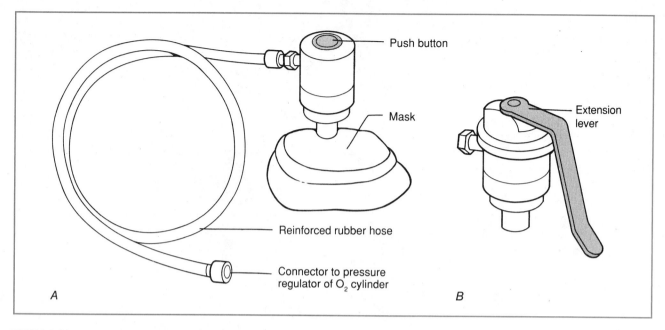

FIGURE 8-23.   DEMAND VALVE.   (A) Demand valve assembly with mask, optimally suited for assisted ventilation. (B) If used for controlled ventilation, the valve should be fitted with an extension lever.

pressing the button, and oxygen will flow into the patient's lungs until the cutoff pressure is reached; then the oxygen flow will stop automatically. The net effect is to increase the volume of each breath the patient takes and to enrich each breath with oxygen. When the demand valve is used in this fashion—triggered by the inhalations of the patient rather than the actions of the rescuer—the process is called **assisted ventilation.**

In fact, it is for assisted ventilation that the demand valve is primarily recommended. It is the method of choice for delivering oxygen to a conscious patient in PULMONARY EDEMA, for the positive pressure delivered to the airways is thought to help drive fluid out of the alveoli.

The demand valve is much *less* useful for controlled ventilation. It should not be used for more than a few minutes in conjunction with a mask in an apneic patient, because the high pressures invariably lead rapidly to gastric distention. Nor should a demand valve be used for very long in conjunction with an endotracheal tube, because prolonged delivery of dry gases directly into the trachea can damage respiratory tissues. Finally, a demand valve should not be used at all in children under 12 years old, except under very special circumstances (e.g., airway obstruction due to croup or epiglottitis). In general, for the nonbreathing patient, bag-valve-mask devices enable finer control of ventilation and better assessment of the patient's pulmonary compliance.

> **USE THE DEMAND VALVE TO *ASSIST* VENTILATIONS OF PATIENTS WHO ARE BREATHING SPONTANEOUSLY BUT INADEQUATELY.**

Automatic Transport Ventilators

A nearly ideal adjunct for providing artificial ventilation to a nonbreathing patient in the prehospital phase is an automatic transport ventilator (ATV). Most ATVs are very small and compact—some no larger than the portable tape players that joggers carry on their belts—and usually weigh between 2 and 5 kg. The ATV is hooked up to an oxygen cylinder and gives pulses of oxygen at selected volumes and rates. Advantages of ATVs in prehospital care include the following:

- ATVs can be set to deliver a specific tidal volume at a specific rate. Thus one can control the patient's minute ventilation with considerable accuracy.
- When using an ATV to ventilate a patient who has not yet been intubated, the rescuer has both hands free to seal the mask to the patient's face and maintain head tilt.

- ATVs have more favorable flow properties than demand valves: ATVs deliver oxygen at flow rates of 15–30 liters per minute over 1–2 seconds; those lower inspiratory flow rates and longer inhalation times decrease the likelihood of producing gastric distention and regurgitation.
- Once the patient has been intubated, the ATV frees up the rescuer for other tasks. The ATV will automatically ventilate the patient through the endotracheal tube according to the settings chosen.

The major limitation of the automatic transport ventilator is that models currently available may not be used for children under 5 years old. Nonetheless, the American Heart Association now regards ATVs as Class I equipment, that is, useful, effective, and always acceptable in advanced life support.

Each commercial brand of automatic transport ventilator is designed a little differently, and the paramedic should become familiar with the specific equipment used in his or her service. As a general rule, most ATVs allow one to set at least the tidal volume and the respiratory rate. (Good average settings for adults are a tidal volume of 10–15 ml/kg and a respiratory rate of 10/min. For children, the rate should be 20/min.) ATVs should be equipped with a low-pressure alarm to alert the rescuer when the oxygen cylinder is nearly empty or if the ATV becomes disconnected.

Percutaneous Translaryngeal Ventilation*

Consider the following scenario: You have been called to the scene of a large fire in a factory 15 miles out of town. As you arrive, firefighters are just rescuing an unconscious man from inside the burning building. They bring him over to you, and you immediately notice that he has extensive burns of the face and that he is making a very high-pitched squeak with each inhalation. You realize that he is developing laryngeal edema and that within a few minutes his upper airway may be closed off altogether. You try to intubate him, but you can't see any landmarks; the whole airway is swollen. Meanwhile, he stops breathing altogether. What can you do to save his life?

You *could* attempt a cricothyrotomy, with the "cut-and-poke" technique described in Chapter 7.

But if you've never done a cricothyrotomy before, trying it out for the first time on a burned patient with a swollen airway may be a little harrowing, at best, especially dealing with unfamiliar equipment like a scalpel and tracheotomy tube.

There is, however, an alternative method, one that utilizes equipment with which prehospital personnel are much more comfortable, namely an intravenous catheter. The method is called *percutaneous* (through the skin) *translaryngeal* (across the larynx) *ventilation* (PTV). (You may find references to the same procedure under the heading "percutaneous trans*tracheal* ventilation," but that, in fact, is a misnomer; the needle puncture is made through the cricothyroid membrane, which, as we all know by now, is part of the larynx, not the trachea.) To carry out PTV, you need to do the following:

- **Assemble the necessary equipment:**
  1. Over-the-needle CATHETER, 12- or 14-gauge, with a 10-ml SYRINGE attached.
  2. Povidone-iodine SWABS for disinfecting the skin.
  3. Adhesive TAPE or tie for securing the catheter in place.
  4. Oxygen TUBING (you can cut the tubing off a standard oxygen mask or nasal cannula).
  5. CONNECTOR WITH THUMB PORT (Fig. 8-24) to join the catheter to the oxygen tubing and permit intermittent ventilation. You will probably have to rig up the connector yourself; and if PVT is authorized in your paramedic service, you should have several connectors prepared ahead of time and stashed with your other airway equipment. As shown in Figure 8-24, a very simple but effective ventilating connector can be fashioned by cutting a thumb port from a suction catheter and the flash site from an IV assembly. Hook up the connector to the oxygen tubing, so it will be ready for use the moment you have attached it to the translaryngeal catheter.
  6. OXYGEN CYLINDER with standard flow control valve.
- **Position the patient** supine, with his head extended.
- **Identify the cricothyroid membrane** by stabilizing the larynx with the thumb and middle fingers of one hand and palpating for the V notch (Adam's apple) with the index finger. (See Fig. 7-44 if you've forgotten where to find the cricothyroid membrane.)
- **Prep the area** over the cricothyroid membrane quickly with povidone-iodine swabs.

---

*Not required by the United States Department of Transportation for certification as a paramedic.

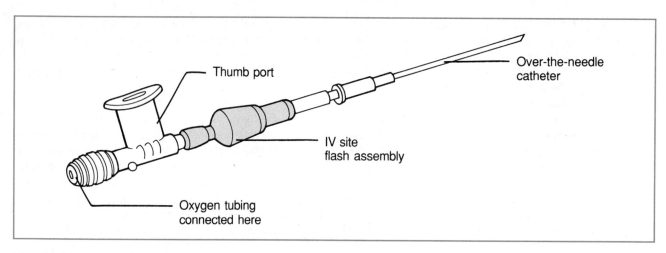

FIGURE 8-24. **PTV VENTILATING DEVICE.** A thumb port cut from a suction unit can be used to permit intermittent ventilation through a translaryngeal catheter.

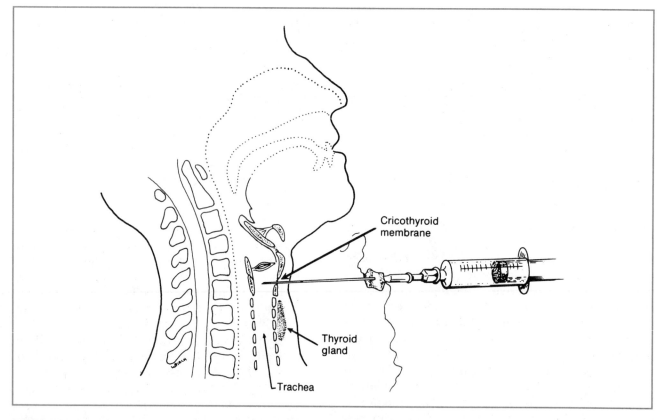

FIGURE 8-25. **CRICOTHYROID MEMBRANE PUNCTURE** with an over-the-needle catheter for percutaneous translaryngeal ventilation (PTV).

- **Puncture the skin** over the cricothyroid membrane with the over-the-needle catheter.
- **Advance the needle** through the skin and cricothyroid membrane, at an angle of approximately 60 degrees to the horizontal (Fig. 8-25). You should feel the needle "pop" into the larynx.

- **Verify the position of the needle** by aspirating the syringe. The return of free air into the syringe confirms that the needle is in the airway and not in the subcutaneous tissue.
- **Advance the plastic catheter** over the needle its full length, so that the catheter hub comes to rest against the skin.

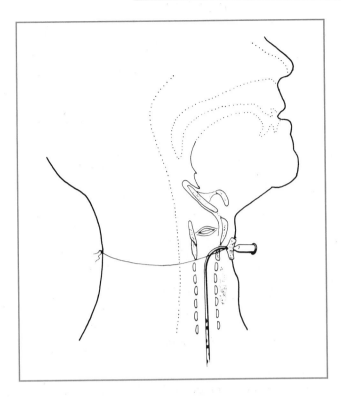

FIGURE 8-26.   CATHETER CORRECTLY PLACED.   Free movement of air in and out of the catheter ensures that it is in the trachea and not in the soft tissues of the neck.

- Hold the catheter securely against the patient's neck, and **remove the needle** from the catheter.
- **Reconfirm the position of the catheter** by aspirating it again with the syringe.
- **Fasten the catheter hub** securely to the skin (Fig. 8-26).
- **Hook up the connector** to the catheter hub.
- **Open the oxygen flow valve** to its maximum, about 15 liters per minute.
- **Occlude the thumb port** for 3 seconds or until you see the patient's chest rise.
- **Release the thumb port** to permit passive exhalation.

Like cricothyrotomy, PTV is a potentially hazardous procedure and should therefore be performed only by those who have been trained and authorized to do so.

MONITORING GAS EXCHANGE

In a number of circumstances it is very useful to know something about the patient's arterial blood gases or the composition of his exhaled air. Two devices have recently been introduced into prehospital emergency care that enable us to obtain some of that information: the pulse oximeter and the end-tidal carbon dioxide monitor.

Pulse Oximetry

Until quite recently, the only means a paramedic had to evaluate a patient's state of oxygenation were direct observations of the patient: the patient's apparent degree of respiratory distress; the color of his mucous membranes; the quality of his breath sounds. While those observations remain very important, they are not always easy to come by under field conditions. Try assessing subtle changes in mucous membrane color in the victim of a nighttime traffic accident trapped inside a wrecked car! Or try listening for abnormal breath sounds while the fire rescue team is deploying hacksaws and prybars to dismantle the wreckage from around the patient. In the prehospital world, nothing is as simple as it sounds in the books.

Hospital-based medical personnel have for years had the option of assessing oxygenation by measuring a patient's blood gases directly. A needle can be introduced into a superficial artery and an arterial blood sample withdrawn and sent for analysis. The apparatus required to measure arterial blood gases, however, is large and cumbersome and not, therefore, practical for prehospital use. So for years, paramedics had to rely entirely on what they could manage to see and hear to get a rough idea of whether the patient was adequately oxygenated.

Pulse oximetry has changed all that—changed it so dramatically that some have called pulse oximetry "the fifth vital sign." While that description may be somewhat exaggerated, pulse oximetry *is* a simple, rapid, safe, and noninvasive method of measuring—minute by minute—how well a person's blood is oxygenated.

What pulse oximetry measures, in fact, is the percentage of hemoglobin in the arterial blood that is saturated with oxygen (the SaO_2). As we shall learn in Chapter 9, hemoglobin is an iron-containing protein within red blood cells that has the ability to combine with oxygen. When it does so, it takes on a bright red color; when it releases oxygen, hemoglobin reverts to a darker, red-blue shade. That property of hemoglobin accounts for the common observation that arterial blood (which is well oxygenated) is bright red while venous blood (less well oxgygenated) is darker and somewhat bluish. Pulse oximetry takes advantage of those color differences to measure the oxygen saturation of arterial blood. A sensor probe, clipped to the patient's finger or ear lobe, uses a light-emitting diode (LED) to transmit light through the vascular bed to a light-*sensing* detector. The amount of light transmitted across the vascular bed will depend on the proportion of hemoglobin that is saturated with oxygen. To ensure that the instrument is measuring *arterial* and not venous oxygen saturation, pulse oximeters are designed to assess only *pulsating* blood vessels. (Question: Why is it important to measure the *arterial* oxygen saturation and not the venous oxygen saturation?) Thus pulse oximeters, as their name suggests, must also measure the patient's pulse—and one way to check the functioning of a pulse oximeter is to compare the pulse reading it gives you with your own measurement of the patient's pulse by palpation.

A normally oxygenated, normally perfused person should have an SaO_2 between 97 and 99 percent. Any reading below 94 percent indicates respiratory compromise, and below 91 percent signals a need for aggressive oxygen therapy.

When Can a Pulse Oximeter Be Helpful?

Pulse oximetry has many potential applications in the field, and paramedics keep finding more uses for the device every day. Among the situations in which pulse oximeters may be useful in prehospital emergency care are the following:

- Monitoring the oxygenation of a patient **during an intubation attempt or during suctioning**. While the rule is to hold your own breath while you intubate, many rescuers neglect to do so and lose track of how long the patient has been without oxygenation. The low-saturation alarm on the pulse oximeter can jolt the paramedic out of his reverie and remind him that it's time to interrupt the intubation attempt and ventilate the patient.
- **Identifying deterioration in a trauma victim**. In the victim of multiple trauma, the signs of a developing tension pneumothorax, for instance, may not be evident until the problem is quite advanced. A declining SaO_2 can alert the rescuer early that something bad is happening and thus prompt a search for the cause of the problem.
- **Identifying deterioration in the cardiac patient**. Pulse oximetry may enable early identification of patients developing congestive heart failure in the wake of a heart attack.
- **Identifying high-risk patients with respiratory problems**, for example those asthmatics having serious attacks or emphysematous patients in severe decompensation.
- **Assessing vascular status in orthopedic trauma**. Pulse oximetry is (or should be) routine practice in fracture of an extremity to evaluate the pulse distal to the fracture (for example, the pulse in

the wrist if the arm is broken). Loss of a pulse means that the limb is in jeopardy and may require urgent action in the field if transport time is long. A pulse oximeter clipped to a finger or toe on a broken limb might therefore provide critical information about the ongoing circulation to the limb.

How to Use a Pulse Oximeter

There are at least 60 pulse oximeters on the market in the United States, varying considerably in design, size, and complexity. All of them, however, have certain features in common, and the general procedure for operating a pulse oximeter usually is as follows:

- **Turn the unit on**. When turned on, most pulse oximeters will first calibrate themselves, then perform an internal check, and finally indicate that they are ready for use.
- **Select a site for the probe**. The site should be highly vascular so that the oximeter can easily locate an arterial pulsation. Usually the fingertip is the most convenient site, but a toe, the ear lobe, the bridge of the nose, and (in infants) the lateral foot are alternative possibilities.
- **Apply the sensor correctly**, so that the light-emitting diode and the light-receiving sensor are directly opposite one another.
- As soon as the sensor detects a pulse, the pulse rate will be displayed and, ideally, an audible beep should sound with each heart beat. **Verify** the heart rate displayed on the pulse oximeter by palpating the patient's pulse. If the pulse rate you palpate is different from the rate reported by the oximeter, any SaO_2 reading you get may be suspect.
- Within about 10 seconds, the oximeter should display a reading for SaO_2. If it does not, or if the pulse rate shown is not accurate, move the sensor to another site and try again.

Sources of Error in Using a Pulse Oximeter

The usefulness of a pulse oximeter depends on its providing accurate information. The oximeter that gives a reading of 99 percent SaO_2 when the patient is in fact severely hypoxemic is not going to be much help to anyone. So it is important to be aware of circumstances that might produce erroneous readings.

- **Bright ambient light** may enter the spectrophotometer of the pulse oximeter and create an incorrect reading. Protect the sensor clip by covering it with a towel or aluminum foil.
- **Patient motion** can confuse the pulse oximeter,

for it may mistake motion for arterial pulsation and read the oxygen saturation from a vein rather than an artery. (What kind of error would that produce—a reading lower than the actual SaO_2 or a reading higher than the actual SaO_2?)

- **Poor perfusion** makes it difficult for the oximeter to sense a pulse and therefore to make a reading. Poor perfusion occurs in states such as shock, cardiac arrrest, and cold exposure. If the patient's limbs are vasoconstricted and cold, it may be necessary to place the pulse oximeter clip on the patient's ear lobe or nose.
- **Venous pulsations** may occur in some patients with right-sided heart failure (see Chap. 23). As noted, the pulse oximeter uses pulsations to identify *arteries*. If a vein is pulsating, the oximeter may regard the vein as an artery and measure a venous oxygen saturation.
- **Abnormal hemoglobins** may produce a falsely high SaO_2. The abnormal hemoglobin we worry about the most is *carboxy*hemoglobin, which is formed by the attachment of **carbon monoxide** to the hemoglobin molecule. As we shall learn in Chapter 27, carbon monoxide binds to oxygen receptors on hemoglobin far more efficiently than oxygen does; so even small amounts of carbon monoxide in the ambient air can rapidly occupy a significant proportion of a person's hemoglobin. The pulse oximeter cannot distinguish between hemoglobin that is occupied by oxygen and hemoglobin occupied by carbon monoxide. So it may give a high SaO_2 reading for a patient who is in fact severely hypoxemic from carbon monoxide poisoning. The results of pulse oximetry should therefore be interpreted cautiously in victims of smoke inhalation or other circumstances likely to have produced carbon monoxide poisoning.

The above examples underscore the importance of always weighing the information provided by pulse oximetry (or any other device) against clinical observations:

> **WHEN IN DOUBT, LOOK AT THE PATIENT!**

If the patient is turning blue and struggling to breathe, you may ignore the pulse oximeter reading that says the patient is adequately oxygenated.

End-Tidal Carbon Dioxide Monitoring

Inadvertent placement of an endotracheal tube into the patient's esophagus is one of the most frequent causes of failed resuscitation (it is also a very frequent cause of lawsuits against anesthesiologists). The usual methods of checking for proper placement of an endotracheal tube are not, unfortunately, foolproof. (Can you recall what those methods are? If not, review p. 91.) Even seeing the tip of the endotracheal tube pass through the patient's vocal cords does not guarantee that the tube will *stay* in the trachea, for flexion or extension of the patient's head may displace the tube into the esophagus the moment you're not looking.

End-tidal CO_2 monitoring has recently been promoted as a means of detecting inadvertent esophageal intubation. A CO_2 detector is attached in series between the endotracheal tube and the ventilation device (e.g., bag-valve or automatic transport ventilator). The percentage of CO_2 contained in the last few milliliters of the patient's exhaled air—called the **end-tidal carbon dioxide** (because it is exhaled at the end of the tidal volume)—is measured by a special sensor. Electronic end-tidal CO_2 monitors use a photoelectric sensor that relies on absorption of infrared light by CO_2. Much more practical for field use—and much less expensive—is a disposable colorimetric device that changes hue as gas passes through it. The most widely used version consists of a specially treated membrane sensitive to changes in pH (acidity) that result from exposure to CO_2. As the percentage of CO_2 in the patient's exhaled air rises, the color of the detector changes from purple to tan to yellow.

How does measurement of CO_2 help in identifying placement of an endotracheal tube? Air exhaled through an endotracheal tube that has been properly placed in the trachea of a normally perfused patient should contain about 4 to 5% CO_2 (a yellow reading on the colorimetric device). If the tube has been mistakenly placed in the esophagus, on the other hand, there should be virtually no CO_2 in the "exhaled" gas (less than 0.5%—a purple reading). Thus there is no doubt that an end-tidal CO_2 monitor can be useful in detecting esophageal intubation in a *normally perfused* patient.

The problem is that the vast majority of patients requiring endotracheal intubation in the field are patients in cardiac arrest who, by definition, are not well perfused at all. Even during the best CPR, tissue perfusion is very low, and as a consequence, end-tidal CO_2 falls to only 25 to 30 percent of normal. For that reason, end-tidal CO_2 readings obtained during cardiac arrest need to be interpreted with caution:

While a high reading (over 2%) almost certainly indicates successful tracheal intubation, a low reading does not necessarily mean that the tube is in the esophagus. So one must in any case watch for the rise and fall of the chest, check both sides of the chest for breath sounds, and listen over the epigastrium for air bubbling into the stomach.

When CPR is successful, a sudden increase in end-tidal CO_2 may be the first indication of a return of spontaneous circulation, as large quantities of "stale," CO_2-rich blood are returned to the lungs.

The end-tidal CO_2 monitor is probably most useful for monitoring endotracheal tube placement in a *non*-arrested patient—for instance, to assist in blind nasotracheal intubation. It is not yet clear, however, whether end-tidal CO_2 monitoring will prove consistently useful in the advanced life support of cardiac arrest.

GLOSSARY

accessory muscles   Muscles other than the *diaphragm* and *intercostals* that are brought into play to assist breathing when a person is in respiratory distress.

acute myocardial infarction (AMI)   A condition present when an insufficient oxygen supply to the heart muscle leads to death of that segment of the muscle.

alveolar air   That portion of the *tidal volume* that reaches the alveoli and participates in gas exchange there.

assisted ventilation   Use of adjunctive equipment, such as a bag-valve-mask or demand valve, to boost the *tidal volume* of a spontaneously breathing patient.

atelectasis   Collapse of the alveolar air spaces in the lungs.

carbon dioxide (CO_2)   An end product of carbohydrate metabolism, eliminated from the body by respiration.

controlled ventilation   Artificial ventilation of a patient who is not breathing spontaneously.

cyanosis   Blueness of the skin caused by *hypoxemia.*

dead space   That portion of the *tidal volume* that does not participate in gas exchange.

diaphragm   A large skeletal muscle that plays a major role in breathing and that separates the chest cavity from the abdominal cavity.

dyspnea   The sensation of being short of breath.

hemoglobin   Oxygen-carrying pigment of red blood cells.

hypercarbia   Excessive partial pressure of *carbon dioxide* in the blood; an arterial PCO_2 greater than 45 to 50 *torr,* usually the result of *hypoventilation.*

hyperpnea   Abnormally deep breaths.

hyperventilation   An increased rate and/or depth of breathing that results in abnormal lowering of the arterial *carbon dioxide* tension (PCO_2).

hypocarbia   Abnormally low *carbon dioxide* tension in the blood; an arterial PCO_2 less than 35 torr.

hypoventilation   Inadequate *ventilation,* with a resultant rise in the arterial PCO_2 to levels above normal (higher than 45 torr).

hypoxemia   Inadequate *oxygen* in the blood; an arterial PO_2 less than 60 torr.

hypoxic drive   The situation in which a person's stimulus to breathe arises from a fall in arterial PO_2 (rather than the normal stimulus, a rise in PCO_2).

intercostal muscles   The muscles between the ribs, which assist in breathing.

laryngectomee   Person who has undergone partial or total surgical removal of the larynx; a "neck breather."

laryngectomy   Surgical removal of the larynx.

minute volume   The volume of air inhaled or exhaled during 1 minute, calculated by multiplying the *tidal volume* times the respiratory rate.

oxygen (O_2)   A colorless, odorless, tasteless gas essential to life, composing 21 percent of the air we breathe.

partial pressure   The fractional concentration of a gas in a gas mixture.

pleura   The membrane lining the outer surface of the lungs (visceral pleura), the inner surface of the chest wall (parietal pleura), and the thoracic surface of the diaphragm (parietal pleura).

pleural space   Potential space between the two pleural layers.

pneumothorax   Air in the *pleural space.*

psi   Abbreviation for pounds per square inch, a measurement of pressure.

pulmonary arteries   The arteries that carry blood poor in oxygen from the right ventricle of the heart to the lungs.

pulmonary veins   The veins that carry oxygenated blood from the lungs to the left atrium of the heart.

reducing valve   The pressure regulator on an oxygen cylinder, which decreases the high pressures inside the cylinder to much lower pressures that can be delivered safely to the patient.

respiration   The exchange of oxygen and carbon dioxide among the body tissues, the lungs, and the atmosphere.

safe residual   Minimum permissible pressure in an oxygen cylinder, defined as 200 *psi.*

shunt   The situation in which a portion of the output of the right heart reaches the left heart without being oxygenated in the lungs.

singultus   Hiccups.

stoma   A surgically created opening, such as that made for a tracheostomy.

tachypnea   Excessively rapid rate of breathing (over 25/min in adults).

tidal volume   The amount of air inhaled or exhaled during normal, quiet breathing; the volume of one breath.

torr   Units of pressure, equivalent to millimeters of mercury (mm Hg).

total lung capacity   The volume of gas contained in the lung at the end of maximal inhalation.

ventilation   Breathing; moving air in and out of the lungs.

FURTHER READING

OXYGEN THERAPY

Bourn S. Gearing for oxygen delivery. *JEMS* 13(8):58, 1988.

Branson RD. Contamination of multiple-use humidifiers in ambulances (letter). *Ann Emerg Med* 17:761, 1988.

Cameron J et al. Bacterial contamination of ambulance oxygen humidifier water reservoirs: A potential source of pulmonary infection. *Ann Emerg Med* 15:1300, 1986.

Corley M et al. The myth of 100% oxygen delivery through manual resuscitation bags. *J Emerg Nursing* 19(1):45, 1993.

Darin J, Broadwell J, MacDonell R. An evaluation of water-vapor output from four brands of unheated, prefilled bubble humidifiers. *Respir Care* 27:41, 1982.

Doyle JD. The rational use of medical oxygen. *Emerg Med* 24(12):215, 1992.

Feinsilver SH. Oxygen toxicity. *Emerg Med* 23(3):89, 1991.

Gaull ES. Are you overlooking O$_2$? *Emerg Med Serv* 22(6):31, 1993.

Miller K. The ABGs of emergency care. *Emergency* 20(12):29, 1990.

Peters WR, Jolly PC. Gastric rupture from nasal oxygen catheter. *Bull Mason Clin* 26:70, 1972.

Ruple JA, Geronimo P. Inspiring confidence in oxygen therapy. *JEMS* 15(11):24, 1990.

Selinger SR et al. Effects of removing oxygen from patients with chronic obstructive pulmonary disease. *Am Rev Respir Dis* 136:85, 1987.

Shannon TM, Celli B. Oxygen therapy. *Emerg Med* 23 (21):63, 1991.

Tinits P. Oxygen therapy and oxygen toxicity. *Ann Emerg Med* 12:321, 1983.

Waxman K. Oxygen delivery and resuscitation. *Ann Emerg Med* 15:1420, 1986.

MOUTH-TO-MOUTH VENTILATION

American Heart Association, Emergency Cardiac Care Committee. Risk of infection during CPR training and rescue: Supplemental guidelines. *JAMA* 262:2714, 1989.

Berg RA et al. Bystander cardiopulmonary resuscitation: Is ventilation necessary? *Circulation* 88:1907, 1993.

Cummins RO. Infection control guidelines for CPR providers (editorial). *JAMA* 262:2732, 1989.

Emergency Cardiac Care Committee and Subcommittees, American Heart Association. Guidelines for cardiopulmonary resuscitation and emergency cardiac care. *JAMA* 268:2171, 1992.

Melker R. Recommendations for ventilation during cardiopulmonary resuscitation: Time for a change? *Crit Care Med* 13:882, 1985.

Ornato JP. Providing CPR and emergency care during the AIDS epidemic. *Emerg Med Serv* 18(4):45, 1989.

Ornato JP et al. Attitudes of BCLS instructors about mouth-to-mouth resuscitation during the AIDS epidemic. *Ann Emerg Med* 19:151, 1990.

Raviglione MC, Battan R, Taranta A. Cardiopulmonary resuscitation in patients with the acquired immunodeficiency syndrome: A prospective study. *Arch Intern Med* 148:2602, 1988.

Safar P. Ventilatory efficacy of mouth-to-mouth artificial respiration. Airway obstruction during manual and mouth-to-mouth artificial respiration. *JAMA* 167:335, 1958.

ADJUNCTS FOR ARTIFICIAL VENTILATION

Austin DA, Graves JR. Who says EMTs can't operate a bag-valve-mask? *JEMS* 13(9):62, 1988.

Barnes TA, Watson ME. Oxygen delivery performance of four adult resuscitation bags. *Disaster Med* 1:204, 1983.

Bourn S. You can breathe easy. *JEMS* 14(5):59, 1989.

Campbell TP et al. Oxygen enrichment of bag-valve-mask units during positive-pressure ventilation: A comparison of various techniques. *Ann Emerg Med* 17:232, 1988.

Committee on Trauma, American College of Surgeons. Essential equipment for ambulances. *Bull Am Coll Surg* September, 1977.

Corley M et al. The myth of 100% oxygen delivery through manual resuscitation bags. *J Emerg Nursing* 19(1):45, 1993.

Elling R, Politis J. An evaluation of emergency medical technicians' ability to use manual ventilation devices. *Ann Emerg Med* 12:765, 1983.

Finer NN et al. Limitations of self-inflating resuscitators. *Pediatrics* 77:417, 1986.

Goddard JM. Concentrations of oxygen delivered by air entrainment oxygen masks. *Ann R Coll Surg Engl* 67:366, 1985.

Harrison R et al. Mouth-to-mask ventilation: A superior method of rescue breathing. *Ann Emerg Med* 11:74, 1982.

Hess D, Baran C. Ventilatory volumes using mouth-to-mouth, mouth-to-mask and bag-valve-mask techniques. *Am J Emerg Med* 3(4):292, 1985.

Jesudian M et al. Bag-valve-mask ventilation: Two rescuers are better than one: Preliminary report. *Crit Care Med* 13:122, 1985.

Lawrence PJ. Ventilation during cardiopulmonary resuscitation: Which method? *Med J Aust* 143:443, 1985.

Marcum L. Can you ventilate? A study of provider ventilation skills. *JEMS* 17(11):31, 1992.

Rossi R, Lindner KH, Ahnefeld FW. Devices for expired air resuscitation. *Prehosp Disaster Med* 8(2):123, 1993.

Safar P. Pocket mask for emergency artificial ventilation and oxygen administration. *Crit Care Med* 2:273, 1974.

Shade BR. Ventilating via bag-valve device. *Emergency* 29(3):18, 1992.

Stewart RD et al. Influence of mask design on bag-mask ventilation. *Ann Emerg Med* 14:403, 1985.

Terndrup TE, Kanter RK, Cherry RA. A comparison of infant ventilation methods performed by prehospital personnel. *Ann Emerg Med* 18:607, 1989.

Whelan G. Ensuring ventilation. *Emerg Med* 16(15):109, 1984.

PERCUTANEOUS TRANSLARYNGEAL VENTILATION

Campbell CT et al. A new device for emergency percutaneous transtracheal ventilation in partial and complete airway obstruction. *Ann Emerg Med* 17:927, 1988.

Dobbinson TL et al. Needle tracheostomy: A laboratory study. *Anesth Intens Care* 8:72, 1980.

Frame SB et al. Transtracheal needle catheter ventilation in complete airway obstruction: An animal model. *Ann Emerg Med* 18:127, 1989.

Grace TL. The crico-ventilating device: A method for ventilation of the needle cricothyroidotomy. *Emerg Med Serv* 12(4):45, 1983.

Levinson MM et al. Emergency percutaneous transtracheal ventilation (PTV). *JACEP* 8:396, 1979.

Ravussin P et al. A new transtracheal catheter for ventilation and resuscitation. *Can Anaesth Soc J* 32:60, 1985.

Reich DL, Mingus M. Transtracheal oxygenation using simple equipment and a low-pressure oxygen source. *Crit Care Med* 18:664, 1990.

Richtsmeier WJ et al. Transtracheal ventilation with crash cart equipment. *Otolaryngol Head Neck Surg* 102:191, 1990.

Yealy DM, Stewart RD, Kaplan RM. Myths and pitfalls in emergency translaryngeal ventilation: Correcting misimpressions. *Ann Emerg Med* 17:690, 1988.

PULSE OXIMETRY

Aughey K et al. An evaluation of pulse oximetry in prehospital care. *Ann Emerg Med* 20:887, 1991.

Bourn S. Bells and whistles. *JEMS* 18(11):29, 1993.

Cox D. Measuring up to standards: Pulse oximetry making its contribution to prehospital care. *Emergency* 25(7):38, 1993.

Cydulka RK et al. Prehospital pulse oximetry: Useful or misused? *Ann Emerg Med* 21:675, 1992.

Farrell K. Test piloting pulse oximetry. *JEMS* 15(6):61, 1990.

Gramlich T. Pulse oximetry. *Emergency* 24(8):25, 1992

Jay GD. Pulse oximetry. *Emerg Med Serv* 20(5):40, 1991.

Mackreth B. Assessing pulse oximetry in the field. *JEMS* 15(6):56, 1990.

Mardirossian G, Schneider RE. Limitations of pulse oximetry. *Anesth Prog* 39:194, 1993.

Mateer JR et al. Continuous pulse oximetry during emergency endotracheal intubation. *Ann Emerg Med* 22:675, 1993.

Mayefsky JH et al. The usefulness of pulse oximetry in evaluating acutely ill asthmatics. *Ped Emerg Care* 8(5):262, 1992.

Portner RS, Merlin MA, Heller MB. The fifth vital sign. *Emergency* 22(3):37, 1990.

Silverston P. Pulse oximetry at the roadside: A study of pulse oximetry in immediate care. *Br Med J* 298:711, 1989.

END-TIDAL CARBON DIOXIDE MONITORING

Anton WR et al. A disposable end-tidal CO_2 detector to verify endotracheal intubation *Ann Emerg Med* 20:271, 1991.

Goldberg JS. Colorimetric end-tidal carbon dioxide monitoring for tracheal intubation. *Anesth Analg* 70:191, 1990.

Goldfarb B, Cohen H. True colors: Measuring end-tidal carbon dioxide. *JEMS* 15(6):68, 1990.

MacLeod BA et al. Verification of endotracheal tube placement with colorimetric end-tidal CO_2 detection. *Ann Emerg Med* 20:267, 1991.

Ornato JP, Peberdy MA. Prehospital end-tidal carbon dioxide monitoring. *JEMS* 18(3):140, 1993.

Sayah A, Peacock W, Overton D. End-tidal CO_2 measurement in the detection of esophageal intubation during cardiac arrest. *Ann Emerg Med* 19:857, 1990.

Sum Ping ST et al. Accuracy of the FEF CO_2 detector in the assessment of endotracheal tube placement. *Anesth Analg* 74:415, 1992.

White RD, Asplin BR. Out-of-hospital quantitive monitoring of end-tidal carbon dioxide pressure during CPR. *Ann Emerg Med* 23:25, 1994.

Zaleski L et al. The esophageal detector device: Does it work? *Anesthesiology* 79:244, 1992.

PERFORMANCE CHECKLISTS

The following pages contain checklists for correct performance of some of the skills described in this chapter. The checklists can be used as a review and as a guide for practicing the respective skills.

Performance Test
Pocket Mask

Student _____ Date _____

Instructor: Place an "X" in the Fail column beside any step that is done incorrectly, out of sequence, or omitted.

Maximum Time (sec)	Activity	Critical Performance*	Fail
10	Positioning mask	Pointed end of mask over bridge of nose	
		Rescuer at patient's vertex	
		Triple airway maneuver to clamp mask to face	
	Proper head position	Hyperextends patient's head	
	Ventilates	Blows into mask until chest rises	
		Removes mouth from mask; observes chest fall	
		Records volume of at least 500 ml/breath	
10	Addition of oxygen	Attaches tubing to O$_2$ cylinder	
		Attaches other end of tubing to mask	
		Sets flow rate to 10 L/min	
		Resumes ventilations through the mask	
	Interposition of ventilations	Interposes ventilation between every 5 compressions	
		1½ to 2 seconds for ventilations	

*CPR is in progress; second student doing compressions.

Instructor _____

Performance Test
Oropharyngeal Airway and Bag-Valve-Mask Ventilation

Student _____   Date _____

Instructor: Place an "X" in the Fail column beside any element that is done incorrectly, out of sequence, or omitted.

Maximum Time (sec)	Activity	Critical Performance*	Fail
10	Airway selection	Measures airway against face, from lips to angle of jaw	
		Selects appropriate airway	
	Opening victim's mouth	Crossed finger maneuver	
	Airway insertion	Tip of airway faces roof of patient's mouth	
		Rotates airway 180 degrees when halfway in	
		Tongue not pushed back into throat	
		Flange against patient's lips or teeth	
10	Positioning mask	Pointed end of mask over bridge of nose	
		Clamps mask to face with "C" clamp or palm	
		Tight seal	
	Proper head position	Hyperextends patient's head	
	Ventilation (4 times)	Squeezes bag until chest rises	
		Releases bag and observes for chest falling	
		Records volume of at least 500 ml for each breath	
10	Addition of oxygen	Attaches oxygen tubing to O_2 cylinder	
		Attaches other end of tubing to bag-valve-mask	
		Opens oxygen tank	
		Turns on flow to 10–12 L/min	
		Resumes ventilations	
	Interposition of ventilations	Interposes ventilation between every 5 compressions	
		1½ to 2 seconds for ventilations	

*CPR is in progress; second student doing compressions.

Instructor _____

Performance Test
Oropharyngeal Airway and Demand Valve

Student _____   Date _____

Instructor: Place an "X" in the Fail column beside any element that is done incorrectly, out of sequence, or omitted.

Maximum Time (sec)	Activity	Critical Performance[a]	Fail
10	Airway selection	Measures airway against face, from lips to angle of jaw	
		Selects appropriate airway	
	Opening victim's mouth	Crossed finger maneuver	
	Airway insertion	Tip of airway faces roof of patient's mouth	
		Rotates airway 180 degrees when halfway in	
		Tongue not pushed back into throat	
		Flange against patient's lips or teeth	
10	Opening oxygen tank	Face and body not over pressure regulator	
		Regulator fully pressurized	
	Positioning mask	Pointed end of mask over bridge of nose	
		Mask clamped over face correctly	
		Tight seal	
	Proper head position	Hyperextends patient's head	
	Ventilation (4 times)	Depresses button until chest rises[b]	
		Releases button and observes for chest falling	
		Records volume of at least 1,000 ml for each breath	
	Interposition of ventilations	Interposes ventilation between every 5 compressions	
		1½ to 2 seconds for ventilations	

[a]CPR is in progress; second student doing compressions.
[b]Care must be taken when using a demand valve unit with a manikin, lest the lungs of the manikin be blown out. Depress button on demand valve only until gauge or signal light indicates adequate inflation.

Instructor _____

Performance Test
Use of an Oxygen Cylinder

Student _____   Date _____

Instructor: Place an "X" in the Fail column beside any element that is done incorrectly, out of sequence, or omitted.

Activity	Critical Performance	Fail
Proper position	Oxygen cylinder securely upright	
	Rescuer to side of cylinder; no part of body over cylinder valve	
Cracking tank	Slowly opens main cylinder valve until rush of air is audible	
	Rapidly closes main cylinder valve	
Application of pressure regulator	Checks that pressure regulator is correct one for cylinder	
	Checks for intact washer	
	Checks that humidifier bottle contains sterile water	
	Checks that humidifier bottle is tightly closed	
	Applies pressure regulator to cylinder in correct position	
	Tightens regulator securely to cylinder	
Opening cylinder	Opens main cylinder valve slowly to pressurize regulator	
	Turns cylinder valve one-half turn more	
Connection of equipment	Selects oxygen delivery device to be used	
	Connects tubing from cylinder to device	
Flow adjustment	Opens flow regulator	
	Adjusts flow to rate ordered by instructor	
Termination of O_2 therapy	Shuts flow meter to zero	
	Closes main cylinder valve	
	Opens flow meter to bleed system, until indicator is at zero	
	Closes flow meter securely	

Instructor _____

9
Circulation

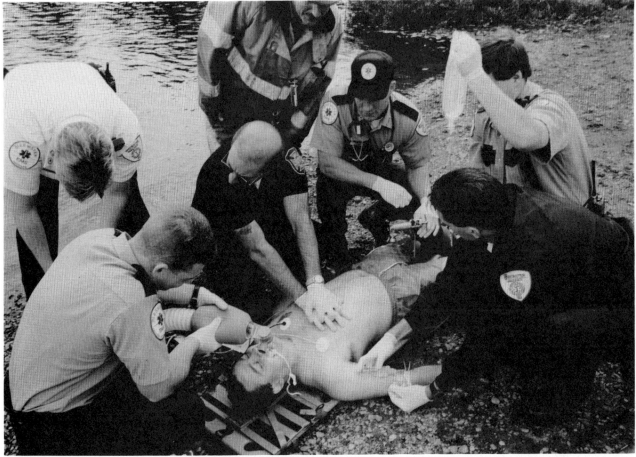

Brewster Ambulance Service, Brewster, Massachusetts. Photo by Brian Clark.

OBJECTIVES

We have reached the third letter of the rescue alphabet: **C** for **circulation.** Having established an *airway* and made sure that the patient is *breathing*, we must now look to the status of his circulatory system; for well-ventilated lungs will scarcely benefit the patient if blood is not flowing through the lungs to pick up oxygen or if blood is not reaching the peripheral tissues to deliver that oxygen. We therefore need to rule out the possibility that either (1) the circulation has stopped altogether (cardiac arrest) or (2) the circulation has become inadequate to perfuse the peripheral tissues (shock).

In this chapter, we shall examine in detail the factors required to maintain normal circulation and the clinical consequences of circulatory failure. We shall, first of all, discuss the ultimate form of pump failure—cardiac arrest—and we shall review the basic life support measures for treating cardiac arrest in adults. (Advanced life support in cardiac arrest will be discussed in Chap. 23, when we consider cardiac emergencies in detail. Cardiopulmonary resuscitation [CPR] in children will be taken up in Chap. 30, dealing with pediatric emergencies.) We shall then look at the other constituents of a circulatory system, fluids and tubing (blood vessels), and consider how shock comes about. Finally, we shall examine the methods used to treat a patient in shock. By the end of this chapter, the student should be able to

1. List the three components required for a functioning circulatory system
2. Identify, given a list of definitions, the correct definition of
   - Acid
   - Anaerobic
   - Asystole
   - Base
   - Colloid
   - Crystalloid
   - Electrolyte
   - Hemoglobin
   - Hypotonic
   - Hypertonic
   - Isotonic
   - Osmosis
   - Shock
   - Ventricular fibrillation
3. Describe or demonstrate on a manikin:
   - How to check for a pulse in an unconscious person
   - How to position a patient for CPR
   - How to locate the correct compression point for CPR
   - How to deliver chest compressions
4. List five measures that can be taken to ensure maximally effective CPR
5. Identify, given a description of several clinical situations, situations in which
   - CPR should (or should not) be started
   - CPR should be terminated
6. List three ways in which CPR for a victim of trauma differs from CPR applied to a medical patient
7. Describe the osmotic effect of infusing
   - A hypotonic intravenous solution
   - A hypertonic intravenous solution
   - A colloid solution
8. List five ways in which fluids can be lost from the body
9. List five symptoms and signs of dehydration, and describe the treatment of dehydration
10. List the most characteristic sign of overhydration
11. Identify, given a description of several patients, a patient with
    - Respiratory acidosis
    - Respiratory alkalosis
    - Metabolic acidosis
    - Metabolic alkalosis
    and describe the appropriate treatment for each
12. Explain the mechanism that produces cyanosis and the clinical significance of cyanosis
13. List the indications for giving
    - Whole blood
    - Packed red blood cells
    - Fresh-frozen plasma
    - Plasma substitutes
    - Salt solutions
    - Glucose solutions
14. Identify a patient having a transfusion reaction, given a description of the patient's clinical findings, and describe how the case should be managed
15. Describe three mechanisms by which shock may occur
16. List four possible causes of hemorrhagic shock
17. List two ways of assessing a patient's perfusion
18. Identify a patient in hypovolemic shock, given a description of the patient's clinical findings, and:
    - Explain the mechanisms behind the patient's signs and symptoms
    - Outline the correct treatment of the patient
19. List the indications and contraindications for applying the military anti-shock trousers (MAST)
20. List the indications for intravenous therapy
21. Identify patients who have developed complications of intravenous therapy, given a description of several patients with different clinical findings, and indicate the appropriate treatment for each

22. List three measures you can take to reduce the likelihood of thrombophlebitis developing from the IVs you start in the field
23. Calculate the flow rate through an IV, given information about the volume to be infused and the properties of the IV administration set
24. List four possible causes of an IV suddenly slowing down or stopping

PREREQUISITES FOR PERFUSION

The circulatory (cardiovascular) system is designed to carry out one crucial job and one job only: to keep a particular fluid (blood) flowing between the lungs and the peripheral tissues. In the lungs, blood dumps the gaseous waste products of metabolism—chiefly carbon dioxide—and picks up life-giving oxygen. In the peripheral tissues, the process is reversed: Blood *unloads* its oxygen and *picks up* the wastes. Were blood flow to stop, therefore, or even to slow down significantly, the results would be catastrophic. The cells of the brain, heart, and all the other organs of the body would, first of all, have nowhere to eliminate their wastes, so they would rapidly be engulfed in the toxic by-products of their own metabolism. But even more serious, if blood flow to the tissues were to be disrupted, *oxygen* delivery would cease with it. For a few minutes, the cells could switch over to an emergency metabolic system—one that does not require oxygen (**anaerobic** metabolism). But that form of metabolism produces even more acids and toxic wastes. So within a very few minutes of circulatory failure, cells throughout the body would begin to suffocate and die, and the body would enter a state known as *shock.*

It is clear, then, that keeping the blood moving continuously through the body is a critical task. To carry out that critical task, the circulatory system requires three intact components:

- A functioning PUMP: the heart
- Adequate fluid VOLUME: the blood and body fluids
- An intact system of TUBING capable of reflex adjustments (constriction and dilatation) in response to changes in pump output and fluid volume: the blood vessels

If any one of those components—the pump, the volume, or the tubing—is damaged or deficient, the whole system is in jeopardy.

We shall look first at what happens when the pump stops functioning.

WHEN THE PUMP STOPS: CARDIAC ARREST

Approximately 360,000 persons in the United States each year experience cardiac arrest secondary to acute myocardial infarction, usually during the first 2 hours of their symptoms and usually *before* they reach the hospital. Cardiac arrest occurs when the heart stops beating effectively. As we shall learn in Chapter 23, that can come about in one of several ways. To begin with, the heart can stop beating altogether and become perfectly still—a condition called **cardiac standstill,** or asystole. In other cases, the heart does not stand still, but its component muscle fibers get "out of synch," so that instead of contracting as a single unit, the heart as a whole simply quivers ineffectually—a condition called **ventricular fibrillation.** Finally, cardiac arrest can come about when the heart is still contracting, but contracting so feebly that it cannot pump blood out into the circulation; that condition is known as **cardiovascular collapse,** and it occurs as a result of severe bleeding, severe damage to the heart muscle, or overdosage of drugs that depress the heart. No matter what the underlying mechanism of cardiac arrest, however, the net effect is the same: The patient is *clinically dead,* and whether or not he continues down the road to irreversible, biologic death will depend significantly on how quickly basic life support is instituted.

If you have passed an EMT-A course, you should by now be able to perform the techniques and procedures of basic life support in your sleep! Those procedures are so important, however, that we shall review them here. The recommendations presented are those in the current guidelines for cardiopulmonary resuscitation (CPR) of the American Heart Association.

It should be emphasized that skills are learned by *doing,* not reading. The other side of the coin is that skills are *lost* by not doing. Studies have shown rapid decay in CPR skills among paramedical personnel who did not participate in frequent refresher training. CPR skills are the paramedic's most important resource for saving lives. *Do not permit those skills to decay!* Make a date with the local manikin at least once every 6 months for the duration of your professional career.

> **DON'T LET YOUR CPR SKILLS GET RUSTY. A PATIENT'S LIFE MAY DEPEND ON THEM.**

Basic Life Support*

Basic life support (BLS) has traditionally been regarded as the technique of recognizing respiratory or cardiac arrest and applying the ABCs (airway, breathing, and circulation) of cardiopulmonary resuscitation until more definitive therapy (advanced life support [ALS]) becomes available. Originally, the concept of basic life support focused primarily on cardiac arrest and its treatment. More recently, however, the concept has been expanded to include *preventive* aspects, since it has become increasingly clear that many sudden deaths can be prevented by early intervention. Thus education in prudent living habits, coronary risk factors, warning symptoms of heart attack, and the method of activating the local EMS system are now included together with CPR as an integral part of all BLS training programs.

The concept of basic life support has also, more recently, been expanded even further. Because of the widespread availability of automatic external defibrillators and the extreme importance of early defibrillation, the American Heart Association now regards defibrillation as part of basic life support.

In this section, though, we shall concentrate on the ABCs of cardiopulmonary resuscitation. It is assumed that students taking a paramedic course already have training and experience in BLS. The following discussion, therefore, is intended primarily to *review* the principles learned during EMT-A training† and to indicate where changes have been made in recommended procedures. We shall postpone discussion of *advanced* life support until Chapter 23, when we consider cardiovascular emergencies, such as heart attack, in detail.

We have already looked at the A and B of CPR: opening the AIRWAY, checking for BREATHING, and instituting artificial ventilation if breathing is absent. In a patient with respiratory arrest only, those steps will be sufficient to support life. But if the patient has both respiratory *and* cardiac arrest, we need to do something to circulate the blood that we have been so conscientiously oxygenating. That is, we need to add the C of the ABCs: checking for CIRCULATION and instituting an artificial circulation if the pulse is absent.

---

*The material in this section is based on Emergency Cardiac Care Committee and Subcommittees, American Heart Association, Guidelines for cardiopulmonary resuscitation (CPR) and emergency cardiac care. *JAMA* 268:2171, 1992.

†For a more detailed discussion of BLS, see N.L. Caroline, *Emergency Medical Treatment: A Text for EMT-As and EMT-Intermediates* (3rd ed.). Boston: Little, Brown, 1991. Chapters 4–7.

Checking for a Pulse

Having opened the airway and given two full lung inflations, you must next determine whether the victim has a pulse. To do so, maintain head tilt with one hand and place the fingers of your other hand on the victim's Adam's apple (Fig. 9-1A). Then slide your fingers toward you down into the groove between the victim's larynx and neck muscles (Fig. 9-1B) to FEEL FOR A CAROTID PULSE. Palpate lightly, without compressing, for 5 to 10 seconds. If the pulse is palpable, simply continue rescue breathing at a rate of about 12 breaths per minute. If, however, you cannot feel a definite carotid pulsation, you must start external chest compressions.

Positioning the Patient

Although it is possible to open a person's airway and even to provide effective artificial ventilation when someone is sitting or is lying down on a soft surface, external chest compressions can be effective *only* if the patient is SUPINE ON A FIRM SURFACE. Even perfectly performed CPR produces only a fraction of the normal cardiac output, and the perfusion pressure generated by CPR is not high enough to compete with gravity. Thus, if the patient's head is elevated above the level of his heart, blood is unlikely to be able to make the trip uphill to his brain. A firm surface is required because effective chest compressions must depress an adult's sternum (breast bone) at least 1½ to 2 inches (4–5 cm). That cannot be accomplished if the surface beneath the victim gives way with every compression. So the victim should be placed on the ground, the floor, a backboard, or a similar unyielding surface. If he is in bed, place a board under his back or, if a board is not immediately available, move the victim quickly to the floor. If possible, ELEVATE THE LOWER EXTREMITIES—for instance, on pillows—to promote the return of venous blood to the heart and thereby improve cardiac output during chest compressions.

Identification of Landmarks

In the adult, chest compressions are delivered over the lower half of the sternum. The objective is to increase the pressure inside the chest (the **intrathoracic pressure**) and thereby drive blood out of the heart. Direct compression of the heart between the sternum and the spine may also contribute to producing net flow of blood.

To locate the correct spot for applying chest compressions, kneel facing the victim, with your

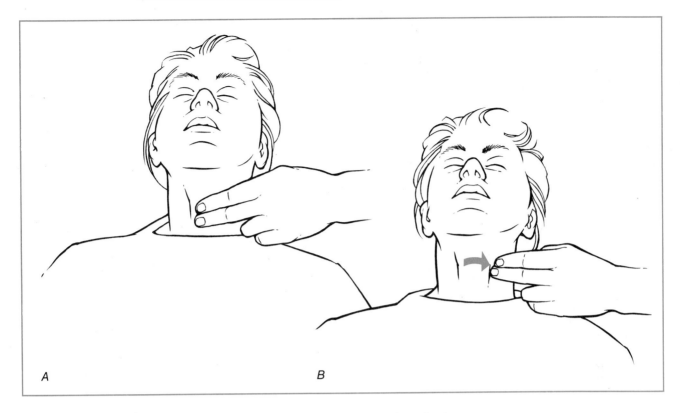

FIGURE 9-1. **PALPATING FOR THE CAROTID PULSE.** (A) Locate the Adam's apple. (B) Slide your fingers toward you, down into the groove between the larynx and the neck muscles.

knees close to his chest. With your hand that is closest to the victim's feet (e.g., your left hand if you are kneeling at his left side), use your middle and index fingers to locate the victim's rib cage on the side nearest you. Then run your fingers up along the rib cage to the notch where the ribs meet the sternum in the center of the lower chest. With your middle finger on that notch, place your index finger beside it on the lower end of the sternum (Fig. 9-2A). Then place the heel of your other hand right next to the index finger on the sternum (Fig. 9-2B). The heel of your hand should be lined up on the long axis of the sternum. Now remove your first hand from the notch, and place it on top of the hand that is in position on the sternum, so that the heels of both hands are parallel, one on top of the other, and your fingers are directed straight away from you. You may hold your fingers interlocked (Fig. 9-3A) or extended (Fig. 9-3B), but in either case, KEEP YOUR FINGERS OFF THE CHEST! Allowing the fingers to rest on the victim's ribs during compressions increases the likelihood of rib fracture or costochondral separation (separation of the ribs from their cartilaginous connections to the sternum).

Delivery of Cardiac Compressions

Once you have established the correct hand position, lock your elbows and POSITION YOUR SHOULDERS DIRECTLY OVER YOUR HANDS, so that the thrust for external chest compressions will be *straight down* (Fig. 9-4). If the thrust is delivered off to a side, the victim's trunk will roll with each compression, and part of the force you apply will be dissipated— so the compression will be less effective. For a normal sized adult, you need to apply enough force with each compression to depress the sternum 1½ to 2 inches (4–5 cm). Then release the pressure completely to allow the heart to refill. THE COMPRESSION PHASE SHOULD OCCUPY AT LEAST HALF OF THE CYCLE. If you are uncertain, err on the side of more sustained compressions and shorter release periods. Avoid bouncing compressions, since they are much less effective and are apt to cause injury. Compressions should be regular, smooth, and uninterrupted. Between compressions, the heel of your hand should rest *lightly* on the sternum, so that it will not move from the correct compression point. Do *not* lift your hands off the chest or change their position

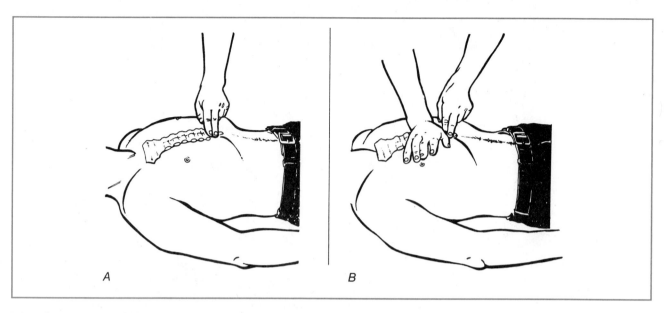

FIGURE 9-2. **LOCATING THE LANDMARKS FOR CHEST COMPRESSIONS.**
(A) Locate the notch at the lower end of the sternum with your middle finger, and place your index finger on the sternum. (B) Place the heel of your
other hand beside the index finger of your first hand. Reproduced courtesy
of Asmund Laerdal, Stavanger, Norway.

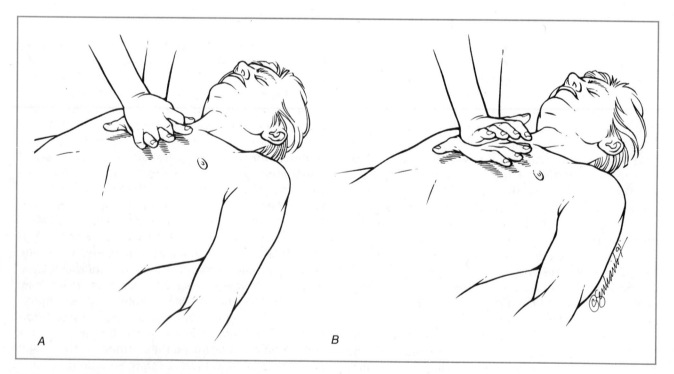

FIGURE 9-3. **KEEP YOUR FINGERS OFF THE CHEST!** Either hold them inter-
laced (A) or extended (B).

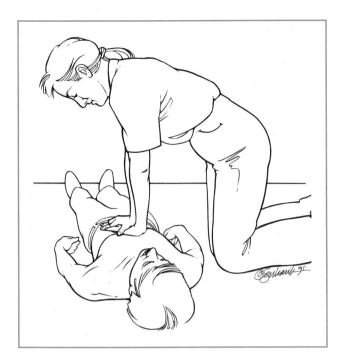

FIGURE 9-4. **PROPER RESCUER POSITION FOR CHEST COMPRESSIONS,** with shoulders directly over the victim's sternum and elbows locked.

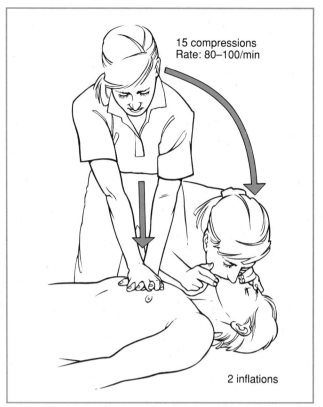

15 compressions
Rate: 80–100/min

2 inflations

FIGURE 9-5. **ONE-RESCUER CPR.** Give 15 compressions followed by 2 full lung inflations.

between compressions. If your hand slips down over the xiphoid (the cartilaginous lower tip of the sternum), compressions may cause laceration of the liver and fatal internal bleeding. Thus you must be sure to maintain proper hand position and to recheck the landmarks if you think your hands may have shifted.

Combining Compressions and Ventilations

Artificial ventilation must *always* be maintained when chest compressions are given. It does precious little good to provide an artificial circulation if the blood being circulated isn't carrying any oxygen! Thus, to carry out full CPR, you must combine rescue breathing with external chest compressions.

When there is ONE RESCUER, chest compressions and artificial ventilation are performed in a ratio of **15 : 2,** that is, 15 CHEST COMPRESSIONS followed by 2 full LUNG INFLATIONS (Fig. 9-5). Because of the interruptions necessary to give the ventilations, you have to deliver the compressions at a rate of **80 to 100 per minute** to ensure that at least 60 compressions are given in a minute's time. The easiest way to keep track of the rate is to count aloud, "One-and-two-and-three-and . . ." up to 15 as you compress. Then give 2 ventilations 1½ to 2 seconds each, and then another 15 compressions, and so forth. After four complete cycles of 15 compressions and 2 ventilations, CHECK FOR THE RETURN OF A SPONTANEOUS PULSE for 3 to 5 seconds. If a pulse

is present, resume ventilations only. If the pulse is absent, resume the entire CPR sequence.

When there are TWO RESCUERS, the first (R1) should be positioned at the victim's head, to maintain the airway and perform rescue breathing, while the second (R2) kneels beside the victim's chest (preferably on the side opposite R1) to perform external chest compressions (Fig. 9-6). The current American Heart Association guidelines recommend that the *compression rate for two rescuers* also be **80 to 100 per minute** (best accomplished by R2 counting out loud, "One-and-two-and-three-and . . ."). In two-rescuer CPR, the ratio of compressions to ventilations is **5 : 1,** and the rescuer performing chest compressions should *pause* for 1½ to 2 seconds after each cycle of 5 compressions to allow for a full ventilation. The pause may be shortened or eliminated once the patient has been intubated; in fact, once the patient is intubated, there is no longer any need to synchronize compressions with ventilations so long as R1 delivers 12 to 15 ventilations per minute and R2 delivers around 80 compressions per minute.

When R2 (the compressor) becomes tired, the rescuers should exchange positions. Doing so will be easier if R1 and R2 are on opposite sides of the victim, for they are less likely to get tangled up in one anoth-

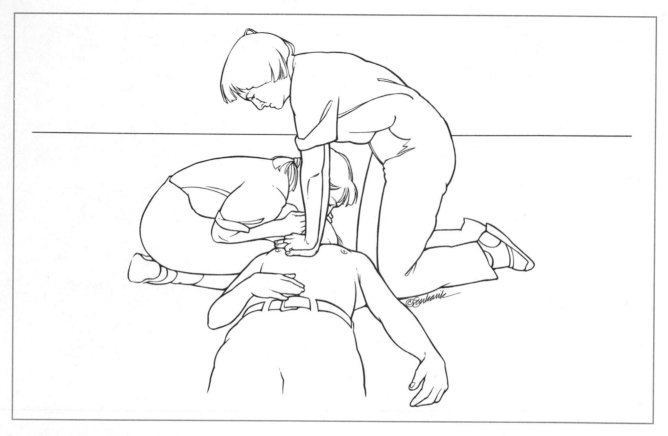

FIGURE 9-6. TWO-RESCUER CPR.   When two rescuers perform CPR, they
should be on opposite sides of the victim so that they do not collide when
changing roles.

er's legs as R1 moves to the victim's chest and R2 moves to the victim's head.

When performing two-rescuer CPR, the rescuer doing ventilations should periodically check the carotid pulse to assess the effectiveness of chest compressions (each compression should produce a palpable pulsation). Every few minutes, CPR should be stopped altogether for a 5-second check for the return of a spontaneous pulse.

The steps of BLS are detailed in the performance checklists at the end of this chapter and are summarized schematically in Figure 9-7. Remember: The most important thing about those steps is that they are ALWAYS PERFORMED IN THE SAME SEQUENCE. That may seem elementary, but in practice it is easy to become distracted from priorities of management when working under pressure in the field. In the unconscious trauma victim, for example, a very dramatic, bloody wound may divert the rescuer's attention from higher priority problems, unless the rescuer consciously reminds himself or herself: "AIRWAY first, *then* BREATHING, *then* PULSE, *then* BLEEDING."

Ensuring Effective CPR

Properly performed CPR may bring a patient back literally from the brink of biologic death. Improperly performed CPR, on the other hand, is likely to be of no benefit whatsoever and may even do harm. Following the guidelines listed below will help to ensure maximally effective CPR with a minimum of complications.

**GUIDELINES FOR EFFECTIVE
CPR**

- Pay attention to the AIRWAY, to keep it fully open.
- AVOID EXCESSIVE INFLATION PRESSURES. Inflate just enough to make the chest rise.
- Maintain PROPER HAND POSITION:
  1. Fingers *off* the chest.
  2. Hands resting *lightly* on the sternum between compressions.

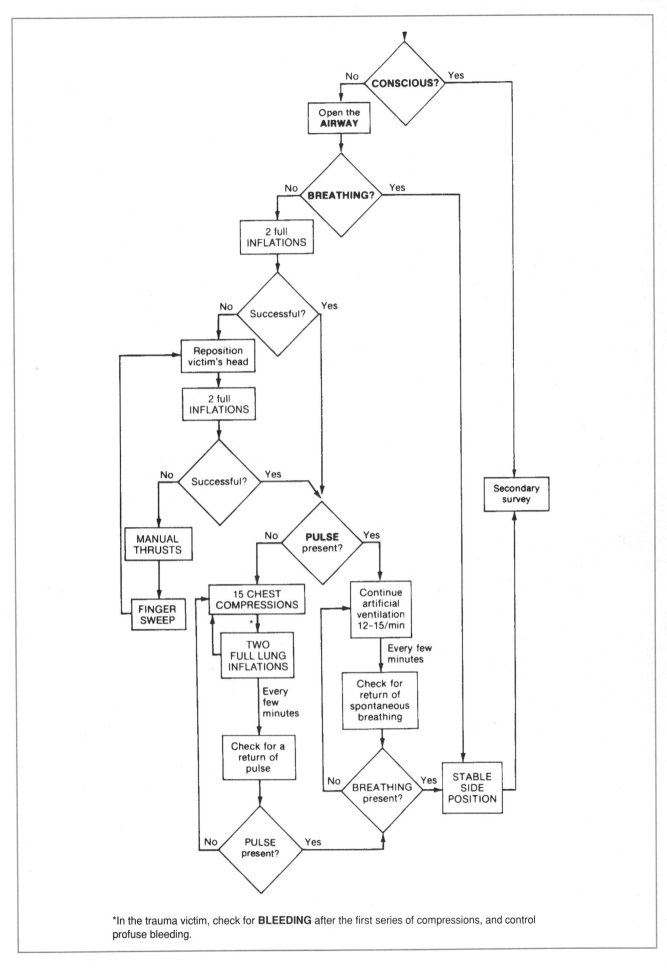

FIGURE 9-7. **BASIC LIFE SUPPORT:** One-rescuer CPR.

- Keep your compressions SMOOTH, REGULAR, AND UNINTERRUPTED.
  1. Maintain each compression for at least half the compression-release cycle.
  2. Avoid bouncing or jerky compressions.
- Keep your SHOULDERS DIRECTLY OVER the victim's STERNUM, and keep your ELBOWS STRAIGHT.
- DO NOT INTERRUPT CPR FOR MORE THAN 7 SECONDS AT A TIME, except for
  1. Endotracheal intubation (may take 20–30 seconds).
  2. Moving the victim, such as up or down stairs (may take 20–30 seconds).

Even properly performed CPR may cause rib fractures or other complications in some patients. Such complications can be minimized by careful attention to details of performance, but they cannot be eliminated altogether. Concern for injuries that might result from properly performed CPR should *never* inhibit a paramedic from carrying out CPR in cardiac arrest. Remember:

> **FOR THE VICTIM OF CARDIAC ARREST, THE ONLY ALTERNATIVE TO CPR IS DEATH.**

When to Deploy CPR

The basic life support techniques described are applicable to *all unconscious victims*, many of whom may require no more than opening the airway. In cases of *respiratory arrest*—as may occur in drowning, stroke, heart attack, airway obstruction, drug overdose, head trauma, electrocution, and so on—artificial ventilation will be required. When there is also *cardiac arrest*, chest compressions must be integrated into the sequence.

CPR is most effective when started immediately after cardiac arrest, and the chances of successful resuscitation decline rapidly as time passes. Therefore there must be a MAXIMUM SENSE OF URGENCY IN STARTING BLS. No more than a few seconds should intervene between recognizing the need for BLS and starting treatment.

It is well established that after a variable period of cardiac arrest (which may be anywhere from 5–30 minutes, depending on the prearrest status of the patient, environmental temperature, and other factors), CPR is unlikely to revive the victim or to restore a useful level of cerebral function. The question therefore arises whether it is worthwhile to start CPR when the victim has been in cardiac arrest for more than a certain amount of time—say, 10 to 15 minutes. The most practical answer to that question is GIVE THE PATIENT THE BENEFIT OF THE DOUBT AND START RESUSCITATION. It is very difficult to know exactly how long a person found unconscious has actually been in cardiac arrest. Even if bystanders can identify the moment of *collapse,* there is no guarantee that the patient's heart stopped beating immediately when he became unconscious. A patient who has been unconscious for 20 minutes may in fact have had a pulse until only a moment before you arrived, and such a patient has every chance of being restored to normal cardiac and cerebral function *if you start CPR.* Thus, the choice boils down to a very simple one:

> **IF YOU START CPR, THE PATIENT MAY OR MAY NOT BE SUCCESSFULLY RESUSCITATED.**
> **IF YOU DO NOT START CPR, THE PATIENT WILL CERTAINLY DIE.**

Does that mean that CPR must be initiated in every person whose heart stops beating? Is no one to be permitted to die peacefully in bed without being assaulted by an army of first aiders or other rescuers? Clearly, that is not the intent of basic life support. CPR is intended for the treatment of SUDDEN, UN-EXPECTED DEATH in persons who might otherwise have many years of productive life ahead. It is not intended for persons known to be in the terminal stages of incurable disease. In general, deciding whether CPR is appropriate is not a major dilemma in the prehospital phase of care; for when an ambulance is summoned, it must be taken for granted that the patient's emergency was unforeseen and that the patient is in need of care. Here again, therefore, give the patient the benefit of the doubt and start CPR. If additional information about the patient's prearrest status becomes available—for instance, that the patient is known to have terminal cancer—that information can be conveyed to the physician who takes over responsibility for the patient at the receiving hospital, and the physician may then decide whether to terminate resuscitation efforts.

"New CPR"

The method of basic life support described above is the method currently recommended by the American Heart Association. It is the method for which we have the most reliable scientific data, and it is the best method we have at the moment. But it is not an ideal method, for even when performed perfectly, standard CPR provides only about 30 percent of normal cerebral perfusion and only 10 percent of normal coronary perfusion. For that reason, there is an ongoing search for more effective ways of doing CPR, and paramedics will no doubt hear about experimental CPR techniques (and may even participate in the research on those techniques). Thus it is useful for the paramedic to be aware of some of the experimental CPR techniques currently being studied. Those include manual techniques that do not require special equipment and mechanical techniques that do require special equipment.

The principal techniques of "new CPR" that do not require special equipment involve giving AB-DOMINAL COMPRESSIONS in addition to chest compressions. The theory is that pressing on the abdomen increases the pressure inside the aorta as well as within the chest, which ought to improve blood flow to vital organs. The abdominal compressions can be applied at the same time as the chest compressions, in which case the technique is called SIMUL-TANEOUS CHEST AND ABDOMINAL COMPRES-SION (CPR-SCAC). Or one can interpose an abdominal compression between every two chest compressions, a technique called, not surprisingly, INTERPOSED ABDOMINAL COMPRESSION (CPR-IAC). Early studies of both techniques have been promising, but there is not yet enough data to warrant recommending either method in place of standard CPR.

Among the techniques of "new CPR" that do require special equipment, two may have potential utility for prehospital care. In the first—called ACTIVE COMPRESSION-DECOMPRESSION (ACD)—a suction device modeled on a household drain plunger ("plumber's helper") is applied to the anterior chest wall. Pushing and pulling rhythmically on the plunger alternately compresses and reexpands the chest. In the first human trials with the device, results were very encouraging, and a good product is now commercially available. (Instructions for use of the ACD device are presented in Chap. 23.) A second device that may have potential field application in the future is the CPR VEST. The vest is fitted around the patient's chest and is then rapidly inflated and deflated by a pneumatic apparatus to create changes in the pressure within the patient's chest. Again, early results look promising, but whether this device, which is quite expensive, will prove effective and practical in the field remains to be seen.

The ABCs in Trauma

Up to this point, we have looked at the ABCs as they apply to a medical patient, that is, a person found unconscious without obvious injury. The cause of unconsciousness may be a cardiac dysrhythmia, drowning, electrocution, or a variety of other problems, but the ABCs of basic life support will be applied in the same way regardless. We need also, however, to consider how the ABCs are applied in the case of the unconscious victim of *trauma*, for there certain modifications in technique (*not* sequence) are required. We shall have a great deal more to say about trauma management in Section IV. For our purposes here, it is sufficient to summarize the special considerations that apply when carrying out CPR in a victim of trauma.

Let us start with the AIRWAY. Every victim of major trauma must be assumed to have sustained an injury to his cervical spine until proved otherwise. Be particularly careful with patients who have been involved in vehicular accidents, falls from a height, or diving accidents or who show injury about the head and face. In such cases, you must AVOID ALL FOR-WARD, BACKWARD, OR LATERAL MOVEMENTS OF THE HEAD. To open the airway, therefore, use **jaw thrust** (Fig. 9-8A), which is basically a modification of the triple airway maneuver *without backward tilt of the head*. Place your hands on either side of the victim's head, so that the head is maintained in a fixed, neutral position without being tilted back. Then use either your thumbs or index fingers to push the mandible forward. If that maneuver is unsuccessful by itself in opening the airway, you may tilt the head back *very slightly*. Alternatively, you may try the **chin lift** (Fig. 9-8B): Place the fingers of one hand under the chin and lift gently upward to bring the chin forward. Use the thumb of the same hand to depress the victim's lower lip lightly and thereby open his mouth. In a variation of the chin lift, the **jaw lift** (Fig. 9-8C), you place your thumb behind the lower incisors rather than beneath the lower lip as you lift gently on the chin with your other fingers. Whichever of those methods you use, be sure to keep the head, neck, and spine in alignment.

The check for BREATHING is carried out in trauma patients just as in other unconscious patients. If breathing is absent, artificial ventilation must be initiated as described in Chapter 8. Trauma to the victim's face may necessitate mouth-to-nose rather than mouth-to-mouth ventilation.

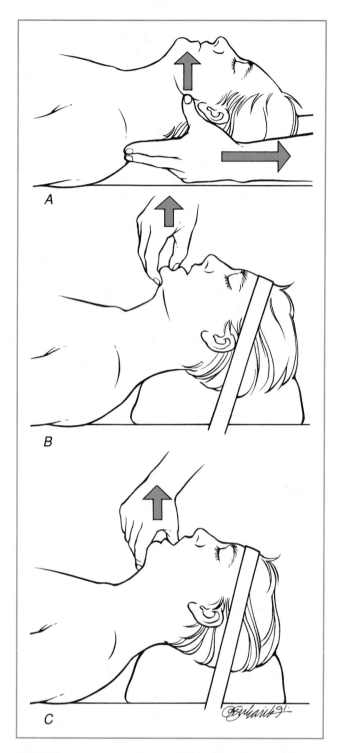

FIGURE 9-8. OPENING THE AIRWAY IN A PATIENT WITH POSSIBLE SPINAL INJURY. (A) Modified jaw thrust. (B) Chin lift. (C) Jaw lift.

Assessing the CIRCULATION in the trauma victim has *two* important elements. First of all, as in any other unconscious victim, you must determine whether there is any circulation at all, that is, whether there is a PULSE. If not, start external chest compressions in the usual fashion. But in the trauma victim, you must also be certain that the patient's circulating blood volume is reaching his tissues and not spilling out of his body with every compression delivered to his chest. Thus, the second element of the circulation that must be checked and attended to as part of the routine ABCs in trauma is BLEEDING. If the patient *is* bleeding profusely, the bleeding must be controlled as soon as possible after chest compressions have been started, lest the patient **exsanguinate** (bleed to death) during the resuscitation.

Unlike the victim of a heart attack or a cardiac dysrhythmia, the victim of trauma found in cardiac arrest is unlikely to be revived solely by CPR in the field. Saving the life of a severely injured person nearly always requires blood replacement and prompt surgery. Therefore, it is of overwhelming importance that the trauma victim in cardiac arrest—or in a condition likely to progress to cardiac arrest (e.g., severe shock)—reach a medical facility as soon as possible. DO NOT DELAY AT THE SCENE. Start basic life support measures, protect the spine from motion, and get on the road! If advanced life support procedures, such as starting an intravenous infusion, are required, do them en route.

> **FOR THE VICTIM OF TRAUMA IN CARDIAC ARREST: START CPR, LOAD, AND GO!**

FLUIDS AND ELECTROLYTES

We have seen that one vital component of the circulatory system is its pump, the heart. In the next two sections, we shall examine a second vital component—the fluids that fill and complement the system and some of the chemicals dissolved in those fluids.

Water and Electrolytes

The human body is composed mostly of water, which provides the environment where the chemical reactions necessary to life take place. Water also serves as a transport medium for nutrients, hormones, and waste materials. The **total body water** (TBW) constitutes 60 percent of the weight of an adult man and is distributed among the following compartments (Fig. 9-9):

- **Intracellular fluid** (ICF) is the water contained inside the cells; it normally accounts for 45 percent of body weight.

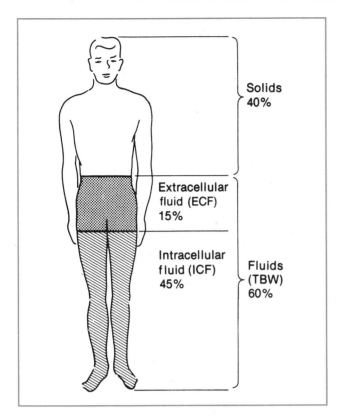

FIGURE 9-9. **BODY FLUIDS.** Sixty percent of body weight is water.

- **Extracellular fluid** (ECF), the water outside the cells, accounts for 15 percent of body weight and is further divided into
  1. **Interstitial fluid,** the water bathing the cells, which accounts for about 10.5 percent of body weight. The interstitial fluid also includes special fluid collections, such as cerebrospinal fluid (CSF) and intraocular fluid.
  2. **Intravascular fluid** (plasma), the water within the blood vessels, which carries red blood cells, white blood cells, and vital nutrients. Intravascular fluid normally accounts for about 4.5 percent of body weight.

Thus, in a man weighing 70 kg (154 lb), there are about 42 liters of water:

ICF = 31.5 liters
ECF = 10.5 liters
   Interstitial fluid = 7.35 liters
   Plasma = 3.15 liters

Water in the body serves as a universal solvent for a variety of solutes. Those solutes can be classified as either electrolytes or nonelectrolytes.

Electrolytes are substances whose molecules dissociate into charged components (**ions**) when placed in water. Ions with a *positive* charge are called *cations*, since they migrate toward the negative pole (cathode) when an electric current is passed through the water. The most important cations in the body are:

CATIONS

Sodium (Na^+)
Potassium (K^+)
Calcium (Ca^{++})
Magnesium (Mg^{++})

Ions with a *negative* charge are called *anions*, since those ions migrate toward the positive pole (anode) when electric current is passed through water. The anions of major significance in the human body include:

ANIONS

Chloride (Cl^-)
Bicarbonate (HCO_3^-)

In physiologic solutions such as the extracellular fluid, the total number of cations always equals the total number of anions.

Let us examine what happens, for example, when ordinary table salt, or sodium chloride (NaCl), is dissolved in water through which an electric current is passed (Fig. 9-10). The NaCl molecules dissociate into Na^+ ions (cations) and Cl^- ions (anions), and each migrates toward the pole of opposite charge.

The unit of measurement for electrolytes is called the **milliequivalent** (mEq), which is the chemical-combining power of the ion and is based on the number of available ionic charges in an electrolyte solution. One milliequivalent of any cation is able to react completely with 1 mEq of any anion. For example, Na^+ is a singly charged (monovalent) cation, and Cl^- is a singly charged anion. Thus 1 mEq of Na^+ will react with 1 mEq of Cl^- to form NaCl (Fig. 9-11). Ca^{++} has *two* positive charges (bivalent cation); thus the Ca^{++} ion represents 2 mEq and requires 2 mEq of a singly charged anion to combine (Fig. 9-12).

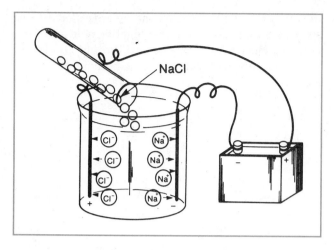

FIGURE 9-10. MIGRATION OF ELECTROLYTES. Positive ions (cations) such as Na^+ migrate toward the negative pole (cathode), while negative ions (anions) such as Cl^- migrate toward the positive pole (anode).

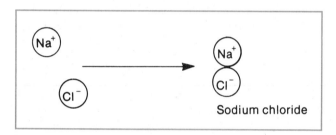

FIGURE 9-11. REACTION OF Na^+ AND Cl^-. When sodium and chloride unite, they form salt (sodium chloride).

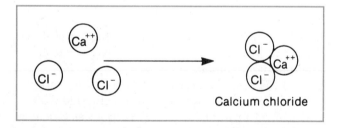

FIGURE 9-12. REACTION OF Ca^{++} AND Cl^-. A doubly charged cation such as Ca^{++} needs two anions.

The body also contains solutes that have no electric charge, **nonelectrolytes**. Those include glucose and urea. Such solutes are usually measured in milligrams (mg). The normal concentration of glucose in the blood, for example, is about 70 to 110 mg per 100 ml. (In the scientific journals, glucose concentration may be expressed in millimoles per liter in accordance with the conventions of the Système International. Using those SI units, the normal concentration of glucose in the blood is 3.9–6.1 mmol/L.)

Osmosis

As noted earlier, the body is made up of several fluid compartments separated from one another by various membranes—cell membranes, the membranes lining blood vessels, and so on. The concentration of fluid in those compartments, that is, the number of solute particles (whether electrolytes or nonelectrolytes) in a given volume, is chiefly influenced by a process called **osmosis.** If two solutions are separated by a semipermeable membrane (e.g., a cell wall), water will flow across the membrane *from* the solution of *lower* concentration *to* the solution of *higher* concentration. The net effect is to equalize the solute concentrations on each side of the membrane.

In Figure 9-13A, a cell has been placed in a solution whose solute concentration is lower than that inside the cell. (The cell is said to be **hypertonic** with respect to the solution in the beaker; conversely, the solution in the beaker is **hypotonic** with respect to the intracellular fluid.) Water moves from the solution of lower concentration (in the beaker) across the cell membrane into the solution of higher concentration (in the cell). The net effect (Fig. 9-13B) is to equalize the solute concentrations inside and outside the cell (to make them **isotonic**). As shown in the figure, the cell must expand its volume to accommodate the extra water.

FIGURE 9-13. OSMOSIS. In osmosis, water moves from the solution of lower concentration to the solution of higher concentration.

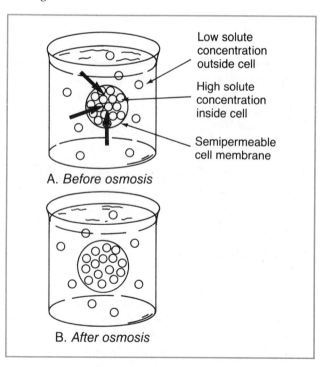

A. *Before osmosis*

B. *After osmosis*

Consider a more clinically relevant situation. Suppose you infused a significant volume of pure water, without any solutes, into a patient's vein. Since the solute concentration inside his red blood cells would be vastly higher than that in the water you infused, water would move in large quantities across the red cell membranes *into* the cells. There is a limit, however, to how far such membranes can be stretched, and eventually the red blood cells would burst from the extra volume inside them. For that reason, intravenous infusions are usually close to isotonic, that is, of approximately the same solute concentration as the blood, in order to minimize such fluid shifts. (Question: What would happen to the red blood cells if you infused a very *hyper*tonic solution into a vein? Would fluid move in or out of the cells? Would extracellular fluid tend to move into or out of the veins?)

In the extracellular fluid, the principal solute exerting osmotic force is sodium (Na^+), which is normally present in a concentration of between 135 and 147 mEq per liter. Normal saline, one of the fluids used for intravenous infusions (see Table 9-3), contains 144 mEq of Na^+ per liter. Thus normal saline is considered to be isotonic with the extracellular fluid.

Diffusion of Solutes

Water passes freely across membranes in the body to produce osmosis. Most membranes, however, limit the passage of *solute* molecules. Some solute molecules cross membranes more readily than others, depending on their size and physical properties. Glucose, for example, rapidly equilibrates across membranes, while sodium has more difficulty passing through the membrane barrier. Large molecules like albumin (one of the plasma proteins) are even more severely restricted. For practical purposes, that means that an intravenous infusion of a glucose solution (e.g., 5% dextrose in water, or D5/W for short) can be expected to equilibrate rapidly between the vascular and extravascular spaces, since glucose can cross membranes quickly and water will follow by osmosis. An infusion of saline (NaCl in water), on the other hand, will stay in the vascular space somewhat longer than a glucose infusion, because Na^+ does not move as rapidly across membranes. After a few hours, however, the Na^+ will also equilibrate between the vascular and extravascular spaces. Solutions of electrolytes, such as saline, or of low-molecular-weight nonelectrolytes, such as D5/W, are referred to as **crystalloids.** Solutions of high-molecular-weight substances, such as albumin or dextran, are called **colloids** and will generally stay in the vascular space for many hours, since their large

molecules do not easily traverse the membranes of cells lining the blood vessels. (Based on that information, which intravenous fluid—D5/W, saline, or albumin—would be *best* for a patient needing intravascular volume expansion, e.g., a patient in hemorrhagic shock? Why?)

Let us review some of the definitions we have learned up to this point:

isotonic solution A solution having a concentration of solute molecules equivalent to that inside the cells (Fig. 9-14). Thus, isotonic solutions administered intravenously into a normally hydrated person will neither draw water out of the cells nor contribute water to the cells. Example: normal saline solution.

hypotonic solution A solution having a solute concentration *lower* than that of the cells (Fig. 9-15). Thus, when a hypotonic solution is infused intravenously into a normally hydrated patient, water will migrate *from* the solution *into* the cells. Example: 1/2 normal saline (72 mEq Na^+/liter).

hypertonic solution A solution having a concentration of solute molecules *higher* than that inside the cells (Fig. 9-16). When a hypertonic solution is administered intravenously to a normally hydrated patient, it will draw water *from* the cells *into* the vascular space. Example: 50% dextrose (D50) or 10% saline solution.

crystalloid solution A solution that does not contain protein or other large molecules. Example: normal saline solution.

colloid solution A solution that does contain protein or other large molecules, hence one that re-

FIGURE 9-14. ISOTONIC SOLUTION. When an isotonic solution is infused into the blood, there is no net movement of water into or out of the cells.

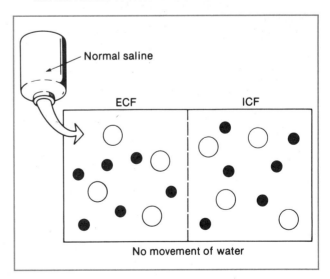

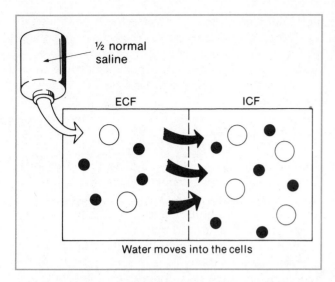

FIGURE 9-15. HYPOTONIC SOLUTION. When a hypotonic solution is infused into the blood, water flows from the plasma into the cells.

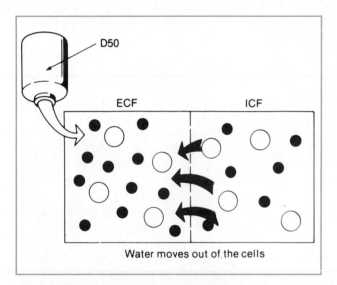

FIGURE 9-16. HYPERTONIC SOLUTION. When a hypertonic solution is infused into the blood, there is net movement of water from the cells into the plasma.

mains in the vascular space longer and is useful in maintaining vascular volume. Example: albumin.

These concepts form the basis for choosing the most appropriate intravenous fluid for any given patient.

A Closer Look at Electrolytes

Each electrolyte serves a specific purpose in the body's work. It is important to know something

about the peculiar characteristics of each, since you will be dealing with patients whose electrolytes may be deranged, and you will be administering solutions with varying electrolyte compositions.

The Principal Cations

Sodium (Na^+) is the most prevalent of the *extracellular* cations and, through its osmotic force, has a primary role in regulating the distribution of water throughout the body. As a general rule, WATER FOLLOWS SODIUM. So if sodium is *lost* from the body, as when a patient takes a diuretic medication, water is lost with it; similarly, when sodium is *retained*, water also is retained. For example, when you eat a bag of potato chips, you ingest a very large quantity of salt ($Na^+ + Cl^-$). Acutely, the body responds by holding onto water (hence urine output temporarily declines). In normal individuals, the kidneys and other regulatory mechanisms soon straighten things out. One of the jobs of the kidneys is to sit and count sodium ions as they circulate by; so sooner or later, the kidneys will detect that there is too much sodium in the body and will excrete the extra sodium along with the retained water. Thus the intake of sodium is balanced by sodium output, and a constant level of sodium is maintained in the body. However, patients with certain illnesses—such as congestive heart failure or some kidney ailments—do not get rid of sodium so readily; they tend instead to *retain* sodium. For such a patient—one with congestive heart failure, for example—who already has an excess of sodium and water aboard, the bag of potato chips may be fatal, for it may cause him to retain so much water that he literally drowns in his own extracellular fluid.

Potassium (K^+) is the chief cation of the *intracellular* fluid and has a critical role in mediating electric impulses in nerves and muscles, including the heart muscle. If the potassium concentration in the body becomes too low or too high, serious cardiac dysrhythmias may develop. An abnormally *high* potassium level (**hyperkalemia**) in the body can sometimes be detected on the electrocardiogram (ECG) by the presence of a tall, peaked T wave (Fig. 9-17). (We shall learn what a T wave *is* in Chapter 23.)

Patients with renal disease tend to have difficulty excreting potassium and may therefore develop hyperkalemia if their dietary intake of potassium is excessive (potassium is found in high concentration in bananas, citrus fruits, tomato juice, and avocados, to name a few). On the other hand, patients taking diuretic medications tend to *lose* significant amounts of potassium and may develop potassium deficiency (**hypokalemia**) if they do not supplement their intake

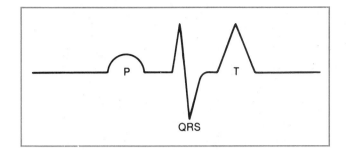

FIGURE 9-17. ECG IN HYPERKALEMIA. An abnormally high serum potassium is sometimes signalled by tall, pointed T waves on the ECG.

with potassium-rich foods or prescribed potassium preparations. (Question: What dietary advice should be given to a patient with chronic heart failure taking diuretic medications? To a patient with chronic renal failure?)

Calcium (Ca^{++}), which we derive largely from milk products and meat in the diet, is a very versatile cation, participating in bone development, blood clotting, and neuromuscular activity. Calcium is required for normal muscle contraction; if a deficit of calcium occurs, muscles become irritable (they start to twitch or go into spasm), and convulsions may result. The heart muscle also depends on calcium for its normal contractility; if calcium is deficient, cardiac contractions will grow feeble.

Magnesium (Mg^{++}), which is contained in many foods, plays an important role as a coenzyme in the metabolism of proteins and carbohydrates. In addition, magnesium acts in a manner similar to calcium in controlling neuromuscular irritability.

The Principal Anions

Chloride (Cl^-) tends to tag along with sodium and thus is found primarily in the extracellular fluid. Since sodium also has an affinity for another anion, bicarbonate, there is a reciprocal relationship between the chloride and bicarbonate concentrations in the extracellular fluid; thus chloride participates indirectly in acid-base balance (discussed later in this chapter).

Bicarbonate (HCO_3^-) is the chief *buffer* in the body, whose job it is to see that the acid-base balance of the body is maintained. If a significant amount of bicarbonate is lost from the body, which may occur in severe diarrhea, a metabolic *acidosis* results. Conversely, if there is an excess of bicarbonate, as may occur when too much bicarbonate is administered during a resuscitation, metabolic *alkalosis* occurs. Those concepts are discussed in more detail later in this chapter.

Other anions include **phosphate** (HPO_4^-), important in cell metabolism; **organic acids,** such as lactic acid; and **proteins.** Plasma proteins play a particularly important role in maintaining vascular volume; because they are large molecules, they stay within the vascular space and thus contribute to the osmotic "pull" of water from the interstitial fluid into the capillaries.

Abnormal States of Fluid and Electrolyte Balance

The healthy body maintains a delicate balance between intake and output of fluids and electrolytes, ensuring that the internal environment is kept fairly constant despite varying inputs and obligatory losses. That constancy of the internal environment is called **homeostasis.** The ill or traumatized body, however, may be unable to maintain homeostasis, and excesses or deficits of fluids and body chemicals may occur. As a medical professional who will be administering intravenous fluids, the paramedic needs to know when parenteral fluids are indicated, what kind of fluids are required for different situations, and when intravenous fluids can be dangerous. Although verbal orders or protocols will largely govern the use of intravenous fluids in the field, it is still necessary for the paramedic to develop judgment in the use of those fluids. At a minimum, the paramedic must know enough about intravenous therapy to question orders that seem inappropriate and to function independently should radio communications fail during an emergency situation.

The normal person loses approximately 2.0 to 2.5 liters of fluid daily through urine output and through the lungs and skin. Those losses are replaced by intake of liquids and by nutrients that are partially converted to water in their metabolism. However, in illness, abnormal states of hydration may occur in which intake and output are no longer in balance.

Dehydration

Abnormal losses of fluids and electrolytes may occur through a variety of mechanisms:

- GASTROINTESTINAL LOSSES, especially through vomiting and diarrhea
- INCREASED INSENSIBLE LOSS (mostly through the lungs), as a consequence of fever, hyperventilation, or high environmental temperatures
- INCREASED SWEATING
- INTERNAL LOSSES ("third space" losses), as occur in peritonitis, pancreatitis, ileus, and other

conditions in which fluid is lost from the vascular space into a body cavity
- PLASMA LOSSES, from burns, drains, and granulating wounds

In each instance, the fluid lost will have a unique electrolyte composition, and long-term therapy will be aimed at restoration of the specific body chemicals that are deficient. For purposes of treatment in the field, however, all excessive fluid losses can be considered to lead to DEHYDRATION.

The *symptoms* of dehydration include loss of appetite (anorexia), nausea, vomiting, and sometimes fainting on standing up (**postural syncope**). On physical examination, the dehydrated patient has *poor skin turgor* (the skin over the forehead or sternum will "tent" when pinched), a *shrunken, furrowed tongue,* and *sunken eyes*. The *pulse* is *weak* and *rapid,* rising more than 15 per minute when the patient is raised from a recumbent to a sitting position (a maneuver that may also cause the patient to feel faint). When fluid and electrolyte depletion are severe, shock and coma may be present.

SYMPTOMS AND SIGNS OF DEHYDRATION: SUMMARY

- Anorexia, nausea
- Postural syncope
- Poor skin turgor
- Furrowed tongue
- Sunken eyes
- Weak, rapid pulse

The dehydrated patient needs REPLACEMENT OF FLUID AND ELECTROLYTES and therefore should be given an intravenous infusion of normal saline or Ringer's solution (see Table 9-3), at a rate usually around 100 to 200 ml per hour for an adult, depending on the circumstances. Keep the patient flat to optimize circulation to the brain. The treatment of associated shock will be discussed later in this chapter.

Overhydration

Overhydration occurs when there is an increase in total body salt and water, as in congestive heart failure or some cases of cirrhosis of the liver.

THE CARDINAL SIGN OF OVERHYDRATION IS EDEMA.

However, edema (swelling) does not become clinically apparent until 2 to 4 kg (5–10 lb) of excess fluid has been retained. Patients with heart disease may also manifest circulatory overload in the form of left heart failure (see Chap. 23), with dyspnea, bubbly noises (crackles) in their lungs, and other signs of pulmonary edema. Obviously, such patients do *not* need any more fluid. Indeed, therapy is directed at RIDDING THE BODY OF EXCESS FLUIDS through salt restriction, diuretic drugs, and occasionally even bloodletting (phlebotomy). Therefore, when you must start an IV on an already overhydrated patient for purposes of keeping a route open for intravenous medications, the goals should be (1) to give as little fluid as possible (use a microdrip fluid administration set, and regulate the rate to "keep open") and (2) to give a type of fluid that will not stay in the vascular space, for example D5/W.

Acid-Base Balance

Acid-base balance refers to the regulation of the amount of **hydrogen ions** (H^+) in body fluids. The body must maintain the concentration of hydrogen ions within strict limits for cells to function optimally. Even slight deviations from the normal hydrogen ion concentration can profoundly disturb vital chemical reactions, such as the release of oxygen from the blood into the tissues. The term **pH** is used to express the hydrogen ion concentration of a fluid.

At a pH of 7.0, a solution is neutral. A fluid with a pH *below* 7.0 has an *increased* concentration of hydrogen ions and is called **acid,** while a fluid with a pH *above* 7.0 has a *decreased* concentration of hydrogen ions and is called **alkaline** or **basic.** (Question: Is a pH of 7.1 more acid or more alkaline than a pH of 7.6? Does the solution of pH 7.1 have a higher or lower hydrogen ion concentration than the solution of pH 7.6?)

The body maintains a slightly alkaline pH, the normal pH range in the extracellular fluid being 7.35 to 7.45. At a pH higher than that range (hydrogen ion concentration decreased), the body is considered to be in a state of **alkalosis.** A pH below that range (hydrogen ion concentration increased) indicates **acidosis.** The latter term is a relative one, since the body fluid rarely becomes truly acid (pH below 7.0), but only relatively more acid than normal.

The extreme limits of pH compatible with life are about 6.9 on the acid side and 7.8 on the alkaline side.

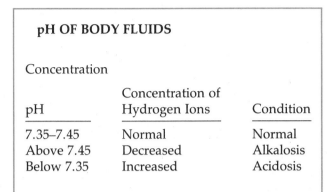

pH OF BODY FLUIDS

Concentration

pH	Concentration of Hydrogen Ions	Condition
7.35–7.45	Normal	Normal
Above 7.45	Decreased	Alkalosis
Below 7.35	Increased	Acidosis

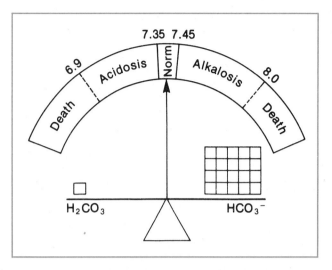

FIGURE 9-18. BICARBONATE BUFFER SYSTEM.
When body fluids are in acid-base balance, the ratio of HCO_3^- to H_2CO_3 is normally 20 : 1 and the pH is between 7.35 and 7.45.

The process of metabolism usually produces an excess of *acid*. The body must rid itself of that acid to maintain acid-base balance; that is, to keep the hydrogen ion concentration within the normal range. For that purpose, the body has three principal lines of defense:

- The BUFFER SYSTEM
- The RESPIRATORY SYSTEM
- The RENAL SYSTEM

The BUFFER SYSTEM is the most rapidly acting of the three defense mechanisms, operating within a fraction of a second to prevent excessive shifts in hydrogen ion concentration. A **buffer** is like a chemical sponge that is able to soak up hydrogen ions when they are present in excess and release them when their concentration is deficient. The most important buffer system in the body is the CARBONATE SYSTEM, which consists of a mixture of carbonic acid (H_2CO_3) and bicarbonate (HCO_3^-) in a normal ratio of 1 : 20 (Fig. 9-18).

Carbonic acid is a weak acid that constantly breaks down and reforms into water (H_2O) and carbon dioxide (CO_2):

$$H_2CO_3 \rightarrow H_2O + CO_2$$

or into hydrogen ions and bicarbonate ions:

$$H_2CO_3 \rightarrow H^+ + HCO_3^-$$

Thus, carbonic acid is in equilibrium with both carbon dioxide and bicarbonate:

$$H_2O + CO_2 \leftrightarrow H_2CO_3 \leftrightarrow H^+ + HCO_3^-$$

The direction in which the reaction proceeds depends in part on what substrates are present in excess. For example, if carbon dioxide is added to the system (as in hypoventilation, with carbon dioxide retention), the reaction will proceed to the right in an attempt to rebalance the system:

$$\boxed{CO_2} + H_2O \rightarrow H_2CO_3 \rightarrow H^+ + HCO_3^-$$

As a consequence, carbonic acid is produced, and the fluid becomes slightly more acid; it is prevented from becoming extremely acid, however, because the carbonic acid generated partially dissociates into bicarbonate. On the other hand, if hydrogen ion is added to the system, as in diabetic acidosis, the reaction proceeds largely to the left:

$$CO_2 + H_2O \leftarrow H_2CO_3 \leftarrow \boxed{H^+} + HCO_3^-$$

In this instance, the excess acid leads to generation of excess CO_2. To help dispose of that excess carbon dioxide, we need another line of defense, that furnished by the respiratory system.

The RESPIRATORY SYSTEM acts as a backup in acid-base regulation. The respiratory mechanism is slower than the buffer mechanism, requiring about 1 to 3 minutes to be effective.

Increased blood levels of CO_2 or H^+ stimulate the respiratory center in the brainstem, which in turn issues orders to the lungs to increase the rate and depth of respiration. That in turn increases the minute volume (remember?) and therefore the rate at which CO_2 is exhaled from the lungs. The CO_2 concentration in the extracellular fluid falls, and consequently there is less CO_2 available to form carbonic acid. As the CO_2 and hydrogen ion concentrations return toward normal, the stimulus to the respiratory center decreases, and the rate and depth of breathing also return toward normal. (Question: Why does a diabetic in ketoacidosis hyperventilate? Hint: What happens when you add H^+ to the system?)

The RENAL SYSTEM, the third line of defense, is a slow mechanism for dealing with changes in hydrogen ion concentration, requiring from several hours to several days to operate. Thus, renal regulation is important chiefly in the long-term maintenance of acid-base balance.

The kidneys play their role in pH regulation by excreting excess hydrogen or bicarbonate ions that have accumulated in the body. The kidneys count hydrogen ions (when they are not busy counting sodium ions). If the pH of the extracellular fluid falls (i.e., hydrogen ion concentration increases), the kidneys eliminate more hydrogen ions; if the pH of the extracellular fluid rises (i.e., hydrogen ion concentration decreases), the kidneys eliminate more bicarbonate ions to restore the balance.

The lines of defense in acid-base regulation are summarized in Figure 9-19.

Let us look at some of the clinical situations in which those concepts are important. Normally, as mentioned, bicarbonate and carbonic acid in the extracellular fluid are in balance, as shown in Figure 9-20. However, there are several clinical conditions in which that balance is disrupted.

Respiratory Acidosis

Any condition that hampers ventilation may result in retention of CO_2 and thus an increase of carbonic acid in the blood.

$$\text{Breathing } \downarrow \rightarrow CO_2 \uparrow \rightarrow H_2CO_3 \uparrow \rightarrow \text{pH} \downarrow$$
$$\text{(acidosis)}$$

Because the *pH falls*, the condition is, by definition, an ACIDOSIS; and because in this instance the primary problem is in the respiratory component of the system—a failure to sustain a sufficient minute volume—it is a RESPIRATORY acidosis (Fig. 9-21). Respiratory acidosis may occur, for example, in chronic bronchitis, where obstruction to gas exchange in the lungs prevents CO_2 from being eliminated normally.

Whenever there is a disturbance in acid-base balance, the body will try to compensate for it by mobilizing one of the lines of defense described earlier. In respiratory acidosis, the respiratory system is the site of the problem, so the respiratory system cannot be

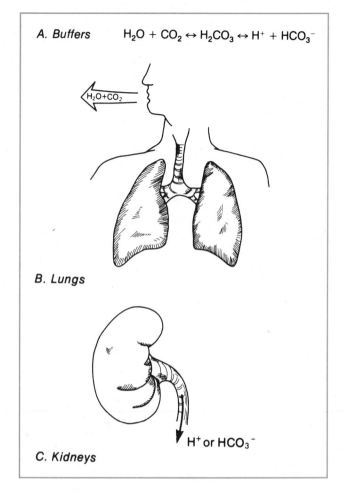

A. Buffers $H_2O + CO_2 \leftrightarrow H_2CO_3 \leftrightarrow H^+ + HCO_3^-$

B. Lungs

C. Kidneys H^+ or HCO_3^-

FIGURE 9-19.   LINES OF DEFENSE IN ACID-BASE BALANCE.   The body has three principal mechanisms for regulating acid-base balance: the bicarbonate buffer system, the lungs, and the kidneys.

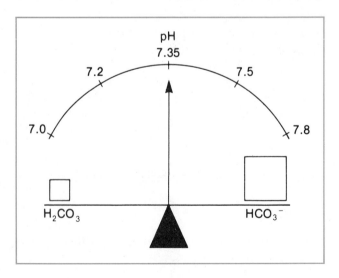

FIGURE 9-20.   NORMAL ACID-BASE BALANCE.

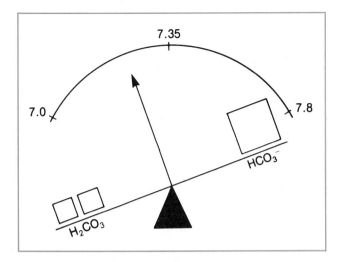

FIGURE 9-21. RESPIRATORY ACIDOSIS. An excess of CO_2 in the body tilts the balance toward acidosis.

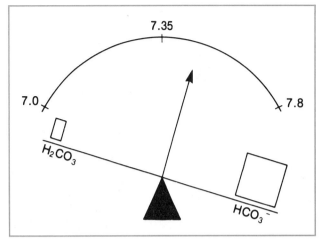

FIGURE 9-22. RESPIRATORY ALKALOSIS. When too much acid is blown off, in the form of CO_2, the balance tilts toward alkalosis.

deployed to compensate for the disturbance. The body's compensation comes instead from the kidneys, which conserve bicarbonate and excrete more hydrogen ions to normalize the pH.

If we want to *treat* a person in respiratory acidosis, we need to attack the underlying defect directly, that is, to improve the patient's breathing so that he will blow off more CO_2. If, for example, we *assist the patient's ventilations* with a bag-valve-mask, we can increase his tidal volume (and therefore his minute volume) and help him excrete more of the retained CO_2 through his lungs.

Respiratory Alkalosis

In respiratory alkalosis, the problem is just the reverse: There is a deficiency of carbonic acid because of excessive CO_2 elimination (Fig. 9-22). Respiratory alkalosis may occur, for example, when an anxious person hyperventilates and thereby blows off more CO_2 than his metabolic processes are producing:

$$\text{Breathing} \uparrow \rightarrow CO_2 \downarrow \rightarrow H_2CO_3 \downarrow \rightarrow \text{pH} \uparrow$$
$$\text{(alkalosis)}$$

Again, because the primary defect is in the respiratory system, *compensation* must come from the kidneys, which in this instance have to excrete bicarbonate ions and retain hydrogen ions to return the pH toward normal.

Theoretically, one could *treat* respiratory alkalosis by administering CO_2 to the patient, to give him back the CO_2 he has blown off. That is, in fact, the principle behind the way we used to manage the hyperventilation syndrome: The patient would be instructed to breathe into a paper bag, which

compelled him to rebreathe his own exhaled CO_2. That method is no longer recommended, since the exhaled air in the paper bag is rapidly depleted of oxygen, and the patient may become hypoxemic long before he is able to normalize his PCO_2. So it is now recommended simply to calm and reassure the hyperventilating patient so that he will slow his respiratory rate.

Metabolic Acidosis

Metabolic acidosis occurs when the metabolic processes of the body produce an excess of acid, as is the case in diabetic ketoacidosis. The acid poured into the extracellular fluid consumes some of the bicarbonate buffer. Thus there is both an increase in acid and a decrease in the available base (Fig. 9-23).

Immediate *compensation* for metabolic acidosis occurs through the lungs. We have already pointed out that a fall in pH stimulates the respiratory center to increase the rate and depth of respiration. As that occurs, more CO_2 is blown off, and the concentration of carbonic acid falls. Over the long term, however, the kidneys also kick in to excrete more hydrogen ions, again to compensate for the excess acid in the extracellular fluid.

To *treat* metabolic acidosis, we need to give the patient back some of the bicarbonate that has been consumed. That is usually done by administering sodium bicarbonate solution intravenously. Definitive treatment of a metabolic acidosis, however, involves eliminating the cause. If a person is in shock, for example, and is churning out lactic acid from anaerobic metabolism, bicarbonate or another buffer may tide him over for a while; but the most important aspect of treatment will be to correct the tissue hypoxia that

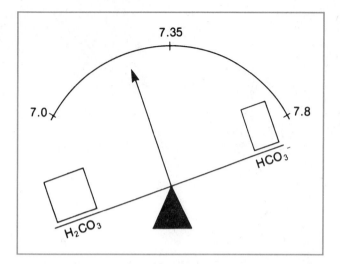

FIGURE 9-23.   METABOLIC ACIDOSIS.   An excess of metabolic acids in the body both consumes bicarbonate and liberates hydrogen ions; the net effect is to tilt the balance toward acidosis.

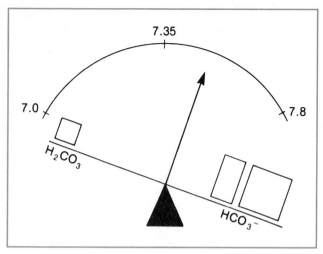

FIGURE 9-24.   METABOLIC ALKALOSIS.   An excess of bicarbonate tilts the balance toward alkalosis.

led to the production of excess lactic acid in the first place.

Metabolic Alkalosis

Metabolic alkalosis may come about from ingesting large amounts of sodium bicarbonate as an antacid; it may also occur when a physician or paramedic administers too much sodium bicarbonate intravenously to a patient (Fig. 9-24).

The lungs make a perfunctory attempt to compensate for metabolic alkalosis by slightly decreasing the respiratory rate and depth in order to retain CO_2. But the lungs are not going to quit breathing altogether just to make the acid-base centers happy; so the kidneys pitch in to retain hydrogen ions and thus balance the excess bicarbonate.

The derangements of acid-base balance are summarized in Figure 9-25.

BLOOD AND ITS COMPONENTS

Blood is the circulating fluid of the cardiovascular system, and it serves a variety of functions:

- *Respiratory* function: Blood transports oxygen from the lungs to the tissues and carbon dioxide from the tissues to the lungs.
- *Nutritional* function: Blood carries nutrients (glucose, proteins, fats) from the digestive tract to cells throughout the body.

- *Excretory* function: Blood ferries the waste products of metabolism from the cells where they are produced to excretory organs.
- *Regulatory* function: Blood brings hormones to their target organs and transmits excess internal heat to the surface of the body to be dissipated.
- *Defensive* function: Blood carries defensive cells and antibodies, which protect the body against foreign organisms.

Composition of Blood

Blood consists of formed elements (cells) and the fluid (plasma) in which the formed elements are suspended.

Formed Elements

RED BLOOD CELLS (RBCs), or **erythrocytes,** lend blood its characteristic color. In the normal adult, red blood cells account for 40 to 45 percent of the blood by volume. The percent of whole blood accounted for by red blood cells is called the **hematocrit** (Fig. 9-26). With severe blood loss or chronic anemia, the hematocrit may fall much lower than 45 percent.

The most important constituent of the red blood cell is a molecule called **hemoglobin,** an iron-containing protein that has the ability to unite with oxygen. In so doing, hemoglobin acquires a bright red color, the color associated with arterial blood. When hemoglobin releases oxygen, its color returns to the darker red-blue shade characteristic of venous blood. Human blood normally contains about 15 gm of hemoglobin per 100 ml of blood. If more than 5 gm of hemoglobin per 100 ml of blood becomes unsaturated, that is, not combined with oxygen, the blood

Condition	pH	H_2CO_3	HCO_3^-	Diagram	Compensation	Examples
Respiratory acidosis	↓	↑	—	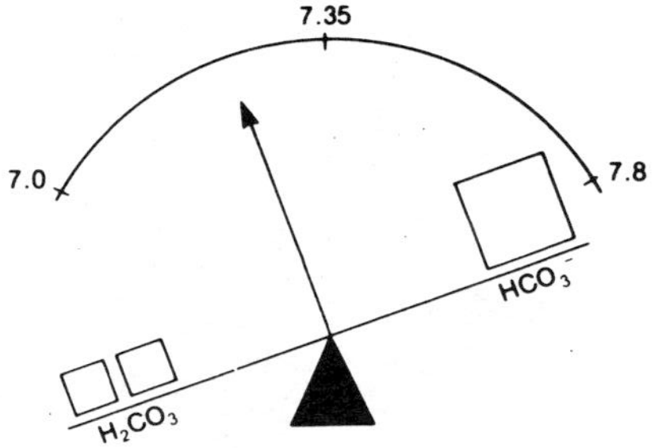	Kidneys excrete H^+, retain HCO_3^-	Respirations depressed by drugs, trauma; emphysema; chronic bronchitis
Respiratory alkalosis	↑	↓	—	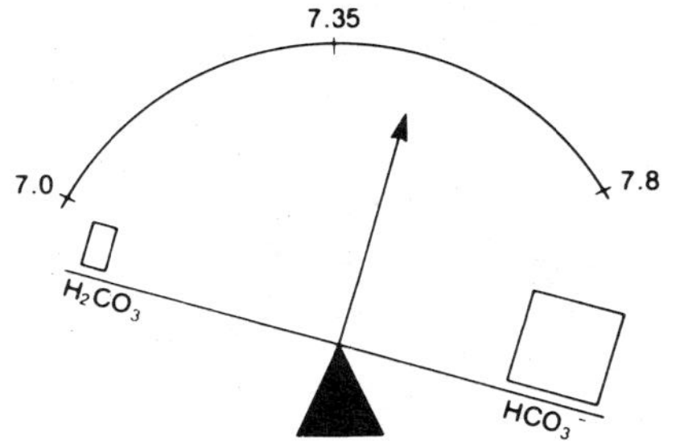	Kidneys excrete HCO_3^-, retain H^+	Hyperventilation syndrome
Metabolic acidosis	↓	↑	↓	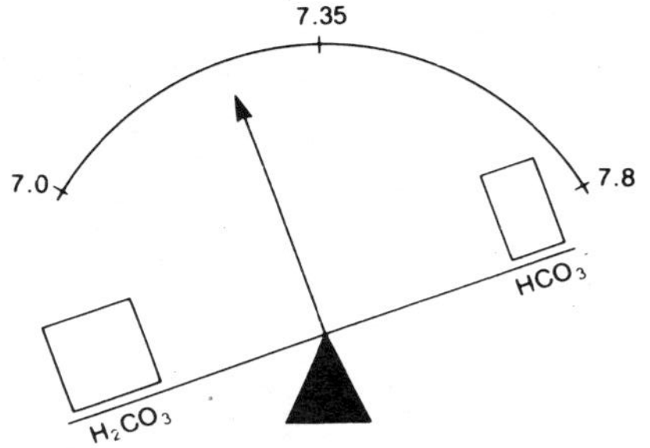	Lungs exhale more CO_2; kidneys excrete H^+	Diabetic ketoacidosis; lactic acidosis in shock
Metabolic alkalosis	↑	—	↑	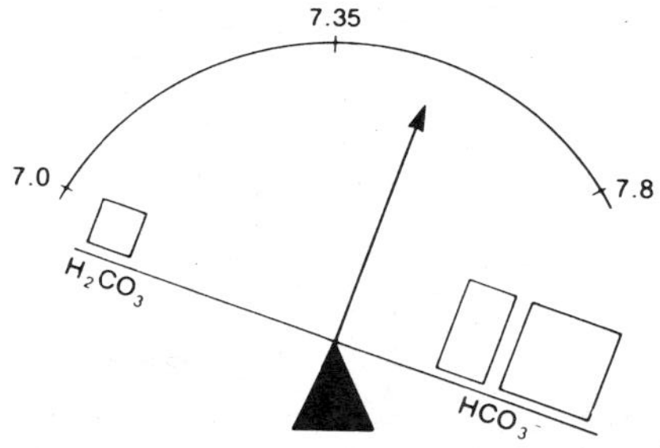	Lungs retain CO_2; kidneys retain H^+	Ingestion of sodium bicarbonate

FIGURE 9-25. SUMMARY: DERANGEMENTS OF ACID-BASE BALANCE.

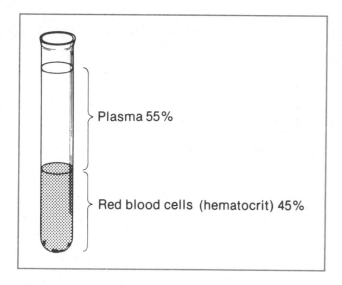

Plasma 55%

Red blood cells (hematocrit) 45%

FIGURE 9-26.　BLOOD COMPOSITION.　Normally, red blood cells account for about 45 percent of the volume of blood.

assumes a bluish color, which is reflected in the skin and mucous membranes as **cyanosis.** It is important to note, however, that a person who is deficient in hemoglobin, such as someone suffering from anemia, may have a large percentage of his hemoglobin unsaturated *without* manifesting cyanosis. For example, if the patient's hemoglobin is 6 gm per 100 ml and 3 gm per 100 ml is not combined with oxygen, he will *not* be cyanotic even though 50 percent of his hemoglobin is unsaturated. Thus, cyanosis is not a reliable guide to the state of a patient's oxygenation. If present, cyanosis does suggest hypoxemia, but the absence of cyanosis does *not* inevitably imply that a person is adequately oxygenated.

WHITE BLOOD CELLS (WBCs), or **leukocytes,** serve a defensive function by engulfing infective organisms, such as bacteria, and by producing antibodies.

PLATELETS, or **thrombocytes,** participate in the process of blood clotting and sealing leaks in injured vessels.

Plasma

Plasma constitutes about 55 percent of the blood by volume and is a complex fluid, containing a variety of proteins (clotting factors, hormones, enzymes, antibodies), inorganic salts, nutrients, waste materials, and gases in solution. Because of its high protein content, pooled human plasma has been used as a replacement for fluid in patients with significant blood loss. As we shall see later, however, there are other fluids that can be used more safely for the same purpose.

Blood Typing

The normal plasma of one individual may contain substances that will cause clumping together (**agglutination**) of the red blood cells of another individual. Such bloods are termed *incompatible,* and if they are mixed together by a transfusion, serious and even fatal reactions may ensue. The safe administration of blood from a donor to a patient requires that the blood of both donor and recipient be typed and cross matched to ensure that the patient receives only blood that is compatible with his own. The compatibility of blood is based on the presence or absence of certain special proteins called **antigens** on the surface of red blood cells and the presence or absence of **antibodies** to those antigens in the plasma. The major classification scheme for blood is known as the *ABO system,* and the blood types are named for the antigen present on the red blood cells.

From Table 9-1, we can see that an individual with type A blood should not receive a transfusion from a type B donor, since the donor's red blood cells would be agglutinated rapidly by the recipient's anti-B antibody. The individual with type A blood could safely receive blood either from another type A person or from a type O donor, whose red cells have no antigens. (Because of that property of his red blood cells, the type O individual is known as a *universal donor;* i.e., he can donate blood to individuals of all blood types. The type AB individual, on the other hand, has no *antibodies* in his plasma; thus he can *receive* blood from any other group. Persons of blood type AB are therefore called universal *recipients.* In practice, however, it is best to cross match every blood donation, even from a type O donor, for minor antigen groups other than the ABO groups may cause incompatibility.)

The relationships among the ABO groups are diagrammed in Table 9-2.

Rh Factor

The red cells of about 85 percent of the population also contain an antigen known as Rh factor (taken from the word *Rhesus,* the type of monkey in which research on this factor has been conducted). When the red cells contain that substance, the blood is called *Rh-positive;* when the red cells lack the antigen, the blood is termed *Rh-negative.* Antibodies (agglutinins) to the Rh antigen do not occur naturally in the body. However, they may develop within a few weeks in the blood of an Rh-negative individual if he receives a transfusion of Rh-positive blood. Once sensitized, the Rh-negative person may have a severe or fatal reaction should he subsequently receive another transfusion of Rh-positive blood. A similar sen-

TABLE 9-1. BLOOD TYPING—ABO SYSTEM

BLOOD TYPE	ANTIGEN PRESENT ON RBC	ANTIBODY PRESENT IN SERUM
A	A	Anti-B
B	B	Anti-A
AB	A and B	None
O	None	Anti-A and Anti-B

TABLE 9-2. COMPATIBILITY AMONG ABO BLOOD GROUPS

CELLS OF DONOR	REACTION WITH SERUM OF RECIPIENT			
	O	A	B	AB
O	−	−	−	−
A	+	−	+	−
B	+	+	−	−
AB	+	+	+	−

+ = agglutination; − = nonagglutination

sitization may occur in a pregnant Rh-negative woman if she is carrying an Rh-positive fetus. As Rh-positive antigens from the fetus cross the placenta into the mother's circulation, she may develop antibodies against the Rh factor. If in a subsequent pregnancy she again carries an Rh-positive baby, the agglutinins in her blood may cause destruction of the red blood cells in the fetus.

Blood Preparations, Derivatives, and Substitutes

Whole Blood

Whole blood is drawn in a special solution to prevent clotting and, after typing, is stored in the cold until needed for use. It can be kept for 2 to 3 weeks, but as it ages the platelets within it deteriorate; therefore if a patient receives a great deal of banked blood, his clotting abilities may be impaired. For that reason, when massive transfusions are necessary, a few units of relatively fresh blood should be given along with the banked blood.

The most important indication for administering whole blood is to restore circulating volume in patients with *acute loss of whole blood,* such as from trauma or massive internal hemorrhage. Whole blood is much less suited to the treatment of shock resulting from loss of plasma alone (e.g., burns) or from loss of extracellular fluid (e.g., massive diarrhea).

Whenever it is given, whole blood should be administered through a special infusion set that contains filters to screen out particulate matter.

Packed Red Blood Cells

Packed red blood cells are obtained by separating the red cells from the plasma in which they are suspended. Packed cells are stored in the cold and remain viable for about 2 to 3 weeks. Like whole blood, packed red cells must be typed and cross matched before administration. (Why?) The use of packed red cells is indicated to *improve the oxygen-carrying capacity of the blood;* thus they are given primarily for various types of severe anemia. In some institutions, packed red blood cells reconstituted in crystalloid or colloid solutions are also favored for the treatment of hemorrhagic shock.

Plasma

Plasma, obtained by taking the supernatant of sedimented whole blood, is available in several forms—liquid, fresh-frozen, and vacuum dried—each of which has certain advantages and disadvantages. The fresh-frozen form is the most commonly used. The primary indication for giving fresh-frozen plasma is to correct coagulation problems due to documented deficiencies in clotting factors. Plasma is also sometimes used as an emergency volume expander in the treatment of shock, since plasma need not be cross matched and thus can be given immediately while waiting for cross-matched blood to become available. There are, however, safer solutions than plasma for volume expansion (plasma, like whole blood and packed cells, may carry the hepatitis virus); so many authorities now feel that plasma should be reserved for patients with proven coagulation problems.

Plasma Substitutes

There are a variety of macromolecular solutions available that have colloidal and osmotic properties similar to those of plasma and that are used to maintain circulatory volume in the emergency treatment of shock. While such solutions do not replace red blood cells, platelets, or plasma proteins lost in hemorrhage, they are more readily available than whole blood or plasma in an emergency, since they do not require typing and can be carried in the ambulance. Furthermore, during mass casualties, the supply of blood and blood products may not be adequate, and substitutes must be used. Plasma substitutes do not carry the risk of hepatitis or AIDS.

Among the various plasma substitutes or volume expanders are dextrans, plasma protein fractions, and polygeline. DEXTRANS are high-molecular-weight glucose polymers that stay in the vascular space because of their large size. Because they tend to coat red blood cells, dextrans may cause clotting problems if given in large quantities, and they can also interfere with the cross matching of blood. For that reason, if dextrans are to be used, blood for type and cross match should be drawn *before* dextran administration. High-molecular-weight dextran also interferes with platelet function, so it may increase bleeding.

PLASMA PROTEIN FRACTION (Plasmanate) contains mainly albumin plus a small amount of serum globulin. It is an excellent plasma substitute, but expensive and reported to produce hypotensive reactions in some patients.

POLYGELINE (Haemaccel), HETASTARCH (Hespan), and other starch solutions are constituted to resemble the osmotic and electrolyte composition of the plasma and do not interfere with clotting or blood typing. Many of these products have a long shelf life and are thus ideally suited for prehospital use.

Crystalloids

Crystalloids, as noted earlier, are solutions that do not contain protein or other large molecules; that is, they are noncolloids. Their effects in restoring volume in shock are usually quite transitory, since the fluid rapidly equilibrates across the capillary walls into the tissues. It has been shown, for example, that approximately 60 percent of infused normal saline, when given as a bolus, will diffuse out of the intravascular space within 20 minutes of administration. Thus, when noncolloid solutions are used in the treatment of hemorrhagic shock, you need to give two to three times the volume of blood lost.

There is no argument that crystalloids are the fluids of choice in situations where only salt and water have been lost, such as dehydration. Where debate continues, however, is in regard to the role of crystalloids versus colloids in the treatment of shock. Despite a great deal of research on the subject, there is still no overwhelming evidence to support one therapeutic approach over the other. Until such evidence *is* forthcoming, practical considerations will continue to favor the use of crystalloids for initial fluid resuscitation in the field.

The crystalloids most commonly used for that purpose are normal saline and Ringer's solution. **Normal saline** is simply sodium chloride (NaCl) in water at a concentration isotonic with the extracellular fluid. **Ringer's solution** is similarly constituted, but has small amounts of potassium and calcium added. **Lactated Ringer's** solution contains 28 mEq of lactate as well, which is added as a buffer (the liver breaks lactate down into bicarbonate). There is no evidence that any one of these solutions is superior to another for acute resuscitation, so the choice among them remains a matter of the physician's preference.

Recently there has been considerable interest in the use of **hypertonic saline solutions** (3–6%) for emergency treatment of blood loss. Infusing a hypertonic solution should, in theory, attract interstitial fluid into the vascular space (why?), so such solutions should, at least temporarily, improve intravascular volume. Early experiments in animals have been promising, but the effectiveness of such fluids in humans remains to be demonstrated.

The compositions of the more commonly used intravenous fluids are summarized in Table 9-3.

Complications of Blood Transfusion

The paramedic will not ordinarily be performing blood transfusions, but he or she may be called on to transport a patient who has a blood transfusion already running. For that reason, the paramedic needs to be aware of possible complications of transfusion and know how to spot the early signs of such complications.

FEVER is the most common transfusion reaction. It may be caused by a sensitivity to the donor's white blood cells or by contamination of transfusion equipment. ALLERGIC REACTIONS are also relatively common and are usually manifested by **urticaria** (hives).

HEMOLYTIC REACTIONS, that is, the disruption of red blood cells due to incompatibility, are less common but very serious. Such reactions usually become evident by the time about 50 ml of donor blood has been infused. The patient may then start to complain of low back pain, throbbing headache, shortness of breath, or substernal pain, and he may become restless and anxious. However, hemolytic reactions may also occur with few symptoms at all, especially in the semiconscious or comatose patient. On physical examination, the patient having a transfusion reaction will often show

- Flushing of the face, followed by cyanosis
- Diaphoresis (sweating), with cold, clammy skin
- Bradycardia, followed by a rapid, thready pulse
- Distended neck veins
- Falling blood pressure

TABLE 9-3.   COMMONLY USED INTRAVENOUS FLUIDS

SOLUTION	GLUCOSE (MG%)	CATIONS (mEq/L)			ANIONS (mEq/L)	
		Na$^+$	K$^+$	Ca^{++}	Cl$^-$	LACTATE
D5/W	5					
D50	50					
0.45% NaCl		77			77	
0.9% NaCl*		154			154	
3% NaCl		513			513	
Ringer's		147.5	4	4.5	156	
Ringer's lactate		130	4	3	109	28
D5/LR	5	130	4	3	109	28

*Also known as normal saline

IF YOU SUSPECT A TRANSFUSION REACTION FOR ANY REASON, STOP THE TRANSFUSION IMMEDIATELY.

Do not wait for further symptoms to occur. To repeat, STOP THE TRANSFUSION IMMEDIATELY! Then take the following steps:

- Keep the intravenous (IV) line open with D5/W.
- Save the remaining donor blood for further testing.
- Draw an unclotted blood sample (purple-top Vacutainer tube) from the patient, from a site other than the IV line.
- Notify the physician, who may instruct you to give furosemide (Lasix), an 80- to 100-mg bolus IV. The furosemide is followed by infusion of D5/W at 100 ml per hour.
- If hypotension (low blood pressure) develops, infuse normal saline or plasma substitutes rapidly.

Another potential complication of transfusion is HEART FAILURE, which may develop in patients with borderline cardiac compensation if they receive an excessive volume load during transfusion.

Complications may also occur on account of faulty transfusion technique or equipment, for example on account of air entering the administration set. Normal adults can tolerate as much as 200 ml of air introduced into a peripheral vein, but in critically ill patients, as little as 10 ml of air may be fatal. The first indication that a patient has suffered an AIR EMBOLISM may be sudden shock with cyanosis, hypotension, tachycardia, and a deteriorating level of consciousness. If you have reason to believe that air has entered the patient's vein (e.g., if the patient's condition suddenly deteriorates and you see air in the IV tubing), immediately clamp off the tubing and turn the patient onto his *left side* with his *head down* and his *legs elevated.* That position enables the air to rise into the right atrium of the heart, where it stays trapped so that it cannot enter the pulmonary arteries.

Finally, medical personnel may themselves suffer complications of blood transfusion through careless handling of blood administration equipment. About 0.5 percent of patients receiving two or more units of blood will develop clinical signs of VIRAL HEPATITIS. Pooled plasma transfusions multiply that risk. There is also a very small but real risk of contracting AIDS from transfused blood. For those reasons, emergency personnel should exercise extreme care in handling blood administration equipment. (For details of precautions against hepatitis and AIDS, see Chap. 28.)

SHOCK

The word *shock* means different things to different people. To most people, shock means an unpleasant surprise or refers to what happens when you stick your finger in a light socket. But in medical parlance, shock has a very precise meaning: Shock occurs when, for any reason, there is **inadequate tissue perfusion,** that is, inadequate blood flow in and out of the body tissues (*per-* = through + *fusus* = to pour).

Mechanisms and Types of Shock

Recall that normal tissue perfusion requires three intact mechanisms (Fig. 9-27A):

- A functioning PUMP: the heart
- Adequate fluid VOLUME: the blood and body fluids
- An intact system of TUBING capable of reflex adjustments (constriction and dilatation) in response to changes in pump output and fluid volume: the blood vessels.

If any one of those mechanisms is damaged, tissue perfusion may be disrupted, and shock will ensue.

We have already considered, in our discussion of cardiac arrest, how PUMP FAILURE (Fig. 9-27B) results in cessation of useful cardiac output and therefore loss of tissue perfusion. When shock comes about because of failure of the pump, or heart, we call it **cardiogenic shock** (*cardio-* = heart + *-genic* = causing). Cardiac arrest is the most drastic form of cardiogenic shock, but not the only form. Cardiogenic shock may also occur secondary to myocardial infarction, cardiac dysrhythmias, pulmonary embolism, severe acidosis, and a variety of other conditions, all of which have one thing in common: They interfere with the ability of the heart to pump normally.

Even if the pump is perfectly intact, shock may occur because of LOSS OF VOLUME from the system (Fig. 9-27C), for perfusion cannot take place if there isn't enough fluid to propel through the system. When shock comes about because of inadequate volume, we call it **hypovolemic shock** (*hypo-* = deficient + *-vol* = volume + *-emia* = in the blood). Volume can be lost as *blood* (hemorrhagic shock), as *plasma* (burns), or as *electrolyte solution* (vomiting, diarrhea, sweating).

FIGURE 9-27.   MECHANISMS OF SHOCK.   Normal perfusion (A) requires a functioning pump, adequate volume, and intact tubing capable of constriction. When the pump fails (B), in cardiogenic shock, flow grows sluggish or stops altogether. In hypovolemic shock (C), there is no longer enough fluid to fill the system. Massive vasodilatation (D) leads to neurogenic shock.

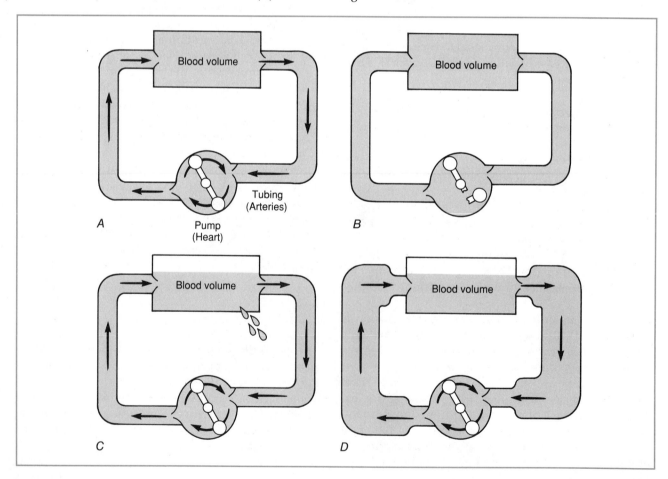

> **SUSPECT A HYPOVOLEMIC COMPONENT OF SHOCK IN ANY PATIENT WITH UNEXPLAINED SHOCK, AND TREAT FOR HYPOVOLEMIA FIRST.**

FAILURE OF VASOCONSTRICTION, that is, a decrease in what is termed peripheral vascular resistance, may lead to **neurogenic shock.** It is called neurogenic because the sympathetic nervous system ordinarily controls the dilatation and constriction of blood vessels. In a healthy person, the caliber of the blood vessels is constantly changing in response to signals from the nervous system, in order to adapt to changes in position, fluid volume, and so forth. The reason that you don't faint every time you stand up, for example, is because blood vessels in your legs reflexly constrict to divert the circulation toward more vital areas, like the brain. Similarly, you don't go into shock every time you donate a pint of blood or sweat a liter of fluid because your blood vessels constrict to accommodate a smaller fluid volume. In certain situations, though, nervous system control over the caliber of blood vessels becomes deranged—for example after spinal cord injury or in some cases of pulmonary embolism or gastric overdistention—and the blood vessels lose their tone and dilate. Thus a given blood volume suddenly has to be accommodated in a much larger container (Fig. 9-27D). The net effect is a *relative* hypovolemia (the volume in the container is now inadequate relative to the increased size of the container), which the body experiences as shock.

In many cases of shock, more than one component of the circulatory system is affected. Thus, a patient in shock after a myocardial infarction is likely to have an element of cardiogenic shock, because his damaged heart can no longer pump efficiently, as

well as an element of hypovolemic shock, if he has been vomiting, sweating, or too nauseated to take in fluids. There are also certain types of shock that by their very nature result from COMBINED DEFICITS. In ANAPHYLACTIC SHOCK, for example, which is a kind of shock resulting from an exaggerated allergic reaction, there is malfunction of both the heart and the blood vessels.

Certain categories of patients are at *high risk* to develop shock, and the paramedic needs to be particularly alert to the possibility of shock when examining patients in those categories:

PATIENTS AT HIGH RISK OF DEVELOPING SHOCK

- Patients known to have suffered TRAUMA or BLEEDING FROM ANY CAUSE
- The ELDERLY, especially men with urinary tract infection
- Patients with MASSIVE MYOCARDIAL INFARCTION
- PREGNANT WOMEN
- Patients with a possible source for SEPTIC SHOCK, including women who have had a back-street abortion, burned patients, and patients with diabetes or cancer

---

The types of shock are summarized in Table 9-4. In the remainder of this chapter, we shall concern ourselves primarily with hypovolemic shock. Cardiogenic shock will be discussed in more detail in Chapter 23, neurogenic shock in Chapter 16, and anaphylactic shock in Chapter 26.

TABLE 9-4. TYPES OF SHOCK

TYPE OF SHOCK	SITE OF MALFUNCTION	EXAMPLES
HYPOVOLEMIC	VOLUME (blood or plasma)	Massive hemorrhage (blood loss) Burns (plasma loss) Severe diarrhea (ECF loss) Profuse sweating (ECF loss)
CARDIOGENIC	PUMP (heart muscle)	Myocardial infarction
NEUROGENIC	TUBING (vascular system)	Spinal cord injury
MIXED TYPES	PUMP AND TUBING	Anaphylaxis Sepsis

Causes of Hypovolemic Shock

Hypovolemic shock occurs when a significant amount of fluid is lost from the intravascular space. As mentioned earlier, that loss may be in the form of blood, plasma, or electrolyte solution. In prehospital emergency care, the form of fluid loss we see most frequently is blood loss due to hemorrhage.

Hemorrhage (profuse bleeding) may be external or internal. **External bleeding** is usually recognized quite readily, but **internal bleeding** may be hidden—and if you don't suspect it, you will not be alert to the possibility of shock. A person who has sustained *blunt trauma to the abdomen,* for example, may bleed to death (exsanguinate) into his abdominal cavity without a single drop of blood being spilled outside the body. *Fractures of the pelvis and long bones* are also often a source of significant internal bleeding. Pelvic fractures sustained in crush injury produce shock in about 40 percent of patients and may lead to exsanguination; a fracture of the femur may result in blood loss of 1,000 to 1,500 ml (about 2–3 pints). A person need not sustain trauma, however, to bleed internally. A duodenal ulcer that erodes into a blood vessel or an ectopic pregnancy (pregnancy outside the womb) that ruptures into the abdomen can also produce severe and even fatal internal hemorrhage. Thus, the paramedic needs to maintain a high index of suspicion whenever there is a clinical picture that looks like shock.

SUMMARY: CAUSES OF HYPOVOLEMIC SHOCK

- Loss of BLOOD (hemorrhagic shock)
  1. External bleeding
  2. Internal bleeding
     a. From trauma: Blunt trauma to the chest, abdomen; fractures of the pelvis and long bones
     b. Nontraumatic sources: bleeding ulcer, ruptured ectopic pregnancy
- Loss of PLASMA (burns)
- Loss of GASTROINTESTINAL FLUIDS (vomiting, diarrhea)
- Loss of SWEAT
- INTERNAL ("third space") LOSSES (peritonitis)

The Body's Response to Blood Loss

The first thing that happens when the circulatory system starts to lose volume is a very slight drop in pressure within the system (Fig. 9-28A). That slight drop in pressure sets off alarms in the form of receptors inside the aorta and carotids that are sensitive to volume and pressure within the vascular space (**baroreceptors**). The alarms activate the sympathetic nervous system, which in turn sends messages back to the blood vessels—at first mainly to arteries supplying "low priority" tissues like skin, fat, and muscles—to constrict. By constricting, the blood vessels decrease their diameter and thus their volume (Fig. 9-28B). So the reduced volume of fluid is now flowing through a smaller container, and blood pressure is maintained. That is why blood pressure does not fall significantly during the early stages of bleeding.

For the tissues out in the periphery, however, the near-normal blood pressure is small consolation. The tissues don't care a whit about blood pressure. All they care about is that their regular oxygen delivery arrives on time; and if blood has been lost from the body, there are fewer red blood cells in the system to carry oxygen, so delivery of oxygen is going to be held up. As things start to become rather stuffy at the tissue level, the tissues clamor for oxygen, again activating the sympathetic nervous system. The only way that the body can improve oxygen delivery under those circumstances is to have each red blood cell make more deliveries by speeding up the trip back and forth from the lungs to the tissues. And the only way to do *that* is for the pump to work faster, that is, for the heart rate to speed up (**tachycardia**), which is precisely what usually happens.

Up to this point, the body is holding its own. Blood pressure is maintained at or near normal by vasoconstriction, and the tissues are getting their oxygen by a more rapid recirculation of the remaining red blood cells. If, however, the person continues to lose blood, the tissues out in the periphery will soon begin to pay a price for the body's compensatory mechanisms. For as blood vessels constrict more and more (i.e., peripheral resistance continues to increase), peripheral tissues are increasingly deprived of blood flow. That fall in tissue perfusion has several detrimental effects:

- Unable to obtain the quantity of oxygen they need for their normal operation, cells *switch from aerobic to anaerobic metabolism.* Anaerobic metabolism produces more acid (lactic and pyruvic acid) than aerobic metabolism, and—again because

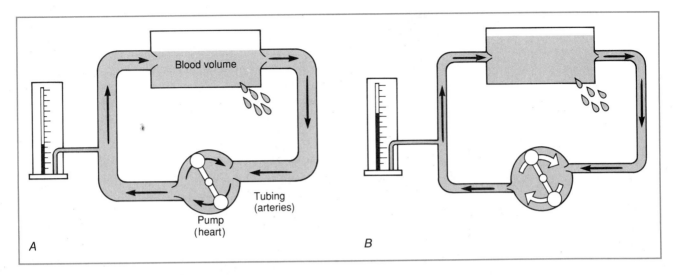

FIGURE 9-28. COMPENSATORY MECHANISMS IN VOLUME LOSS. When the system starts to lose volume (A), there is a slight drop in blood pressure. The body responds with tachycardia and vasoconstriction (B), which help restore blood pressure.

perfusion is poor—the acid accumulates in the fluid around the cell. The upshot is METABOLIC ACIDOSIS, which cannot be fully corrected until adequate circulation has been restored.

- For reasons not completely understood—perhaps because of the accumulation of toxic waste products—CAPILLARY WALLS BECOME LEAKY. Large molecules like albumin that were previously confined inside the capillary walls and helped maintain vascular volume by exerting osmotic pressure now start oozing out into the surrounding tissue. That leads to both a further fall in intravascular volume and the development of EDEMA (swelling) in the extravascular tissues.
- Meanwhile, as red blood cells creep along through the narrowed tubes, they tend to clump together, forming a kind of sludge.

Clearly, then, as blood loss continues, the system will start to fail. Blood vessels can constrict only so far. The heart can beat only so fast. And the peripheral tissues can survive only so long on anaerobic metabolism in an increasingly acidotic milieu. Once those limits are exceeded, the *blood pressure will start to fall* (i.e., **hypotension** will occur). Blood pressure is the driving force that moves blood out to the peripheral tissues. So as blood pressure falls, peripheral perfusion declines even further.

How much blood loss are we talking about? In an adult, loss of about 15 to 20 percent of blood volume (2–3 pints of blood) will produce moderate shock; by the time a person has lost 30 percent of his circulating blood volume (more than 3 pints of blood) he will be in severe shock and his life will be in danger.

Hemorrhage is sometimes classified according to the estimated blood loss (Table 9-5).

Symptoms and Signs of Hypovolemic Shock

Most of the typical symptoms and signs of shock come about because of inadequate tissue oxygenation and the body's attempts to compensate for volume loss. Probably the earliest signs of shock are REST-LESSNESS and ANXIETY: The patient looks scared! The decline in tissue perfusion may not yet be enough to produce outright asphyxia, but it *is* setting off all sorts of alarms all over the body, to which the patient responds with a feeling of apprehension—a "gut" knowledge that something isn't quite right. If he is conscious, he may complain of THIRST, reflecting the deficit of fluids in the body, but at the same time he may feel NAUSEATED and even VOMIT. The diversion of blood flow by vasoconstriction, away from "low priority" peripheral tissues will cause the skin to become PALE, COLD, AND CLAMMY (Fig. 9-29A); sometimes it has a MOTTLED appearance. Meanwhile, as we have learned, the heart has to speed up in order to circulate the

TABLE 9-5. CLASSIFICATION OF HEMORRHAGE

CLASS	BLOOD LOSS	SYMPTOMS AND SIGNS
I	<800 ml	Usually none (equivalent to donating one unit of blood)
II	800–1500 ml (15–30%)	Anxiety and restlessness Pulse >100* Systolic pressure unchanged Diastolic pressure ↑ Urine output ↓
III	2000 ml (30–40%)	Pulse >120* Respirations >30 Systolic pressure ↓ Mental status ↓
IV	>2500 ml (>40%)	Pulse >120* Respirations >30 Narrow pulse pressure (= systolic − diastolic) Cold, clammy skin

*In some cases of abdominal trauma, there is shock without a rapid pulse.

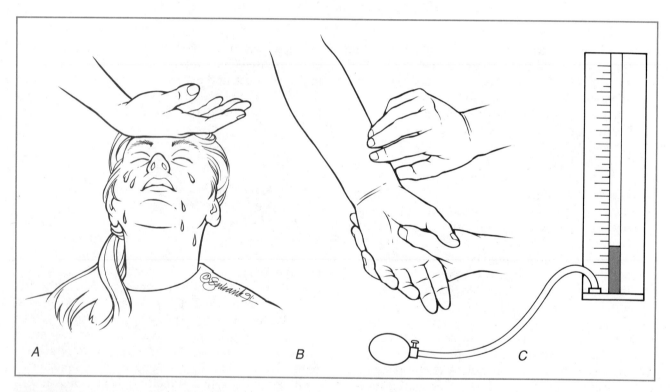

FIGURE 9-29.   CLINICAL SIGNS OF SHOCK.   (A) The skin becomes pale or mottled, cold, and sweaty. (B) The pulse is usually rapid and weak. (C) A *late* sign is a falling blood pressure.

remaining red blood cells more rapidly, so what we find clinically is a RAPID, WEAK PULSE (Fig. 9-29B)—rapid because the heart is beating faster, weak because the blood vessels are now very narrow and the volume moving through them is decreased.

While the arteries are constricting and the heart is speeding up, the brain, alone in its ivory tower, is trying to figure out why it has gotten so stuffy up there. The brain doesn't know that the blood volume has decreased on account of hemorrhage; all the brain knows is that it is not getting enough oxygen, and it figures that the lungs must be falling down on the job. So the respiratory center in the brainstem sends urgent word to the respiratory muscles to speed up their activity, and the result is RAPID, SHALLOW BREATHING (tachypnea).

As bleeding continues, the BLOOD PRESSURE finally FALLS (Fig. 9-29C).

> **DON'T WAIT UNTIL THE BLOOD PRESSURE FALLS BEFORE YOU SUSPECT SHOCK AND BEGIN TREATMENT!**

Falling blood pressure is a *late* sign in shock, signalling the collapse of all compensatory mechanisms. By the time the blood pressure falls, the ball game is nearly over. Furthermore, the blood pressure measured at the arm gives little information about perfusion of vital organs; it tells only about perfusion of the arms, with which the rescuer (as well as the patient's vital organs) is relatively unconcerned. The name of the game in treating shock is to SAVE THE BRAIN AND THE KIDNEYS. Those are the organs that must remain perfused if the patient is to survive and return to a healthy life.

The best indication of *brain perfusion* is the patient's **state of consciousness.** If he is conscious and alert, his brain is being perfused adequately no matter what the sphygmomanometer (blood pressure measuring device) says. If he is CONFUSED, DISORIENTED, OR UNCONSCIOUS, perfusion of the brain is likely to be inadequate.

Kidney perfusion can be gauged by urine output in a catheterized patient. Adequately perfused kidneys put out at least 30 to 50 ml of urine per hour; poorly perfused kidneys shut down and stop putting out urine altogether.

In the field—where patients will not ordinarily have urinary catheters—you can get an estimate of the patient's *peripheral* perfusion by testing for **capillary refill.** To do so, press on one of the patient's fingernails until it blanches (turns white; Fig. 9-30A); then release the pressure (Fig. 9-30B). If the skin under the nail doesn't "pink up" within 2 seconds (about as long as it takes to say "good capillary refill"), *peripheral* perfusion is compromised. But to determine how well a patient is perfusing his *vital* organs, you can rely only on the patient's state of consciousness.

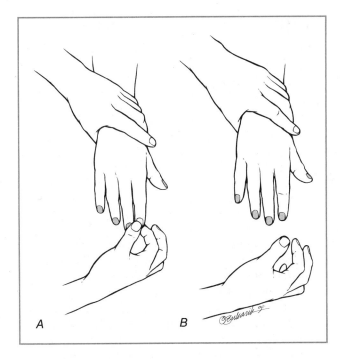

A   B

FIGURE 9-30.   CAPILLARY REFILL TEST. Press on the fingernail (A) until it blanches. Then release the pressure (B). The skin under the nail should "pink up" within 2 seconds if the patient is normally perfused.

> **SUMMARY: SYMPTOMS AND SIGNS OF SHOCK**
>
> - Restlessness and anxiety
> - Thirst
> - Nausea and sometimes vomiting
> - Cold, clammy, pale (or mottled) skin
> - Weak, rapid pulse (tachycardia)
> - Shallow, rapid breathing (tachypnea)
> - Changes in the state of consciousness (confusion, disorientation, coma)
> - Fall in blood pressure (hypotension)

Those signs and symptoms together give us a clinical picture of shock, which was described very accurately by Billroth writing in 1870:

The face becomes pale, lips blue, pulse is smaller, the temperature falls in the extremities, the patient is subject to fainting spells, nausea and vomiting, vision is obscured; with continuous hemorrhage, the countenance grows waxy, the eyes dull, the body temperature is lower, the pulse small, thready, and very frequent, respiration is incomplete, the patient constantly grows more feeble and anxious; at last he remains unconscious and there is twitching of the arms and legs which is renewed at the slightest irritation, and then death.

Billroth was describing the natural course of death from exsanguination. The task of emergency care personnel is to try to alter that course by providing early, appropriate treatment.

Treatment of Hypovolemic Shock

In this section, we shall consider some general principles in the management of hypovolemic shock. Later on in the book, after we have learned a good deal more about trauma, we shall return to the topic of hypovolemic shock and how its detection and treatment fit into the overall assessment and management of the trauma victim.

The *priorities* in treating a patient in shock are the same as in treating any other patient: ABC.

- Establish and maintain an **open airway.** Keep suction at hand to clear the mouth and pharynx of a semiconscious patient if he should vomit.
- Administer **oxygen.** Assist ventilations as needed.
- **Control bleeding** if present. Use direct pressure over the site of external bleeding. (For other methods to control external bleeding, see Chap. 15.)
- Apply **military anti-shock trousers (MAST)** (see next section of this chapter), if they are part of your local protocol.
- Start **transport.**
- Start at least one, and preferably two **large bore peripheral IVs** (14- to 16-gauge), using an over-the-needle catheter. (If the patient is in critical condition, you may have to start the IV while en route to the hospital.) Draw blood (two red-top Vacutainer tubes and one purple-top tube), so that the emergency room team may obtain a hematocrit, type and cross match, and other tests immediately on your arrival. Unless local medical policy favors a different resuscitation fluid, give normal saline or lactated Ringer's solution. Run in the first 300 to 500 ml as fast as it will flow or according to local protocol.
- Give the patient **nothing by mouth;** he is very likely to vomit.
- Keep the patient at **normal temperature.** Usually that means covering the patient with a **blanket,** since victims of hypovolemic shock are often unable to conserve body heat effectively and are easily chilled.
- Place the patient in a **physiologic position,** with his head elevated about 15 to 30 degrees and his extremities propped up about 30 degrees on pillows (injuries permitting). Do *not* use the Trendelenburg position (30-degree head-down tilt). That position simply makes it harder for the patient to breathe and increases the work of the heart, without appreciably improving the central circulation.
- **Monitor cardiac rhythm.** *Any* critically ill or injured patient is apt to suffer dysrhythmias.
- **Monitor** the **state of consciousness, pulse,** and **blood pressure.** In a patient who is very vasoconstricted, the blood pressure sounds may be difficult to hear, especially under field conditions. If so, use the pulses as a rough guide, as detailed in Table 9-6. Thus, for example, if you can feel a pulse over the femoral artery but not over the radial artery, the systolic blood pressure is probably somewhere between 70 and 80 mm Hg.
- Depending on local practice, the base physician may order one or both of the following:
  1. *Sodium bicarbonate,* to treat acidosis.
  2. A *vasopressor* (such a dopamine, Aramine, or Levophed) to enhance vasoconstriction.

Know the protocols for shock in your EMS system, and have the appropriate medications drawn up and ready to administer.

SUMMARY: TREATMENT OF SHOCK

- Maintain an AIRWAY.
- Give OXYGEN.
- Control BLEEDING.
- MAST, according to protocol.
- IV FLUIDS; nothing by mouth.
- Keep the patient WARM and recumbent, legs elevated.
- MONITOR cardiac rhythm, state of consciousness, and vital signs.
- DO NOT DELAY AT THE SCENE. Start the ABCs, load up, and *move!*

TABLE 9-6. ESTIMATING THE BLOOD PRESSURE BY THE SITE OF A PALPABLE PULSE

PULSE SITE	ESTIMATED MINIMUM BLOOD PRESSURE
Carotid	60 mm Hg
Femoral	70 mm Hg
Radial	80 mm Hg

MILITARY ANTI-SHOCK TROUSERS (MAST)

Military anti-shock trousers (MAST), also known as pneumatic anti-shock garments (PASG), are inflatable garments that surround the legs and abdomen of a patient and can generate up to around 100 mm Hg of pressure. The idea of a pneumatic pressure suit has been around for a long time, since George Crile reported on "the resuscitation of the apparently dead and a demonstration of the pneumatic blood pressure" in 1903. That early work led Crile to develop the G suit for the U.S. Army Air Corps in 1942. In the 1960s, a U.S. Army researcher, Dr. Burt Kaplan, modified the G suit for medical use, and the prototype of the MAST was tested by the army in the Viet Nam conflict, with apparently favorable results. The MAST made its civilian debut with the Miami Fire Department in the early 1970s, and by 1977, experience with the device had been so favorable that the Committee on Trauma of the American College of Surgeons included the MAST in their list of essential equipment for ambulances.

What the MAST Can and Cannot Do

In the 1980s, various researchers began to question whether the MAST was really effective in the treatment of shock. The "MAST controversy" that has sputtered back and forth since then has, on the whole, generated more heat than light. At the time of this writing, it is still not possible to state with certainty what the MAST can and cannot accomplish, but the current evidence would seem to support the following statements:

- By applying uniform pressure to sources of bleeding, the MAST—especially when pumped up only to relatively low pressures (around 30–40 mm Hg)—may CONTROL BLEEDING and PROMOTE HEMOSTASIS (the natural cessation of bleeding, through sealing off of damaged blood vessels). That is the same principle used in applying pressure over a wound to control hemorrhage manually.
- The MAST RAISES THE BLOOD PRESSURE of a patient in shock. Whether elevating the blood pressure is, in fact, of benefit to the patient has not been proved, and some researchers believe that raising the blood pressure before bleeding has been controlled may have harmful effects on the patient. But there is no doubt that raising the patient's blood pressure is useful to the *paramedic*, for often veins that were collapsed and invisible

magically pop up after the MAST has been inflated, making the job of starting IVs immeasurably easier.
- The inflated MAST provides a good SPLINT for a fractured pelvis and also helps in splinting fractures of the lower extremities. (Ideally, fractures of the femur should be traction-splinted after application of the MAST.)

What we do *not* know as of this time is whether the MAST improves the overall outcome for a seriously injured patient. Recent research at Baylor College of Medicine in Houston suggests that, at least in certain types of injuries, the MAST does not improve the patient's chances of survival and may indeed adversely affect the outcome. It will therefore be up to the medical directors of local EMS systems to stay abreast of the research in this area and to make their decisions regarding deployment of the MAST accordingly. In those EMS systems that are still using the MAST, the current evidence would support the following guidelines:

WHEN TO USE THE MAST

- To control DIFFUSE BLEEDING OF THE LOWER EXTREMITIES (inflate to 30–40 mm Hg)
- To stabilize PELVIC FRACTURES
- For cases of NEUROGENIC SHOCK, with systolic blood pressure below 80–90 mm Hg and signs of poor perfusion
- For cases of HYPOVOLEMIC SHOCK, with systolic blood pressure below 50 mm Hg and signs of poor perfusion
- For HEMORRHAGIC SHOCK when not contraindicated

WHEN NOT TO USE THE MAST

- For patients with CHEST INJURY or any injury above the level of the MAST when applied
- For patients with HEAD INJURY
- For patients in heart failure with PULMONARY EDEMA

Application of the MAST

The steps in applying the MAST are shown in Figure 9-31.

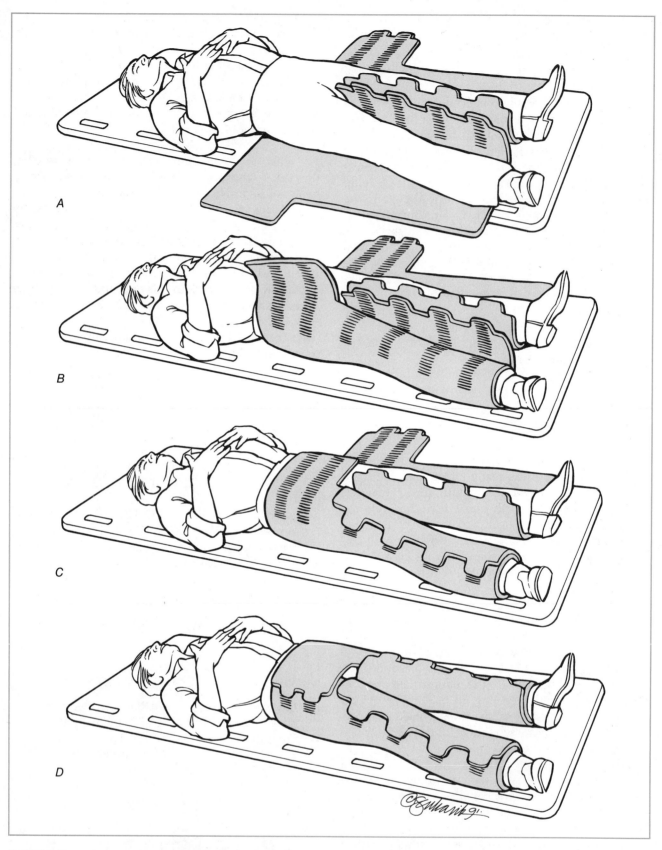

FIGURE 9-31.   APPLICATION OF THE MAST.   (A) Logroll the patient onto the
MAST, which has been spread out flat on a backboard. (B) Fasten one leg
section. (C) Fasten the other leg section. (D) Fasten the abdominal section.

- **Spread the MAST out flat on a backboard,** so that it is free of wrinkles. Attach the foot pump and open the stopcock valves.
- **Logroll the patient** onto the garment. The patient should be placed such that the top of the MAST garment is just below his lowest rib (Fig. 9-31A). If the patient is a victim of trauma, use full spine precautions in moving him onto the backboard (see Chapter 16).
- **Wrap the left leg of the MAST around the patient's left leg,** and secure the Velcro fasteners (Fig. 9-31B).
- **Wrap the right leg of the MAST around the patient's right leg,** and secure the Velcro fasteners (Fig. 9-31C).
- **Secure the abdominal segment** of the MAST around the patient's abdominal region (Fig. 9-31D).
- **Check with medical command** whether to inflate the MAST. If you receive the go-ahead:
- Recheck that all the stopcock valves are open.
- Use the foot pump to **inflate the MAST** *to the lowest pressure required to produce a clinical response.* If you have a pressure gauge in the system, inflate to about 30–40 mm Hg.
- **Close the stopcock valves.**

The entire process outlined above should not take more than 60 to 90 *seconds!* Most patients who need the MAST are seriously injured, so they also need to reach a trauma care facility as quickly as possible. Application of the MAST should never delay transport.

Deflation of the MAST

The simplest rule to remember regarding deflation of the MAST is:

> **DO NOT DEFLATE THE MAST IN THE FIELD.**

To the extent that the MAST supports the blood pressure, provides hemostasis, and so forth, all of those effects will be reversed when the MAST is deflated. It is desirable, therefore, to have restored at least some of the patient's circulating blood volume before releasing the pressure provided by the MAST.

Before the MAST is deflated in the hospital, then, the patient should have at least two good IV infusions running, with adequate volumes of typed and cross-matched blood on standby. If the patient's vital signs are relatively stable, and the physician so instructs, one may then begin cautious deflation of the MAST as follows:

- **Record** the patient's **pulse and blood pressure.**
- Slowly **deflate the abdominal section** *only.*
- **Recheck** the patient's **vital signs** over 5 to 10 minutes. If the blood pressure drops by 5 mm Hg or more, infuse 100 to 200 ml of volume over 10 minutes until the blood pressure stabilizes again.
- When the patient's vital signs are again stable, slowly **deflate one leg section.**
- Again, **recheck the vital signs** over 5 to 10 minutes. If there is another blood pressure drop, again infuse volume until the blood pressure comes back up.
- If vital signs are stable, it is then permissible to go ahead and **deflate the other leg section,** again slowly, with careful monitoring of blood pressure at 2- to 3-minute intervals.

In severely injured patients, the deflation procedure, which can take between 20 and 60 minutes, will usually not be feasible, and the patient must be taken straight to the operating room with the MAST still on and inflated.

PRINCIPLES OF INTRAVENOUS THERAPY

Intravenous (IV) lines are inserted for one of two general purposes:

- To provide a ROUTE FOR REPLACEMENT OF FLUID in patients who have lost significant volumes of fluid or blood or are *at risk* to lose significant volumes of fluid or blood. For patients in this category, the intravenous fluid of choice will be *normal saline* or *lactated Ringer's.*

PATIENTS WHO NEED IVs FOR FLUID REPLACEMENT

- All patients in HYPOVOLEMIC SHOCK
- Patients who are LIKELY TO DEVELOP HYPOVOLEMIC SHOCK from
  1. Profuse external bleeding
  2. Internal bleeding
     a. Ulcer (patient vomiting blood or having blood in his stool)
     b. Vaginal bleeding
     c. Blunt trauma to the abdomen
     d. Fracture of the pelvis or femur

3. Severe or widespread burns
4. Heat exhaustion
5. Intractable vomiting and/or diarrhea
- Patients in NEUROGENIC SHOCK and SEPTIC SHOCK
- Any patient who needs the MAST

- To provide a LIFELINE for emergency administration of drugs (i.e., to "keep the vein open," or KVO). As we learned earlier, when a patient has poor cardiac output (as in shock), blood is shunted away from the skin and skeletal muscles. Thus, drugs administered subcutaneously or intramuscularly are absorbed at a low and unpredictable rate. Giving a drug directly into the vein ensures that the desired dose of the drug reaches the circulation. The intravenous fluid usually used to "keep the vein open" is *D5/W*.

PATIENTS WHO NEED KEEP-OPEN IVs

- Patients AT RISK OF CARDIAC ARREST (It's easier to start the IV *before* the arrest!)
- Patients who need or may need PARENTERAL MEDICATION, for example those with:
  1. Seizures
  2. Congestive heart failure
  3. Coma

When to Start the IV

Timely intravenous therapy is an important part of the management of many life-threatening conditions; but intravenous therapy undertaken at an inappropriate time may become part of the problem rather than part of the solution. In a critically ill or injured patient,

---

STARTING AN IV SHOULD NOT DELAY THE TRANSPORT OF A PATIENT TO THE HOSPITAL.

Starting an IV should not interfere with more urgent priorities either. Where, then, does the IV fit into the greater scheme of things? We return, as always, to the ABCs.

PRIORITIES IN THE CRITICALLY INJURED

- Ensure an adequate AIRWAY:
  1. Manual methods (e.g., head tilt-chin lift).
  2. Endotracheal intubation as soon as possible.
- Ensure adequate BREATHING:
  1. Oxygen.
  2. Assisted or controlled ventilation, as needed.
- Support the CIRCULATION:
  1. CPR as needed.
  2. Control bleeding.
  3. MAST.
  4. IV (en route to hospital, if necessary).

Selecting an Intravenous Cannula

Intravenous cannulas come in four types:

- HOLLOW NEEDLE, for example, a "butterfly" needle, which is a hollow needle with two plastic wings to facilitate its handling—but even a standard hypodermic needle can be used in an emergency. A butterfly needle is easy to insert, but also easy to dislodge; and any steel needle is more likely than a flexible catheter to perforate the vein.
- Plastic catheters that are inserted OVER a hollow needle (e.g., Angiocath or Medicut).
- Plastic catheters that are inserted THROUGH a hollow needle (e.g., Intracath).
- WIRE-GUIDED (Seldinger-type) catheters, in which a steel guide wire is introduced into the vein *through* a needle, then—after the needle is withdrawn—the catheter is introduced *over* the guide wire.

As a general rule, the *over-the-needle catheter* is preferred for use in the field, since it is more readily secured than a butterfly needle and less cumbersome than a through-the-needle catheter. The over-the-needle catheter, furthermore, is less likely than the through-the-needle catheter to be partially sheared off during insertion and transformed into a catheter embolus. Finally, the over-the-needle catheter is usually shorter than the through-the-needle catheter, so it enables faster flow, because resistance to flow through a catheter is directly proportional to the catheter's length: the longer the catheter, the slower the flow; the shorter the catheter, the faster the flow. (Don't trash all your through-the-needle catheters, though; you may need them for decompressing a pneumothorax—see Chap. 17.)

Whatever type of catheter is chosen, it should be of large caliber if it is intended for replacement of fluids. Again, this is a matter of fundamental physics: The rate of flow through any pipe is proportional to the radius of the pipe; thus, the larger the caliber of the catheter (the smaller the gauge number), the faster fluid can flow through it. A 16- or even a 14-gauge catheter—inserted over a needle or over a guide wire—is appropriate for an adult, especially if massive quantities of fluid must be infused. (For a *keep-open line*, an 18- or 20-gauge catheter will do.) It should be pointed out that not all catheters of the same gauge have the same flow rates. The flow through a 2-inch 16-gauge Argyle Medicut, for example, is 50 percent faster than that through a 2-inch 16-gauge Deseret Angiocath, perhaps because the end of the Medicut is tapered to permit greater laminar flow.

Other factors that influence the flow rate through an intravenous catheter include the length and diameter of the administration set tubing, the height of the IV bag above the patient, and pressure applied on the IV bag. A pressure infuser can triple the flow rate of IV fluids. (The size of the vein chosen for venipuncture does *not* significantly influence the flow rate.) Taking all of those considerations into account, we can formulate the following recommendations for selecting IV catheters and equipment for rapid infusion of large volumes of fluid:

**GUIDELINES FOR RAPID
IV INFUSIONS**

- Use a SHORT, LARGE-BORE CATHETER (preferably 2-inch 14- or 16-gauge Medicut).
- Use a LARGE-DIAMETER, SHORT-LENGTH ADMINISTRATION SET.
- Apply CIRCUMFERENTIAL PRESSURE around the IV bag: Use a blood pressure cuff or specially-designed pressure unit to generate up to 300 mm Hg pressure.

Potential Complications of Intravenous Therapy

Like every invasive procedure, intravenous therapy may be attended by complications, most of which can be avoided with proper attention to technique.

Thrombophlebitis

Infection and **thrombophlebitis** (inflammation of the vein)—both of them most frequently due to lapses in aseptic technique—occur too often in association with IVs started in the field. One study found that the incidence of fever was seven times greater and the incidence of phlebitis five times greater in patients whose IVs were started in the field than in patients whose IVs were started in the emergency room. Even taking into account the more difficult conditions in the prehospital setting, those figures do not speak well for the intravenous placement techniques of paramedics!

In the hospital, phlebitis is usually associated with prolonged intravenous therapy or with the use of intravenous solutions that are particularly irritating to veins (e.g., dextrose solutions, which have a very low pH, or hypertonic solutions of any sort). Thrombophlebitis can also be produced by mechanical factors, such as excessive motion of the IV needle or catheter. It is manifested by *pain and tenderness* along the course of the vein and *redness and edema* at the venipuncture site. Those signs generally do not appear until after several hours of intravenous therapy, so you are unlikely to see a case of phlebitis unless you are doing an interhospital transport of a patient who already has an established IV. If you do detect the signs and symptoms of phlebitis in a patient, stop the infusion and DISCONTINUE THE IV at that site. Warm compresses applied to the site may provide some relief.

It is far better, however, to prevent thrombophlebitis or infection than to treat it afterward. Taking a little bit of care in starting an IV need not take a lot of time:

**PREVENTING
THROMBOPHLEBITIS AT
IV SITES**

- Use a povidone-iodine preparation to SCRUB AND DISINFECT the skin over the venipuncture site; then do a final wipe with an alcohol swab.
- Don sterile GLOVES after disinfecting the skin.
- After inserting the catheter, cover the puncture site with a STERILE DRESSING.
- ANCHOR THE CATHETER and tubing securely to prevent any motion of the catheter within the vein.

Pyrogenic Reactions

Pyrogens are foreign proteins capable of producing fever. Their presence in the infusion solution or administration set may induce a reaction characterized by an abrupt temperature elevation (as high as 106°F, or 41°C) with severe chills, backache, headache, weakness, nausea, and vomiting; occasionally vascular collapse occurs, with all the signs and symptoms of shock. The reaction usually begins about half an hour after the infusion has been started.

If there are *any* signs of such a reaction—for example, if the patient starts to complain of headache or backache after you've started running in fluids—STOP THE INFUSION IMMEDIATELY! Start a new IV in the other arm with a *fresh infusion solution,* and remove the first IV. If the patient is showing signs of shock, treat as any other case of shock.

Pyrogenic reactions can be largely avoided by inspecting the IV bag carefully before use. If there are any leaks in the bag, or if the fluid inside looks at all cloudy, do not use that bag.

Local Infiltration

Infiltration of intravenous solution into the subcutaneous tissues at the venipuncture site is a common complication of IV therapy and occurs when the needle or catheter is dislodged from the vein, especially when a small, thin-walled vein is used. The signs of infiltration are not usually difficult to detect:

- *Edema* and *pain* at the venipuncture site
- A significant *decrease in the infusion rate,* or the complete cessation of flow through the IV
- *Failure to elicit a blood return* into the catheter when the infusion bag is lowered below the level of the patient and the clamp is opened wide

If you detect any of those signs, DISCONTINUE THE INFUSION IMMEDIATELY, and remove the needle or catheter from the vein. Cold compresses over the venipuncture site help reduce the swelling and diminish pain.

Circulatory Overload

Circulatory overload may occur when excessive volumes of fluid are administered intravenously as a result of miscalculating the rate, miscalculating the patient's fluid needs, or allowing a "runaway IV" to flow out of control. The symptoms of circulatory overload are those of congestive heart failure—distention of the neck veins, tachypnea, bubbly respiratory noises (crackles)—and are discussed in more detail in Chapter 23. If any of those symptoms occur, immediately SLOW THE IV TO A KEEP-OPEN RATE, and place the patient in a SITTING POSITION WITH LEGS DANGLING. Radio your medical director for instructions regarding further measures, which may include the administration of diuretic drugs.

Air Embolism

Air embolism (an air bubble in the circulation) may occur with any intravenous infusion, although it is most likely to happen when blood is administered under pressure. The symptoms and management of air embolism were already discussed in an earlier section. Here again, however, it is preferable to *prevent* air embolism than to treat it:

PRECAUTIONS AGAINST AIR EMBOLISM

- Inspect tubing for defects before using.
- Make sure all connections are fitted tightly.
- Discontinue the infusion before the bag is completely empty.
- Avoid circumstances that will increase negative pressure in the tubing, such as:
  1. Elevation of the IV site above the level of the heart.
  2. Placement of the flow-regulating clamp too high on the tubing; it should be at about the level of the patient's heart.

Catheter Shear

Plastic catheters advanced over or through a needle (particularly those advanced *through* a needle) are subject to shearing. If, for example, a catheter is withdrawn *through* a needle, it may get hung up on the sharp beveled edge of the needle and be severed off, thus becoming a plastic embolus kayaking through the circulation toward the lungs. For that reason, once a catheter has been advanced over or through a needle, NEVER, NEVER, NEVER pull the catheter back. If it is necessary to remove the catheter, *first* withdraw the needle, *then* withdraw the catheter.

ONCE A CATHETER HAS BEEN ADVANCED OVER OR THROUGH A NEEDLE, NEVER, NEVER, NEVER PULL IT BACK!

Arterial Puncture

You may accidently puncture the wrong sort of blood vessel if the vein you selected for cannulation lies close to an artery. If you do insert a catheter into an artery by mistake, you'll know it pretty quickly because bright red blood will come spurting back at you through the catheter. The color of the blood and its flow characteristics should alert you to your error. Immediately WITHDRAW THE CATHETER or needle, and APPLY FIRM PRESSURE over the puncture site for at least 5 minutes, or until bleeding stops.

INSERTION OF A PERIPHERAL INTRAVENOUS LINE

Skilled paramedics can get a peripheral IV started in 2 to 3 minutes. To do so takes not only practice but also an organized approach to the task.

Getting Ready

Probably the most time-consuming part of starting an IV is getting set up. Since getting set up does not require fine-tuned manual dexterity, it can be done in a moving vehicle—and it can be done relatively quickly if you have a fixed routine.

1. **Explain the procedure to the patient.** Few people are entirely without anxiety about getting stuck with needles, and in the context of illness or injury, such anxieties may be magnified. Try to allay the patient's anxiety by explaining (a) why the IV line is necessary and (b) what is involved in the procedure. (You need to explain those things in any case, in order to obtain informed consent!) Remember that although starting an IV may be routine for *you*, it is not routine for the patient. An unhurried, informative, and confident attitude on your part will go a long way to quiet the patient's fears.

2. **Assemble all the necessary equipment:**
   - Select the **intravenous fluid** ordered by the physician, and inspect the container. Plastic bag infusion sets are preferable to bottles in the field, since bottles break. Whatever container is used, check it for leakage, cloudiness, and the manufacturer's expiration date. *Never use an intravenous fluid that is cloudy, outdated, or suspect in any other way.*
   - Select the appropriate **infusion set** (Fig. 9-32)— a standard macrodrop set for fluid replacement, a microdrip set for a keep-open lifeline—and attach it to the solution container. Close the flow regulator and squeeze the reservoir of the infusion set until it is about half full. Then open the flow regulator and flush the air from the tubing.
   - Select the **catheter** you will insert, according to the considerations mentioned earlier.
   - Antiseptic cleaning solution, preferably **povidone-iodine swabs** and alcohol swabs.
   - **Sterile dressing** (4- by 4-inch gauze).
   - Adhesive **tape** cut into strips of 3 to 4 inches in length.
   - A 20-ml **syringe** in which to collect a blood sample.
   - **Armboard** if you are using a hand vein.
   - **Pen** and **labels** for writing identifying information.
   - **Vacutainer tubes** for blood samples (two red-tops, one purple-top).
   - **Tourniquet.** The tourniquet may be soft rubber tubing, a commercial tourniquet, or a blood pressure cuff. The blood pressure cuff permits the best control and often enables you to find a vein when other means have failed. To use a blood pressure cuff as a tourniquet, first determine the systolic pressure; then inflate the cuff to about 20 mm Hg *below* the systolic pressure, and clamp the tubing of the sphygmomanometer with a Kelly forceps. When ready to release the tourniquet, simply unclamp the Kelly.

3. **Select a suitable vein.** Let the patient's arm hang dependent for a few minutes; then apply the tourniquet at midarm, above the antecubital fossa (the hollow of the elbow). Check to make sure the radial pulse is still present after you have placed the tourniquet; if the pulse is not palpable, the tourniquet should be loosened. Inspect the hand and forearm for a vein that appears fairly straight and lies on a flat surface. The vein should be well fixed, it should not roll, and it should feel springy when palpated. *Avoid* the following:
   - Veins overlying joints. When you put an IV over a joint, you have to immobilize the joint, which is both cumbersome and uncomfortable for the patient.
   - Veins that lie close to arteries (check for pulsations nearby).
   - Veins near injured areas.
   - Veins of the lower extremities.
   In general, the forearm (Fig. 9-33A) is the preferred site and the dorsum (back) of the hand (Fig. 9-33B) second choice.

4. **Don rubber gloves.**

5. **Prepare the venipuncture site.** *Scrub* the area chosen for venipuncture with several iodine swabs, one after another. Start from an area just above the vein and wipe vigorously in widening circles around it, allowing a broad margin around the

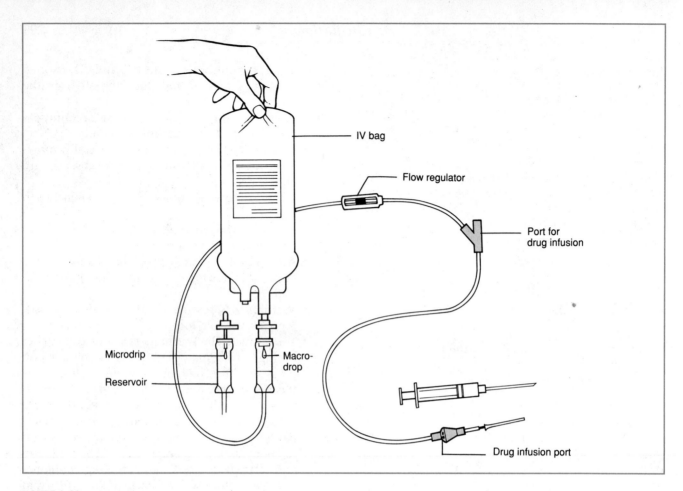

FIGURE 9-32. INTRAVENOUS BAG AND ADMINISTRATION SET.

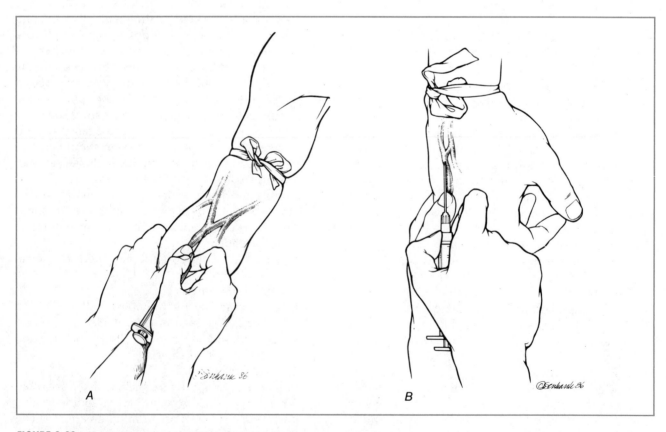

FIGURE 9-33. PREFERRED SITES FOR PERIPHERAL IVs. The antecubital
fossa (A) is first choice, the dorsum of the hand (B) second choice.

site you plan to puncture. Just dabbing the skin daintily with a swab won't do: Scrub! Since some patients may react to iodine left on the skin, give a final wipe with an alcohol swab to remove the iodine.

If you are working in an ambulance, all of the steps just outlined can be carried out while the vehicle is moving. It is a good idea, however, to have the driver slow or stop the vehicle for the 30 seconds or so that it takes to do the actual venipuncture and secure the catheter. For even if you're slick enough to whip in an IV in a bouncing ambulance, the extra motion of the catheter within the vein will predispose the patient to later complications, especially phlebitis.

Inserting the IV

The technique of inserting the IV depends on which type of IV catheter you have selected. With any type of catheter, you will have to **stabilize the vein** by applying light traction on the skin distal to the point of entry, as shown in Figure 9-33. Then proceed according to the instructions for the catheter you are using.

Over-the-Needle Catheter

1. **Align the catheter.** It should enter the *skin* at a 45-degree angle, about 1 to 2 cm distal to the vein, bevel facing *up*. As soon as the catheter has punctured the skin, lower it to about a 15-degree angle to enter the vein (Fig. 9-34A).
2. **Enter the vein** from the side or from above. You should be able to feel the needle "pop" through into the vein, and blood should then return through the needle.
3. Gently **advance the needle** another few millimeters beyond the point where blood return was first encountered—to be certain that the catheter tip is securely inside the lumen of the vein.
4. **Slide the catheter over the needle** into the vein (Fig. 9-34B).
5. Carefully **withdraw the needle,** while holding the catheter stable.
6. Stabilize the catheter with one hand, and use your other hand to attach a 20-ml syringe. **Draw the blood sample,** and hand it to an assistant to distribute among the Vacutainer tubes (or set it aside, to fill the tubes yourself after the IV has been secured). If you have difficulty in drawing the blood sample, abandon the attempt. It is better to draw the sample afterward, from another site, than to risk blowing the IV.
7. **Release the tourniquet.**

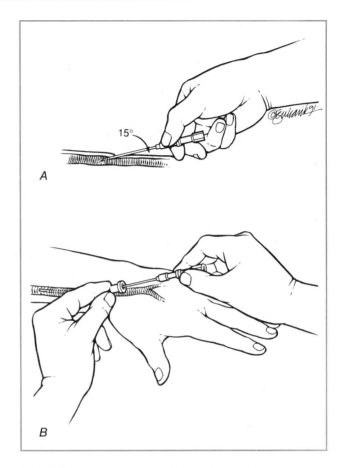

FIGURE 9-34. INSERTING AN OVER-THE-NEEDLE CATHETER. (A) Once the needle has penetrated the skin, align it at a 15-degree angle to enter the vein. (B) When the needle is securely in the vein, slide the catheter over it into the vein.

8. **Attach the IV tubing,** and open the clamp wide to permit unimpeded flow. The fluid should flow through the infusion reservoir in a steady stream; if it does not, the catheter tip may be resting up against the wall of the vein, so pull back very slightly on the catheter.

Through-the-Needle Catheter

1. Hold the unit by the hub of the needle, and **align the needle.** It should enter the *skin* at a 45-degree angle, about 1 to 2 cm distal to the vein, bevel facing *up*. As soon as the needle has punctured the skin, lower it to about a 15-degree angle to enter the vein (Fig. 9-35A).
2. **Enter the vein** from the side or from above. Blood will appear in the catheter when the needle has entered the vein.
3. **Release the tourniquet.**
4. **Advance the catheter** into the vein by using one hand to stabilize the hub of the needle while pushing the catheter, within its plastic sheath,

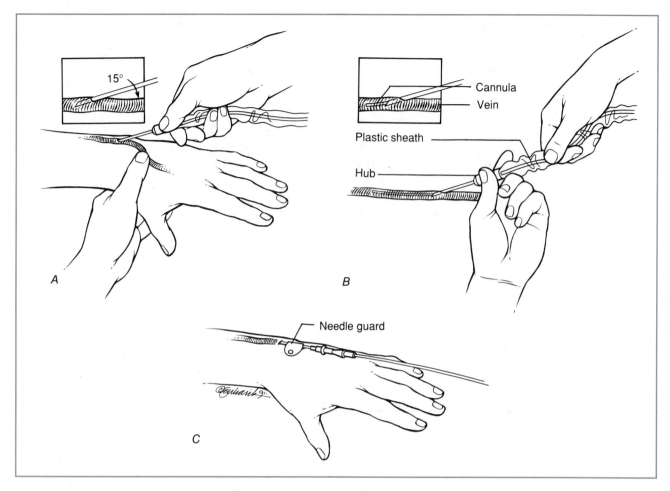

FIGURE 9-35.   INSERTING A THROUGH-THE-NEEDLE CATHETER.   (A) Once the catheter has pierced the skin, align it at a 15-degree angle to enter the vein. (B) Grip the catheter through its plastic sheath and advance it through the needle. (C) Snap on the needle guard.

through the needle with the other hand (Fig. 9-35B). DO *NOT* PULL BACK ON THE CATHETER! Keep advancing the catheter until the catheter hub rests against the needle hub.

5. **Withdraw the needle** completely from the skin.
6. **Snap on the needle guard** at the point where the catheter emerges from the needle, to prevent the catheter being bent against the sharp bevel of the needle and sheared off (Fig. 9-35C).
7. Stabilize the catheter with one hand and use your other hand to attach a 20-ml syringe. **Draw the blood sample,** and hand it to an assistant to distribute among the Vacutainer tubes.
8. **Attach the IV tubing,** and open the clamp wide to permit unimpeded flow. The fluid should flow through the infusion reservoir in a steady stream; if it does not, the catheter tip may be resting up against the wall of the vein, so pull back very slightly on the catheter.

Wire-Guided (Seldinger) Catheter

1. **Attach the introducer needle to a syringe,** and align the needle as described for the previous two techniques.
2. **Enter the vein,** confirming the position of the needle by blood return into the syringe (Fig. 9-36A).
3. **Release the tourniquet.**
4. **Detach the syringe** from the introducer needle.
5. **Insert the guide wire** through the needle into the vein (Fig. 9-36B).
6. **Withdraw the needle,** leaving just the wire inside the vein (Fig. 9-36C).
7. **Thread the catheter over the guide wire** into the vein (Fig. 9-36D).
8. Holding the catheter steady, **withdraw the guide wire** (Fig. 9-36E).
9. Stabilize the catheter with one hand and use your

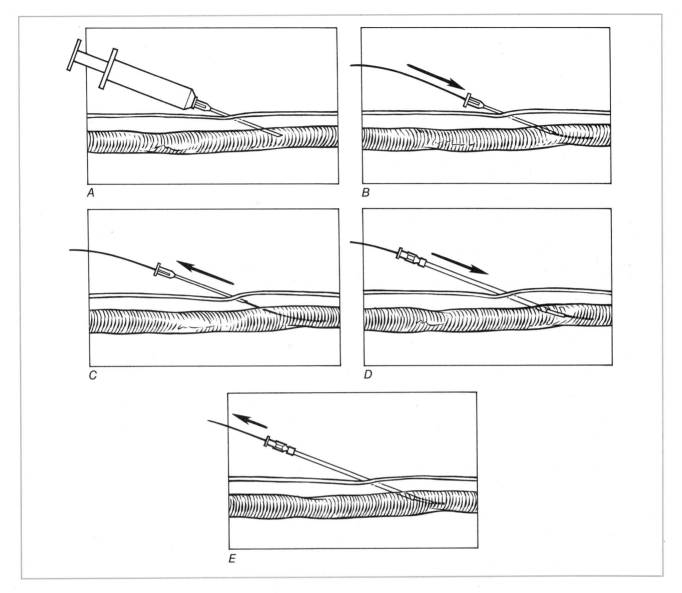

FIGURE 9-36. **SELDINGER TECHNIQUE.** (A) Attach the introducer needle to a syringe, and use the needle to enter the vein. (B) Thread the guide wire through the needle. (C) Remove the needle. (D) Thread the catheter over the guide wire. (E) Remove the guide wire.

other hand to attach a 20-ml syringe. **Draw the blood sample,** and hand it to an assistant to distribute among the Vacutainer tubes.

10. **Attach the IV tubing,** and open the clamp wide to permit unimpeded flow.

Whichever type of catheter you have inserted, when good flow has been established, put a dab of povidone-iodine ointment over the puncture site and **cover the puncture site with a sterile dressing.** Then **tape the catheter securely** in place. Loop the IV tubing, and tape it to the arm as well so that an accidental pull on the tubing will not yank out the catheter.

Be generous with adhesive tape! However, exclude the point of connection between the catheter and the infusion set from your tape job. On the tape, write the type of cannula used, the gauge, and the date (e.g., "14-gauge Angiocath, 10/10/94"). If the IV is in a hand vein or near a joint, immobilize the extremity on an armboard.

Calculating the Flow Rate

Once the catheter is in place, you need to adjust the infusion to the flow rate ordered by the physician or called for by your protocol. To do so, you must know

- The VOLUME to be infused
- The TIME PERIOD over which it is to be infused
- The PROPERTIES OF THE ADMINISTRATION SET you are using, that is, how many drops (gtt) per milliliter (ml) it delivers

The rate is then calculated as follows:

$$\text{gtt/min} = \frac{\text{volume to be infused} \times \text{gtt/ml of administration set}}{\text{total time of infusion in minutes}}$$

For example, suppose the physician orders an infusion of 1 liter (1,000 ml) of normal saline to be run in over 4 hours, and the macrodrop administration set being used provides 10 gtt per milliliter:

Total volume to be infused = 1,000 ml
gtt/ml = 10
Time of infusion (minutes) = 240

$$\text{gtt/min} = \frac{1,000 \text{ ml} \times 10 \text{ gtt/ml}}{240 \text{ min}} = \text{approximately } 42 \text{ gtt/min}$$

Sometimes the IV order is given in a different fashion; the physician may request, for example, an infusion of normal saline at 120 ml per hour. Again, you must know the properties of the infusion set, and you calculate the drops per minute exactly as before:

$$\text{gtt/min} = \frac{\text{volume to be infused} \times \text{gtt/ml of infusion set}}{60 \text{ min}}$$

In the above example, the volume to be infused over 1 hour is 120 ml, and let us say the infusion set again delivers 10 gtt per milliliter:

$$\text{gtt/min} = \frac{120 \text{ ml} \times 10 \text{ gtt/ml}}{60 \text{ min}} = 20 \text{ gtt/min}$$

(Suppose you were asked to speed up the rate to 200 ml/hr using the same infusion set. How many drops per minute would that require?)

Troubleshooting

To be skilled in intravenous therapy, the paramedic needs to know not only how to insert an IV but also how to keep it running. It should become second nature to glance every few minutes at the drip chamber and make sure the IV is still running at the rate you set. If it has slowed down, or stopped, make a *system-*atic search for the cause, starting at the patient's arm and working back toward the IV bag; after each maneuver, recheck what is happening in the drip chamber. Needless to say, if the first or second maneuver you try solves the problem, you needn't continue down the whole checklist.

- Check the forearm to make certain the tourniquet isn't still secured there! (It may be hidden under a shirt sleeve.)
- Straighten out the patient's arm if it is bent.
- Examine the venipuncture site for signs of infiltration (swelling and coolness). If you have any doubts, open the flow regulator clamp wide, and lower the bag below the level of the patient's heart. If blood does not flow back into the IV tubing, the line has probably infiltrated and will need to be removed.
- Check the administration set tubing for kinks.
- Raise the IV bag.
- Close the regulator clamp, and "milk" the tubing toward the patient's arm. Then reopen the clamp and see if flow has improved.

If none of those maneuvers produce a free flow through the IV, discontinue the IV and start a new infusion at another site with a new administration set and a fresh bag of IV solution.

CENTRAL INTRAVENOUS LINES

In some EMS systems, paramedics are authorized to cannulate the internal jugular, external jugular, or subclavian veins. The U.S. Department of Transportation does *not* require skill in central venous cannulation for certification as a paramedic and, indeed, discourages the prehospital insertion of central lines for several reasons:

DISADVANTAGES OF CENTRAL VENOUS LINES IN PREHOSPITAL CARE

- They take too long to establish (5–10 minutes).
- They require strict sterile technique (e.g., gloves, drapes, sterile prep).
- They require a lot of practice, and skill decay is rapid.
- They have a high complication rate (pneumothorax, air embolism, arterial injury).

• A chest x-ray should be obtained *immediately* after placement to ensure correct position and rule out complications.

This author concurs with the U.S. Department of Transportation that central venous lines are neither necessary nor desirable in the prehospital phase of emergency care. In view of the reality that paramedics *are* performing those techniques, however, the correct procedures for doing so are outlined here.

Preparation for central venous cannulation is essentially the same as described earlier for cannulation of a peripheral vein, except that as a general rule, the through-the-needle catheter or wire-guided catheter is easier to use, especially for the internal jugular and subclavian veins.

External Jugular Vein Cannulation

The external jugular vein (Fig. 9-37) runs downward and obliquely backward behind the angle of the jaw until it pierces the deep fascia of the neck just above the middle of the clavicle; the external jugular vein ends in the subclavian vein, where valves retard backflow of blood. To cannulate the external jugular:

1. Place the patient in a **supine, head-down position** to fill the jugular vein; turn the patient's head to the side opposite the intended venipuncture site.
2. **Disinfect** and, preferably, anesthetize **the skin.**
3. **Align the catheter** in the direction of the vein, with the point aimed toward the shoulder on the side of the venipuncture (Fig. 9-38).
4. **Make the puncture** midway between the angle of the jaw and the midclavicular line; stabilize the vein by placing a finger lightly on top of it just above the clavicle.
5. Proceed as described for cannulation of a peripheral vein (see p. 205). TAKE CARE NOT TO LET AIR ENTER THE CATHETER ONCE IT IS IN THE VEIN. Attach the infusion set as soon as there is blood return through the catheter.
6. **Tape the line** securely, but do *not* put circumferential dressings around the neck.

Internal Jugular Vein Cannulation

The internal jugular vein (Fig. 9-39) emerges from the base of the skull, enters the carotid sheath behind the internal carotid artery, then runs posteriorly and lat-

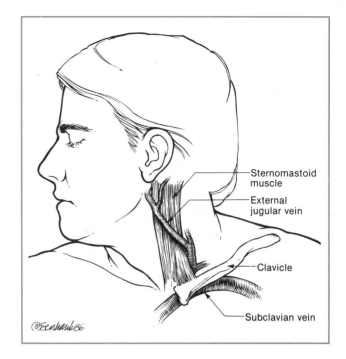

FIGURE 9-37. ANATOMY OF THE EXTERNAL JUGULAR VEIN.

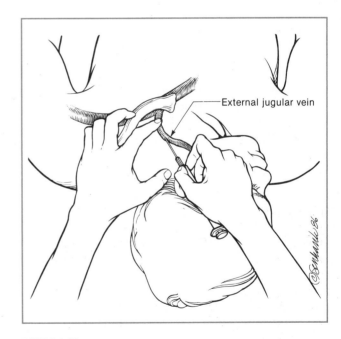

FIGURE 9-38. CANNULATION OF THE EXTERNAL JUGULAR VEIN.

erally to the internal carotid and common carotid. Finally, near its termination, the internal jugular is lateral to and slightly in front of the common carotid artery. To cannulate the internal jugular:

1. Place the index and middle fingers of one hand about 3 cm lateral to the midsternal line, and re-

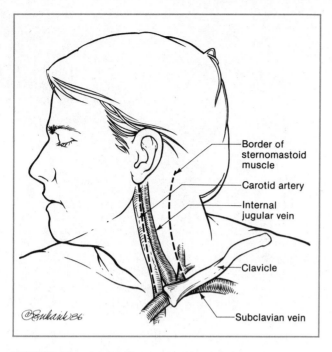

**FIGURE 9-39.   ANATOMY OF THE INTERNAL
JUGULAR VEIN.**

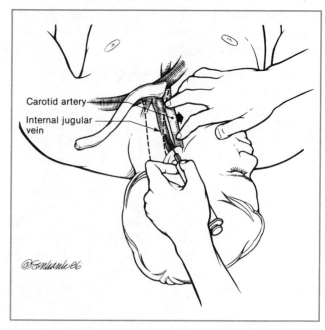

**FIGURE 9-40.   CANNULATION OF THE INTERNAL
JUGULAR VEIN.**

tract the carotid artery medially, away from the anterior border of the sternomastoid muscle (Fig. 9-40).

2. **Introduce the needle** at the midpoint of that anterior border, halfway between the clavicle and the angle of the jaw.
3. Direct the needle toward the nipple at a 30- to 45-degree angle with the frontal plane.
4. Proceed as for a peripheral IV (see p. 205).

Subclavian Vein Cannulation

The subclavian vein (Fig. 9-41) is a short vein that begins as an extension of the axillary vein at the lateral border of the first rib; it crosses over the first rib and passes in front of the anterior scalene muscle, which separates the subclavian vein from the subclavian artery running behind it. The subclavian vein continues behind the medial third of the clavicle, where it is immobilized by small attachments to the rib and clavicle. Then it unites with the internal jugular to form the innominate vein. The apical pleura of the lungs are in contact with the subclavian vein at its junction with the internal jugular. To cannulate the subclavian vein:

1. Insert the needle 1 cm below the junction of the medial and middle thirds of the clavicle.

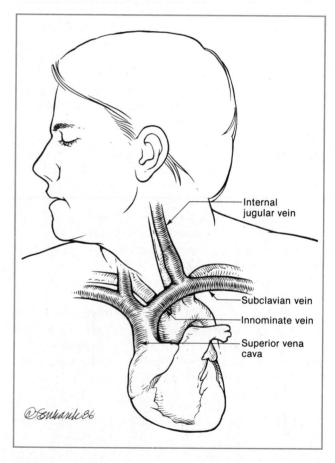

FIGURE 9-41.   ANATOMY OF THE SUBCLAVIAN VEIN.

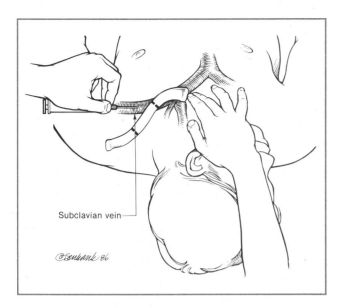

FIGURE 9-42. CANNULATION OF THE SUBCLAVIAN VEIN.

2. Hold the syringe and needle parallel to the back of the patient.
3. Direct the needle *toward the opposite shoulder.* Establish a point of reference by firmly pressing the fingertip into the suprasternal notch and directing the course of the needle slightly behind the fingertip (Fig. 9-42).
4. When the lumen of the subclavian vein has been entered, rotate the needle so that it is facing more toward the feet, since the catheter will have to make a turn into the innominate vein.

Hazards and Complications of Central Venous Cannulation

Cannulation of the jugular and subclavian veins, as noted earlier, entails several dangers, and the rescuer who uses these techniques must know how to recognize the potential complications, which can be fatal if undetected:

- HEMATOMA (a collection of blood beneath the skin) may occur in the neck, either from the venipuncture itself or from accidental puncture of an adjacent artery. The veins, nerves, arteries, and lymphatic ducts in the neck all lie very close to one another, so it is not difficult to puncture the wrong structure. IF A HEMATOMA DOES OCCUR ON ONE SIDE OF THE NECK, DO NOT ATTEMPT VENIPUNCTURE ON THE OP-

POSITE SIDE! A bilateral hematoma in the neck can strangle the patient!
- PNEUMOTHORAX is a very common complication of these procedures. Be alert for any sign of respiratory distress in a patient who has had cannulation of the internal jugular or subclavian vein. Chest x-ray should be performed on all such patients when they reach a medical facility.
- HEMOTHORAX (blood in the thoracic cavity) may be caused by leakage of blood from a punctured vessel into the chest cavity; like pneumothorax, hemothorax will be signalled by respiratory distress. If blood loss is massive, signs of shock may be evident as well.
- AIR EMBOLISM occurs when air is sucked into the jugular or subclavian vein and can be rapidly fatal in a critically ill or injured patient.
- INFILTRATION OF FLUID INTO THE PLEURAL OR MEDIASTINAL CAVITY occurs when the catheter breaks through the wall of the vein. A liter of fluid poured rapidly into the pleural space has the same harmful effect on respiration as the equivalent hemothorax.

All of the above are good reasons to stick to peripheral IVs in the field!

GLOSSARY

acidosis A disturbance in the body's acid-base balance due to CO_2 retention or overproduction of organic acids and characterized by a *pH* less than 7.35.

aerobic metabolism Metabolism that can proceed only in the presence of oxygen.

agglutination Clumping together of red blood cells.

air embolism An air bubble introduced into the circulation.

alkalosis A disturbance in the body's acid-base balance that occurs from hyperventilation, loss of acids (vomiting), or excessive intake of alkalis and characterized by a *pH* greater than 7.45.

anaerobic metabolism Metabolism that takes place in the absence of oxygen.

anion A negatively charged ion, e.g., Cl⁻ (chloride ion).

antecubital fossa The hollow in the front side of the elbow.

antibody A protein produced in the body in response to a specific *antigen* that destroys or inactivates the antigen.

antigen An agent that, when taken into the body, stimulates the formation of specific protective proteins called *antibodies*.

asystole Absence of ventricular contractions; *cardiac standstill*.

baroreceptor Special sensing device located in the aortic arch and carotid sinus that detects changes in pressure (volume) within the vascular system.

base A compound that dissociates to form hydroxyl ions (OH^-); a solution having a pH greater than 7.0.

buffer A substance in a fluid that tends to minimize changes in *pH* that would otherwise result from the addition of *acid* or *base* to the fluid.

cardiac standstill *Asystole*; absence of cardiac contractions.

cardiovascular collapse Failure of the heart and blood vessels; *shock*.

cation A positively charged ion, e.g., Na^+ (sodium ion).

colloid An intravenous solution containing protein or another high-molecular-weight solute, e.g., albumin.

crystalloid An intravenous solution that does not contain protein or other high-molecular-weight solutes, e.g., 5% dextrose in water (D5/W), normal saline, or Ringer's solution.

diaphoresis Profuse sweating.

edema Condition in which excess fluid accumulates in body tissues, manifested by swelling.

electrolyte A substance whose molecules dissociate into charged components (ions) when placed in water.

erythrocyte Red blood cell.

exsanguinate To bleed to death.

extracellular fluid (ECF) The portion of the total body water outside the cells, comprising the interstitial fluid and the plasma.

hematocrit The percentage of a sample of whole blood occupied by red blood cells.

hematoma A localized collection of blood in the tissues.

hemoglobin The oxygen-carrying pigment in red blood cells.

hemolysis The disruption of red blood cells that results from some adverse factor, such as a transfusion reaction or immersion in hypotonic solution.

hemorrhage Profuse bleeding.

hemostasis Stopping hemorrhage.

hemothorax Bleeding into the pleural cavity.

homeostasis A tendency to constancy or stability in the body's internal environment.

hyperkalemia Excessive amount of potassium in the blood.

hypertonic Having an *osmotic pressure* greater than a solution to which it is being compared, usually the *intracellular fluid*.

hypokalemia Abnormally low concentration of potassium in the blood.

hypotension Low blood pressure.

hypotonic Having an *osmotic pressure* lower than a solution to which it is being compared, usually the *intracellular fluid*.

infiltration Leakage of intravenous fluid outside of the vein and into the surrounding tissues; extravasation.

intracellular fluid (ICF) The portion of the total body water contained within the cells, usually about 45 percent of body weight.

intrathoracic pressure Pressure within the chest cavity.

ion An electrically charged molecule, e.g., Na^+ or Cl^-.

leukocyte White blood cell.

MAST Abbreviation for military anti-shock trousers.

osmosis The passage across a semipermeable membrane of pure solvent from a solution of lower solute concentration to one of higher concentration.

osmotic pressure The pressure exerted by a solution of greater solute concentration on water in a solution of lower solute concentration.

PASG Abbreviation for pneumatic anti-shock garment.

perfusion The flow of blood through tissues.

peripheral vascular resistance The resistance to blood flow in the systemic circulation that depends on the degree of constriction in the network of peripheral blood vessels.

pH A measure of the hydrogen ion (H^+) concentration, hence the acidity or alkalinity, of a fluid.

phlebotomy The withdrawal of blood from a vein.

plasma The fluid portion of the blood from which the cells have been removed.

postural syncope Fainting on standing up.

pyrogen A foreign protein capable of inducing fever.

Rh factor An *antigen* present on the red blood cells of some individuals.

shock A state of inadequate tissue perfusion.

sternum Breast bone.

tachycardia A rapid heart rate (over 100 per minute).

thrombocyte Platelet.

thrombophlebitis Condition in which inflammation of a vein leads to the formation of a clot (thrombus) in the vein.

urticaria Hives.

vasoconstriction   Narrowing of the diameter of a blood vessel.

ventricular fibrillation   Form of cardiac arrest characterized by rapid, tremulous, and ineffectual contractions of the cardiac ventricles.

xiphoid   Small cartilaginous and bony portion of the sternum attached to the lower end of the body of the sternum.

FURTHER READING

BASIC LIFE SUPPORT

Barranco F et al. Cardiopulmonary resuscitation with simultaneous chest and abdominal compression: Comparative study in humans. *Resuscitation* 20(1):67, 1990.

Bieber RM. CPR in transportation: A vital link. *EMT J* 3(3):59, 1979.

Brody GM, Beckerman B. CPR: A review of "new" techniques. *Emerg Med* 22(17):119, 1990.

Chandra N et al. Contrasts between intrathoracic pressures during external chest compression and cardiac massage. *Crit Care Med* 9:789, 1981.

Cohen TJ et al. Active compression-decompression: A new method of cardiopulmonary resuscitation. *JAMA* 267:2916, 1992.

Cohen TJ et al. A comparison of active compression-decompression cardiopulmonary resuscitation with standard cardiopulmonary resuscitation for cardiac arrests occurring in the hospital. *N Engl J Med* 329:1918, 1993.

Criley JM. The heart is a conduit in CPR. *Crit Care Med* 9:373, 1981.

DeBard ML. The history of cardiopulmonary resuscitation. *Ann Emerg Med* 9:273, 1980.

Emergency Cardiac Care Committee and Subcommittees, American Heart Association. Guidelines for cardiopulmonary resuscitation and emergency cardiac care. *JAMA* 268:2171, 1992.

Fisher JM. ABC of resuscitation: Recognising a cardiac arrest and providing basic life support. *Br Med J* 292:1002, 1986.

Halperin HR et al. A preliminary study of cardiopulmonary resuscitation by circumferential compression of the chest with use of a pneumatic vest. *N Engl J Med* 329:762, 1993.

Johnson LM. Giving a CPR form new life. *Am J Nurs* 86:60, 1986.

Kern KB et al. A study of chest compression rates during cardiopulmonary resuscitation in humans: The importance of rate-directed chest compressions. *Arch Intern Med* 152:145, 1992.

Knopp RK. CPR: Separating the wheat from the chaff (editorial). *Ann Emerg Med* 12:547, 1983.

Kouwenhoven WB, Knickerbocker GG. Closed-chest cardiac massage. *JAMA* 173:1064, 1960.

Lee RV et al. Cardiopulmonary resuscitation of pregnant women. *Am J Med* 81:311, 1986.

Lewinter JR et al. CPR-dependent consciousness: Evidence for cardiac compression causing forward flow. *Ann Emerg Med* 18:1111, 1989.

Liss HP. A history of resuscitation. *Ann Emerg Med* 15:65, 1986.

Luna GK et al. Hemodynamic effects of external cardiac massage in trauma shock. *J Trauma* 29:1430, 1989.

Mahoney BD et al. Efficacy of pneumatic trousers in refractory prehospital cardiopulmonary arrest. *Ann Emerg Med* 12:8, 1983.

Maier GW et al. The physiology of external cardiac massage: High-impulse cardiopulmonary resuscitation. *Circulation* 70:86, 1984.

Marsden AK. Basic life support. *Br Med J* 299:442, 1989.

McDonald JL. Systolic and mean arterial pressures during manual and mechanical CPR in humans. *Crit Care Med* 9:382, 1981.

McIntyre KM. CPR: Old problems, new techniques. *Cardiovasc Med* 10(9):16, 1985.

McNail EL. Re-evaluation of cardiopulmonary resuscitation. *Resuscitation* 18:1, 1989.

Melker RJ. Recommendation for ventilation during cardiopulmonary resuscitation: Time for a change? *Crit Care Med* 13:882, 1985.

Melker RJ, Banner MJ. Ventilation during CPR: Two-rescuer standards reappraised. *Ann Emerg Med* 14:397, 1985.

Niemann JT. Cardiopulmonary resuscitation. *N Engl J Med* 327:1075, 1992.

Newton JR et al. A physiologic comparison of external cardiac massage techniques. *J Thorac Cardiovasc Surg* 95:892, 1988.

Ornato JP et al. Measurement of ventilation during cardiopulmonary resuscitation. *Crit Care Med* 11:79, 1983.

Rudikoff MJ et al. Mechanisms of blood flow during cardiopulmonary resuscitation. *Circulation* 61:345, 1980.

Sack JB et al. Interposed abdominal compression: Cardiopulmonary resuscitation and resuscitation outcome during asystole and electromechanical dissociation. *Circulation* 86:1692, 1992.

Safar P, Bircher N. *Cardiopulmonary Cerebral Resuscitation* (3rd ed.). Philadelphia: Saunders, 1988.

Sanders AB, Meislin HW, Ewy GA. The physiology of cardiopulmonary resuscitation. *JAMA* 252:3283, 1984.

Swenson RD et al. Hemodynamics in humans during conventional and experimental methods of cardiopulmonary resuscitation. *Circulation* 78:630, 1988.

Taylor GJ et al. Importance of prolonged compression during cardiopulmonary resuscitation in man. *N Engl J Med* 296:1515, 1977.

Warren ET et al. External cardiopulmonary resuscitation augmented by the military antishock trousers. *Am Surg* 49:651, 1983.

Yatsu FM. Cardiopulmonary-cerebral resuscitation. *N Engl J Med* 314:440, 1986.

FLUIDS AND ELECTROLYTES

Geiderman JM, Goodman SL, Cohen DB. Magnesium—the forgotten electrolyte. *JACEP* 8:204, 1979.

Lindeman RD, Papper S. Therapy of fluid and electrolyte disorders. *Ann Intern Med* 82:64, 1975.

Rund DA. Fluid and electrolyte disorders. *Emerg Med Serv* 17(6):31, 1988.

Travenol Laboratories. *The Fundamentals of Body Water and Electrolytes*. Deerfield, Ill: Travenol, 1973.

Wilson RF, Sibbald WJ. Fluid and electrolyte problems in the emergency department. *JACEP* 5:339, 1976.

ACID-BASE BALANCE

Abbot Laboratories. *Acid-Base Balance* (pamphlet). North Chicago: Abbot, 1974.

Flomenbaum N. Acid-base disturbances. *Emerg Med* 16(3): 59, 1984.

Hazard PB, Griffin JP. Sodium bicarbonate in the management of systemic acidosis. *South Med J* 73:1339, 1980.

Hazard PB et al. Calculation of sodium bicarbonate requirement in metabolic acidosis. *Am J Med Sci* 283:18, 1982.

Kassirer JP. Serious acid-base disorders. *N Engl J Med* 291:773, 1974.

Mennen M, Slovis CM. Severe metabolic alkalosis in the emergency department. *Ann Emerg Med* 17:354, 1988.

Miller WC. The ABCs of blood gases. *Emerg Med* 16(3):37, 1984.

Stein JM. Interpreting arterial blood gases. *Emerg Med* 18(1):61, 1986.

Sun JH et al. Carbicarb: An effective substitute for $NAHCO_3$ for the treatment of acidosis. *Surgery* 102:835, 1987.

BLOOD AND FLUID THERAPY

Aeder MI et al. Technical limitations in the rapid infusion of intravenous fluids. *Ann Emerg Med* 14:307, 1985.

Berkman SA. The spectrum of transfusion reactions. *Hosp Pract* 19(6):205, 1984.

Better OS et al. Early management of shock and prophylaxis of acute renal failure in traumatic rhabdomyolysis. *N Engl J Med* 322:825, 1990.

Bickell WH, Shaftan GW, Mattox KL. Intravenous fluid administration and uncontrolled hemorrhage (editorial). *J Trauma* 29:409, 1989.

Blood products. *Med Lett Drugs Ther* 21:93, 1979.

Brzica SM. Trouble with transfusions. *Emerg Med* 15(20):115, 1983.

Collins ML, Kafer ER. Using blood components: I. *Emerg Med* 17(11):131, 1985.

Cone JB et al. Beneficial effects of a hypertonic solution for resuscitation in the presence of acute hemorrhage. *Am J Surg* 154:585, 1987.

Cross JS et al. Hypertonic saline attentuates the hormonal response to injury. *Ann Surg* 209:684, 1989.

Dula DJ et al. Rapid flow rates for the resuscitation of hypovolemic shock. *Ann Emerg Med* 14:303, 1985.

Gervin AS et al. Resuscitation of trauma patients with type-specific uncrossmatched blood. *J Trauma* 24:327, 1984.

Gould SA et al. Red cell substitutes: An update. *Ann Emerg Med* 14:798, 1985.

Greenfield RH, Bessen HA, Henneman PL. Effect of crystalloid infusion on hematocrit and intravascular volume in healthy, nonbleeding subjects. *Ann Emerg Med* 18:51, 1989.

Iserson KV. Whole blood in trauma resuscitations. *Am J Emerg Med* 3:358, 1985.

Jones WT. Managing hypovolemia. *JEMS* 17(7):48, 1992.

Kafer ER, Collins ML. Using blood components: II. *Emerg Med* 17(14):46, 1985.

Kaweski SM et al. The effect of prehospital fluids on survival in trauma patients. *J Trauma* 30:1215, 1990.

Kruskall MS et al. Transfusion therapy in emergency medicine. *Ann Emerg Med* 17:327, 1988.

Landow L et al. Efficacy of large-bore intravenous fluid administration sets designed for rapid volume resuscitation. *Crit Care Med* 18:540, 1990.

Levy DB, Peppers MP. IV fluids used in shock. *Emergency* 23(4):22, 1991.

Maningas PA et al. Hypertonic sodium chloride solutions for the prehospital management of traumatic hemorrhagic shock: A possible improvement in the standard of care? *Ann Emerg Med* 15:1411, 1986.

Martin RR et al. Prospective evaluation of preoperative fluid resuscitation in hypotensive patients with penetrating truncal injury: A preliminary report. *J Trauma* 33:354, 1992.

Mattox KL et al. Prehospital hypertonic saline-dextran infusion for post-traumatic hypotension. *Ann Surg* 213: 482, 1991.

Mazzoni MC et al. The efficacy of iso- and hyperosmotic fluids as volume expanders in fixed-volume and uncontrolled hemorrhage. *Ann Emerg Med* 19:350, 1990.

Moss GS et al. Colloid or crystalloid in the resuscitation of hemorrhagic shock: A controlled clinical trial. *Surgery* 89:434, 1981.

Muller-Suur N. Blood volume substitutes in emergency care. *Disaster Med* 1:173, 1983.

Peters RM et al. Comparison of isotonic and hypertonic fluids in resuscitation from hypovolemic shock. *Surg Gynecol Obstet* 163:219, 1986.

Schwab CW et al. Immediate trauma resuscitation with type O uncrossmatched blood: A two-year prospective experience. *J Trauma* 26:897, 1986.

Shackford SR et al. Whole blood versus packed-cell transfusions: A physiologic comparison. *Ann Surg* 193:337, 1981.

Shoemaker WC. Comparison of emergency resuscitation with colloids and crystalloids. *Disaster Med* 1:10, 1983.

Traverso LW et al. Fluid resuscitation after an otherwise fatal hemorrhage: I. Crystalloid solutions. *J Trauma* 26:168, 1986.

Traverso LW et al. Fluid resuscitation after an otherwise fatal hemorrhage: II. Colloid solutions. *J Trauma* 26:176, 1986.

Vassar MJ et al. 7.5% sodium chloride/dextran for resuscitation of trauma patients undergoing helicopter transport. *Arch Surg* 126:1065, 1991.

Weil MH, Rackow EC. A guide to volume repletion. *Emerg Med* 16(8):101, 1984.

West HC et al. Immediate prediction of blood requirements in trauma victims. *South Med J* 82:186,1989.

White SJ et al. A comparison of field techniques used to pressure-infuse intravenous fluids. *Prehosp Disaster Med* 6(4):429, 1991.

LEG-RAISING AND TRENDELENBURG POSITION

Bivens HG, Knopp R, dos Santos PA. Blood volume distribution in the Trendelenburg position. *Ann Emerg Med* 14:641, 1985.

Gaffney FA et al. Passive leg raising does not produce a significant or sustained autotransfusion effect. *J Trauma* 22:190, 1982.

Reich DL et al. Trendelenburg position and passive leg raising do not significantly improve cardiopulmonary performance in the anesthetized patient with coronary artery disease. *Crit Care Med* 17:313, 1989.

Sibbald WJ et al. Trendelenburg position: Hemodynamic effects in hypotensive and normotensive patients. *Crit Care Med* 7:218, 1979.

Stern SA et al. Effect of blood pressure on hemorrhage volume and survival in a near-fatal hemorrhage model incorporating vascular injury. *Ann Emerg Med* 22:155, 1993.

Wong DH et al. Acute cardiovascular response to passive leg raising. *Crit Care Med* 16:123, 1988.

SHOCK

Adams SL et al. Absence of a tachycardic response to intraperitoneal hemorrhage. *J Emerg Med* 4:383, 1986.

Caroline NL. *Emergency Medical Treatment: A Text for EMT-As and EMT-Intermediates* (3rd ed.). Boston: Little, Brown, 1991. Chaps. 8 and 9.

Diprose P, Sleet RA. How well do doctors resuscitate patients with haemorrhagic shock? *Arch Emerg Med* 10(3):135, 1993.

Garvin JM. Keeping shock simple. *Emerg Med Serv* 9(5):49, 1980.

Geelhoed GW. Shock and its management. *Emerg Med Serv* 5(6):42, 1976.

Parillo JE. Pathogenetic mechanisms of septic shock. *N Engl J Med* 328:1471, 1993.

Rackow ER. Of shock and vasoactive drugs. *Emerg Med* 16(1):115, 1984.

Sander-Jensen K et al. Vagal slowing of the heart during haemorrhage: Observation from 20 consecutive hypotensive patients. *Br Med J* 292:364, 1986.

Schriger DL, Baraff LJ. Capillary refill: Is it a useful predictor of hypovolemic states? *Ann Emerg Med* 20:601, 1991.

Schumer W. Septic shock. *JAMA* 242:1906, 1979.

Secher NH et al. Bradycardia during reversible hemorrhagic shock: A forgotten observation? *Clin Physiol* 5:315, 1985.

Snyder HS et al. Lack of a tachycardic response to hypotension in penetrating abdominal injuries. *J Emerg Med* 7:335, 1989.

Vayer JS. Absence of a tachycardic response to shock in penetrating intraperitoneal injury. *Ann Emerg Med* 17:227, 1988.

Weil MH, Desai V. Measuring the severity of shock. *Emerg Med* 24(5):207, 1992.

Wilson RF. Science and shock: A clinical perspective. *Ann Emerg Med* 14:714, 1985.

MILITARY ANTI-SHOCK TROUSERS

Abraham E et al. Effect of pneumatic trousers on pulmonary function. *Crit Care Med* 10:754, 1982.

Abraham E et al. Cardiorespiratory effects of pneumatic trousers in critically ill patients. *Arch Surg* 119:912, 1984.

Ali J et al. Pneumatic antishock garment decreases hemorrhage and mortality from splenic injury. *Can J Surg* 34:496, 1991.

Aprahamian C et al. Effect of circumferential pneumatic compression devices on digital flow. *Ann Emerg Med* 13:1092, 1984.

Bartlett L. An overview of military antishock trousers. *Emerg Med Serv* 14(6):23, 1985.

Bass RR et al. Thigh compartment syndrome without lower extremity trauma following application of pneumatic antishock trousers. *Ann Emerg Med* 12:382, 1983.

Bickell WH, Dice WH. Military antishock trousers in a patient with adrenergic-resistant anaphylaxis. *Ann Emerg Med* 13:189, 1984.

Bickell WH et al. Effect of antishock trousers on the trauma score: A prospective analysis in the urban setting. *Ann Emerg Med* 14:218, 1985.

Bickell WH et al. Randomized trial of pneumatic antishock garments in the prehospital management of penetrating abdominal injuries. *Ann Emerg Med* 16:653, 1987.

Bircher N, Safar P, Stewart RD. A comparison of standard, MAST-augmented, and open chest CPR in dogs. *Crit Care Med* 8:147, 1980.

Bivens HG et al. Blood volume displacement with inflation of antishock trousers. *Ann Emerg Med* 11:409, 1982.

Brotman S, Browder B, Cox E. MAS trousers improperly applied causing a compartment syndrome in lower extremity trauma. *J Trauma* 22:598, 1982.

Brown K et al. Trauma rounds: The case of the penetrating chest wound. *JEMS* 16(3):83, 1991.

Cayten CG et al. A study of pneumatic antishock garments in severely hypotensive trauma patients. *J Trauma* 34:728, 1993.

Chipman CD. The MAST controversy. *Emerg Med* 15(3):206, 1983.

Chisholm CD, Clark DE. Effect of pneumatic antishock garment on intramuscular pressure. *Ann Emerg Med* 13:581, 1984.

Christiansen KS. Pneumatic antishock garments (PASG): Do they precipitate lower-extremity compartment syndromes? *J Trauma* 26:1102, 1986.

Civetta JM et al. Prehospital use of the military antishock trouser (MAST). *JACEP* 5:581, 1976.

Cogbill TH et al. Pulmonary function after military antishock trouser inflation. *Surg Forum* 32:302, 1981.

Crile GW. *Hemorrhage and Transfusion: An Experimental and Clinical Research.* New York: Appleton, 1909. P.139.

Flint LM et al. Definite control of bleeding from severe pelvic fracture. *Ann Surg* 189:709, 1979.

Gaffney FA et al. Hemodynamic effects of medical antishock trousers (MAST garment). *J Trauma* 21:931, 1981.

Goldsmith SR. Comparative hemodynamic effects of antishock suit and volume expansion in normal human beings. *Ann Emerg Med* 12:348, 1983.

Gustafson RA et al. The use of the MAST suit in ruptured abdominal aortic aneurysms. *Am Surg* 49:454, 1983.

Hanke BK et al. Antishock trousers: A comparison of inflation techniques and inflation pressures. *Ann Emerg Med* 14:636, 1985.

Hauswalk M, Greene ER. Aortic blood flow during sequential MAST inflation. *Ann Emerg Med* 15:1297, 1986.

Honigman B et al. The role of pneumatic antishock garment in penetrating cardiac wounds. *JAMA* 266:2398, 1991.

Lee HR et al. MAST augmentation of external cardiac compression: Role of changing intrapleural pressure. *Ann Emerg Med* 10:560, 1981.

Lee HR et al. Venous return in hemorrhagic shock after application of military anti-shock trousers. *Am J Emerg Med* 1:7, 1983.

Lilja GP, Long RS, Ruiz E. Augmentation of systolic blood pressure during external cardiac compression by the use of the MAST suit. *Ann Emerg Med* 10:182, 1981.

Lilja GP et al. MAST usage in cardiopulmonary resuscitation. *Ann Emerg Med* 13:833, 1984.

Lloyd S. MAST and IV infusion: Do they help in prehospital trauma management? *Ann Emerg Med* 16:565, 1987.

Ludewig RM, Wangensteen SL. Effect of external counterpressure on venous bleeding. *Surgery* 65:515, 1969.

Mahoney BD, Mirick MJ. Efficacy of pneumatic trousers in

refractory prehospital cardiopulmonary arrest. *Ann Emerg Med* 12:8, 1983.

Mannering D et al. Application of the medical anti-shock trouser (MAST) increases cardiac output and tissue perfusion in simulated mild hypovolaemia. *Intensive Care Med* 12:143, 1986.

Mattox KL. Prospective randomized evaluation of anti-shock MAST in post-traumatic hypotension. *J Trauma* 26:779, 1986.

Mattox KL et al. Prospective MAST study in 911 patients. *J Trauma* 29:1104, 1989.

McBride G. One caution in pneumatic anti-shock garment use. *JAMA* 247:112, 1982.

McCabe JB, Seidel DR, Jagger JA. Antishock trouser inflation and pulmonary vital capacity. *Ann Emerg Med* 12:290, 1983.

McSwain NE. Pneumatic anti-shock garment: State of the art 1988. *Ann Emerg Med* 17:506, 1988.

McSwain NE. Pneumatic anti-shock garment: Does it work? *Prehosp Disaster Med* 4(1):42, 1989.

McSwain NE. PASG: Holding on for dear life. *Emergency* 22(8):39, 1990.

Oertel T, Loehr M. Bee-sting anaphylaxis: The use of medical antishock trousers. *Ann Emerg Med* 13:459, 1984.

Pepe PE, Bass RR, Mattox KL. Clinical trials of the pneumatic antishock garment in the urban prehospital setting. *Ann Emerg Med* 15:1407, 1986.

Polando G et al. PASG use in pelvic fracture immobilization. *JEMS* 15(3):48, 1990.

Pricolo VE et al. Trendelenburg versus PASG application: Hemodynamic response in man. *J Trauma* 26:718, 1986.

Ransom KJ, McSwain NE. Physiologic changes of antishock trousers in relationship to external pressure. *Surg Gynecol Obstet* 158:488, 1984.

Rockwell DD et al. An improved design of the pneumatic counterpressure trousers. *Am J Surg* 143:377, 1982.

Sanders AB, Meislin HW. Alterations in MAST suit pressure with changes in ambient temperature. *J Emerg Med* 1:37, 1983.

Sanders AB, Meislin HW. Effect of altitude change on MAST suit pressure. *Ann Emerg Med* 12:140, 1983.

Savino JA et al. Overinflation of pneumatic antishock garments in the elderly. *Am J Surg* 155:572, 1988.

Tandberg D et al. Successful treatment of paroxysmal supraventricular tachycardia with MAST. *Ann Emerg Med* 13:1068, 1984.

Wangensteen SL et al. The effect of external counterpressure on arterial bleeding. *Surgery* 64:922, 1968.

Wasserberger J, Ordog G. MAST in profound hemorrhagic shock (letter). *Prehosp Disaster Med* 8(2):206, 1993.

Wayne MA, MacDonald SC. Clinical evaluation of the antishock trouser: Prospective study of low-pressure inflation. *Ann Emerg Med* 12:285, 1983.

Wayne MA, MacDonald SC. Clinical evaluation of the antishock trouser: Retrospective analysis of five years of experience. *Ann Emerg Med* 12:342, 1983.

Williams TM, Knopp R, Ellyson JH. Compartment syndrome after antishock trouser use without lower extremity trauma. *J Trauma* 22:595, 1982.

INTRAVENOUS LINES

Abbot Laboratories. *Venipuncture and Venous Cannulation.* North Chicago: Abbot, 1971.

Abraham E et al. Central venous catheterization in the emergency setting. *Crit Care Med* 11:515, 1983.

Armstrong P et al. Ethyl chloride and venepuncture pain: A comparison with intradermal lidocaine. *Can J Anaesth* 37:656, 1990.

Dailey RH. Lines into veins. *Emerg Med* 15(13):167, 1983.

Dailey RH. Use of wire-guided (Seldinger-type) catheters in the emergency department. *Ann Emerg Med* 12:489, 1983.

Emerman CL et al. A prospective study of femoral versus subclavian vein catheterization during cardiac arrest. *Ann Emerg Med* 19:26, 1990.

Falk JL. On entering veins and arteries. *Emerg Med* 14(8):22, 1982.

Fares LG et al. Improved subclavian cannulation technique. *Surg Gynecol Obstet* 162:277, 1986.

Feliciano DV et al. Major complications of percutaneous subclavian vein catheters. *Am J Surg* 138:869, 1979.

Goldman DA et al. Guidelines for infection control in intravenous therapy. *Ann Intern Med* 79:848, 1973.

Haynes BE et al. Catheter introducers for rapid fluid resuscitation. *Ann Emerg Med* 12:606, 1983.

Heimbach LJ. Accessing the external jugular vein. *Emergency* 25(11):53, 1993.

Iserson KV, Reeter AK. Rapid fluid replacement: A new methodology. *Ann Emerg Med* 13:97, 1984.

Iserson KV et al. Comparison of flow rates for standard and large-bore blood tubing. *West J Med* 14:183, 1985.

Jesseph JM et al. Patient positioning for subclavian vein catheterization. *Arch Surg* 122:1207, 1987.

Jones SE, Nesper TP, Alcouloumre E. Prehospital intravenous line placement: A prospective study. *Ann Emerg Med* 18:244, 1989.

Lawrence DL. Prehospital IV therapy: Are we contributing to patient complications? *JEMS* 15(1):51, 1990.

Lawrence DW, Lauro AJ. Complications from IV therapy: Results from field-started and emergency department-started IVs compared. *Ann Emerg Med* 17:314, 1988.

Lewis FR. Ineffective therapy and delayed transport. *Prehosp Disaster Med* 4:129, 1989.

Maki DG. Preventing infection in intravenous therapy. *Hosp Pract* 11(4):95, 1976.

Maki DG, Goldman DA, Rhame FS. Infection control in intravenous therapy. *Ann Intern Med* 79:867, 1973.

Maki DG, Ringer M. Evaluation of dressing regimens for prevention of infection with peripheral intravenous catheters. *JAMA* 258:2396, 1987.

Mateer JR et al. Rapid fluid resuscitation with central venous catheters. *Ann Emerg Med* 12:149, 1983.

Millikan JS, Cain TL, Hansbrough J. Rapid volume replacement for hypovolemic shock: A comparison of techniques and equipment. *J Trauma* 24:428, 1984.

Nott MR et al. Relief of injection pain in adults: EMLA cream for 5 minutes before venepuncture. *Anaesthesia* 45:772, 1990.

O'Gorman M, Trabulsy P, Pilcher DB. Zero-time prehospital IV. *J Trauma* 29:84, 1989.

Orebaugh SL. Venous air embolism: Clinical and experimental considerations. *Crit Care Med* 20:1169, 1992.

Plumer AL. *Principles and Practice of Intravenous Therapy* (3rd ed.). Boston: Little, Brown, 1982.

Pons PT et al. Prehospital venous access in an urban paramedic system: A prospective on-scene analysis. *J Trauma* 28:1460, 1988.

Rottman SJ. Prehospital fluid administration in trauma. *Prehosp Disaster Med* 4:127, 1989.

Schwartzman P, Rottman SJ. Prehospital use of heparin locks: A cost-effective method for intravenous access. *Am J Emerg Med* 5:475, 1987.

Steele BF. Intravenous therapy. *EMT J* 2(3):55, 1978.

Swanson RS et al. Emergency intravenous access through the femoral vein. *Ann Emerg Med* 13:244, 1984.

Verdile VP. Trends in IV therapy. *Emergency* 22(4):44, 1990.

Wears RL, Winton CN. Load and go versus stay and play: Analysis of prehospital IV fluid therapy by computer simulation. *Ann Emerg Med* 19:163, 1990.

Westreich M. Preventing complications of subclavian vein catheterization. *JACEP* 7:368, 1978.

PERFORMANCE CHECKLISTS

The following pages contain checklists for correct performance of some of the skills described in this chapter. The checklists can be used as a review and as a guide for practicing the respective skills.

Performance Test
One-Rescuer CPR: Adult

Student _____ Date _____

Instructor: Place an "X" in the Fail column beside any element that is done incorrectly, out of sequence, or omitted.

Step	Activity	Critical Performance	Fail
Assessment	Determine unresponsiveness	Taps or gently shakes shoulder	
		Shouts, "Are you O.K.?"	
Airway	Position the victim	Turns victim supine if needed, supporting head and neck (4–10 sec)	
	Open the airway	Uses head tilt–chin lift maneuver	
	Determine breathlessness	Maintains open airway	
		Ear over mouth, observes chest	
		Looks, listens, and feels for breathing	
Breathing	Ventilate twice	Maintains open airway	
		Seals mouth and nose properly	
		Ventilates twice, 1½–2 sec/ventilation	
		Observes chest rise	
		Ventilation volume adequate	
		Allows deflation between breaths	
Circulation	Determine pulselessness	Palpates carotid pulse on near side of manikin	
		Maintains head tilt with other hand	
	Begin chest compressions	Rescuer's knees by victim's shoulder	
		Landmark check prior to hand placement	
		Proper hand position throughout	
		Rescuer's shoulders over victim's sternum	
		Equal compression-relaxation times	
		Compress 1½–2 in.	
		Keeps hands on sternum during upstroke	
		Complete chest relaxation on upstroke	
		Says any helpful mnemonic	
		Compression rate: 80–100/min	
Compression-ventilation cycles	Do 4 cycles of 15 compressions and 2 ventilations	Proper compression-ventilation ratio = 15 : 2 per cycle	
		Observes chest rise 1–1½ sec/ventilation	
		Completes 4 cycles in 52–73 sec	
Reassessment	Recheck pulse If no pulse:	Palpates carotid pulse (5 sec)	

Continue CPR	Ventilate twice	Ventilates 2 times	
		Observes chest rise	
		1½ sec/ventilation	
		Resumes cardiac compressions	

Instructor _____

Based on the recommendations in Emergency Cardiac Care Committee and Subcommittees, American Heart Association. Guidelines for cardiopulmonary resuscitation and emergency cardiac care. *JAMA* 268:2172, 1992.

Performance Test
Two-Rescuer CPR: Adult

Student _____ Date _____

Instructor: Place an "X" in the Fail column beside any element that is done incorrectly, out of sequence, or omitted.

Step	Activity	Critical Performance	Fail
Assessment	Rescuer #1 (ventilator): Determines unresponsiveness	Taps or gently shakes shoulder Shouts, "Are you O.K.?"	
Airway	Positions victim	Turns victim supine if necessary	
	Opens the airway	Uses head tilt–chin lift to open airway	
	Determines breathlessness	Looks, listens, feels for breathing (3–5 sec)	
		Says, "Not breathing."	
Breathing	Rescuer #1 ventilates twice	Observes chest rise	
		1½ sec/ventilation	
Circulation	Rescuer #1 determines pulselessness	Palpates carotid artery (5–10 sec)	
	States results	Says, "No pulse."	
	Rescuer #2 locates landmark notch	Locates landmark on victim's chest	
	Gets into position	Hands, shoulders in correct position	
Compression-ventilation cycles	Rescuer #2 begins chest compressions	Correct ratio compressions-ventilations = 5 : 1	
		Compression rate = 80–100/min	
		Says any helpful mnemonic	
	Rescuer #1 ventilates and checks for compression effectiveness	Stops compressing for each ventilation	
		Ventilates 1 time (1½–2 sec) after every 5 compressions	
		Checks pulse to confirm compressions	
		Time for 10 cycles = 40–53 sec	
Call for switch	Rescuer #2 calls for switch when tired	Says, "Switch after next cycle."	

Switch	Simultaneously: Rescuer #1 moves to chest	Moves to chest	
		Locates landmark on victim's chest	
		Gets into position for compressions	
	Rescuer #2 moves to head	Moves to head	
		Checks carotid pulse (5 sec)	
		Says, "No pulse."	
		Opens airway	
		Ventilates once*	
		Switch accomplished with minimum delay	

*During practice and testing, only one rescuer actually ventilates the manikin. The other rescuer simulates ventilation.

Instructor _____

Based on the recommendations in Emergency Cardiac Care Committee and Subcommittees, American Heart Association. Guidelines for cardiopulmonary resuscitation and emergency cardiac care. *JAMA* 268:2172, 1992.

10
Overview of Pharmacology

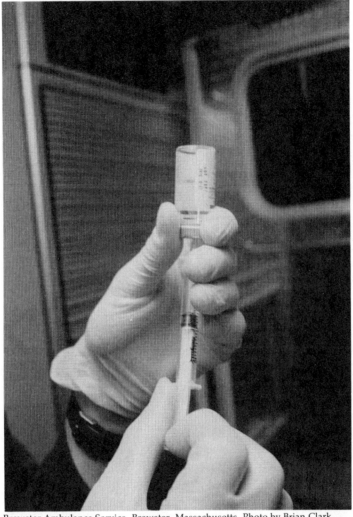

Brewster Ambulance Service, Brewster, Massachusetts. Photo by Brian Clark.

OBJECTIVES

One of the principal areas in which the activities of the EMT-paramedic differ from those of the EMT-A (ambulance) is in the administration of pharmacologic agents. Such agents have both lifesaving and life-endangering potential, depending on how they are used. The wrong drug or the wrong dosage or technique of administration of the right drug can kill a patient as effectively as a lethal weapon. Therefore, the paramedic must be intimately familiar with the pharmacologic agents used in the field—their indications and contraindications, their side effects, their dangers. Nowhere in emergency care can ignorance or carelessness on the part of the paramedic do so much harm as in the administration of drugs.

In this chapter, we shall learn some of the basic principles of the administration of drugs—what drugs are, how they are delivered to the body, and what one has to know about a drug before one may administer it. Detailed information about *specific* drugs can be found in the Drug Handbook at the end of this textbook. It is recommended that the student refer to the appropriate section of the Drug Handbook to learn about each specific drug when it is first mentioned in the text and to review the information each time the drug is mentioned thereafter. By the end of *this* chapter, the student should be able to

1. Explain the difference between a drug's generic name and its trade name
2. Identify the meaning of terms for different forms of drugs, given a list of terms and a list of definitions, and indicate which drug forms are used in prehospital emergency care
3. List five factors that can affect the actions of a drug
4. List the routes by which drugs can be given, and indicate the relative speed with which drugs are absorbed through each route
5. Identify, given a list of definitions, the definition of
   - Indication
   - Contraindication
   - Depressant
   - Stimulant
   - Physiologic action
   - Therapeutic action
   - Untoward reaction
   - Antagonism
   - Cumulative action
   - Tolerance
   - Synergism
   - Potentiation
   - Habituation
   - Idiosyncrasy
   - Hypersensitivity
6. List the types of information a paramedic must know about every drug he or she uses in the field
7. Calculate a person's weight in kilograms, given his or her weight in pounds
8. Convert dosages from grams to milligrams and vice versa
9. Convert volumes from liters to milliliters and vice versa
10. Calculate the correct drug dosage for a patient, given the patient's weight in kilograms or pounds and the usual dosage of the drug in milligrams per kilogram
11. List the steps in administering a drug to a conscious patient
12. List at least eight safety precautions in giving medications
13. Describe or correctly demonstrate
    - How to use a standard syringe
    - How to use a Tubex syringe
    - How to use a prefilled syringe
    - How to draw up a solution from a vial or ampule
    - How to give medications via an intravenous line
    - How to add medications to an IV bag
    - How to give an intramuscular injection
    - How to give a subcutaneous injection

DRUG INFORMATON

A drug is a chemical compound administered as an aid in the diagnosis, treatment, or prevention of a disease or other abnormal condition; drugs may be given in an attempt to alter the disease process itself or to relieve the symptoms of the process.

The drugs we use are derived from four principal *sources*: animal, vegetable, mineral, and synthetic. For example, insulin, a medication taken by diabetics, is usually prepared from the pancreas of ANIMALS (cattle or pigs). A variety of roots, leaves, flowers, and seeds provide VEGETABLE sources of drugs; digitalis, used in the treatment of heart failure, is a drug of vegetable origin prepared from the dried leaves of a wildflower called purple foxglove. MINERALS such as calcium, iron, and magnesium are also used in the treatment of various medical problems. Finally, many of the drugs on the market today are manufactured synthetically; SYNTHETIC forms of vitamins, steroids, narcotics, and many other drugs are widely available.

Drug Names

Most drugs have several names. The names of a drug fall into four broad categories:

- OFFICIAL NAME: The name under which the drug is listed in the *United States Pharmacopeia* (USP) and other official publications.
- CHEMICAL NAME: An exact description of the drug's chemical makeup, of interest mainly to chemists and others involved in the manufacture of drugs.
- GENERIC NAME: Usually the name given to the drug by the company that first manufactures it, before the drug has become official. The generic name is generally derived from the chemical name but is shorter and simpler.
- TRADE NAME: The brand name, proprietary name, or trademark. A trade name has the symbol ® in the upper righthand corner, indicating that the name has been registered as a trademark by a particular manufacturer. The first letter of a trade name is capitalized. Since a given drug may be marketed by a number of manufacturers, it may have several different trade names.

Let us consider, for example, tetracycline, a widely used antibiotic medication:

- Official name: tetracyline USP
- Chemical name: 4-dimethylamino-1,4,4a,5,5a,6,11,12a-octahydro-3,6,-10,12,12a-pentahydroxy-6-methyl-1,11-dioxo-2-naphthacenecarboxamide
- Generic name: tetracycline
- Trade names: Achromycin®, Cyclopar®, Mysteclin®, Sumycin®

In this text, we shall refer to drugs by their generic names. When a drug is widely known by its trade name, we shall note the trade name in parentheses, for example, diazepam (Valium), norepinephrine (Levophed), furosemide (Lasix), naloxone (Narcan), and oxytocin (Pitocin).

Drug Standards and Legislation

The manufacture of pharmaceuticals in the United States and most other countries is subject to a variety of legal standards. Those standards are necessary to ensure that drugs issued by different manufacturers are of uniform strength and purity. In the United States, drug standards are published in the *United States Pharmacopeia* and the *National Formulary*. In addition, several federal laws have been enacted since the beginning of the century to protect the consumer (the patient) from unsafe substances and unscrupulous manufacturers or distributors.

Laws Regulating the Sale and Administration of Drugs

The *Pure Food Act* of 1906 was the first federal legislation in the United States aimed at protecting the public from mislabelled, poisonous, or otherwise harmful foods, medications, and alcoholic beverages. It required little more than the labelling of drugs, and it was replaced by the more comprehensive legislation of 1938.

The federal *Food, Drug and Cosmetic Act* (1938, amended in 1952 and 1962) added several important provisions that were not contained in the earlier law, among them:

- It requires that labels list the possible habit-forming drugs contained within and also give warning regarding possible side effects.
- It authorizes the federal Food and Drug Administration (FDA) to determine the safety and efficacy of drugs before they are marketed.
- It requires that dangerous drugs be issued only on prescription of a physician, dentist, or veterinarian.

Enforcement of the Food, Drug and Cosmetic Act is the responsibility of the FDA, an arm of the Department of Health and Human Services.

The *Harrison Narcotic Act* (1914) regulates the import, manufacture, sale, and prescription of opium, cocaine, and their derivatives, as well as several nonnarcotic drugs. This act requires precise record-keeping in the dispensing of controlled drugs and in the registration of distributors, such as pharmacists, within the Department of Internal Revenue. The act specifies fines and imprisonment for the illegal possession or distribution of controlled drugs.

The *Narcotic Control Act* (1956) amended the Harrison Act by increasing the penalties for violation of the Harrison Act and, further, by making the possession of heroin unlawful. Under this act, in addition, the acquisition and transportation of marijuana is illegal.

In 1970, Congress enacted the federal *Controlled Substances Act*, a comprehensive document that specifies requirements for registration, procurement, storage, distribution, record-keeping, and the penalties for noncompliance with respect to all narcotic and nonnarcotic drugs that have a potential for abuse. Those drugs are classified into five categories, or *schedules*, according to their abuse potential:

- Schedule I: Drugs that have the highest abuse potential and no legal medical use. Schedule I drugs are *outlawed altogether*. *Examples:* heroin, lysergic acid diethylamide (LSD), marijuana.
- Schedule II: Legal drugs of high abuse potential, which may lead to severe dependence. *Examples:* amphetamines, opiates, cocaine, meperidine hydrochloride (Demerol), short-acting barbiturates.
- Schedule III: Drugs that may lead to moderate dependence. *Examples:* codeine combinations, paregoric, amphetamine combinations.
- Schedule IV: Drugs that may lead to limited dependence. *Examples:* phenobarbital, chloral hydrate, diazepam (Valium), meprobamate (Miltown).
- Schedule V: Drugs with the least abuse potential among the controlled substances. *Examples:* cough syrups containing codeine.

Some states have passed their own legislation and set up additional schedules. When state laws are more stringent than the federal law, the state law takes precedence. Paramedics should become familiar with the laws pertaining to controlled substances in the state in which they are practicing.

Federal Agencies Involved in the Regulation of Drugs

Because of the way in which drug legislation evolved, regulation of drugs in the United States falls under the jurisdiction of several agencies, among them:

- The *Drug Enforcement Agency* (DEA), formerly the Bureau of Narcotics and Dangerous Drugs (BNDD), which came into being with the Federal Controlled Substances Act of 1970. The DEA is a division of the Justice Department and is responsible for executing all the provisions of the Controlled Substances Act, including the registration of physicians who are permitted to dispense controlled substances.
- The *Food and Drug Administration* (FDA), which, as noted, is charged with the enforcement of the federal Food, Drug and Cosmetic Act.
- The *Public Health Service* (PHS), which regulates biologic products, such as vaccines and antitoxins.
- The *Federal Trade Commission* (FTC), which is empowered to suppress misleading drug advertising.

Drug Forms

Drugs come in many different forms, both solid and liquid, each of which has special properties. The following list is intended only to familiarize you with the spectrum of drug forms; in the field, you will be using only a very limited subset of the drug forms described.

Solid Drugs

extract A concentrated preparation of a drug made by putting the drug into solution (in alcohol or water) and evaporating off the excess solvent to a prescribed standard. *Example:* liver extract, which has been used in the treatment of anemia, is prepared by dissolving ground mammalian liver and allowing the solvent to evaporate. The extract may then be incorporated into a tablet or capsule.

powder A drug that has been ground into pulverized form. *Example:* mixtures of powdered sodium bicarbonate and calcium carbonate, used as an antacid in the treatment of ulcers. *Example in prehospital care:* activated charcoal powder.

pill A drug shaped into a ball or oval to be swallowed; pills are often coated to disguise an unpleasant taste. *Example:* ferrous sulfate (iron), often given in the form of coated pills to patients with anemia.

capsule A cylindrical gelatin container enclosing a dose of medication. *Example:* theophylline with glyceryl guaiacolate (Quibron).

pulvule A pulvule resembles a capsule, but it is not made of gelatin and it does not separate. Pulvules are usually proprietary forms of a drug. *Example:* propoxyphene hydrochloride (Darvon).

tablet A powdered drug that has been molded or compressed into a small disc. *Example:* aspirin tablets. *Example in prehospital care:* nitroglycerin tablets.

suppository A drug mixed in a firm base that melts at body temperature and is shaped to fit the rectum or vagina. Suppositories may be used for their local action (*example:* glycerin suppositories, used to promote evacuation of the rectum) or for their systemic effect (*example:* aminophylline suppositories, used for bronchodilation).

ointment A semisolid preparation for external application to the body, usually containing a medicinal substance. *Example:* neomycin ointment, used as a topical antibiotic.

patch A medication impregnated into a membrane or adhesive that is applied onto the surface of the skin. *Example:* nitroglycerin patch.

Liquid Drugs

solution A liquid containing one or more chemical substances entirely dissolved, usually in water. *Example:* normal saline solution. The majority of medications used in prehospital care are solutions.

suspension Preparation of a finely divided drug intended to be (or already) incorporated in a suitable liquid. (Note: All bottles containing suspensions must be shaken thoroughly before use, since their ingredients tend to separate on standing.) *Example:* aqueous penicillin, supplied as a powder requiring the addition of sterile water.

fluidextract Concentrated form of a drug prepared by dissolving the crude drug in the fluid in which it is most readily soluble. Fluidextracts are standardized such that 1 milliliter (ml) contains 1 gram (gm) of the drug. *Example:* aromatic cascara fluidextract.

tincture Dilute alcoholic extract of a drug. *Example:* tincture of iodine, used as a skin antiseptic.

spirits Preparation of a volatile substance dissolved in alcohol. *Example:* spirits of ammonia, formerly used to rouse people from a faint through its noxious odor.

syrup Drug suspended in sugar and water to improve its taste. *Example:* cough syrup. *Example in prehospital care:* syrup of ipecac.

elixir Syrup with alcohol and flavoring added. *Example:* terpin hydrate elixir, a cough medicine.

milk Aqueous suspension of an insoluble drug. *Example:* milk of magnesia.

emulsion Preparation of one liquid (usually an oil) distributed in small gobules in another liquid (usually water). Emulsions are often used as lubricants. *Example:* hydrophilic petrolatum in water.

liniments and **lotions** Preparations of drugs for external use, usually to relieve some discomfort (e.g., pain, itching) or to protect the skin. *Example:* calamine lotion.

FACTORS AFFECTING THE ACTION OF DRUGS

Drugs may produce their effects locally, systemically, or both. *Local effects* are those that result from the direct application of a drug to a tissue, as for example when lotions are applied to the skin to relieve itching. *Systemic effects* occur after the drug is absorbed by any route and distributed by the bloodstream; systemic effects almost invariably involve more than one organ, although the response of one or another organ may predominate.

The action of a drug is rarely a completely fixed property of the medication. The effect of any given drug, to the contrary, may vary depending on the patient, the dosage of the drug, the route by which the drug is given, and the drug's metabolic fate.

Factors Relating to the Patient

One of the chief variables affecting the action of a drug is the patient himself. Patients differ from one another in several ways with respect to how they react to medications:

- AGE. Patients of different ages may have very different responses to the same drug. The elderly, for example, tend to be much more sensitive to the effects of drugs and often, therefore, require smaller doses than younger patients. It is not, however, solely a matter of dosage. Some drugs actually have different effects altogether in different age groups. Barbiturates, for instance, act as sedatives in most adults, but in elderly patients they may have precisely the opposite effect, producing excitement or agitation.

- WEIGHT. Many drugs are formulated for an average adult, usually considered to be a 70-kg (154-lb) man. Clearly, however, the ultimate concentration in the body of a given dose of a drug is going to be quite different if that drug is taken instead by a 48-kg (106-lb) fashion model or a 136-kg (300-lb) weight lifter. For that reason, when specifying drug dosages for emergency prehospital care, we shall usually give the dosage in milligrams of the drug per kilogram of the patient's body weight (mg/kg)—to correct for differences in weight between patients.

- CONDITION OF THE PATIENT. The patient's overall state of health will also affect his response to many drugs. If his kidneys are not working properly, for example, he may not be able to excrete medications efficiently, so the concentration of a drug may build up inside his body until it reaches toxic levels. If the patient is in shock and therefore, by definition, his peripheral tissues are not normally perfused, it may take many hours before he will absorb a drug that has been given by injection.

- INDIVIDUAL VARIATION. All biologic responses show individual variability, and the response of any given patient to a drug will also be subject to the same variability. A dosage that is therapeutic for one person may not have any effect at all on another, while it may produce symptoms of toxicity in a third. The "recommended dosage" of a drug is, in fact, a statistical average from which the individual dose varies according to the statistical curve for normal distribution.

- IDIOSYNCRATIC AND ALLERGIC REACTIONS. Finally, a patient may react badly to an otherwise innocuous drug because of some peculiarity in his own biochemical makeup or because he has been sensitized to the drug by prior exposure (i.e., because he is allergic to the drug).

Routes of Administration

The action of a drug, most particularly the speed with which it works, is also influenced by the way it enters the body, that is, the route of administration. The route of administration appropriate for one drug may be entirely inappropriate for another, so for any given drug, it is essential to know the routes by which it may be given.

Oral

Most patients take their daily medications at home by the oral route (*per os,* or PO), for that route is painless, convenient, and economical. Drugs taken by mouth are absorbed at an unpredictable but generally slow rate from the stomach and intestines—usually somewhere between 30 and 90 minutes. Because absorption is slow and unpredictable, drugs are rarely given by the oral route in emergency situations. The major exceptions are syrup of ipecac, used to induce vomiting, and activated charcoal, used to bind ingested poisons, both of which are given orally in certain poisoning and overdose emergencies.

Rectal

Drugs may be administered rectally for their local effect; they may also be given rectally because they are irritating if given orally or because the patient is unable to take an oral medication (e.g., if he is vomiting). In the field, rectal administration is almost never indicated. However, certain medications, such as the bronchodilator aminophylline, are available in suppository form, and under unusual circumstances, the paramedic might be called upon to administer them. Absorption across the rectal mucosa is rapid but unpredictable.

The oral and rectal routes of administration are *enteral* routes; that is, they involve passage of the drug across membranes of the gut (*entero*-). All of the routes of administration that follow are **parenteral** routes, that is, routes that do *not* require absorption across an enteral membrane.

Intravenous (IV)

The intravenous route is the most rapidly effective and also the most dangerous route of administration. Drugs given intravenously go directly into the bloodstream and thence to the target organs, without any appreciable delay in absorption. Thus IV injection enables you to deliver a known quantity of drug over a known period; that is, it allows the most accurate control of dosage. It is a dangerous route, however, precisely because the entire dose of the drug is delivered in one blast, so a toxic reaction is much more likely.

Absorption of a drug given intravenously normally takes about 12 seconds. The absorption rate will be slowed in heart failure (because of the longer circulation time). In cardiac arrest with cardiopulmonary resuscitation (CPR) in progress, a drug given intravenously will take 3 to 4 times longer than normal to reach its target organ because the cardiac output is only one-fourth to one-third normal. Therefore it will take at least 1 or 2 minutes after giving an emergency drug during CPR to ensure that the drug has circulated adequately.

In general, drugs given intravenously should be given SLOWLY, unless you receive contrary orders. In the field, it is preferable to give intravenous medications through an established IV line rather than by direct venipuncture, as the latter technique may result in infiltration of the drug.

Intramuscular

Drugs given by the intramuscular (IM) route take longer to act than those given intravenously, since they must first be absorbed from the muscle into the bloodstream. By the same token, medications given intramuscularly have a longer duration of action than those given intravenously, since they are absorbed gradually over a period of minutes to hours. Obviously, *absorption of medications given by the intramuscular route or the subcutaneous route depends on adequate blood flow to muscles and peripheral tissues,* which is not the case in shock or cardiac arrest. Therefore, intramuscular injections should be given only to patients with adequate perfusion.

DO NOT GIVE INTRAMUSCULAR OR SUBCUTANEOUS INJECTIONS TO PATIENTS WITH IMPAIRED PERIPHERAL PERFUSION.

An intramuscular injection usually involves volumes of about 1 to 5 ml and is given into the deltoid muscle of the upper arm (the preferred site for prehospital applications) or into the upper outer quadrant of the gluteus muscle of the buttocks. (The technique for intramuscular injection is described later in this chapter.) The use of the deltoid muscle of the arm has the advantage that the rate of drug absorption can be slowed in the event of an adverse reaction. Should the patient develop dyspnea, dizziness, itching, edema, urticaria, wheezing, or any other sign of an allergic reaction following an intramuscular (or subcutaneous) injection in the arm, you should immediately fasten a venous tourniquet proximal to the injection site and then manage the patient as described in Chapter 26, on anaphylactic reactions.

Subcutaneous

Subcutaneous (SC or SQ) injections are given beneath the skin into the fat or connective tissue immediately underlying it. Subcutaneous injections are usually limited to small volumes (less than 2 ml) of nonirritating substances. Medications administered by the subcutaneous route are also absorbed more slowly and over a more prolonged period than when given intravenously; peak drug effect usually occurs within about 30 minutes. The subcutaneous route is used to administer epinephrine in asthmatic attacks of mild to moderate severity. The injections are usually given under the skin of the upper outer arm, anterior thigh, or abdomen.

Inhalation

Inhalation is used primarily for administration of aerosolized bronchodilators, such as Bronkosol or the Medihalers prescribed to some asthmatics. Paramedics may on occasion administer *nebulized* drugs, such as racemic epinephrine or isoetharine, by inhalation.

Endotracheal

Some drugs are very rapidly absorbed across the bronchial membranes and thus may take effect nearly as quickly when sprayed down an endotracheal tube as when administered intravenously. Among the drugs used by paramedics, those that may be given endotracheally can be remembered by the mnemonic NAVEL:

Narcan
Atropine
Valium
Epinephrine
Lidocaine

> **DO NOT GIVE ANY DRUGS OTHER THAN THOSE JUST LISTED BY THE ENDOTRACHEAL ROUTE!**

The lungs will be very unhappy indeed if they are suddenly inundated with sodium bicarbonate, furosemide, and so forth.

The technique of endotracheal drug administration is described later in this chapter.

Sublingual

Sublingual (SL) administration refers to giving a medication under the tongue. That is the way in which nitroglycerin is most often administered. Drugs given sublingually are usually rapidly absorbed, with effects apparent within a few minutes.

Drugs may also be *injected* into the network of veins (venous plexus) under the tongue (strictly speaking, that is actually just another form of intravenous injection)—a technique that is especially useful for giving narcotic antagonists to patients who have overdosed on heroin, for finding a suitable vein in such patients is often nearly impossible.

Topical

Drugs may be applied topically, that is, on the surface of the body. Ordinarily, the intact skin is an effective barrier to absorption of drugs. But some drugs have been specially prepared to cross that barrier at a very slow rate, so the route is useful for sustained release of drugs over a long period. Thus some patients take nitroglycerin in the form of a cream rubbed into the skin or a patch pasted onto the skin. Estrogens (female hormones) are also sometimes given in the form of a patch.

Intracardiac

Intracardiac administration refers to the direct injection of drugs through the chest wall into the heart. We have listed it last here because we consider it the last choice. While in some medical facilities the intracardiac route is used to administer epinephrine during cardiac arrest, that route has *no* advantages over intravenous or endotracheal instillation, and it has several potential hazards. The hazards include laceration of a coronary artery, pneumothorax, and inadvertent injection into the cardiac muscle rather than one of its chambers—in which case the epinephrine may cause intractable ventricular fibrillation. In addition, intracardiac injection requires interruption of cardiac compressions and artificial ventilation. For all of those reasons, the intracardiac route should be used only as a last resort when all efforts to establish an IV and insert an endotracheal tube have failed.

Rates of Absorption

The speed at which a drug is absorbed is related to the route by which it is given. Obviously, drugs injected directly into the circulation, as in intravenous injections, gain access to the bloodstream fastest. Nearly as rapid is the absorption across the respiratory mucosa when drugs are sprayed down an endotracheal tube or breathed in from an inhaler. Other mucosal surfaces, such as that in the rectum, also provide rapid absorption, although at an unpredictable rate. Intramuscular injection is slower, for the drug must be picked up from the muscles by the circulating blood; the same is true of subcutaneous injections, which are absorbed more slowly than intramuscular. Down near the slowest end of the scale are drugs administered orally. The slowest absorption of all is across intact skin. The rates of absorption are summarized in Table 10-1.

Distribution of the Drug Within the Body

Once a drug has been absorbed into the bloodstream, where does it go from there? In general, drugs pass freely and quickly out of the vascular space and into the interstitial fluid. Therefore the amount of a drug reaching a particular part of the body will be determined by the blood flow to that part of the body. There are, however, some body compartments less accessible to certain drugs than others. Some drugs, for example, because of their physical properties, do not reach the central nervous system (we say that such drugs cannot pass the "blood-brain barrier"). Similarly there are drugs that pass easily between a mother's circulation and the placental circulation of her fetus, and there are other drugs that do not enter the fetal circulation.

TABLE 10-1.   RATES OF ABSORPTION BY DIFFERENT ROUTES

ROUTE OF ADMINISTRATION	TIME UNTIL DRUG TAKES EFFECT*
Topical	Hours to days
Oral	30–90 minutes
Rectal	5–30 minutes (unpredictable)
Subcutaneous injection	15–30 minutes
Intramuscular injection	10–20 minutes
Sublingual tablet	3–5 minutes
Sublingual injection	3 minutes
Inhalation	3 minutes
Endotracheal	3 minutes
Intravenous	30–60 seconds
Intracardiac	15 seconds

*In a healthy person with normal perfusion.

Inactivation and Elimination of the Drug

When a drug is taken into the body, by any route, it acts only for a certain amount of time. Clearly, something must happen to that drug, to eliminate it or inactivate it, for otherwise it would continue to act forever. In fact, the body has two principal ways of terminating the action of a drug: It can excrete the drug as it is, or it can change the drug into an inactive substance.

Excretion of unaltered drugs usually takes place either through the lungs or through the kidneys. Gases and volatile liquids used for general anesthesia, for example, are excreted primarily through the *lungs*. A certain proportion of ingested alcohol is also eliminated via the lungs, a fact that provides the basis for the Breathalyzer test. Drugs may also be excreted unchanged by the *kidneys*, a process that can be altered by changing the pH of the urine. Thus, for example, the excretion of weak acids, like aspirin or barbiturates, can be enhanced by making the urine alkaline—a fact of importance in treating patients who have overdosed with those agents. Clearly, drugs that depend on the kidneys for their excretion will remain in the body longer if there is any impairment in renal function.

The body's second important mechanism of terminating the action of the drug is by metabolizing the drug to an inactive compound (*biotransformation*). A large majority of the metabolic reactions involved take place in the liver, so if there is disease of the liver, inactivation of drugs may be impaired.

Interactions Among Different Drugs

When administering medications, it is important to know not only how they affect the patient but also how they may affect one another. An interaction between drugs occurs whenever the actions (therapeutic or toxic) of one drug on the body are in some way modified by another chemical substance (which may be a prescription drug but may also be the nicotine from cigarette smoke, something in the diet, or any other substance to which a person is exposed). Drugs can interact with one another in four ways:

- **addition**   The increased effect that may occur when two drugs that have the same action are given together. We take advantage of the additive effects of drugs when we give certain combination painkillers, such as Darvocet (Darvon plus acetaminophen).
- **synergism**   Combined effect of two drugs that is greater than the sum of their individual effects.

Synergism seems to be at work between some of the drugs used against tuberculosis: They are more effective in combination than one would predict from simple addition of their actions.

- **potentiation** The enhancement of the action of a drug by another substance that does not have that action at all. Probenecid, for example, a medication used to treat gout, can potentiate the action of penicillin by blocking the excretion of penicillin by the kidneys.
- **antagonism** Decrease in the action of a drug by the administration of another drug. We make use of drug antagonism when we give naloxone to reverse the effects of narcotics.

As is clear from the examples cited, not all interactions among drugs are harmful. Some interactions enable us to make more effective use of drugs. But there *are* harmful or undesirable interactions between drugs, and it is important to know, when giving any particular drug, with what other drugs it may be incompatible.

There are, in fact, tens of thousands of possible drug interactions, particularly in a society like ours, in which people take a lot of pills. The books on drug interactions are often the size of the Manhattan telephone directory, and no human brain could be expected to absorb all that information. Fortunately, however, the number of *clinically significant* drug interactions is quite limited, and the number of those interactions that involve drugs the paramedic will be using in the field is even more limited. In this text, whenever we present a new drug, we shall list its clinically important interactions with other drugs, and the paramedic should learn those interactions along with the correct dosage of the drug and other vital drug facts.

Special Terminology

Before we conclude this section, we need to learn a few more special terms used to describe drugs and their actions:

indications The conditions for which the drug is recommended (e.g., hypoglycemic coma is an *indication* for 50% dextrose).

contraindications Conditions that preclude the use of the drug (e.g., asthma is a *contraindication* to morphine; that is, morphine must *not* be given to a patient with asthma).

depressant A substance that lessens the activity of the body or any of its organs. Morphine, for example, is a respiratory depressant.

stimulant A drug that increases the activity of the body or any of its organs (e.g., caffeine, epinephrine).

physiologic action Action caused by the drug when given in the concentrations normally present in the body (applies to drugs that are derived from normal body chemicals, such as epinephrine and norepinephrine).

therapeutic action Beneficial action of a drug to correct a bodily dysfunction.

untoward reaction Side effect regarded as harmful to the patient; a toxic reaction.

irritation Action that produces slight or temporary damage to tissues.

cumulative action Action of increased intensity after administration of several doses of a drug.

tolerance Progressive decrease in susceptibility to the effects of a drug after repeated doses.

habituation Situation in which the effects produced by a drug are necessary to maintain a person's feeling of well-being. Habituation is common, for example, with the nicotine from cigarettes.

idiosyncrasy An abnormal susceptibility to a drug, peculiar to an individual.

hypersensitivity Allergy to a drug, occurring after previous exposure to the drug.

WEIGHTS, MEASURES, AND DOSAGES

To determine the correct dosage of a drug, you must be familiar with the units in which the drug is measured. There are two systems of measurement applicable to drug therapy. The first, the *apothecary system,* is the older of the two and is seldom used anymore. The apothecary system measures solids in units such as grains, drams, ounces, and pounds; liquid apothecary measures include minims, fluidrams, ounces, pints, and gallons. The second system, the *metric system,* is the most frequently used in the official listing of drugs, and it is the system that we shall use throughout this text. The primary unit of weight in the metric system is the gram, and the primary volume, or liquid, measurement is the liter.

One can convert units from the metric system to the apothecary system and vice versa. The conversions are usually approximations only. Some of the more common conversions are as follows:

FROM METRIC TO APOTHECARY

Metric	Apothecary
1 ml (milliliter)	15 minims
10 ml	2.5 fluidrams
100 ml	3.5 fluidounces
1,000 ml (1 liter)	1 quart

1 gm (gram)	15 grains
10 gm	2.5 drams
100 gm	3.3 ounces
1,000 gm (1 kilogram)	2.2 lbs

FROM APOTHECARY TO METRIC

Apothecary	Metric
1 minim	0.06 ml
1 fluidram	4 ml
1 fluidounce	30 ml
1 pint	500 ml
1 quart	1,000 ml (1 liter)
1 grain	60 mg
1 dram	4 gm
1 ounce	30 gm
1 pound	500 gm

The only conversion that you are likely to have to make in the field is that from pounds (apothecary) to kilograms (metric), since most patients will give their weight in pounds and most dosages are calculated on the basis of drug weight or concentration *per kilogram* of body weight. *To convert pounds to kilograms,* simply divide the weight in pounds by 2.2:

$$\text{Weight in kilograms} = \frac{\text{weight in pounds}}{2.2}$$

Thus a 150-pound man would weigh approximately 70 kilograms (kg)—68.2 kg to be exact.

Metric Units

The metric system is based on multiples or derivatives of 10, that is, the *decimal system.* If you feel rusty about manipulating decimals, turn first to Chapter 10 of the Study Guide accompanying this text for a review of the decimal system.

As noted earlier, the primary unit of *weight* in the metric system is the GRAM. The secondary unit is the MILLIGRAM, which is derived from the primary unit; *milli-* means "thousandth," and therefore a milligram is one one-thousandth of a gram (i.e., there are 1,000 milligrams in a gram).

$$\frac{1}{1,000} \text{ gram} = 0.001 \text{ gram} = 1 \text{ milligram}$$

Note that to convert grams to milligrams, one multiplies by 1,000, which is the same as moving the decimal point three places to the *right.* Conversely, to convert milligrams to grams, one must divide by 1,000, that is, move the decimal point three places to the *left.*

$$\frac{2,000}{\text{milligrams}} = \frac{2,000 \text{ milligrams}}{1,000 \text{ milligrams/gram}} = 2 \text{ grams}$$

Suppose a physician orders 1,000 milligrams of a certain drug, and that drug is dispensed in 0.5-gram tablets; how many tablets should be given? To find the answer, you first have to convert milligrams to grams:

$$\frac{1,000}{\text{milligrams}} = \frac{1,000 \text{ milligrams}}{1,000 \text{ milligrams/gram}} = 1 \text{ gram}$$

Then divide the desired dose (1 gram) by the concentration in each tablet (0.5 grams per tablet):

$$0.5 \text{ gram} \overline{\smash{)}1.0 \text{ gram}} \overset{2.0 \text{ (tablets)}}{= 5 \text{ gram} \overline{\smash{)}10.0 \text{ gram}}}$$

Hence one would have to administer two 0.5-gram tablets to give the dose of 1,000 milligrams orally.

The units of *volume,* or liquid measure, in the metric system are also based on decimal fractions. The primary unit of volume is the LITER, and the secondary unit is the MILLILITER. We have already noted that *milli-* means "thousandth." Thus a milliliter is one one-thousandth of a liter (i.e., there are 1,000 milliliters in a liter).

$$\frac{1}{1,000} \text{ liter} = 0.001 \text{ liter} = 1 \text{ milliliter}$$

To convert liters to milliliters, multiply by 1,000, which is the same as moving the decimal point three places to the *right.*

$$4 \text{ liters} = 4 \times 1,000 \text{ milliliters} = 4,000 \text{ milliliters}$$

Conversely, to convert milliliters to liters, divide the milliliters by 1,000, which is the same as moving the decimal point three places to the *left.*

$$\frac{3,000}{\text{milliliters}} = \frac{3,000 \text{ milliliters}}{1,000 \text{ milliliters/liter}} = 3 \text{ liters}$$

Another measure sometimes used is the *cubic centimeter* (cc). One milliliter of water weighs one gram and occupies one cubic centimeter of volume. Thus a milliliter and a cubic centimeter both express one-thousandth of a liter and can be considered equivalent expressions. In this text, we will use the milliliter in describing liquid measures.

In the remaining discussion, we shall refer to the metric units by their *abbreviations*.

METRIC ABBREVIATIONS

Term	*Abbreviation*
kilogram	kg (= 1,000 gm)
gram	gm
milligram	mg
microgram	μg (= 0.001 mg)
liter	L
milliliter	ml

Drug Concentrations and Calculation of Dosage

Administration of the correct dose of a drug requires, first of all, knowing the *concentration of the drug*, that is, how many milligrams of the drug are contained in the liquid in which it is suspended. Sometimes that information is printed on the label of the drug container (e.g., "Drug X at a concentration of 5 mg/ml"). Other ampules or vials may simply list the total volume and total amount of drug inside, and you have to figure out the concentration per milliliter. That can be done relatively easily, using the formula:

$$\text{Concentration} = \frac{\text{total mg}}{\text{total ml}}$$

Thus, if an ampule contains, for example, 50 mg of Drug Y in 5 ml, the concentration is:

$$\text{Concentration} = \frac{50 \text{ mg}}{5 \text{ ml}} = 10 \text{ mg/ml}$$

Things become a bit trickier when the label of the drug lists the drug concentration as a percent, for example, "1% Xylocaine." What *percent* means in terms of drug concentration is the number of **grams** present **in 100 ml**. Thus, 1% Xylocaine contains 1 gram of drug in every 100 ml; dividing the numerator and denominator by 100, we arrive at a concentration of 10 mg per milliliter.

$$\frac{1 \text{ gm}}{100 \text{ ml}} = \frac{1,000 \text{ mg}}{100 \text{ ml}} = 10 \text{ mg/ml}$$

(Question: What is the concentration of a 20% solution of magnesium sulfate? If you have an ampule containing 10 ml of that solution, what is the total amount of magnesium sulfate, in milligrams, in the ampule?)

When a physician issues an order for a given drug, the order will be given in terms of the number of milligrams (or grams) of the drug to be administered. Then you have to translate that dose in milligrams into a *volume* of the drug containing that dose, so that you can draw up the correct amount into the syringe. Once you know the concentration of the drug preparation, it's easy to figure out the volume corresponding to a given dose:

$$\frac{\text{Volume to be}}{\text{administered}} = \frac{\text{desired dose (in mg)}}{\text{concentration on hand (mg/ml)}}$$

Suppose, for example, you are instructed to administer 20 mg of Drug Z (desired dose), which is supplied in a concentration of 10 mg per milliliter (concentration on hand). How many milliliters of the drug should you draw up in the syringe?

$$\begin{aligned}\frac{\text{Volume to be}}{\text{administered}} &= \frac{\text{desired dose (in mg)}}{\begin{array}{c}\text{concentration}\\ \text{on hand (mg/ml)}\end{array}}\\[2mm] &= \frac{20 \text{ mg}}{10 \text{ mg/ml}}\\[2mm] &= 2 \text{ ml}\end{aligned}$$

Thus, you will have to draw up 2 ml of Drug Z to give the 20-mg dose ordered.

Let us practice these calculations with some more examples:

EXAMPLE 1: The physician orders you to administer 4 mg of diazepam (Valium) slowly IV. Diazepam is supplied in a concentration of 5 mg per milliliter. How many milliliters should you administer?

$$\frac{4 \text{ mg (desired dose)}}{5 \text{ mg/ml (concentration on hand)}} = ? \text{ ml}$$

EXAMPLE 2: The physician instructs you to administer 80 mg of lidocaine, which is supplied in a concentration of 20 mg per milliliter. How many milliliters of lidocaine should you administer?

Desired dose = ?

Concentration on hand = ?

$$\frac{\text{Desired dose (mg)}}{\text{Concentration on hand (mg/ml)}} = ?$$

Now we will make it a little more complicated. The therapeutic dosage of morphine sulfate is 0.1 mg per kilogram of body weight. Morphine is supplied in a concentration of 10 mg per milliliter. How many milliliters should you give a 70-kg man?

STEP 1: Calculate the dosage, that is, how many *milligrams* you should give a 70-kg man.

0.1 mg/kg × 70 kg = 7 mg

STEP 2: Calculate the volume containing 7 mg. (Hint: 7 mg is the desired dose, and 10 mg/ml is the concentration on hand.)

For more practice in doing these calculations, turn to Chapter 10 of the Study Guide that accompanies this textbook.

ADMINISTRATION OF DRUGS

The administration of medications by a paramedic under orders from a physician requires that both parties be as well-informed as possible. That means, first of all, that the paramedic must know as much as possible about the drugs he or she is permitted to give.

What You Need to Know About Any Drug You Give

For any drug used in the field, the paramedic *must* know the following information:

- What are the THERAPEUTIC EFFECTS of the drug? That is, what is the desired effect that giving the drug is supposed to accomplish?
- What are the INDICATIONS for the drug? That is, for what condition(s) is the drug properly used?
- What are the CONTRAINDICATIONS to use of the drug? That is, under what conditions should the drug *not* be used?
- What is the correct DOSAGE of the drug, given the patient's age and weight, and how is the drug usually supplied (i.e., in what concentration)?
- What SIDE EFFECTS may be expected secondary to the drug? (Side effects are to be distinguished from idiosyncratic or allergic reactions; *side effects* are *predictable* effects, sometimes undesirable, that occur in addition to the drug's therapeutic effects. *Idiosyncratic reactions* are completely *un*predictable. *Allergic reactions* are also unpredictable—unless the patient has had an allergic reaction to the same drug in the past—and may lead

to life-threatening anaphylaxis. Allergic reactions should be anticipated with ANY drug, whereas side effects are usually fairly specific to a given drug.)
- What is the MODE OF ADMINISTRATION? Drugs may be given, as noted earlier, through a variety of routes—orally, subcutaneously, intravenously, and so forth. A drug that is therapeutic when given by one route may be lethal when given by another.
- Is the drug INCOMPATIBLE with any other medication you might give or that the patient might be taking?

Let us take, for example, the diuretic agent furosemide (Lasix):

THERAPEUTIC EFFECTS	• Potent diuretic, causing the excretion of large volumes of urine within 5 to 30 minutes of administration, thus useful in ridding the body of excess fluid in conditions such as congestive heart failure (CHF). • Vasodilator allowing temporary "internal phlebotomy" in conditions of fluid overload.
INDICATIONS	To reverse fluid overload associated with CONGESTIVE HEART FAILURE and PULMONARY EDEMA.
CONTRA-INDICATIONS	• Should not be given to **pregnant women**. • Should not be given to patients with **hypokalemia** (low potassium). Hypokalemia may be suspected in a patient who has been on chronic diuretic therapy or whose ECG shows prominent P waves, diminished T waves, and the presence of U waves. • **Hypovolemic states**.
SIDE EFFECTS	Immediate side effects may include *nausea* and

vomiting, potassium depletion (with attendant cardiac dysrhythmias), and *dehydration*. Acute urinary retention may occur in an uncatheterized male.

HOW SUPPLIED	• Prefilled syringes of 2 ml, 4 ml, and 10 ml containing 10 mg per milliliter. • Ampules of 2 ml, 4 ml, and 10 ml containing 10 mg per milliliter.
ADMINISTRATION AND DOSAGE	In the field, furosemide is given **intravenously**. If at all possible, the patient should have a urinary catheter in place. *Dosage:* **20 to 40 mg** SLOWLY IV (injected over 1–2 min). If a response is not obtained, a second dose of 60 to 80 mg may be given, not sooner than 2 hours after the first dose.
INCOMPATIBILITY	Furosemide should not be given to patients taking **lithium** (it may block the renal excretion of lithium and thereby cause lithium toxicity).

Each time a new drug is encountered in this text, turn to the Drug Handbook at the back of the text, where the drug's characteristics will be summarized in the format used above; you will be expected to learn those characteristics by heart. For those interested in learning more about a particular drug, a list of references is provided after the description of the drug. It is also a good idea to become familiar with one or more of the books that provide information on prescription drugs or on general pharmacology. The following are among the many good references:

Gilman AG, Goodman LS, Gilman A. Goodman and Gilman's *The Pharmacologic Basis of Therapeutics* (8th ed.). New York: McGraw, 1990. An excellent comprehensive textbook of pharmacology.

Physicians' Desk Reference (PDR), issued annually by Medical Economics Company, Oradell, New Jersey. This book contains information on proprietary drugs, cross-referenced by generic name, proprietary name, and therapeutic use. It also contains a valuable product identification section, with full-size, color pictures of more than 1,000 drug products, which can be very helpful in identifying the medications that a patient is taking.

One other source of information about the drugs you use is the package insert that accompanies each vial or ampule of a drug. Those inserts provide detailed information regarding the indications, precautions, contraindications, dosages, and adverse reactions to the drug.

Steps in Administering a Drug

The danger of something going wrong in administering a drug—for example, administering the wrong drug or the wrong dose of a drug—can be minimized by following a set procedure that incorporates a number of safety precautions:

1. MAKE SURE THE BASE PHYSICIAN UNDERSTANDS THE SITUATION. As we have seen, the decision whether to order the administration of any given drug is a complex one, involving such considerations as the patient's age, signs and symptoms, overall condition, allergic history, coexisting medical problems, and other drugs he may be taking. Thus it is critical that the paramedic gather complete and accurate information about the patient to enable the physician to make prudent decisions about drug administration.

2. MAKE SURE YOU UNDERSTAND THE PHYSICIAN'S ORDERS CLEARLY. If those orders are unclear or seem—on the basis of your knowledge—to be in some way mistaken (e.g., dosage above the usual range, an unusual route of administration), *ask the physician to repeat the order.* Do not take for granted that the doctor is infallible, especially at three o'clock in the morning.

> **NEVER GUESS WHAT THE PHYSICIAN HAS ORDERED. WHEN IN DOUBT, ASK.**

3. Always REPEAT ORDERS BACK TO THE PHYSICIAN before administering a medication, to confirm that you received the order accurately. In

the repetition, state the *name of the drug*, the *dose*, and the *route* by which it is to be given. Remember, as a paramedic you are as much responsible for the administration of the drug and its possible consequences as the physician giving the order, so be absolutely certain what drug is to be administered, in what dosage, and by what route.

4. If the patient is conscious, or if there is another reliable source of information, CONFIRM THAT THE PATIENT IS NOT ALLERGIC TO THE DRUG THAT HAS BEEN ORDERED.

5. READ THE LABEL CAREFULLY as you take the vial or syringe from its box and again before you give the drug. Make a note of the *drug concentration* printed on the label and also of the drug's *date of expiration*.

6. CHECK FOR DEFECTS in the vial or ampule, and make sure that the fluid inside is not cloudy, discolored, or precipitated. If the medication is suspect in any way, do *not* use it.

7. If you have orders to administer more than one drug, MAKE SURE THAT THE DRUGS ARE NOT INCOMPATIBLE. Some drugs will not mix with others; for example, if sodium bicarbonate is mixed with calcium chloride, an insoluble precipitate of calcium carbonate will form in the solution. Should any cloudiness occur after a drug has been injected into IV tubing, *clamp the tubing immediately* and replace it with a new administration set.

8. NOTIFY THE PHYSICIAN WHEN THE MEDICATION HAS BEEN ADMINISTERED.

9. MONITOR THE PATIENT FOR POSSIBLE ADVERSE SIDE EFFECTS.

10. DISPOSE OF THE SYRINGE AND NEEDLE SAFELY. Do *not* try to recap the needle, for the likelihood is quite high of sticking yourself in the

process; rather, dispose of the needle and syringe in a container designed for that purpose.

One word of caution. Even though, by the time you finish your paramedic course, you should be able to recite in your sleep the dosages of the drugs your service uses, DO NOT TRUST YOUR MEMORY IN AN EMERGENCY!! Whether you are giving medications according to voice orders or protocols,

> **ALWAYS RECHECK THE CORRECT DOSAGE BEFORE YOU ADMINISTER A DRUG.**

The most convenient way to do so is to make a file card listing all of the drugs in your drug box and their correct dosages and keep the list taped inside the drug box, so that the dosages will be right there in front of you when you need them.

Syringes

A STANDARD HYPODERMIC ASSEMBLY (Fig. 10-1) consists of a *syringe* (a hollow barrel plus a plunger that fits inside the barrel) and a needle. Syringes come in different sizes, from those that will hold only 0.5 ml of fluid to those that will hold 50 ml of fluid. Along the barrel of the syringe is the *scale*, a series of gradations indicating how much volume has been drawn up into the syringe. To assemble a standard syringe, it is necessary only to connect the needle (which is supplied with a protective cap) to

FIGURE 10-1. STANDARD HYPODERMIC ASSEMBLY.

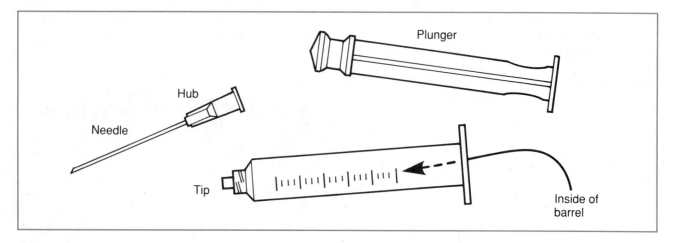

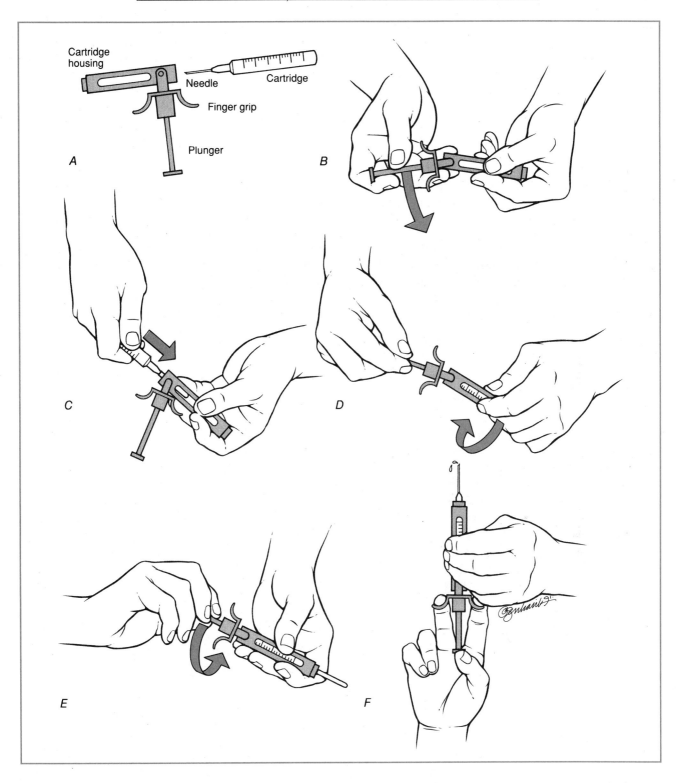

FIGURE 10-2. **TUBEX SYSTEM.** (A) Components. (B) Swing handle down to load. (C) Insert cartridge. (D) Screw cartridge into housing. (E) Screw plunger into cartridge. (F) Evacuate air from cartridge.

the syringe tip, taking care not to touch the surfaces that are to be connected together.

A TUBEX system (Fig. 10-2A) consists of a stainless steel housing and a prefilled, disposable cartridge. The system is used most often for the injection of controlled substances, such as morphine. To assemble a Tubex syringe:

1. Swing the plunger handle of the syringe down (Fig. 10-2B).
2. Check the label on the cartridge to make sure it is the drug you want to give and to determine the concentration. Insert the cartridge into the cartridge housing (Fig. 10-2C).
3. Screw the cartridge into the housing (Fig. 10-2D).
4. Bring the plunger back into alignment with the cartridge housing, and screw it into the cartridge (Fig. 10-2E).
5. Expel any air from the dead space in the cartridge (Fig. 10-2F).

A third type of syringe in very widespread use for prehospital emergency care is the PREFILLED SYRINGE, which is supplied as a plastic barrel/needle assembly and a glass cartridge containing the medication. To use a prefilled syringe:

1. Check the label on the cartridge to make certain it is the drug you want. Inspect the contents of the cartridge for discoloration, cloudiness, or particulate matter (if any of those are present, discard the cartridge and take another).
2. Pop off the caps from both the medication cartridge and the plastic barrel (Fig. 10-3A).
3. Insert the cartridge into the barrel and twist it into place (Fig. 10-3B).
4. Hold the cartridge with the needle pointing up and tap on it to bring any air inside it to the top (Fig. 10-3C). Then briefly uncap the needle, expel the air, and *carefully* recap the needle.

FIGURE 10-3.   PREFILLED SYRINGE.   (A) Pop off caps with your thumbs. (B) Insert cartridge into barrel and twist into place. (C) Evacuate air from cartridge.

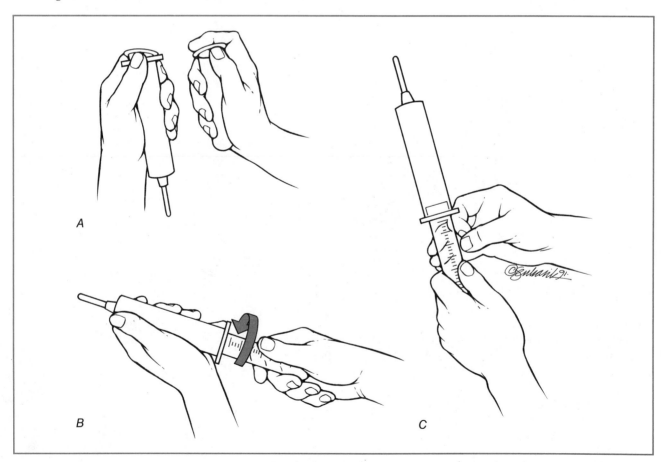

Drawing Up Solutions from an Ampule or Vial

An **ampule** is a glass container in which a *single dose* of a sterile drug preparation, either in a powdered or liquid form, is sealed (in this section, we shall discuss ampules containing the *liquid* form of a drug). Ampules are used to store drugs given by injection, such as epinephrine or furosemide. To draw up medication from an ampule into a syringe, the procedure is as follows:

1. Prepare a syringe of the appropriate volume with a needle of the appropriate gauge (see sections on IV, IM, and SQ injections).
2. Read the *name and concentration* of the medication printed on the ampule, and inspect the solution for discoloration, cloudiness, or particles (Fig. 10-4A). Compute the *volume* of the drug you need to draw up according to the formula described earlier.
3. Snap your finger sharply against the stem of the ampule (Fig. 10-4B) to move the solution down into the well of the ampule.

FIGURE 10-4.   DRAWING UP A DRUG FROM AN AMPULE.   (A) Inspect the ampule. (B) Tap solution down into the well. (C) Break off the stem. (D) Draw up the medication into a syringe. (E) Evacuate air from the syringe.

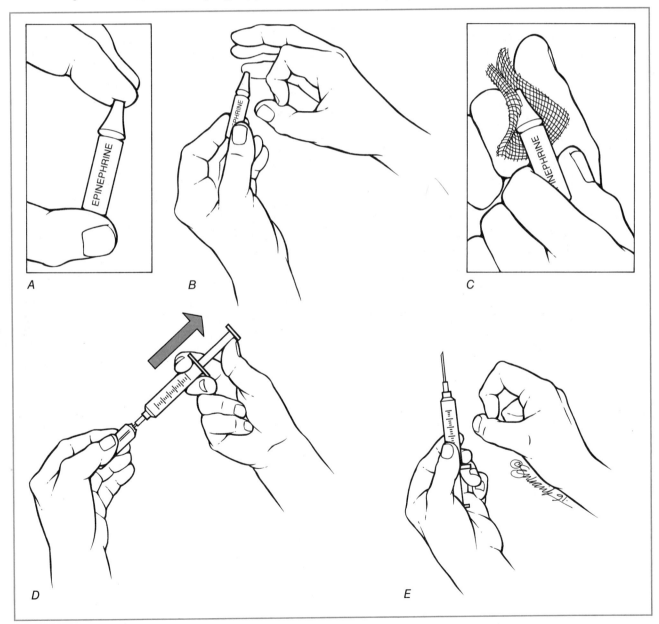

4. Grasp the top of the ampule in a 4- by 4-inch gauze pad, to protect your fingers from injury, and break off the top of the ampule at the stem. Some ampules must first be scored with a sharp piece of metal that will be supplied in the box with the ampule; others, which are designated by a colored ring painted around the neck of the ampule, are already scored and will break along the colored line.

5. Insert the needle into the ampule (Fig. 10-4D), taking care that the needle does not touch the ampule's rim. Pull back on the plunger of the syringe to draw up the specified volume of medication, according to the dosage you calculated.

6. Expel any air present in the syringe (Fig. 10-4E), and *carefully* recap the needle.

A **vial** is a glass container storing sterile powdered or liquid drugs for parenteral use. It differs from an ampule in that a vial is sealed with a rubber stopper and may contain multiple doses. To draw up a solution from a vial:

1. Prepare a syringe of the appropriate volume with a needle of the appropriate gauge (see sections on IV, IM, and SQ injections).

2. Read the *name and concentration* of the medication printed on the vial, and inspect the solution for discoloration, cloudiness, or particles. Compute the *volume* of the drug you need to draw up according to the formula described earlier.

3. Disinfect the rubber stopper of the vial with an alcohol wipe.

4. Draw *air* into the syringe in a volume equal to that of the solution to be withdrawn.

5. Insert the needle at an angle through the rubber stopper, and *inject the air* into the vial.

6. Invert the vial, and draw up the specified volume of medication, according to the dosage you calculated (Fig. 10-5). Withdraw the needle from the vial.

7. Expel any air present in the syringe, and *carefully* recap the needle.

Giving Drugs Through an Intravenous Line

When ordered to give a medication by "IV push," it is preferable to do so through an established intravenous line rather than directly into a vein, for the chances of the drug infiltrating are greater if you are trying to hold a needle steady inside a vein while pushing on the plunger of the syringe. The proce-

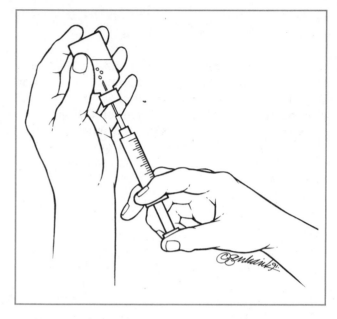

FIGURE 10-5. DRAWING UP A DRUG FROM A VIAL. Invert the vial, inject a volume of air equivalent to the volume of medication you need, and withdraw the medication into the syringe.

dure for giving a medication through an IV line is as follows:

1. Disinfect the drug administration port on the IV line with an alcohol swab (Fig. 10-6A).

2. Uncap the needle from your syringe.

3. Insert the needle into the drug administration port, taking care not to jam it straight through and out the other side!

4. Pinch the tubing distal to the port (i.e., farther from the patient) to prevent the drug from flowing backward into the IV bag, and inject the medication SLOWLY (Fig. 10-6B).

5. Remove the needle, and dispose of the needle and syringe in a safe receptacle.

6. Open the control clamp wide (Fig. 10-6C) to flush any remaining medication from the line. Then readjust the clamp so that the IV is running at the rate ordered.

7. Monitor the patient carefully for signs of an adverse reaction.

Adding Drugs to an IV Bag

Certain drugs are added to the intravenous solution itself, rather than administered directly to the patient, particularly drugs whose effects must be carefully titrated (such as lidocaine when given as a drip

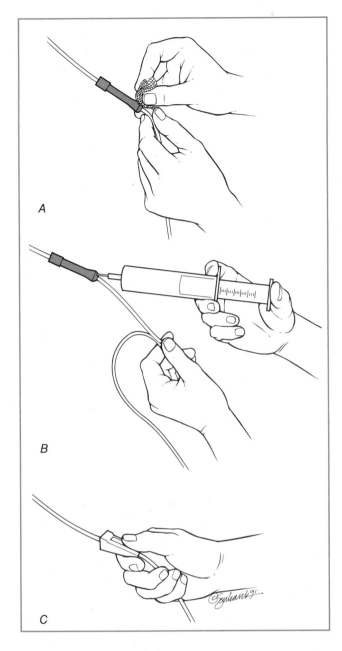

FIGURE 10-6. GIVING DRUGS IV. (A) Prep the drug administration port. (B) Pinch off the tubing, and inject the drug. (C) Open the regulator clamp to flush the system.

or norepinephrine). The method of adding medications to an IV bag is as follows:

1. Set up the IV bag and administration set in the usual manner.
2. Check the *drug name* on the vial, ampule, or prefilled syringe. Check the *concentration of the drug* it contains (mg/ml).
3. *Compute the volume* of the drug to be added to the

IV bag. Draw up that amount in a syringe (if a prefilled syringe is used, note what proportion of the volume of the syringe is required).
4. Close the control clamp on the administration set (Fig. 10-7A).
5. Disinfect the rubber stopper or sleeve on the IV bag with an alcohol swab.
6. Puncture the stopper with the needle, and inject the desired volume of medication into the bottle or bag (Fig. 10-7B).
7. Withdraw the needle, and discard the needle and syringe in an appropriate container. Agitate the IV bag gently to be sure that the added drug is well mixed in the solution.
8. *Label the bag* with the *name* of the medication added, the date and time, the *amount* added, the resulting *concentration* of medication in the IV bag, and your name (e.g., "Lidocaine, 500 mg added, November 3, 1994, 8:45 A.M., concentration now 2 mg/ml, Harvey Mantooth).
9. *Calculate the rate* at which the IV must be run (drops/min) in order to deliver the desired dose of medication (see p. 233), and regulate the flow accordingly.

Intramuscular Injections

Intramuscular (IM) injections are not used frequently in the field, although in some EMS systems, morphine is administered to well-perfused patients by the intramuscular route. The intramuscular route is best *avoided* in patients with chest pain, for injection directly into a muscle may cause elevation of the circulating muscle enzymes and thereby confuse the patient's subsequent laboratory picture (some of the same enzymes are measured in order to determine whether the *heart* muscle has been damaged). Intramuscular injections are also relatively contraindicated in shock; for so long as the patient remains in shock, the injected medication will not be mobilized from his muscles (and if the shock should be reversed, a large dose of the medication may suddenly be absorbed all at once, when it is no longer needed or desirable). Nonetheless, the intramuscular route may be useful in some situations, for example to give morphine for pain relief to a patient with an uncomplicated fracture whose transport to hospital will take a long time.

The technique for intramuscular injection is as follows:

1. *Explain the procedure to the patient*, and *obtain consent*. Verify that the patient is not allergic to the drug you plan to administer.

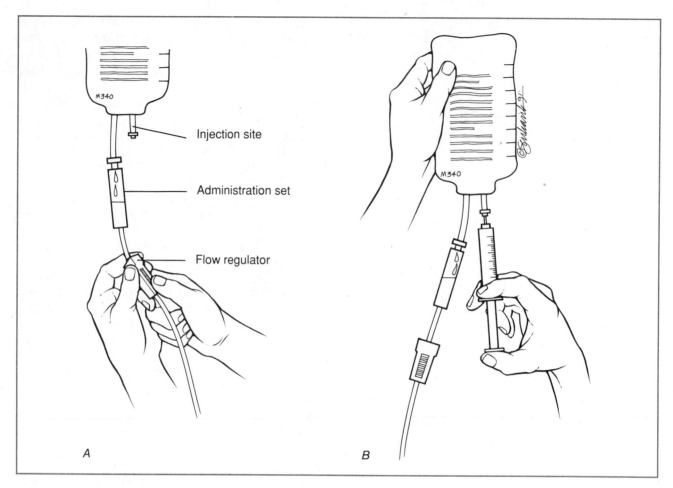

A

B

FIGURE 10-7.   ADDING DRUGS TO AN IV BAG.   (A) Clamp the flow regulator shut. (B) Inject the medication into the injection port on the bag.

2. Prepare a syringe (2–5 ml), and attach a *21-gauge needle*.
3. *Check the label* on the medication container, *compute the dosage,* and draw up the desired volume in a syringe as previously described.
4. Locate the deltoid muscle (Fig. 10-8A).
5. Disinfect the injection site with an alcohol swab (Fig. 10-8B).
6. With one hand, bunch the deltoid muscle together. Hold the syringe in your other hand like a dart, and quickly thrust the needle into the tissue at a 90-degree angle (Fig. 10-8C).
7. Pull back slightly on the plunger of the syringe to be sure that the needle has not accidently entered a blood vessel (Fig. 10-8D).
8. If there is no blood return into the syringe, inject the medication (Fig. 10-8E).
9. Quickly withdraw the syringe, and apply firm pressure over the injection site (Fig. 10-8F). Dispose of the needle and syringe in an appropriate receptacle.

10. Monitor the patient for adverse reactions to the medication.

Subcutaneous Injections

Subcutaneous injections are used in prehospital care chiefly for the administration of epinephrine to patients with mild to moderately severe asthmatic or anaphylactic reactions. The technique is as follows:

1. *Explain the procedure to the patient,* and *obtain consent.* Verify that the patient is not allergic to the drug you plan to administer.
2. Prepare a 1-ml syringe, and attach a *25-gauge needle.*
3. *Check the label* on the medication container, *compute the dosage,* and draw up the desired volume in a syringe as previously described.
4. Locate the deltoid muscle.
5. Disinfect the injection site with an alcohol swab.

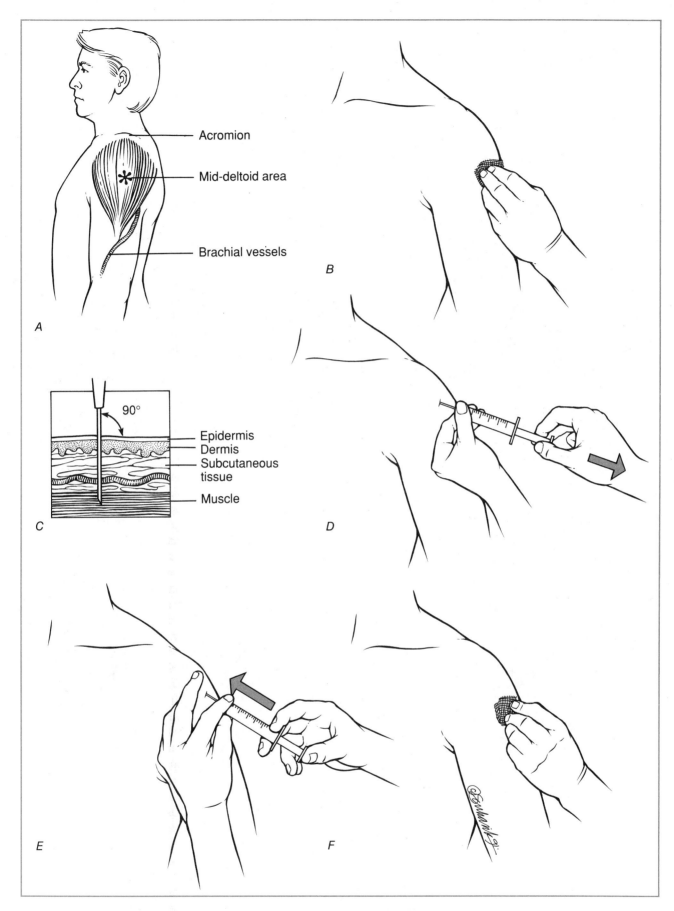

FIGURE 10-8. **INTRAMUSCULAR INJECTION.** (A) Injection site in the deltoid muscle. (B) Prep the skin over the site. (C) Insert the needle at a 90-degree angle to the muscle. (D) Aspirate for blood. (E) If there is no blood return, inject. (F) Apply pressure to the injection site.

243

6. Gently grasp the skin over the injection site, and pull it away from the underlying muscle. Insert the needle into the subcutaneous tissue at a 45-degree angle to the skin (Fig. 10-9).

7. Pull back slightly on the plunger of the syringe to be sure that the needle has not accidently entered a blood vessel.

8. If there is no blood return into the syringe, inject the medication.

9. Quickly withdraw the syringe, at the same angle as it was inserted, and apply firm pressure over the injection site. Dispose of the needle and syringe in an appropriate receptacle.

10. Monitor the patient for adverse reactions to the medication.

Giving Medications Through an Endotracheal Tube

The endotracheal route is indicated primarily for patients in cardiac arrest when an intravenous line cannot be established. In such cases, **atropine, lidocaine,** and **epinephrine** (and *only* those drugs) may be given down the endotracheal tube, with absorption nearly as rapid as via the intravenous route. Use 2.0 to 2.5 times the intravenous dosage. To give a medication through an endotracheal tube, proceed as follows:

1. While someone else ventilates the patient with 100% oxygen, dilute the required dosage of the medication in a syringe containing 10 ml of sterile water.

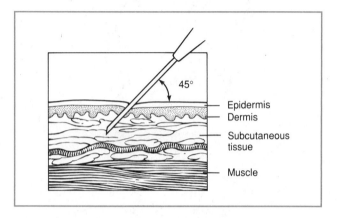

FIGURE 10-9. SUBCUTANEOUS INJECTION. Insert the needle at a 45-degree angle into the fatty tissue beneath the skin.

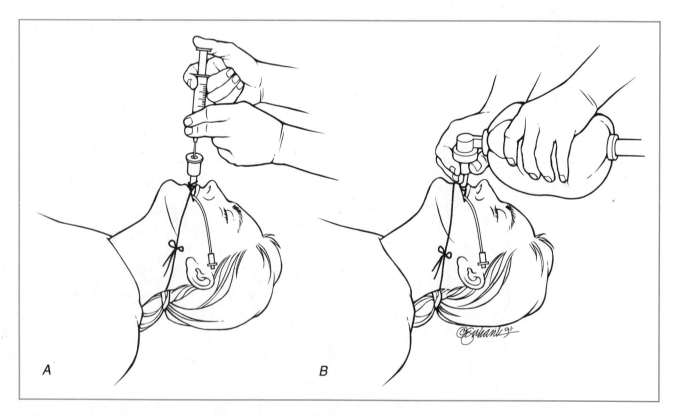

FIGURE 10-10. GIVING DRUGS THROUGH AN ENDOTRACHEAL TUBE.
(A) After a period of preoxygenation, inject the drug down the endotracheal tube. (B) Immediately reconnect the bag and ventilate vigorously.

2. Disconnect the bag-valve device from the endotracheal tube, and rapidly squirt the contents of the syringe down the tube (Fig. 10-10A).
3. Immediately reconnect the bag to the endotracheal tube, and ventilate the patient briskly to facilitate passage of the medication down the trachea (Fig. 10-10B).

Alternatively, you can inject the medication through the *wall* of the endotracheal tube without interrupting ventilations by piercing the endotracheal tube gently with the needle of the drug syringe. However, while that method works nicely in theory, under field conditions it may result in your stabbing yourself or your partner!

GLOSSARY

additive effect   Increased effect that may occur when two drugs that have the same action are given together.

allergic reaction   Hypersensitivity on reexposure to a substance that does not ordinarily cause adverse symptoms in the average person.

ampule   A sealed glass container of a single dose of a sterile medication.

antagonism   Decrease in the action of a drug by the administration of another drug.

biotransformation   The metabolic process by which a drug is inactivated.

contraindications   Conditions that preclude the use of a drug.

cumulative action   Action of increased intensity after administration of several doses of a drug.

depressant   A substance that lessens the activity of the body or any of its organs.

generic name   The name given to a drug by the company that first manufactures it; usually a simplified version of the drug's chemical name.

habituation   Situation in which the effects produced by a drug are necessary to maintain a person's feeling of well-being.

hypersensitivity   Allergy.

idiosyncratic reaction   Abnormal sensitivity to a drug, peculiar to an individual.

indications   The conditions for which a drug is recommended.

irritation   Action of a drug that produces slight or temporary damage to tissues.

parenteral   By a route *other than* through the digestive tract.

physiologic action   Action caused by a drug when given in the concentrations normally present in the body.

potentiation   Enhancement of the action of a drug by another substance that does not have that action at all.

side effect   An expected and predictable effect of a drug that is not part of its therapeutic effect.

stimulant   A drug that increases the activity of the body or any of its organs.

synergism   Combined effect of two drugs that is greater than the sum of their individual effects.

therapeutic action   Beneficial action of a drug to correct a bodily dysfunction.

tolerance   Progressive decrease in susceptibility to the effects of a drug after repeated doses.

untoward reaction   Side effect regarded as harmful to the patient; a toxic reaction.

vial   A glass container storing a sterile powdered or liquid drug for parenteral use, sealed with a rubber stopper, and often containing multiple doses.

FURTHER READING

Bogner PH. *Handbook of Pharmacologic Therapeutics*. Boston: Little, Brown, 1988.

Garrison H et al. Paramedic skills and medications. *J Prehosp Disaster Med* 6:29, 1991.

Greenblatt DJ, Koch-Weser J. Intramuscular injection of drugs. *N Engl J Med* 295:542, 1976.

Holliman CJ et al. Medication mishaps: Avoiding inappropriate use of prehospital meds. *Emerg Med Serv* 21(11):21, 1992.

Jahns BE, Levy DB. Common drug reactions and interactions. *Emergency* 23(11):22, 1991.

Langille DB et al. Contamination of multiple-dose vials due to repeat use of syringes. *Can Med Assoc J* 140:539, 1989.

Moss RL. Therapeutic agents utilized in urban/rural prehospital care. *Prehosp Disaster Med* 8:161, 1993.

Ordog GJ et al. Efficacy of absorption of sublingual and intravenous cardio-green. *Ann Emerg Med* 13:426, 1984.

Peppers MP. Understanding pharmacology. *Emergency* 25(1):18, 1993.

Reed JS, Anderson AC, Hodges GR. Needlestick and puncture wounds: Definition of the problem. *Am J Infect Control* 8(4):101, 1980.

Shuster M, Chong J. Pharmacologic intervention in prehospital care: A critical appraisal. *Ann Emerg Med* 18:192, 1989.

Valenzuela TD, Criss EA. Can your ALS drugs withstand the summer heat? *Emerg Med Serv* 19(8):53, 1990.

Valenzuela TD et al. Thermal stability of prehospital medications. *Ann Emerg Med* 18:173, 1989.

III

THE SECONDARY SURVEY

In prehospital emergency care, the priorities of evaluation and treatment of a patient are based upon the degree of threat to the patient's life. The more immediate the danger to the patient, the higher the priority in detecting the problem and taking corrective measures. Up to this point, we have considered only the highest priority problems, those that jeopardize the airway, breathing, and circulation; that is, we have so far learned only the *primary* survey, the rapid assessment of a patient to identify (and start the treatment of) conditions that pose an immediate threat to life.

Once the primary survey has been completed—whether at a glance (for the conscious, alert patient) or after several steps of treatment (for the unconscious patient)—we can move on to the **secondary survey.** The overall purpose of the secondary survey is to detect problems that do *not* pose an immediate threat to life but that may become more serious, or even life-threatening, if they are not promptly managed. More specifically, the *objectives of the secondary survey* are

- To win the patient's confidence and thereby alleviate some of the anxiety contributing to his discomfort
- To identify the patient's problem(s) rapidly and establish which problem(s) require immediate care in the field
- To obtain information about the patient that may not be readily available to those caring for him later in the hospital, for example through observations of the environment in which the patient is found

The secondary survey in fact consists of two phases: an INFORMATION-GATHERING PHASE, called **history-taking,** in which we try to determine the nature of the patient's problems by asking questions and observing the setting in which the patient was found; and an EXAMINATION PHASE, called **physical assessment,** in which we make a rapid but complete hands-on evaluation of the patient to determine his vital signs and detect injuries or signs of illness.

The value of the information obtained through history-taking and physical examination will be largely dependent on the manner in which those procedures are conducted. Patient assessment must be rapid, but unhurried, and SYSTEMATIC; a hasty, shotgun approach inevitably leads to omissions. Thus the paramedic must learn to carry out the assessment of each patient in a specific order, lest a step be skipped and important findings be missed. Both the history and physical assessment should be *orderly* and *thorough.*

In the next three chapters we shall, for teaching purposes, first present the method of obtaining a medical history (Chap. 11), then the method of physical assessment (Chap. 12), and finally the format for communicating medical information by voice and in writing (Chap. 13). In the field, however, circumstances will dictate the order in which the first two of those phases are accomplished. Urgent treatment may be required before you can stop to ask questions or do a thorough examination, as in the case of a patient with severe chest pain, who should receive oxygen immediately. Or it may be more expedient to obtain parts of the history while carrying out the physical assessment (certainly communication with the patient should not lapse during the physical examination!). Furthermore, different categories of patients will require different approaches. The approach to a victim of trauma will not be the same as the approach to a "medical" patient (a patient suffering from illness). What we wish to do in the next three chapters is simply to provide an *overall framework* for conducting the secondary survey.

We shall cover a lot of material in these chapters. Don't panic! We shall go back over that material several times in the course of this book, as we deal with illnesses and injuries affecting specific body systems.

When we conclude the section on trauma, for example, we shall go over in detail both the primary and secondary surveys of the injured patient. When we learn about illnesses affecting the cardiovascular system, we shall examine the characteristic stories and physical signs of patients with such illnesses. So there will be ample time to master the details of patient assessment. These three chapters, then, are intended as an overview, so that you can see the various elements of patient assessment in context—what comes *first*, what comes next, and so forth. Do not try to memorize the material now, but come back and review this section when you have finished studying the rest of the book. You may be surprised to find that you have, by then, already learned everything in these three chapters.

11
Obtaining the Medical History

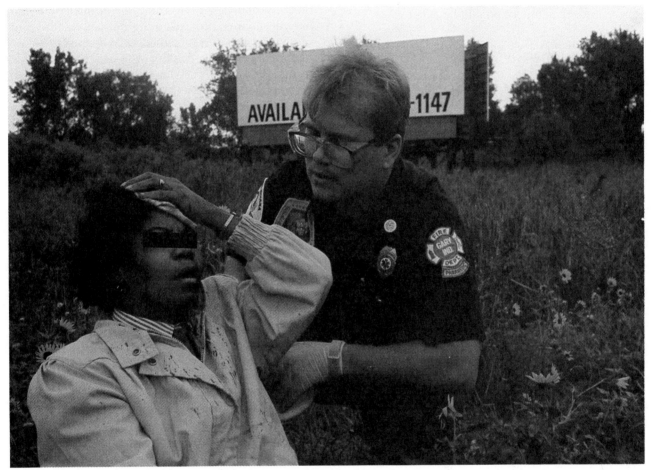

Gary Fire Department, Gary, Indiana. Photo by Michael S. Kowal.

OBJECTIVES

Taking a history in the field is not like taking a history in a doctor's office. In the difficult, often chaotic conditions in which a paramedic works, it is nearly impossible to obtain a detailed account of the patient's entire medical background, nor would it be desirable to collect all that information even if it *were* possible. Nonetheless, one can obtain important—sometimes critically important—information about the patient during the prehospital phase of care, and in this chapter we shall learn how to do so. By the end of this chapter the student should be able to

1. List four reasons for obtaining the medical history
2. List four potential sources of information about what has happened to the patient
3. Give four examples of information that can be obtained by observations of the scene
4. List the preliminary steps that should be taken before obtaining a history from a conscious patient
5. Identify questions from a patient interview that are improperly phrased, given a list of questions
6. Define "chief complaint," and identify the chief complaint in a patient's history
7. Differentiate between symptoms and signs, given a list containing both symptoms and signs
8. State the questions one would ask to elucidate the history of the patient's present illness, given his chief complaint
9. List the information about a person's past medical history that is relevant to prehospital emergency care
10. Identify the chief complaint, information from present illness, and information from the past medical history, given the medical history of a patient

WHY TAKE A HISTORY?

The fundamental reason for taking a history is to find out WHAT HAPPENED to the patient. Even when that information may seem obvious—for example, in the case of a person injured in a vehicular accident—taking the history may yield information that changes the picture altogether. Let's take that accident victim, for instance. If you simply examine him, you may find that he has only minor injuries, perhaps not even serious enough to warrant transport to a hospital. But if you take the history, you may learn that the *reason* he swerved off the road was that he sud-

denly blacked out for a few moments—information that hints at a serious cardiac dysrhythmia for which the patient definitely *does* need evaluation in the hospital.

A second reason to take a history is to determine WHAT HURTS or what it is that is bothering the patient. As we shall see shortly, that may or may not be obvious, and what is obvious may or may not be the problem.

Yet another reason for taking a history is to find out WHAT ELSE IS WRONG, that is, to learn about the patient's *underlying medical problems* that may bear on the seriousness of his condition or the kind of care he will require. It makes a big difference, for example, whether a person pulled from a smoky fire was previously perfectly healthy or whether he had a history of severe asthma, for the asthmatic is likely to suffer serious and even fatal complications of smoke inhalation. If you don't know about the asthma, you won't be prepared to deal with the complications.

Finally, a very important reason for collecting information about the patient in the field is to obtain DATA THAT MIGHT OTHERWISE BE UNAVAILABLE TO THE DOCTOR who will care for the patient later, in the hospital. An unconscious patient who is simply deposited in the emergency room, for example, constitutes a complete mystery to the medical staff there. But if the paramedic who transports the patient also brings the three empty pill bottles that were found at the patient's side, the emergency room staff are already a long way toward solving the mystery. Similarly, a patient injured in a vehicular accident represents an unknown combination of injuries when he arrives in the emergency room. Information from the paramedic about the accident scene—that the patient was the driver of the vehicle, that the steering column was bent and the front windshield was smashed, that the patient was found 15 feet away from the vehicle—immediately alerts the doctors in the emergency room to look for injuries to the head, chest, and spine and therefore assists the emergency room staff enormously in their search for the most serious injuries.

SOURCES OF INFORMATION

The process of taking a history and performing a physical examination is basically detective work—collecting clues in order to solve the mystery of what is wrong with the patient. No detective relies on a single source of information, nor should a paramedic do so. There are, in fact, several potential sources of information—both inanimate and animate—about what happened to the patient.

The Scene

The very first source of information that will confront you, before a single word is spoken, is the scene in which you find the patient. An observant paramedic can learn a great deal about the patient from the patient's surroundings. Let us consider separately the clues in the surroundings of a medical patient and those in the the surroundings of a trauma patient.

The Scenario of Illness

Suppose you are called to the home of a person found unconscious. What secrets can the walls tell you? Look around as you enter the home. What does it tell you about the person who lives there? Is it clean and orderly? Is it in total disorder? What about the patient's immediate surroundings? Are there empty pill bottles nearby? A suicide note by the bedside? Empty bottles of alcohol? Cigarettes? Drug paraphernalia? Is there a home oxygen setup? A wheelchair in the corner? A white cane by the front door?

In the bathroom cabinet, are there medications that give clues to the patient's underlying illnesses? Is there a doctor's name printed on any of the medicine bottles?

Use your *nose* as well as your eyes. Is there a smell of gas, smoke, vomitus?

The Scenario of Injury

The scene in which the patient was found is perhaps of even more importance when evaluating the victim of injury; for even if the patient is unconscious and cannot tell you anything about what happened, the scene can provide a great deal of the story.

The first thing one can often determine from the scene of an accident is the **mechanism of injury,** that is, the way in which an injury occurred and the forces that were involved in producing the injury. Consider the scenarios pictured in Figure 11-1, for example. The woman who fell down the stairs (Fig. 11-1A) can be suspected to have sustained impact to her hip, shoulder, and possibly her head. (One also needs to ask *why* she fell down the stairs. Did she trip? Did she first have a dizzy spell, which would suggest an underlying medical problem?) The casualty pictured in Figure 11-1B evidently fell from a ladder onto a concrete floor and landed on his back, so probably the head and spine hit the floor first; then the ladder came down on the victim's chest and abdomen. Injuries to the head, spine, chest, and abdomen are all highly likely in this situation. The *position* of the vehicle in Figure 11-1C tells you a lot about the forces that were involved in the accident, even before you've had a chance to examine the people who were inside the vehicle. In a head-on collision, any unrestrained occupant within the vehicle will be thrown forward, so you'll need to look for injuries to the head, chest, knees, and (by transmission of forces along the femur) hips. Notice also whether there are skid marks on the road, suggesting that the driver tried to apply his brakes, as one would normally expect. If there are no skid marks, consider the possibility that the driver lost consciousness *before* the accident. The driver pictured in Figure 11-1D was in a car that was hit from behind. The broken windshield should alert you to the possibility of serious head injury. We shall consider the mechanisms of injury in more detail in Chapter 14.

The accident scene can give you information not only about the mechanisms of injury but also about the potential *seriousness of the injury.* A large pool of blood on the driver's seat, for example, suggests the possibility of hemorrhagic shock, and you should try to form an estimate of how much blood was lost—a few teaspoonfuls? a cup? a quart? The precise location and position of the patient may also be informative. Finding an injured driver unconscious 50 yards down the road from his wrecked vehicle suggests that he was *not* unconscious immediately after the accident, but rather lost consciousness only after a few minutes, during which he managed to get out of the vehicle and wander down the road. Information of that sort may help the neurosurgeon at the hospital decide whether it is necessary to take the patient to the operating room at once or whether there is time to wait and observe the patient's condition.

The Patient

Probably the most important source of information is, of course, the patient, for no one is more qualified than the patient to tell you where it hurts, what the pain feels like, and so forth. Furthermore, directing your questions first to the patient establishes the fact that he is the center of your interest and that he still has some control over his own situation. One of the most frightening things about illness or injury is the feeling that one has lost control of one's destiny. It is, in addition, extremely irritating for anyone—sick or well—to be talked about in the third person as if he were not present ("When did he start having these fainting spells?"), for it makes a person feel as if his opinions are of no consequence. What you *want* to convey is precisely the opposite—that the patient is the most important person present. Thus, whenever you are dealing with a conscious patient, direct your questions *first* to the patient, even if he appears confused or uncommunicative. A disturbed person may calm down considerably if you address him in an as-

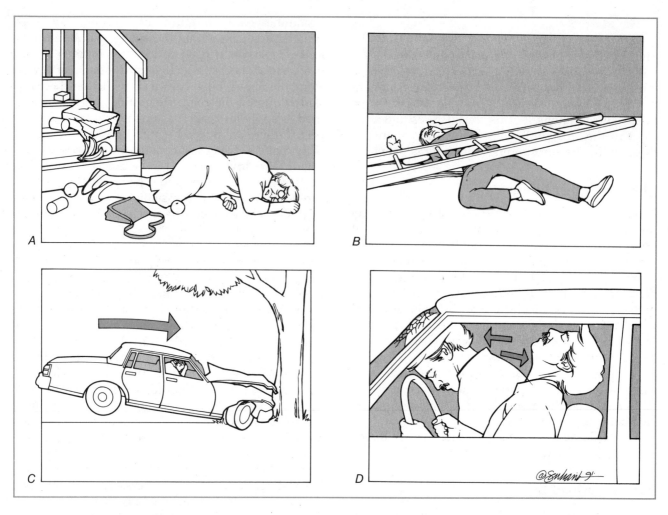

FIGURE 11-1.   MECHANISMS OF INJURY. (A) Fall down a flight of stairs. (B) Fall from a height. (C) Head-on collision, with massive deceleration forces. (D) Rear-end collision; broken windshield attests that driver was initially thrown forward.

sured, friendly manner. A child old enough to talk should be able to tell you a lot about where it hurts. Even a person robbed of speech by a stroke may be able to nod or shake his head in response to questions.

> **NEVER ASSUME THAT IT IS IMPOSSIBLE TO TALK TO A PATIENT UNTIL YOU HAVE TRIED.**

There may, however, be circumstances in which the patient cannot give you any information (e.g., if he is unconscious) or situations in which the information he does give is of questionable reliability (e.g., the patient with chest pain who tries to mini-

mize his symptoms). In such situations, you may need to turn to other informants.

Other Informants

When you do question others, interview them one at a time, for it is difficult to get a clear idea of what happened from a chorus of voices. It is usually best to start with any FIRST RESPONDERS who might be present, such as firefighters, police officers, or others who may have reached the patient ahead of you and started first aid. Find out from the first responders:

- What happened
- In what position the patient was found, and what condition he was in at the time
- What the first responder has done for the patient up to now

It can also be very helpful to talk to BYSTAND-ERS—family, friends, or people who just happened to be on the scene. Family members may be able to provide important information about the patient's medical history—for example, that he is a dialysis patient or that he suffered a heart attack a year ago. Or they may be able to fill in parts of the story omitted by the patient, especially when the patient tends to deny or minimize his symptoms. Bystanders may be able to describe what happened just before an incident ("I saw him walking down the street sort of funny and then he just keeled over and his arms and legs started jerking back and forth.").

Medical Identification Devices

Finally, one may learn important information about the patient from a medical identification device. One of the most commonly used such devices in the United States is the MEDIC ALERT TAG (Fig. 11-2), which is worn as a necklace, bracelet, or anklet. On the front of the tag is the Medic Alert logo, and on

FIGURE 11-2. **MEDIC ALERT TAG.**

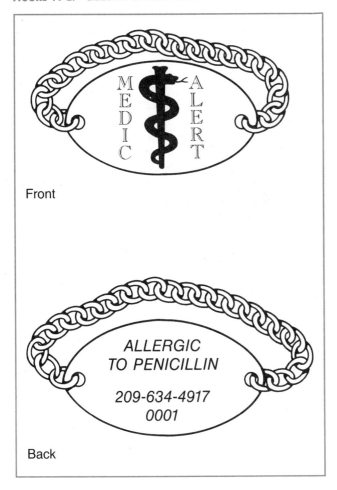

Front

ALLERGIC
TO PENICILLIN

209-634-4917
0001

Back

the back is engraved a brief statement of the patient's problem (e.g., "Allergic to penicillin" or "Diabetic"). A similar bracelet, in use in several European countries, is issued by an organization called SOS. The SOS bracelet has a small compartment that can be unscrewed, and inside is a strip of paper containing information about the wearer's identity and medical history. In addition to identification devices worn as jewelry, there are others that are carried as wallet cards or even stored in the home. The VIAL OF LIFE, for example, is a small cylinder containing information about the patient and is usually stored in the refrigerator. A label on the refrigerator door indicates that there is a "vial of life" inside.

Let us consider a hypothetical patient to illustrate just how much valuable information a paramedic can gather in the field—information to which the emergency room personnel would not otherwise have access. Suppose you arrive at the scene of a road accident. The patient, who was the driver of the vehicle, is unconscious, so you have to gather all your information from observations of the scene and interviews with bystanders. You notice that skid marks lead to the place where the car is accordioned up against a tree; the car's windshield is smashed, and the steering column is bent. There is about a quart of blood in the passenger compartment. A police officer who reached the scene ahead of you says that the driver was conscious when the squad car pulled up, but he lost consciousness about 5 minutes later. A bystander who was waiting for a bus across the street tells you that the car was weaving back and forth across the road before it plowed into the tree. Here is the information you have collected and what that information can tell the doctors who will care for the patient in the hospital:

ACCIDENT SCENE INFORMATION	WHAT THAT TELLS THE DOCTOR
Observations of the scene:	
Skid marks	Patient was conscious before the accident
Car accordioned against tree	Powerful deceleration forces involved
Steering column bent	Look for sternal/rib fractures, myocardial contusions
Windshield smashed	Look for head/cervical spine injury
About a quart of blood inside the car	Anticipate shock if not already present

Report from first responder:

Patient was conscious at first, lost consciousness afterward	"Lucid interval" suggests an epidural hematoma—call the neurosurgeons!

Report from bystander:

Vehicle was weaving down the road erratically	Driver may have been intoxicated with drugs or alcohol

Clearly, that is a lot of information, and it is information that could—by enabling speedier diagnosis and treatment—save the patient's life. Obtaining that information, therefore, may be one of the most important things that you will do for the patient.

SOURCES OF INFORMATION: SUMMARY

- The SCENE
  1. Clues to underlying illnesses
  2. Mechanisms of injury
  3. Severity of injury
- The PATIENT
- OTHER INFORMANTS
  1. First responders
  2. Bystanders (family, friends, passersby)
- MEDICAL IDENTIFICATION DEVICES

THE APPROACH TO THE PATIENT

You have reached the scene of a "possible heart attack" in a downtown department store, and you have duly made note of the patient's surroundings. Your primary survey was accomplished at a glance by observing that the patient is conscious and alert. Where do you go from there?

1. JETTISON any PRECONCEIVED IDEAS from your mind. Just because the call came in to the dispatcher as a "possible heart attack" does not mean it *is* a heart attack. Keep an open mind, or you will miss something.
2. INTRODUCE YOURSELF, and explain your role ("My name is George Goodfellow, and I'm a paramedic. Can I be of help?").

3. FIND OUT THE PATIENT'S NAME AND AGE, and use the name periodically throughout the interview to convey the message that you regard him or her as an individual. Unless the patient is a child, using the patient's name means using the *family name*. All adults should be addressed as Mister, Miss, or Mrs. (address John Jones as "Mr. Jones," not "John"), for addressing an adult stranger by his first name implies disrespect.
4. Try to POSITION YOURSELF AT THE PATIENT'S LEVEL. If the patient is sitting, pull up a chair beside him. If he is lying on the floor, kneel beside him. Do *not* tower over him.
5. Initiate some PHYSICAL CONTACT, as a way of indicating that you are caring and willing to help. Simply taking the patient's wrist in your hand can provide comfort to the patient and, at the same time, enable you to make a quick assessment of the patient's radial pulse.
6. MAINTAIN EYE CONTACT WITH THE PATIENT to indicate that you are giving your full attention to what he or she is saying.

Now you are ready to start asking some questions.

ASKING QUESTIONS

Unlike interviewing in a doctor's office or hospital, where questioning can be lengthy and entirely open-ended, interviewing in the field under emergency circumstances must be selective and direct. If the situation truly *is* an emergency, there simply isn't time to find out whether the patient had chickenpox as a child, nor would such information have much bearing on his immediate care. Nor is there time to permit the patient to give an exhaustive and detailed account of everything that led up to the emergency. Once you have a general idea of the patient's problem, you will need to ask some relatively direct questions to elucidate that problem further. Nonetheless, your questions should not be phrased in such a way as to put words into the patient's mouth. In particular, avoid asking questions that can be answered with a "yes" or "no." It is better, for example, to ask, "What makes the pain better?" than to suggest an answer to the patient by asking, "Does the pain get better if you stop and rest?" If you are trying to pin down a specific piece of information, present the patient with alternatives rather than with a yes-or-no question. For example, if you are trying to get a feeling for the constancy of a patient's pain, you might ask, "Is the pain there all the time, or does it come and go?"

| DO NOT ASK QUESTIONS THAT CAN BE ANSWERED WITH A "YES" OR "NO." |

Whenever circumstances permit, obtain the history *before* examining the patient. If that is not possible, at least ask your questions about a given part of the body *before* you examine that part of the body; otherwise the patient is likely to get the impression that you have found something terribly wrong in the course of your examination. If, for instance, you take your stethoscope from the patient's chest and chirp, "Tell me, Ma'am, have you ever had a heart attack?" the unfortunate woman is very likely to conclude that you have just detected some telltale sign of heart disease.

The information you need to obtain from the patient falls into three categories: (1) the patient's *chief complaint*; (2) the *history of the present illness*; and (3) the patient's *other medical history.*

THE CHIEF COMPLAINT

The first piece of information you need to obtain is the patient's **chief complaint,** that is, the problem that prompted him to call for help. In many instances, that will seem obvious without asking, as, for example, in the case of a patient who lies bleeding in the street after being struck by an automobile. Even in that circumstance, however, it is useful to find out what is bothering the patient most, for his report may lead to unexpected findings. Our patient in the street, for example, may have a dramatically obvious compound fracture of the leg, yet when you inquire what is bothering him most, he may report, "I can't breathe"—leading you to discover an unsuspected pneumothorax.

| IF YOU DON'T ASK, YOU WON'T FIND OUT. |

The chief complaint is elicited by asking an open-ended question such as, "What seems to be the trouble?" or, if the patient is injured, "What is bothering you the most?" When reporting the patient's chief complaint, it is customary to state it in a word or phrase, preferably in the patient's own words, such as "squeezing in my chest" or "twisted ankle." Most chief complaints are characterized by pain, abnormal function, some change from a normal state, or an observation made by the patient. From that initial statement, one then proceeds to develop a line of questioning to learn more about the chief complaint. That amplification of the chief complaint is called the "history of the present illness."

THE HISTORY OF THE PRESENT ILLNESS

The patient's present "illness" may be a medical problem (e.g., a heart attack) or an injury (e.g., trauma sustained in an automobile accident), but in either instance you will need to gather further information. In doing so, it is important to understand the distinction between a symptom and a sign. A **symptom** is SOMETHING THE PATIENT FEELS and that, therefore, only he can tell you about—for example, dizziness, itching, nausea. A **sign** is SOMETHING YOU CAN OBSERVE, whether or not the patient is aware of it. When you take a medical history, you are gathering information about *symptoms.* Signs are discovered only when you perform the physical examination.

One of the most frequent chief complaints in a medical patient is PAIN, which is usually evaluated in the prehospital phase by the PQRST format, to which we would add an "A":

PQRST FORMAT FOR EVALUATING PAIN

P What PROVOKES the pain? Did something in particular bring it on? Does anything make it worse? Does anything make it better?

Q What is the QUALITY of the pain? Dull? Sharp? Cutting? Throbbing? Crushing? Squeezing?

R Does the pain RADIATE to any other area, or does it stay in one place?

S What is the SEVERITY of the pain? Ask the patient to grade it on a scale of 1 (insignificant) to 10 (unbearable).

T What is the TIMING of the pain? When did it start? What has happened to it over time (gotten worse? gotten better?)? If there are associated symptoms, what is their relative timing (e.g., did the pain come on before or after the nausea?)?

| A | Are there any ASSOCIATED SYMPTOMS? Nausea? Dizziness? Other unusual or unpleasant feelings? |

Let us look, for example, at a middle-aged patient with classic symptoms of myocardial infarction (heart attack). The information elicited in the history of the present illness might be as follows:

CHIEF COMPLAINT: Chest pain.
- PROVOCATION: Nothing seemed to bring it on. The patient was just sitting watching television when the pain came on. Nothing seems to make it better or worse (he took 2 nitroglycerin, but they didn't help).
- QUALITY: The pain is crushing, "as if an elephant is sitting on my chest."
- RADIATION: The pain starts just beneath the sternum and radiates into the jaw and down the left arm.
- SEVERITY: The pain is very severe (the patient rates it 8 on a scale of 10); he feels as if he could die from the pain.
- TIMING: The pain started 2 hours ago, and it has gotten progressively worse ever since.
- ASSOCIATED SYMPTOMS: The patient also complains of feeling nauseated, weak, and dizzy.

Thus, by exploring the patient's chief complaint with a few further questions, we have been able to obtain a quite clear picture of the patient's problem. As we learn more about specific illnesses and injuries, we shall learn other questions that can be asked to clarify a given problem. We shall learn, for example, to find out whether a patient with chest pain has experienced any shortness of breath, which might signal heart failure, or any palpitations, which would suggest he experienced a disturbance of cardiac rhythm.

If time permits, it's a good idea to conclude this part of your history-taking by briefly summarizing what you have heard the patient say. You could comment, for instance, "Let's see if I've got this right. Your pain started about 2 hours ago, while you were watching TV, and two nitroglycerins didn't help." A summary of that sort gives the patient a chance to correct any misunderstandings or to add something that was left out. Equally important, your summary conveys the message that you've really been *listening*—and someone who listens is someone who cares.

OTHER MEDICAL PROBLEMS

After the inquiries into the patient's present illness are complete, it is still necessary to obtain some further information about the patient's medical background. In the field, we are primarily interested in those aspects of the patient's past medical history that may in some way bear on his current problem or on the treatment he will receive. For example, in the burned patient, it is important to know whether he has underlying cardiac problems, because such problems might influence the way he responds to intravenous fluids. It is not particularly relevant, on the other hand, to learn whether he had measles as a child or underwent a hernia operation 5 years previously. In general, the following information should be gathered about the patient's other medical problems:

- Does the patient have any MAJOR UNDERLYING MEDICAL PROBLEMS (e.g., cardiac, respiratory, renal)? Is he a diabetic? Is he currently under a doctor's care for any serious condition?
- Does the patient take any MEDICATIONS regularly? If so, what medications? Medications may provide important clues to the patient's underlying conditions when he himself is not fully aware of the nature of his problem. Did he take his medications today? When? Has he taken any other drugs or alcohol during the past several hours? If so, what, when, and how much?
- Does the patient have any known ALLERGIES? Ask specifically about Novocain (or "numbing medicine" in the dentist's office), since patients with certain cardiac dysrhythmias may require the related drug, lidocaine.
- Is the patient regularly seen by a particular DOCTOR? At a particular hospital? Generally speaking, it is preferable to bring the patient to the hospital where his medical records are on file, provided that hospital is near enough and has the facilities necessary to deal with the patient's current problem.

In the doctor's office, it is also customary to question the patient regarding his *family history*. That information is rarely of immediate importance in the field and in most instances is not worth taking the time to elicit. The patient with crushing chest pain will be treated as a possible myocardial infarction irrespective of whether his parents both died in their 40s of heart attacks or whether they both lived to a ripe old age. However, the information the patient *volunteers* about his family may provide useful clues as to what is worrying him. The patient with shortness of breath who relates that his father died at age 40 of a heart attack is clearly wondering whether the same fate is about to befall him, and it is worth pursuing that line of inquiry—if for no other reason than to enable the patient to talk about what is worrying him. You might ask him straight out, "Are you worrying that the same thing will happen to you?" If he answers in the affirmative, try to learn why he has that worry. What symptoms has he had that he associates with a heart attack? That type of questioning may give the patient an opportunity to discuss symptoms that he has not mentioned previously.

The current family medical situation may provide useful information in instances where you suspect that the patient is suffering from a communicable disease. If, for example, the chief complaint is vomiting and diarrhea, it is useful to know whether anyone else in the household has had a similar problem.

Now, let's take it from the top and see how the whole history might sound as elicited by an experienced paramedic in the field. In the dialogue below, paramedic Wanda Warmheart has responded to a call for a "man down." Arriving at the scene, she finds an elderly man lying at the foot of a flight of stairs at the entrance to an apartment building. He is conscious and alert.

Wanda: *Hello, I'm Wanda Warmheart. I'm a paramedic. What's happened here?*
Patient: *Oh, those kids left their skates on the stairs again, and I fell over them, fell right down the stairs, I did. I'm so upset.*
Wanda: *I guess this wasn't on your program for the day.*
Patient: *No, it certainly wasn't.*
Wanda: *[Kneeling beside him and taking hold of his wrist] Can you tell me your name, sir?*
Patient: *William Fremont.*
Wanda: *And how old are you, Mr. Fremont?*
Patient: *85 years old this week.*
Wanda: *Can you tell me where it hurts, Mr. Fremont?*
Patient: *Right here, in my hip. I'm so afraid I may have broken it—you know, at my age.*
Wanda: *Well, it's a possibility we'll have to consider. But tell me, what is the pain like?*
Patient: *It's just throbbing away in my leg.*
Wanda: *How bad is it?*
Patient: *Not so bad if I keep real still, but it hurts like the dickens if I try to move my leg.*
Wanda: *Anything else bothering you, Mr. Fremont?*
Patient: *Well, I've got these pins-and-needles in my foot, maybe from not moving it.*
Wanda: *I see.*
Patient: *And a real splitting headache. I banged my head good on the way down those stairs.*
Wanda: *Are you under a doctor's care, Mr. Fremont?*

Patient: *Yeah, Dr. Goodwrench, over at Mercy Hospital, he takes care of my plumbing, don't you know.*
Wanda: *Besides your, uh, plumbing, do you have any other medical problems?*
Patient: *No, no. Always been healthy as a horse.*
Wanda: *Do you take any medications regularly?*
Patient: *Only the little white heart pills.*
Wanda: *What are those for?*
Patient: *To keep the engine running regular, don't you know, the old ticker.*
Wanda: *Are you allergic to anything that you know of?*
Patient: *No, no I don't think so.*
Wanda: *O.K., Mr. Fremont, now I need to take a look at you, and then my partner and I are going to put that leg in a splint to keep it from moving around on the way to the hospital.*

There are several things worth noting in that interview. The first thing is that when the patient expresses his dismay over what has happened, the paramedic acknowledges that she is aware of that dismay ("I guess this wasn't on your program for the day."). By doing so, she sends the message that (1) it is all right to have such feelings and (2) she is on the patient's side. She elicits the patient's name very early on, and thereafter she uses it frequently during the interview, to convey the fact that she regards the patient as an individual. She establishes physical contact early as well, by checking the patient's radial pulse. When the patient is describing his pain, she encourages him to go on by saying, "I see" (sometimes a nod of the head or saying, "uh huh" will accomplish the same thing). And when she finishes her questions, she explains to the patient what is going to happen next. Meanwhile, in the space of about one and a half minutes, she has established a good rapport with the patient and has learned that the patient tripped down the stairs, that the blood supply to his leg may be compromised (pins-and-needles feelings in his foot), that he may have an accompanying head injury, that he sees a urologist regularly, and that he apparently has been treated for cardiac dysrhythmias.

We left Wanda Warmheart about to carry out a physical assessment of the patient, which is what we shall do in the next chapter.

GLOSSARY

chief complaint The problem for which the patient is seeking help, usually expressed in a word or phrase.
history of the present illness (HPI) Elaboration of the patient's chief complaint.

mechanism of injury   Way in which an injury occurred and the forces involved in producing the injury.

secondary survey   Evaluation of the patient to detect problems that are not immediately life-threatening but that could become more serious or even life-threatening if not managed promptly.

sign   Indication of illness or injury that the *examiner* can see, hear, feel, smell, and so on.

symptom   Pain, discomfort, or other bodily abnormality that the patient *feels*.

FURTHER READING

Bourn S. Lessons from history. *JEMS* 15(4):78, 1990.

Caroline NL. Hidden at the scene: Clues to social emergencies. *Emerg Med Serv* 11(4):83, 1982.

Kinney B. Assessment: The key to quality patient care. *Emerg Med Serv* 18(4):30, 1989.

Stewart C. Mechanisms of injury. *Emerg Med Serv* 18(1):21, 1989.

12
Physical Assessment

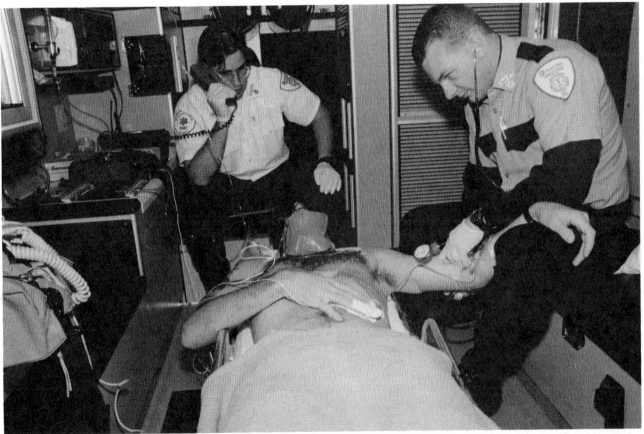

Brewster Ambulance Service, Brewster, Massachusetts. Photo by Brian Clark.

OBJECTIVES

As we learned in the previous chapter, taking a history is all about *symptoms*—the patient's subjective account of what happened to him and what it feels like. Physical assessment, on the other hand, involves assessing the patient's *signs*, the objective data about the patient's body that we can detect through the use of our senses: sight, hearing, touch, smell. In this chapter, we shall learn how to deploy our senses to find signs of serious illness or injury. By the conclusion of this chapter, the student should be able to

1. List the observations to be made about the patient's general appearance
2. Explain how the state of consciousness is assessed and how it should be described
3. Identify behavior that should alert the paramedic to the possibility of hypoxia or impending shock, given a description of several patients with different behaviors
4. Explain the reason for making a quick check for obvious injuries before beginning the head-to-toe survey
5. Indicate the possible significance of a given skin condition (color, temperature, moisture), given a description of a patient's skin condition
6. List the aspects of the pulse that should be evaluated, and state how the pulse is described
7. List the aspects of respiration that should be assessed, and indicate how the respirations should be described
8. Describe the method of measuring the respiratory rate
9. Indicate the significance of abnormal respiratory sounds, given a list of abnormal sounds
10. Describe the usual method of measuring the blood pressure, and indicate what alternative method(s) can be used under noisy field conditions
11. Identify normal vital signs for an adult, given a list containing different sets of vital signs
12. Explain the significance of various abnormal physical signs in an injured patient, given a list of signs
13. Explain the significance of various abnormal physical signs in a medical patient, given a list of signs
14. List the differences between the examination of an injured patient and the examination of a patient with a medical problem with respect to examination of
    • the head
    • the neck
    • the chest
    • the abdomen
    • the extremities and back

FIRST THINGS FIRST: A REMINDER

Physical assessment in fact begins before the secondary survey. It begins at the moment you encounter the patient, when you ask the basic questions that make up the *primary* survey:

PRIMARY SURVEY: REVIEW

• Is the patient CONSCIOUS? If not,
• Does he have an open AIRWAY?
• Is he BREATHING?
• Is his CIRCULATION in immediate jeopardy?
  1. Does he have a PULSE?
  2. Is there SEVERE BLEEDING?

The primary survey is *always* the first step in patient assessment, taking precedence over all other aspects of history-taking and physical examination. In many instances, you will complete the primary survey at a glance, as when you encounter an alert, communicative patient with minor medical problems. In other instances, however, as when the patient is unconcious or the victim of major trauma, close examination will be required to accomplish the primary survey. If that survey elicits any positive findings, such as an obstructed airway or massive hemorrhage, you must attend to those problems immediately, before proceeding further in the assessment of the patient.

When the primary survey is complete and any problems detected therein have been brought under control—only *then* should you take a closer look at the patient and *systematically* examine him from head to toe, to detect less obvious injuries or signs that may give clues to underlying medical problems. The first thing you will inevitably observe is the patient's general appearance.

GENERAL APPEARANCE

Each of us, without even trying and without being conscious of doing so, makes dozens of observations about the appearance of others during the first few seconds of an encounter. We notice if the other person is sitting or standing, fat or thin, smiling or frowning, dressed neatly or sloppily. Instinctively, we take in those observations and form judgments based upon them. In assessing a patient, we must make similar observations, but in a much more conscious, objective, and *systematic* fashion, looking for very specific things that will give us an immediate sense of how serious the situation might be.

The Position of the Patient

The position in which the patient is found can tell us a great deal. In the victim of trauma, the position may enable us to figure out what were the mechanisms of injury or what type of injury was sustained. A patient who walks toward you supporting his wrist with his other hand has almost certainly suffered a Colles' fracture; the patient lying supine with his arms flexed across his chest is very likely to have suffered injury to the cervical spine.

Position can be similarly informative in assessing medical patients. A person who is having difficulty breathing, for any reason, will almost invariably sit bolt upright or even pace about, but will not voluntarily assume a recumbent position. A patient with a kidney stone will thrash about, seeking a position of comfort, while someone with peritonitis (an inflammation of the abdominal cavity) will lie absolutely still, because the slightest movement is painful.

Level of Consciousness

The next thing we need to observe about a patient is his level of consciousness. Changes in the state of consciousness are often the first clue to an alteration in the patient's condition, so we want to establish a baseline as soon as we encounter the patient.

When describing a patient's level of consciousness, avoid words like *lethargic, obtunded, torpid*, and the like. Such terms are not very informative, since people seldom agree on what they mean. What you consider "obtundation," the doctor in the emergency room may consider only "lethargy," and he may therefore conclude that the patient's condition has improved when in fact his condition has not changed at all. Therefore, describe the patient's state of consciousness in terms of his REACTIONS TO SPECIFIC STIMULI or his responses to specific inquiries, for example, "The patient responds to deep pain, but not to shouting his name," or "The patient was drowsy but easily awakened by verbal stimuli," or "The patient knew his name and address, but could not remember the date." That type of report provides the listener with information that he can recheck very precisely later on to determine whether there has been any genuine change in the patient's status.

As you speak with the patient, make a note of whether he is ALERT OR CONFUSED. Is he ORIENTED to *time* (time of day, day of the week, and date), to *place* (where he is), and to *person* (who he is). Note the patient's SPEECH. Progressive slurring of words or vagueness in answering questions, especially when the patient formerly spoke clearly and coherently, indicates a decreasing level of consciousness. Garbled words may indicate a stroke. If the patient cannot speak at all, try to determine WHETHER HE CAN UNDERSTAND by giving a simple command (e.g., "Squeeze my hand."). With young children or infants, estimate their alertness by noting their interest in their surroundings and by observing their voluntary movements. If the patient is unconscious or sleeping, determine WHAT STIMULUS IS REQUIRED TO WAKE HIM UP: Can he be roused by your voice? Does it require a painful stimulus, such as a pinch, to wake him? Or is it impossible to wake him no matter what you do?

If the patient moves in response to a given stimulus, observe the NATURE OF HIS MOVEMENT. Is it purposeful? That is, does the patient try to move away from a painful stimulus or to remove the noxious stimulation (e.g., by pushing your hand away)? Or does he respond with *abnormal movements* such as decortication (flexion of the arms and extension of the legs) or decerebration (extension and internal rotation of the arms and extension of the legs)? Does he move at all?

When we study injuries to the central nervous system, in Chapter 16, we shall learn about some of the scoring systems that have been devised to quantitate the observations mentioned, and in your work in the field, you will undoubtedly use whatever neurologic scale is standard in your EMS system. For our purposes here, it is sufficient to become aware of the things one must observe to evaluate a person's state of consciousness.

Behavior and Degree of Distress

At the same time that you are assessing the patient's level of consciousness, you will inevitably be taking note of his behavior and the degree of his distress. Again, this is something everyone does quite naturally, without being consciously aware of doing it. If, for example, you find your patient engrossed in the Game of the Week on television, his feet propped up on a hassock, a beer in one hand and a cigarette in the other, you will not be terribly impressed by his statement, "Hey, fellas, I think I'm having a heart attack." If, on the other hand, he is sitting at the edge of his chair, his face ashen and shiny with sweat, his fist clenched over his chest, you will have a different impression altogether. What you need to do as a medical professional, as opposed to an ordinary observer, is to start becoming aware of the data that you are unconsciously recording and the judgments you are basing on that data.

If the patient is conscious, observe his posture, his movements, and his facial expression. Is he sitting quietly, in no apparent discomfort? Is he struggling to breathe? Is his face contorted in pain? Does he look frightened?

Be particularly alert for RESTLESSNESS. Restlessness is common in many types of injuries and some illnesses. It may indicate nothing more than a general discomfort, a full bladder, a reaction to restraints, or some other small problem of that sort. *However*, RESTLESSNESS IS ALSO ONE OF THE EARLIEST SIGNS OF HYPOXEMIA OR INTERNAL BLEEDING, and its presence should alert the rescuer to the possibility of serious underlying problems. The point is important enough to repeat:

> **RESTLESSNESS IS A DANGER SIGNAL!**

It may be the only early sign of massive internal bleeding or critical oxygen deprivation. Never dismiss restlessness as insignificant until all potentially serious causes have been ruled out.

Obvious Wounds or Deformities

As you quickly form your initial impressions of the victim of trauma, you will also be able to observe whether there are any obvious signs of injury—for example, a bloodstained shirt, a leg splayed out at a strange angle. Do not stop to deal with such things at this point in your assessment (you should, in any case, have already taken care of any *serious* bleeding during the primary survey!). The reason for making a mental note of obvious injuries at the outset is chiefly to alert you to parts of the patient's body that should not be moved pending closer examination.

Assessment of the Skin

Observe the patient's skin for color, temperature, and moisture. The *color* of the skin (Table 12-1), especially in white patients, reflects the circulation immediately underlying the skin as well as the oxygen saturation of the blood. In darker individuals, those changes may not be readily evident in the skin but may be assessed by examining the mucous membranes (e.g.,

the lips, the conjunctivae of the eyes). When the blood vessels supplying the skin are fully dilated, so that blood flow to the periphery is increased, the skin becomes warm and pink. If, on the other hand, the blood vessels supplying the skin constrict or if cardiac output drops, the skin becomes *pale, mottled*, or *cyanotic*. **Pallor** also occurs if arterial blood flow ceases to a part of the body (e.g., when there is a clot in an artery) or when there has been a lot of bleeding.

Skin *temperature* (Table 12-2) rises as peripheral blood vessels dilate and falls as blood vessels constrict. Fever and high environmental temperatures usually stimulate vasodilatation, while shock usually elicits vasoconstriction. Normal skin is moderately warm and dry. The dryness or the *moisture* of the skin is largely determined by the sympathetic nervous system. Stimulation of the sympathetic nervous system, as in shock or any other severe stress, causes sweating, so the skin becomes moist. Depression of the sympathetic nervous system, which may result from injury to the thoracic or lumbar spine, can cause the skin in the affected areas to be abnormally dry and cool.

Use the back of your hand to assess the warmth and moisture of a patient's skin (Fig. 12-1).

Within the first few moments of encountering the patient, then, we have already managed—simply by

TABLE 12-1. INSPECTION OF THE SKIN

SKIN COLOR	POSSIBLE CAUSE
Red	Fever
	Allergic reactions
	Carbon monoxide poisoning
White (pallor)	Excessive blood loss
	Fright
Blue (cyanosis)	Hypoxemia
	Peripheral vasoconstriction from cold or shock
Mottled	Cardiovascular embarrassment (as in shock)

TABLE 12-2. PALPATION OF THE SKIN

SKIN TEMPERATURE	POSSIBLE CAUSE
Hot, dry	Excessive body heat (heat stroke)
Hot, wet	Reaction to increased internal or external temperature
Cool, dry	Exposure to cold
Cool, clammy	Shock

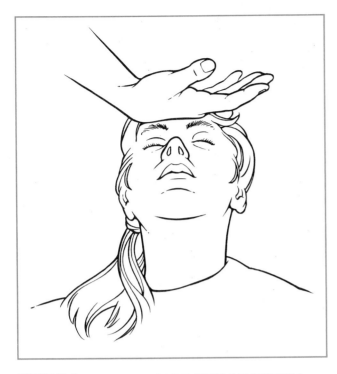

FIGURE 12-1.   ASSESSING THE SKIN CONDITION.
Use the back of your hand to assess the temperature and moisture of the skin.

pausing to observe his general appearance—to get a good general impression of the seriousness of his problem. And while it will require a closer examination to find out precisely what that problem is, the patient's general appearance can often help us at least to rule in or out certain possibilities. The man engrossed in the Game of the Week on television, for example, is very unlikely to have sustained a significant myocardial infarction; a victim of a vehicular accident who is alert and in no observable distress almost certainly has not suffered a tension pneumothorax or a torn aorta; however, an unconscious victim of the same accident who shows no visible sign of injury but whose skin is cold and clammy can be presumed to be bleeding internally. The patient's general appearance, therefore, will very often dictate the urgency with which we must proceed with the rest of the patient's assessment and care.

To summarize the assessment of a patient's general appearance:

GENERAL APPEARANCE

- Position
- Level of consciousness
- Behavior and degree of distress

- Obvious wounds or deformities
- Skin color, temperature, moisture

VITAL SIGNS

When you have finished the appraisal of the patient's general appearance, the next thing to do is to measure the patient's vital signs—the pulse, respirations, blood pressure, and temperature. They are called "vital" signs because they measure vital functions and thereby provide a quick assessment of the integrity of the cardiovascular, respiratory, and central nervous systems. And in the secondary survey, just as in the primary survey, it is those systems that receive highest priority. It is also worth noting that being *vital* signs (i.e., characteristic of life), they are *dynamic*; they *change over time*. The implication is clear:

MEASURE THE VITAL SIGNS FREQUENTLY.

Pulse

Assessing the pulse gives us our first rapid check on the patient's *cardiovascular status*. The pulse is best palpated over the radial or carotid artery, using the tips of your index and middle fingers (*not* your thumb). Feeling the pulse gives us information about the rate, strength, and regularity of the heart beat.

First measure the pulse RATE by counting the number of beats during 15 seconds and then multiplying that number by 4 to get beats per minute (if the pulse is irregular or very slow, however, count it for a full minute). The normal pulse rate for an adult at rest is **60 to 80 per minute,** but in a well-trained athlete the resting pulse may be in the range of 50 per minute without implying any abnormality.

As you are counting the pulse rate, make a note of the FORCE of the pulse beat. A normal pulse feels "full," as if a strong wave had passed beneath the fingertips. When there is severe vasoconstriction, the pulse will often feel weak, or "*thready*," while a heart beat that is more forceful than usual will produce a strong, "*bounding*" pulse.

Finally, note the RHYTHM of the pulse beat. A normal rhythm is regular, like the ticking of a clock. If some beats seem to come early or late, the rhythm is regarded as irregular.

Report your findings by describing the rate, force, and rhythm of the pulse, for example, "The patient's pulse was 72, full, and regular," or "The pulse was 120, thready, and regular."

Respirations

Assessment of *respiratory status* begins with the measurement of the respiratory RATE. Without taking your fingers from the patient's radial pulse (why not?), shift your gaze to his chest and count the number of breaths he takes in 30 seconds; multiply by 2 to get the respiratory rate per minute. (If you let the patient's wrist rest on his upper abdomen, as the rescuer in Figure 12-2 is doing, you will be able to feel as well as see the rise and fall of the chest.) The normal respiratory rate in an adult is about **16 per minute** (the normal range is about 12–20).

While you are counting the respirations, make a note of the respiratory RHYTHM. Normal breathing is fairly regular, but certain illnesses and injuries may produce irregular or otherwise abnormal breathing patterns. Two such abnormal patterns that are common in disturbances of the central nervous system are Cheyne-Stokes respiration and central neurogenic hyperventilation.

Cheyne-Stokes respiration may arise from a variety of neurologic or metabolic derangements, many of which are reversible. In the Cheyne-Stokes pattern (Fig. 12-3), periods of rapid, irregular breaths—starting shallow, becoming deeper, then becoming shallower—alternate with periods of nonbreathing (apnea); the cycle repeats every 30 to 120 seconds, with 5- to 30-second periods of apnea.

FIGURE 12-2.   COUNTING THE RESPIRATIONS. Without taking your hand from the radial pulse, shift your gaze to the patient's chest.

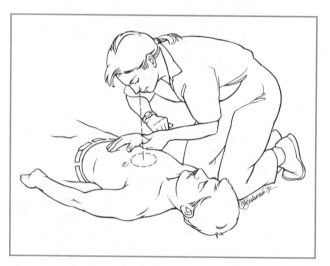

Central neurogenic hyperventilation (Fig. 12-4) often predicts a grave outcome. It is characterized by very deep, rapid respirations (*hyperpnea* and *tachypnea*). The breathing of a diabetic patient in ketoacidosis may also be characterized by hyperpnea and tachypnea and is referred to as **Kussmaul's respiration.**

Note the EASE of respirations. In a healthy person, breathing is relatively effortless, while a person with respiratory problems may have labored or gasping respirations. Be alert for SIGNS OF RESPIRATORY DISTRESS:

SIGNS OF RESPIRATORY DISTRESS

- Flaring of the nostrils on inhalation
- "Tugging" of the trachea
- Use of accessory muscle in the neck and abdomen to assist breathing
- Retraction of the intercostal and suprasternal spaces during inhalation
- Tachypnea
- Anxiety

Evaluate the DEPTH of respiration (the tidal volume). A person with a broken rib may breathe shallowly to minimize the pain that motion of the chest wall causes him. Shallow respirations also characterize patients with cervical spine injuries or those who have overdosed on narcotic drugs, while unusually deep respirations may signal acidosis or injury to the brain.

Listen for ABNORMAL RESPIRATORY NOISES. A healthy person breathes quietly at rest, and his breathing is scarcely audible at all. **Snoring** indicates partial obstruction of the upper airway by the tongue, which can usually be corrected by head tilt. **Gurgling** respirations betoken *fluid* in the upper airway, while **stridor**—a high-pitched, squeaking noise on inhalation—indicates *narrowing* of the upper airway, usually as a result of swelling (laryngeal edema). Stridor is a particularly ominous sound, for it may signal imminent closure of the airway altogether.

Finally, note any ABNORMAL ODORS ON THE BREATH, such as the smell of alcohol. A diabetic in ketoacidosis will often have a fruity odor to his breath. Certain poisons, such as cyanide, also produce a characteristic breath odor.

When reporting on the patient's respirations, in-

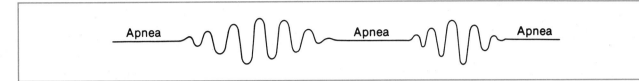

FIGURE 12-3. CHEYNE-STOKES RESPIRATION.

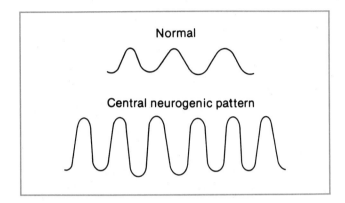

FIGURE 12-4. CENTRAL NEUROGENIC HYPERVENTILATION.

clude all of the observations mentioned above, for example: "The patient's respirations were regular, deep, gurgling, and slightly labored at 30 per minute, with a fruity odor to her breath."

Blood Pressure

The blood pressure is the pressure that circulating blood exerts against the walls of arteries, and it gives us yet another assessment of the patient's cardiovascular status. To measure the blood pressure, wrap the sphygmomanometer snugly around the patient's arm above the elbow. Locate the brachial pulse (Fig. 12-5A), and place the diaphragm of your stethoscope over it (Fig. 12-5B) as you inflate the cuff until the needle on the pressure gauge stops bouncing with each beat—usually somewhere between 150 and 200 mm Hg. Then *slowly* release the pressure in the cuff and note the point at which you first hear the Korotkoff sounds (the **systolic pressure**) and the point where those sounds become muffled or disappear altogether (**diastolic pressure**).

Often field conditions do not permit one to hear the Korotkoff sounds at all. If that is the case, there are two other methods of assessing at least the *systolic* pressure. The more accurate of the two is to palpate the patient's radial artery as you inflate the sphygmomanometer cuff (Fig. 12-5C). Keep inflating the cuff about 20 mm Hg beyond the point where you can

no longer feel a radial pulse. Then slowly release the pressure from the cuff, noting at what pressure the radial pulse becomes palpable—that is approximately the systolic pressure. A less accurate method of estimating the systolic pressure is simply to inflate the cuff to a pressure that you think is higher than the patient's systolic pressure and then to *watch the needle on the pressure gauge* as you slowly let the air out of the cuff. The needle should move smoothly until it reaches the systolic pressure, at which point it usually starts to "jump" with each pulse beat.

Normal blood pressure varies with age and sex. In a healthy adult man, the normal *systolic* pressure is between about 120 and 150 mm Hg, and the normal *diastolic* pressure is between 65 and 90 mm Hg. The corresponding figures for an adult woman of the same age are about 8 mm Hg lower. (One can get a rough idea of the normal systolic pressure for any given age group by adding 100 to the patient's age, up to a total of 150.)

Temperature

Measurement of the patient's temperature is classically a part of taking the vital signs. In the field, however, it will ordinarily be sufficient simply to estimate the patient's temperature by placing a hand on his forehead, as described earlier. The temperature *should* be measured accurately, though, when it is relevant to the patient's chief complaint (e.g., heat stroke, high fever, cold exposure), and ambulance services operating in areas where cold exposure is a possibility should be equipped with special low-reading thermometers.

VITAL SIGNS: SUMMARY

- PULSE
  1. Assess rate, force, and rhythm
  2. Normal value at rest: 60 to 80 per minute*
- RESPIRATIONS
  1. Assess rate, rhythm, ease, depth, abnormal noises, abnormal odors

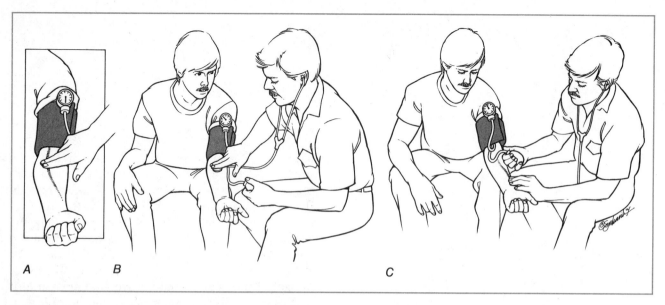

A   B   C

FIGURE 12-5. MEASURING THE BLOOD PRESSURE. (A) Locate the brachial artery. (B) Listen with the diaphragm of your stethoscope over the brachial artery as you deflate the cuff. (C) When conditions do not permit you to hear Korotkoff sounds, palpate for the return of the radial pulse.

2. Normal value at rest: 12 to 20 per minute*
- BLOOD PRESSURE: normally 120/65 to 150/90*
- TEMPERATURE: normally 98.6°F (37°C)

*In adults (for normal vital signs in children, see Chapter 30)

HEAD-TO-TOE SURVEY

In the remainder of the secondary survey, we employ several techniques of examination that are already familiar from basic life support, for they derive from the three methods of observation used in cardiopulmonary resuscitation (CPR): Look, listen, and feel. In the secondary survey, we give each of those methods a special name.

- **Inspection** means LOOKING at an area of the body. To inspect something, it must be visible; so *expose* the area to be examined. Use the best light available. Look for colors, contours, symmetry.
- **Auscultation** is LISTENING for sounds, and it is aided by the use of a stethoscope. The flat diaphragm of the stethoscope applied firmly to the skin best detects sounds of high frequency, like those of the lungs. The bell of the stethoscope conducts low-frequency sounds, like certain heart sounds. However, if the bell is applied too firmly, the skin beneath it may be stretched

and act as a diaphragm; the bell will then pick up only high-frequency sounds.
- **Palpation** is FEELING with the hands. The fingertips are best suited for detecting textures and consistency, while the back of the hand, as noted, is best suited for noting temperature.

In medicine, we use one additional technique of examination, besides the three we learned as part of basic life support:

- **Percussion** is the act of striking a part of the body with short, sharp blows to produce a sound. In the usual method of percussion, the middle finger of one hand is placed against the patient's body wall and is struck a quick blow with the end of the bent middle finger of the other hand. The sound produced, or the *percussion note*, gives information about the consistency of the underlying tissue. Percussion may be very difficult in the field, since it is rarely quiet enough under field conditions to appreciate the quality of the percussion note. Nonetheless, percussion can be a valuable technique in assessing, for example, the patient with a possible hemothorax or pneumothorax. If one side of the chest is filled with air (pneumothorax), the affected side will have a more hollow, or resonant percussion note than the uninjured side; if, on the other hand, one side of the chest is filled with blood (hemothorax), the percussion note over that side will be dull with respect to the normal side.

In describing the head-to-toe survey, we shall proceed first through the survey of an injured patient, then repeat the survey for a patient with a medical problem. The *sequence* in which the survey is carried out will be the same in both instances, but there are significant differences in emphasis.

The Injured Patient

Examining the victim of trauma immediately involves a constraint that is not operative when examining a medical patient:

> **THE VICTIM OF TRAUMA SHOULD NOT BE MOVED UNLESS INJURY TO THE SPINAL CORD HAS BEEN DEFINITIVELY RULED OUT.**

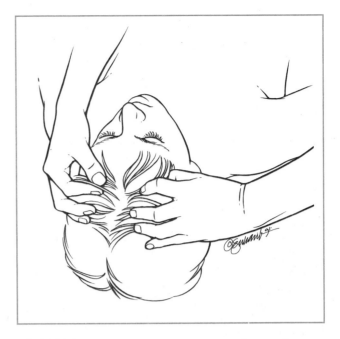

FIGURE 12-6. CHECKING THE SCALP. Inspect for blood; palpate for bumps or depressions.

A little common sense is required in applying that dictum. Clearly a person who simply twisted his ankle, while technically a victim of trauma, is unlikely to have suffered significant spinal cord injury. But in any patient who has suffered massive trauma, especially involving the head, one must assume the possibility of spinal cord injury and avoid any unnecessary movement of the patient.

Examination of the Head

Don gloves, and inspect the *scalp* for lacerations or contusions (Fig. 12-6). Is there blood in the hair? Where is it coming from? Check the back of the head in the supine patient by gently sliding a hand beneath it and feeling for blood. Palpate the *skull* for tenderness or depressions indicative of fracture.

Inspect the *ears*. Pay particular attention to the area just behind the ear, over the mastoid bone. Bluish discoloration (**ecchymosis**) over the mastoid bone is called **Battle's sign** and signals probable basilar skull fracture. Inspect the ears themselves and the nose for discharge of clear fluid or blood. Blood draining from the ears may be a sign of skull fracture; clear fluid from the nose or ears may be cerebrospinal fluid, again an indication of probable skull fracture. (If fluid *is* draining from the ears or nose, do *not* attempt to dam up the leak.)

Inspect the *eyes*. Is there trauma or swelling above the orbits? Ecchymoses around the eyes ("**coon's eyes**") without evidence of direct injury are a clue to skull fracture. Look at the *pupils*. Are they equal in size? Do they react to light? Briskly or sluggishly? Pupils are normally round, equal, and briskly reactive to light. Unequal pupils (**anisocoria**) are normal in about 2 to 4 percent of the population, but in the context of head trauma they suggest the presence of cerebral edema. (Cataract surgery on one eye may also cause inequality of pupil size; the pupil of the operated eye will be unreactive.)

Observe the *motions of the eyes*. Normally, the eyes gaze straight ahead unless focused on something. When the eyes move, they move together (conjugately). In head injury or direct trauma to the eyes, the gaze may be abnormal; that is, the eyes may turn in different directions or may not move in unison. That is known as **dysconjugate gaze.** If the patient is conscious, have him follow your finger with his eyes 90 degrees up, down, left, and right, and note whether gaze is paralyzed in any direction. Patients with fractures of the orbit may show *paralysis of upward gaze.*

Inspect the *face* for symmetry, and palpate the facial bones—including the zygomata (cheek bones) and maxilla (upper jaw) for instability or tenderness.

Inspect the *mouth* for blood, loose teeth, or foreign materials, such as broken dentures, that might be aspirated if not promptly removed. Observe the *lips* for cyanosis. Palpate the mandible (lower jaw) for stability.

Examination of the Neck

Expose the neck completely to examine it (i.e., unbutton the collar, remove any scarf, and so forth). Inspect the neck for obvious bruises, for open wounds (which must be covered immediately), and for the presence of a stoma. Observe the neck during respirations for retraction of the suprasternal muscles, a sign of respiratory distress.

Inspect and palpate the *trachea* to determine whether it is in the midline and whether it shifts in one direction or the other during the respiratory cycle. Deviation of the trachea suggests the presence of a pneumothorax or obstruction of a bronchus. If the patient is sitting or semisitting (i.e., at 45 degrees), note whether the *jugular veins* are distended, which may signal the presence of blood in the pericardium or a condition that has raised the intrathoracic pressure (such as tension pneumothorax).

Slide your hand gently behind the patient's neck to palpate for deformity, blood, or tenderness. Once you have completed this part of the examination, stabilize the patient's head and neck with sandbags or some other quick, temporary measure before you proceed further.

Examination of the Chest

Expose the chest (open the patient's shirt entirely), and observe the motions of the chest as the patient breathes. Does the chest move symmetrically? Does part of the chest bulge outward with exhalation and retract with inhalation ("flail" chest)? Are there any bruises of the chest wall? Are there open wounds of the chest wall? If so, put your ear close to the wound and listen: Can you hear air being sucked into the chest through the wound? (Open chest wounds should be closed immediately with a one-way-valve dressing—see Chap. 17.)

Palpate the chest wall for tenderness and instability over the ribs. Compress the rib cage as another check for tenderness. Palpate also for air crackling beneath the skin (**subcutaneous emphysema**), which is often associated with pneumothorax.

Auscultate the chest to determine the equality of breath sounds in the two lungs and the presence of abnormal sounds. Listen first to be certain breath sounds are *present* at all and are *equal on both sides* of the chest. To do so, compare symmetric areas on opposite sides of the chest (Fig. 12-7), listening to each spot first on one side, then the other. The absence of breath sounds on one side may signal a pneumothorax, hemothorax, or—in the intubated patient—passage of the endotracheal tube down the main bronchus of the other lung. Also listen over the left side of the chest for *heart sounds*, which should be

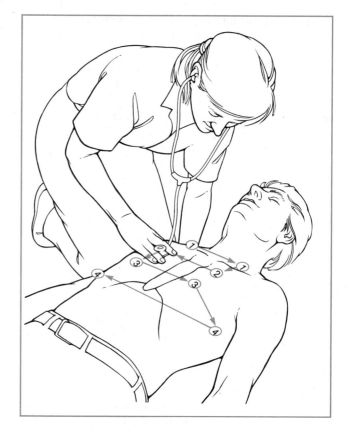

FIGURE 12-7.   AUSCULTATION OF THE CHEST.   Listen over comparable areas, right and left.

clear and regular. Muffling of the heart sounds suggests that blood has accumulated in the sac surrounding the heart (the pericardium); an irregular heart beat may be a sign that the heart was bruised (myocardial contusion) in an impact injury, such as steering wheel trauma.

If there is reason to suspect a pneumothorax or hemothorax, *percuss* symmetric areas on both sides of the chest and compare the percussion notes: Does one side sound more hollow than the other?

Examination of the Abdomen

Expose the abdomen to examine it, but keep the patient warm, lest he tense his abdominal muscles from shivering. Always examine the abdomen with the patient supine. First, *inspect*. Look for *distention*. If the abdomen is distended, it is very likely to be filled with blood, so you had better anticipate shock. Are there localized *ecchymoses* over the flank or around the navel, suggestive of internal hemorrhage? Are any abdominal organs protruding through an open wound (**evisceration**)? Note also whether the abdominal muscles are being used to assist respirations.

Next, *listen* with the diaphragm of the stethoscope to determine whether *bowel sounds* are present. In a healthy person, one can usually hear at least a gurgle or two from the gut by listening for about 30 seconds. If there has been significant trauma to the abdomen, however, the intestines may go into a sort of paralysis, and bowel sounds may cease altogether. Adequate examination for bowel sounds requires listening for a full minute under quiet conditions with the diaphragm of the stethoscope resting lightly on the abdomen—something that may not be feasible in the field. If the patient is seriously injured, do not take time in the field to try to hear bowel sounds.

Palpate the abdomen GENTLY. Avoid sudden pokes and cold hands. Use the pads of your fingers, and hold your hand almost parallel to the patient's abdomen. If there is reason to suspect injury or pain in any area of the abdomen, palpate that area last. In trauma, the most important thing to note is the consistency of the abdomen: Is it soft? Is there muscular guarding? Is it rigid? A truly rigid abdomen feels wooden or boardlike, and it generally indicates serious internal injury.

Examination of the Back

Without moving the patient, slide your hands beneath the small of the patient's back and palpate for deformity or tenderness. Withdraw you hands, and inspect them for blood.

Examination of the Pelvis

Place your hands over the two iliac crests (the wide bones of the patient's hips) and compress them firmly together to test for tenderness and instabililty of the pelvis. If compressing the pelvis causes pain, suspect a pelvic fracture.

Examination of the Genitals

If there is blood on the patient's clothing suggestive of injury to the genital region, you must expose the area and examine it. The patient should be properly shielded from the gaze of bystanders, and if at all possible, a female patient should be examined by a female paramedic. Note the source of bleeding and any other wounds or bruises. In the male, check for **priapism** (sustained erection of the penis), which is a sign of spinal cord injury.

Examination of the Extremities

Start with the lower extremities, since you're already positioned beside them when you complete your examination of the pelvis. It may be necessary to cut away a trouser leg or a sleeve to get a clear look at an extremity (do not try to *pull* clothes off, as that may jar an injured limb); use your heavy-duty scissors to cut along the seam of the pant leg or shirt sleeve.

Inspect the extremity for bruises, bleeding, swelling, or deformity, and make a note of any *abnormal position*, which suggests fracture or dislocation. In evaluating an injured extremity, compare it to the uninjured one.

Whenever there is injury to an extremity, EVALUATE THE PULSE DISTAL TO THE INJURY. In the upper extremities, that means checking the radial pulse (Fig. 12-8A). In the lower extremities, it means checking either the dorsalis pedis pulse (Fig. 12-8B), the posterior tibial pulse (Fig. 12-8C), or both. When you have difficulty feeling a pulse, note the relative warmth of the extremity compared to its opposite number and check for capillary refill, as described in a previous chapter.

Neurologic function in an injured extremity should also be assessed, by TESTING SENSATION AND STRENGTH DISTAL TO THE INJURY. To test *sensation*, touch the patient's toes or fingers lightly and ask him to report when he feels the touch. If sensation is absent in the toes, keep moving up the legs until you reach the point where the patient *is* able to feel your touch, and make a record of where that point is. To test *motor function*, first ask the patient simply to wiggle his fingers and toes. Test strength in the upper extremity by asking the patient to grasp two or three of your fingers in each of his hands and to squeeze as hard as he can (Fig. 12-9A). Assess the strength in his lower limbs by asking him to push down with his feet against your hand (Fig. 12-9B). If the patient is unconscious, test for movement by applying a painful stimulus (e.g., pinprick) to the sole of each foot and the palm of each hand and noting whether the patient withdraws each extremity in response to pain. Paralysis of the lower extremities is referred to as **paraplegia;** paralysis involving all four extremities is called **quadriplegia.**

Whether checking pulses, warmth, sensation, or strength, ALWAYS COMPARE THE INJURED EXTREMITY TO THE UNINJURED EXTREMITY.

In an unconscious patient, one can obtain further information about the integrity of his spinal cord by testing *deep tendon reflexes*. In the field, it is sufficient to test the *biceps* tendon (Fig. 12-10A), which assesses spinal level C5–C6, and the *patellar* tendon (Fig. 12-10B), which assesses spinal level L2–L4.

Finally, in examining the extremities, don't forget to look for a *medical identification bracelet* or anklet, which may give important information about the patient's medical background.

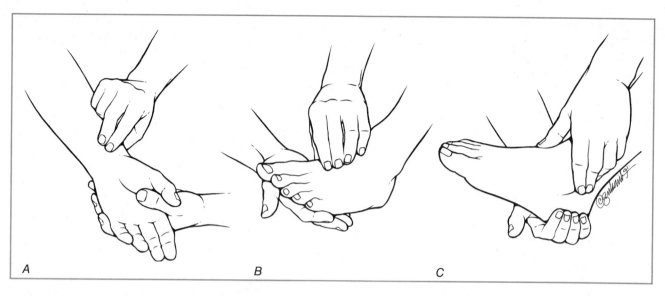

FIGURE 12-8.   CHECKING THE DISTAL PULSES.   (A) The radial pulse. (B) The dorsalis pedis pulse. (C) The posterior tibial pulse.

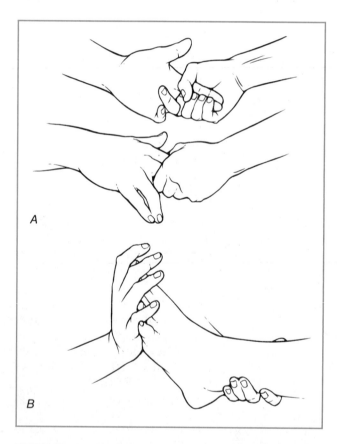

FIGURE 12-9.   TESTING DISTAL MUSCLE STRENGTH. (A) To test upper extremity strength, ask the patient to squeeze the fingers of each of your hands. (B) To test lower extremity strength, have the patient push down with his foot against resistance from your hand.

The Patient with a Medical Problem

As noted earlier, the sequence in which we conduct the assessment of a medical patient is the same as that for a victim of trauma, but of necessity, we are looking for different signs. Thus, while we do not ordinarily have to search the medical patient for bruises and lacerations, we do have to check for the stigmata of various physiologic processes gone awry.

Examination of the Head

First, examine the patient's *face* for asymmetry, which may be the first clue to a stroke. Does one side of the mouth seem to droop? Does one side of the face look somehow flatter than the other? Inspect the *eyes*. First note the color of the **sclerae** (the whites of the eyes). Yellow discoloration (**icterus**) may signal disease of the liver or gallbladder. Examine the *pupils* (Table 12-3) to determine whether they are equal in size and reactive to light. As noted, pupils are normally round, equal, and briskly reactive to light—both directly (i.e., when you shine a light straight at the eye) and consensually (i.e., when you shine a light at the *other* eye). Pupils may become *constricted* because of bright light, central nervous system disease, some narcotics (including propoxyphene [Darvon]), or stimulation of the parasympathetic nervous system. The pupils *dilate* with fright, pain, hypoxemia, brain injury, and certain drugs (e.g., atropine). Unequal pupils in a medical patient may signal a stroke, but may also be due to cataract surgery or normal variation.

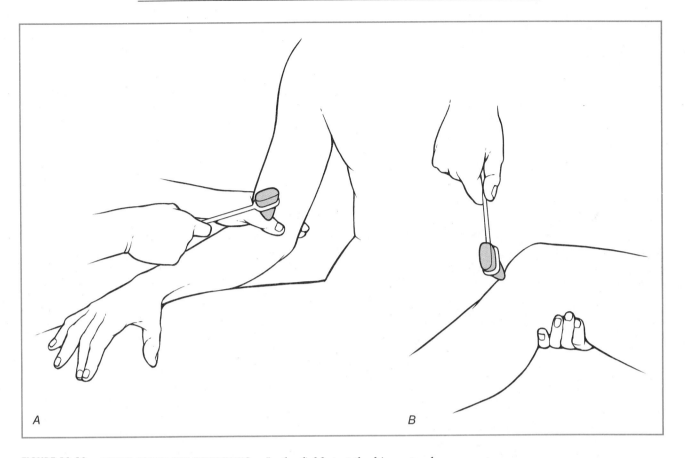

A

B

FIGURE 12-10. DEEP TENDON REFLEXES. In the field, test the biceps tendon reflex (A) and the patellar tendon reflex (B).

TABLE 12-3. EXAMINATION OF THE PUPILS

PUPILLARY SIGN	POSSIBLE CAUSES
Dilated	Fright
	Brain ischemia
	Drugs (atropine)
Constricted ("pinpoint")	Narcotics overdose
	Disorders affecting the CNS
	Bright light
Unequal	May be normal (2–4% of the population)
	Head injury, stroke
	Cataract surgery on one side

If there is any reason to suspect a stroke, check the patient's *extraocular motions* as described earlier—by having the patient follow your finger with his gaze as you move your finger 90 degrees up, down, left, and right. In some cases of stroke, the gaze will be paralyzed to the right or left. If the patient is unconscious, check for the **doll's eyes** phenomenon: When the head of an unconscious person is turned rapidly to one side, the eyes move together toward the opposite side. If there is significant damage to the brain, however, the doll's eyes phenomenon may be lost, and the eyes will then move in the same direction that the head is turned.

Examine the **conjunctivae** (the pink membrane of the eyes) for pallor or cyanosis, and inspect the lips for cyanosis as well.

Examination of the Neck

In taking the vital signs, we measured the pressure in the arterial system (the "blood pressure"). It is also useful, especially in patients with cardiac problems, to get an estimate of the pressure within the *venous* system, for that tells us how efficiently the heart is pumping blood out of the right ventricle. The height of the blood in the *jugular veins* of the neck is an indirect measure of the pressure in the right side of the heart. To get an impression of the venous pressure, place the patient in a semisitting position at a 45-degree angle (if his condition permits). Shine a light along the neck at an angle so that the jugular vein stands out in relief. Describe the venous pressure by determining the distance from the sternal angle to the top of the jugular column; for example, "The jugular veins are distended 10 cm (4 inches) above the sternal angle with the patient at 45 degrees." Marked distention of the jugular veins usually indicates elevated pressure in the right side of the heart, as in right heart failure or pericardial tamponade (blood in the pericardium).

Examination of the Chest

Inspect the chest to determine its shape and symmetry. Is the chest barrel-shaped, suggesting chronic obstructive pulmonary disease? Is the spine abnormally curved? Those deformities point to possible respiratory difficulties.

Observe the *respiratory cycle.* Normally, inhalation is active while exhalation is passive. In diseases such as emphysema, the lungs are overinflated, and the patient must use accessory muscles in the neck and abdomen to assist in exhalation. Exhalation also becomes active when airway obstruction is present, and the patient uses his abdominal muscles to force the diaphragm upward.

Look for *signs of respiratory distress,* as described on page 264. Listening to the patient speak can also provide a rough gauge of respiratory function, for a patient with severe dyspnea from any cause will usually speak only in short phrases, pausing after every few words to catch his breath.

Listen to the chest, front and back, with your stethoscope—always comparing a spot on the left to a comparable spot on the right—for the presence of *abnormal breath sounds.* When listening for abnormal sounds, recall that fluid transmits sound better than air does. In most of the older medical literature, abnormal lung sounds are referred to as

- **Rales,** fine, crackling sounds that were once thought to indicate the presence of fluid in the alveoli because they are often associated with conditions that produce fluid-filled alveoli. In pulmonary edema, for example, rales may be so loud that they can be heard without a stethoscope. In fact, however, rales are probably caused by the popping open of air spaces. You can get an idea of what rales sound like by rolling a few strands of hair between your fingers right next to your ear.
- **Rhonchi,** harsher sounds than rales that were thought to be produced by collections of fluid in the larger airways or a solid, partially obstructing object in the bronchus.
- **Wheezes,** high-pitched, whistling sounds made by air flowing through narrowed airways. Diffuse wheezing on exhalation is prominent in

asthma and may be heard in left heart failure or pulmonary embolism as well. Wheezes localized to one section of the chest suggest obstruction of a smaller bronchus.

During the past 10 to 15 years, physiologists have urged that the terms "rales" and "rhonchi" be abandoned, since they are not physiologically accurate. The tendency now is to refer to all gurgles, rasps, crunches, and other *discontinuous* noises in the lungs as **crackles** and to call any *continuous,* whistling noises **wheezes.** But one still encounters mention of rales and rhonchi among physicians, so it is worthwhile to know what the terms refer to.

Note whether the patient is *coughing.* Cough is a response to bronchial irritation. Simple chemical irritation from aspirated material or smoke may cause cough. A nonproductive cough suggests either that the cause is irritation only or that the cough is ineffective in clearing the airways. If the cough produces *sputum,* note the color, consistency, amount, and odor. Mucus is white or clear. A **purulent** (infected) sputum is usually yellow or green. Coughing up blood (**hemoptysis**) may be indicative of cardiac or pulmonary disease.

Auscultate over the *heart* to determine the *apical heart rate* (the heart rate heard over the lower tip of the heart), and note any discrepancy between the apical rate and the pulse rate you measured at the wrist. Listen also for the presence of an *irregular rhythm;* any patient whose rhythm is irregular should be monitored, regardless of his chief complaint.

Of the many extra sounds that can occur in normal or diseased hearts, the *third heart sound* (S_3) is probably the most significant for prehospital care, but it may be very difficult to hear if the surroundings are not quiet. In adults, the presence of the S_3 usually indicates congestive heart failure. Listen for this sound with the bell of the stethoscope pressed lightly over the apex of the heart; if present, the S_3 will be heard as a soft, extra sound immediately following the "dubb" of the normal "lub-dubb" sequence. The rhythm of the S_3 can be mimicked by repeating the word *Kentucky* rapidly.

Examination of the Abdomen

Examine the abdomen of a medical patient if his chief complaint relates to that part of the body (e.g., vomiting, abdominal pain). The patient should be lying supine for this part of the examination, preferably with his legs flexed at the hips and knees, to loosen the abdominal muscles. First, expose the abdomen and inspect it for *distention.* Then place your stethoscope lightly on the abdomen and listen for a full minute for *bowel sounds*. Normal bowel sounds are low-pitched, gurgling noises that occur only once or twice in a minute. When there is a bowel obstruction, bowel sounds initially become much more frequent and high pitched as peristalsis increases in an attempt to overcome the obstruction. Late in bowel obstruction, or in peritonitis from any cause, bowel sounds may disappear altogether.

Palpate the abdomen gently with the pads of your fingers. Check for the presence of abnormal masses or pulsations. A vigorously pulsating mass in the abdomen may be an aortic aneurysm and requires rapid, deliberate transport to the hospital. The patient who has tenderness in the abdomen may guard the painful area by tightening the abdominal muscles. Distracting the patient can overcome voluntary guarding but will not affect true rigidity.

The attempt to elicit what is called *rebound tenderness* is mentioned here only to be condemned. Rebound tenderness is elicited by putting firm pressure on the patient's abdomen with one hand and then suddenly releasing that pressure. In the patient with peritoneal irritation, that maneuver will evoke severe pain, and it is cruel and unnecessary. You will obtain the same information sooner or later when the stretcher is inadvertently jolted or the ambulance goes over a bump, for the patient with peritoneal inflammation will usually cry out in pain from any unexpected movement.

Examination of the Back and Extremities

Check the patient's back and lower extremities for **edema** (swelling), indicative of fluid retention. Press

TABLE 12-4. PRIORITIES OF ASSESSMENT IN INJURY AND ILLNESS

THE INJURED PATIENT	THE PATIENT WITH AN ILLNESS
PRIMARY SURVEY:	PRIMARY SURVEY:
GENERAL APPEARANCE	GENERAL APPEARANCE
Position	Position
Level of consciousness	Level of consciousness
Degree of distress	Degree of distress
Obvious wounds/deformities	
Skin condition	Skin condition
VITAL SIGNS:	VITAL SIGNS:
HEAD-TO-TOE SURVEY	HEAD-TO-TOE SURVEY
Scalp: Bleeding, deformity	
Ears: Blood, fluid	
Nose: Deformity, discharge	Face: Asymmetry
Eyes: Injury, pupils, eye movements, conjunctivae	Eyes: Jaundice, pupils, conjunctivae
Mouth: Foreign material, blood, vomitus, cyanosis of the lips	Mouth: Cyanosis of the lips
Neck: Tracheal deviation, tenderness, deformity, jugular distention	Neck: Jugular distention
Chest: Bruises, asymmetry, unequal breath sounds	Chest: Abnormal shape, abnormal breath sounds (crackles, wheezes)
Heart: Muffled heart beat; rate and regularity	Heart: Rate and regularity
Abdomen: Distention, masses, ecchymoses, presence of bowel sounds	Abdomen: Distention, bowel sounds, tenderness, rigidity
Pelvis: Stability, tenderness	
Genitalia: Bruises, wounds	
Back: Bruises, wounds, spinal tenderness	Back: Edema
Extremities: Deformity, bruises, pulses, movement, sensation, capillary refill	Extremities: Edema, equality of pulses, strength and sensation

gently but firmly over the anterior tibia (shin bone); if your pressure leaves an indentation, *pitting* edema is present.

Check for the equality of *peripheral pulses*. The acute absence of a pulse in one extremity, together with sharp, sudden, severe pain in the limb, may indicate occlusion of the artery in that extremity. Numbness, weakness, and tingling follow the pain, and the skin gradually turns mottled, blue, and cold.

Test each extremity for *movement, strength,* and *sensation*. Weakness on one side of the body (**hemiparesis**) or paralysis on one side of the body (**hemiplegia**) suggests the patient may have suffered a stroke.

In the unconscious patient, examine the arms for *needle tracks* along the veins that may give evidence of drug abuse. Check as well for needle marks over the anterior thighs that indicate a diabetic insulin user. And, once again, don't forget to look for a medical identification bracelet or anklet.

PUTTING IT ALL TOGETHER

Circumstances will inevitably dictate which aspects of the physical examination are most relevant and merit most emphasis in any given case. The priorities in the physical examination will, as we have noted, be influenced primarily by whether the patient is suffering from a medical problem or is the victim of trauma. The emphasis will also be affected by the patient's chief complaint; the patient who complains of shortness of breath, for example, will merit more attention to his chest than the patient complaining of severe pain in the left elbow. The differences between the approach to a victim of trauma and the approach to a medical patient are summarized in Table 12-4. Please note, however, that in EVERY patient, THE PRIMARY SURVEY COMES FIRST.

One further word. We have covered considerable ground in this chapter and have made reference to a great many physical signs. DON'T PANIC! We shall return again and again to those signs as we learn about specific injuries and illnesses. Indeed, we shall review the entire physical assessment of the trauma victim, from start to finish, when we conclude Part IV of this text and know more about specific injuries.

Finally, a reminder. All patients have some feelings about being examined. Undressing in front of another person is ordinarily something one does in situations of intimacy and trust. Indeed, in our language, *naked* is often used as a synonym for *defenseless*. Thus every person will feel some anxiety about being examined by a stranger, and some may even regard the physical examination as a humiliating in-

vasion of privacy. Whenever circumstances permit, take the history *before* you examine the patient, to establish some relationship with the patient before examining his or her body. Furthermore, the fully clothed paramedic should always be aware of the unclothed patient's feelings of embarrassment and see to it that the patient is properly draped and shielded from the stares of bystanders. Conduct the examination in an efficient, businesslike manner, and maintain your conversation with the patient as you do so.

GLOSSARY

anisocoria   Inequality of the size of the pupils.

apical pulse   Pulse obtained by auscultating over the apex of the heart (normally at the level of the fifth intercostal space in the left midclavicular line).

auscultation   The technique of listening for (with a stethoscope) and interpreting sounds that occur within the body.

Battle's sign   Bluish discoloration over the tip of the mastoid bone behind the ear, signifying basilar skull fracture.

central neurogenic hyperventilation   An abnormal breathing pattern seen in severe illness and injury involving the brain, characterized by marked tachypnea and hyperpnea.

Cheyne-Stokes respiration   An abnormal breathing pattern characterized by rhythmic waxing and waning of the depth of respiration, with regularly occurring periods of apnea.

conjunctiva   The delicate membrane that lines the eyelids and covers exposed surfaces of the eyeball; normally pink, it may be pale in anemia or bright red in infection (conjunctivitis).

consensual reaction   A similar reaction of both pupils (e.g., constriction) to a stimulus applied to only one of them (e.g., bright light).

coon's eyes   Also called "raccoon sign"; bilateral, symmetric, periorbital ecchymoses seen with some skull fractures.

crackles   Any discontinuous adventitious sounds in the lungs, caused by the popping open of air spaces.

dysconjugate gaze   A gaze in which the two eyes are not aligned but rather stare in different directions.

ecchymosis   "Black-and-blue mark" caused by extravasation of blood under the skin.

edema   The condition in which excess fluid accumulates in body tissues, which may be manifested as crackles in the lung or swelling in the peripheral tissues.

evisceration Disembowelment; protrusion of abdominal organs through an open abdominal wound.

hemiparesis Weakness on one side of the body.

hemiplegia Paralysis on one side of the body.

hemoptysis Coughing up blood from the lungs.

icterus The yellow appearance of the *sclerae* and other tissues caused by an accumulation of bile pigments; jaundice.

inspection The first part of the examination of any part of the body, involving a careful visual examination.

Kussmaul breathing Respiratory pattern characteristic of the diabetic in ketoacidosis, with marked hyperpnea and tachypnea.

mastoid A large, spongy bone behind the ear.

pallor Paleness of the skin.

palpation Feeling a part of the patient's body with the hand to assess the consistency of the parts beneath.

paraplegia The loss of both motion and sensation in the legs and lower part of the body, most commonly caused by damage to the spinal cord.

percussion Striking a part of the patient's body with short, sharp blows to produce a sound that will indicate the condition of the structures within.

pericardial tamponade Accumulation in the pericardial sac of blood or excess fluid that interferes with cardiac function.

priapism Sustained erection of the penis, which may be a sign of spinal cord injury.

purulent Full of pus.

quadriplegia Paralysis of all four extremities.

rales Fine, crackling sounds once thought to indicate the presence of fluid in the alveoli.

rhonchi Rattling or gurgling breath sounds.

sclera Tough white covering of the eyeball.

snoring Noise made on inhalation when the upper airway is partially obstructed by the tongue.

sphygmomanometer Device for measuring blood pressure.

stridor Harsh, high-pitched respiratory noise associated with severe upper airway obstruction, such as that caused by laryngeal edema.

subcutaneous emphysema Condition in which trauma to the lung or airway results in the escape of air into tissues of the body, especially the chest wall, neck, and face, causing a crackling sensation on palpation of the skin.

wheezes High-pitched, whistling sounds made by air flowing through narrowed airways.

FURTHER READING

Bull G. Strip and flip. *Emerg Med Serv* 14(6):13, 1985.

Caroline NL. *Emergency Medical Treatment: A Text for EMT-As and EMT-Intermediates* (3rd ed.). Boston: Little, Brown, 1991. Chap. 11.

DeGowin EL. *Bedside Diagnostic Examination.* New York: Macmillan, 1973.

Donelan S. Patient assessment: Training rescuers to find the problems. *Rescue* 3(3):28, 1990.

Kennedy WC. Vital signs: Reading the essentials. *JEMS* 15(5):26, 1990.

McConnell WE. Orderly assessment. *Emergency* 22(10):34, 1990.

Murphy PM. Minding your P's and Q's with the ABCs. *JEMS* 18(5):67, 1993.

O'Carroll BM. Taking blood pressure: A critical measure of health. *Rescue* 2(6):45, 1989.

Schriger DL, Baraff L. Defining normal capillary refill: Variation with age, sex, and temperature. *Ann Emerg Med* 17:932, 1988.

Shanaberger CJ. Thorough assessments: Giving patients a fighting chance. *JEMS* 15(9):81, 1990.

13
Medical Reporting and Record Keeping

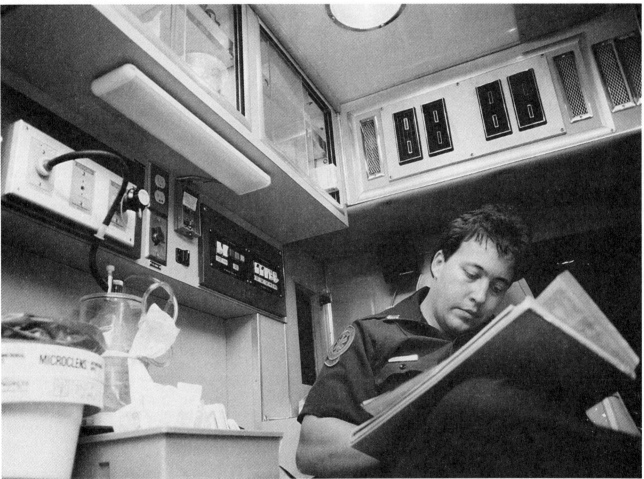

Baton Rouge Parrish Emergency Medical Services, Baton Rouge, Louisiana. Photo by Michael S. Kowal.

Objectives
Reporting Your Findings
Keeping Records

Glossary
Further Reading

OBJECTIVES

In taking the patient's history and in examining him, we have obtained a lot of valuable and perhaps even crucial information. If that information is to be useful to those who take over the care of the patient, it will have to be organized concisely and logically, for no one has time—especially in an emergency—to listen to a long, rambling story. In this chapter, therefore, we shall review how to organize the information we acquired about the patient into a brief, orderly report. By the end of this chapter, the student should be able to

1. Select the information that constitutes part of the patient's history and the information that belongs in the report of his physical assessment, given a list of information about the patient
2. Label the following in a sample case history:
   • The chief complaint
   • The history of the present illness
   • Other medical history
   • The description of the patient's general appearance
   • The vital signs
   • Pertinent negatives
3. Arrange the data from a patient's history and physical examination in the correct reporting sequence, given a list of information about the patient in random order
4. List the additional information, besides the patient's history and physical findings, that should be recorded on the trip sheet
5. State two reasons for making certain that the medical record of each case is accurate, legible, and complete

REPORTING YOUR FINDINGS

In reporting the findings of your history and physical assessment, whether by radio to the base physician or in person, when handing over the patient to emergency room personnel, the first guideline to remember is:

ALWAYS REPORT YOUR FINDINGS IN THE SAME SEQUENCE, REGARDLESS OF THE SEQUENCE IN WHICH THEY WERE ACTUALLY OBTAINED.

Thus, for example, in responding to a call for a middle-aged man with chest pain, probably the first thing you will do upon reaching the patient is to start oxygen by nasal cannula and put two fingers on his radial pulse, to make sure he is not having a serious dysrhythmia. Only afterward will you get his story and perform a more detailed physical assessment. But when you *report* on the patient, the information that he was given oxygen will be presented *last*, along with any other treatment he received. The assessment of the patient's pulse will be reported along with his other vital signs, after the account of his history. The reason for sticking rigidly to a single sequence of case presentation is twofold: First of all, if you always recite the information in the same sequence, you are less likely to leave anything out. In the second place, doctors are also trained to present medical information in that same sequence. They are accustomed to *hearing* medical information presented that way. So as soon as a doctor hears the patient's sex and age, for example ("The patient is a 45-year-old male. . . ."), the next item of information he or she is listening for is the chief complaint ("who called for an ambulance because of chest pain."). If the chief complaint doesn't materialize at that point, the doctor will immediately feel that something is missing from the report; and if the chief complaint does pop up later on in the report, the doctor is very likely not to "hear" it, because it isn't where it belongs in the story. The same is true for the details of the physical examination. One expects to hear the vital signs before the head-to-toe survey; if they are reported at some other point, they may not register. So what will ensue is a series of questions like, "What did you say the vital signs were? Did you mention his state of consciousness?" The doctor will think you are awfully disorganized, you will think the doctor is awfully stupid, tempers will grow short, and everyone will be unhappy—no one more so than the patient who is supposed to benefit from the interaction.

In prehospital care, it is customary to report medical information in four parts:

• The HISTORY: what other people told you
• The PHYSICAL FINDINGS: what you saw for yourself
• The TREATMENT GIVEN TO THE PATIENT SO FAR
• Any CHANGES IN THE PATIENT'S CONDITION while under your care

The History

For purposes of reporting, the history consists of all the information that you acquired by talking to the patient and bystanders. It is a report of what *happened* and how the patient *feels* (**symptoms**). The sequence in which that report is given is designed to sketch a progressively clearer picture of the patient, starting with a few very broad brush strokes, then drawing in more and more details.

Age and Sex

The very first statement about the patient should indicate the patient's age and sex: "The patient is a 70-year-old woman . . ." or "The patient is a 15-year-old boy. . . ." As soon as you have transmitted only those two facts about the patient, the doctor listening at the other end of the radio can already start to form a picture of the patient and to rule in or out various diagnostic possibilities. When you report, for example, "The patient is a 25-year-old male . . . ," the doctor can already dismiss the possibility of an obstetric problem and assign a very low probability to problems such as heart attack, stroke, and so forth.

Chief Complaint

Immediately after giving the patient's age and sex, state the chief complaint, the reason for which an ambulance was called. As we learned in Chapter 11, the chief complaint should be expressed in a word or short phrase, such as "twisted ankle" or "couldn't breathe." So the first sentence of your report might sound like this:

"The patient is a 78-year-old man who called for an ambulance because he couldn't get his breath."

"The patient is a 12-year-old boy who fell off a skateboard and twisted his leg."

"The patient is a 35-year-old woman who was involved in a vehicular accident."

History of the Present Illness

Now we need to know more about the chief complaint: how? when? where? how much? If the chief complaint is pain, report the results of your "PQRST" inquiries. If the problem is trauma, indicate the possible mechanisms of the accident.

It is important to point out that the history of the *present* illness may, in fact, contain information about the patient's past medical history—*if* that information is relevant to the patient's current chief complaint. For example, if the patient's chief complaint is chest pain, it is relevant to mention, as part of the history of the present illness, that the patient had a heart attack a year ago and that he regularly takes nitroglycerin for angina. On the other hand, the fact that he had major surgery for a bowel obstruction last year belongs in the "other medical history," for it has no direct bearing on his present chief complaint.

Let us consider the 78-year-old man who couldn't get his breath, and listen to what the history of his present illness might sound like:

The patient felt well when he went to bed, but he wakened about two hours later with the feeling that he couldn't breathe. He had to get up and walk around in order to get his breath. He did not cough up any fluid or blood. He did not experience any chest pain. He is not a smoker. He has no known history of cardiac or lung problems.

There are two points to note about the history of the present illness just presented. First of all, as mentioned, it contains information about the patient's past history—the fact that there is no *history* of cardiac or lung problems (the paramedic making the report has apparently concluded, with some justification, that the patient is *now* suffering from a cardiac or lung problem). Secondly, note that there are a number of statements about things the patient did *not* experience: He did not cough up blood. He did not experience chest pain. He is not a smoker. He does not have a cardiac history. Statements of that sort are called **pertinent negatives,** that is, symptoms (or, in the physical examination, signs) that a patient with a certain chief complaint might be *expected* to have but does *not* have. We shall return to the matter of pertinent negatives when we discuss the reporting of the physical examination.

Other Medical History

As we learned in Chapter 11, the information about the patient's medical history that will be important for prehospital care is the following:

- MAJOR UNDERLYING MEDICAL PROBLEMS, other than those related to the chief complaint
- MEDICATIONS the patient is currently taking (or supposed to be taking!)
- ALLERGIES, especially to medications
- Name of the patient's DOCTOR or the HOSPITAL where he usually gets his care.

As we shall see in Chapter 20, there are some minor variations in the medical history that we collect from a victim of trauma as opposed to a medical patient, but the essentials are as noted above.

Returning, then, to our 78-year-old patient with shortness of breath, his other medical history might sound like this:

The patient had surgery last year at Mercy Hospital for cancer of the colon. He takes 6 to 8 aspirin per day for arthritis. He has no known allergies and is not seen regularly by any doctor.

With that information, we have completed the first part of our report, the part that is chiefly hearsay, that is, the patient's history. We then proceed to the more objective part of the report—the account of what we actually observed in examining the patient.

Physical Findings

As we begin to describe what we found on examining the patient, the doctor at the other end of the radio can begin to form a clearer picture of the patient. Up to this point, the doctor simply has a vague impression of an elderly man who says he can't breathe. Now we shall bring that picture into focus.

General Appearance

The first thing the doctor wants to hear about is the potential seriousness of the situation. How sick is this old man? Is he in a lot of distress? Is he conscious at all? The answers to such questions can be furnished in one or two sentences summarizing our assessment of the patient's general appearance. Recall that in evaluating the general appearance, we made note of:

- The POSITION in which we found the patient
- The patient's LEVEL OF CONSCIOUSNESS
- The patient's BEHAVIOR and DEGREE OF DISTRESS
- The condition of the patient's SKIN

In victims of trauma, we also made note of obvious wounds and deformities, which may be mentioned at this point if they are relevant to the patient's major problem; otherwise, postpone the information until the report of the head-to-toe survey.

Returning to our elderly gentleman with shortness of breath, the description of his general appearance might sound like this:

We found the patient sitting bolt upright at the edge of his bed, in considerable respiratory distress. He is conscious, alert, and fully oriented but can speak only in short gasps. He is sweating heavily, and the skin is cool and wet.

Vital Signs

Immediately after the description of the patient's general appearance come the vital signs, the first objective measurement of the status of his vital systems:

The patient's pulse was initially 96, thready, and irregular. Respirations were 28, noisy, and labored. Blood pressure was 180/110.

Head-to-Toe Survey

Next come the findings from the head-to-toe examination of the patient, in head-to-toe sequence:

The patient's pupils were round, regular, midposition, and reactive to light. There was slight cyanosis of the lips. The jugular veins were distended to 4 inches with the patient sitting upright. Crackles were audible halfway up the chest bilaterally. The apical heart rate was 96 and irregular. There was no edema of the back or extremities.

Again, note the pertinent negatives: "There was no edema of the back or extremities." Why bother at all to mention pertinent negatives? Why spend time talking about symptoms the patient doesn't have or physical findings that aren't there? The reason is that if you *don't* mention the pertinent negatives, the doctor at the other end of the radio has no way of knowing whether you even bothered to check that particular detail. Suppose, for instance, you didn't mention the fact that the patient does not have edema. The doctor doesn't know whether (1) edema really isn't present or (2) you forgot to check whether edema is present. Including the pertinent negatives in your report would eliminate that confusion.

The hooker, of course, is the word *pertinent*. Clearly there are an infinite number of negative observations one could make about a patient ("His hair isn't green," or "His eyes aren't crossed."). To know precisely what *is* pertinent to a given chief complaint, one needs to know about specific illnesses and injuries and how they commonly present themselves. Thus, as you proceed through this book and learn more about different illnesses and injuries, your skills in identifying pertinent negatives will increase proportionally.

When you finish reporting the results of your head-to-toe survey, describe the patient's ECG FINDINGS, if he was monitored:

The ECG showed atrial fibrillation.

You have now finished describing the objective findings—the things you observed directly. Your description has been so clear that by now the doctor—even though he has not seen the patient himself—is nearly certain that the patient is suffering from congestive heart failure. The next step is to tell the doctor what you have done for the patient so far.

Treatment So Far

Describe whatever measures you have taken to relieve the patient's symptoms or stabilize his condition:

The patient was placed on a stair-chair, sitting upright with his legs dangling, and given 100% oxygen by demand valve.

Changes in Condition

Finally, indicate whether the patient's condition has changed in any way since he has been under your care:

The patient "pinked up" on oxygen, and his respiratory rate has slowed somewhat, to 24 per minute.

At this point, if you are reporting in by radio, you would request orders for further treatment measures.

Now, let's take the whole report from the beginning and hear how it would sound as the paramedic delivered it:

The patient is a 78-year-old man who called for an ambulance because he couldn't get his breath. The patient felt well when he went to bed, but he wakened about 2 hours later with the feeling that he couldn't breathe. He had to get up and walk around in order to get his breath. He did not cough up any fluid or blood. He did not experience any chest pain. He is not a smoker. He has no known history of cardiac or lung problems. The patient had surgery last year at Mercy Hospital for cancer of the colon. He takes 6 to 8 aspirin per day for arthritis. He has no known allergies and is not seen regularly by any doctor.

We found the patient sitting bolt upright at the edge of his bed, in considerable respiratory distress. He is conscious, alert, and fully oriented but can speak only in short gasps. He is sweating heavily, and the skin is cool and wet. His pulse was initially 96, thready, and irregular. Respirations were 28, noisy, and labored. Blood pressure was 180/110. The patient's pupils were round, regular, midposition, and reactive to light. There was slight cyanosis of the lips. The jugular veins were distended to 4 inches with the patient sitting upright. Crackles were audible halfway up the chest bilaterally. The apical heart rate was 96 and irregular. There was no edema of the back or extremities. The ECG showed atrial fibrillation.

The patient was placed on a stair-chair, sitting upright with his legs dangling and given 100% oxygen by demand valve. He "pinked up" on oxygen, and his respiratory rate has slowed somewhat, to 24 per minute.

Sometimes students learning to report a patient's findings tend to mix up elements of the history with elements of the physical examination. You will not confuse the information that belongs in the history with that belonging in the physical examination if you bear in mind that you can take a history over the telephone, without seeing the patient—for the history consists entirely of hearsay information. A physical examination, on the other hand, cannot be performed without seeing the patient, but it *can* be performed on a patient who is unable to communicate.

> **SYMPTOMS BELONG IN THE HISTORY.**
> **SIGNS BELONG IN THE PHYSICAL EXAMINATION.**

The correct sequence for presenting medical information is summarized in Table 13-1.

TABLE 13-1.   PRESENTING MEDICAL INFORMATION

- AGE and SEX of the patient
- CHIEF COMPLAINT: The reason the patient called for help (e.g., chest pain)
- History of the PRESENT ILLNESS: An elaboration of the chief complaint (e.g., What was the pain like? Where did it radiate? How long did it last?)
- OTHER MEDICAL HISTORY
  1. Significant other illnesses
  2. Medications
  3. Allergies
  4. Usual doctor or hospital

INFORMATION FROM PATIENT OR BYSTANDERS

- PHYSICAL FINDINGS
  1. General appearance
     a. Position
     b. Level of consciousness
     c. Degree of distress
     d. Skin condition
  2. Vital signs
  3. Head-to-toe survey
- ECG FINDINGS, if the patient was monitored

DIRECT OBSERVATION

- TREATMENT given in the field
- CONDITION while in your care
  1. Position in which patient was transported (e.g., supine, semisitting)
  2. Any changes in vital signs or other aspects of patient's condition

PARAMEDIC RUN REPORT

No.   Date: _____

PATIENT INFORMATION

Family name: _____   First name: _____

Age: _____   Sex: _____   Telephone: _____

Address: _____

Insurance _____

Site: [1] Home   [2] Industrial   [3] Vehicular

EMERGENCY DETAILS

Times	Requested by:
Call received _____	[4] Family
Ambulance left _____	[5] Bystanders
At scene _____	[6] Police
Left scene _____	[7] Other
At hospital _____	Site of Incident
Back in service _____	Location _____

DIAGNOSTIC INFORMATION

[8]   Medical problem   [17]   Trauma

[9]   Dyspnea

[10]   Pain in _____

[11]   Coma

[12]   Fever

[13]   Seizures

[14]   Stroke

[15]   Obstetric

[16]   Other: _____

_____

Area involved _____

[18]   Hemorrhage

[19]   Burns

[20]   Shock

[21]   Open wound

[22]   Closed wound

[23]   Fracture of

[24]   Pneumothorax

[25]   Animal/snake bite

TRAUMA CHART
(Areas affected)

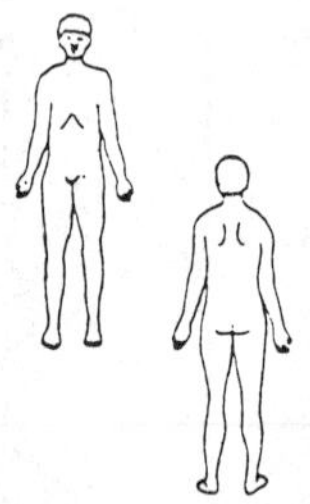

HISTORY OF THE PRESENT ILLNESS

LEVEL OF CONSCIOUSNESS

[26]   Alert   [27]   Semi-conscious   [28]   Unconscious

VITAL FUNCTIONS

Airway: [29] Open   [30] Obstructed

Breathing: [31] Spontaneous   [32] Absent   [33] Labored

Pulse: [34] Present   [35] Absent

       [36] Regular   [37] Irregular

       [38] Full   [39] Thready

VITAL SIGNS

Time	Pulse	BP	Resp.	Level of consciousness

PHYSICAL FINDINGS

Skin:

[40]   Warm   [41]   Cold

[42]   Dry   [43]   Wet

Mucous Membranes:

[44] Pink   [45] Pale   [46] Blue

Pupils:

[47] Normal   [48] Pinpoint   [49] Dilated

[50] Equal   [51] Unequal

[52] Reactive   [53] Unreactive

Neck Veins:

[54] Flat   [55] Distended

Breathing:

[56] Normal   [57] Labored

Breath Sounds:

[58] Equal   [59] Unequal

Abdomen:

[60] Soft   [61] Rigid

Bowel Sounds:

[62] Present   [63] Absent

Extremities:

[64] Normal   [65] Edema

[66] Moving   [67] Paralyzed

If paralyzed, which one(s):

_____

_____

_____

Other Findings:

ECG Findings:

TREATMENT

A, B, Cs	For Trauma
[68] Opened airway manually	[83] **MAST**
[69] Oropharyngeal airway	[84] Bandage/dressing(s)
[70] Endotracheal tube	[85] Pressure dressing
[71] Oxygen _____ %	[86] Tourniquet
[72] Mask	[87] Chest tube
[73] Nasal prongs	[88] Padded board splint
[74] Bag valve mask	[89] Traction splint
[75] Suctioning	[90] Air splint
[76] CPR	[91] Vacuum splint
Intravenous	[92] Sling
[77] Successful [78] Unsuccessful	[93] Cervical collar
[79] Central [80] Peripheral	[94] Backboard
[81] D5W [82] Ringer's	[95] Other: _____
Amount given _____	_____

DRUGS

	Dose		Dose
[96] Atropine _____		[105] Steroids _____	
[97] Diazepam _____		[106] Others: _____	
[98] Dopamine _____		_____	
[99] Epinephrine _____		_____	
[100] Furosemide _____		_____	
[101] Lidocaine _____		_____	
[102] Morphine _____		_____	
[103] Naloxone _____		_____	
[104] Nitroglycerin _____			

EVACUATION DETAILS

Crew	Evacuation to
Paramedic _____	Hospital _____
Paramedic _____	Ward _____
Doctor _____	Doctor _____
Other(s) _____	Discharge date _____

Mileage	Condition on Transfer
Odometer Reading	[107] Unchanged
At dispatch _____	[108] Improved
Back in service _____	[109] Worsened
	[110] Dead

FIGURE 13-1.   **AMBULANCE TRIP SHEET.**

KEEPING RECORDS

All the information that you gave orally to the doctor also has to be written down—legibly, accurately, and in as much detail as possible. Making your run reports complete and accurate is for the good of the patient and also for your own good. The patient benefits because those who take over his care have a detailed record of his initial findings, which can then serve as a baseline against which later findings can be compared. *You* benefit because a detailed medical record is your best protection in the event that the case is ever the subject of a court proceeding. Remember:

> ## IF YOU DON'T DOCUMENT IT, YOU CAN'T PROVE YOU DID IT.

Most ambulance services use preprinted trip sheets that are designed to facilitate both the recording of important information and the analysis of data. In each ambulance service, there will be slightly different priorities regarding the data that should be recorded. At a minimum, however, all trip sheets should include at least the following information:

AMBULANCE TRIP SHEET: MINIMUM INFORMATION

- DATE and TIMES (time call was received, time of arrival at the scene, time of departure from the scene, time of arrival at the hospital)
- Dispatch information on NATURE OF THE CALL
- Patient's NAME, AGE, and SEX
- The patient's HISTORY, including any pertinent statements by the patient
- Observations of the SCENE, where relevant
- Findings on PHYSICAL EXAMINATION
- Any TREATMENT given, described as precisely as possible
- Any ON-LINE ADVICE from Medical Control
- Any CHANGES IN THE PATIENT'S CONDITION while under your care
- NAMES of those providing prehospital care (paramedics; doctor or nurse contacted by radio)
- Any UNUSUAL CIRCUMSTANCES arising during the call

In the sample trip sheet shown in Figure 13-1, a great deal of information can be recorded simply by checking off the appropriate boxes and marking a body diagram. A trip sheet of that type can be filled out relatively quickly but still enables the administrative and medical supervisors to gather important information for evaluating the service. Trip sheets should be filled out at least in duplicate—one copy to accompany the patient to the hospital, where it can be incorporated into the patient's medical record; the other copy or copies to be retained by the ambulance service for systems evaluation.

Always keep in mind that the trip sheet, like any other medical record, is a LEGAL DOCUMENT. It may not be erased or changed with correction fluid. If you have made a mistake in something you wrote, draw a single line through the error, make a note that it was an error, and explain. Sign the explanation.

GLOSSARY

pertinent negative A symptom or sign that the patient might be expected to have, given his or her chief complaint, but does not have.

trip sheet The written record of an ambulance call; also referred to as a run report.

FURTHER READING

Ball RA. Documentation: The overlooked aspect of emergency care. *JEMS* 15(5):31, 1990.

Briese G. SIFRA: A standard information reporting form for ambulances. *Emerg Med Serv* 5(2):58, 1976.

Boyd DR. Record keeping. *EMT J* 1(1):54, 1977.

Brown-Nixon C. Field documentation myths. *Emerg Med Serv* 19(8):18, 1990.

Colletta SJ et al. For a more efficient medical record. *Emerg Med* 22(13):153, 1990.

Clark LA. Documentation: A lingering impact. *Emergency* 20(4):42, 1988.

Griffin PM. An audit method for ambulance calls. *Emergency* 11(2):9, 1979.

Henry GL. Legal rounds: About the medical record. *Emerg Med* 22(2):47, 1990.

Henry GL. Legal rounds: Just for the record. *Emerg Med* 22(13):141, 1990.

Henry GL. Legal rounds: The medical record reappraised. *Emerg Med* 22(10):47, 1990.

Hirsch HL. Legal implications of patient records. *South Med J* 72:726, 1979.

Holder AR. The importance of medical records: Medicolegal rounds. *JAMA* 228:119, 1974.

Lazar RA, Schappert RJ. Presumed insufficient: The importance of the prehospital care report. *JEMS* 16(1):101, 1991.

Payne BC. The medical record as a basis for assessing physician competence. *Ann Intern Med* 91:623, 1979.

Shanaberger CL. The legal file: If it isn't written down. . . *JEMS* 15(6):79, 1990.

Shanaberger CL. The legal file: The unrefined art of documentation. *JEMS* 17(1):155, 1992.

Strange JM. Does your documentation reflect your care? *Emerg Med Serv* 19(8):23, 1990.

The ultimate run sheet (editorial). *Emerg Med Serv* 13(10):142, 1984.

IV

TRAUMA

The history of modern ambulance services in the United States has been dominated by a tug-of-war between two groups of medical specialists, each championing the cause of a different population of patients. One of those groups was composed of surgeons—at first, mostly orthopedic surgeons—who were concerned that the way trauma victims were handled before reaching the hospital might be worsening their injuries. So the first thrust to improve ambulance services in the United States, in the early 1960s, came primarily from the surgeons, who placed emphasis on control of bleeding, splinting of fractures, and moving the patient expeditiously to the hospital.

Meanwhile, however, revolutionary happenings were afoot in internal medicine. The technique of cardiopulmonary resuscitation (CPR) had been developed, and early studies already indicated that CPR could be deployed effectively by nonphysicians. Defibrillation came into widespread use within hospitals. Technology developed for the space program made it possible to transmit a patient's electrocardiogram (ECG) by radio over long distances (telemetry). And across the ocean, in Belfast, Northern Ireland, Dr. Frank Pantridge was demonstrating the effectiveness of his "Flying Squad," a mobile coronary care unit, staffed by a doctor, nurse, and medical student, that brought the facilities of the emergency room *to* the patient suffering a heart attack.

It did not take long for that idea to cross the ocean to the United States, where the late Dr. William Grace, of St. Vincent's Hospital in New York City, set up a mobile heart unit in 1965. Similar units soon sprang up across the United States, at first mostly physician-staffed. The introduction of ECG telemetry into ambulances, by Dr. Eugene Nagel working with the Miami Fire Department in 1967—which enabled ambulance personnel to transmit their patient's ECG to doctors at a base hospital—opened the door for paramedic staffing of mobile intensive care units.

In the decade of the 1970s, then, a different group of doctors—mostly cardiologists, internists, and anesthesiologists—gained ascendancy in the world of prehospital care, and the victims of heart attack displaced the victims of trauma as the principal target population for prehospital intervention. In Los Angeles, Dr. Walter Graf established the CART (Coronary Ambulance Rescue Team); in Seattle, Dr. Leonard Cobb and the Seattle Fire Department set up Medic I; in Long Island, Dr. Costas Lambrew started Cardiac Alert. Emphasis in training programs shifted to dysrhythmia recognition and treatment, CPR, and *stabilizing the patient at the scene.*

That strategy worked well for patients with cardiac problems. It did not work so well for patients who had suffered serious trauma. And by the early 1980s, the surgeons were clamoring for changes in the approach to the injured patient. By the end of the decade, the tug of war had pulled EMS back in their direction, and the emphasis in paramedic training shifted to advanced trauma life support (ATLS). The old credo, "Stabilize the patient before leaving the scene," which had replaced "Swoop and scoop," was in turn being superceded by the ATLS battle cry: "Load and go!"

The fact is that *both* groups of doctors—the internists championing the cause of cardiac patients and the surgeons championing that of trauma victims—were correct. The internists were correct to assert that it is possible to stabilize the condition of a critically ill person in the field and even begin to reverse the pathologic process by giving appropriate medications. The surgeons were correct to insist that, in a victim of trauma, the pathologic process cannot be reversed in the field, for even stabilization requires, at the very least, provision of IV fluid with oxygen-carrying capacity (i.e., blood) and usually surgical repair of the injury as well.

Hopefully, the decade of the 1990s will see a truce in the old tug-of-war between surgeons and internists so that everyone involved in prehospital care can pull together for the greatest good to the greatest number of patients. For what we are beginning to appreciate is that providers of prehospital care need to be trained in two quite distinct approaches—the approach to a person who has fallen ill (a "medical patient") and the approach to a person who has sustained injury (a "trauma patient"). The two approaches are—or should be—complementary, *not* mutually exclusive.

Up to this point, we have studied mostly the approach to the medical patient. In the eight chapters that make up this unit on trauma, we shall be concerned exclusively with the approach to patients who have been injured. We shall look first at some general principles of how injury occurs. We shall then examine in detail the effects of trauma on different regions and systems of the body. Finally, we shall sum up by reviewing the entire sequence of assessment and treatment in the patient with multiple injuries, and we shall learn the priorities that govern situations in which there is more than one casualty.

FURTHER READING

Alexander RH et al. The effect of advanced life support and sophisticated hospital systems on motor vehicle mortality. *J Trauma* 24:486, 1984.

Alyono D, Perry JF Jr. Impact of speed limit. I. Chest injuries: Review of 966 cases. *J Thorac Cardiovasc Surg* 83:519, 1982.

American College of Emergency Physicians. Guidelines for trauma care systems. *Ann Emerg Med* 22:1079, 1993.

Aprahamian C et al. Traumatic cardiac arrest: Scope of paramedic services. *Ann Emerg Med* 14:583, 1985.

Border JR. Panel discussion. Prehospital trauma care—stabilization or scoop and run. *J Trauma* 23:708, 1983.

Centers for Disease Control. Deaths resulting from firearm- and motor-vehicle-related injuries—United States, 1968–1991. *MMWR* 43:37, 1994.

Compton J et al. Role of the intensive care ambulance in the transport of accident victims. *Aust NZ J Surg* 53:435, 1983.

Copass MK et al. Prehospital cardiopulmonary resuscitation of the critically injured patient. *Am J Surg* 148:20, 1984.

Emerman CL et al. A comparison of EMT judgment and prehospital trauma triage instruments. *J Trauma* 31:1369, 1991.

Gallaher M et al. Effects of 65-mph speed limit on rural interstate fatalities in New Mexico. *JAMA* 262:2243, 1989.

Gervin AS et al. The importance of prompt transport in salvage of patients with penetrating heart wounds. *J Trauma* 22:443, 1982.

Gratton MC et al. Effect of standing orders on paramedic scene time for trauma patients. *Ann Emerg Med* 20:1306, 1991.

Ivatury RR et al. Penetrating thoracic injuries: In-field stabilization vs. prompt transport. *J Trauma* 27:1066, 1987.

Jacobs LM et al. Prehospital advanced life support: Benefits in trauma. *J Trauma* 24:8, 1984.

Marzuk PM, Tardiff K, Hirsch CS. The epidemiology of murder-suicide. *JAMA* 267:3179, 1992.

Nagel E et al. Telemetry-medical command in coronary and other mobile emergency care systems. *JAMA* 214:332, 1970.

Pantridge JF, Geddes JS. A mobile intensive care unit in the management of myocardial infarction. *Lancet* ii:271, 1967.

Pepe PE, Stewart RD, Copass MK. Prehospital management of trauma: A tale of three cities. *Ann Emerg Med* 15:1484, 1986.

Pons PT et al. Prehospital advanced trauma life support for critical penetrating wounds to the thorax and abdomen. *J Trauma* 25:828, 1985.

Potter D et al. A controlled trial of prehospital advanced life support in trauma. *Ann Emerg Med* 17:582, 1988.

Reines HD et al. Is advanced life support appropriate for victims of motor vehicle accidents? The South Carolina highway trauma project. *J Trauma* 28:563, 1988.

Sampalis JS. Impact of on-site care, prehospital time, and level of in-hospital care on survival in severely injured patients. *J Trauma* 34:252, 1993.

Siegel JH et al. Causes and costs of injuries in multiple trauma patients requiring extrication from motor vehicle crashes. *J Trauma* 35:920, 1993.

Smith JP et al. Prehospital stabilization of critically injured patients: A failed concept. *J Trauma* 25:65, 1985.

Spaite DW et al. The impact of injury severity and prehospital procedures on scene time in victims of major trauma. *Ann Emerg Med* 20:1299, 1991.

Summers S, Summers B. Beat the clock. *Emerg Med Serv* 21(9):27, 1992.

Trunkey DD. Is ALS necessary for pre-hospital trauma care? *J Trauma* 24:86, 1984.

Warm H. Tomorrow's ambulance: An emergency room on wheels. *Am J Surg* 120:66, 1970.

Waters JM, Wells CH. The effects of a modern emergency medical care system in reducing automobile crash deaths. *J Trauma* 13:645, 1973.

14
Mechanisms of Trauma

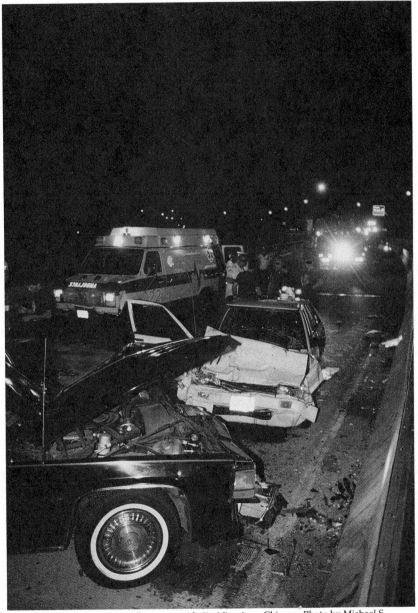

Chicago Fire Department and Emergency Medical Services, Chicago. Photo by Michael S. Kowal.

Objectives
A Little Physics
Blunt Trauma
Penetrating Injuries

Blast Injuries
Glossary
Further Reading

OBJECTIVES

During the past 30 years, as death rates from stroke and heart disease have been declining, trauma—both accidental and intentional—has emerged as one of the major public health problems in the United States.

Accidents are now the leading cause of death for Americans between the ages of 1 and 37 years and the fourth leading cause of death overall. In 1992, accidents claimed the lives of approximately 88,000 persons in the United States, nearly half of the fatalities (39,235) occurring in motor vehicle accidents. Among the victims of vehicular trauma, the majority were drivers or occupants of automobiles; however, 10 percent of the fatalities occurred in motorcyclists, 10 to 15 percent in pedestrians, and about 2 percent in bicyclists.

Second only to motor vehicles as the most important cause of trauma deaths in the United States are firearms, which killed 33,000 people in 1982 (including 16,575 suicides, 13,841 homicides, and 1,756 accidents).

Accidents in the home are also a very important source of trauma mortality. Forty percent of the 12,200 fatal falls that occur each year happen at home, along with about 75 percent of the 4,200 fatal burn injuries.

Finally, a fact of considerable significance to EMS providers: 70 percent of trauma deaths occur in rural areas, that is, in areas likely to be remote from medical facilities.

All of the statistics just cited point to the importance of trauma as a cause of disability and death in our society and, therefore, underline the necessity for paramedics to become as skilled as possible in trauma management.

In this chapter, we will begin our study of trauma by learning a bit of the physics of injury, that is, the forces that produce injury, and the types of injury that result. By the end of this chapter, the student should be able to

1. Describe the effects on an object's kinetic energy of
   - Increasing the object's mass
   - Increasing the object's velocity
   - Having the object collide with another object
2. Identify the three distinct collisions that occur when a moving car strikes an immovable object
3. Identify, given a list of injuries, the injuries most characteristic of
   - A head-on collision
   - A lateral collision
   - A rear-end collision
   - Pedestrian trauma
4. List the injuries apt to be associated with
   - A dented dashboard
   - A bent steering column
   - A cracked front windshield
   - A stoved-in front door
   - Seat belts
5. List at least four things you need to find out about a patient who has fallen from a height
6. List the injuries you are likely to encounter in
   - A small child who fell from a second-story balcony
   - An adult who jumped from the second-story window of a burning building
7. List the important points to look for
   - In taking the history of a gunshot wound victim
   - In examining the victim of a gunshot wound
8. List the four categories of injuries that can be produced by an explosion, and give an example of each
9. Identify injuries likely to be associated with a blast, given a list of injuries

A LITTLE PHYSICS

While drivers of motor vehicles may or may not obey the community's traffic laws, they must—whether they wish to or not—obey the physical laws that govern all objects on our planet.

To understand those physical laws, we first of all need to define a few terms:

- **velocity (V)** The speed of an object, measured in feet per second (fps), meters per second (mps), miles per hour (mph), and so forth.
- **acceleration (a)** The rate of *change* of velocity. When the rate of change in velocity is negative, that is, when the velocity *decreases*, we usually speak of **deceleration.**
- **gravity (g)** The acceleration of a body by the attraction of the earth's gravitational force, normally 32.2 feet/second². It is often convenient to express acceleration in multiples of the gravitational force, or "G" forces.
- **kinetic energy (KE)** The energy associated with bodies in motion, expressed mathematically as:

$$KE = \frac{mV^2}{2}$$

where m = the *mass* of the body
  V = the velocity

(According to this equation, which will be more important in determining the kinetic energy generated by a collision—the mass of the vehicle or the speed at which it is travelling?)

The first physical law of interest to us as students of trauma is the *law of conservation of energy*, which says that energy cannot be created or destroyed, but only changed in form. Thus when two objects collide—say an automobile and a utility pole—the kinetic energy (the energy of the moving vehicle and its contents) does not just disappear; it must be absorbed. The amount of energy absorbed by each object involved in the impact will be determined from the changes in velocity and the masses involved. We know intuitively that if there is a big difference in mass between the two objects, the smaller object will absorb the greater amount of energy. For example, if a 12-ton truck strikes a pedestrian, clearly the pedestrian, having the smaller mass, will sustain greater damage (absorb more kinetic energy). Similarly, when a person falls from a height and hits the ground, the person, having a much smaller mass than the earth he struck, will absorb a much greater proportion of the kinetic energy generated by the fall.

That brings us to another physical law of importance in understanding trauma, **Newton's first law** of motion: A body will remain at rest or in motion at a constant velocity unless acted upon by an outside force. Thus, for example, an automobile travelling at 55 mph will continue travelling at that velocity unless some outside force acts to speed it up (e.g., a tail wind) or slow it down (e.g., road friction, wind resistance, a sudden encounter with a utility pole).

When a car travelling 55 mph hits a utility pole, there are, in fact, three separate impacts, each involving the transfer of kinetic energy. The first impact occurs when the *vehicle* is brought to an abrupt stop (Fig. 14-1A). In that first collision, kinetic energy is absorbed by deformation of the vehicle, and the motion of the car is arrested by bending of its frame. The second impact occurs when the *occupants* of the vehicle, who were also travelling 55 mph, collide with part of the vehicle's structure (Fig. 14-1B), such as the steering wheel, windshield, or dashboard. Their motion continues until energy is absorbed by the structure of the car (denting of the dashboard, for example) or by bending of the occupants' bodies. Finally, the third impact occurs when the *organs* within the occupant's body are hurled against body structures as the body decelerates—for example, the brain thrown forward and back within the skull, the heart and lungs colliding violently with the chest wall.

BLUNT TRAUMA

The physical laws just described are exemplified in blunt trauma, which occurs when the transfer of kinetic energy produces tissue damage without disrupting the skin. In examining blunt trauma, let us look first at several types of vehicular accidents, since such accidents account for the majority of trauma cases that you are apt to see as a paramedic. The mechanisms of injury in motor vehicle injuries are summarized in Table 14-1.

Frontal (Head-on) Collision

Frontal impact accounts for approximately 70 percent of all vehicular collisions. When there is a frontal impact, the unrestrained occupant is hurled forward and brought to a sudden halt against objects within the vehicle—either by sliding *down and under* the dashboard or sailing *up and over* it.

Down-and-Under Injuries

When the unrestrained front-seat occupant slides forward, the first impact is often that of the knee against the DASHBOARD, which may produce a **fracture of the patella** (knee cap). If the impact occurred at high velocity (and therefore involved high kinetic energy), the kinetic energy of the impact may, in addition, be transmitted back along the shaft of the femur to cause **fracture of the femur** itself or a **posterior dislocation of the hip.**

After the knee hits the dashboard, the top of the driver's body continues moving forward until it is brought to a halt against the STEERING WHEEL, perhaps the most lethal object in the vehicle. The steering assembly is composed of a semirigid metal ring (the wheel) fixed to a rigid post (the column), and together they constitute an exceptionally efficient battering ram. Whenever there is structural evidence of steering wheel impact—front-end deformity of the vehicle, displacement of the steering column, or damage to the steering wheel ring—be alert for any of the "ring of injuries" that impact with the steering wheel may have produced:

STEERING WHEEL INJURIES

- Lacerations of the mouth or chin
- Bruises of the anterior neck; if present, consider:
  1. Tracheal fracture

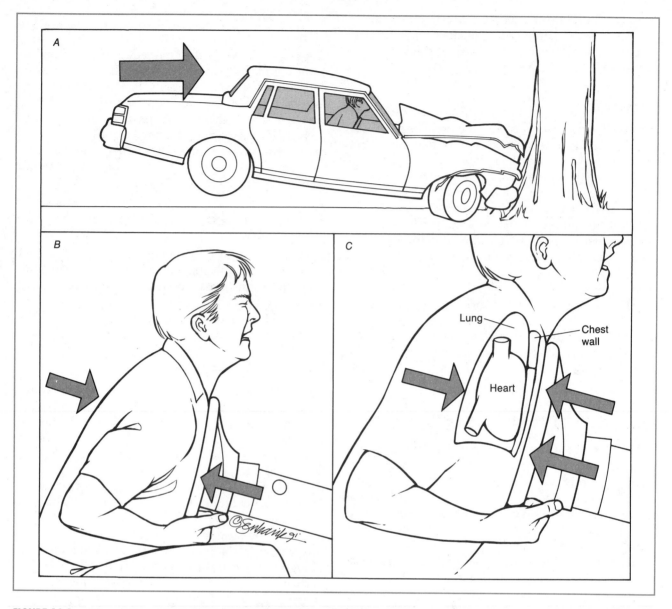

FIGURE 14-1.   THE THREE COLLISIONS THAT OCCUR IN A COLLISION.
(A) Collision 1: The *auto* collides with the tree. (B) Collision 2: The *occupant*
collides with structures inside the auto. (C) Collision 3: The *organs* of the
body collide with body walls.

2. Cervical spine injury
- Fracture of the sternum, with underlying
  1. Myocardial contusion
  2. Pericardial tamponade
- Rib fractures/flail chest, with underlying
  1. Pulmonary contusion
  2. Pneumothorax
  3. Hemothorax
- Shearing of the aorta, with rapid exsanguination
- Shearing or compression of abdominal organs:
  liver, spleen, pancreas, duodenum

Clearly, steering wheel injuries have lethal potential,
but often such injuries are not evident from a cursory
examination of the patient. If you don't also examine
the *vehicle*, you may not suspect the injury.

**WHEN THERE IS DAMAGE TO THE STEERING
ASSEMBLY, THERE IS CRITICAL INJURY TO THE
DRIVER UNTIL PROVED OTHERWISE.**

TABLE 14-1. MECHANISMS OF INJURY IN MOTOR VEHICLE ACCIDENTS

TYPE	STRUCTURAL CLUES	BODY CLUES	LOOK FOR THESE INJURIES
HEAD-ON COLLISION	Deformed front end Cracked windshield	Bruised head	Brain injury Scalp, facial cuts Cervical spine injury
	Deformed steering column	Bruised neck Bruised chest	Tracheal injury Sternal/rib fracture Flail chest Myocardial contusion Pericardial tamponade Pneumothorax/hemothorax Exsanguination from aortic tear
	Deformed dashboard	Bruised abdomen Bruised knee	Ruptured spleen/liver/bowel/diaphragm Fractured patella Dislocated knee Femoral fracture Dislocated hip
LATERAL COLLISION	Deformed side of car	Bruised shoulder	Clavicular fracture Fractured humerus Multiple rib fractures
	Door smashed in	Bruised pelvis	Fractured hip Fractured iliac wing
	"B" pillar deformed	Bruised temple	Brain injury Cervical spine fracture
	Broken door/window handles	Bruised arms	Contusions
	Broken window glass	Dicing lacerations	Multiple square or angulated injuries
REAR-END COLLISION	Posterior deformity of the auto Headrest not adjusted Check for secondary anterior deformity		"Whiplash" injuries Deceleration injuries of a head-on collision

Up-and-Over Injuries

The second route that an unrestrained front-seat occupant can take is up and over the dashboard. Children, because of their high center of mass and large head, are particularly likely to take the up-and-over route, almost always head-first. Thus the first impact is likely to be that of the head against the WIND-SHIELD. That impact often produces injuries to the head itself—simple or depressed **skull fractures**, cerebral contusions, **lacerations** of the scalp and face, fracture of facial bones. Meanwhile, as the skull comes to an abrupt halt against the windshield, the trunk is still moving forward, and the kinetic energy may well be absorbed by the cervical spine as it is forced into rapid hyperflexion and hyperextension. The potential for **cervical spine** injury is therefore considerable.

> **WHEN THE WINDSHIELD IS CRACKED OR BROKEN, THE FRONT SEAT OCCUPANT HAS SUFFERED CERVICAL SPINE INJURY UNTIL PROVED OTHERWISE.**

Restrained Passengers

Restrained passengers—those wearing some form of seat belt—are much less likely to suffer severe injury in a head-on collision because they are largely protected from the secondary collision (occupant against dashboard, windshield, etc.) as well as from being ejected from the vehicle. Indeed, if the seat belt is perfectly designed and worn, the occupant should experience only the vehicle's deceleration forces. Seat belts in standard passenger cars are not perfectly designed, however, nor are they invariably worn correctly. A person wearing only a LAP BELT, for example, will be restrained from sliding forward at the time of a head-on collision, but not from folding forward at the waist, like a jackknife, allowing the head to strike the dashboard or steering wheel. **Lacerations of the chin** are particularly common in such cases, occurring when the driver's face hits the steering wheel. If the belt has been improperly secured, over the waist rather than over the iliac crests of the pelvis, there may also be **compression injuries of the abdomen.**

Three-point or combination LAP/SHOULDER BELTS restrain the body much more securely than a lap belt alone and thus significantly increase a person's chances of surviving a major head-on collision. However, even the lap/shoulder belts leave the head free to move forward, so the neck is subject to enormous stresses, and **fractures of the low cervical and upper thoracic spine** are not uncommon. **Clavicular fractures** are also seen in restrained passengers, at the point where the chest strap crosses the the clavicle.

Lateral (T-Bone) Collisions

A lateral impact collision occurs, as the term implies, when the vehicle is hit from the side. Such collisions produce injury both from secondary impact and from direct intrusion of the deformed part of the car (usually the door) into the passenger space. Seat belts do not help a great deal in a lateral impact collision and may, in fact, trap the passenger in the path of an incoming car door. Examine the vehicle closely as you approach it, and you may be able to predict the injuries you will encounter in its occupants.

Usually, the first impact is between the shoulder girdle and the "B" pillar of the car, which may result in **fracture of the clavicle, fracture of the humerus,** or even **multiple rib fractures** and underlying **injury to the lung** as the humerus is driven against the chest wall. If the car door has been rammed into the occupant's pelvis, one is also likely to see **fracture of the pelvis or hip** as the head of the femur is rammed through the acetabulum (hip socket).

When the shoulder and pelvis are brought to a halt, the head is still moving, so the next impact will be of the head against the door post, leading to a variety of **head injuries.** The kinetic energy of the impact is usually absorbed by the neck, and **cervical spine fractures** are seen with some frequency in lateral impact collisions.

Rear-end Collisions

Rear-end collisions typically occur when a stationary vehicle, such as a car stopped at a traffic light, is struck from behind by a moving vehicle. The impact produces a sudden acceleration in the stationary vehicle, which in turn pushes the occupants posteriorly. If they are properly restrained, with correctly adjusted headrests, injury should be minimal. If the headrest is not properly adjusted, however, the relatively heavy head will accelerate more slowly than the body, allowing the neck to hyperextend over the top of the seat. The result is often a tearing of cervical ligaments, and a so-called **whiplash** injury.

A vehicle that has been struck from behind may, in fact, suffer two collisions—the first when it is hit from behind, the second if it subsequently plows into an object in front of it (e.g., another stationary car). In that case, one may see any of the deceleration injuries just described under the heading of frontal collisions. Once again, it is necessary to take a good look at the vehicle if you want to understand the forces to which the patient was exposed.

Rollover Collisions

When a vehicle rolls over, the unrestrained passenger has a high probability of being ejected from the vehicle; the risk of death for an occupant ejected from a vehicle is anywhere from 10 to 25 times higher than that for occupants who are not ejected. Even those who remain in the car, however, are subject to multiple impacts in multiple directions as they collide with various surfaces within the car. Almost any injury is possible under such circumstances, and spinal injury must be assumed to have occurred. Examine the car and its surroundings carefully for clues that it turned over (scratches, dents in the roof, marks along the road or in the brush).

Pedestrian Injuries

Of the 47,093 traffic fatalities recorded in the United States in 1988, 6,869 were pedestrians, and a large percentage of those pedestrians were children.

Pedestrian injuries have a high mortality rate, and the reason is not hard to understand if we recall the kinetic energy equation we learned earlier. When a pedestrian is struck by a vehicle, the mass of the vehicle is so much greater than that of the pedestrian that there will inevitably be a large transfer of energy from the vehicle to the pedestrian, even when the vehicle is moving quite slowly.

In the vast majority of pedestrian accidents, the pedestrian is struck by the car's bumper. If the pedestrian is an *adult*, the most likely site of initial impact will be the lower leg, so **open fractures of the tibia and fibula** are very common in this situation. A second impact may then occur as the pedestrian is thrown against the hood of the car, which is likely to result in **fractures of the pelvis and femur**. Finally, when the pedestrian rebounds off the car onto the ground, **head injury** commonly occurs. When the pedestrian is a child (Fig. 14-2), the first impact will be between the car bumper and the child's abdomen, pelvis, or femur (depending on his height); the second impact occurs when he is thrown against the hood, usually causing a thoracic injury; the final injury occurs when he is thrown to the ground in a head-down position, resulting in severe and often fatal trauma to the head.

Falls from Heights

Falls from heights (i.e., greater than about 10 feet) most commonly involve children under 5 years old who are left unsupervised near a window or on a porch with inadequate railings. Adult falls from heights usually occur in the context of criminal activity, attempted suicide, or use of alcohol, narcotics, or hallucinogens.

A fall produces a vertical deceleration injury. The severity of that injury will depend on a number of factors, all of which will be important in assessing the patient:

- The HEIGHT from which the victim has fallen, for that will determine the *velocity* of the fall. A person falling one story (12 feet) onto concrete, for example, will fall at about 28 feet per second (fps) and experience an impact force of about 48 G. A person falling from the second story (24 feet) will reach a velocity of 39 fps and experience an impact force of 95 G on the same surface. It is usually assumed that falls from greater than six stories (72 feet) are not survivable.

- The POSITION OF THE BODY at the moment of impact. Children tend to fall head-first, owing to the relatively greater mass of a child's head, so **head injuries** are common in children, as are injuries to the **wrists** and **upper extremities** when the child attempts to break his fall with outstretched arms. Adults, on the other hand, usually try—at least when not intoxicated—to land on their feet.

- The AREA OVER WHICH THE IMPACT IS DISTRIBUTED—the larger the area, the greater the dissipation of the force.

- The SURFACE onto which the person has fallen, and the degree to which that surface can deform ("give") under the force of the falling body. Deep snow, for example, has a relatively large capacity to deform, while concrete has scarcely any "give" at all; contrary to what many people believe, water also has very little give. And, according to the physical laws we have already learned, if the surface does not deform, the body will! The surface may also present hazards because of irregularities or protruding structures; it is far more dangerous to fall onto a wrought-iron picket fence, for example, than onto the grass beside it.

- The PHYSICAL CONDITION OF THE VICTIM. Internal injuries sustained in falls seem to be at least partially dependent on preexisting medical problems—such as ulcer disease or an enlarged spleen—which render one or another organ more vulnerable to injury.

FIGURE 14-2. PEDESTRIAN INJURY PATTERN. First the *leg* is struck by the car bumper; next the *chest* is struck by the grill; finally the *head* hits the ground.

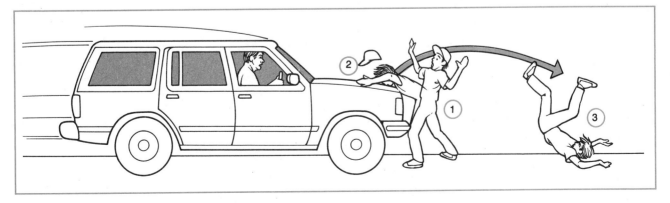

Two types of injury occur as a result of falls from heights: those due to direct impact and those due to deceleration. Let us consider the awake adult who has fallen two stories and landed on his feet (Fig. 14-3). The injuries resulting from *direct impact* are most likely to be *fractures*—first of all **fractures of both calcaneus bones** (heel bones), as the feet hit the ground; then, as the weight of the body is slammed against the spinal column, there are likely to be **compression fractures of the L1 and L2 vertebrae.** If the fall is from a greater height, the **femur** or **pelvis** may be fractured as the femurs are jammed upward into the acetabula.

FIGURE 14-3.   VERTICAL DECELERATION INJURY. The impact is absorbed by the *heels* and transmitted up the legs to the *lumbar spine*.

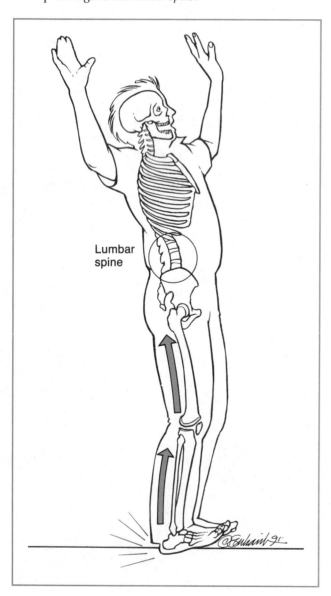

Lumbar spine

Meanwhile, *internal deceleration forces* are likely to produce *injury to internal organs.* When the body comes to an abrupt stop against the ground, the organs within continue to fall before they too come to an abrupt stop. The results are shearing forces that may produce **pulmonary contusions, laceration of the spleen and liver, rupture of the bladder,** and a variety of other internal injuries.

PENETRATING INJURIES

Penetrating injuries are injuries that involve a disruption of the skin. While a variety of objects may cause penetrating injuries—various tools, knives, and so forth—in the United States by far the most common sources of penetrating injuries are firearms of one sort or another. Firearms are responsible for approximately 33,000 deaths and an estimated 120,000 nonfatal injuries in the United States each year. We shall therefore confine our discussion here to the mechanisms of injury produced by firearms.

The amount of damage a firearm produces will depend on a number of factors:

- The type of firearm (pistol, shotgun, rifle)
- The velocity of the missile
- The physical properties of the missile
- The distance from the muzzle of the firearm to the victim
- The tissue that is struck

Types of Firearms

There are three general categories of firearms: shotguns, rifles, and handguns.

Shotguns fire round pellets ("shot")—anywhere from about half a dozen to several hundred at a time, depending on the gauge of the shelling containing the pellets and the size of each individual pellet. When the shell discharges, the pellets are sprayed out the shotgun barrel in a V pattern. The density of pellets at a given distance will, needless to say, depend on the amount of shot in the shell; it will also depend on the length of the shotgun barrel and the "choke" of the barrel (the constriction at the end of the barrel). The longer the barrel and the tighter the choke, the greater the tendency of the pellets to remain together. At very close range (under 10 yards), then, the shotgun can be the most devastating of all guns, producing injuries very much like blast injuries (see next section). Entrance and exit wounds can be very large, with shotgun wadding, bits of clothing, skin, and hair all driven into the wound to cause massive contamination.

Rifles are so named because of the grooves ("rifling") cut into the inside of the barrel to spin the bullet as it passes through and thereby give the bullet more gyroscopic stability. That makes the bullet travel straighter and thus more accurately.

Handguns are of two types, revolvers and pistols ("automatics"). Like rifles, handguns have grooves cut into their bore to impart a spin to the bullet.

The Velocity of the Missile

Recall once again the equation for kinetic energy:

$$KE = \frac{mV^2}{2}$$

where m = the mass of the object
V = the velocity of the object

It is clear from that equation that the velocity of the bullet will play a much larger role than the size of the bullet in determining its destructive capability. If you double the mass of the bullet, for example, you will double its kinetic energy; but if you double the *velocity* at which the bullet is travelling, you will quadruple its kinetic energy.

Any penetrating missile, regardless of its velocity, produces its damage through two mechanisms: *crushing* the tissue in its path and *stretching* the surrounding tissues. As a bullet penetrates into tissue (Fig. 14-4), it produces a **permanent cavity** of crushed tissue that may be a cylinder of the same diameter of

the bullet. At the same time, however, the kinetic energy of the moving bullet pushes tissues rapidly away from the bullet and forms a large **temporary cavity,** whose volume may be 30 times that of the bullet passing through it. The temporary cavity compresses immediately after the bullet passes through the tissue but then reforms and collapses several more times, until all of the kinetic energy transferred from the bullet to the tissue has dissipated. Furthermore, the *pressure* produced within the temporary cavity may approach 100 times atmospheric pressure. The higher the velocity of the bullet, the larger the cavity and thus the greater the stretch on surrounding tissues.

The production and collapse of the temporary cavity also produce a sort of vacuum along the path of the bullet—a vacuum powerful enough to suck bits of the victim's clothing and other debris from the skin into the wound.

Another point about the bullet's velocity: As the speed of the bullet increases, its stability in flight decreases—especially at speeds above 3,000 fps—so instead of travelling in a straight line, the bullet tends to **yaw** (oscillate around its axis) or **tumble** (roll end over end). The result is to increase the size of the permanent cavity and therefore to increase the area of tissue destruction.

Table 14-2 summarizes the velocities associated with some commonly encountered firearms. Low-velocity weapons are those that propel missiles at

FIGURE 14-4. WOUND BALLISTICS.   A bullet travelling through tissue produces a temporary cavity of stretched tissue and a permanent cavity of crushed tissue.

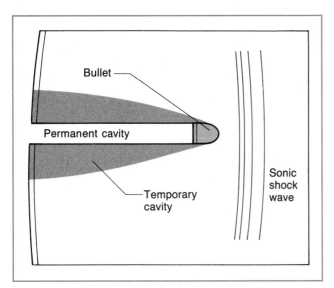

TABLE 14-2.   VELOCITIES OF VARIOUS FIREARMS

TYPE OF FIREARM	VELOCITY (FEET PER SECOND)	
	AT THE MUZZLE	AT 100 YARDS
HANDGUNS		
25 automatic pistol	810	700
32 Colt	690	595
357 Magnum	1,550	—
38 Special	855	790
45 automatic	850	775
SPORTING RIFLES		
.22 short	1,125	920
.22 long rifle	1,335	1,045
222 Remington	3,200	2,690
270 Winchester	3,480	3,070
30-06 Springfield	2,410	2,120
444 Marlin	2,400	1,845
MILITARY RIFLES		
U.S. M-16 5.56 mm	3,200	2,630
U.S. M-14 7.62 mm (NATO)	2,860	2,570
Russian 7.62 mm	2,810	2,570
British .303	2,540	2,340

speeds of under 1,000 fps and include most hand-guns. Some handguns and most sporting rifles fall into the category of medium velocity firearms (1,000–2,000 fps), while military rifles such as the M-16 are considered high-velocity weapons (over 2,000 fps).

Physical Properties of the Missile

The wounding capability of the bullet also depends critically on its physical properties. The Hague Convention of 1906 specified that all bullets used in war must be copper-jacketed, to keep the bullet intact as it passes through tissue. That reduces the kinetic energy transferred to the tissue and thereby reduces the amount of resulting injury. Unfortunately, there is no Hague Convention regulating the use of bullets in civilian life, where bullets are often modified to increase their destructiveness. The soft-point bullet, for example, is designed so that its tip flattens on impact, causing its diameter to increase by 200 to 250 percent. Thus it makes a much bigger hole to begin with (the **entrance wound**), a much larger permanent cavity, and a very large **exit wound** (up to about 5 inches in diameter when a bullet has traversed the thigh). Furthermore, soft-tip bullets *fragment* within the body, and each fragment then takes its own path, creating its own channel of crush injury. Other alterations in the configuration of the bullet—hollow noses, vertical cuts in the nose, and so forth—have similar effects.

Firing Distance

As a bullet moves through the air, it expends kinetic energy and slows down—until eventually it will not have sufficient energy left to counteract gravity and it will fall to the ground. Clearly, then, the closer the firearm is to the victim, the greater the kinetic energy of the bullet and the greater the damage. That is, in fact, usually a rather academic consideration, since the majority of gunshot wounds are inflicted by bullets fired at close range. Powder marks tattooed onto the skin around the wound are a good indication of a bullet fired at close range.

Target Tissue

Finally, a very important factor influencing the seriousness of a gunshot wound is the type of tissue through which the bullet passes. Tissue of high elasticity like muscle, for example, is better able to tolerate stretch (temporary cavitation) than tissue of low elasticity, like liver. A high velocity bullet fired

through a fleshy part of the leg may do much less damage than a relatively low velocity bullet that punctures the aorta.

> **SUMMARY: WHAT TO ASK AND WHAT TO LOOK FOR IN GUNSHOT WOUNDS**
>
> WHAT TO ASK:
> - *What kind of weapon* was used (handgun, rifle, or shotgun; type and caliber, if known)?
> - At *what range* was it fired?
> - *What kind of bullet* was used? (Ideally, see if you can find an unfired cartridge.)
>
> WHAT TO LOOK FOR:
> - Powder residue around the wound
> - Entrance and exit wounds (the exit wound is usually larger and more ragged)

BLAST INJURIES

Strictly speaking, blast injuries refer to the injuries produced when the pressure waves generated by an explosion strike body surfaces. Although most commonly associated with military conflict, blast injuries are also seen in civilian practice in mines, shipyards, chemical plants, and increasingly in association with terrorist activities.

People who are injured in explosions may, in fact, be injured by any of four different mechanisms (Fig. 14-5):

- **Primary blast injuries** are those due entirely to the blast itself, that is, to the impact against the body of the wave of pressure generated by the explosion.
- In **secondary blast injuries,** damage results from being struck by flying debris, such as glass or splinters, that has been set in motion by the explosion.
- **Tertiary blast injuries** occur when the victim is hurled by the force of the explosion against a stationary object.
- Finally, **miscellaneous blast injuries** include burns from hot gases or fire started by the blast; respiratory injury from inhaling toxic gases; crush injury from the collapse of buildings, and so forth.

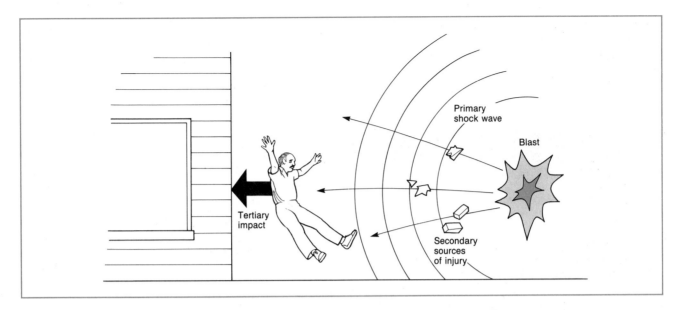

FIGURE 14-5. **INJURIES IN AN EXPLOSION.**

The vast majority of patients who survive an explosion will have some combination of the four types of injury mentioned above. We will confine our discussion here to *primary* blast injuries, since those are the most easily overlooked.

The Physics of an Explosion

When an explosion occurs, a relatively small volume of explosive material is transformed into gaseous products that expand very rapidly. As they do so, they assume the shape of a sphere whose pressure is much higher than that of the air around it. That very high pressure is propagated as a pressure wave, or shock wave, that travels out in all directions from the point of explosion. The speed, duration, and pressure of the shock wave are affected by

- The SIZE of the explosive charge. The larger the explosion, the faster the shock waves and the longer they will last.
- The nature of the SURROUNDING MEDIUM. Pressure waves travel much more rapidly in *water*, for example, and are effective at greater distances in water.
- The DISTANCE from the explosion. The farther one is from the explosion, the slower the shock wave velocity and the longer its duration.
- The presence or absence of REFLECTING SURFACES. If the pressure wave is reflected off a solid object, its pressure may be multiplied several times. Thus, for example, a shock wave that

might cause minimal injury in the open can cause devastating trauma if the victim is standing beside a wall or similar solid object.

Those, then, are factors of which you need to take note when assessing the blast victim: How big was the explosion? Was the victim on land or in water? How far was he from the explosion? Was he near any reflecting surfaces? Include all such information in your report to the base physician.

The changes in pressure produced by the shock wave are accompanied by transient *winds*, sometimes of very high velocity, that can accelerate small objects to speeds of hundreds of feet per second. A missile travelling at 50 fps can easily penetrate human skin; at 400 fps, a missile can enter any of the major body cavities and cause serious internal injury. Blast winds can also send the human body flying against larger, more stationary objects.

Primary Blast Injuries

Injuries due to the primary blast are almost exclusively confined to *gas-containing organs*: the ear, the respiratory system, and the gastrointestinal tract.

The EAR is the most sensitive to blast injuries because it was designed precisely to *detect* weak pressure waves in the air. The **tympanic membrane will rupture** at pressures of 5 to 7 pounds per square inch (psi) above atmospheric pressure. Thus the tympanic membranes are a sensitive indicator of the possible presence of other blast injuries. The patient may complain of **tinnitus** (ringing in the ears), **otalgia** (pain in the ears), or some loss of hearing, and blood may be visible in the ear canal.

> **WHEN THERE IS EVIDENCE OF EAR PROBLEMS AFTER AN EXPLOSION, LOOK FOR SERIOUS INJURY TO THE LUNGS.**

The primary blast injury to the LUNGS is basically similar to a pulmonary contusion sustained in blunt chest trauma, for the pressure wave of the blast drives the chest wall inward against the lungs. The patient may complain of tightness or pain in his chest and may cough up blood; on physical examination you are apt to find tachypnea and other signs of respiratory distress. (What are the signs of respiratory distress? Do you remember?) There may also be subcutaneous emphysema over the chest. The underlying injuries may include **pneumothorax** or **pulmonary edema** (or both!). If there is *any* reason to suspect lung injury in a blast victim (even just the presence of a ruptured eardrum), administer oxygen. Avoid giving oxygen under positive pressure, however (i.e., by demand valve), for that may simply increase the damage to the lung. Be cautious as well with intravenous fluids, which may be poorly tolerated in patients with this sort of lung injury. Consult your base physician before setting the flow rate of the IV.

One of the most dreaded complications of blast injury to the lung, and the one that poses the most immediate threat to life, is **arterial air embolism,** which may occur when alveoli are torn and air bubbles enter the tiny pulmonary blood vessels alongside them. If those air bubbles enter a coronary artery, they may produce electrocardiographic signs of myocardial infarction or even cause sudden death. If they enter a cerebral artery, they can produce disturbances in vision, changes in behavior, changes in state of consciousness, or a variety of other neurologic signs.

> **IF THE VICTIM OF A BLAST INJURY HAS ANY NEUROLOGIC ABNORMALITIES, NOTIFY THE BASE PHYSICIAN AT ONCE!**

Optimal treatment of arterial air embolism requires decompression in a hyperbaric chamber, and arrangements will need to be made to get the patient to such a facility, which may be many miles distant.

Primary blast injury to the GASTROINTESTINAL TRACT most commonly involves the large bowel and is more apt to occur in underwater blast injuries than in those sustained in air. Clues to bowel injury include abdominal pain, tenderness, and rigidity.

The most important thing to remember about primary blast injuries is that they often have few if any external signs. They are, therefore, very easy to overlook, especially if a patient has dramatic secondary and tertiary blast injuries, such as bleeding from multiple lacerations or a fracture sustained when hurled against a wall. IF YOU DON'T LOOK FOR PRIMARY BLAST INJURIES, YOU WON'T FIND THEM! Check the ear canals first; if there is blood or if the patient reports difficulty in hearing, assume there is a primary blast injury until proved otherwise.

GLOSSARY

acceleration   The rate of change in velocity.

deceleration   A negative acceleration, i.e., a slowing down.

entrance wound   The point at which a penetrating object enters the body.

exit wound   The point at which a penetrating object leaves the body, which may or may not be in a straight line with the entrance wound.

gravity   The acceleration of a body by the attraction of the earth's gravitational force, normally 32.2 feet/second^2.

kinetic energy   The energy associated with bodies in motion, expressed mathematically as half the mass times the square of the velocity.

otalgia   Pain in the ear.

permanent cavity   The path of crushed tissue produced by a missile traversing part of the body.

temporary cavity   A transient hollow produced by the stretching of tissues around the path of a missile traversing part of the body.

tinnitus   A ringing, or sometimes a buzzing or roaring noise, in the ears.

velocity   The speed of an object in a given direction.

yaw   Oscillation around the vertical axis.

FURTHER READING

Barbara J, Kunkle R. Shattering the myths about crush syndrome. *JEMS* 17(1):52, 1992.

Barlow B et al. Ten years of experience with falls from a height in children. *J Pediatr Surg* 18:509, 1983.

Brainard BJ. Injury profiles in pedestrian motor vehicle trauma. *Ann Emerg Med* 18:881, 1989.

Butcher T. Explosive emergencies: Treating blast injuries in the field. *JEMS* 16(6):50, 1991.

Daffner RH et al. Patterns of high-speed impact injuries in motor vehicle occupants. *J Trauma* 28:498, 1988.

Fackler ML. Ballistic injury. *Ann Emerg Med* 15:110, 1986.

Forry S. Mechanisms of injury: Making a vital assessment tool work. *JEMS* 17(3):73, 1992.

Greenberg MI. Falls from heights. *JACEP* 7:300, 1978.

Hamit HF. In the wake of a blast. *Emerg Med* 16(2):115, 1983.

Hill JF. Blast injury with particular reference to recent terrorist bombing incidents. *Ann R Coll Surg Engl* 61:4, 1979.

Huller T, Bazini Y. Blast injuries of the chest and abdomen. *Arch Surg* 100:24, 1970.

Hunt RC et al. Comparison of motor vehicle damage documentation in emergency medical services run reports compared with photographic documentation. *Ann Emerg Med* 22:651, 1993.

Lindsey D. The idolatry of velocity, or lies, damn lies, and ballistics. *J Trauma* 20:1068, 1980.

Lowenstein SR et al. Vertical trauma: Injuries to patients who fall and land on their feet. *Ann Emerg Med* 18:161, 1989.

Lucas GM et al. Injuries sustained from high velocity impact with water: An experience from the Golden Gate Bridge. *J Trauma* 21:612, 1981.

Phillips YY. Primary blast injuries. *Ann Emerg Med* 15:1446, 1986.

Stanford TM. Taking a shot at ballistics. *Emergency* 22(3):45, 1990.

Stapczynski JS. Blast injuries. *Ann Emerg Med* 11:687, 1982.

Stewart C. Mechanisms of injury. *Emerg Med Serv* 18(1):21, 1989.

Thygerson AL. Gunshot wounds. *Emergency* 13(8):14, 1981.

15
Wounds and Burns

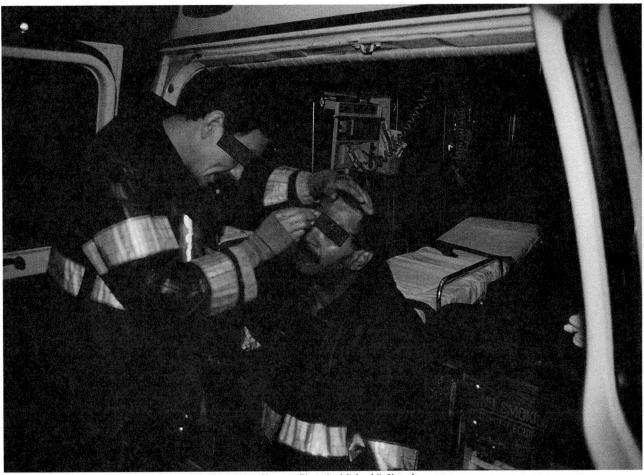

Chicago Fire Department and Emergency Medical Services, Chicago. Photo by Michael S. Kowal.

OBJECTIVES

The skin is the largest organ of the human body and serves as the interface between the body and the outside world. For that reason, injuries involving the skin are common. Furthermore, injuries to the skin are usually the most immediately obvious of a person's injuries, even if not necessarily the most serious. An inexperienced rescuer is therefore apt to be distracted by dramatic external wounds and neglect to check for higher priority problems, such as an obstructed airway.

In this chapter, we shall take a closer look at the skin and the soft tissues immediately beneath it. We shall examine the ways in which the skin and soft tissues can be injured and the measures we can take in the field to prevent such injuries from progressing in severity. By the end of this chapter, the student should be able to

1. Label the structural components of the skin, given a drawing of a magnified section of skin in cross section
2. List the functions performed by intact skin
3. Arrange the steps of treatment in order of priority, given a patient with multiple injuries including soft tissue injuries and a list of treatment steps in random order
4. Outline the correct treatment for
   • A contusion
   • An abrasion
   • A laceration
   • A wound with an impaled object
   • A partial avulsion
   • An amputation
5. List five methods of controlling external bleeding, and indicate which is the most effective method
6. Indicate which pressure point is used to control bleeding of
   • The scalp
   • The forearm
   • The leg
7. Identify correct and incorrect procedures in the application of a tourniquet, given a description of the steps in application
8. List in the correct order of priorities the steps in assessing and managing the victim of flame burns
9. List at least six clues to the possible presence of respiratory injury in a burn victim
10. List two indications for endotracheal intubation in a burn victim
11. Describe the IV fluid therapy (i.e., the type of fluid, the flow rate) for an adult burn victim given his weight and the extent of his burn

12. List five questions you need to have answered in taking the history of a patient burned in a fire
13. Given a description of several burns, identify and describe the correct treatment of each of the following:
    • A first-degree burn
    • A second-degree burn
    • A third-degree burn
14. Calculate the extent of a burn using the Rule of Nines, given a description of the victim's burns
15. Identify patients who have suffered critical burns, given a description of several patients with different burn injuries
16. Identify a patient whose limb is in jeopardy from a burn, given a description of the patient, and outline the appropriate management
17. Identify correct and incorrect procedures in the treatment of chemical burns, given a description of the various procedures
18. List three types of burn that a person may suffer as a result of electric injury
19. List six nonburn injuries that a person may suffer as the result of contact with a high-voltage electric source
20. Describe the correct approach to a victim of high-voltage injury and list the steps of management, given a description of the patient and his findings
21. List three ways one can avoid being struck by lightning
22. Describe the correct steps to take at the scene of a lightning strike, given a description of the scene and of the lightning victim(s)
23. Describe the therapeutic effects, indications, contraindications, side effects, administration, and dosage of the following, after studying the relevant sections of the Drug Handbook at the end of this textbook:
    • Morphine sulfate
    • Mannitol
    • Sodium bicarbonate

STRUCTURE AND FUNCTION OF THE SKIN

The human skin is much more than just a pretty wrapping that keeps the inside of the body from falling out. The skin, or **integument,** is in fact a complex organ that plays a crucial role in maintaining the constancy of the internal environment (**homeostasis**). Among the most important *functions* of the skin are the following:

• The skin acts as an all-purpose fortress to PROTECT underlying tissue FROM INJURY, including that caused by extremes of temperature, ultraviolet radiation, mechanical forces, toxic chemicals, and invading microorganisms.

- The skin aids in TEMPERATURE REGULATION, preventing heat loss when the core body temperature starts to fall and facilitating heat loss when core temperature rises.
- As a watertight seal, the skin PREVENTS EXCESSIVE LOSS OF WATER FROM THE BODY and drying of tissues, thereby helping to maintain the chemical stability of the internal environment. Without skin, a person would become waterlogged after the first rain and would resemble a prune after the first hot day of summer.
- The skin serves as a SENSE ORGAN, keeping the brain informed about a whole host of features of the external environment. Changes in temperature, touch, and bodily position as well as sensations of pain are all mediated through the sense receptors within the skin.

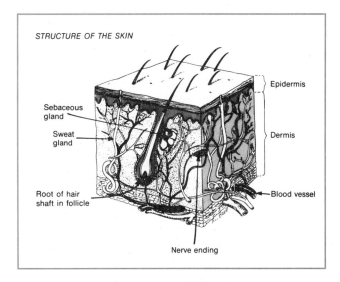

FIGURE 15-1. STRUCTURE OF THE SKIN.

It follows from the functions described above that significant damage to the skin may render the body vulnerable to bacterial invasion, temperature instability, and major disturbances of fluid balance. As we shall see later in this chapter, that is precisely what happens when a significant area of the skin suffers thermal injury.

To carry out its functions, the skin needs a specialized *structure* (Fig. 15-1). Accordingly, the skin is composed of two principal layers, the epidermis and the dermis. The **epidermis,** or outermost layer, is the body's first line of defense, the principal barrier against water, dust, microorganisms, and mechanical stress. The epidermis is itself composed of several layers: an outermost layer (stratum corneum) of hardened, nonliving cells, which are continuously shed through a process called desquamation; and three inner layers of living cells that constantly divide to give rise to the cells of the stratum corneum. Those deeper layers of the epidermis also contain variable numbers of cells bearing **melanin** granules; the darkness of a person's skin is directly proportional to the amount of melanin present.

Underlying the epidermis is a tough, highly elastic layer of connective tissues called the **dermis.** The dermis is a complex material composed chiefly of collagen fibers, elastic fibers, and a mucopolysaccharide gel. **Collagen** is a fibrous protein with a very high tensile strength, so it gives the skin a high resistance to breakage under mechanical stress. **Elastin,** as the name implies, imparts elasticity to the skin, allowing the skin to spring back to its usual contours. The **mucopolysaccharide gel,** for its part, gives the skin resistance pe compression.

Enclosed within the dermis are several specialized skin structures:

- NERVE ENDINGS, which mediate the senses of touch, temperature, pressure, and pain.
- BLOOD VESSELS, which—like blood vessels elsewhere in the body—carry oxygen and nutrients to the skin and bear away carbon dioxide and metabolic waste products. Cutaneous blood vessels in addition serve a crucial role in *regulating body temperature,* by regulating the volume of blood that flows from the body's warm core to its cooler surface.
- SWEAT GLANDS, which produce sweat and discharge it through ducts passing to the surface of the skin. Sweat consists of water and salts, and sweating is regulated through the action of the sympathetic nervous system. The average volume of sweat lost during 24 hours under normal conditions is from 500 to 1,000 ml; during strenuous exercise, however, sweat glands may secrete as much as 1,000 ml in an hour's time. As we shall learn in Chapter 31, evaporation of water from the skin surface is one of the body's major mechanisms for shedding excess heat.
- HAIR FOLLICLES, structures that produce hair and enclose the hair roots. Each follicle contains a single hair. Attached to the hair follicle is a small muscle that, on contraction, causes the follicle to assume a more vertical position. Sensations such as cold and fright stimulate the autonomic nervous system, which in turn brings about contraction of those muscles; the result is the appearance of the skin called "gooseflesh." Hairs in each part of the body have definite pe-

riods of growth, after which they are shed and replaced; scalp hair, for example, has a life span of 2 to 5 years and grows at an average rate of 1.5 to 3.9 mm per week.

- At the neck of each hair follicle is a SEBACEOUS GLAND, a specialized secretory mechanism that produces an oily substance called *sebum*. The secretions of the sebaceous glands are emptied into the hair follicles and from there reach the surface of the skin. The precise function of sebum is not well understood, although it has been suggested that sebum keeps the skin supple so that it doesn't crack.

The layer of tissue beneath the dermis is, by definition, the **subcutaneous layer,** and it consists mainly of **adipose tissue** (fat). Subcutaneous fat serves as insulating material to protect underlying tissues from extremes of heat and cold. It also provides a substantial cushion (in some people, that cushion is more substantial than in others!) for underlying structures, while serving as an energy reserve for the body.

Finally, beneath the subcutaneous layer are the muscles and bones.

WOUNDS

Broadly speaking, a wound is any injury to the soft tissues, that is, an injury to the skin with or without involvement of the subcutaneous tissues and muscle beneath.

Probably the most important thing to remember about soft tissue injuries in general is that they are relatively *low-priority injuries*. Soft tissue injuries may be the most obvious and the most dramatic of a patient's injuries, but they are seldom the most serious unless they compromise the airway or are associated with massive bleeding. Therefore, you should always search systematically and thoroughly for other injuries or life-threatening conditions before tending to soft tissue trauma.

DON'T LET DRAMATIC SOFT TISSUE INJURIES DISTRACT YOU FROM THE PRIMARY SURVEY!

It is customary to classify wounds according to whether they are closed or open.

Closed Wounds

In a **closed wound,** there is damage to the soft tissues beneath the skin surface, but there is no break in the continuity of the epidermis. The characteristic closed wound is a **contusion,** or bruise. In a contusion, the skin is intact, but damage has occurred beneath the epidermis. Trauma to the nerve endings there produces PAIN, while leakage of edema fluid into the spaces between the damaged cells produces SWELLING. If small blood vessels in the dermis have been disrupted, there will be a black-and-blue mark (**ecchymosis**) over the injured area; if large blood vessels have been torn beneath the contused area, a **hematoma,** or collection of blood beneath the skin, will be evident as a lump with a bluish discoloration.

Small contusions do not require any special treatment. When there is extensive closed injury, however, bleeding beneath the skin may reach significant proportions, and swelling may compromise vital structures. Therefore, when there are extensive contusions, measures should be taken to minimize the bleeding and swelling. The easiest way to remember the measures used to treat closed injury is by thinking of the mnemonic **ICES:**

TREATMENT OF EXTENSIVE CONTUSIONS

I   Apply **ice** or cold packs to the injured area. Cold will stimulate blood vessels to constrict, thereby slowing the bleeding.

C   Apply firm **compression** over the injured area, to decrease bleeding. Compression may be manual initially, but is most effectively applied with an air splint thereafter (see p. 308).

E   **Elevate** the injured part to a level above the heart, to encourage drainage and decrease swelling.

S   Apply a **splint** to an injured extremity. By preventing motion, a splint decreases bleeding. If you use an air splint, you will get a double benefit—splinting *and* compression.

Open Wounds

An open wound is one in which there is disruption in the continuity of the skin. Open wounds are therefore potentially much more serious than closed wounds for two reasons:

- Open wounds have a greater potential for serious BLOOD LOSS. When the skin is unbroken, there is a limit to how much blood can pour out of a disrupted blood vessel. Granted, a significant volume of blood—up to about 2 units—can be lost into the soft tissues of the leg; but at a certain point, the increasing pressure within the leg will prevent further bleeding. If, however, the wound in the leg is open, there is nothing to prevent further bleeding, and one can lose one's entire blood volume through any significant open wound.
- Open wounds are vulnerable to INFECTION. So long as the skin remains intact, it provides an amazingly effective barrier against the hordes of bacteria in the environment as a whole and on the surface of the skin itself. The moment that barrier is breached, however, a wound becomes **contaminated**; that is, microorganisms enter. Whether the contamination goes on to produce infection will depend in large measure on how the wound is managed.

Accordingly, there are two general principles that govern the treatment of *all* open wounds, regardless of type:

TREATMENT OF OPEN WOUNDS: GENERAL PRINCIPLES

- CONTROL BLEEDING by whatever method is most effective (see p. 308).
- KEEP THE WOUND AS CLEAN AS POSSIBLE. *Cut* away any clothing covering the wound. Irrigate out loose dirt and debris by pouring sterile water or even tap water over the area. Do *not*, however, try to pick out foreign matter embedded in a wound. Simply irrigate copiously, and then cover the wound with a dry, sterile dressing.

Open wounds are usually classified into four categories: abrasions, lacerations, puncture wounds, and avulsions.

Abrasions

An **abrasion** (Fig. 15-2A) is a superficial wound that occurs when the skin is rubbed or scraped over a rough surface so that part of the epidermis is lost. So-called brush burns or mat burns are good examples. Abrasions typically ooze small amounts of blood and may be quite painful. They may also be embedded with dirt and debris.

Do not try to clean up an abrasion in the field; you don't have the means to do so properly. If you feel impelled to do *something*, just cover the wound lightly with a sterile dressing. If, as is often the case, the patient is a child who fell off a bicycle, and if his injuries are limited to the abrasions, give him a lollipop in addition to a dressing.

Lacerations

A **laceration** (Fig. 15-2B) is a cut inflicted by a sharp instrument, such as a knife or razor blade, producing a clean or jagged incision through the skin surface and underlying structures. Sometimes the word *laceration* is reserved for jagged or irregular cuts, while *incision* is used to refer to a clean cut. The seriousness of a laceration will depend on its depth and the structures that have been damaged. Lacerations may also be the source of significant bleeding if the sharp instrument also disrupted the wall of a blood vessel, particularly in regions of the body where major arteries lie close to the surface (as in the wrist).

Almost invariably, the first priority in treating a laceration will be to *control bleeding*, initially by applying direct manual pressure over the wound.

Puncture Wounds

A **puncture wound** is a stab from a pointed object, such as a nail or a knife (in the old days, the ice pick was the weapon of choice for inflicting puncture wounds, but the ice pick apparently went out with the icebox). Technically speaking, a bullet wound is also a puncture wound. As a general rule, puncture wounds do not cause significant *external* bleeding, but they may cause extensive and even fatal *internal* bleeding as well as all sorts of other havoc that cannot be seen from the outside of the body.

A special case of the puncture wound is the IMPALED FOREIGN OBJECT (Fig. 15-2C), in which the instrument that caused the injury remains embedded in the wound. When an impaled object is present, observe the following guidelines:

MANAGEMENT OF AN IMPALED OBJECT

- DO NOT TRY TO REMOVE AN IMPALED OBJECT. Efforts to do so may cause severe hem-

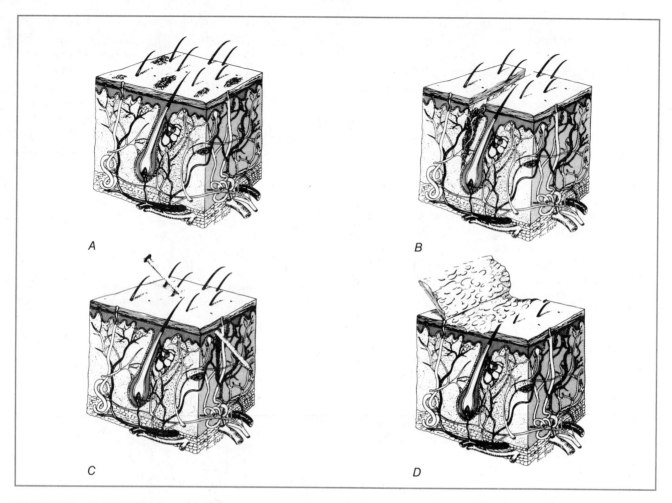

FIGURE 15-2. **TYPES OF OPEN WOUNDS.**   (A) Abrasion. (B) Laceration.
(C) Puncture wound with impaled object. (D) Avulsion.

orrhage and further injury to underlying structures.

- Control hemorrhage by direct compression, but do not apply pressure on the impaled object itself or on immediately adjacent tissues.
- DO NOT TRY TO SHORTEN AN IMPALED OBJECT unless it is extremely cumbersome (e.g., a fence post impaled in the chest); any motion of the object may damage surrounding tissues.
- STABILIZE THE OBJECT IN PLACE with a bulky dressing, and immobilize the extremity (if the object is impaled in an extremity) with a splint to prevent motion (Fig. 15-3).

Avulsions

An **avulsion** occurs when a flap of skin has been torn loose, either partially (Fig. 15-2D) or completely. (When a part of the body has been completely avulsed, we say it has been **amputated.**) Depending

on where the avulsion occurs, it may or may not be accompanied by profuse bleeding. The principal danger in an avulsion—beside the usual dangers of blood loss and contamination—is loss of the blood supply to the avulsed flap. If the part of the flap that connects it to the body (the **pedicle**) is folded back or kinked in any way, circulation to the flap will be compromised and that piece of skin will die if the circulation to it is not quickly restored. Therefore, in treating a partially avulsed piece of skin, quickly irrigate any dirt or debris out of the wound and then gently fold the skin flap back onto the wound so that it is more or less normally aligned. Hold the flap in place with a dry, sterile compression dressing.

When a part of the body is completely avulsed, that is, amputated—whether a section of skin or an entire limb—it is important to try to PRESERVE THE AMPUTATED PART in optimum condition, to maximize the chances of its being successfully reimplanted. Once the victim's injuries have been stabilized, turn your attention to the amputated part, which will also require meticulous care.

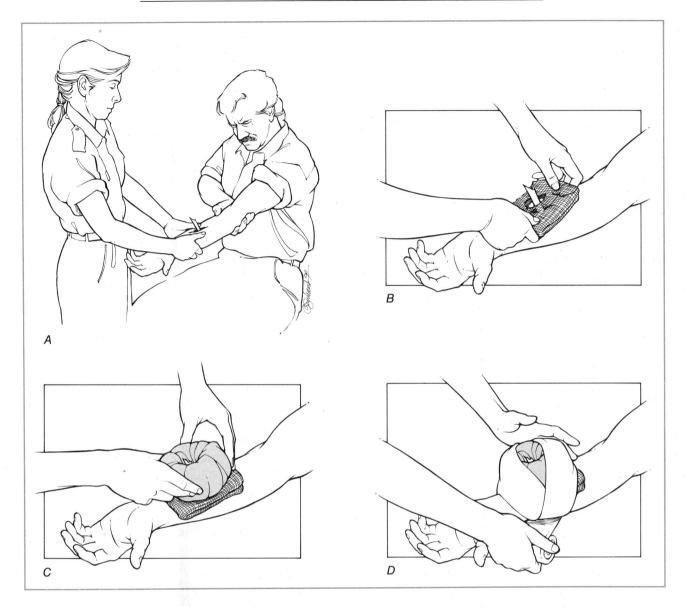

FIGURE 15-3.   STABILIZING AN IMPALED OBJECT.   (A) Apply direct pressure at the wound edges to control bleeding. (B) Cut a hole through several layers of gauze and gently slip them over the impaled object. (C) Use triangular bandages to build a "doughnut" around the object. (D) Secure the "doughnut" and gauze pads with a triangular bandage. (Question: What's wrong with this picture? See Question 13 in Chap. 28 of the *Study Guide for Emergency Care in the Streets, Fifth Edition*.)

PRESERVATION OF AMPUTATED PARTS

- RINSE the amputated part free of debris with cool, sterile saline.
- WRAP the part loosely in saline-moistened sterile gauze.
- SEAL the amputated part inside a plastic bag, and place it in a cool container (e.g., a styro-foam cooler). Keep it cold, but do not allow it to freeze.
- NEVER WARM AN AMPUTATED PART.
- NEVER PLACE AN AMPUTATED PART IN WATER.
- NEVER PLACE AN AMPUTATED PART DIRECTLY ON ICE.
- NEVER USE DRY ICE TO COOL AN AMPUTATED PART.

Transport of the patient and his amputated part should be as expeditious as possible. When the amputated part is a limb or part of a limb, notify the emergency room in advance of the type of case you are transporting and your estimated time of arrival, so that a surgical team can be mobilized while you are en route.

CONTROL OF EXTERNAL BLEEDING

External bleeding is bleeding that can be seen coming from a wound, when the integrity of the skin has been violated. Theoretically, bleeding can be characterized according to the type of blood vessel that has been damaged. ARTERIAL BLEEDING occurs in spurts, and the blood is usually bright red (why?). VENOUS BLEEDING, on the other hand, is more likely to be slow and steady, and the color of the blood is darker. In fact, most open wounds show a combination of arterial and venous bleeding, so the distinction is usually rather academic.

There are fundamentally five methods of controlling external bleeding in the field: direct pressure, elevation, pressure point control, immobilization, and a tourniquet.

Direct Pressure

Application of pressure over a bleeding wound (Fig. 15-4A) stops blood from flowing into the damaged

FIGURE 15-4. METHODS TO CONTROL EXTERNAL BLEEDING. (A) Direct manual pressure. (B) Air splint. (C) MAST. (D) Pressure point control. (E) Splint. (F) Tourniquet.

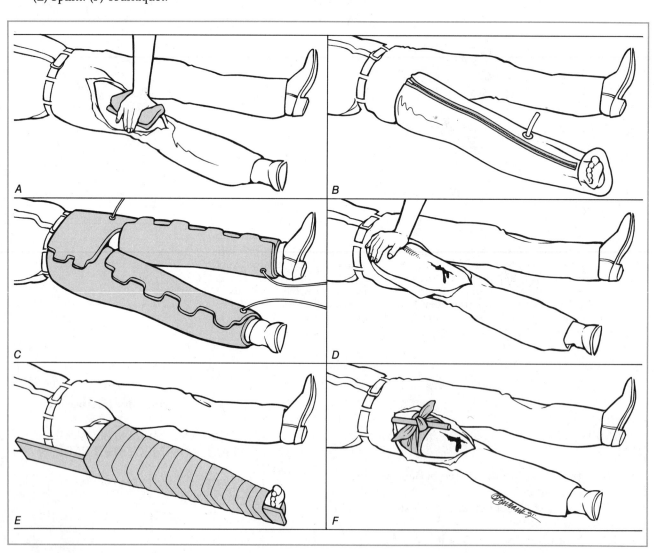

vessel(s) and thereby allows the platelets to do their job of sealing up the vascular walls.

> **STEADY, DIRECT PRESSURE AGAINST THE BLEEDING SITE IS THE MOST EFFECTIVE MEANS TO CONTROL BLEEDING.**

If possible, use a sterile dressing to exert pressure, otherwise a clean cloth or handkerchief. If there aren't any dressings or clean cloths available, then use your gloved hand to apply pressure over the bleeding site. To maintain pressure, apply a pressure dressing over the site. On an extremity, one effective way of maintaining uniform pressure on a bleeding site is to apply an AIR SPLINT (Fig. 15-4B) over the dressed wound. If one or both of the *lower* extremities are bleeding, the MAST can also be used to apply pressure (Fig. 15-4C). Pressure over the bleeding site should be maintained until the bleeding stops or until the patient reaches the hospital and other personnel take responsibility for his care.

Elevation

When venous bleeding occurs from an extremity, the rate of bleeding can be substantially slowed by elevating the extremity above the level of the heart. Elevation of the extremity will not by itself control bleeding, but it may be helpful in conjunction with other measures, such as direct pressure.

Pressure Point Control

When direct pressure by itself is not sufficient to control bleeding, or when there are a number of bleeding points supplied by the same artery, pressure point control (Fig. 15-4D) may help slow the bleeding. The artery chosen must be fairly superficial and overlie a hard structure against which it can be compressed. Thus, the pressure points most frequently used are

- The **temporal artery,** which overlies the temporal bone of the skull and is used to control bleeding from the SCALP
- The **brachial artery,** which overlies the humerus and is used to control bleeding from the FOREARM
- The **femoral artery,** which can be compressed against the pelvis and is used to control bleeding from the LEG

Splinting

Any movement of an extremity, even an uninjured extremity, promotes blood flow within the extremity. When, in addition, the extremity is injured, motion may also disrupt the clotting process and lacerate more blood vessels. It follows, therefore, that *preventing* motion of an injured extremity will have the opposite effects. That is the reason for splinting a bleeding extremity. Any kind of splint will do, such as the padded board splint shown in Figure 15-4E. Use of an air splint, however, once again gives a double benefit—splinting *and* direct pressure.

Tourniquet

It is rarely, if ever, necessary to use a tourniquet, for control of external hemorrhage can almost always be achieved by one or more of the methods already described. Furthermore, use of a tourniquet is associated with several potential *hazards*, including damage to nerves and blood vessels and, when the tourniquet is in place for an extended period, loss of the distal extremity. A tourniquet applied too loosely, on the other hand, may actually increase bleeding if venous return has been occluded without hampering arterial inflow. For all those reasons,

> **USE A TOURNIQUET ONLY AS A LAST RESORT, WHEN IT IS THE ONLY WAY TO SAVE THE PATIENT'S LIFE.**

Having said all that, it is true that there are rare cases in which a tourniquet may be lifesaving, particularly in patients who have suffered a traumatic partial amputation of a limb. If a tourniquet *is* required, observe the following guidelines in its application (Fig. 15-4F):

> **GUIDELINES FOR USE OF A TOURNIQUET**
>
> - Use WIDE, FLAT MATERIALS ONLY, such as a cravat or folded handkerchief. Never use rope, wire, or other narrow materials that might cut into the skin and damage underlying tissues.
> - Apply a PAD over the artery to be compressed.
> - Wrap the tourniquet TWICE around the ex-

tremity, at a point about 4 inches distal to the axilla or groin, and tie a half-knot.

- Place a stick, pencil, or similar object on top of the half knot, and complete the square knot above the stick (Fig. 15-5A).
- Twist the stick to tighten the tourniquet UNTIL THE BLEEDING STOPS AND NO FURTHER. Secure the stick in that position.
- NEVER COVER A TOURNIQUET with a bandage or anything else, lest it escape notice when the patient arrives at the hospital. To make doubly sure that the tourniquet is not overlooked, write "TK" on the patient's forehead with a grease pencil.
- RECORD on the patient's trip sheet THE TIME that the tourniquet was applied.

THERMAL BURNS

Thermal burns are burns caused by exposure to more heat energy than the body can absorb without damage. That exposure can take place in one of several ways. Most commonly, thermal burns are caused by OPEN FLAME, from careless handling of matches or flammable materials, residential fires, and sometimes industrial fires. Flame burns are very often deep burns, especially if a person's clothing caught fire, and are apt to be associated with inhalation injuries as well. HOT LIQUIDS produce *scald injuries*. The victims are most often children, who are apt to overturn a cup of coffee from the table or a pot of boiling liquid from the stove. Scald injuries usually are not as deep as those caused by open flame (although boiling grease or boiling water *can* produce deep burns), and they are less likely than other types of burns to be associated with nonburn injuries. Coming in contact with HOT OBJECTS, such as the burner of an electric stove, produces *contact burns*. Ordinarily, reflexes protect a person from prolonged exposure to a very hot object, so contact burns are not usually deep unless the victim was somehow prevented from drawing away from the hot object (e.g., unconscious, intoxicated). Finally, a relatively rare source of burns is the FLASH produced by some explosions, which may briefly expose a person to very intense heat. Victims of flash burns nearly always have other injuries from the explosion.

The Primary Survey in the Burned Patient

Burns are soft tissue injuries, and soft tissue injuries are, as noted earlier, relatively low-priority injuries. A whole host of other considerations must precede our attention to the burn itself. As always, the primary survey comes first.

Hazards: Dealing with the Fire

The very first step in dealing with the victim of a flame injury, once both you and the victim are in a safe environment, is to PUT OUT THE FIRE! That may seem obvious, but it is remarkable how many patients still arrive by ambulance at hospital emergency departments with clothes smoldering. A person whose clothing is on fire should not be permitted to run, since that serves to fan the flames; nor should he remain standing, since he is more apt to inhale flame or to ignite his hair in the upright position. Rather, place him on the floor or ground, and use the most expeditious means to smother the flames: Roll him in a blanket or douse him with large quantities of water. Be sure to remove all smoldering clothing and any articles that may retain heat. If bits of smoldering cloth are adhered to the skin, *cut* them away, do not pull them away. Melted synthetic fabrics adhered to the skin prolong the duration of exposure to

FIGURE 15-5. APPLICATION OF A TOURNIQUET. (A) Cravat is wrapped twice around the arm, over padded artery; (B) cravat is twisted with a stick until bleeding slows and can be controlled thereafter by direct pressure.

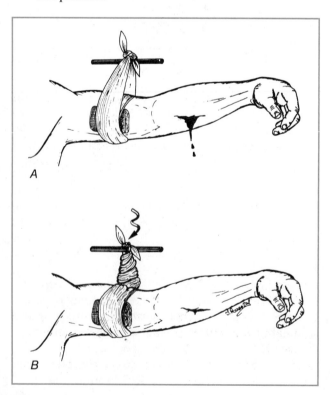

high heat, so if the fabric cannot be easily removed, quickly soak it in cold water to terminate its burning effect.

Ensure an Open AIRWAY

As in any other seriously ill or injured patient, in the burned patient, the airway comes first. In the burned patient, furthermore, the airway may be in particular jeopardy, for the same heat and flames that caused his external burn may have produced potentially life-threatening damage to the airway. Laryngeal edema can develop with alarming speed in burn victims, especially in infants and children, and early endotracheal intubation, before the airway has closed off altogether, may be lifesaving in such cases. To intervene early, however, you need to spot the problem early, and to do that, you need to be alert for the *clues to respiratory involvement:*

SUSPECT RESPIRATORY TRACT INJURY IN BURNS WHEN:

- There is a HISTORY of
  1. Exposure to smoke or hot gases
  2. Confinement in a closed space when the burn occurred
  3. Loss of consciousness in a burning area
- PHYSICAL EXAMINATION reveals
  1. Facial burns
  2. Singed nasal hairs
  3. Blistering or redness inside the mouth
  4. Hoarseness, stridor, or brassy cough
  5. Sooty sputum
  6. Wheezing

If any of those clues are present, notify the base physician at once with a full report, so that a decision can be made about early nasotracheal intubation. Bear in mind that intubation of an awake, scared patient in the field is no picnic, and considerable further damage can be inflicted on the airway if the patient is struggling. If intubation does become necessary under such circumstances, explain carefully to the patient what is to be done, why it is necessary, and how he can best cooperate. Have all the equipment set up at your side so that intubation, once begun, can proceed rapidly and smoothly.

Even if there is no evidence of airway involvement, early intubation should also be considered in any fire victim who is stuporous or comatose.

Acute gastric dilatation occurs commonly in severely burned patients. Distention of the stomach may interfere with the patient's breathing and, more importantly, may lead to regurgitation of stomach contents. An awake patient can usually protect his airway against aspiration of stomach contents; a stuporous or comatose patient cannot. So the airway of a comatose burn victim needs to be secured with an endotracheal tube, after which (and *only* after which) a nasogastric (NG) tube may be passed to decompress the stomach.

Given the risks of gastric dilatation and regurgitation in burned patients, it is clear that a patient with significant burns should be given NOTHING BY MOUTH.

Ensure Adequate BREATHING

The vast majority of deaths from fires are not from the burn wound but rather related to pulmonary injury or the inhalation of toxic gases. Direct pulmonary injury may occur from the inhalation of very hot *steam*, which can conduct heat all the way down into the smaller airways and produce damage at the bronchiolar and alveolar level. At the same time, carbon monoxide and other toxic products of combustion can displace oxygen from both the alveolar air and the blood hemoglobin. We shall deal with toxic inhalations in greater detail in Chapter 22. For our purposes here, it is sufficient to emphasize that

---

EVERY PERSON BURNED IN A FIRE SHOULD RECEIVE OXYGEN.

Ensure Adequate CIRCULATION

When a severely burned person is treated in a burn unit, a great deal of emphasis is given, during the first 24 to 48 hours of his care, to fluid resuscitation, to try to prevent what is called **burn shock.** Burn shock occurs partly because of fluid loss across the damaged skin, but also because of a series of volume shifts within the body itself. Capillaries become leaky, so intravascular volume oozes out of the circulation into the interstitial spaces. Meanwhile, cells of normal tissues take in increased amounts of salt and water from the fluid around them.

While those changes take place rapidly, they do not take place as rapidly as bleeding. So it is a reasonably safe general rule that:

IF A BURNED PATIENT IS IN SHOCK IN THE PREHOSPITAL PHASE, LOOK FOR ANOTHER INJURY AS THE SOURCE OF SHOCK.

The Secondary Survey in the Burned Patient

Only when you have completed the primary survey as described should you take time to obtain the more detailed information that the secondary survey provides.

Taking the History

In questioning the burn victim or others at the scene, it is important to obtain at least the following information:

- What is the patient's CHIEF COMPLAINT? *You may think it's the burn, but you could be in for a surprise ("I think I broke my leg when I jumped out of the window. . . .").*
- WHEN precisely did the burn occur (i.e., how long before your arrival)?
- With WHAT was the patient burned? Open flame? Hot liquids? A hot object?
- What, if anything, has the patient or bystanders done for the injury?
- Was the patient in a CLOSED SPACE with smoke, steam, or other products of combustion? If so, for how long? Did he LOSE CONSCIOUSNESS at any point?
- Does the patient have any significant UNDERLYING MEDICAL PROBLEMS? Ask specifically about *heart disease* and *kidney disease*, which could complicate fluid therapy, and about *pulmonary problems*, which could cause a more severe reaction to smoke inhalation.

It is a good idea, in any case, to START INTRAVENOUS FLUIDS as early as possible in any patient who has been severely burned. Do not delay transport to do so, but try to get a large-bore (16- to 18-gauge) IV catheter into an antecubital vein (it's OK to use the burned extremity if you can't find another site; an IV in a burned upper extremity is still preferable to an IV in a lower extremity). The IV fluid of choice in burns is LACTATED RINGER'S solution. According to most of the experts, you can approximate the amount of fluid the burned patient will need by using the **Parkland formula,** which states that *during the first 24 hours*, the burned patient will need

4 ml/kg body weight/% of body surface burned

Half of that amount needs to be given during the first 8 hours. Thus, for example, if a 70-kg man has sustained burns to 30 percent of his body, his fluid needs over the first 8 hours will be

$$\tfrac{1}{2} \times 4 \text{ ml} \times 70 \text{ kg} \times 30 = 4{,}200 \text{ ml}$$

which works out to about 525 ml per hour.

You will doubtless need to know the Parkland formula for your certification examinations. In actual practice in the field, however, where both the patient's weight and the precise extent of his burns may be difficult to establish with any accuracy, the following general guidelines are usually adequate:

Physical Assessment

Proceed through the steps of physical assessment in the usual sequence, starting with the patient's general appearance, then his vital signs. Take particular note of the pulse and respirations, and repeat the measurements frequently. A rising PULSE may be one of the first indications of hypoxemia or impending shock. An increasing rate of RESPIRATIONS suggests compromise of the airway or problems developing within the lungs.

It is only when we reach the head-to-toe survey that we actually take a look at the burn itself. In assessing the burn, we want to establish three things:

- How *deep* is the burn?
- How *extensive* is the burn?
- How *critical* is the burn?

PREHOSPITAL FLUID RESUSCITATION IN BURNS

- ADULTS: Start at 500 to 1,000 ml per hour.*
- CHILDREN:
  Age 5 and over: Start at 500 ml per hour.
  Under 5: Start at 150 ml per hour.

*Check with base physician if patient is known to have cardiac or renal disease.

How Deep Is the Burn?

It is customary to classify burns, first of all, according to the depth of damage they have inflicted (Fig. 15-6).

- A **first-degree burn** is limited to the *epidermis*. The skin is fiery red and very painful, but usually there are no blisters. First-degree burns ordinarily heal in 3 to 7 days, often with peeling of the outer epidermal layer but without permanent scarring. Sunburn is a typical example of first-degree burn.
- A **second-degree burn** (also called a partial-thickness burn) penetrates more deeply than a first-degree burn, involving destruction of all the epidermal layers and extending into the dermis. Second-degree burns are sometimes subclassified as either superficial or deep. *Superficial second-degree burns* involve only the outermost part of the dermis and are characterized by extreme pain and hypersensitivity to touch. The skin looks MOIST and MOTTLED pink or red, and it BLANCHES ON PRESSURE. Hairs on the skin are intact. There are usually BLISTERS. Superficial second-degree burns usually heal by themselves in 10 to 18 days without leaving permanent scars. *Deep second-degree burns,* on the other hand, involve tissue destruction down to the deepest layers of the dermis. Such burns may be moist and blistered like more superficial second-degree burns, but more often they tend to be DRY, with areas of mottled red mixed with whitish patches. The skin does not blanch on pressure. It may or may not be painful. Healing may take weeks and leave bad scars. Furthermore, deep second-degree burns are easily infected; and, by definition,

if a second-degree burn becomes infected, it converts to a third-degree burn.

- A **third degree burn,** or full-thickness burn, involves destruction of all the epidermal *and* dermal layers, right down to the subcutaneous tissue. The skin in a third-degree burn may appear charred and leathery or may be pale and dry. Sometimes thrombosed veins are visible through a translucent, pearly surface. Pain is usually absent because the nerve endings in the dermis have been destroyed. Healing can occur only by skin grafting or with scarring.
- Some sources also refer to an additional category of burns, **fourth-degree burns,** to denote involvement of even deeper tissues, such as muscle and bone. For field purposes, such additional distinctions are probably not necessary. As is, the depth of a burn is usually quite difficult to determine precisely during the first few hours, and a really accurate assessment requires repeated observation over 2 to 3 days. What we are after in the field is a rough initial estimate that will enable us to make appropriate decisions about where to evacuate the patient.

How Extensive Is the Burn?

The next thing you need to determine is how large an area of the body the burn covers. To do so, you will have to remove the patient's clothing, which also provides a good opportunity for removing jewelry, belt buckles, boots, and other items that can both retain heat and obscure burned areas.

For burns covering very small areas, the **Rule of Palms** can help us estimate the extent of the burn. The Rule of Palms is based on the observation that the palm of a person's hand constitutes about 1 per-

FIGURE 15-6. THE DEPTH OF A BURN. (A) First-degree burn. (B) Second-degree burn. (C) Third-degree burn.

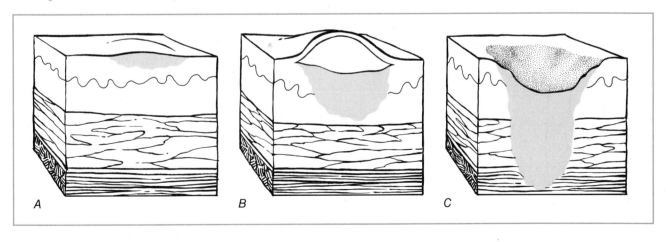

cent of his body surface area (BSA). So if a person has a burn that covers an area about three times the size of his palm, for example, we would estimate it to involve approximately 3 percent of his body surface area.

For more extensive burns, it is customary to use the **Rule of Nines** (Fig. 15-7) to estimate the percent BSA involved. Strictly speaking, calculations of the extent of a burn are based only on second- and third-degree burns present, but for practical purposes in the field, *include all burned areas* in your assessment. As noted earlier, it is very difficult to determine the ultimate depth of a burn during the first hours after injury, and generally first- and second-degree burns are so intermingled that it is impossible to sort out which is which under field conditions.

You will no doubt encounter other, more accurate systems for determining the extent of burn injury, such as the Lund and Browder chart, which corrects for changes in body dimensions due to growth. Such systems are very useful in hospital burn units; they are not so useful, and not at all necessary, in the pre-hospital phase of treatment. Once again, what we are after in the field is a *quick estimate* of the extent of the burn, which one ought to be able to make in about 15 to 30 seconds without recourse to a pocket calculator.

FIGURE 15-7. RULE OF NINES.

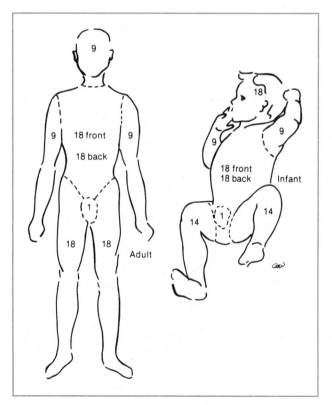

How Critical Is the Burn?

Finally, we need to come to some assessment of the overall severity of the burn (and the patient's other injuries) in order to choose the hospital best suited to care for this particular patient's problem. The following should be considered critical burns that warrant transport to a major burn treatment center:

CRITICAL BURNS

- Burns of any degree involving MORE THAN 25 percent BSA
- THIRD-DEGREE burns involving MORE THAN 10 percent BSA
- Burns complicated by RESPIRATORY INJURY
- Almost all burns of the FACE, HANDS, FEET, or GENITALIA
- Burns complicated by FRACTURE or MAJOR SOFT TISSUE INJURY
- ELECTRIC burns and DEEP CHEMICAL BURNS
- Burns occurring in patients with SERIOUS UNDERLYING DISEASE (e.g., heart disease, diabetes)
- Burns in INFANTS (see Chap. 30) and in the ELDERLY

The Rest of the Head-to-Toe Survey

When you have finished your brief inspection of the patient's skin, you have only just begun the head-to-toe survey. Remember, the burn is a low-priority injury. The purpose of doing the head-to-toe survey is to make sure there are no other injuries that have higher priority for treatment. Often such injuries may be obscured by the burn itself, so you need to pay attention to the circumstances of the burn and the possible mechanisms of injury. If the patient jumped from a second-story window, for example, there may be fractures beneath the obvious burns of his legs.

Look for injuries to the EYES, and cover injured eyes with moist, sterile pads. Check the NECK, CHEST, and EXTREMITIES for *circumferential burns.* Progressive edema beneath a circumferential burn—especially when the burned skin has become leathery and unyielding—may act as a tourniquet. In the neck, a circumferential burn may strangle the patient; in the chest, it may restrict his respirations; and in an extremity, it may cut off the circulation and put the extremity in jeopardy. Patients with circumferential burns must therefore reach a medical facility quickly, for it may be necessary to make an incision into the burned area to decompress it. CHECK THE DISTAL PULSES IN BURNED EXTREMITIES. Any limb without a pulse should be cooled with towels soaked in cold water while the patient is transported urgently to the hospital.

Management of the Burned Patient

General Management

Management of the burned patient in fact begins with the steps taken during the primary survey to extinguish the fire and ensure an adequate airway, breathing, and circulation. Only when the ABCs are under control should you turn your attention to the burn itself.

Management of the Burn Wound

First-Degree Burns

Although first-degree burns can be very painful, they rarely pose a threat to life unless they involve nearly the whole surface of the body. If you reach the patient with first-degree burns within about the first hour of the injury, immerse the burned area in cool water or apply cold compresses to the burn. Burned hands or feet may be soaked directly in cool water, while towels soaked in cold water may be applied to burns of the face or trunk. The object of the exercise is twofold: to stop the burning process and to provide relief of pain. The Water-Jel dressing is a commercially available product that does both those things very well and also provides a good burn dressing in the bargain. However you cool the burn, take care not to cool the whole patient; that is, don't let the patient get chilled. A dry sheet or blanket applied over the wet dressings will help prevent systemic heat loss.

Whatever you put on the burn, DO NOT USE SALVES, OINTMENTS, CREAMS, SPRAYS, OR ANY SIMILAR MATERIALS ON ANY TYPE OF BURN. They will just have to be scrubbed off in the emergency department, causing the patient further pain.

> **NEVER PUT GOO ON A BURN!**

No further treatment should be necessary in the field for the uncomplicated first-degree burn; simply transport the patient in a comfortable position to the hospital.

Second-Degree Burns

Treatment of second-degree burns in the field is very similar to that of first degree. Again, immersion of the burned area in cold water or application of wet or Water-Jel dressings within the first hour can diminish edema and provide significant pain relief. Burned extremities should also be elevated, again to minimize edema formation.

DO NOT ATTEMPT TO RUPTURE BLISTERS OVER THE BURN; they are the best burn dressing God or man ever devised. If second-degree burns cover more than 15 percent of the body, or if accompanied by first-degree burns covering more than about 30 percent of the body, start *intravenous fluids* with Ringer's lactate as described earlier.

Pain in second-degree burns may be very severe. If wet dressings do not provide sufficient pain relief, give *morphine*, 2 to 4 mg slowly *IV*. Do not give any narcotic drugs, however, until after fluid resuscitation is well established (i.e., until after you have run in at least 200 ml and the patient's vital signs are stable).

Third-Degree Burns

Third-degree burns will not require analgesics or any other special measures other than those already instituted (e.g., intravenous fluids). The burns themselves should simply be covered with dry sterile dressings (if the burned area is extensive, cover the whole patient with a sterile sheet), and the patient should be protected from extremes of temperature.

SUMMARY: APPROACH TO THE BURNED PATIENT

1. PUT OUT THE FIRE!
2. Safeguard the AIRWAY: Be alert for clues to an airway in jeopardy.
3. Help the patient to BREATHE: Give *oxygen*.
4. Ensure the CIRCULATION: Start *intravenous fluids*.
5. Do the SECONDARY SURVEY:
   a. Find out the *circumstances* of the burn.
   b. Check VITAL SIGNS often.
   c. Be alert for
      (1) Injuries sustained in falls (fractures, spine injury).
      (2) Circumferential burns.
      (3) Absence of distal pulses.

6. Treat the burns
   a. No goo!
   b. Cold, wet dressings covered by dry dressings.
   c. Elevate burned extremities; remove constricting jewelry.
   d. Give morphine, 2 to 4 mg IV *after* IV therapy is established.
7. Splint fractures.
8. Give nothing by mouth.
9. Keep the patient warm.

For special considerations in burned children, see Chapter 30.

CHEMICAL BURNS

Chemical burns occur when the skin comes in contact with strong acids, alkalis, or other corrosive materials; the burn will progress so long as the corrosive substance remains in contact with the skin. Thus, the cornerstone of therapy is removal of the chemical from contact with the patient's body.

SPEED IS ESSENTIAL. Begin flushing the exposed area of the patient's body immediately with copious quantities of water. If the patient is in or near the home, the shower or a garden hose is ideal. In an industrial setting, use the decontamination shower or a hose. After an initial flushing of at least 5 minutes, rapidly remove the patient's clothing, especially shoes and socks, that may have become contaminated with the offending agent, taking care not to get any of the hazardous chemicals on your own clothing or skin. Do not waste time looking for specific antidotes; copious flushing with water is more effective and more immediately available. Furthermore, so-called neutralizing agents often work by combining with the chemical that caused the burn in an exothermic reaction, that is, a reaction that produces heat. Thus, the very process of neutralizing the offending chemical may cause further burns to the patient.

Flushing should be continued for a *minimum* of 30 minutes before moving the patient; for chemical burns caused by strong alkalis (e.g., oven and drain cleaners), 1 to 2 *hours* of flushing is recommended. When flushing is complete, cover the burned area with a sterile dressing, or cover the whole patient with a sterile sheet, and transport the patient to the hospital.

> **THE TREATMENT FOR A CHEMICAL BURN IS WATER, WATER, AND MORE WATER.**

Special Cases

In alkali burns caused by DRY LIME, combination with water will produce a highly corrosive substance. For that reason, when a patient has been in contact with dry lime, *first* remove his clothing and *brush* as much lime as you can from his skin (wear gloves!!). *Then* start flushing copiously with a garden hose or shower, and continue flushing for at least 30 minutes.

SODIUM METALS produce considerable heat when mixed with water and may explode. Cover the burn with oil, which will stop the reaction by preventing the sodium from coming in contact with the atmosphere.

HYDROFLUORIC ACID (HF) is used in drain cleaners in the home; industrially it is used for etching glass and plastic. The patient burned with HF will complain bitterly of pain, and the pain won't get any better even with continuous flushing—a sign that the process of tissue destruction is still ongoing. Treatment of HF burns requires injection of calcium gluconate into the burn wound, a procedure that should be undertaken in the emergency room, not in the field. The patient with HF burns, therefore, should be moved to the hospital after an initial 5 to 10 minutes of flushing to remove surface chemical.

HOT TAR BURNS are, strictly speaking, thermal burns, not chemical burns, although they tend to get classified with chemical burns. The most important treatment in the prehospital phase is to IMMERSE THE AFFECTED AREA IN COLD WATER to dissipate the heat from the tar and speed up the hardening process. Once the tar has cooled, it will not do any further damage, and there is no need to try to remove it in the field.

IF YOU DON'T KNOW the identity of the chemical that caused the burn, assume it is *not* a special case, and flush the burn wound with water for at least 30 minutes as described.

Chemical Burns of the Eye

If chemicals have splashed into the patient's eyes, the eyes too must be flushed with copious amounts of water. The most efficient way to do so is simply to support the patient's head under a faucet, directing a steady stream of lukewarm tap water into the affected eye (Fig. 15-8). If the patient wears contact lenses and the stream of water does not flush them out, pause after a minute or two of irrigation to allow the patient to remove his contact lenses, for if they remain in place, they will prevent water from reaching the cornea underneath. Be sure to irrigate well underneath the eyelids. NEVER USE ANY CHEMICAL ANTIDOTES (e.g., vinegar, baking soda) IN THE EYES. Irrigate with water only. After a *minimum* of 30 minutes, irrigation, patch the patient's eyes with lightly applied dressings and transport him to the hospital for evaluation.

ELECTRIC BURNS

High-voltage electric injuries account for approximately 3 percent of hospital admissions for burns, and there are about 1,200 accidental deaths by electrocution in the United States each year. In one recent survey of electric injuries, the majority of victims were found to have been electrocuted in the course of their work (one third of them were linemen or electricians). Domestic injuries, on the other hand, are most likely to involve children.

Electric burns may produce devastating internal injury with little external evidence. The degree of tissue injury in an electric burn is related to the resistance of various body tissues, the intensity of current that passes through the victim, and the duration of exposure.

FIGURE 15-8. CHEMICAL BURNS TO THE EYES.
Flush the affected eye under a gentle stream of water for at least 20 minutes (hold the eyelids open if necessary).

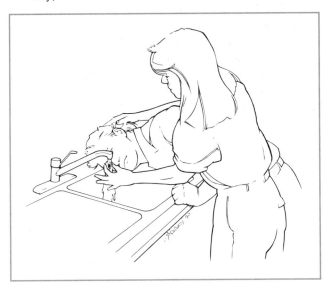

When a person comes in contact with an electric source, the amount of current delivered to the inside of the body will depend to some extent on the resistance of his skin; wet, thin, clean skin offers less resistance than dry, thick, dirty skin; thus a moist inner surface of the forearm will have much less resistance than a dry, calloused palm.

As electric current travels from the contact site into the body, it is converted to *heat*, which follows the current flow—usually along blood vessels and nerves—causing extensive damage to the tissues in its wake. When the voltage is low (i.e., under 1,000 volts, as in household sources), current follows the path of least resistance, generally along blood vessels, nerves, and muscles; when the voltage is high, as that from high tension lines, current takes the shortest path. In either case, the greater the current flow, the greater the heat generated.

Alternating current is considerably more dangerous than direct current because the alternations cause repetitive (*tetanic*) muscle contractions, which may "freeze" the victim to the conductor until the current source is turned off. Furthermore, alternating current is more likely than direct current to induce ventricular fibrillation. The direction of current flow is also significant. Current moving from one hand to the other is particularly dangerous, since current may then flow across the heart; a current of only 0.1 ampere to the heart can provoke ventricular fibrillation.

Burn Injuries from Electricity

Electricity can cause three types of burns. The most common is the type I burn, or **contact burn,** a true electric injury in which the current is most intense at the entrance and exit sites. At those points, you may see a characteristic *bull's-eye lesion*, with a central, charred zone of third-degree burns; a middle zone of cold, gray, dry tissue; and an outer, red zone of coagulation necrosis. The contact burn, while usually not in itself very serious, is an important marker, for it may signal devastating injury inside the body.

The type II burn, or **flash burn,** is really an electrothermal injury and is caused by the arcing of electric current. If a person passes close enough to a source of high voltage current, he will reach a point where the resistance of the air between the current source and himself is sufficiently low that current arcs through the air, from the current source to the passerby. An arc of that sort has a temperature anywhere from 3,000 to 20,000°C—high enough to produce significant charring.

The type III electric burn, or **flame burn,** is another thermal injury; it occurs when electricity ignites a person's clothing or surroundings.

Nonburn Injuries from Electricity

Burns may be only one of the problems of a patient who has come in contact with an electric source—and not necessarily the most serious.

The two most common causes of death from electric injury are asphyxia and cardiac arrest. ASPHYXIA may occur when prolonged contact with alternating current induces tetanic contractions of the respiratory muscles; asphyxia may also be the result of current passing through the respiratory center in the brain and knocking out the impulse to breathe. CARDIAC ARREST may occur either secondarily, from hypoxia, or as a direct result of the electric shock. As noted earlier, currents as small as 0.1 ampere can trigger ventricular fibrillation if they pass directly through the heart, which is particularly likely when current travels across the body from hand to hand. In cases where cardiac arrest does not occur, cardiac damage may nonetheless be manifest in various rhythm disturbances seen on the electrocardiogram.

A whole host of NEUROLOGIC COMPLICATIONS have been reported in connection with electric injury, including seizures, delirium, confusion, coma, and temporary quadriplegia.

DAMAGE TO THE KIDNEYS is common after electric injury and resembles the syndrome seen after a crush injury, which is due to the breakdown products of damaged muscle (myoglobin) being liberated into the circulation.

Severe tetanic muscle spasms may lead to FRACTURES and DISLOCATIONS, which are often overlooked because of preoccupation with the electric injury itself. Posterior dislocation of the shoulder and fracture of the scapula—both otherwise rather rare injuries—have been reported in a number of cases of electrocution. And don't forget the CERVICAL SPINE, especially in a lineman who has fallen from a utility pole.

Approach to the Patient Who Has Suffered Electric Injury

In dealing with the victim of an electric injury, the usual priorities apply.

Hazard Control

The first priority at the scene of an electric injury is to protect yourself and bystanders from becoming the next victims. Do *not* use a rope, wooden pole, or any other object to try to dislodge the victim from the current source. Do *not* try to cut the wire. Do not go anywhere near a high-tension line. There is only one safe way to deal with a live high-tension wire and that is:

> ## CALL THE ELECTRIC COMPANY.

Wait until a qualified person has shut off the power before you approach the victim.

Primary Survey

As soon as the electric hazard has been neutralized, proceed to the ABCs. As you open the airway, bear in mind the possibility of cervical spine injury, and avoid hyperextension of the head. Start cardiopulmonary resuscitation (CPR) as indicated. If the electrocution occurred in a relatively inaccessible place, such as on a utility pole, it will be necessary to start rescue breathing at once, while the victim is still on the pole, and then lower the victim to the ground as quickly as possible.

Secondary Survey

Make careful note of the patient's state of consciousness, and record his vital signs. Try to determine the path the current has taken through the body by looking for an ENTRANCE WOUND and an EXIT WOUND and by carefully palpating the skin and soft tissues. When deep tissues have been seriously damaged by heat, the surrounding muscle swells and becomes rock-hard. Thus, if you find a rigid abdomen or rigid extremity, there is a high probability of serious internal injury. Be alert for FRACTURES or DISLOCATIONS, and check the distal pulses on all four extremities.

Treatment at the Scene

If the patient is in cardiac arrest, CPR with advanced life support will, of course, have priority; there is usually a very good chance of successfully resuscitating the victim of an electric injury, but it may require prolonged CPR to do so. If the patient is not in cardiac arrest, observe the following treatment guidelines:

**TREATMENT OF
ELECTRIC INJURIES**

- Administer oxygen.
- MONITOR cardiac rhythm.
- Start at least one IV and run in lactated Ringer's solution wide open, to keep the kidneys flushed out.
- Contact base physician for orders, which may include:
  1. SODIUM BICARBONATE, 1 to 2 ampules, to alkalinize the urine (which promotes excretion of myoglobin).
  2. MANNITOL, 0.5 gm per kilogram, to induce an osmotic diuresis, which also helps clear myoglobin from the kidneys.
- Cover any surface burns with dry, sterile dressings.
- Splint any fractures.
- If the patient has fallen, immobilize the cervical spine.

LIGHTNING INJURIES

One special case of electric injury deserves specific mention, and that is the injury sustained from lightning. It is estimated that approximately 1,000 persons are injured by lightning in the United States each year, of whom between 250 and 300 die. Those figures indicate that the majority of those injured by lightning do survive, and indeed there have been several instances reported in which lightning victims who seemed to be quite "dead" recovered after prolonged resuscitation. Therefore, victims of lightning injury deserve intensive rescue efforts, even when the situation seems hopeless.

Lightning strikes when there is a massive discharge of electricity between two bodies that have different charges, as, for example, between a thundercloud and the earth. The stream of current will take the path of least resistance from its origin to its destination; thus, if there is any object projecting above the surface of the earth that is a better conductor of electricity than the air—such as a building, light pole, antenna, flagpole, or tree—that object will "attract" the lightning bolt. Even a person running across an open field may be the highest object in the area, thereby "attracting" a lightning bolt. Golfers standing on the open fairway with a metal golf club

in hand are at particular risk during an electric storm.

The best treatment for lightning injuries is prevention, and all health professionals have a responsibility to educate the public in preventive measures. Clearly, the most effective prevention of all is to come in out of the rain, but that is not always possible. So one must know what to do if caught in a sudden electric storm:

**PREVENTION OF
LIGHTNING INJURIES**

- STAY LOW. If out in the open, as in a field, lie flat on the ground. Do *not* run across open areas.
- Stay away from objects that project from the ground; do not stand alongside trees, poles, fences, or high buildings.
- Get away from open water.
- Do not hold onto fishing poles, golf clubs, or any other potential lightning rods. Do not fly a kite in the rain, Ben Franklin notwithstanding.
- If in a car, keep the windows shut.

Injuries Produced by Lightning

A lightning strike differs in several important respects from a high-voltage electric current, so the damage it produces is also somewhat different. To begin with, lightning carries enormous electric power—its energy can reach 100 *million* volts and peak currents can be in the range of 200,000 amps. It is, however, *direct*, not alternating current, and the duration of exposure is measured in milliseconds. Thus lightning injuries tend to resemble blast injuries more than they do high-voltage injuries, with damage to the tympanic membranes of the ears and to air-containing internal organs. Muscle damage does occur, however, and the release of myoglobin from injured muscle may, as in high-voltage injury, jeopardize the kidneys.

For the cardiovascular system, lightning acts as a cosmic defibrillator, delivering a massive direct current countershock that depolarizes the entire heart. As in the case of conventional countershock, the heart may resume beating spontaneously a few seconds after the shock or after a couple of minutes of CPR. *Respiratory* arrest, however, is apt to persist for quite a while in lightning victims, so continued artificial ventilation is often needed for hours after the pulse is restored.

The central nervous system is almost invariably affected by a lightning strike. At least 70 percent of victims will *lose consciousness* for some period, and nearly 90 percent will have some confusion or amnesia (loss of memory). Temporary paralysis of the legs is common. Permanent paralysis and quadriplegia have been reported in some cases.

A person need not sustain a direct hit from lightning to be injured; in fact most victims are not struck directly. Much more commonly, the victim is "splashed" by lightning striking a nearby tree or other projecting object. Ground current produced by lightning striking the ground near the victim can also cause severe injury and accounts for incidents in which there are multiple casualties over an extended area, such as on a golf course.

The cutaneous *burn* produced by lightning does not have the charred, bull's-eye appearance of the high-voltage burn; rather, a lightning burn usually has a feathery or zigzag appearance caused by the splash effect.

Nonetheless, the immediate threats to life caused by a lightning strike are the same as those caused by a high-voltage power line injury: airway obstruction, respiratory arrest, and cardiac arrest.

Assessment and Management of Lightning Injuries

When you reach the scene of a lightning strike, all the usual priorities apply, but there are two special considerations to keep in mind:

- HAZARD CONTROL: If the electric storm is still going on, the first priority will be to get the victim(s) and rescuers to a safe place, preferably indoors, or at least inside the ambulance. Lightning *can* strike twice in the same place, and often does. There is, however, *no hazard whatsoever* in touching the victim of a lightning strike; contrary to what your grandmother may have told you, electricity does not remain within the body of a person who has been hit by lightning.
- TRIAGE: A lightning strike is very apt to involve more than one victim. Therefore, the very first thing you need to do on arrival at the scene, before you even leave the safety of the ambulance, is to MAKE A RAPID SURVEY OF THE ENTIRE SCENE TO DETERMINE THE NUMBER OF VICTIMS.

> **IN A LIGHTNING STRIKE WITH MULTIPLE VICTIMS, PRIORITY GOES TO THE VICTIMS WHO ARE NOT BREATHING.**

Carry out the *primary survey* as usual, and start CPR where necessary. In establishing an airway, bear in mind the possibility of CERVICAL SPINE INJURY, and do not hyperextend the neck; use chin lift with the head in neutral position.

Victims of cardiac arrest caused by lightning strike deserve aggressive, continuing CPR, because the chances of a successful resuscitation are excellent, even when the patient looks very dead initially and even when there is a long delay in the return of spontaneous breathing.

> **DON'T GIVE UP QUICKLY ON THE PATIENT IN CARDIAC ARREST DUE TO LIGHTNING.**

If the patient *is* breathing, proceed to the *secondary survey,* and take particular note of

- The patient's STATE OF CONSCIOUSNESS. As noted, confusion, amnesia, and even coma are common. Document the state of consciousness carefully, as described in a previous chapter.
- The VITAL SIGNS. A weak, rapid pulse suggests there is internal bleeding from injury to internal organs.
- The ABDOMEN, for rigidity that may signal injury to abdominal viscera.
- The EXTREMITIES, for deformity (suggesting fracture or dislocation), loss of pulses (suggesting muscle injury and edema within the limb), or paralysis.

Treatment of lightning injuries is very similar to that of injuries sustained from high-voltage lines:

> **TREATMENT OF LIGHTNING INJURIES: SUMMARY**
>
> - EVALUATE THE ENTIRE SCENE FIRST: Priority for treatment goes to victims who are not breathing.

- Establish an AIRWAY, with cervical spine precautions. Perform CPR as needed.
- Administer oxygen.
- MONITOR cardiac rhythm.
- Start a large-bore IV and run in lactated Ringer's solution wide open, to keep the kidneys flushed out.
- If there is evidence of muscle damage, contact the base physician for orders, which may include
    1. SODIUM BICARBONATE, 1 to 2 ampules, to alkalinize the urine (which promotes excretion of myoglobin).
    2. MANNITOL, 0.5 gm per kilogram, to induce an osmotic diuresis, which also helps clear myoglobin from the kidneys.
- Cover any surface burns with dry, sterile dressings.
- Splint any fractures.
- If the patient has fallen, immobilize the cervical spine.

GLOSSARY

abrasion   A portion of the body denuded of epidermis by scraping or rubbing.

adipose   Referring to fat tissue.

amnesia   Loss of memory.

amputation   Injury in which part of the body is completely severed.

avulsion   Injury that leaves a piece of skin or other tissue either partially or completely torn away from the body.

collagen   Protein that gives tensile strength to the connective tissues of the body.

contact burn   Burn produced by touching a hot object.

contusion   A bruise; an injury that causes bleeding beneath the skin but does not break the skin.

dermis   The inner layer of skin, containing hair follicle roots, glands, blood vessels, and nerves.

ecchymosis   Extravasation of blood under the skin to produce a "black-and-blue mark."

elastin   A protein that gives the skin its elasticity.

epidermis   The outermost layer of the skin.

first-degree burn   Burn involving only the epidermis, producing very red, painful skin.

flash burn   Electrothermal injury caused by arcing of electric current.

full-thickness burn   Third-degree burn.

hematoma   A localized collection of blood in the soft tissues as a result of injury or a broken blood vessel.

homeostasis   Tendency to constancy or stability in the body's internal environment.

impaled object   Object that has caused a puncture wound and remains embedded in the wound.

incision   A wound usually made deliberately, as in surgery; a clean cut, as opposed to a laceration.

integument   The skin.

laceration   A wound made by tearing or cutting tissues.

melanin   The pigment that gives skin its color.

myoglobin   A protein found in muscle that is released into the circulation after crush injury or other muscle damage and whose presence in the circulation may produce renal damage.

partial-thickness burn   Second-degree burn.

pedicle   Narrow strip of tissue by which an avulsed piece of tissue remains connected to the body.

scald   Burn produced by hot liquids.

sebaceous gland   Gland located in the dermis that secretes sebum.

sebum   Oily substance secreted by sebaceous glands.

second-degree burn   Burn that involves the epidermis and part of the dermis, characterized by pain and blistering.

subcutaneous   Beneath the skin.

tetany   Sustained contraction of a muscle group.

third-degree burn   Burn that extends through the epidermis and dermis into the subcutaneous tissues beneath.

FURTHER READING

WOUNDS

Angeras MH et al. Comparison between sterile saline and tap water for the cleaning of acute traumatic soft tissue wounds. *Eur J Surg* 158:347, 1992.

Bledsoe B, Bundick K. Cultivating the prehospital care of agricultural emergencies. *JEMS* 17(5):66, 1992.

Connolly JF. Managing cuts and bruises. *Emerg Med* 20(19):78, 1988.

Prasad N. The unkindest cut of all. *Emerg Med Serv* 21(10):55, 1992.

Stueland D, McCarty J, Stamas P Jr. Prehospital care of agricultural injuries. *Prehosp Disaster Med* 8(2):193, 1993.

VanGiesen PJ et al. Storage of amputated parts prior to replantation. *J Hand Surg* 8:60, 1983.

Westreich M, Binns JH, Posch JL. Emergency care of the reimplantation patient. *JACEP* 6:194, 1977.

CONTROL OF EXTERNAL BLEEDING

Porter RS, Verdile VP. Control of external hemorrhage. *Emergency* 22(7):23, 1990.

THERMAL BURNS

Ayvazian BH, Monafo WW. Initial management of the burned patient. *Emerg Med Serv* 5(5):11, 1976.

Ball R. Hot stuff: Assessing and treating burns. *JEMS* 18(2):30, 1993.

Baxter CR, Waeckerle JF. Emergency treatment of burn injury. *Ann Emerg Med* 17:1305, 1988.

Bingham HG. Early management of the burned patient. *Emerg Med Serv* 6(5):9, 1977.

Bloch M. Cold water for burns and scalds. *Lancet* 1:695, 1968.

Bose B, Tredget T. Treatment of hot tar burns. *Can Med Assoc J* 127:21, 1982.

Bourn MK. Fire and smoke: Managing skin and inhalation burns. *JEMS* 14(9):62, 1989.

Cavallo J et al. Sunburn. *Dermatol Clin* 4:181, 1986.

Cemling RH et al. Management of hot tar burns. *J Trauma* 20:242, 1980.

Dimick AR. The burn at first sight. *Emerg Med* 15(15):130, 1983.

Dimick AR, Drabeck T. Respiratory burns. *Emergency* 11(1):49, 1979.

Dimick AR, Wagner R. A matter of burns and breath. *Emergency* 22(13):123, 1990.

Duda J. Burn wise. *Emergency* 21(6):44, 1989.

Edlich RF et al. Emergency department treatment, triage and transfer protocols for the burn patient. *JACEP* 7:152, 1978.

Gillespie RW. The burn at first sight. *Emerg Med* 16(4):141, 1984.

Gursel E, Tintinalli J. Emergency burn management. *JACEP* 7:209, 1978.

Hammond JS, Ward G. Transfers from emergency room to burn center: Errors in burn size estimate. *J Trauma* 27:1161, 1987.

Keswani MH et al. The boiled potato peel as a burn wound dressing: A preliminary report. *Burns* 11:220, 1985.

Lloyd JR. Comprehensive burn care. *Emerg Med Serv* 8(1):9, 8(2):16, 1979.

Luterman A, Talley MA. Field management of burn injuries. *Emerg Med Serv* 17(7):30, 1988.

McKinley JC, Jelenko C, Lasseter MC. Call for help: An algorithm for burn assessment, triage and acute care. *JACEP* 5:13, 1976.

Merrell SW et al. Fluid resuscitation in thermally injured children. *Am J Surg* 152:664, 1986.

Nordberg M. Questions and controversies in burn care. *Emerg Med Serv* 17(9):24, 1988.

Ofeigsson DJ. First-aid treatment of scalds and burns by water cooling. *Postgrad Med* 30:4, 1961.

Raine TJ et al. Cooling the burn wound to maintain microcirculation. *J Trauma* 21:394, 1981.

Rodeheaver GT et al. Extinguishing the flaming burn victim. *JACEP* 8:307, 1979.

Rose A. Continuous water baths for burns. *JAMA* 47:1042, 1906.

Rose HW. Initial cold water treatment for burns. *Northwest Med* 35:267, 1936.

Schreiber MM. Acute sunlight damage to the skin. *Ariz Med* 37:254, 1980.

Shulman AG. Ice water as primary treatment of burns. *JAMA* 173:1916, 1960.

Stewart CE. Sunburn. *Emerg Med Serv* 19(5):81, 1988.

Stratta RG et al. Management of tar and asphalt injuries. *Am J Surg* 146:766, 1983.

Thygerson AL. Burn treatment. *Emergency* 15(6):18, 1983.

Wachtel TL. Major burns: What to do at the scene and en route to the hospital. *Postgrad Med* 85(1):178, 1989.

Waymack JP et al. Acute upper airway obstruction in the postburn period. *Arch Surg* 120:1042, 1985.

CHEMICAL BURNS

Binns H, Gursel E, Wilson N. Gasoline contact burns. *JACEP* 7:404, 1978.

Hansbrough JF et al. Hydrocarbon contact injuries. *J Trauma* 25:250, 1985.

Jelenko C. Chemical burns. *Emerg Med* 5(6):33, 1973.

Luterman A, Fields C, Curreri W. Treatment of chemical burns. *Emerg Med Serv* 17(9):36, 1988.

Salisbury R. A burn primer. *Emerg Med* 20(14):155, 1988.

Skiendzielewski JJ. Cement burns. *Ann Emerg Med* 9:316, 1980.

Tintinalli JE. Hydrofluoric acid burns. *JACEP* 7:24, 1978.

ELECTRIC BURNS

Beswick DR, Morse SD, Barnes AU. Bilateral scapular fractures from low-voltage electrical injury. *Ann Emerg Med* 11:676, 1982.

Bingham H. Electrical burns. *Clin Plast Surg* 13:75, 1986.

Budnick LD. Bathtub-related electrocutions in the United States, 1979 to 1982. *JAMA* 252:918, 1984.

Caroline NL. *Emergency Medical Treatment: A Text for EMT-As and EMT-Intermediates* (3rd ed.). Boston: Little, Brown, 1991. Chap. 13.

Dixon GF. The evaluation and management of electrical injuries. *Crit Care Med* 11:384, 1983.

Fatovich DM et al. Household electrical shocks: Who should be monitored. *Med J Austr* 155:301, 1991.

Fish R. Electric shock, Part II: Nature and mechanisms of injury. *J Emerg Med* 11:457, 1993.

Fontanarosa PB. Taking charge of patients with electrical injuries. *JEMS* 17(3):50, 1992.

Fontanarosa PB. Electrical shock and lightning strike. *Ann Emerg Med* 22:378, 1993.

Hammond JS, Ward G. High-voltage electrical injuries: Management and outcome of 60 cases. *South Med J* 81:1351, 1988.

Housinger TA et al. A prospective study of myocardial damage in electrical injuries. *J Trauma* 25:122, 1985.

Hunt JL, Sato RM, Baxter CR. Acute electric burns. *Arch Surg* 115:434, 1980.

Jensen PJ et al. Electrical injury causing ventricular arrhythmias. *Br Heart J* 57:279, 1987.

Kinney TJ. Myocardial infarction following electrical injury. *Ann Emerg Med* 11:622, 1982.

Kobernick M. Electrical injuries: Pathophysiology and management. *Ann Emerg Med* 11:633, 1982.

Mortenson ML. ELectricity sparks multi-system assessment. *Emerg Med Serv* 12(1):15, 1983.

Purdue GF et al. Electrocardiographic monitoring after electrical injury: Necessity or luxury. *J Trauma* 26:166, 1986.

Reichl M et al. Electrical injuries due to railway high tension cables. *Burns* 11:423, 1985.

Salisbury R. High-voltage electrical injuries. *Emerg Med* 21(13):86, 1989.

Seward PN. Electrical injuries: Trauma with a difference. *Emerg Med* 24(8):157, 1992.

Solem L, Fischer RP, Strate RG. The natural history of electric injury. *J Trauma* 17:487, 1977.

Thygerson AL. Electric burns. *Emergency* 12(4):35, 1980.

Wilkinson C, Wood M. High voltage electric injury. *Am J Surg* 136:693, 1978.

Yang JY et al. Electrical burn with visceral injury. *Burns* 11:207, 1985.

LIGHTNING INJURIES

Amey BW et al. Lightning injury with survival in five patients. *JAMA* 253:243, 1985.

Caroline NL. *Emergency Medical Treatment: A Text for EMT-As and EMT-Intermediates* (3rd ed). Boston: Little, Brown, 1991. Chap. 13.

Cherington M et al. Lightning strikes: Nature of neurological damage in patients evaluated in hospital emergency departments. *Ann Emerg Med* 21:575, 1992.

Cooper MA. Lightning injuries: Prognostic signs for death. *Ann Emerg Med* 9:134, 1980.

Cooper MA. Of volts and bolts. *Emerg Med* 15(8):99, 1983.

Craig SR. When lightning strikes: Pathophysiology and treatment of lightning injuries. *Postgrad Med* 79:109, 1986.

Kirstenson S et al. Lightning-induced acoustic rupture of the tympanic membrane. *J Laryngol Otol* 99:711, 1985.

Kotagal S et al. Neurologic, psychiatric and cardiovascular complications in children struck by lightning. *Pediatrics* 70:190, 1982.

Moran KT et al. Lightning injury: Physics, pathophysiology, and clinical features. *Irish Med J* 79:120, 1986.

Ravitch MM et al. Lightning stroke. *N Engl J Med* 264:36, 1961.

Redleaf MI, McCabe BF. Lightning injury of the tympanic membrane. *Ann Otol Rhinol Laryngol* 102:867, 1993.

Taussig HB. "Death" from lightning—and the possibility of living again. *Ann Intern Med* 68:1345, 1968.

Taylor CO, Carr JC, Rich J. EMS system in action: Survival of two girls after direct lightning strikes. *EMT J* 5(6):419, 1981.

16

Injuries to the Head, Neck, and Spine

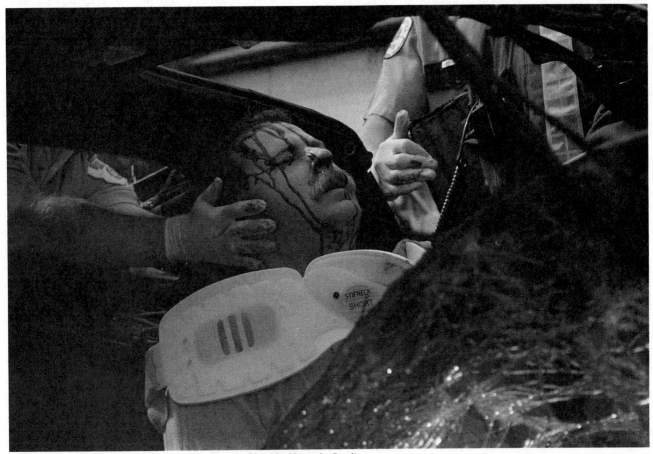

Brewster Ambulance Service, Brewster, Massachusetts. Photo by Nancy L. Caroline.

OBJECTIVES

Nearly half of all victims of serious trauma have injury to the head, and approximately 25 percent of trauma deaths—as many as 40,000 deaths per year in the United States—are due to head injury. Spinal cord injury is somewhat less common—approximately 12,000 cases per year in the United States of traumatic damage to the spinal cord—but the effects are devastating. Facial injuries, which often accompany head injury, may be not only disfiguring but also life-threatening if the airway is jeopardized. All told, the head and neck house uniquely vulnerable and uniquely important structures, and for that reason, injuries to the head and neck must be taken very seriously. In this chapter, we shall first review the anatomy and function of the central nervous system in order to understand how injury to the head and neck may affect vital functions. We shall then look separately at injuries to the head, to the face, to the soft tissues of the neck, and to the spinal cord—considering in each case how best to assess the patient and what treatment measures need to be taken. By the end of this chapter, the student should be able to

1. List the structures that enclose and protect the brain
2. List the major functions of the
   • Cerebrum
   • Cerebellum
   • Brainstem
3. Identify the five segments of the spinal column, given a drawing or description of the spinal column
4. Explain how head injury may lead to increases in intracranial pressure, and describe the possible adverse consequences of an elevated intracranial pressure
5. List three things that may jeopardize the airway of an unconscious, head-injured patient
6. Describe a patient's level of consciousness in terms of the AVPU Scale, given a description of the patient's clinical findings
7. List five questions that need to be answered in taking the history of a head-injured patient
8. Identify vital signs consistent with (a) neurogenic shock, (b) hypovolemic shock, and (c) increased intracranial pressure, given several sets of vital signs
9. Rate a patient's level of consciousness according to the Glasgow Coma Scale, given the patient's findings on examination
10. List at least three signs of skull fracture that may be detected on physical examination of a head-injured patient, and describe the prehospital treatment of a skull fracture
11. List the steps of treatment of a scalp laceration
12. Given a description of several patients with different clinical findings, identify a patient with
    • A concussion
    • A cerebral contusion
    • An epidural hematoma
    • A subdural hematoma
    and describe the treatment of a head-injured patient
13. List five signs of increasing intracranial pressure
14. List three potentially serious or life-threatening conditions that may be associated with maxillofacial injuries
15. List five clues to maxillofacial fracture
16. Describe the prehospital treatment of a patient with
    • Epistaxis
    • Maxillary fracture
    • An avulsed tooth
17. Identify the major structures of the eye, given a diagram of the eye or a description of the structures
18. Describe the examination of an injured eye, and state which part of the examination is the most important
19. Describe the correct steps in managing a patient with an impaled object
    • In the skull
    • In the cheek
    • In the eye
20. Identify a patient with a laryngeal injury, given a description of the patient's clinical findings, and list the steps in treating the patient
21. State the principal danger(s) associated with bleeding from the neck, and list the steps in treating an open neck wound
22. List eight circumstances in which spinal injury should be assumed to have occurred
23. List the special considerations in the spine-injured patient regarding
    • Maintaining an airway
    • Assessing breathing
    • Supporting the circulation
    and describe the steps in treating a patient with possible spinal cord injury
24. Identify the approximate level of a spinal cord injury, given the findings of a patient's neurologic examination

ANATOMY AND FUNCTION OF THE CENTRAL NERVOUS SYSTEM

When we consider injuries to the head and neck, what we are most concerned about, in fact, is the **cen-**

tral nervous system, or CNS, which consists of the brain and spinal cord.

Few would disagree that the brain is the most important organ in the human body, the organ ultimately responsible for all vital functions as well as for who we are, what we do, what we say, what we feel. The brain is also an organ that, unlike skin or bone or many other tissues, cannot repair itself. Once brain cells are destroyed, from whatever cause, they cannot be regenerated. Clearly, then, it is of enormous importance to provide the brain with maximum protection from harm. The human body does so by housing the brain within several layers of soft and hard wrappings. Each of those protective layers, though, is itself vulnerable to its own special kinds of injuries.

If we start from the outside and proceed inward toward the brain, the first protective layer we encounter is the SCALP. The scalp is itself composed of five layers, which can be most easily remembered by the mnemonic "SCALP":

- **S**kin, with hair.
- **S**ubcutaneous tissue, highly vascular tissue that bleeds profusely when lacerated.
- **G**alea **a**poneurotica, a tough, tendinous layer.
- **L**oose connective tissue (areolar tissue), which is easily stripped from the layer beneath in "scalping" injuries. The looseness of the areolar layer also provides room for blood to accumulate after blunt trauma (subgaleal hematoma).
- **P**eriosteum.

Immediately beneath the scalp is the SKULL, the hard, inflexible box that encloses the brain. As we shall see later on, having one's brain inside a hard box is a mixed blessing. On the plus side, a hard box provides significant protection to the delicate brain tissue, and it spares the brain the direct effects of many small bumps that are part of everyday life. However, because it is a rigid structure, the skull permits little if any expansion of its contents; thus accumulations of blood within the skull or swelling of brain tissue can rapidly lead to a rise in intracranial pressure. Elevated pressure inside the skull in turn squeezes the brain against various bony prominences within the cranium, and the brain does not like to be squeezed. The skull, in addition, provides a hard and, in some places, rather irregular surface against which brain tissue and its blood vessels can be contused when the head receives a blow or is exposed to rapid acceleration-deceleration forces. Ordinarily, then, the hard box of a skull serves us very well, but in head trauma, the inflexible nature of that box may create serious and even lethal problems.

The skull (Fig. 16-1) in fact consists of 29 bones, which can be categorized as either cranial bones or facial bones. The bones of the **cranium**—the frontal, occipital, temporal, and parietal bones—enclose and protect the brain. They are fused together at immovable joints called **sutures.** In infancy, the bones of the cranium are not yet fully fused, and the sutures are still soft; but as the baby grows, the cranial bones knit firmly together, so that they become for all intents

FIGURE 16-1. **MAJOR BONES OF THE SKULL.**

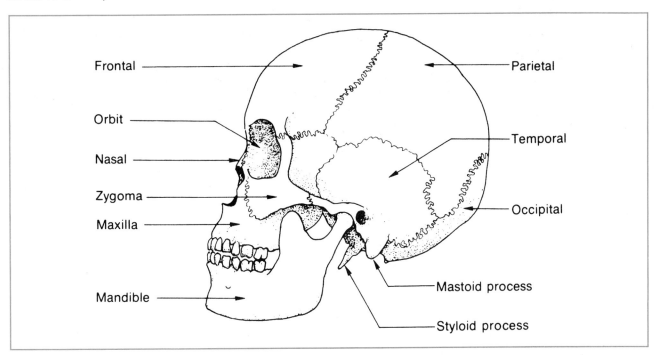

and purposes a single bone that permits no expansion of its contents.

Among the *facial* bones, those most important to us in emergency medicine include the upper jaw, or **maxilla;** the lower jaw, or **mandible;** and the cheek bones (**zygomata**). The mandible is attached to the skull by hinge joints, which permit the lower jaw to move up and down.

The skull is not, in fact, completely closed. It does have an opening at its base, the **foramen magnum,** where the brainstem is continuous with the beginning of the spinal cord.

Continuing inward from the skull, we next encounter three layers of fibrous coverings of the brain, the MENINGES (Fig. 16-2). The outermost meningeal layer is a strong, fibrous wrapping called the **dura mater,** which literally means "tough mother." The dura covers the entire brain, folding in to form the **tentorium,** a structure that separates the cerebral hemispheres from the cerebellum and brainstem. The dura mater is firmly attached to the internal wall of the skull, but in certain places—usually just beneath the suture lines of the skull—it splits into two surfaces and forms venous sinuses. When those venous sinuses are disrupted in head injury, blood can collect beneath the dura to form a *subdural hematoma.* The meningeal *arteries* are located between the dura and the skull, so when one of those arteries (usually the middle meningeal artery) is disrupted, bleeding occurs *above* the dura (*epi*dural hematoma).

Beneath the dura, one finds the second meningeal layer, a delicate, transparent membrane called the **arachnoid.** The third meningeal layer, the **pia mater** ("soft mother"), is a thin, highly vascular membrane firmly adherent to the surface of the brain.

Yet another protective "cushion" for the brain is provided by the CEREBROSPINAL FLUID, or CSF, that flows within the subdural and subarachnoid spaces to bathe both the brain and spinal cord. CSF is produced within the brain, and it serves not only as a shock absorber against mechanical injury but also as a source of nutrients for the central nervous system.

Finally, within all of the protective layers described, we come to the brain itself (Fig. 16-3), the quarterback of the central nervous system that calls the plays for the rest of the body. Specifically, the brain carries out the following functions:

- The brain serves as a *regulatory center,* through which the activities of the whole body are integrated and controlled. The brain receives sensory impulses that provide information about the body's internal state ("There's an infection in my

FIGURE 16-2. THE MENINGES: Dura mater, arachnoid, and pia mater.

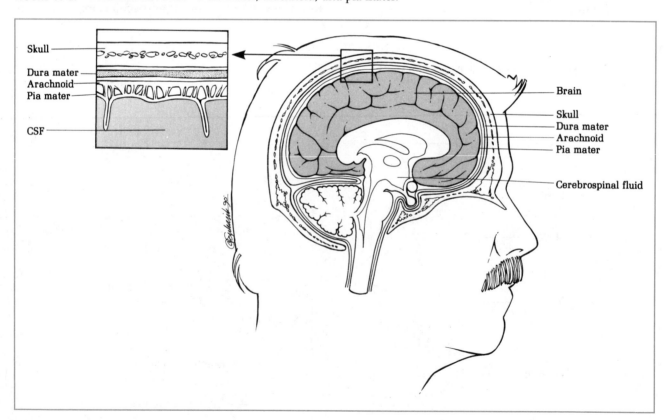

bladder.") and external environment ("Ouch! It's hot!"). In response, the brain sends out messages to enable the appropriate responses ("White blood cells, please proceed to bladder," or "Take your hand off the stove!").

- The brain is also a *center of sensations*. The brain interprets our perceptions of the environment received from sensory organs (eyes, ears, nose, taste buds, skin) and generates sensations such as sight, hearing, smell, taste, and touch.
- The brain is the *seat of consciousness*, that is, the state of awareness of oneself and one's surroundings.
- The brain is the *source of voluntary acts*.
- The brain is the *seat of the emotions*. It is the brain that decides whether we feel happiness, sadness, rage, and all the other emotions that affect our behavior.
- The brain is the *source of higher mental processes*, including thought, reasoning, judgment, memory, and learning.

FIGURE 16-3. **THE BRAIN AND UPPER SPINAL CORD.**

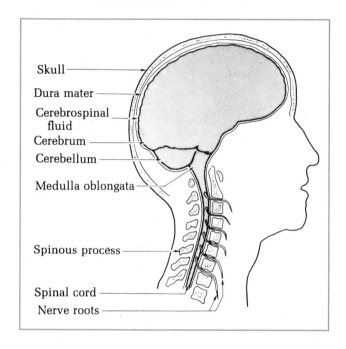

Anatomically, the brain consists of millions of nerve cells complexly interconnected. The bulk of the human brain is occupied by the **cerebrum,** the part of the brain responsible for higher functions, such as reasoning. The cerebrum consists of two sides, or *hemispheres*, that are not entirely equivalent functionally. In a right-handed person, for example, the speech center is usually located in the left cerebral hemisphere, which is then said to be the *dominant* hemisphere. Recent research suggests that a person's dominant hemisphere is more concerned not only with language but also with rational, analytic, abstract thinking, while the nondominant side of the brain deals in intuition, imagination, and insight.

Each cerebral hemisphere is divided functionally into various specialized areas (Fig. 16-4). The *frontal*

FIGURE 16-4. **THE BRAIN** is divided functionally into specialized areas.

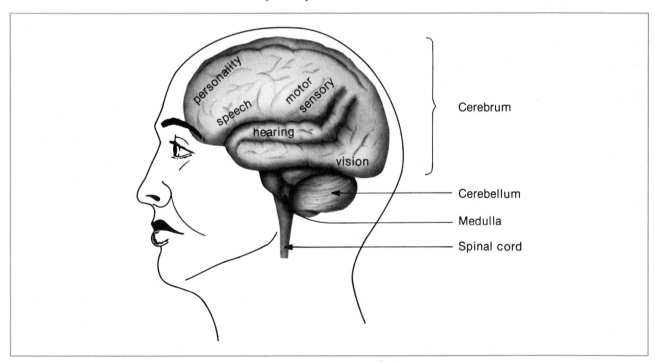

area, for example, is concerned with emotions, while vision is controlled in the *occipital* lobe of the brain. Most people are familiar with the phenomenon of "seeing stars" after a blow to the back of the head; those "stars" are in fact produced by the occipital poles of the brain—the vision centers—banging against the back of the skull. The speech centers are primarily in the *temporal* lobe of the dominant hemisphere (i.e., the left hemisphere in a right-handed person). The *parietal* lobes house the motor and sensory centers for the opposite (contralateral) side of the body; that is, the motor and sensory centers for the right side of the body are in the left side of the brain and vice versa.

Beneath the cerebral hemispheres, in the inferoposterior part of the brain, is found the CEREBELLUM. The cerebellum is sometimes called the "athlete's brain" because it is concerned with maintenance of posture and equilibrium as well as coordination of skilled movements.

The BRAINSTEM, at the base of the brain, houses many structures critical to the maintenance of vital functions. High in the brainstem, for example, is the **reticular activating system,** which is responsible for maintaining the awake state. In the lower brainstem, or **medulla,** are the control centers for regulating respiration and heart beat. An increase in intracranial pressure, as may occur in head injury, can squeeze the cerebellum down through the foramen magnum and in the process squash the medulla against the bones of the skull; the resulting injury to the medulla in turn leads to cardiovascular derangements and respiratory arrest.

Continuous with the brainstem is the second component of the central nervous system, the spinal cord. Like the brain, the spinal cord is enclosed within several protective layers. The outermost layers are, of course, the skin, subcutaneous tissue, and musculature of the neck and back. The bony protection of the spinal cord is furnished by the VERTEBRAL COLUMN, or spinal column, which also serves as the main axis of the body, providing rigidity but permitting some degree of movement. The spinal column consists of 33 bones, called **vertebrae.** At the top of the spinal column rests the skull, from whose base exit the long nerve tracts that make up the spinal cord. Ribs articulate with 12 of the vertebrae to form the thorax, while the pelvis articulates with the lower part of the spinal column, or **sacrum,** to form the pelvic girdle. The spine consists of five sections (Fig. 16-5):

- CERVICAL SPINE, comprising the first 7 vertebrae in the *neck* region
- THORACIC SPINE, consisting of 12 vertebrae in

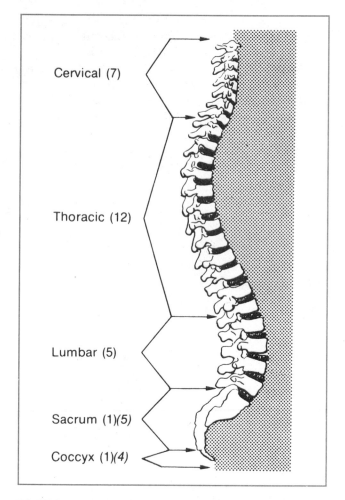

FIGURE 16-5. THE VERTEBRAL COLUMN. Note that the five sacral vertebrae are fused together, as are the four vertebrae that make up the coccyx.

the *upper back* with which the 12 pairs of ribs articulate
- LUMBAR SPINE, made up of 5 vertebrae in the *lower back*
- SACRUM, 5 fused vertebrae, which articulate with the pelvis at the sacroiliac joint to form part of the pelvic girdle
- COCCYX, 4 fused vertebrae that make up the tail bone

The VERTEBRAE (Fig. 16-6) each consist of a body, or solid portion, and a vertebral arch, which surrounds the opening (foramen) through which the spinal cord passes. The vertebrae are separated from one another by **intervertebral discs,** flexible, elastic connections of cartilage that cushion the vertebrae and permit a limited degree of motion in the spine.

The vertebral openings (foramina) are lined up one on top of another to form a vertical canal through which the SPINAL CORD passes. Like the brain, the

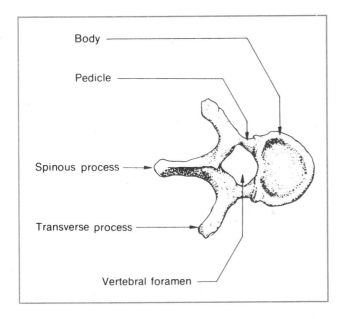

FIGURE 16-6. A VERTEBRA. The spinal cord runs through the central vertebral foramen.

spinal cord is further protected by three meningeal layers and a CSF shock absorber. The spinal cord itself consists of numerous nerve tracts connecting the brain with all the other organs in the body. Three of the most important of those tracts are

- The *posterior columns*, which mediate POSITION and vibratory sense
- The *lateral spinothalamic tracts*, which mediate PAIN and temperature sense
- The *corticospinal tract*, which controls MOVEMENT

It is not important to remember the names of those tracts; but it *is* important to check the spine-injured patient for the three modalities of function that those tracts represent: position sense, pain sense, and movement.

The thoracic and lumbar portions of the spinal cord also supply the ganglia (nerve collections) of the SYMPATHETIC NERVOUS SYSTEM. We shall learn a great deal more about that system in Chapter 23. For our purposes here, it is sufficient to know that injury to the thoracolumbar spine may paralyze not only the voluntary nervous system but the sympathetic nervous system as well. Sympathetic nerves, as we shall learn, mediate changes in arterial caliber. It is through the sympathetic nervous system that arteries receive the signals ordering them to constrict. When sympathetic nerves are damaged or interrupted, therefore, arteries will no longer constrict in response to changes in posture, core body tempera-

ture, and so forth. As a result, there may be dramatic pooling of blood within the suddenly dilated blood vessels, with an associated fall in blood pressure (neurogenic shock). Temperature regulation may also become disordered, for ordinarily vasoconstriction is one of the body's chief mechanisms for conserving heat, by shunting blood away from the surface of the body.

HEAD INJURIES

Each year in the United States nearly 50,000 lives are lost in motor vehicle accidents. Head injuries occur in more than two-thirds of those accidents and are a major cause of mortality in most of them. Head injuries also occur commonly in victims of assault, in elderly people suffering falls, and in a variety of accidents involving children. When head injuries are fatal, it is invariably because of associated injury to the brain.

How the Brain Is Injured

The brain can be injured directly by a penetrating object, such as a bullet. But more commonly injury to the brain occurs indirectly, as a result of external forces exerted on the skull. Consider the most common source of brain injury, the motor vehicle accident. We learned in Chapter 14 that when a moving vehicle comes in contact with an immovable object, there are in fact three collisions involved: the collision of the vehicle with the object, the collision of the passenger with the vehicle, and the collision of the passenger's internal organs with the skeletal structures of the body. Thus, when a car's forward motion is suddenly arrested by a utility pole, the front-seat passenger continues to move forward until *his* forward motion is arrested by the impact of his head with the windshield. That impact causes a sudden deceleration of the skull, but the brain continues to move forward until *its* forward motion is arrested by impact with the inside of the skull. In fact, the brain is likely to crash into the skull twice—first in the original direction of motion, then, on rebound, against the opposite inner surface of the skull. So deceleration injuries to the brain may occur in either or both of two places: the point of initial impact (called "coup") or the side opposite ("contrecoup"). In either case, the response of the bruised brain will be similar to that of any other bruised tissue: It will start to *swell*, initially because cerebral blood vessels dilate to increase blood flow to the injured areas. After several hours, an increase in cerebral water (cerebral edema) also starts to contribute to the swelling.

Now we can appreciate the problem of having one's brain inside a closed box. When swelling occurs in an extremity, it is not ordinarily a critical problem, because the soft tissues have a lot of "give." But when swelling occurs within a rigid, closed box like the skull, there is no room in which the brain can expand. Therefore any increase of *volume* within the skull leads rapidly to an increase in *pressure* within the skull (**intracranial pressure**).

A rising intracranial pressure can have several deleterious and ultimately fatal effects. To begin with, there is the effect on the **cerebral perfusion pressure,** that is, the pressure of blood flowing through the brain:

$$CPP = MAP - ICP$$

where CPP = cerebral perfusion pressure
       MAP = mean arterial pressure
       ICP = intracranial pressure

If we examine the above equation, it becomes clear that as the intracranial pressure increases, the cerebral perfusion pressure inevitably falls, which means that blood flow to the brain decreases. Clearly a decreasing cerebral blood flow is a potential catastrophe, for the brain is dependent on a constant supply of blood to furnish the oxygen and glucose it needs to survive. So the body attempts to restore cerebral perfusion pressure by raising the mean arterial pressure. Thus what we see clinically is that as the intracranial pressure increases, the blood pressure rises (and, as a reflex response, the pulse rate decreases). That protective response will work only up to a certain point, however; and if intracranial pressure continues to rise, the resulting damage to brain structures will become irreversible and death will shortly follow.

Another possible consequence of increasing intracranial pressure is a condition known as **herniation.** Herniation occurs when the pressure within the skull is so great that it forces parts of the brain downward, through the tentorium or foramen magnum, causing severe damage to the brain structures that are squeezed against the skull. Depending on which part of the brain has herniated, the patient may show dilation of the pupil on the side of the injury, paralysis of the contralateral arm and leg, decerebrate posturing (see p. 336), or cardiorespiratory arrest.

In the following sections, we shall consider a variety of head injuries that may or may not lead to brain injury and increased intracranial pressure.

Assessment of the Head-Injured Patient

The assessment of a patient who has suffered head injury begins, of course, with the *primary survey.*

Primary Survey

As for any other patient, the primary survey of the head-injured patient starts with the ABCs. And in the victim of trauma, the ABCs are specifically geared to early detection of injuries or their complications that have life-threatening potential:

- AIRWAY: If the patient is unconscious, his airway is in jeopardy. In opening the airway, however, bear in mind that

> **ANY PATIENT WITH SIGNIFICANT HEAD INJURY ALSO HAS CERVICAL SPINE INJURY UNTIL PROVED OTHERWISE.**

If the forces that produced the head injury were powerful enough to cause loss of consciousness, they were powerful enough to damage the cervical spine and the spinal cord within it. Act accordingly, and secure the airway without hyperextending the head or neck (**jaw thrust or chin lift alone**). In the unconscious patient, an oropharyngeal airway may be useful to maintain the airway while you proceed with the evaluation, but definitive airway protection requires endotracheal intubation.

In the head-injured patient, the airway may also be in jeopardy from *vomiting,* from *bleeding* in the mouth or nose, or from *"foreign" objects* such as broken teeth. Therefore it is necessary to make a quick inspection of the patient's mouth as part of the primary survey and to suction out any blood, vomitus, secretions, or foreign materials you find there.

- BREATHING: Assess the adequacy of the patient's breathing, and observe the chest during one or two respiratory cycles. If there is any respiratory distress, expose the chest immediately for a more thorough examination, for chest injuries may kill very quickly. In any case, start *oxygen* administration as soon as possible, since the most common cause of death from head injury is cerebral anoxia, and cerebral anoxia ought to be largely preventable. If the patient's breathing is abnormally slow or shallow, assist ventilations with a bag-valve mask. Many authorities now recommend maintaining a moderate degree of *hyperventilation* by giving about 20 to 25 breaths per minute. The theory is that hyperventilation lowers the arterial PCO_2, which in turn causes cerebral vasoconstriction and may thereby help minimize cerebral edema. (Recall that in the early stages, cerebral edema occurs because of dilatation of cerebral blood vessels.) Recently that theory has been called into question. It is best, therefore, to follow the protocols established by your local medical director regarding ventilation of a head-injured patient.

- CIRCULATION: Check for a pulse at the neck and at the wrist, and control major bleeding. Recall that if a pulse is present at both the neck and the wrist, the systolic blood pressure is at least 80 mm Hg. If the pulse is present at the neck but *absent* at the wrist, the systolic blood pressure is probably between 60 and 70 mm Hg, a sign of late shock.

In seriously injured patients, it is now customary to add two more letters to the ABCs of the primary survey—*D* for "disability," a quick assessment of the patient's neurologic status, and *E* for "expose," that is, undressing the patient to facilitate thorough examination.

- DISABILITY: Immediately following the ABCs, it is desirable to make a quick assessment of the patient's level of consciousness and pupillary signs. If the patient's condition permits, a more complete neurologic examination will be carried out during the secondary survey, but when the patient's condition is critical, the quick "disabililty" assessment may be all that is possible in the field. The patient's *level of consciousness* is assessed at this point using the "AVPU Scale":

AVPU SCALE

A The patient is **alert**. He knows his name, where he is, what day it is, and so forth.

V The patient responds to **voice**. He may not be alert or open his eyes spontaneously, but he does respond in an appropriate way when spoken to.

P The patient responds only to a **painful** stimulus, such as a pinch or a pinprick.

U The patient is completely **unresponsive**, even to a painful stimulus.

At the same time, quickly check the *pupils*, and note their size, whether they are equal, and whether they constrict when a light is directed at them. Record your findings and the time. Then stabilize the patient's head and neck temporarily, for example with sandbags, to minimize motion as you proceed through the rest of the examination.

- EXPOSE: Undress the patient to enable a thorough physical examination. While you are doing so, you can start looking around and asking a few questions.

The History

Taking a history does not begin until the primary survey has been completed and any problems detected in the primary survey have been managed. At that point, try to find out—from the patient, if he is conscious, or from bystanders—a few details of what happened and of the patient's medical background:

- Inspect the scene to try to determine the MECHANISMS OF INJURY. Look for telltale signs such as a cracked windshield. If the patient is conscious, ask him how the injury occurred.
- If the patient is conscious now, find out WHETHER HE LOST CONSCIOUSNESS at any point. If so, *when* with respect to the time of the injury (immediately or after some delay)? *How long* was he unconscious?
- DID THE PATIENT VOMIT? (Almost every child will vomit after a head injury; vomiting in adults after head injury is more significant, and it may indicate serious intracranial pathology.)
- What are the patient's CURRENT SYMPTOMS? Does he have *headache*? *Dizziness*? *Double vision*? *Nausea*? *Weakness* (if so, where)? *Pain elsewhere* in the body, particularly in the neck or over any other part of the spine? Does he have any *numbness* or pins-and-needles sensations (**paresthesias**) anywhere in his body?
- Has the patient ingested any DRUGS OR ALCOHOL during the past several hours? Drugs or alcohol may produce changes in the level of consciousness that could be mistakenly attributed to a head injury.

- Find out about SIGNIFICANT UNDERLYING ILLNESSES. Stupor or coma in the victim of a road accident may take on a quite different meaning and be amenable to very fast, effective treatment if it turns out that the accident victim is an insulin-dependent diabetic.

By the time you have gathered the answers to those questions, you should be ready to proceed through the steps of the secondary survey.

General Appearance

As usual, we begin the secondary survey by getting a general feeling for the patient's overall condition. In the victim of trauma, we shall be looking specifically for clues to underlying injury.

- Note the POSITION IN WHICH THE PATIENT WAS FOUND for clues to the mechanisms of injury.
- Now is the time to make a more careful assessment of the patient's LEVEL OF CONSCIOUSNESS. One widely used method of evaluating the level of consciousness along with a few other neurologic parameters is the **Glasgow Coma Scale** (Table 16-1), which assigns a numerical score to the patient's responses in three categories: eye opening, best motor response, and best verbal response. Whatever method you use to assess the level of consciousness, repeat your assessment frequently:

> **THE MOST IMPORTANT SINGLE SIGN IN THE EVALUATION OF A HEAD-INJURED PATIENT IS A CHANGING STATE OF CONSCIOUSNESS.**

- If the patient is conscious, make note of his BEHAVIOR AND DEGREE OF DISTRESS. Unfortunately, many victims of head trauma are not very cooperative and are often under the influence of alcohol besides, so the patient's behavior may pose a problem. You must not, however, lose sight of your objective: to give the best care possible.
- Observe the SKIN CONDITION. Cold, clammy skin suggests hypovolemic shock, which in turn suggests that there is a major injury in addition to the head injury. In *neurogenic* shock, from spinal cord injury, the skin is usually of normal color and temperature because of peripheral vasodilatation.
- If you have not done so already, while you were undressing the patient, make a quick check for OBVIOUS WOUNDS OR DEFORMITIES.

Vital Signs

The vital signs may provide very valuable information about the patient's underlying injuries. Get a full

---

TABLE 16-1. GLASGOW COMA SCALE

	TEST	PATIENT'S RESPONSE	SCORE
Eye opening	Spontaneous speech	Opens eyes on own	4
		Opens eyes when asked to in a loud voice	3
	Pain	Opens eyes when pinched	2
	Pain	Does not open eyes	1
Best motor response	Commands	Follows simple commands	6
	Pain	Pulls hand away when pinched	5
	Pain	Pulls a part of body away when examiner pinches him	4
	Pain	Flexes body inappropriately to pain (decorticate posturing)	3
	Pain	Body becomes rigid in an extended position when examiner pinches victim (decerebrate posturing)	2
	Pain	No motor response to pain	1
Verbal response (talking)	Speech	Carries on a conversation correctly and tells examiner where he is, who he is, month, and year	5
	Speech	Confused and disoriented	4
	Speech	Speech is clear but makes no sense	3
	Speech	Makes garbled sounds that examiner cannot understand	2
	Speech	Makes no sounds	1

- Assess the patient's score in each category, and total the scores of the three categories. A total score of 7 or less indicates coma.
- Assess the patient's score in each category frequently, and record each observation and the time it was made. Keep a parallel record of vital signs.

set of vital signs early in your assessment of the patient, and repeat them at 5-minute intervals.

- Assess the rate, rhythm, and force of the PULSE. A rapid, thready pulse suggests hypovolemic shock. In *neurogenic* shock, the pulse is usually normal or slow. The pulse will also slow down in response to rising intracranial pressure.
- Note the rate and quality of the RESPIRATIONS. Is there an abnormal respiratory pattern? Head injury may produce several types of abnormal respirations. Initially, a rising intracranial pressure is usually reflected by a *slowing* of the respiratory rate; but as the pressure inside the skull continues to rise and the respiratory center in the medulla is progressively squeezed, tachypnea occurs. Be particularly alert for sudden apnea, and be prepared to start artificial ventilation. Look for *diaphragmatic breathing*, an indication of intercostal muscle paralysis. (Question: What sort of injury produces intercostal muscle paralysis?)
- Measure the BLOOD PRESSURE, and note any changes over time. In general, the blood pressure will rise as intracranial pressure rises, particularly the systolic blood pressure—so the net effect is a widening of the pulse pressure (systolic minus diastolic pressure). If the blood pressure is *falling*, you need to look for an injury somewhere besides the patient's head. The skull is a very small box, and it is nearly full of brain, so there is scarcely any room inside for blood. Thus, if the patient is in hypovolemic shock, he is bleeding somewhere else. To repeat:

HYPOTENSION IN A HEAD-INJURED ADULT IS SCARCELY EVER CAUSED BY THE HEAD INJURY. LOOK FOR A SOURCE OF MAJOR HEMORRHAGE ELSEWHERE IN THE BODY.

The vital signs, then, can often help to distinguish between an injury to the head that is causing increased intracranial pressure and an injury elsewhere that is causing hypovolemic shock (Table 16-2).

Head-to-Toe Survey

In conducting the head-to-toe survey of the head-injured patient, you will, as usual, be looking for other injuries in addition to the head injury. In this section, however, we will review only the possible clues to the head-injury itself.

- Examine the HEAD (Fig. 16-7) for
  1. Lacerations of the scalp.
  2. Signs of skull fracture, including
     a. Depression of the skull.
     b. Ecchymoses behind the ears ("Battle's sign").
     c. Bilateral, symmetric, periorbital ecchymoses ("coon's eyes," or "raccoon sign").
     d. Blood or clear fluid draining from the nose or ear. (If there *is* leakage of clear fluid from the ears or nose, do NOT attempt to dam it up with cotton or gauze; place a sterile gauze lightly over the nose or external ear, allowing flow to continue freely.)
  3. Instability of the facial bones.
- Inspect the PUPILS (Fig. 16-8) for
  1. Size (dilated? constricted? midposition?). When you describe the pupils, do not simply state that the pupils were "moderately dilated," because no one will know just how dilated moderately dilated is. Describe the pupils in terms of their actual size (e.g., "The pupils were approximately 7 mm."). Better still, *draw* the approximate size of the pupils on the neurologic examination record.
  2. Equality.
  3. Reaction to light.

The size of the pupils is controlled by the third cranial nerve, which may get squeezed against

TABLE 16-2. DETECTING HYPOVOLEMIC SHOCK IN A HEAD-INJURED PATIENT

	INCREASING INTRACRANIAL PRESSURE	SHOCK (HEMORRHAGE ELSEWHERE)
Blood pressure	Rising	Falling
Pulse	Slow	Rapid
Respirations	Initially slow, later rapid or irregular	Rapid
Skin	May be hot	Cold, clammy

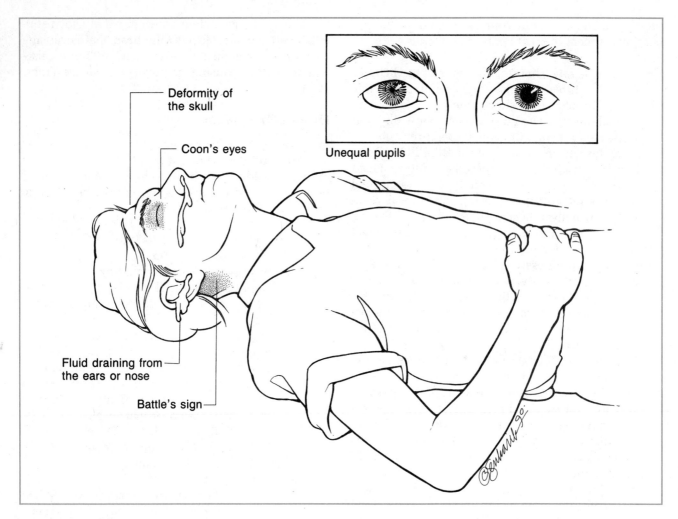

Deformity of
the skull

Coon's eyes

Unequal pupils

Fluid draining from
the ears or nose

Battle's sign

FIGURE 16-7.   SIGNS OF HEAD INJURY.

the tentorium when intracranial pressure increases. If that happens, the pupil on the same
side of the body will dilate. A unilaterally dilated
pupil in an *alert* patient is *not* due to head injury.
But the development of a unilaterally dilated
pupil in a patient with a depressed level of consciousness is a *dire emergency* and demands immediate transport of the patient.

4. Before turning your attention from the eyes,
   check the EXTRAOCULAR MOTIONS in a
   conscious patient by having him follow your
   moving finger up, down, right, and left with
   his gaze. Paralysis of upward gaze may signal
   a fracture of the orbit of the eye, while paralysis of gaze to the right or left suggests pathology in the brain.

• Examine the FACE for lacerations, bruises, and
  stability of the facial bones (Fig. 16-9). Make sure
  to check the MOUTH for blood, broken teeth or
  dentures, and other foreign materials.

• Assess the NECK for irregularities or tenderness
over the vertebrae. The fully conscious patient
will be able to report discomfort in the neck and
will be partially protected from undue motion in
an injured neck by paravertebral muscle spasm.
The comatose or confused patient, on the other
hand, will not be able to report what hurts and
may seriously aggravate a neck injury by thrashing around. As soon as you have finished your
examination of the neck, apply a *cervical collar*.

• Complete the head-to-toe survey. Remember, the
head injury may not be the patient's most serious
injury. When you come to the EXTREMITIES,
test for *movement* and *sensation* in both hands and
both feet. If the patient is unconscious, note *how*
(if at all) he responds to a painful stimulus. Is the
response purposeful (e.g., does he try to pull
away from the painful stimulus)? Does he show
a **decerebrate response** (arms and legs extended, Fig. 16-10A) or a **decorticate response**
(arms flexed, legs extended, Fig. 16-10B)?

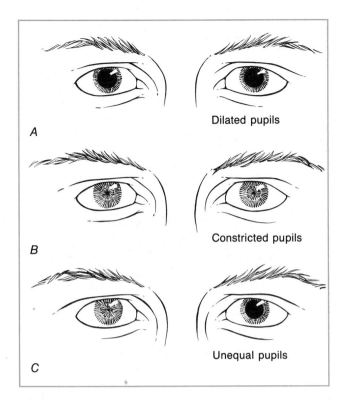

FIGURE 16-8. **EXAMINATION OF THE PUPILS.** (A) Dilated pupils. (B) Constricted pupils. (C) Unequal pupils.

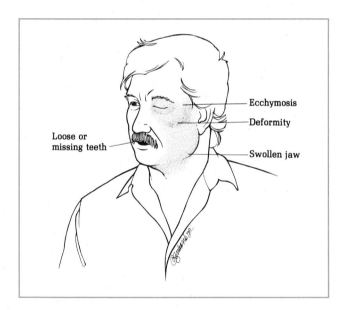

FIGURE 16-9. **SIGNS OF FACIAL TRAUMA.**

Record the findings of your examination along with the time, and repeat key examinations at frequent intervals. For the purpose of remembering what to reassess and for recording the data, it is useful to carry a checklist of neurologic signs. A sample

of one such checklist, that developed by the Committee on Trauma of the American College of Surgeons, is illustrated in Figure 16-11. Your local EMS system may employ a different checklist, such as the Glasgow Coma Scale described earlier, but some means should be developed to record *sequential* observations of vital signs and neurologic function. That is because

> **THE MOST IMPORTANT ASPECT OF NEUROLOGIC ASSESSMENT IS WHETHER THE PATIENT'S FINDINGS ARE CHANGING AND IN WHAT DIRECTION.**

Thus it is necessary to make repeated evaluations in the field and in transit, each time recording the time of the evaluation and the findings, so that emergency department personnel can rapidly determine whether the patient's condition is improving or deteriorating. The patient who is improving is much less likely to have significant intracranial pathology and can safely be kept under observation. The patient who shows deterioration, on the other hand, is of great concern and may require urgent surgery. The observations you make in the field, if precise and detailed, will therefore be of enormous value to those who must render definitive care to the patient. BE OBSERVANT. BE THOROUGH. BE PRECISE. KEEP DETAILED RECORDS.

Let us now consider some of the specific types of head injury that you may encounter.

Scalp Injuries

The scalp has a very rich blood supply and therefore tends to bleed profusely when lacerated. In children, the volume of blood loss from a scalp wound may be sufficient to produce shock; in adults, shock is usually *not* due to a scalp wound but rather to an injury elsewhere. Nonetheless, bleeding from a scalp wound should be rapidly controlled. To do so, palpate the skull with a gloved finger in the area of the scalp wound to be sure there isn't a depressed skull fracture beneath the wound. If the skull is stable, press your fingertips firmly against the edges of the scalp wound for a few minutes, then apply a pressure dressing. If the skull is unstable, apply pressure to the scalp close to the wound but beyond the unstable section.

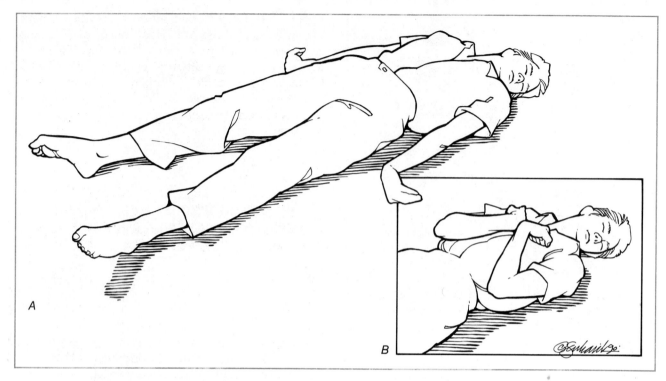

FIGURE 16-10. RESPONSES SUGGESTIVE OF BRAIN INJURY.   (A) Decerebrate response. (B) Decorticate response.

Skull Injuries

Obvious injuries to the skull, such as depressed fractures or signs of basilar skull fracture, should be
noted in the head-to-toe survey. There is no specific
treatment in the field, but the presence of such an
injury bespeaks significant forces involved in producing the injury and should therefore alert you to the
possibility of other serious injuries, especially those
involving the spine.

When the patient is a child, obtain a complete
and detailed history of how the head injury occurred,
and observe the accident scene closely. If the story of
the incident seems inconsistent with the observed injuries or mechanisms of injury, suspect child abuse,
and report your suspicion privately to the receiving
physician in the emergency room.

If there is an *impaled object* in the skull, leave it in
place. In the case of a *gunshot wound*, look for both
the entrance wound and the exit wound; if they are
not in a straight line, or if there is no exit wound, it
means that the bullet has ricocheted within the skull,
and you have to assume that the cervical spinal cord
was damaged until proved otherwise.

Brain Injuries

While the management of various brain injuries will
be more or less the same in the field, it is useful to

understand some of the underlying pathologic processes, in order to appreciate the potential urgency in
managing a head-injured patient.

Concussion

A concussion is the mildest form of head injury and
does not involve any permanent damage. The patient
may lose consciousness for a short period after the
injury and even have a brief period of apnea. Very
often he will have some loss of memory (**amnesia**) for
the events immediately surrounding the accident;
and he is likely to complain of headache, dizziness,
nausea, or ringing in the ears. There will not, however, be any significant findings on neurologic examination, and the patient's level of consciousness
will remain stable or improve. Needless to say, the
only way you will be able to determine that the level
of consciousness is stable or improving is to maintain
a neurologic checklist and make repeated observations.

Contusion

A cerebral contusion, as the name implies, is a bruise
of the brain. And as in any bruise, the reaction of the
injured tissue will be to *swell*. As described earlier,
swelling of the brain inevitably leads to an increase
in intracranial pressure and all that goes along with
it. A patient who has sustained a cerebral contusion

NEUROLOGIC EXAMINATION RECORD

INSTRUCTIONS. Record vital signs in Unit I. If the patient can talk, check (✔) one subdivision in units II, III, and IV. An oriented patient should know his name, age, etc. A moan can be checked as "garbled" speech. If unable to talk, check (✔) "none" in Unit III and one block in Unit V. In an "inappropriate" response, the patient is not effective in removing the painful stimulus; when "decerebrate," the extremities reflexly extend and/or hyperpronate. In Unit VI, draw the size and shape of each pupil and check (✔) for a reaction to light. Under Unit VII, normal strength is scored as "4," slight weakness "3," a 50 percent reduction in strength "2," marked weakness and without spontaneous movement "1," and complete paralysis "0."

UNIT	TIME:					
I Vital Signs	blood pressure					
	pulse					
	respirations					
	temperature					
II Conscious and	oriented					
	disoriented					
	restless					
	combative					
III Speech	clear					
	rambling					
	garbled					
	none					
IV Will awaken to:	name					
	shaking					
	light pain					
	strong pain					
V Nonverbal reaction to pain	appropriate					
	inappropriate					
	"decerebrate"					
	none					
VI Pupils	size of right					
	size of left					
	reacts on right					
	reacts on left					
VII Ability to move	right arm					
	left arm					
	right leg					
	left leg					

FIGURE 16-11. **NEUROLOGIC CHECKLIST.** Reproduced courtesy of the American College of Surgeons.

is likely to have been unconscious for some time or to have a deteriorating level of consciousness while under your care. If he is still conscious, he may complain of nausea or may vomit without warning. The danger of a cerebral contusion resides in the danger of increasing intracranial pressure.

Intracranial Hemorrhage

Increased intracranial pressure is also likely to develop when there is *bleeding* inside the skull; for just as the closed box of the skull has no extra room to accommodate a swollen brain, so too it has no extra room to accommodate blood clots. In either case, the net effect is to raise the pressure inside the skull.

Bleeding may occur either between the skull and the dura (**epidural hematoma**) or beneath the dura (**subdural hematoma**).

An EPIDURAL HEMATOMA (Fig. 16-12) is nearly always the result of a blow to the head that produces a linear fracture of the thin temporal bone. The middle meningeal artery courses along within a groove in that bone, so it is apt to be disrupted when the temporal bone is fractured. If so, there will be

brisk arterial bleeding into the epidural space, so symptoms may develop very rapidly. Often the patient loses consciousness at the time of the injury, then wakes up for a while ("lucid interval"), but after about an hour lapses back into unconsciousness. Meanwhile, as intracranial pressure increases, the third cranial nerve gets compressed against the tentorium, and the pupil on the side of the hematoma becomes fixed and dilated. Death will follow very rapidly if surgery to evacuate the hematoma is not performed immediately at this point.

SUBDURAL HEMATOMA (Fig. 16-13) occurs after falls or injuries involving strong deceleration forces. In subdural hematoma, the bleeding is *venous*, not arterial, so the hematoma may develop more gradually. Clinically, one sees a fluctuating level of consciousness and focal neurologic signs, such as weakness of one extremity or slurred speech.

In the field, it is generally not possible, or necessary, to distinguish between a cerebral contusion with edema and a cerebral hematoma. What is important is to recognize the signs of increasing intracranial pressure and to appreciate that those signs indicate a dire emergency.

FIGURE 16-12. **EPIDURAL HEMATOMA** is usually the result of a blow to the head that produces a linear fracture of the temporal bone. Blood collects between the dura and the skull.

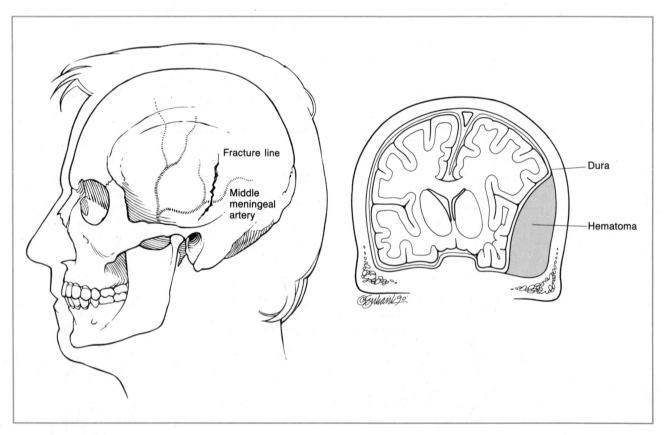

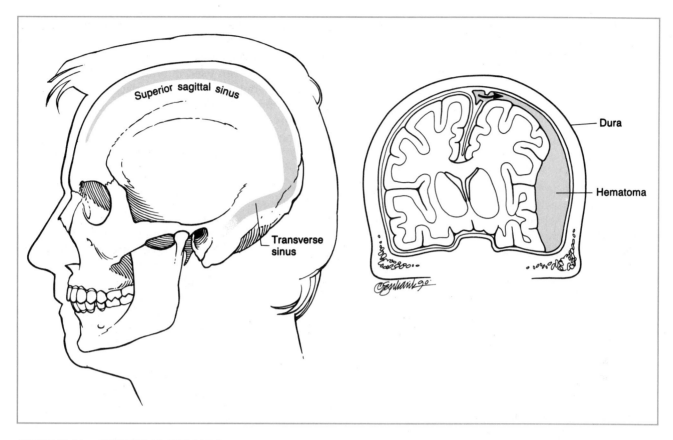

FIGURE 16-13. **SUBDURAL HEMATOMA** occurs when there is venous bleeding beneath the dura.

**SIGNS OF INCREASING
INTRACRANIAL PRESSURE:
SUMMARY**

- Deteriorating level of consciousness
- Hemiplegia (rarely, quadriplegia)
- Vomiting
- Unilateral pupillary dilatation
- Rising blood pressure with slowing pulse
- Abnormal respirations or apnea

Management of the Head-Injured Patient

Management of the patient who has suffered a head injury begins with the primary survey, already described. To summarize the ABCs:

- The importance of maintaining an open AIRWAY cannot be overemphasized. So long as the patient is not intubated, be prepared to take immediate

action at the first sign of vomiting—turn the patient onto his side and suction the mouth. In the unconscious patient, the trachea should be intubated at the earliest opportunity. Endotracheal intubation of a head-injured patient requires special precautions or it may precipitate dangerous increases in intracranial pressure. Therefore, intubation of the head-injured patient is best carried out under controlled conditions in the emergency room. If intubation *must* be undertaken in the field (long transport time, difficulty in maintaining the airway manually), observe the following guidelines:

**ENDOTRACHEAL INTUBATION
OF THE HEAD-INJURED
PATIENT: GUIDELINES**

- Preoxygenate with 100% OXYGEN for at least 5 minutes.
- Meanwhile, give LIDOCAINE, 1.5 mg per kilogram IV; then wait 2 minutes.

- Intubate, keeping the patient's head in neutral position.

Do *not* use succinylcholine to paralyze the patient for intubation (succinylcholine given without prior administration of a nondepolarizing blocking agent will raise intracranial pressure).

- If the respirations are depressed, assist BREATHING with a bag-valve-mask or bag-valve-endotracheal tube and 100% oxygen. Maintain a ventilation rate of about 20 breaths per minute to prevent hypercarbia, for an elevated PCO_2 can worsen cerebral edema.
- Stabilize the CIRCULATION, which means *control bleeding*. Unless there are signs of shock, *fluids should be restricted* in a head-injured patient, for excessive fluids may worsen cerebral edema. If you start an IV lifeline, therefore, run it at a keep-open rate only (no more than 30 ml/hr). Use normal saline for the keep-open line, NOT D5/W, which may also worsen cerebral edema.

In addition to the ABCs, there are a few other supportive measures that should be taken for the head-injured patient:

- DO NOT ALLOW THE PATIENT TO BECOME OVERHEATED. Patients with head injury, as contrasted to those with spinal cord injury, tend to develop a very high temperature (**hyperpyrexia**), which in turn may worsen the condition of the brain. Do *not* cover the patient with blankets if the ambient temperature is 70°F (21°C) or above.
- COVER WOUNDS as needed. If there is an open fracture of the skull with brain tissue oozing out (it tends to resemble toothpaste), cover it *lightly* with a sterile dressing that has been moistened with sterile saline. The same goes for leakage of blood or CSF from the ears—loose sterile dressings, just to keep the area clean. As noted earlier, objects impaled in the skull should be left where they are and protected from being jarred.
- MONITOR THE CARDIAC RHYTHM, which may be disturbed if there is brainstem damage or associated chest injury. Head-injured patients are prone to cardiac dysrhythmias such as ventricular tachycardia. *Bradycardia* should raise the suspicion of increasing intracranial pressure.
- There is usually no need to give any MEDICATIONS to a head-injured patient in the field. Formerly, it was recommended to give steroid drugs,

such as dexamethasone, but the effectiveness of such drugs has not been established on a scientific basis. Osmotic diuretics such as mannitol have also been used in brain injury, to reduce cerebral edema and thereby decrease intracranial pressure. While mannitol may be temporarily effective for that purpose, it can have a dangerous rebound effect. Thus mannitol and other diuretics should be given in the prehospital phase only to buy time during a prolonged transport, and preferably after the base physician has consulted with a neurosurgeon. If diuretics *are* ordered, the usual dosages are:

1. MANNITOL, 0.5 gm per kilogram slowly IV (the patient should have a urethral catheter in place).
2. Furosemide (Lasix), 40 to 80 mg IV.

- Be prepared to deal with SEIZURES. If they occur, they must be controlled as rapidly as possible, lest the seizures provoke further increases in intracranial pressure. Draw up 10 mg of DIAZEPAM (Valium) in a syringe, and tape the syringe to the stretcher. If the patient begins to convulse, notify the base physician immediately and request orders to administer the diazepam.
- Since every head-injured patient must be presumed to have a spinal injury as well, IMMOBILIZE THE PATIENT ON A BACKBOARD for transport.

TRANSPORT should be smooth and expeditious. As noted, conscious head-injured patients may not be entirely cooperative and may not wish to go to the hospital. As a general rule, however,

> **EVERY HEAD-INJURED PATIENT WHO HAS HAD A PERIOD OF UNCONSCIOUSNESS MUST BE EVALUATED IN THE HOSPITAL.**

It is your job to persuade the reluctant patient of the importance of a thorough evaluation.

If the patient is unconscious or has a deteriorating level of consciousness, transport him *directly* to a hospital that has neurosurgical facililties if at all possible, even if that means bypassing the nearest hospital. Delay in surgery for certain conditions, such as subdural hematoma, may be fatal; the extra time it takes to move the patient from one hospital to another could mean the difference between life and death. So if there is a neurosurgical facility in or near your community, transport directly to that facility, and notify the receiving hospital of your patient's status. Remember to keep repeating the assessment of vital and neurologic signs en route and to record all of your observations fully and accurately.

HEAD INJURY: SUMMARY

Assessment
- The most important sign in evaluating head injury is a CHANGING STATE OF CONSCIOUSNESS.
- Hypertension and bradycardia mean rising intracranial pressure.
- SHOCK MEANS INJURY ELSEWHERE.
- A head-injured patient has a CERVICAL SPINE INJURY UNTIL PROVED OTHERWISE.

Treatment
- Establish an AIRWAY (jaw thrust; early intubation). Be alert for vomiting. Have suction at hand.
- Assist BREATHING as needed to prevent hypercarbia; aim for about 20 breaths per minute.
- Administer 100% OXYGEN.
- Control BLEEDING.
- Cover open WOUNDS. Exposed brain tissue or CSF leakage should be covered *lightly* with loose, sterile dressings.
- Start an IV LIFELINE: normal saline at a keep-open rate.
- DO NOT OVERHEAT the patient.
- MONITOR cardiac rhythm.
- Keep rechecking NEUROLOGIC AND VITAL SIGNS, and record each finding accurately.
- IMMOBILIZE THE SPINE.
- Be prepared to deal with SEIZURES. Have diazepam drawn up in a syringe and ready.
- TRANSPORT directly to a neurosurgical facility.

FACIAL INJURIES

Facial injuries occur commonly. Approximately three-quarters of all patients who require hospital evaluation after motor vehicle accidents, for example, have some degree of facial injury. Injuries to the face and its structures may appear very dramatic but ordinarily are not in themselves life-threatening. Facial injuries are worrisome, however, for three reasons:

(1) They may be associated with AIRWAY OBSTRUCTION; (2) they may signal the presence of a CLOSED HEAD INJURY; indeed, in one study, 55 percent of patients admitted to hospital because of facial fractures were found to have closed head injury; and (3) approximately 10 percent of all patients with facial fracture have CERVICAL SPINE INJURY as well. Furthermore, even when not associated with a threat to life or limb, facial injuries are extremely distressing to the person who sustained them. A person's face is the most "public" part of his body, the part he uses to present himself to the world, and no one wants his face disfigured.

Soft Tissue Injuries to the Face

Facial LACERATIONS are treated as lacerations anywhere else, with direct pressure to control bleeding and sterile dressings.

When a FOREIGN OBJECT IS IMPALED IN THE CHEEK, the object *should be removed*, because massive bleeding associated with cheek injuries may obstruct the airway. This is probably the only instance in which an impaled object should be removed in the field rather than stabilized in place. (The other possible exception to the general rule for impaled objects is an object impaled in the airway that obstructs breathing.) Gently palpate the inside the cheek to determine whether the impaled object has penetrated all the way through. If that is the case, carefully pull the object out from the same side that it entered; if you have difficulty removing the impaled object, however, don't try to force it—just leave it in place.

When the object has been removed, pack the inside of the cheek (between the teeth and the cheek) with sterile gauze, and apply counterpressure with a dressing and bandage secured firmly over the outside of the wound. If bleeding is still profuse, position the patient so that blood will drain out of his mouth rather than down his throat, and suction the mouth as needed.

A HEMATOMA anywhere on the face needs to be treated in the emergency room, lest it lead to permanent deformity. An untreated hematoma of the ear, for example, will result in "cauliflower ear." In the field, the only treatment feasible is application of a cold pack, to minimize swelling and discomfort.

EPISTAXIS (nosebleed) without fracture is one of the most common emergencies requiring first aid or more extensive treatment. Simple, unilateral epistaxis in young adults and children usually arises from the *anterior* part of the nose, sometimes without any history of injury. It is best controlled simply by pinching the nostrils together. (A clothespin will work very nicely if you happen to carry one in your jump kit!) Such bleeding is rarely massive unless it is associated with a fracture, and it tends to be self-limited. There is rarely any need to insert any sort of pack into the nose for an anterior nosebleed, as compression accomplishes the same purpose.

Severe epistaxis is more frequently encountered among the elderly, especially if there is associated hypertension, and the bleeding often originates in the *posterior* part of the nose, so that bleeding may not even be visible through the nares. Inspection of the back of the patient's throat, however, will reveal blood dripping down the posterior oropharynx if the source of bleeding is posterior. A severe posterior nosebleed can be a life-threatening emergency, and the patient should be treated initially as any other patient with exsanguinating hemorrhage; that is, get the IV line in quickly, and infuse normal saline or lactated Ringer's at the rate ordered by the physician. If signs of shock are present, keep the patient flat, with his head or whole body turned to the side to facilitate drainage of blood. If vital signs are stable, on the other hand, have him sit upright, bending over a bowl, with his mouth propped open by a bite-block. Instruct the patient to breathe only through his mouth and to resist the temptation to swallow, for swallowing blood may lead to vomiting. If he has blood in his mouth, he should spit it out.

If those maneuvers fail to slow the bleeding and if transit time to the hospital will be prolonged, you may have to insert a posterior and anterior *nasal pack,* the former used to buttress the latter. In the field, that is most easily accomplished by passing a Foley catheter with a 30-ml balloon into the posterior nasopharynx. Before you start, protect yourself and the patient from blood with large sheets or gowns. Don gloves. Have the patient sit up and give him a large bowl. Instruct him to evacuate as much clot as he can by blowing hard out of each nostril, one after the other. Meanwhile, prepare the Foley catheter.

Before you insert the catheter, cut off the tip distal to the balloon, to prevent the tip from bumping against the posterior pharynx and causing the patient to gag. Then lubricate the catheter with a water-soluble jelly or lidocaine jelly, and, while your partner holds the patient's head steady, pass it into the more patent nostril until its tip is visible in the back of the throat. Inflate the balloon about 15 ml, and pull the catheter gently forward until you feel resistance; at that point inflate the balloon with another 5 to 7 ml of air (Fig. 16-14A). Holding the Foley catheter under slight tension, pack the bleeding nostril anteriorly, using the balloon of the Foley to provide a solid posterior wall against which the anterior packing can be applied. Use petrolatum gauze specially designed for nasal packing. When the nostril is firmly packed, pad

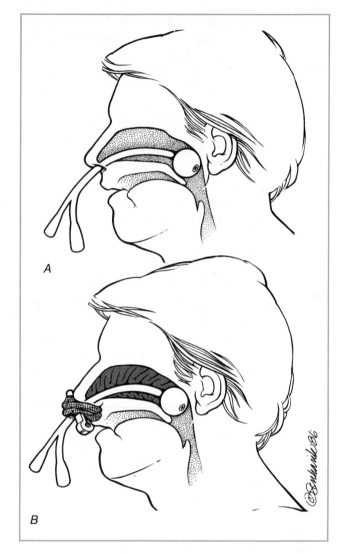

FIGURE 16-14. NASAL PACKS. (A) A Foley catheter is placed in the posterior nasopharynx. (B) Petrolatum gauze is packed against the Foley balloon, and a clamp holds the catheter in tension against the nares.

the external nares with a folded 4- by 4-inch gauze pad, and place a plastic umbilical clamp across the catheter to secure it against the nares and maintain tension (Fig. 16-14B). Merely taping the catheter to the cheek is not sufficient. Adjust the tension so that the balloon is snug but not painful.

Maxillofacial Fractures

Maxillofacial fractures occur when the face absorbs the energy of a strong impact. The forces involved may be massive. It requires forces of up to 150 G, for example, to fracture the maxilla, and forces of that magnitude can be expected to produce cerebral contusions and cervical spine injuries as well. Thus the first thing to remember about maxillofacial fractures is

WHEN YOU FIND A MAXILLOFACIAL FRACTURE, IMMOBILIZE THE SPINE AND MONITOR NEUROLOGIC SIGNS.

The first clue to the presence of a maxillofacial fracture is usually *ecchymosis*, so a black-and-blue mark anywhere over the face should alert you to the possibility of facial fracture. A deep facial laceration is also a tip-off that underlying bone may have been injured, and pain on palpation over a bone tends to support the suspicion of fracture.

The most common facial fracture is a BROKEN NOSE, which can be recognized by swelling, tenderness, and sometimes displacement from the normal position. Usually there is **crepitus,** a crackling feeling on palpation, and often there is epistaxis.

Next most common are FRACTURES OF THE MANDIBLE. When the mandible is fractured, there is at least a 50:50 chance that it is fractured in more than one place and will therefore be unstable to palpation. Furthermore, the patient will have an abnormal bite (**malocclusion**), and there is likely to be ecchymosis and swelling over the fracture site. Teeth may be partially or completely avulsed in association with mandibular fracture.

MAXILLARY FRACTURES are seen primarily in accidents involving massive forces, such as motor vehicle accidents. Maxillary fractures produce massive facial swelling, instability of the mid-facial bones, and malocclusion. There may be a "black eye," and the patient's face appears elongated.

When one of the cheekbones (ZYGOMATA) is fractured, that side of the patient's face looks flattened, and there is loss of sensation over the cheek, nose, and upper lip.

The characteristics of common maxillofacial fractures are summarized in Table 16-3. In the field, it is probably not necessary to try to distinguish among the various maxillofacial injuries. What *is* important is to safeguard the airway and the cervical spine. The following general principles of TREATMENT apply to all patients with significant maxillofacial injury:

- Establish an AIRWAY, which may be in particular jeopardy in patients who have sustained maxillary fractures. An S tube or nasopharyngeal airway can be useful in such a situation if the patient is not conscious. (Use a nasopharyngeal airway *only* if there is no evidence of trauma to the nose and if there is no bleeding or CSF leak from the nose.) Inspect the mouth for small fragments of teeth or dentures that might be aspirated, and remove them. Suction any blood from the mouth and throat.
- Examine the mouth for broken or missing TEETH. If a tooth has been lost, try to find it! If a tooth has been avulsed and cannot be found, the physician must assume it has been aspirated until proved otherwise. Should you find an intact missing tooth at the scene of an accident, pick it up by the crown, not the root, and place it in a container of refrigerated, fresh, whole milk for storage en route to the emergency room. Keep

TABLE 16-3. SUMMARY OF MAXILLOFACIAL INJURIES

SITE	SIGNS AND SYMPTOMS	TREATMENT IN THE FIELD
Multiple facial bones	Massive facial swelling Malocclusion of the teeth Palpable deformities	Ensure an open AIRWAY Control external BLEEDING Cervical spine precautions If shock is present, look for other injuries
Zygoma (cheek bone)	Loss of sensation below the orbit Palpable flattening Loss of upward gaze Trismus	Ice bag to injured area
Nose	Crepitus and instability Swelling, tenderness, displacement	Pressure to control bleeding Cold packs
Maxilla	Mobility of the facial skeleton Malocclusion; facial swelling	Ensure an open AIRWAY
Mandible	Malocclusion	Preserve loose or avulsed teeth Four-tailed bandage

the tooth from banging against the sides of the container by cushioning it with sterile gauze. Notify the receiving hospital to have an oral surgeon standing by, for he may be able to reimplant the avulsed tooth if the patient and his tooth arrive at the hospital promptly. If arrival at the hospital will be delayed more than about 20 minutes, and if you are not occupied with more critical problems, try to reimplant the tooth yourself. Flush it clean with sterile saline, and likewise flush out the socket. Then line up the tooth in its correct position, and press it *slowly* and *gently* into the socket, allowing fluid to escape from the socket as you do so. Once the tooth is in place, have the patient bite down firmly on a gauze roll for 15 to 20 minutes.

- If there is swelling or ecchymosis associated with the fracture, a COLD PACK may help minimize further swelling and alleviate pain.
- Firmly apply a self-adhering roller bandage (Kerlix, Kling) to hold a FRACTURED MANDIBLE stable during transport. Make sure, however, that you do not compromise the airway by splinting the mandible.
- Assume that there is a cervical spine injury, and IMMOBILIZE THE SPINE (cervical collar, backboard).

Temporomandibular Joint Dislocation

One of the most distraught patients one can encounter is the patient who has dislocated his mandible and is, as a result, unable to close his mouth. Typically, he will run toward the rescuer, wild-eyed, gesturing frantically toward his wide-open mouth and making incomprehensible noises. When obtaining the history, which will not be possible until after the problem has been successfully treated, you will probably learn that the patient had been yawning extravagantly or eating something of unusually large dimensions (e.g., a "Whopper"), when he felt a "pop" and was suddenly unable to shut his mouth. The experience is not only embarrassing but can also be quite painful, for the jaw muscles go into spasm soon after the jaw is dislocated.

In the field, try at least once to replace the mandible into its proper position, since it becomes progressively more difficult to do so as time passes and muscle spasm increases. Don gloves, wrap your thumbs in gauze to protect them, and place both thumbs in the patient's mouth, one on each side over the lower molars. Your fingers meanwhile grasp the lower jaw near the angle. Apply gentle but firm pressure *downward* to open the joint and stretch the muscles; *then* direct your force toward the back of the patient's head to move the joint back into its normal

slot. Watch your thumbs! The jaws may snap shut as the dislocation is reduced. Do not use undue force. If the dislocation cannot be reduced with moderate pressure, sedation or general anesthesia may be required to accomplish reduction, and the patient should be brought to the hospital. Even if you do succeed in reducing the dislocation, the patient will require evaluation to rule out an associated mandibular fracture.

Injuries to the Eye

Approximately 1.5 million eye injuries occur in the United States each year, of which around 50,000 result in some degree of visual loss. Since trauma to the eyes is so common, and since the potential consequences are so serious, it is important for paramedics to know how to assess and manage ocular injuries.

Anatomy and Function of the Eye

The **globe,** or eyeball, is a spherical structure measuring about 1 inch in diameter that is housed within a bony cavity of the skull called the eye socket, or **orbit.** The structures of the globe (Fig. 16-15) include the following:

- The **sclera,** or "white of the eye," is a tough, fibrous coat that helps maintain the shape of the eye and also helps protect the contents of the eye. In some illnesses, such as hepatitis, the sclera may become yellow ("icteric") from staining by bile pigments.
- The **cornea** is the crystal-clear anterior segment of the sclera overlying the pupil and iris. In old age, the cornea may become cloudy in a condition known as *cataract.*
- The **conjunctiva** is a delicate mucous membrane that covers the sclera and undersurfaces of the eyelids. Often cyanosis can be detected in a patient's conjunctiva when it is not easily seen on the rest of his skin.
- The **iris** is the pigmented tissue made up of muscles and blood vessels that can contract or expand to regulate the size of the pupil.
- The **pupil** is the adjustable opening within the iris. A normal pupil dilates in dim light, to permit more light to enter the eye, and constricts in bright light to decrease the light entering the eye.
- Behind the iris and pupil is a **lens,** a transparent structure that can alter its thickness in order to focus light on the retina at the back of the eye.

Two special fluids help give the eye its shape and structure. The **aqueous humor** fills the space (the **an-**

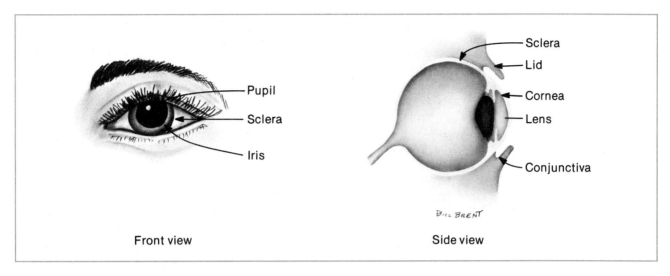

FIGURE 16-15. **STRUCTURE OF THE EYE.**

terior chamber) between the cornea and the lens. Aqueous humor is produced behind the iris, and if lost through a penetrating injury to the eye, it will gradually be replenished. Filling the posterior chamber, behind the lens, is the **vitreous humor,** a jelly-like substance that maintains the shape of the globe. If the vitreous is lost, it cannot be replenished, and blindness will result.

Assessment of the Patient with an Eye Injury

In taking the HISTORY of an eye injury, we want to find out how the injury happened and what symptoms the patient is experiencing. Find out precisely *what happened. When* did the injury occur? Did the patient have any *previous eye problems?* Does he take any *medications* for his eyes? Ask about the patient's *symptoms.* There are a variety of symptoms that may indicate serious ocular injury:

- VISUAL LOSS that does not improve when the patient blinks is probably the most important symptom of eye injury; it may indicate damage to the globe itself or to the optic nerve.
- DOUBLE VISION usually points to trauma involving the extraocular muscles, such as a fracture of the orbit.
- Severe PAIN IN THE EYE is another symptom of significant eye injury.
- A FOREIGN BODY SENSATION usually indicates superficial injury to the cornea or the presence of a foreign object trapped behind the eyelids.

In the PHYSICAL EXAMINATION of the eyes, evaluate each of the visible ocular structures and ocular function:

- ORBITS: for ecchymoses, swelling, lacerations, tenderness.
- LIDS: for ecchymoses, swelling, laceration.
- CONJUNCTIVAE: for redness, pus, foreign bodies.
- GLOBES: for redness, abnormal pigmentation, laceration.
- PUPILS: for size, shape, equality, reaction to light, tenting.
- EYE MOVEMENTS in all directions: for paralysis of gaze or discoordination between the movements of the two eyes (**dysconjugate gaze**).
- Most important of all, VISUAL ACUITY. Make a rough assessment by asking the patient to read a newspaper or a handheld visual acuity chart. Test each eye separately. Document your results carefully (e.g., "The patient was able to read a newspaper held at a distance of 10 inches from each eye."), for this information will be of enormous importance to the physicians who subsequently reassess the patient.

Injury to the Orbits

Trauma to the face may result in fracture of one or several of the bones of the skull that form the orbits. A patient with an orbital fracture may complain of *double vision* and may lose sensation above the eyebrow or over the cheek from associated nerve damage. Sometimes there is massive nasal discharge, and vision is often impaired. Fractures of the inferior orbit are the most common type and can cause paralysis of upward gaze (i.e., the patient's injured eye will not be able to follow your finger *above* the midline). For that reason it is important to CHECK EYE MOVEMENTS IN ALL PLANES IN THE PATIENT WITH POSSIBLE FACIAL FRACTURES.

Orbital fractures require hospitalization and sometimes surgery. Transport the patient in a sitting position. If there is no associated injury to the globe, apply cold packs gently over the traumatized area to diminish swelling. If you suspect injury to the eye itself, however, do *not* apply any sort of compress.

Lid Injuries

The eyelid may suffer closed injury, such as contusion ("black eye") or burns, or open injury, such as a laceration. In general, there is little that can be done for such injuries in the field beyond gentle irrigation of a laceration and gentle patching. No lid injury is trivial, for there may be damage to the eye beneath. Therefore, every patient with eyelid trauma must be evaluated in the emergency room.

Injuries to the Globe

Most injuries to the globe—including contusions, lacerations, foreign bodies, and abrasions—are best treated in the emergency department, where specialized equipment is available. Aluminum eye shields (not gauze patches) applied over BOTH eyes are all that are necessary in the field. But bear in mind that as soon as you cover both of the patient's eyes, he can no longer see—so *you* will have to serve as his eyes, keeping him reassured and oriented to where he is, what you are doing, and so forth.

One type of injury to the globe that definitely *does* require treatment to begin in the field is a CHEMICAL BURN TO THE EYE, especially an alkali burn, which may lead rapidly to total blindness. As we learned in the previous chapter, the most important measure in treating a chemical burn to the eye is to begin IMMEDIATE CONTINUOUS IRRIGATION with copious amounts of saline, lactated Ringer's solution, or tap water. The eyelids must be held open to allow the irrigating solution to flush all the chemical from behind the lids, and contact lenses must be removed. The affected eye should be *continuously* irrigated for *at least* 30 minutes before moving the patient to the hospital.

Another type of "burn" commonly sustained in the eye occurs after exposure to ultraviolet light, the so-called ARC WELDER'S BURN. Any source of ultraviolet light can cause this kind of damage, including various "psychedelic" lighting systems popular in some discos. The patient typically presents with severe pain in his eyes, photophobia (inability to tolerate bright light), and spasm of the eyelids about 5 to 10 hours after exposure to ultraviolet radiation. Proper evaluation requires a slit-lamp examination in the emergency room. The only treatment feasible in the field is to apply cool compresses *lightly* over the eyelids, which may afford considerable relief of pain to a patient in extreme distress.

When there is a FOREIGN OBJECT IMPALED IN THE GLOBE *do not remove it*! Stabilize it in place. For that purpose, use several layers of sterile 4- by 4-inch gauze and a paper cup. Cut a hole in the center of the gauze dressings large enough to pass over the impaled object without difficulty. Slide the dressings over the impaled object, taking care not to jar the object, and position the dressings lightly over the injury site. Then take a paper cup large enough to fit over the impaled object without touching it, and position the cup over the dressings. Fasten the cup in place with a self-adhering roller bandage (Kling, Kerlix). Finally, *patch the other eye* to reduce eye movements (when one eye moves, the other moves with it).

General Principles of Eye Care

The eyes are delicate structures and are subject to injury even when they are not directly traumatized. When blinking reflexes are absent, for example, as in the comatose patient, the surface of the eye may dry out or may accumulate foreign material. Similarly, contact lenses left in place for extended periods in the comatose patient may cause corneal abrasion and edema—as any contact lens wearer who has gone to bed with his hard lenses can attest. Thus,

> ## PROTECT THE EYES OF EVERY COMATOSE PATIENT.

If transport time will be short, simply tape or patch the eyes closed. If, however, extended transport (several hours) will be required, remove the patient's contact lenses.

Contact lenses are of two types, hard and soft. Hard lenses are the most likely to cause irritation to the eyes if left in place for extended periods. To check for the presence of hard lenses, shine your penlight obliquely across the patient's eye, from the outer angle of the eye toward the nose. If a hard lens is present, you'll see a reflection on its edge. The best method for removing a hard contact lens is with a rubber suction cup specially designed for that purpose, and one or two of those suction cups should be part of the standard equipment of every ambulance. Gently separate the patient's eyelids, and moisten the suction cup in sterile eye-irrigation solution. Then squeeze the rubber bulb of the suction cup, and apply the cup to the center of the contact lens. Slowly release the pressure on the cup, so that it grips the lens, and simply lift the lens out of the eye.

If you do not carry one of those suction cups, you can irrigate the contact lens out of the eye. That method is also useful for removing contact lenses after chemical spills in the eye. Place the patient supine, with his head turned toward the side to be irrigated. Fill a rubber bulb syringe with sterile normal saline solution, and holding the tip of the syringe close to the inner (nasal) angle of the eyelid, irrigate the eye gently. The lens should simply float out. Then turn the head to the other side, and irrigate the other eye.

In cases of chemical burns, it may be necessary to remove *soft* contact lenses, in order to irrigate beneath them. If the patient is unable to remove the lenses himself, first scrub your hands and dry them on a lint-free towel. Gently separate the patient's eyelids with the thumb and index finger of one hand; then place the thumb and index finger of the other hand on each end of the soft lens, and pinch it gently out of the eye. Place each lens in a separate container of sterile *normal saline solution*. Don't worry if they shrivel a bit; they will return to their normal shape when they are rehydrated.

If you leave the contact lenses of a comatose patient in place, put a piece of tape on the patient's forehead and write "contact lenses" on it, so that the emergency room staff will be aware of their presence. When you do remove contact lenses in the field, *take good care of them*! Put them in a safe place, and make sure they are entrusted to a responsible person in the emergency room when the patient is transferred there.

NECK INJURIES

The neck is a very vulnerable stretch of anatomy, for it houses (1) a critical portion of the AIRWAY (the larynx), (2) the MAJOR BLOOD VESSELS to and from the head, and (3) the SPINAL CORD, with its nerve supply to the whole body. Clearly injury to any of those structures can be disastrous. So soft tissue injuries to the neck must be considered *critical until proved otherwise.*

Blunt Injury to the Neck

Blunt trauma to the neck may cause collapse of the larynx or trachea with consequent airway obstruction. When, therefore, the patient complains of pain in the anterior neck, or when you see bruising or swelling in that area, look immediately for evidence of trauma to the larynx that may compromise air exchange. Patients with significant laryngeal trauma will often complain of *shortness of breath*, and most will be unable to tolerate lying down supine. On physical examination, the most common finding is *hoarseness* of the voice (sometimes the patient loses his voice altogether). There will be *tenderness* over the anterior neck in nearly all cases, and a majority of patients with significant laryngeal trauma will have *subcutaneous emphysema*. The trachea may be deviated to the right or left. Some patients will cough up blood.

Assess the patient for *signs of respiratory distress*. If ventilation is inadequate, you will have to assist the patient's breathing with a bag-valve-mask and 100% oxygen. Bear in mind as you do so that any force powerful enough to disrupt the larynx is powerful enough to produce cervical spine injury, so handle the patient accordingly.

Most patients with serious laryngeal trauma will need a tracheotomy as soon as possible. Orotracheal intubation may be hazardous in such patients, because one cannot see where the tip of the endotracheal tube is going once it passes the vocal cords, and it may pass straight through a defect in the laryngeal wall. Therefore, if the patient has *any* signs of laryngeal injury, give 100% oxygen; stabilize the cervical spine; assist ventilations gently (bag-valve-mask only, *not* demand valve); and GET MOVING TO THE HOSPITAL. Notify the receiving hospital to set up for emergency tracheotomy.

Penetrating Injuries to the Neck

Penetrating injuries to the neck may sometimes become apparent, if the trachea has been disrupted, by the presence of *subcutaneous emphysema* of the neck and anterior chest and by a frothy mixture of air and blood blowing through the penetrating wound. Such wounds must be sealed off, and if possible, the trachea should be intubated from above (i.e., through the mouth, as opposed to tracheotomy), with the aim of placing the cuff of the endotracheal tube below the area of the trachea that has been penetrated. To accomplish that with any certainty, one needs to use a fiberoptic laryngoscope, which is not standard equipment on most ambulances. Thus considerations such as the patient's overall condition and the distance to the hospital will determine whether you attempt intubation in the field for such cases.

Penetrating injuries to the neck also carry a hazard of exsanguinating hemorrhage from the jugular veins, carotid arteries, or their branches. One special danger associated with bleeding wounds of the neck is the possibility of a fatal AIR EMBOLISM. If a major vein of the neck is disrupted, air can be sucked into the vein and, from there, be swept along with the blood flow into the heart, causing dysrhythmias and death.

When there is significant bleeding from the neck, therefore, the wound must be sealed immediately with petrolatum gauze. Apply a bulky dressing (e.g., a composite pad) over the petrolatum gauze, and hold pressure over the dressing by hand. DO NOT USE CIRCUMFERENTIAL BANDAGES TO HOLD A DRESSING IN PLACE ON THE NECK, as such bandages may interfere with blood flow on the other side of the neck and may also impair breathing. So use manual pressure only, applied over the bleeding site.

Position the patient on his left side in about 15 degrees of Trendelenburg (head down, feet elevated). (Question: Why is the patient placed in that position? Hint: Air bubbles float in blood.) If bleeding is profuse or signs of impending shock are present, treat for shock as outlined in Chapter 9, and move quickly to the hospital.

SPINAL INJURY

It is estimated that approximately 12,000 people sustain spinal cord injury in the United States each year, about one-third to one-half of whom die before reaching the hospital. For the most part, spinal cord trauma affects the 15- to 35-year age group. More than half of the cases are a result of vehicular accidents; about 20 percent result from falls, 12 percent from gunshot wounds and other penetrating injuries, and the remainder from diving accidents, contact sports, and other causes. Some degree of injury to the spinal cord occurs in about 10 percent of all victims of multiple trauma. That fact dictates the first principle of caring for patients with potential spinal cord injuries:

> **EVERY VICTIM OF MULTIPLE TRAUMA HAS A SPINAL CORD INJURY UNTIL PROVED OTHERWISE.**

The initial care of a patient with spinal injury will in many cases determine whether that patient regains normal function or is crippled for the rest of his life. In few other areas of emergency care will the rescuer have as much potential influence on a patient's whole future existence, and it is thus the paramedic's responsibility to be knowledgeable and skilled in the care of patients with possible spinal cord trauma.

The spinal cord connects the brain to all of the other organs in the body. If the cord is interrupted, all connections between the brain and muscle groups or organs *below* the level of cord damage are severed. The part of the body involved becomes functionally incommunicado, as useless as if it had been amputated. A man who has suffered paraplegia secondary to transection of the spinal cord in the lumbar region is, for all practical purposes, a man without legs (as well as a man without bladder control, without sexual function, and so forth). If the injury is higher in the spinal cord—say around the sixth cervical vertebra (C6)—the hands will be affected in addition to the legs. Furthermore, intercostal muscles will be paralyzed, severely compromising respiration. A bit higher in the spinal cord—C4 or above—injury will paralyze the diaphragm as well, making breathing virtually impossible. In such an injury, the patient, if he survives, becomes for the rest of his life a prisoner in his own body, totally dependent on machines and on other people for every need. Once that kind of paralysis has set in, it cannot be cured. The only treatment is *prevention*, and prevention starts, as far as the paramedic is concerned, at the accident scene.

When to Suspect a Spinal Cord Injury

To prevent further damage to a patient with spinal cord injury or potential spinal cord injury, one must first of all be aware that such an injury may have occurred; for if you wait for signs and symptoms of spinal cord injury to develop, it will generally be too late to prevent permanent damage. It is important, therefore, to be familiar with the circumstances that commonly produce spinal cord injuries and to try to determine, through history-taking and examination of the accident scene, whether any of those circumstances are applicable in any given case.

The *history* of the accident is very important. Maintain a high index of suspicion in any case where the *mechanisms of injury* suggest the possibility of spinal cord injury (Fig. 16-16). For example, any accident involving significant acceleration-deceleration forces, such as VEHICULAR TRAUMA, is likely to have snapped the victim's neck violently back and forth. Compression injuries, such as those that might be sustained in DIVING headfirst into a shallow pool or JUMPING FROM A HEIGHT and landing on one's feet, are also a likely source of spinal trauma. Indeed, any fall from a height should immediately alert the paramedic to the possibility of spinal injury.

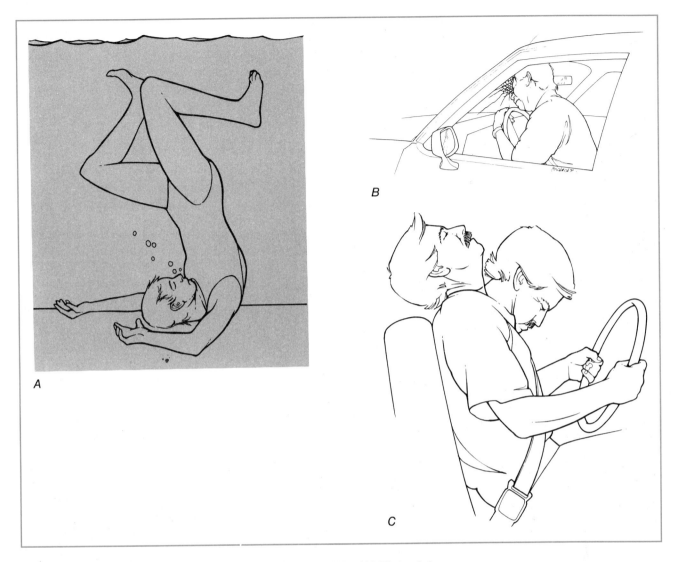

FIGURE 16-16. **MECHANISMS OF SPINAL CORD INJURY.** (A) Diving injury. (B) Forward impact of head. (C) Whiplash.

Associated injuries, especially those that bespeak massive forces involved in the injury, may also provide clues to the presence of spinal cord injury. The majority of cervical spine injuries are associated with head injury, so any patient with HEAD TRAUMA, including FACIAL TRAUMA, or any other MAJOR TRAUMA ABOVE THE CLAVICLES must be assumed to have a cervical spine injury until proved otherwise. CRUSHING INJURIES, such as those that occur in a cave-in, are apt to produce spine injuries, as are injuries due to LIGHTNING, which causes violent muscle contractions. And don't forget GUNSHOT WOUNDS, especially to the head, neck, chest, back, and abdomen. Finally, any victim of MULTIPLE TRAUMA or any patient found UNCONSCIOUS AFTER TRAUMA should be assumed to have a spinal cord injury until proved otherwise.

SUSPECT SPINAL CORD INJURY IN

- Vehicular trauma
- Diving accidents (shallow pools)
- Jumps or falls from a height
- Significant injury above the clavicles (head, face, neck)
- Crush injuries
- Lightning injuries
- Gunshot wounds of the head, neck, chest, back, abdomen
- Multitrauma victims
- Patients who are unconscious after trauma

It should be mentioned that not every patient with injury to the spinal *column* (the vertebrae) has injury to the spinal *cord*. However, the potential for spinal cord injury is always present in a patient who has sustained trauma to the vertebral column, so for practical purposes there is no point in trying to distinguish between the two types of injury in the field.

Try to determine as precisely as possible the circumstances of the accident. Was it a flexion injury, such as occurs in the classic diving accident? Was there torsion on the neck? Find out the exact *time* of the injury; if it has been more than 6 hours since the accident, the chances of restoring lost function are greatly reduced. If the patient is conscious, instruct him not to move. Ask him whether he has pain anywhere in the neck or back. Is there numbness or tingling in any extremity? Are the extremities weak? If the patient cannot move at all, find out whether anyone saw him move at any time after the accident; a patient who has any demonstrable motion whatsoever after spinal injury has a 75-percent chance of recovering functional ambulation at a later date, and it is important for the physician to be able to identify which patients fall into that category. Has the patient been moved in any way since the accident? Have his symptoms changed between the time of the injury and the time that you arrived?

Assessment of the Patient with Possible Spinal Cord Injury

When the circumstances of injury suggest the possibility of spinal cord damage, it will be necessary to apply some means of temporary stabilization to the cervical spine as you perform the primary survey. If there are a sufficient number of rescuers, the most efficient and readily available means of temporary stabilization are a pair of hands or a pair of knees! The object is to KEEP THE HEAD AND NECK IN NEUTRAL POSITION and prevent any flexion, extension, or movement to the side. A cervical collar may be applied (Fig. 16-17) as soon as you have completed your assessment of the airway and the neck, but some means, such as sandbags or manual stabilization, will still have to be used to prevent lateral motion until the patient can be fully immobilized on a backboard.

The Primary Survey

In the victim of trauma, as we learned earlier, the alphabet of the primary survey is expanded to A B C D E:

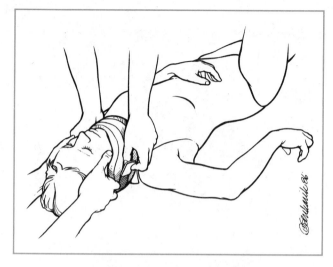

FIGURE 16-17.   APPLICATION OF A CERVICAL COLLAR.   While one rescuer holds the head steady in neutral position, another rescuer applies the collar.

A   If the patient is unconscious, the first priority, as always, is to ensure an open AIRWAY. Use jaw thrust (Fig. 16-18A), chin lift (Fig. 16-18B), or jaw lift (Fig. 16-18C) *without backward tilt of the head*, and insert a nasopharyngeal airway. Keep SUCTION readily available to clear the airway of secretions, blood, or vomitus.

Opinion is divided regarding whether and how to intubate the trachea of a patient with possible cervical spine injury in the prehospital phase. Some authorities feel that nasotracheal intubation is the only safe method for patients who might have spinal cord damage, while others believe that orotracheal intubation with the head held stable is equally safe. Yet other experts argue that there is *no* safe way to intubate a patient who has a cervical spine injury except using special equipment in the hospital. At this time, there are no clinical data that unequivocally resolve the issue one way or the other. The bottom line is that if you cannot maintain a patent airway without an endotracheal tube, the patient should be intubated, using the method you do best. Whether you choose the oral or nasal route, have an assistant stabilize the patient's head and neck to minimize flexion and extension.

B   Evaluate the patient's BREATHING. An injury involving the lower cervical or upper thoracic spinal cord may result in paralysis of the

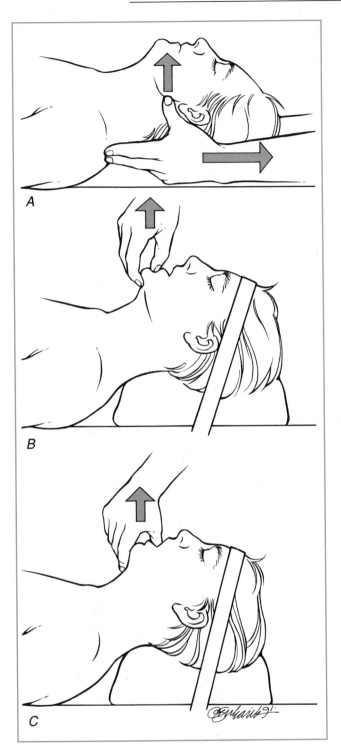

FIGURE 16-18.   OPENING THE AIRWAY IN A SPINE-INJURED PATIENT.   (A) Jaw thrust. (B) Chin lift. (C) Jaw lift. All maneuvers are performed with the head in neutral position.

intercostal muscles. Injury around C4 or higher will paralyze the diaphragm as well, causing severe impairment of respiration. What you will see clinically is *abdominal breathing* and use of accessory muscles in the neck. If breathing is shallow, you will need to assist ventilations. The conscious patient can be instructed in the use of the demand valve, so that each of his spontaneous breaths can be given a little boost. Ventilate the unconscious patient with a bag-valve-mask at about 20 breaths per minute, making sure to keep the head and neck steady (Fig. 16-19).

C   Proceed rapidly to assess the CIRCULATION. That means, at this stage, *control of bleeding*. Further steps to manage shock, if present, will be carried out subsequently.

D   Use the AVPU Scale described earlier to make a rough initial estimate of DISABILITY, that is, the patient's neurologic status. Record your findings along with the time.

E   EXPOSE the patient for closer examination. *Cut* away his clothes to minimize motion of the spine.

FIGURE 16-19.   VENTILATING A PATIENT WITH POSSIBLE CERVICAL SPINE INJURY.   Stabilize the victim's head and neck between your knees as you give artificial ventilation.

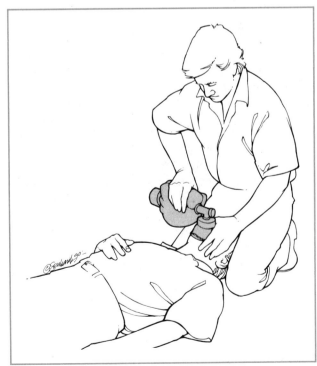

In a severely injured victim of multiple trauma, you may at this point simply have to immobilize the patient on a backboard, load him into the ambulance, and start moving toward the hospital—with any other interventions, such as intravenous therapy, or other examinations performed en route. In the patient who is stable, however, you may proceed directly to the secondary survey.

The Secondary Survey

Even as you were approaching the patient to start the primary survey, you should have been observing his GENERAL APPEARANCE and the POSITION IN WHICH HE WAS FOUND. Do not try to change the patient's position unless his airway is jeopardized. There are some positions quite characteristic of spinal cord injury. A patient with an injury around C6, for example, will often lie with his forearms flexed across his chest and his hands half-closed. If you try to straighten out his arm, it will spring right back to the flexed position as soon as you let go. Another position seen in some cervical spine injuries is the "stick 'em up" position, in which the patient holds his hands above his head.

Measure the patient's VITAL SIGNS. Be alert for HYPOTENSION WITHOUT OTHER SIGNS OF SHOCK, that is, hypotension with a normal or slow pulse and warm skin. That combination is highly suggestive of neurogenic shock ("spinal shock"). Spinal shock occurs immediately after a significant injury to the spinal cord, as a result of widespread dilatation of blood vessels. The systolic blood pressure is usually in the range of 75 to 80 mm Hg. The cord injury responsible for spinal shock also generally produces a flaccid paralysis and complete loss of sensation below the level of the injury. If you find hypotension in association with pale, cold, clammy skin, on the other hand, suspect *hypovolemic*—not neurogenic—shock, and start looking for the source.

Proceed to the HEAD-TO-TOE SURVEY, and check the HEAD and FACE carefully for cuts and bruises. Remember, most patients with cervical spine injuries have head or facial injuries as well. In examining the NECK, palpate gently over the cervical spine for deformity (ask the conscious patient to report any tenderness as you palpate). Examine the CHEST and ABDOMEN for signs of internal injury. Remember, spinal cord injury may mask injuries in the abdomen or lower extremities, for the patient may not be able to feel pain.

In the male, check for **priapism** (sustained erection of the penis), which, when present, is a characteristic sign of spinal cord injury. Note also any signs of *loss of bowel or bladder control*. Slide your gloved

hands beneath the small of the patient's BACK and palpate for deformity or tenderness. Withdraw your hands and inspect them for blood.

Combine your assessment of the EXTREMITIES with a brief NEUROLOGIC EXAMINATION, paying particular attention to the modalities of the major spinal nerve tracts, that is, *position sense, pain,* and *movement.* Can the patient tell when someone is moving his finger or toe up or down? Does he feel pain in response to pinprick? The level at which the spinal cord has been damaged may sometimes be identified by checking for response to pinprick, starting at the toes and moving upward (Fig. 16-20). Use a ball-point pen or grease pencil to mark on the patient's body the level at which he first reports that he can feel the pin. A knowledge of the distribution of spinal nerves will then enable the examiner to estimate at approxi-

FIGURE 16-20. DERMATOMES. The level of sensory deficit may be determined by checking for sensation, starting with the toes, and noting precisely where the patient first begins to feel the pinprick.

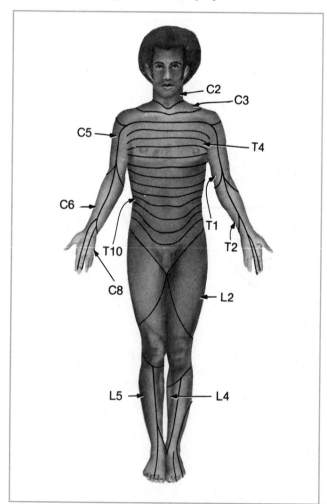

mately what nerve level the damage occurred. A rough guide to remember is as follows:

Rough Guide to the Dermatomes

L3	Knee	T4	Nipples
T10	Umbilicus	C3	Clavicles

Thus, for example, if a patient has intact sensation at the nipples but absent sensation at the umbilicus, his injury is probably somewhere between the fifth and tenth thoracic vertebrae (i.e., between T5 and T10). Like all other neurologic findings, the level of sensation must be rechecked periodically and documented after each check.

To check the patient's MOTOR FUNCTION, first ask him to wiggle his toes, then his fingers. If he cannot move his toes or fingers, can he flex his wrist? His elbow? Make a precise record of what the patient can and cannot do, for once again, the type of function lost will help pinpoint the level of injury in the spinal cord (Table 16-4). In an unconscious patient, test for paralysis by applying a painful stimulus first to each foot, then to each hand, and observe whether the patient pulls the limb away.

It must be emphasized that

A NORMAL NEUROLOGIC EXAMINATION DOES NOT RULE OUT THE POSSIBILITY OF SPINAL CORD INJURY.

Victims of vehicular trauma have been known to walk away from the accident only to become totally paralyzed hours later, when an incautious nod of the head squeezed an unstable vertebral column down against the spinal cord. Thus, when the mechanisms of injury are such that the patient *could* have sustained spinal cord injury, treat him as a spine injury regardless of the neurologic findings. The purpose of the neurologic assessment is *not* to determine whether the patient should be immobilized; it is to furnish data to the neurosurgeons about the precise condition of the patient when first seen, so that they may evaluate any changes in that condition and thereby determine if immediate surgery is necessary.

TABLE 16-4. SEGMENTAL INNERVATION OF SELECTED MUSCLES

REGION	MUSCLE(S)	FUNCTION	SPINAL LEVEL
NECK	Trapezius	Raises and adducts scapula	C3
	Sternomastoid	Shrugging	C1–C2
	Diaphragm	Breathing	C4
SHOULDER	Deltoid	Abduct and rotate upper arm	C5
	Supra- and infraspinatus		C5–C6
ARM	Biceps	Flexion of forearm	C5–C6
	Triceps	Extension of forearm	C7
FOREARM	Multiple muscles	Wrist extension	C6–C7
		Wrist flexion	C8
		Supination of wrist	C5
		Pronation of wrist	C7
HAND	Lumbricals and interossei	Extension of fingers	C7
		Flexion of fingers	C8
		Opposition of thumb	T1
PELVIC GIRDLE	Gluteus	Extends and rotates thigh	L5
THIGH	Quadriceps	Flexes thigh	L3
		Extends leg	
	Biceps femoralis	Extends leg	L5
	Semitendinosus	Flexes leg	L4–S1
LEG AND FOOT		Knee flexion	S1
		Ankle dorsiflexion	L5–S1
BLADDER		Bladder control	S2–S3

Treatment of the Patient with Suspected Spinal Cord Injury

Treatment in cases of possible spinal cord injury is aimed at supporting vital functions and preventing further spinal cord damage. In fact, treatment begins during the primary survey, before assessment is complete, as shown in Figure 16-21. Besides the measures of the primary survey, described earlier, treatment consists of the following:

- Dress wounds, and splint fractures.
- Move the patient to a backboard, keeping his head, neck, and back in alignment. If the MAST device is used in your EMS system, lay the MAST out on the backboard before you transfer the patient to the board.
- If there are signs of *shock,* apply and inflate the MAST (if used in your system), and establish an IV with lactated Ringer's solution.
- Cover the patient with a BLANKET, especially if there are signs of spinal shock. Remember, without the ability to constrict peripheral blood vessels, a person cannot conserve body heat.
- BE PREPARED FOR SEIZURES, and be ready to restrain the patient if he seizes before he has been immobilized to the backboard. Ordinarily, we do not restrain a patient during a seizure; but when there is a question of spinal cord injury, we don't want the patient's head and neck flapping wildly in all directions, so restraint of the patient is necessary. Have a syringe of DIAZEPAM drawn up and ready to administer, taped to the backboard.
- Before moving the patient to the ambulance, IMMOBILIZE THE PATIENT ON A LONG BACKBOARD, so that his head and neck are held securely in alignment with his trunk (see next section). If the patient is unconscious and not intubated, and if you have secured him so that he cannot slip to a side, tilt the backboard onto its side for transport—such that the patient is in a lateral recumbent position, tipped slightly toward the prone position (facing the paramedic in the ambulance). That position will permit drainage of secretions out of his mouth rather than down his throat into the airway.
- At this time, there is no consensus regarding prehospital MEDICATIONS for suspected spinal cord injury. Recent work suggests that very high doses of corticosteroids given within 8 hours of the injury may permit some recovery of nerve function, and in some EMS systems, steroid treatment is being started in the field. If ordered to administer corticosteroids to a spine-injured

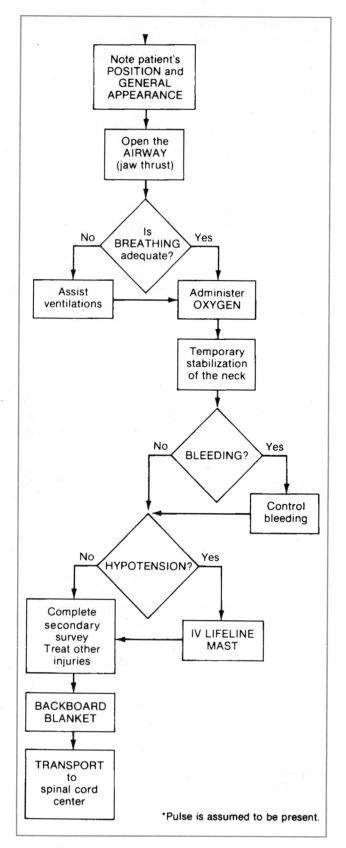

FIGURE 16-21.   MANAGEMENT OF THE PATIENT WITH SUSPECTED SPINAL INJURY.

patient, the dosage is **methylprednisolone, 30 mg/kg** given as an **IV bolus** (methylprednisolone is listed under Hydrocortisone and Other Corticosteroids in section A of the Drug Handbook).

- REASSESS VITAL SIGNS AND NEUROLOGIC STATUS frequently, and record your findings accurately after each assessment, using a neurologic checklist like that in Figure 16-11.

Spinal Immobilization

The most common cause of spinal injury is trauma sustained in automobile accidents, so in this section we will look first at stabilization of the spine-injured patient found in an automobile, as a model for spinal immobilization. The use of backboards and the techniques of spinal immobilization should have been learned during EMT-A training, and we will review this material only briefly here. For a more detailed presentation of the subject, the student is referred to *Emergency Medical Treatment* (see Further Reading) or any other EMT-A text. Like any other skills, skills in backboarding and extrication are subject to decay. Thus, this review of information about spinal immobilization should be accompanied by skill practice sessions.

The problem facing rescuers when an injured patient is found in a wrecked vehicle is how to move the victim out of the vehicle without aggravating possible damage to his spinal cord. The best way to do so is by packaging the patient onto SHORT AND LONG SPINE BOARDS. The advent of basic trauma life support (BTLS) protocols has created some controversy over whether short boards should be used at all. Proponents of the short board argue that it is the safest way to remove an injured person from a wrecked vehicle; opponents of the short board point out that a seriously injured patient's chances of survival decrease about 1 percent per minute of delay between the injury and arrival in the operating room. Application of short boards, they argue, takes too much time—if it takes 5 minutes, that means a 5 percent decrease in the patient's chances of survival.

In reality, both arguments are correct. The use of a short board *is* the safest way to remove an injured patient from a wrecked vehicle, but it *does* take time. So you will have to make a judgment call at every accident scene. If the patient is conscious and alert and has stable vital signs, take the extra minute or two to use a short board. If the level of consciousness is depressed or there are signs of shock or respiratory distress, do a quick extrication with a long board only.

Packaging and Removal of the Injured from an Automobile

We shall assume here that there are two rescuers and that the patient's overall condition is stable:

- The first rescuer positions himself behind the patient, if possible in the back seat for a front-seat patient, and HOLDS THE HEAD STEADY IN NEUTRAL POSITION (Fig. 16-22).
- The second rescuer completes the primary survey and examination of the neck and applies a CERVICAL COLLAR, preferably a Philadelphia collar. The cervical collar *helps* to prevent flexion and extension of the neck; it does *not* provide complete stabilization of the cervical spine. So the second rescuer should continue stabilizing the victim's head until the head has been fully immobilized to a backboard.
- While the first rescuer keeps the head and neck steady, the second rescuer slides the SHORT BACKBOARD or KED (Kendrick Extrication Device) behind the patient, so that the patient's head is lined up with the head extension on the board. If the car seat is curved, it may be necessary to move the patient slightly forward to get the board behind him; if so, the first rescuer should keep his motions coordinated with those of the second rescuer, so that the patient's head and neck remain in alignment with the long axis of his body.
- When the short board is in position, the second rescuer inserts a NECK ROLL to fill the gap be-

FIGURE 16-22.   STABILIZING THE HEAD AND NECK. One rescuer gets behind the patient and holds his head in neutral position.

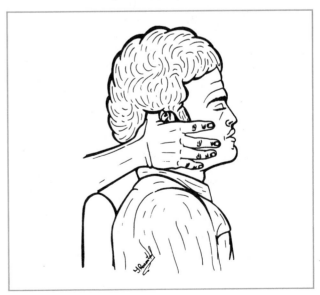

tween the patient's neck and the board. A folded towel or air splint may be used for this purpose. An air splint has the advantage that its size may be adjusted to conform to the patient's anatomy. Take care just to fill in the dead space between the cervical collar and the board; an excessively large neck roll will cause the patient's head and neck to be hyperextended when the head is secured to the board.

- The second rescuer STRAPS THE patient's TORSO to the board. If you are using straps with quick-release buckles, be sure that the buckles are taped to prevent inadvertent release. Also, adjust the straps so that the buckles are high on the chest, near the shoulders; buckles placed over the mid-chest will get in the way should cardiopulmonary resuscitation become necessary.
- The second rescuer secures the patient's forehead to the board with a self-adhering (Kling, Kerlix) bandage. A second bandage can be used to secure the cervical collar to the board. Be careful not to cover the patient's mouth.
- Once the patient has been securely strapped to the short backboard, he may be removed from the vehicle. Probably the safest way to do so is to rotate him carefully and slide him onto a LONG BACKBOARD. The long board is positioned so that one end is resting firmly on the seat, and the other is held parallel to the ground. Then the patient is carefully lowered until he is supine, and the short board is slid gently along the long board. The straps on the short board will have to be loosened momentarily in order to lower the patient's legs.
- Whatever procedure is used to remove the patient from the vehicle, the patient should always be lifted by two rescuers grasping the patient by the trunk and armpits. NEVER LIFT A PATIENT BY PULLING UP ON THE SHORT BACKBOARD; the slots are not intended to be used for lifting but only to provide a passage for the straps.
- Secure the patient, short board and all, to the long backboard.

When the patient's condition is unstable and time does not permit the use of a short board, use the rapid extrication procedure:

- The first rescuer positions himself behind the patient, if possible in the back seat for a front-seat patient, and HOLDS THE HEAD STEADY IN NEUTRAL POSITION (Fig. 16-22).
- The second rescuer completes the primary survey and examination of the neck and applies a CERVICAL COLLAR.
- Coordinating their actions, the two rescuers then pivot the patient on the seat and lower him onto a long backboard that is resting on the seat beneath his buttocks. Basically, that is the same motion that is used in the standard extrication, but in this case the patient's head, neck, and trunk are supported by the rescuers' hands rather than by a short backboard.
- As soon as the patient has been removed from the vehicle, a blanket roll or specially designed blocks should be applied to both sides of his head to prevent lateral motion, and the patient should be securely strapped to the backboard. One of the most efficient ways to accomplish that is with the Spider Strap assembly (Fig. 16-23), which was devised by some resourceful Idaho EMTs to provide

FIGURE 16-23. "SPIDER STRAPS" provide a very quick and efficient way to secure a patient to a long backboard. The head is stabilized with a blanket roll.

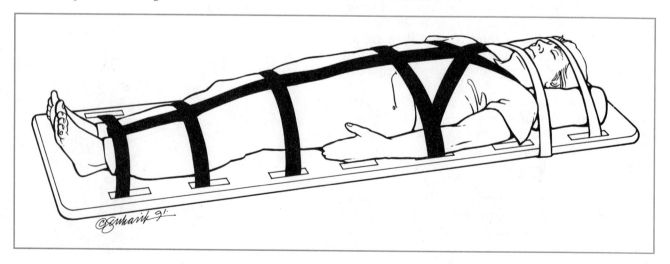

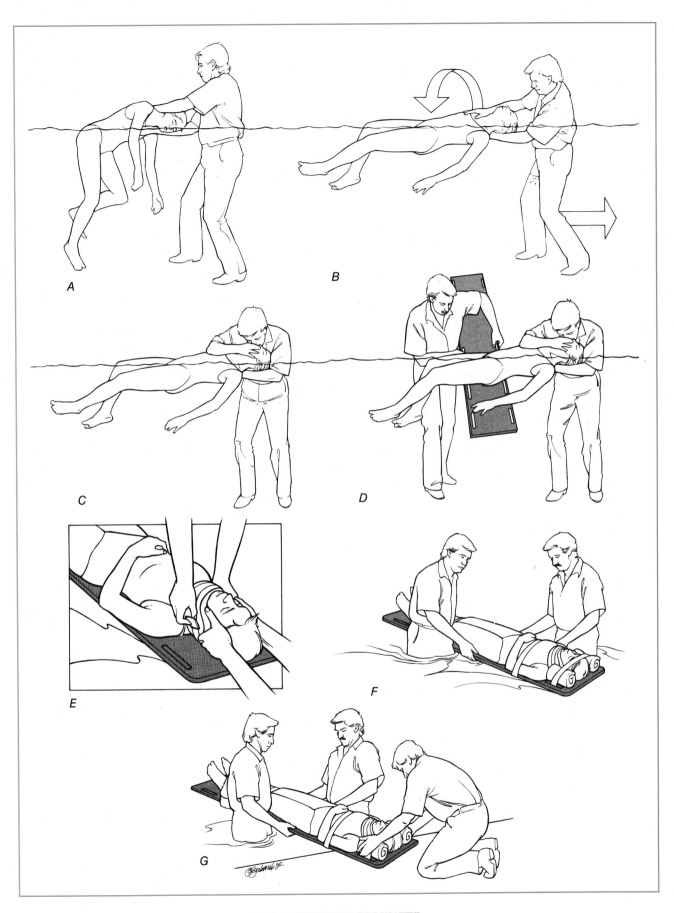

FIGURE 16-24. EXTRICATING A VICTIM FOUND IN SHALLOW WATER (presumed diving accident). (A) Splint victim's head and neck between your arms. (B) Pull and rotate. (C) Start mouth-to-mouth ventilation. (D) With artificial ventilation ongoing, slide backboard beneath victim. (E) Apply cervical collar. (F) Float backboard to edge of water. (G) Lift victim from water.

up to 10 points of attachment to the backboard in as little as 15 seconds.

Packaging and Removal of the Injured from the Water

Clearly, patients injured in different types of accidents will require different measures, but the principles of packaging and removal are the same in all cases—to keep the head, neck, and trunk in alignment. When the patient has sustained possible spinal cord injury in a diving accident, spinal immobilization must begin even before the patient is removed from the water:

- If the patient is prone, approach him from the top of the head, and place one arm under his body so that his head is supported on your arm and his chest on your hand (Fig. 16-24A). Place your other arm across his head and back to splint his head and neck between your arms.
- Continuing to support the patient's head and neck in that fashion, take a step backward and smoothly turn him to the supine position (Fig. 16-24B). If he is not breathing, immediately begin mouth-to-mouth ventilation, before making any further attempts to remove him from the water (Fig. 16-24C).
- A second rescuer slides a rigid device (e.g., a wooden backboard, surfboard, door, wooden plank) under the patient's body while you continue to support the patient's head and neck (Fig. 16-24D). The second rescuer may then apply a cervical collar (Fig. 16-24E).
- Float the board to the edge of the water (Fig. 16-24F) and lift it out, while stabilizing the patient on the board, preferably with straps, to prevent undue motion.

The techniques described above require extensive training and practice *in the water,* for what looks easy in the pictures is in fact usually quite difficult in practice—with rescuers stumbling over slippery rocks and the victim sliding all over the backboard. Paramedics working near recreational waterways should therefore receive special training in aquatic rescue techniques.

GLOSSARY

amnesia   Loss of memory.

anterior chamber   The portion of the eye between the *cornea* and the *lens.*

aqueous humor   The fluid in the *anterior chamber* of the eye.

arachnoid   Middle meningeal membrane.

brainstem   Portion of the brain inferior to the *cerebrum* and continuous with the spinal cord.

central nervous system (CNS)   The brain and spinal cord.

cerebellum   Portion of the brain, located behind and below the *cerebrum,* whose general function is coordination of movement.

cerebral perfusion pressure (CPP)   The pressure of blood flowing through the brain, equivalent to the mean arterial pressure minus the *intracranial pressure.*

cerebrospinal fluid (CSF)   The fluid that bathes the brain and spinal cord.

cerebrum   The portion of the brain that controls higher functions, such as memory, perception, thought, and judgment.

conjunctiva   Delicate membrane that lines the eyelids and covers exposed surfaces of the eyeball.

contralateral   On the side opposite.

contrecoup   Injury resulting from a blow at another site.

cornea   Transparent structure covering the *pupil.*

coup   In reference to head injury, an injury at the site of a blow.

cranium   Part of the skull that encloses the brain.

crepitus   Grating or crackling sound and sensation produced by the rubbing together of fractured bone ends.

decerebrate posture   Posture assumed by patients with severe brain dysfunction, characterized by extension and internal rotation of the arms and extension of the legs.

decorticate posture   Posture assumed by patients with severe brain dysfunction, characterized by extension of the legs and flexion of the arms.

dura mater   The tough, outermost meningeal layer.

dysconjugate gaze   Gaze in which the two eyes are not aligned but instead stare in different directions.

epidural hematoma   Collection of blood between the dura mater and the skull.

epistaxis   Nosebleed.

foramen magnum   The large opening in the inferoanterior part of the occipital bone, through which the brainstem passes.

galea aponeurotica   Tendinous structure of the scalp that connects various facial muscles.

globe   Eyeball.

herniation   In head injury, the extrusion of part of the brain through the *tentorium* or *foramen magnum* as a result of increased intracranial pressure.

hyperpyrexia   Abnormally high fever.

intervertebral disc   Fibrocartilaginous plate that acts as a cushion between adjacent vertebrae.

intracranial pressure (ICP) Pressure within the skull.

iris The pigmented portion of the eye surrounding the *pupil*.

lens The portion of the eye that focuses light rays on the retina.

malocclusion Failure of proper alignment of the upper and lower teeth.

mandible Lower jaw bone.

maxilla Upper jaw bone.

medulla (medulla oblongata) Lower portion of the brainstem that contains the centers for control of respiration and heart beat.

meninges The three membranes covering the brain and spinal cord.

orbit Eye socket.

paresthesia Abnormal sensation, often of the pins-and-needles variety, indicating disturbance in nerve function.

pia mater Innermost layer of the meninges.

priapism Sustained erection of the penis.

pupil The small opening in the center of the *iris* of the eye.

reticular activating system Center in the brainstem that controls the state of wakefulness.

sacrum A part of the lower spine formed by five fused vertebrae, which articulate with the pelvis.

sclera Tough, white covering of the eyeball.

subdural hematoma Collection of blood between the dura and the arachnoid.

suture Type of joint in which the articulating surfaces are permanently fused together, as in the skull.

tentorium The extension of *dura mater* that forms a partition between the *cerebrum* and *cerebellum*.

vertebra One of the 33 bones of the spinal column.

vitreous humor A jellylike, transparent substance filling the inside of the eye.

zygoma Cheek bone.

FURTHER READING

HEAD INJURY

Baxt WG et al. The impact of advanced prehospital emergency care on the mortality of severely brain-injured patients. *J Trauma* 27:365, 1987.

Bouzarth WF. Early management of acute head injury (a surgeon's viewpoint). *EMT J* 2(2):43, 1978.

Braakman R et al. Megadose steroids in severe head injury: Results of a prospective study. *J Neurosurg* 58:326, 1983.

Braughler JM et al. Current application of "high-dose" steroid therapy for CNS injury: A pharmacologic perspective. *J Neurosurg* 62:806, 1985.

Clifton GL et al. Cardiovascular response to severe head injury. *J Neurosurg* 59:447, 1983.

Cold GE. Does acute hyperventilation provoke cerebral oligaemia in comatose patients after acute head injury? *Acta Neurochir* (Wien) 96:100, 1989.

Cottrell JE et al. Furosemide and head injury. *J Trauma* 21:805, 1981.

Davidoff G et al. The spectrum of closed head injuries in facial trauma victims: Incidence and impact. *Ann Emerg Med* 17:6, 1988.

Deardon NM. Effect of high-dose dexamethasone on outcome from severe head injury. *J Neurosurg* 64:81, 1986.

Desai BT et al. Seizures in relation to head injury. *Ann Emerg Med* 12:543, 1983.

Doberstein CE, Hovda DA, Becker DP. Clinical considerations in the reduction of secondary brain injury. *Ann Emerg Med* 22:993, 1993.

Domaingue CM et al. Hypotensive effect of mannitol administered too rapidly. *Anaesth Intensive Care* 13:134, 1985.

Fessler RD, Diaz FG. The management of cerebral perfusion pressure and intracranial pressure after severe head trauma. *Ann Emerg Med* 22:998, 1993.

Freshman SP et al. Hypertonic saline (7.5%) versus mannitol: A comparison for treatment of acute head injuries. *J Trauma* 35:244, 1993.

Giannatta SL et al. High dose glucocorticoids in the management of severe head injury. *Neurosurgery* 15:497, 1984.

Javid M. Head injuries. *N Engl J Med* 291:890, 1974.

Jones PW et al. Hyperventilation in the management of cerebral oedema. *Intensive Care Med* 7:205, 1981.

Kelly JP et al. Concussion in sports: Guidelines for the prevention of catastrophic outcome. *JAMA* 266:2867, 1991.

Kenning JA et al. Upright patient positioning in the management of intracranial hypertension. *Surg Neurol* 15:148, 1981.

Kolin A et al. Myocardial damage from acute cerebral lesions. *Stroke* 15:990, 1984.

Lehman LB. To stanch a scalp bleed. *Emerg Med* 21(13):71, 1989.

Lillehei KO, Hoff JT. Advances in the management of closed head injury. *Ann Emerg Med* 14:789, 1985.

McGraw CP, Howard G. Effect of mannitol on increased intracranial pressure. *Neurosurgery* 13:269, 1983.

McLeod AA et al. Cardiac sequelae of acute head injury. *Br Heart J* 47:221, 1982.

Molofsky WJ. Steroids and head trauma. *Neurosurgery* 15:424, 1984.

Muizelaar JP et al. Adverse effects of prolonged hyperventilation in patients with severe head injury: A randomized clinical trial. *J Neurosurg* 75:731, 1991.

Nissenson AR et al. Mannitol. *West J Med* 13:277, 1979.

Pfenninger EG et al. Arterial blood gases in patients with acute head injury at the accident site and upon hospital admission. *Acta Anaesthesiol Scand* 35:148, 1991.

Popp AJ et al. Cardiac dysfunction following severe head injury. *Surg Forum* 35:479, 1984.

Raphaely RC et al. Management of severe pediatric head trauma. *Pediatr Clin North Am* 27:715, 1980.

Robertson CS et al. Treatment of hypertension associated with head injury. *J Neurosurg* 59:455, 1983.

Rockswold GL, Pheley PJ. Patients who talk and deteriorate. *Ann Emerg Med* 22:1004, 1993.

Rosner MJ et al. Cerebral perfusion pressure, intracranial pressure, and head elevation. *J Neurosurg* 65:636, 1986.

Sacks JJ et al. Bicycle-associated head injuries and deaths in the United States from 1984–1988: How many are preventable? *JAMA* 266:3016, 1991.

Saul TG, Ducker TB. Management of acute head injuries. *Emergency* 12(2):59, 1980.

Scali VJ et al. Handling head injuries. *Emergency* 21(11):22, 1989.

Seelig JM et al. Traumatic acute subdural hematoma: Major mortality reduction in comatose patients treated within four hours. *N Engl J Med* 304:1151, 1981.

Shields CB. Early management of head injuries. *J Ky Med Assoc* 78:9, 1980.

Smith S. A blow to the head. *Emergency* 22(6):16, 1990.

Sosin DM, Sacks JJ, Smith SM. Head injury-associated deaths in the United States from 1979 to 1986. *JAMA* 262:2251, 1989.

Steedman DJ. CSF rhinorrhoea: Significance of the glucose oxidase strip test. *Injury* 18:327, 1987.

Stone JL et al. Acute subdural hematoma: Direct admission to a trauma center yields improved results. *J Trauma* 26:445, 1986.

Turner E et al. Metabolic and hemodynamic response to hyperventilation in patients with head injuries. *Intensive Care Med* 10:128, 1984.

Walls RM. Rapid-sequence intubation in head trauma. *Ann Emerg Med* 22:1008, 1993.

Weiss MH. Head trauma and spinal cord injuries: Diagnostic and therapeutic criteria. *Crit Care Med* 2:311, 1974.

Wilkinson HA et al. Furosemide and mannitol in the treatment of acute experimental intracranial hypertension. *Neurosurgery* 12:405, 1983.

FACIAL INJURY

Amsterdam JT. Dental emergencies: Pain and trauma. *Emerg Med* 25(15):27, 1993.

Barrs DM, Kern EB. Acute nasal trauma: Emergency room care of 250 patients. *J Fam Pract* 10:225, 1980.

Chamberlain JH, Goerig AC. Rationale for the treatment and management of avulsed teeth. *J Am Dent Assoc* 101:471, 1980.

Cook PR et al. A comparison of nasal balloons and posterior gauze packs for posterior epistaxis. *Ear Nose Throat J* 64:78, 1985.

Fairbanks DN. Complications of nasal packing. *Otolaryngol Head Neck Surg* 94:412, 1986.

Fanous NL. The absorbable nasal pack. *J Otolaryngol* 9:462, 1980.

Hendler BH. The sites and signs of maxillofacial trauma. *Emerg Med* 16(6):23, 1984.

Kalish M. Airway management in maxillofacial trauma. *Emerg Med Serv* 18(6):42, 1989.

Kirchner JA. Epistaxis. *N Engl J Med* 307:1126, 1982.

Krasner PR. Management of avulsed teeth. *Emerg Med Serv* 18(6):31, 1989.

Landeen JM. Emergency management of the maxillofacial-injured patient. *Emergency* 10(6):42, 1978.

Lapeyrolerie FM. Emergency dental considerations. *Emergency* 10(12):50, 1978.

Lee MJ, Martinez AJ. Focusing on facial and ocular injuries. *JEMS* 17(2):28, 1992.

Lind GL, Spiegel EH, Munson ES. Treatment of traumatic tooth avulsion. *Anesth Analg* 61:469, 1982.

Lingeman RE. Epistaxis. *Am Fam Physician* 14:79, 1976.

Liston SL, Cortez EA, McNabney WK. External ear injuries. *JACEP* 7:233, 1978.

MacAfee KA. Saving face: Prioritizing the assessment and treatment of maxillofacial trauma. *Emergency* 24(6):39, 1992.

Manson PN, Kelly KJ. Evaluation and management of the patient with facial trauma. *Emerg Med Serv* 18(6):22, 1989.

McCabe MJ. Use of Histacryl tissue adhesive to manage an avulsed tooth. *Br Med J* 301:4, 1990.

McSwain NE. Nasal hemorrhage. *Emerg Med* 21(5):120, 1989.

Medford HM, Curtis JW. Acute care of severe tooth fractures. *Ann Emerg Med* 12:364, 1983.

Nosebleed: An everyday challenge to medical ingenuity. *Emerg Med* 20(8):169, 1988.

Porter M et al. The effect of ice packs upon nasal mucosal blood flow. *Acta Otolaryngol* (Stockh) 111:1122, 1991.

Reducing the dislocated jaw. *Emerg Med* 22(3):61, 1990.

Sarri P. Emergency care of dento-facial injuries. *J Prehosp Med* 2(2):35, 1988.

Scheer B. Emergency treatment of avulsed incisor teeth (editorial). *Br Med J* 301:20, 1990.

Schultz RC, deCamara DL. Athletic facial injuries. *JAMA* 252:3395, 1984.

Wender RW, Swerdloff M, Alexander SA. Prehospital treatment of dental injuries. *Emerg Med Serv* 8(5):10, 1979.

Winspur I. Facial fractures and the ED physician. *Emerg Med Serv* 8(3):31, 1979.

EYE EMERGENCIES

Abrahamson IA. Management of ocular foreign bodies. *Am Fam Physician* 14:81, 1976.

American Academy of Ophthalmology. The eye emergency:
1. Basic procedures. *Emerg Med* 14(16):163, 1982.
2. Burns about the eye. *Emerg Med* 14(17):232, 1982.
3. Corneal abrasion. *Emerg Med* 14(18):126, 1982.
4. Nonpenetrating foreign bodies. *Emerg Med* 14(19):225, 1982.
6. Blunt trauma. *Emerg Med* 14(21):196, 1982.
7. Radiation injuries. *Emerg Med* 15(1):111, 1983.

Casey TA. Examination of the eye. *Hosp Med* 7:20, 1971.

Havener WH. The injured eyeball. *Emerg Med* 6(2):355, 1974.

Hoffman JR, Neuhaus RW, Baylis HI. Penetrating orbital trauma. *Am J Emerg Med* 1:22, 1983.

Jenkins HS, Marcus DF. Central retinal artery occlusion. *JACEP* 8:363, 1979.

Karesh JW. Ocular and periocular trauma. *Emerg Med Serv* 18(6):46, 1989.

Lee MJ, Martinez AJ. Focussing on facial and ocular injuries. *JEMS* 17(2):28, 1992.

Levitsky LR. Ocular examination and contusion injuries. *Emerg Med Serv* 4(1):26, 1975.

Melamed MA. A generalist's guide to eye emergencies. *Emerg Med* 16(3):99, 1984.

Shingleton BJ. A clearer look at ocular emergencies. *Emerg Med* 21(9):52, 1989.

Shingleton BJ. Early management of ocular trauma. *Emerg Med* 24(4):257, 1992.

Soll DB, Oh KT. Industrial ocular injuries. *Am Fam Physician* 14:115, 1976.

Thygerson AL. Focus on eye injuries. *Emergency* 13(11):52, 1981.

Weinstock FJ. Blackout. *Emerg Med* 8(12):23, 1976.

NECK INJURY

Carducci B, Lowe RA, Dalsey W. Penetrating neck trauma: Consensus and controversies. *Ann Emerg Med* 15:208, 1986.

Champion HC. The penetrated neck. *Emerg Med* 15(14):259, 1983.

DeLorenzo R, Mayer D. Laryngeal trauma. *JEMS* 16(9):77, 1991.

Frame SB. Stab wound to the larynx. *Emerg Med* 20(9):62, 1988.

Fuhrman GM et al. Blunt laryngeal trauma: Classification and management protocol. *J Trauma* 30:87, 1990.

Guertler A. Blunt laryngeal trauma associated with shoulder harness use. *Ann Emerg Med* 17:838, 1988.

Gussack GS, Jurkovich GJ, Luterman A. Laryngotracheal trauma: A protocol approach to a rare injury. *Laryngoscope* 96:660, 1986.

Line Jr WS et al. Strangulation: A full spectrum of blunt neck trauma. *Ann Otol Rhinol Laryngol* 94:542, 1985.

Martinez JA et al. Trauma rounds. Problem: Laryngeal injury. *Emerg Med* 16(13):45, 1984.

Orobello P, Myer CM. Don't overlook a traumatized larynx. *Emerg Med* 18(19):54, 1986.

Roberge RJ et al. Tracheal transection following blunt trauma. *Ann Emerg Med* 17:47, 1988.

SPINAL INJURY

Albin MS. Resuscitation of the spinal cord. *Crit Care Med* 6:270, 1978.

American College of Surgeons. Techniques of helmet removal from injured patients. *Bull Am Coll Surg*, October 1980.

Anast GT. Management of cervical spine fracture using Gardner-Wells tongs. *Emergency* 10(4):52, 1978.

Anderson DK, Hall ED. Pathophysiology of spinal cord trauma. *Ann Emerg Med* 22:987, 1993.

Anderson DK et al. Spinal cord injury and protection. *Ann Emerg Med* 14:816, 1985.

Aprahamian CA, Thompson BM, Darin J. Recommended helmet removal techniques in a cervical spine injured patient. *J Trauma* 24:841, 1984.

Aprahamian CA et al. Experimental cervical spine injury model: Evaluation of airway management and splinting techniques. *Ann Emerg Med* 13:584, 1984.

Armstrong TA. In-flight administration of methylprednisolone to patients with spinal cord injury (letter). *Am J Hosp Pharm* 50:2058, 1993.

Ball RA. Don't add insult to injury: Proper handling of head and neck trauma. *JEMS* 15(10):40, 1990.

Batchelor TM. The five most common errors of spinal immobilization. *JEMS* 17(3):84, 1992.

Bayless P, Ray VG. Incidence of cervical spine injuries in association with blunt head trauma. *Am J Emerg Med* 7:139, 1989.

Bicknell JM et al. Unrecognized incomplete cervical spinal cord injury: Review of nine new and 28 previously reported cases. *Am J Emerg Med* 10:336, 1992.

Bivins HG et al. The effect of axial traction during orotracheal intubation of the trauma victim with an unstable cervical spine. *Ann Emerg Med* 17:25, 1988.

Bourn S. Tell the spinal fanatics to "back off." *JEMS* 15(5):73, 1990.

Bracken MB et al. Efficacy of methylprednisolone in acute spinal cord injury. *JAMA* 251:45, 1984.

Bracken MB et al. A randomized, controlled trial of methylprednisolone or naloxone in the treatment of acute spinal-cord injury. *N Engl J Med* 322:1405, 1990.

Bracken MB et al. Methylprednisolone or naloxone treatment after acute spinal cord injury: 1-year follow-up data. *J Neurosurg* 76:23, 1992.

Butman AM, Vomacka RW. Spine immobilization: Part 1. *Emergency* 23(9):48, 1991.

Butman AM, Vomacka RW. Spine immobilization: Part 2. *Emergency* 23(10):46, 1991.

Byun HS et al. Severe cervical injury due to break dancing: A case report. *Orthopedics* 9:550, 1986.

Caroline NL. *Emergency Medical Treatment: A Text for the EMT-A and EMT-Intermediate* (3rd ed.). Boston: Little, Brown, 1991. Chap. 14.

Chan D et al. The effect of spinal immobilization on healthy volunteers. *Ann Emerg Med* 23:48, 1994.

Chandler DR et al. Emergency cervical-spine immobilization. *Ann Emerg Med* 22:1185, 1992.

Chandramohan K. The emergency care of spinal trauma. *Emerg Med* 24(15):203, 1992.

Cline JR et al. A comparison of methods of cervical immobilization used in patient extrication and transport. *Trauma* 25:649, 1985.

Davidson JSD, Birdsell DC. Cervical spine injury in patients with facial skeletal trauma. *J Trauma* 29:1276, 1989.

Dean DF. The child with possible spinal cord injury. *Emerg Med* 14(9):122, 1982.

Dick T. Spider's embrace: The Idaho answer to backboard straps. *JEMS* 14(8):26, 1989.

Dick T. Big hug: Octopus is a better way. *JEMS* 18(2):73, 1993.

Dula DJ. Trauma to the cervical spine. *JACEP* 8:504, 1979.

Dulaney RA. Backboarding the standing patient. *Emergency* 24(12):58, 1992.

Faden AI et al. Megadose corticosteroid therapy following experimental traumatic spinal injury. *J Neurosurg* 60:712, 1984.

Flamm ES et al. Experimental spinal cord injury: Treatment with naloxone. *Neurosurgery* 10:227, 1982.

Gopalakrishnan KC, El Masri WS. Fractures of the sternum associated with spinal injury. *J Bone Joint Surg [Br]* 68B:178, 1986.

Graziano AF et al. A radiographic comparison of prehospital cervical immobilization methods. *Ann Emerg Med* 16:1127, 1987.

Grundy D et al. ABC of spinal cord injury: Early management and complications. *Br Med J* I.292:44, 1986; II.292:123, 1986.

Guthkelch AN et al. Patterns of cervical spine injury and their associated lesions. *West J Med* 147:428, 1987.

Hadley MN et al. Pediatric spinal trauma: Review of 122 cases of spinal cord and vertebral column injuries. *J Neurosurg* 68:18, 1988.

Hauswald M et al. Cervical spine movement during airway management: Cinefluoroscopic appraisal in human cadavers. *Am J Emerg Med* 9:535, 1991.

Herzenberg JE et al. Emergency transport and positioning of young children who have an injury of the cervical spine. *J Bone Joint Surg [Am]* 71A:15, 1989.

Hillard R et al. Spinal immobilization: Practice holds the line. *Rescue* 4(2):21, 1991.

Hills MW et al. Head injury and facial injury: Is there an increased risk of cervical spine injury? *J Trauma* 34:549, 1993.

Hite PR et al. Injuries resulting from bungee-cord jumping. *Ann Emerg Med* 22:1060, 1993.

Holley J, Jorden R. Airway management in patients with unstable cervical spine fractures. *Ann Emerg Med* 18:1237, 1989.

Howell JM et al. A practical radiographic comparison of

short board technique and Kendrick extrication device. *Ann Emerg Med* 18:943, 1989.

Huerta C, Griffith R, Joyce SM. Cervical spine stabilization in pediatric patients: Evaluation of current techniques. *Ann Emerg Med* 16:1121, 1987.

Jackson DW et al. Cervical spine injuries. *Clin Sports Med* 5:373, 1986.

Joyce SM. Cervical immobilization during orotracheal intubation in trauma victims (editorial). *Ann Emerg Med* 17:88, 1988.

Knopp RK. The safety of orotracheal intubation in patients with suspected cervical-spine injury (editorial). *Ann Emerg Med* 19:603, 1990.

Little NE. In case of a broken neck. *Emerg Med* 21(9):22, 1989.

Majernick TG et al. Cervical spine movement during orotracheal intubation. *Ann Emerg Med* 15:417, 1986.

Marsden AK. Emergency cervical splints: Their value and limitation. *Disaster Med* 1(2):197, 1983.

McCabe JB, Angelos MG. Injury to the head and face in patients with cervical spine injury. *Am J Emerg Med* 2:333, 1984.

McCabe JB, Nolan DJ. Comparison of the effectiveness of different cervical immobilization collars. *Ann Emerg Med* 15:50, 1986.

McGuire RA et al. Spinal instability and the log-rolling maneuver. *J Trauma* 27:525, 1987.

Meyer RD, Daniel WW. The biomechanics of helmets and helmet removal. *J Trauma* 25:329, 1985.

O'Malley KF, Ross SE. The incidence of injury to the cervical spine in patients with craniocerebral injury. *J Trauma* 28:1476, 1988.

Podolsky S et al. Efficacy of cervical spine immobilization methods. *J Trauma* 23:461, 1983.

Reiss SJ et al. Cervical spine fractures with major associated trauma. *Neurosurgery* 18:327, 1986.

Rhee KJ et al. Oral intubation in the multiply injured patient: The risk of exacerbating spinal cord damage. *Ann Emerg Med* 19:511, 1990.

Rimel R et al. Prehospital treatment of the patient with spinal cord injuries. *EMT J* 3(4):49, 1979.

Rosen PB et al. Comparison of two new immobilization collars. *Ann Emerg Med* 21:1189, 1992.

Ruge JR et al. Pediatric spinal injury: The very young. *J Neurosurg* 68:25, 1988.

Rural Affairs Committee, National Association of Emergency Medical Services Physicians. Clinical guidelines for delayed or prolonged transport: III. Spine injury. *Prehosp Disaster Med* 8(2):176, 1993.

Scannell G et al. Orotracheal intubation in trauma patients with cervical fractures. *Arch Surg* 128:903, 1993.

Schriger DL et al. Spinal immobilization on a flat backboard: Does it result in neutral position of the cervical spine? *Ann Emerg Med* 20:878, 1991.

Seaman PJ. Logroll technique. *Emergency* 24(5):18, 1992.

Smith M. All aboard! *JEMS* 16(12):24, 1991.

Smith M, Bourn S, Larmon B. Ties that bind: Immobilizing the injured spine. *JEMS* 14(4):28, 1989.

Soicher E, Demetriades D. Cervical spine injuries in patients with head injuries. *Br J Surg* 78:1013, 1991.

Swain A et al. ABC of spinal cord injury: At the accident. *Br Med J* 291:1558, 1985.

Swain A et al. ABC of spinal cord injury: Evacuation and initial management at hospital. *Br Med J* 291:1623, 1985.

Walter J, Doris PE, Shaffer MA. Clinical presentation of patients with acute cervical spine injury. 13:512, 1984.

Wertz EM. Immobilized. *Emergency* 23(8):33, 1991.

Williams J et al. Head, facial, and clavicular trauma as a predictor of cervical-spine injury. *Ann Emerg Med* 21:719, 1992.

Wolf AL. Initial management of brain- and spinal-cord injured patients. *Emerg Med Serv* 18(6):35, 1989.

Wright SW et al. Cervical spine injuries in blunt trauma patients requiring emergent endotracheal intubation. *Am J Emerg Med* 10:104, 1992.

17
Chest Injuries

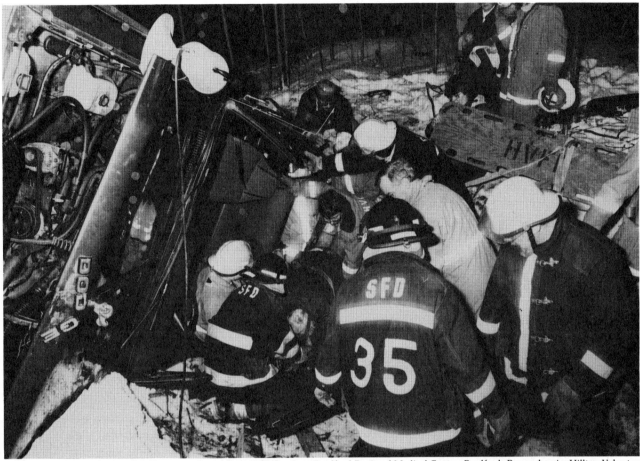

Bradford Township Volunteer Fire Department, and Paramedic Services, Bradford Regional Medical Center, Bradford, Pennsylvania; Hilltop Volunteer Fire Department and Ambulance Service, Cyclone, Pennsylvania; Rew Volunteer Fire Department, Rew, Pennsylvania; Smethport Volunteer Fire Department, Smethport, Pennsylvania. Photo by Jay K. Bradish.

OBJECTIVES

Injuries to the chest are the major cause of mortality in 25 percent of deaths due to trauma; in another 25 percent, chest injuries contribute significantly to the fatal outcome. Those statistics should not be surprising in view of the fact that the chest houses some of the most vital structures in the body: the heart, the lungs, and the great vessels. Thus any significant injury to the chest is apt to lead rapidly to hypoxia, circulatory insufficiency, or both, and thereby to threaten the whole organism. In this chapter, we shall first review the anatomy of the thoracic cavity, in order to better understand the ways in which the chest can be injured. We shall then survey the various injuries that may affect the chest and its contents—looking first at injuries detectable in the primary survey that pose an immediate threat to life, then at injuries assessed during the secondary survey that may also have life-threatening potential. Finally, we shall consider a third category of chest injuries, those that are not a threat to life but that may nonetheless be serious. By the conclusion of this chapter, the student should be able to

1. List four things that may jeopardize the airway in a victim of chest trauma
2. List the parameters to be evaluated, during the primary survey of a patient with chest injury, in the assessment of
   • Breathing
   • Circulation
3. List the symptoms and signs of an open pneumothorax, and describe the correct prehospital management of open pneumothorax
4. Given a description of several patients with different clinical presentations, identify a patient with
   • Tension pneumothorax
   • Massive hemothorax
   • Flail chest
   • Cardiac tamponade
   and describe the correct prehospital management of each
5. List five signs of traumatic asphyxia, and describe the correct prehospital management of traumatic asphyxia
6. List the steps in carrying out
   • Chest decompression for tension pneumothorax
   • Emergency pericardiocentesis
7. Indicate under what circumstances one should anticipate or suspect the presence of
   • Traumatic aortic rupture
   • Bronchial tear
   • Myocardial contusion
   • Pulmonary contusion
   • Diaphragmatic tear
8. Given a description of several patients with different clinical presentations, identify a patient with
   • Rib fracture
   • Simple pneumothorax
   and describe the correct prehospital management of each
9. Explain the significance of
   • Rib fracture in a young person
   • Fracture of the first or second rib
10. List in order the steps in treating a patient with critical thoracic trauma when the precise nature of the injuries is not known

REVIEW OF THORACIC ANATOMY

The thorax (Fig. 17-1) is a hollow cavity formed by the 12 pairs of RIBS that join posteriorly with the THORACIC SPINE and anteriorly with the STERNUM to form a protective bony ring around the organs of the chest. There are three important points to remember about the rib cage:

• The first four ribs are relatively protected by the shoulder girdle and are less likely to be fractured than ribs 5 to 10. Indeed, ribs 1 and 2 are so well protected that when they *are* fractured, one has to assume that massive forces were involved.
• The rib cage becomes stiffer with age. Thus a blunt force applied to the chest of an older person is more likely to fracture ribs than the same force applied to the chest of a younger person. For that same reason, though, blunt trauma is *more* likely to injure the internal organs of a young person's chest, for the pliable rib cage of a young person is more easily compressed against the lungs and heart.
• The inferior border of the thoracic cavity is formed by the diaphragm, which together with the intercostal muscles constitute the main muscles of respiration. The diaphragm is a domed muscle that arches up into the chest. Thus some "abdominal" organs, such as the liver and spleen, are in fact located beneath the ribs and can be injured by trauma to the rib cage. For practical purposes, that means that

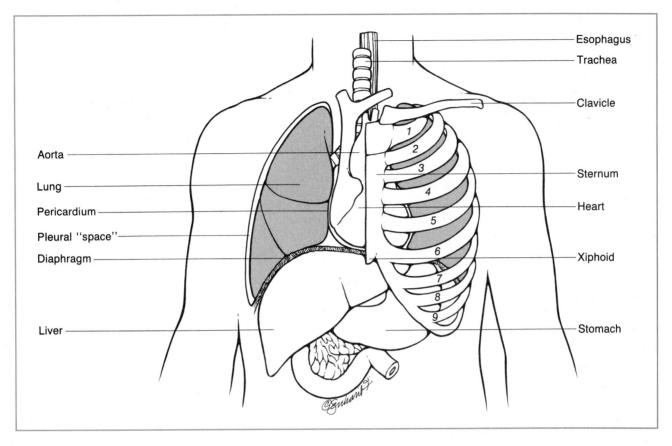

FIGURE 17-1.   ANATOMY OF THE THORACIC CAVITY.

ANY INJURY BELOW THE LEVEL OF THE NIPPLES IS AN ABDOMINAL INJURY AS WELL AS A CHEST INJURY.

Nearly the entire volume of the thoracic cavity is occupied by the LUNGS. Covering each lung is a smooth, slippery membrane called the VISCERAL PLEURA; a similar membrane, the PARIETAL PLEURA, lines the inner wall of the thoracic cavity. Between the two pleural membranes is a *potential* space, the PLEURAL SPACE. Normally, the visceral and parietal pleurae are closely applied one to the other, and no actual pleural space exists. But if the negative pressure within the thoracic cavity is somehow disrupted, by a hole in the lung surface or in the chest wall, the potential pleural space becomes an actual space that can hold up to 2 or 3 liters of air or fluid in each side of the adult chest.

Between the two lungs, in the middle of the thoracic cavity, is the MEDIASTINUM, which contains the heart, the great vessels, the trachea, main bronchi, and esophagus.

The HEART lies just behind and slightly to the left of the sternum, so the heart is subject to injury when there is a direct blow to the sternum or when deceleration forces cause the heart to collide against the sternum. Surrounding the heart is a tough, fibrous sac, the PERICARDIUM, which holds the heart in place and provides it with a certain degree of protection. Normally, the pericardium contains between 20 and 60 ml of fluid that acts as a lubricant to enable the heart to contract freely within it. As we shall see later in this chapter, the accumulation of blood in the pericardial sac, as a result of blunt or penetrating trauma, may have disastrous consequences.

The GREAT VESSELS enter and exit the heart within the mediastinum—the VENAE CAVAE emptying into the right atrium and the AORTA leaving from the left ventricle. The venae cavae, being relatively thin-walled, low-pressure vessels, are subject to compression as the pressure within the chest (intrathoracic pressure) becomes elevated, as in tension pneumothorax (see p. 369). The aorta for its part may suffer tears from violent twisting forces in blunt trauma or deceleration injuries.

THE PRIMARY SURVEY IN CHEST TRAUMA

In the patient who has suffered thoracic trauma, as in any other patient, the object of the primary survey is to detect and manage injuries that pose an immediate threat to life. In patients with significant chest trauma, there is no shortage of such injuries, for, as we have observed, the chest houses some of the structures that are most vital to life. It is now the practice among trauma experts to refer to the "deadly dozen" thoracic injuries (Table 17-1). Among those deadly dozen, the first six can be identified and their management can be initiated in the primary survey, following the usual sequence of ABC.

Injuries That Jeopardize the Airway

The **airway** in any victim of trauma may be jeopardized not only by head position but also by blood, mucus, foreign objects, and trauma to the structures of the airway itself. Chest trauma may disrupt the trachea or a bronchus, leading to airway problems that cannot be definitively managed in the field. We have already covered, in previous chapters, the principles of airway management. It remains to stress here that airway obstruction in trauma may be an insidious problem, developing gradually. Therefore the paramedic must be alert for signs that the airway has become compromised. Even when you are attending to something else, such as the control of bleeding or

TABLE 17-1. THE DEADLY DOZEN THORACIC INJURIES

Immediately life-threatening chest injuries that must be detected and managed during the primary survey:
 1. Airway obstruction
 2. Open pneumothorax
 3. Tension pneumothorax
 4. Massive hemothorax
 5. Flail chest
 6. Cardiac tamponade

Potentially lethal chest injuries that may be identified in the secondary survey:
 7. Thoracic aortic disruption
 8. Bronchial disruption
 9. Myocardial contusion
 10. Diaphragmatic tear
 11. Esophageal injury
 12. Pulmonary contusion

starting an IV, keep an ear tuned for stridor or any other respiratory sounds. Remember:

> **NOISY BREATHING IS OBSTRUCTED BREATHING.**

If there is any difficulty maintaining a patent airway by manual methods in the unconscious victim of chest trauma, intubate the trachea as soon as the patient has been well-oxygenated.

Injuries That Jeopardize Breathing

To evaluate the patient's **breathing,** expose his chest completely, and *look, listen,* and *feel:*

- LOOK for signs of respiratory distress (intracostal or supraclavicular muscle retractions, nasal flaring, tachypnea); deviation of the trachea; asymmetry of chest movements; obvious bruises or open wounds; paradoxical movements of any part of the chest.
- LISTEN without a stethoscope for air being sucked into an open chest wound. Listen with a stethoscope just under each armpit and over the anterior chest (second intercostal space, midclavicular line) bilaterally for presence and equality of breath sounds. If breath sounds are *not* equal, quickly PERCUSS to determine if there is unusual *dullness* or *hyperresonance* on either side.
- FEEL for subcutaneous emphysema, unstable ribs or sternum, tracheal deviation.

Any abnormalities detected in this part of the primary survey should prompt the administration of 100% OXYGEN, even before you have determined the specific source of the problem.

Open Pneumothorax

An open pneumothorax is the result of a penetrating injury to the chest. Small penetrating injuries, such as entrance wounds from small-caliber bullets, usually seal themselves off. But larger defects, such as shotgun wounds, may remain open. If the defect in the chest wall is about two-thirds the diameter of the trachea or larger, air will move preferentially through the chest defect with each respiratory effort rather than into the trachea, creating a so-called sucking chest wound (Fig. 17-2). With the entrance of air into the pleural space on the involved side, the lung on

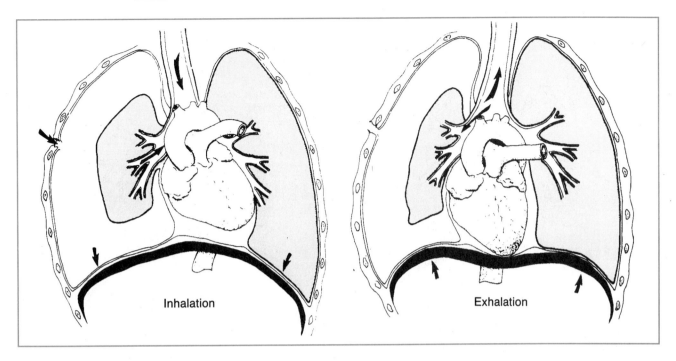

FIGURE 17-2.   OPEN PNEUMOTHORAX.   In open pneumothorax, air enters the affected side of the chest through a hole in the chest wall rather than through the airway. On exhalation, some air from the normal lung is blown into the collapsed lung; on inhalation, the same air is inhaled back into the normal lung.

that side collapses and cannot expand normally on inhalation; so the lung on the damaged side is soon depleted of its oxygen. Meanwhile, during exhalation, some air from the normal lung is exhaled into the lung on the injured side; then the same air is drawn back into the normal lung with the next inhalation. Thus ventilation of the normal lung is also impaired. The net result is both increasing hypoxemia and inadequate movement of air (hypoventilation with consequent hypercarbia).

The SYMPTOMS AND SIGNS of open pneumothorax can be predicted from the nature of the injury. The patient will nearly always be in *respiratory distress* from both hypoxemia and hypercarbia. The *open wound* will be visible on the chest wall, and it will be possible to hear *air being sucked into the wound* on inhalation. There is no need to take further time to listen with a stethoscope, for urgent treatment is required; but if one *were* to auscultate the chest, one would find breath sounds reduced on the affected side (why?), and percussion would reveal hyperresonance.

An open pneumothorax must be treated as soon as it is detected. Immediate TREATMENT consists of applying a sterile OCCLUSIVE DRESSING, such as petrolatum gauze or plastic wrap, over the wound. The dressing should be at least 3 or 4 times the size of the defect so that it covers the open wound com-

pletely and does not itself get sucked into the wound. If the patient is able to cooperate, ask him to cough, then immediately slap the dressing tightly in place as he does so. Tape the occlusive dressing *on three sides only* so that it will serve as a flutter valve to vent any buildup of pressure within the chest. As the patient inhales, the dressing will be sucked against the chest wound, sealing it against the entry of any more air; but as the patient exhales, the open end of the dressing will allow air to escape from the chest. If the dressing is sealed completely by taping all four sides, air can accumulate within the thoracic cavity and lead to tension pneumothorax.

Tension Pneumothorax

Tension pneumothorax is usually the result of blunt chest trauma in which a damaged area of lung tissue does not seal itself off. The tension pneumothorax itself is caused by air leaking into the pleural space through a hole in the lung that acts as a *one-way valve* (Fig. 17-3). Air enters the pleural space during inhalation but cannot escape during exhalation, so pressure builds up in the affected pleural cavity. As the pressure in the affected side of the chest increases, it pushes the mediastinum in the opposite direction (as evidenced by tracheal deviation *away* from the side of the tension pneumothorax), squeezing the opposite

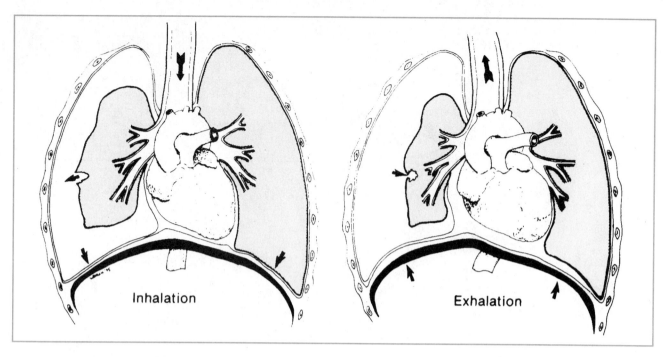

FIGURE 17-3.   ONE-WAY VALVE EFFECT IN TENSION PNEUMOTHORAX.
Air escapes from the lung into the pleural space during inhalation but cannot
reenter the lung during exhalation.

lung and thereby compromising its ventilation as well. Furthermore, as the mediastinum is pushed away from the tension pneumothorax, the superior and inferior venae cavae lying within the mediastinal cavity become kinked and compressed, which in turn hinders the return of blood to the right side of the heart. As a result, cardiac output falls, and blood backs up in the systemic veins.

The patient with tension pneumothorax presents with extreme *dyspnea, restlessness,* and *anxiety.* The *pulse* is *rapid and weak,* reflecting reduced cardiac output. If the venae cavae are being compressed, backup of blood within the systemic veins will be reflected in marked *distention of the jugular veins. Breath sounds* are *diminished* on the side of the pneumothorax, and there is *hyperresonance* to percussion on that side. In addition, the affected side of the chest may appear more expanded than the normal side and will move less with respiratory efforts. In many instances, *subcutaneous emphysema* is present, sometimes involving the entire chest, neck, and face to give the patient a grotesque, bloated appearance.

TREATMENT of tension pneumothorax is extremely urgent and requires immediate *decompression of the affected side of the chest:*

- Equipment needed: 14-gauge through-the-needle catheter (Intracath) preferred, but in an extreme emergency, use any large-bore needle or catheter.

- Cut a slit in the end of the Intracath's plastic sleeve so that the sleeve can serve as a one-way valve once the catheter has been introduced.
- Remove the wire stylet from the catheter.
- Identify the site for puncture into the chest (Fig. 17-4). The preferred site is the second intercostal space (i.e., the space between the second and third ribs) in the midclavicular line (Fig. 17-4B). An alternative is the fourth intercostal space in the midaxillary line (Fig. 17-4C).
- Quickly prepare the site by wiping it with an antibacterial swab (povidone-iodine).
- Insert the needle along the *upper* border of the rib (the intercostal nerve and artery run along the lower border of the rib, and you don't want to puncture either of those structures). You should be able to feel the needle "pop" into the pleural space. When the needle has entered the pleural space, air under pressure should be vented out through the catheter.
- Advance the catheter 1 to 2 inches, hold it securely, and withdraw the needle from the chest wall. Tape the catheter in place.

If you used a standard needle instead of a through-the-needle catheter to vent the chest, you can rig up a flutter valve from a condom (which, we are told, no one should be without in this age of AIDS); or you may leave the needle open to the air, for the diameter

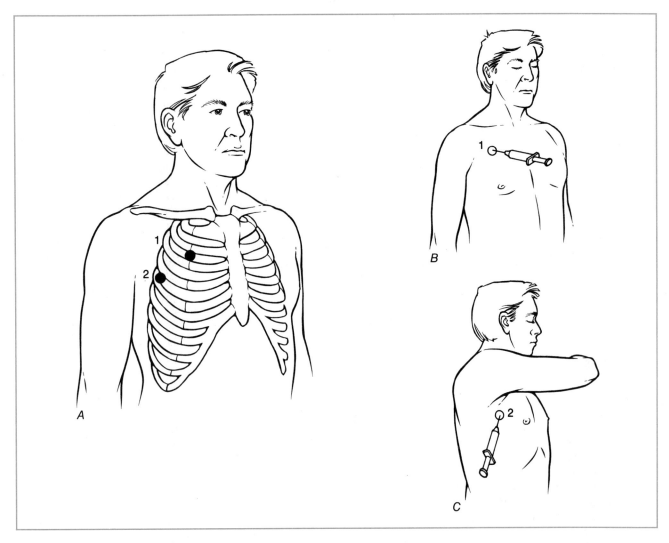

FIGURE 17-4. **(A) SITES FOR CHEST DECOMPRESSION IN TENSION PNEU-MOTHORAX.** Site 1 (preferred) is in the second intercostal space, midclavicular line, shown topographically in B. Site 2 is in the fourth intercostal space, midaxillary line, shown topographically in C.

of the needle is very small compared to that of the trachea, so the amount of air that will *enter* the chest through the needle will be negligible.

Flail Chest

When several ribs, the sternum, or both are fractured in two or more places, an unstable, or flail, chest may result. The portion of the chest wall that is no longer in continuity with the rest of the thoracic cage moves in a *paradoxical* fashion (often best appreciated by palpation)—expanding or bulging out during exhalation and collapsing during inhalation (Fig. 17-5). Whenever the forces involved in an accident are sufficient to produce a flail chest, they are also sufficient to cause pneumothorax and serious injury to the under-

lying lung. In addition, the collapse of a segment of the rib cage during each inhalation leads to repeated contusion and further collapse of the lung beneath, with consequent impairment of oxygenation. (Why is oxygenation impaired? Hint: Think about the mechanisms of shunt.) At the same time, the severe pain characteristic of rib fractures prevents the patient from taking deep breaths. Tidal volume falls, so blood levels of carbon dioxide rise. The net effect is *hypoxemia* and *hypercarbia*, so immediate TREATMENT is aimed at correcting those two defects:

- Administer 100% OXYGEN.
- If the patient is unable to take deep breaths on his own, ASSIST VENTILATIONS with a bag-valve-mask.

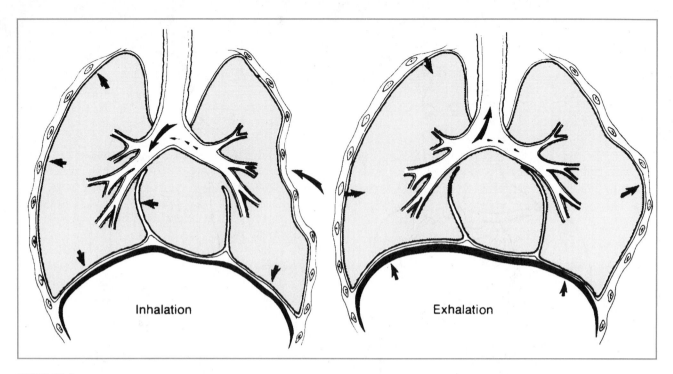

FIGURE 17-5.   PARADOXICAL MOTION OF THE CHEST WALL IN FLAIL CHEST.   The flail segment is pulled in during inhalation and bulges out during exhalation.

> **BE ALERT FOR THE DEVELOPMENT OF PNEUMOTHORAX.**

Positive pressure ventilation of an injured lung can cause pneumothorax or convert a simple pneumothorax into a tension pneumothorax. If the patient develops typical signs of tension pneumothorax or if vital signs start to deteriorate suddenly, decompress the chest immediately.

- STABILIZE THE FLAIL SEGMENT by (1) applying constant, firm manual pressure, (2) buttressing the segment with sandbags or pillows, or (3) having the patient lie with the injured side down (the last method will not be practical if the flail segment is on the anterior chest or if the patient has to be immobilized on a backboard).
- Start TRANSPORT.
- Start an IV en route, but RESTRICT INTRAVENOUS FLUIDS unless there are signs of shock, for excess fluid may be sequestered in the contused lung and lead to worsening shunt.
- MONITOR cardiac rhythm. Flail chest is frequently associated with trauma to the myocardium.

Injuries That Jeopardize the Circulation

To assess the **circulation** of the patient with chest injury, first check the PULSE for quality, rate, regularity, and any marked weakening or loss of the pulse on inhalation (**pulsus paradoxus**). Assess peripheral circulation by noting the SKIN CONDITION (color, moisture, temperature) and checking CAPILLARY REFILL. And evaluate pressure in the venous system by checking the NECK VEINS for distention. Needless to say, any significant EXTERNAL BLEEDING must be controlled as soon as it is detected.

Massive Hemothorax

Massive hemothorax, that is, the accumulation of more than about 1,500 ml of blood within the pleural cavity, is most commonly caused by a penetrating wound, although it can also occur with blunt chest trauma. The *first* signs produced by massive hemothorax are signs of *shock*. Indeed, massive hemothorax is most likely to be detected WHEN SHOCK IS ASSOCIATED WITH THE ABSENCE OF BREATH SOUNDS AND DULLNESS TO PERCUSSION on one side of the chest. As the affected side of the chest begins to fill with blood, respiratory impairment will also become evident in *signs of hypoxemia*—restlessness, anxiety, respiratory distress. *Neck veins* are usually flat because of hypovolemia, but they may be distended if very large volumes of blood compress the mediastinum. The trachea is usually *not* deviated. The differences in clinical presentation between hemothorax and tension pneumothorax are summarized in Table 17-2.

TREATMENT of massive hemothorax will require restoring lost blood volume and draining the blood that has accumulated in the chest—neither of which can be accomplished in the field. The steps to take in the field, therefore, are

- Give 100% OXYGEN.
- Start TRANSPORT.
- Insert at least one LARGE-BORE IV en route and start aggressive fluid therapy with lactated Ringer's.
- Be alert for the development of tension pneumothorax. If you have reason to think that tension pneumothorax is developing, insert a needle into the chest as described earlier.

Cardiac Tamponade

Cardiac tamponade occurs when there is an accumulation of blood in the pericardial sac (Fig. 17-6). Tamponade most commonly results from penetrating injuries, such as stab wounds to the heart, but blunt chest trauma and even acute myocardial infarction with cardiac rupture may cause the myocardium to fill with blood. On rare occasions, overly aggressive cardiopulmonary resuscitation has led to this complication.

As blood begins to fill the pericardial sac, the function of the heart is progressively compromised. Since the pericardial sac is a fibrous and relatively inelastic structure, it does not take a great deal of blood to restrict cardiac activity. As the pressure within the pericardium increases, the ventricles of the heart are prevented from expanding and therefore prevented from filling completely during their relaxation phase (**diastole**). As a consequence, the amount of blood they pump out with each beat (**stroke volume**) is reduced, so cardiac output as a whole decreases. The *blood pressure* also *falls*, owing to the reduced cardiac ouput; but the *venous pressure rises*, because the right heart is compressed and hindered from filling adequately (hence the neck veins become distended). Heart sounds become more and more distant on auscultation, as they are muffled by the insulating blood in the pericardial sac. (Those three signs—muffled heart sounds, falling blood pressure, and elevated venous pressure—are known as **Beck's triad** and are considered classic signs of cardiac tamponade; but they may not always be present in tamponade. Pulsus paradoxus is also considered a classic sign of tamponade but also not invariably present.)

As the stroke volume declines, the **pulse pressure** (difference between the systolic and diastolic pressures) narrows. The heart tries to compensate for the decrease in cardiac output by increasing the heart rate; thus there is *tachycardia*, with a feeble pulse reflecting small stroke volume. The sympathetic nervous system responds with vasoconstriction, in a last-ditch attempt to maintain the blood pressure, so the skin becomes pale, cool, and moist. Nonetheless, the blood pressure usually does fall, and shock is frequently way out of proportion to the amount of blood lost. The signs of cardiac tamponade are summarized in Table 17-3.

The major problem in differential diagnosis in the field will be between cardiac tamponade and tension pneumothorax, both of which may present with deteriorating vital signs and distended neck veins. Some features that distinguish the two conditions are summarized in Table 17-2.

TABLE 17-2. DIFFERENTIATING AMONG TENSION PNEUMOTHORAX, HEMOTHORAX, AND CARDIAC TAMPONADE

	TENSION PNEUMOTHORAX	MASSIVE HEMOTHORAX	CARDIAC TAMPONADE
Presenting sign or symptom	Respiratory distress	Shock	Shock
Neck veins	Distended	Flat	Distended
Trachea	Deviated	Midline	Midline
Breath sounds	Decreased or absent on side of injury	Decreased or absent on side of injury	Equal on both sides
Percussion of chest	Hyperresonant on side of injury	Dull on side of injury	Normal
Heart sounds	Normal	Normal	Muffled

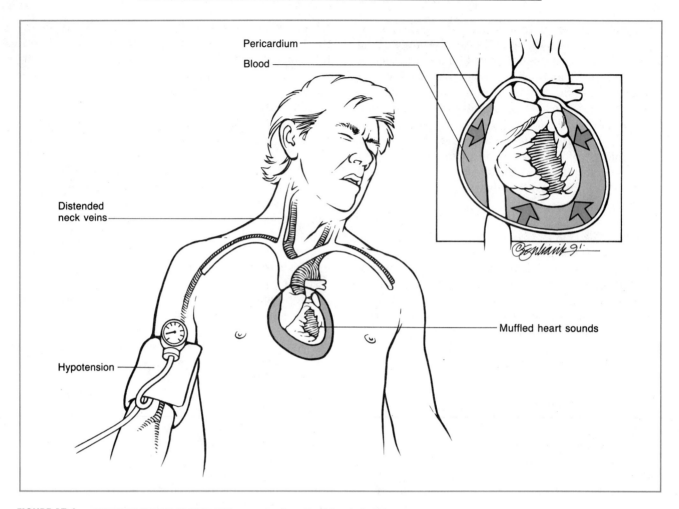

FIGURE 17-6. **CARDIAC TAMPONADE** may produce Beck's triad of hypotension, distended neck veins, and muffled heart sounds.

TABLE 17-3.   SIGNS OF CARDIAC TAMPONADE

PATHOPHYSIOLOGY	CLINICAL SIGN
Insulating effect of blood in the pericardial sac	Muffled heart sounds*
Restriction of ventricular filling during diastole, leading to	
• Decreased stroke volume	Narrowed pulse pressure Pulsus paradoxus
• Decreased cardiac output	Falling blood pressure* with hypotension out of proportion to blood loss
• Backup of blood in the venous circuit	Distended neck veins*
Sympathetic nervous system response	Pale, cool, sweaty skin Tachycardia

*Beck's triad.

Cardiac tamponade is a *dire* emergency. It will lead very quickly to cardiac arrest if not treated by **pericardiocentesis,** the evacuation of blood from the pericardial sac. That procedure should, if at all possible, be carried out in a hospital, under controlled conditions. Only if you are very far from the hospital should you attempt to perform pericardiocentesis in the field, and then only at the express order of the base physician. Pericardiocentesis is carried out as follows:

- Place the patient on the stretcher in a SEMISITTING POSITION, with his upper body elevated to approximately 30 degrees. Attach the four limb leads of an electrocardiograph (ECG) to the patient's extremities.
- Locate the xiphoid, and PREP THE SKIN around the xiphoid thoroughly with povidone-iodine swabs. Give a final wipe with an alcohol swab.
- If time permits, anesthetize the skin and subcutaneous tissue just to the left of the xiphoid by infiltrating 1 to 2 ml of 1% lidocaine.
- Attach a long (spinal or cardiac) 18-gauge needle to a 20-ml syringe.
- Use an alligator clip to attach the hub of the needle to the V lead of an electrocardiograph. The ECG machine should be properly grounded!
- Introduce the needle in the left costosternal angle, just to the left of the xiphoid. The needle should be inserted at a 90-degree angle to the chest and advanced until its tip is past the sternum, then angled upward so that the tip points toward the left shoulder (Fig. 17-7).
- While pulling back slightly on the plunger, advance the needle slowly. Usually you will feel a "pop" when the needle enters the pericardium, and nonclotting blood should immediately flow into the syringe. As soon as that happens, place a clamp on the needle at the point where it emerges from the skin, to prevent it from being accidently advanced further (Fig. 17-8).
- During the whole of this procedure, someone should be keeping an eye on the ECG. Should the needle come in contact with the myocardium, the ECG will show a "current of injury," that is, sudden changes in the T wave and S–T segment (see Chap. 23). If that happens, withdraw the needle very slightly until the ECG complex returns to normal. (Note: If you don't have a wire with alligator clips to attach the V lead to the pericardiocentesis needle, simply monitor the ECG in the usual fashion. If there is any sudden change in the ECG complexes, chances are that your pericardial needle has hit the heart, and you need to draw it back.)

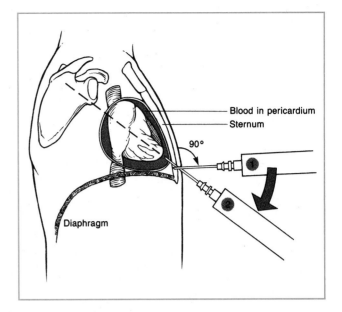

FIGURE 17-7. **LANDMARKS FOR PERICARDIOCENTESIS.** Introduce the needle at a right angle to the chest; once it has advanced past the sternum, angle it upward toward the left shoulder.

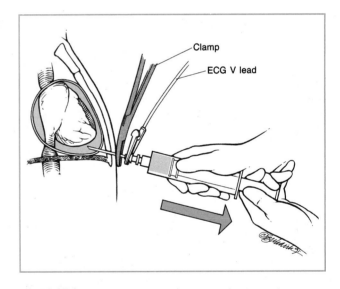

FIGURE 17-8. **PERICARDIOCENTESIS.** Once the needle has entered the pericardium and there is blood return into the syringe, clamp the needle next to the skin to prevent its being advanced any farther.

In acute cardiac tamponade, the aspiration of as little as 20 to 50 ml of blood from the pericardium should produce an immediate improvement in cardiac output and blood pressure. As soon as the procedure has been completed, start TRANSPORT. Establish an IV en route.

Traumatic Asphyxia

The term *traumatic asphyxia* refers to a specific combination of findings that result from severe compression injuries to the chest, such as those caused by severe impact against a steering wheel. Multiple fractures of the ribs and sternum are associated with a "caved-in" chest wall. As the sternum is forced inward, it exerts sudden pressure on the heart beneath; blood in the right heart is rammed back into the veins of the neck with such force that there is bleeding into the subcutaneous tissues of the upper chest and neck. The *signs* of traumatic asphyxia follow from the pathophysiology just described:

- *Caved-in chest*, usually with flail
- Profound *shock*, from both blood loss and cardiac injury
- *Cyanosis* and *swelling* of the head, neck, and shoulders, resembling that seen in victims of strangulation (which is probably how the syndrome got its somewhat inaccurate name of traumatic *asphyxia*, despite the fact that there is no asphyxia involved)
- Bloodshot, protruding eyes
- Swollen, cyanotic tongue and lips
- Often, bloody vomiting (**hematemesis**)

The presence of those findings signals major thoracic trauma that will be rapidly fatal without optimal management (and may indeed be rapidly fatal even *with* optimal management). TREATMENT in the field should be aimed at swiftly managing the ABCs, loading the patient into the ambulance, and getting to a trauma center:

- Ensure an adequate AIRWAY. If you can't keep the airway open manually, intubate the trachea; otherwise don't take the time in the field for intubation.
- Administer 100% OXYGEN by bag-valve-mask. Be alert for signs of developing tension pneumothorax, and be ready to stick a needle in the chest for decompression.
- IMMOBILIZE THE PATIENT on a long backboard.
- Start TRANSPORT.
- Start at least one IV en route and run fluids as rapidly as you can.

THE SECONDARY SURVEY IN CHEST TRAUMA

In patients who have suffered life-threatening chest injuries, such as those described in the previous section, it will not be possible to do much more than a primary survey, for the patient must be transported as rapidly as possible from the site of injury to a trauma center. On the other hand, when the primary survey has failed to detect immediately life-threatening problems, you should proceed to the secondary survey.

This is the time to take a quick look around and try to establish the MECHANISMS OF INJURY. In *vehicular trauma*, try to determine the speed at which the vehicle was travelling at the time of the accident. Note whether the victim(s) used seat belts; if so, what type (lap belts only, shoulder harness)? For each victim, make a note of his location in the car. Also observe the condition of the vehicle, and look for telltale signs such as a smashed windshield or damaged steering wheel. In victims of *gunshot wounds*, try to find out what sort of weapon inflicted the wound and from what distance. RECORD ALL YOUR FINDINGS on the patient's trip sheet.

As you observe the mechanisms of injury, you can start to develop some suspicions regarding the type of injuries to be especially alert for. Finding associated injuries should also increase your index of suspicion (Table 17-4).

Traumatic Aortic Rupture

Traumatic rupture of the aorta is the most common cause of sudden death after deceleration injuries such as vehicular accidents or falls from a height. The aorta has three areas of attachment within the body: at the aortic valve, at the ligamentum arteriosum (just beyond the origin of the subclavian artery), and at points along the thoracic spine. When the body is in motion and brought to a sudden halt, as when it is flung forward against a steering wheel after a head-on collision, the heart and aortic arch continue moving forward until *their* motion is arrested by the sternum and ribs (Newton's first law—remember?). The thoracic portion of the aorta is restrained by its attachments to the thoracic spine. The aortic arch therefore twists forward, and rupture occurs at the ligamentum arteriosum.

About 80 to 85 percent of patients who suffer aortic rupture will die almost instantly, before you even reach the scene. In the remaining 15 to 20 percent, however, the aortic tear will be temporarily sealed by surrounding tissues, and salvage will be possible if the diagnosis is made promptly and the patient reaches the operating room in time. While the patient is likely to complain of pain in the area of the shoulder blade or pain on swallowing, there are *no specific symptoms* to help you identify a ruptured aorta. You

TABLE 17-4. MECHANISMS OF CHEST INJURY IN VEHICULAR ACCIDENTS

IF YOU FIND:		
STRUCTURAL CLUES	BODY CLUES	BE ALERT FOR:
Deformed side of car	Bruised pelvis	Ruptured diaphragm
Deformed front end		Aortic rupture
Deformed steering column	Steering wheel imprint on chest	Myocardial contusion Pneumothorax Thoracic aorta injury
	Sternal fracture	Myocardial contusion Flail chest Pulmonary contusion
Miscellaneous	Scapular fracture	Injury to the descending aorta
	Fractures of the first or second rib	Major vascular injury
	Multiple rib fractures	Hemothorax, pneumothorax, pulmonary contusion
	Thoracic spine fracture	Injury to thoracic aorta

must simply have a high index of suspicion in any accident involving powerful deceleration forces and act with appropriate urgency in such cases.

SUSPECT AORTIC RUPTURE IN ANY ACCIDENT INVOLVING POWERFUL DECELERATION FORCES.

Tracheobronchial Injuries

We have already considered injuries to the larynx and trachea in Chapter 16. Injuries to a major *bronchus* are unusual but may be fatal. The majority result from blunt trauma and occur within about an inch of the carina. The tip-off to the presence of bronchial injury may be *subcutaneous emphysema* involving the chest, face, or neck. Sometimes there will be an associated pneumothorax. If a needle or catheter placed in the chest to decompress a pneumothorax continues to leak air for more than a few minutes, consider that the patient has a bronchial tear until proved otherwise.

Endotracheal intubation may be hazardous in a patient whose tracheobronchial tree has been disrupted; for using a standard laryngoscope, one cannot see where the tip of the endotracheal tube is going, and it may head straight into an injured

part of the bronchus. For that reason, if you suspect tracheobronchial injury, try to AVOID ENDOTRACHEAL INTUBATION. Give the patient 100% OXYGEN by nonrebreathing mask, and encourage him to INHALE SLOWLY, which will lessen the tendency of the bronchus to collapse on inhalation. Do not delay at the scene, but proceed at once to a trauma center.

Myocardial Contusion

One of the most frequently overlooked complications of blunt chest injury is trauma to the heart. Although the heart is a fairly resilient organ, its superficial location just behind the sternum renders it particularly vulnerable to injury from blunt impact. Blunt myocardial trauma most commonly occurs in steering wheel injury, and clinically significant myocardial contusions have resulted from automobile collisions at speeds as low as 25 miles per hour. However, any accident involving blunt injury to the chest may also result in myocardial contusion. Indeed, myocardial injury may occur when the trauma is apparently confined to the abdomen; the heart is, after all, only inches from the abdominal cavity.

Myocardial injuries are often missed because there may be few signs or symptoms of cardiovascular problems on initial examination. However, the potential complications of myocardial trauma are very serious, and therefore it is wise to assume that ALL PATIENTS WHO HAVE SUFFERED MAJOR

CHEST WALL TRAUMA HAVE MYOCARDIAL IN-JURY UNTIL PROVED OTHERWISE.

Myocardial contusion occurs more frequently among younger patients, for, as noted earlier, the thorax is more mobile and pliable in the young. An older individual may have significant calcification in the articulations of the thoracic cage, and thus his thorax is not as prone to depression from blunt impact. When the young person is pinned behind a steering wheel, on the other hand, his sternum can be compressed sharply against his spine, with the heart squeezed in between.

Automobile accidents are the most common cause of blunt myocardial trauma. In observing the scene of the accident and making inquiries of the patient, try to determine how fast the vehicle was moving and against what type of barrier it impacted. Note also the direction of impact. *Frontal impact injuries* are particularly dangerous, since the impact depresses the sternum posteriorly, ramming it straight back into the heart.

The major potential complications of blunt myocardial trauma are cardiac tamponade, which we have already discussed, and myocardial contusion. A myocardial contusion behaves in all respects like an acute myocardial infarction (see Chap. 23) and carries all the same potential risks. Chief among those risks are cardiac dysrhythmias, some of them life-threatening. The location of the injury influences the type of dysrhythmia that occurs; right-sided chest trauma frequently results in atrial dysrhythmias and heart block, while left-sided and frontal injuries are more apt to cause ventricular fibrillation. Early in the course of myocardial contusion, the most dangerous dysrhythmias are ventricular, but fortunately those are not common. When ventricular dysrhythmias do occur, treat them exactly as if they had occurred in the context of acute myocardial infarction (see under Cardiac Dysrhythmias, Chap. 23), giving lidocaine to control premature ventricular contractions and countershock for ventricular fibrillation.

The principles of prehospital TREATMENT of myocardial contusions are basically the principles of treatment for all serious chest injuries:

- Administer 100% OXYGEN.
- MONITOR cardiac rhythm in all victims of chest trauma, and treat life-threatening dysrhythmias, if they arise, as in acute myocardial infarction.
- TRANSPORT expeditiously.
- Establish an IV LIFELINE en route.

Diaphragmatic Tears

Tears in the diaphragm are usually the result of a blow to the *abdomen* that produces a sudden increase in intra-abdominal pressure. The vast majority of cases are the result of automobile accidents. Very strong forces are usually required to rupture the diaphragm, so there will almost invariably be other major injuries accompanying a diaphragmatic tear, and the diaphragmatic injury is unlikely to be detected in the prehospital phase. The only possible tip-off may be hearing bowel sounds in the chest (usually the left chest). If a significant proportion of the abdominal viscera has herniated through the diaphragm into the chest, the abdomen may look caved-in as well.

Since the patient will almost certainly have other serious injuries, treat for the injuries you do detect. If there is reason to suspect a diaphragmatic tear, DO NOT USE A MAST GARMENT.

Esophageal Injury

Esophageal injury is usually caused by penetrating trauma. Blunt trauma to the esophagus is very rare, but liable to be lethal when it occurs. You will not be able to differentiate esophageal injury in the field, nor will it be important to do so.

Pulmonary Contusion

Pulmonary contusion is the most common potentially lethal chest injury seen in the United States. As the name implies, pulmonary contusion is a bruise of the lung, and its lethal potential derives from bleeding and leakage of fluid into the alveoli. As we learned in Chapter 8, when fluid occupies the alveoli, oxygen does not. So blood passing an alveolus that is filled with fluid will not pick up any oxygen but will, rather, return to the left heart as if it had never made the trip through the lungs at all—a situation called *shunt*.

The adverse effects of pulmonary contusion usually do not become clinically evident until 2 or 3 days after the injury, when the amount of fluid sequestered in the lungs increases to the point that it interferes with oxygenation. Aggressive fluid therapy in patients with pulmonary contusion can increase the amount of fluid that ends up in the alveoli and worsen the shunt. Therefore, it is best to *restrict* fluids in patients who are likely to have suffered pulmonary contusion, that is, patients who have suffered steering wheel trauma, blast injuries, or falls from a height.

> **IF THE MECHANISMS OF INJURY SUGGEST PULMONARY CONTUSION, BE STINGY WITH IV FLUIDS UNLESS THERE ARE SIGNS OF SHOCK.**

Other Chest Injuries

In addition to the "deadly dozen" thoracic injuries we have already described, there are a few other chest injuries that are regarded as serious even though not in themselves life-threatening.

Simple Pneumothorax

Pneumothorax results from the entry of air into the pleural space, and it may result from either blunt or penetrating trauma (or from no trauma at all—see below). *Simple* pneumothorax designates a pneumothorax resulting from a one-time leak of air into the pleural cavity—as opposed to the continuing entry of air characteristic of tension pneumothorax. Simple pneumothorax occurs in about 40 percent of all cases of chest trauma, most commonly secondary to rib fractures (the jagged ends of the ribs lacerate lung tissue). The lung may be partially or totally collapsed, depending on how much air entered the pleural space. A healthy person can tolerate quite substantial amounts of air in the pleura; but the victim of serious trauma may have very little respiratory reserve, so even a simple pneumothorax may aggravate his situation considerably. There is, in addition, always the possibility that a simple pneumothorax will turn into a tension pneumothorax.

The major physiologic problem in simple pneumothorax is *shunt*. For just as fluid-filled alveoli cannot participate in gas exchange, so too alveoli that are collapsed cannot furnish oxygen to the adjacent capillaries. The net result, as in shunt from any cause, is *hypoxemia.*

The SYMPTOMS AND SIGNS of simple pneumothorax include dyspnea, pleuritic chest pain (i.e., chest pain that is made worse by a cough or deep breath), and tachypnea. Breath sounds will be diminished or absent on the affected side, and that side will be hyperresonant to percussion.

TREATMENT of a simple pneumothorax consists simply of giving 100% oxygen by nonrebreathing bag. Recheck vital signs frequently, however, to make certain that the simple pneumothorax has not progressed to a tension pneumothorax. If tension pneumothorax develops, or if the patient shows hypotension, tachycardia, and marked respiratory distress, decompress the chest as described earlier.

It should be mentioned that pneumothorax occasionally occurs in otherwise perfectly healthy individuals without any antecedent trauma. Pneumothorax occurring in such circumstances is called **spontaneous pneumothorax,** and it is most frequently seen in young, tall, thin males. Typically, the patient complains of a sudden, sharp chest pain and sudden dyspnea following strenuous exertion, coughing, or sometimes air travel. He may give a history of previous episodes of pneumothorax. Physical findings are the same as those for simple pneumothorax. Usually no treatment other than oxygen is necessary in the field.

Hemothorax

Hemothorax is the presence of blood in the pleural cavity, usually as a result of laceration of the lung or laceration of an intercostal vessel. In the vast majority of cases, bleeding into the pleural space is self-limiting. Small amounts of blood in the pleural space (less than 300 ml) may cause few symptoms and probably will not be detected in the field. As more blood accumulates in the pleural space, however, the patient experiences dyspnea due to lung compression. The affected side will be dull to percussion, with breath sounds somewhat muffled.

TREATMENT for simple hemothorax is essentially similar to that for massive hemothorax but need not be as aggressive.

Rib Fractures

Simple rib fracture is the most common thoracic injury and is significant chiefly because the pain involved inhibits the patient from taking adequate breaths. Whenever a person breathes shallowly, for any reason, the alveoli do not get fully inflated; little by little, they begin to collapse, and the progressive atelectasis makes the lung more vulnerable to pneumonia.

Rib fractures are usually caused by direct blows to the chest and most commonly involve the fifth through the ninth ribs. The first four ribs are relatively protected by the shoulder girdle, and the lowest ribs (the "floating ribs") are less exposed and more mobile, so also relatively protected. As noted earlier, a young patient with a more flexible chest wall is less likely to suffer rib fracture, so when rib fracture does occur in a young person, one must assume that the forces involved were sizable and that there is considerable damage to the lung beneath. In elderly patients with osteoporosis ("thinning" of the bones), on the other hand, ribs may be broken from minimal trauma, such as a fit of coughing.

Because the ribs are part of a ring, when a rib breaks from a direct blow, it often does so at more than one point or separates at the costal margins.

The principal *symptom* of rib fracture is PAIN, which is usually well localized to the site of the injury and which is made worse by deep breathing, coughing, or movement. On examination of the chest, there *may* be deformity or contusion over the painful area; the involved rib will be tender to palpation and may be unstable. The patient will usually lean toward the fracture, to relieve muscular tension on the site. Subcutaneous emphysema implies damage to the underlying lung, which may occur if the end of a fractured rib has penetrated the lung. In any case, be sure to listen and percuss over both sides of the chest to check for pneumothorax or hemothorax.

TREATMENT of uncomplicated rib fracture is aimed at minimizing the patient's pain while at the same time trying to ensure adequate ventilation:

- Administer OXYGEN.
- SPLINT the fracture to enable the patient to breathe more comfortably. A hand or pillow held firmly against the fracture site is often sufficient. Alternatively, the patient's arm can be bound to his chest on the injured side with a series of swaths; the swaths should not, however, be applied so tightly as to interfere with inhalation.
- Encourage the patient to take DEEP BREATHS. That may be easier for him if the fracture is splinted by a hand or pillow.

SUMMARY: GENERAL PRINCIPLES OF MANAGEMENT IN CHEST INJURIES

If in proceeding through the "deadly dozen" you began to feel confused, you are in good company. Experts in chest trauma also sometimes find the clinical picture of a given patient confusing, and it may require a number of sophisticated tests, such as computed tomography (CT) scans, to sort out the precise diagnoses. Fortunately, however,

> **IT IS NOT NECESSARY TO MAKE A SPECIFIC DIAGNOSIS IN ORDER TO APPRECIATE THAT A PATIENT IS CRITICALLY INJURED.**

Your primary survey will tell you if there is an immediate threat to life. If a life-threatening chest injury is detected, the most important thing you can do for the patient is to get him to a trauma center as fast as possible and in the best condition possible. The following general principles apply to all patients with serious chest injuries:

- Maintain an appropriate SENSE OF URGENCY. A sense of urgency is *not* a sense of panic. Know what you have to do in the field, and do it methodically but rapidly.

- Administer 100% OXYGEN at the earliest opportunity.
- ASSIST VENTILATIONS whenever necessary, but bear in mind that positive pressure ventilation may induce a tension pneumothorax in an injured lung, so AVOID HIGH INFLATION PRESSURES and KEEP ALERT FOR SIGNS OF PNEUMOTHORAX.
- For the reason just mentioned, DO NOT USE THE DEMAND VALVE IN A PATIENT WHO HAS SUSTAINED CHEST INJURY, since the high pressures a demand valve generates are more likely to induce pneumothorax.
- MONITOR cardiac rhythm in every patient who has sustained chest injury.
- When a patient with chest injury suddenly begins to deteriorate, check for signs of tension pneumothorax. If deterioration is rapid and you are in doubt, put a needle in the chest as described earlier.
- When the patient is severely injured, LOAD AND GO as soon as you have established an airway and immobilized the spine. Further treatment, such as intravenous therapy, should be initiated en route.
- Patients with serious chest trauma should be transported DIRECTLY TO A TRAUMA CENTER.
- Always consider the MECHANISMS OF INJURY and ASSOCIATED INJURIES, so that you can anticipate potentially life-threatening problems in patients who initially appear stable.

GLOSSARY

Beck's triad   Muffled heart sounds, hypotension, and neck vein distention, characteristic of *cardiac tamponade*.

cardiac tamponade   Restriction of cardiac contraction, diminution of cardiac output, and shock caused by the accumulation of fluid or blood in the pericardium.

diastole   The period of ventricular relaxation, when the ventricles passively fill with blood.

flail chest   The condition in which several ribs are broken, each in at least two places, or in which there is sternal fracture or separation of the ribs from the sternum, producing a free or floating segment of the chest wall that moves paradoxically with respiration.

hematemesis   Vomiting blood.

hemothorax   The presence of blood in the pleural cavity.

pericardiocentesis Aspiration of blood or fluid from the pericardium.

pneumothorax The presence of air in the pleural cavity.

pulse pressure The difference between the systolic and diastolic blood pressures, reflecting the *stroke volume.*

pulsus paradoxus Weakening or loss of the palpable pulse on inhalation, characteristic of cardiac tamponade.

stroke volume The amount of blood pumped forward with each ventricular contraction.

sucking chest wound Open pneumothorax; injury in which air passes in and out of the thoracic cavity through a hole in the chest.

traumatic asphyxia Syndrome resulting from a very severe compression injury of the chest, with cyanosis of the face and neck, bulging of the eyes, and a caved-in chest.

FURTHER READING

CHEST TRAUMA

Archer GJ et al. Results of simple aspiration of pneumothoraces. *Br J Chest Dis* 79:12, 1985.

Barone JE et al. Indications for intubation in blunt chest trauma. *J Trauma* 26:334, 1986.

Bayne CG. Pulmonary complications of the McSwain Dart. *Ann Emerg Med* 11:136, 1982.

Cannon WB, Mark JBD, Jamplis RW. Pneumothorax: A therapeutic update. *Am J Surg* 142:26, 1981.

Chaignaud BE. Uncomplicated rib fractures. *Emerg Med* 22(7):31, 1990.

Champion HR. Trauma score. *Crit Care Med* 9:672, 1981.

Clevenger FW, Yarbrough DR, Reines HD. Resuscitative thoracotomy: The effect of field time on outcome. *J Trauma* 28:441, 1988.

Cowley RA. Managing steering wheel injuries. *Emergency* 11(11):65, 1979.

Delius RE et al. Catheter aspiration for simple pneumothorax. *Arch Surg* 124:833, 1989.

Ferko JG, Singer EM. Injuries to the thorax. *Emergency* 22(4):20, 1990.

Frame SB, McSwain NE. Chest trauma. *Emergency* 21(7):22, 1989.

Gauthier RK. Thoracic trauma. *Emerg Med Serv* 13(3):28, 1984.

Guyton SW, Paull DL, Anderson RP. Introducer insertion of mini-thoracostomy tubes. *Am J Surg* 155:693, 1988.

Hagman J et al. Diaphragmatic rupture following blunt trauma. *Ann Emerg Med* 13:49, 1984.

Hansbrough JF, Chandler JE. Lung laceration following catheter insertion into the chest for pneumothorax. *Emerg Med Serv* 8(2):48, 1979.

Ivatury RR et al. Penetrating thoracic injuries: In-field stabilization vs. prompt transport. *J Trauma* 27:1066, 1987.

Jacobs LM et al. Prehospital advanced life support: Benefits in trauma. *J Trauma* 24:8, 1984.

Johnson I et al. Sternal fracture: A modern review. *Arch Emerg Med* 10:24, 1993.

Kearney PA, Rouhana SW, Burney RE. Blunt rupture of the diaphragm: Mechanism, diagnosis, and treatment. *Ann Emerg Med* 18:1326, 1989.

Kirsh MM, Sloan H. *Blunt Chest Trauma: General Principles of Management.* Boston: Little, Brown, 1977.

Lazcano A, Cougherty JM, Kruger M. Use of rib belts in acute rib fractures. *Am J Emerg Med* 7:97, 1989.

Lucas C, Tintinalli JE. Flail chest. *JACEP* 8:380, 1979.

Markos J et al. Penumothorax: Treatment by small-lumen catheter aspiration. *Austral NZ J Med* 20:775, 1990.

Markowitz I. Trauma rounds. Problem: Pulmonary contusion. *Emerg Med* 17(13):32, 1985.

McGahan JP, Rab GT, Dublin A. Fractures of the scapula. *J Trauma* 20:880, 1980.

McSwain NE Jr. A thoracostomy tube for field and emergency department use. *JACEP* 6:324, 1977.

Miller HAB et al. Management of flail chest. *Can Med Assoc J* 129:1104, 1983.

Mines D, Abbuhi S. Needle thoracostomy fails to detect a fatal tension pneumothorax. *Ann Emerg Med* 22:863, 1993.

Mukherjee D et al. A simple treatment for pneumothorax. *Surg Gynecol Obstet* 156:499, 1983.

Murphy P, McCammon L. Chest trauma: Managing blunt and pentrating injuries. *JEMS* 18(9):33, 1993.

Neclerio EA. Chest trauma. *Clin Symp* 22:75, 1980.

Newman RJ. Chest wall injuries and the seat belt syndrome. *Injury* 16:110, 1984

Nowack RM, Tomlanovich MC. Subcutaneous emphysema. *JACEP* 6:269, 1977.

Ochsner MG et al. Pelvic fracture as an indicator of increased risk of thoracic aortic rupture. *J Trauma* 29:1376, 1989.

Raja OG et al. Simple aspiration of spontaneous pneumothorax. *Br J Dis Chest* 75:207, 1981.

Semrad N. A new technique for closed thoracostomy insertion of chest tube. *Surg Gynecol Obstet* 166:171, 1988.

Smith MG. Penetrating the complexities of chest trauma. *JEMS* 14(8):50, 1989.

Smith SB et al. Spontaneous pneumothorax: Special considerations. *Am Surg* 49:245, 1983.

Treasure RL. Management of flail chest. *Milit Med* 144:588, 1979.

Vallee P et al. Sequential treatment of a simple pneumothorax. *Ann Emerg Med* 17:936, 1988.

Wayne MA, McSwain NE. Clinical evaluation of a new device for treatment of tension pneumothorax. *Ann Surg* 191:760, 1980.

Wilson RF. Averting the worst in chest trauma. *Emerg Med* 14(12):23, 1982.

Wilson RF et al. Hemoptysis in trauma. *J Trauma* 27:1123, 1987.

Wojcik JB, Morgan AS. Sternal fractures: The natural history. *Ann Emerg Med* 17:912, 1988.

Woodring JH, Lee C, Jenkins K. Spinal fractures in blunt chest trauma. *J Trauma* 28:789, 1988.

Wright SW. Myth of the dangerous sternal fracture. *Ann Emerg Med* 22:1589. 1993.

MYOCARDIAL TRAUMA

Arena AA, Martinez JA, McNulty PA. Problem: Acute cardiac tamponade. *Emerg Med* 16(15):51, 1984.

Baxter BT et al. A plea for sensible management of myocardial contusion. *Am J Surg* 158:557, 1989.

Bayer MJ, Burdick D. Diagnosis of myocardial contusion in blunt chest trauma. *JACEP* 6:238, 1977.

Beresky R et al. Myocardial contusion: When does it have clinical significance? *J Trauma* 28:64, 1988.

Cachecho R et al. The clinical significance of myocardial contusion. *J Trauma* 33:68, 1992.

Callahan M. Acute traumatic cardiac tamponade: Diagnosis and treatment. *JACEP* 7:306, 1978.

Conn AKT. Cardiac arrest due to trauma. *Emergency* 11(12):42, 1979.

Dreifus LS. Dysrhythmias related to cardiac trauma. *Chest* 61:294, 1972.

Dubrow TJ et al. Myocardial contusion in the stable patient: What level of care is appropriate? *Surgery* 106:267, 1989.

Fabian TC et al. Myocardial contusion in blunt trauma: Clinical characteristics, means of diagnosis, and implications for patient management. *J Trauma* 28:50, 1988.

Forrester JS. Pericardial tamponade. *Emerg Med* 16(4):108, 1984.

Gervin AS, Fischer RP. The importance of prompt transport in salvage of patients with penetrating heart wounds. *J Trauma* 22:443, 1982.

Green ED et al. Cardiac concussion following softball blow to the chest. *Ann Emerg Med* 9:155, 1980.

Guillot TS, Frame SB. Trauma rounds. Problem: Myocardial contusion. *Emerg Med* 20(3):157, 1988.

Healey MA et al. Blunt cardiac injury: Is this diagnosis necessary? *J Trauma* 30:137, 1990.

Helling TS et al. A prospective evaluation of 68 patients suffering blunt chest trauma for evidence of cardiac injury. *J Trauma* 29:961, 1989.

Honigman B et al. Prehospital advanced trauma life support for penetrating cardiac wounds. *Ann Emerg Med* 19:145, 1990.

Janeira LF. Cardiac tamponade. *Emergency* 12(2):44, 1980.

Jones JW, Hewitt LW, Drapanas T. Cardiac contusion: A capricious syndrome. *Ann Surg* 181:567, 1975.

Kron IL, Cox PM. Cardiac injury after chest trauma. *Crit Care Med* 11:624, 1983.

Kunar SA et al. Myocardial contusion following nonfatal blunt chest trauma. *J Trauma* 23:327, 1983.

Luna GK et al. Hemodynamic effects of external cardiac massage in trauma shock. *J Trauma* 29:1430, 1989.

Mattox KL et al. Five thousand seven hundred sixty cardiovascular injuries in 4459 patients: Epidemiologic evolution 1958–1987. *Ann Surg* 209:698, 1989.

McGahan JP, Rab GT, Dublin A. Fractures of the scapula. *J Trauma* 20:880, 1980.

McSwain NE. Pericardiocentesis. *Emerg Med* 20(22):102, 1988.

Miller FB, Shumate CR, Richardson JD. Myocardial contusion: When can the diagnosis be eliminated? *Arch Surg* 124:805, 1989.

Nelson RM et al. Journal club: Myocardial contusion. *Am J Emerg Med* 3:588, 1985.

Ramp J, Harkins J, Mason G. Cardiac tamponade secondary to blunt trauma. *J Trauma* 14:767, 1974.

Snow N, Richardson JD, Flint LM Jr. Myocardial contusion: Implications for patients with multiple traumatic injuries. *Surgery* 92:744, 1982.

Sturaitis M et al. Lack of significant long-term sequelae following traumatic myocardial contusion. *Arch Intern Med* 146:1765, 1986.

Sutherland GR et al. Frequency of myocardial injury after blunt chest trauma as evaluated by radionuclide angiography. *Chest* 84:1099, 1983.

Weisz GM, Blumenfeld Z, Barzilai A. Electrocardiographic changes in traumatized patients. *JACEP* 5:329, 1976.

18

Injuries to the Abdomen and Genitourinary Tract

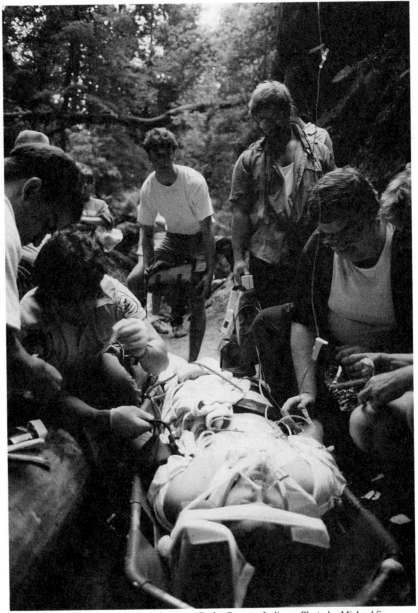

Parke County Emergency Medical Services, Parke County, Indiana. Photo by Michael S. Kowal.

OBJECTIVES

Significant abdominal injury may sometimes be obvious, as when the victim of a stabbing is found with half his intestines hanging out of the stab wound. More often, however, the presence of potentially serious injury within the abdominal cavity may be very difficult to detect, even in the hospital. Nonetheless, it is possible to *suspect* significant abdominal trauma based on the mechanisms of injury and the location of bruises or penetrating wounds on the abdominal wall. In this chapter, we shall first of all review the anatomy—topographic and internal—of the abdomen, in order to understand better what organs may be injured by different types of trauma. We shall then go over the steps in assessing a patient who may have sustained abdominal trauma. Finally, we shall look at some of the injuries—blunt and penetrating—that may involve the abdomen and genitourinary tract. By the end of this chapter, the student should be able to

1. List the organs found in
   • Each of the four abdominal quadrants
   • The intrathoracic abdomen
   • The true abdomen
   • The retroperitoneum
   and indicate which are hollow organs and which are solid organs
2. List the organs that make up
   • The digestive system
   • The genitourinary system
3. Identify the abdominal injuries likely to be present given the mechanisms of injury and the clinical findings in various patients
4. Describe the steps in evaluating the abdomen of a seriously injured patient
5. Given a description of several patients, identify a patient with
   • Penetrating trauma to the abdomen
   • Blunt trauma to the abdomen
   • Trauma to the genitourinary system
   and describe the correct treatment of each

REVIEW OF ABDOMINAL ANATOMY

Although it is important to know what is inside the abdomen—and we shall proceed to that shortly—in fact what we ordinarily *see* when we examine a patient is the outside of his body. It is necessary, therefore, to start our review of anatomy with a look at the *topography* of the abdomen.

Topographic Anatomy of the Abdomen

Viewed from the outside, the abdomen is bounded superiorly by the lowest ribs (the **costal arches**). The region just inferior to the costal arches is called the **epigastrium.** It is important to remember, however, that looks are deceiving. For although from the outside the abdomen appears to begin below the ribs, in fact, as we shall see shortly, there are several important abdominal organs housed *within* the ribs, as high as the fourth intercostal space. Thus once again we must emphasize that

PART OF THE ABDOMEN IS IN THE CHEST!

The most prominent abdominal landmark is probably the **umbilicus,** or navel, which is used as a reference point to divide the abdomen into four quarters (**quadrants**), as shown in Figure 18-1: the right upper quadrant (RUQ), left upper quadrant (LUQ),

FIGURE 18-1.   QUADRANTS OF THE ABDOMEN. RUQ = right upper quadrant; LUQ = left upper quadrant; RLQ = right lower quadrant; LLQ = left lower quadrant.

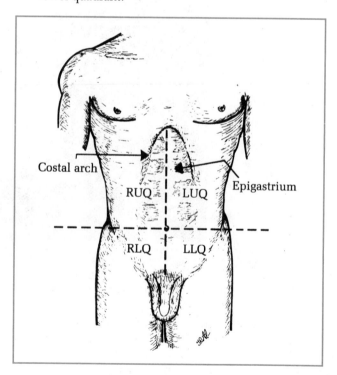

right lower quadrant (RLQ), and left lower quadrant (LLQ). As always, the point of reference is the patient, so the right upper quadrant, for example, refers to the *patient's* right side. Often knowing which quadrant is involved in an injury can help in figuring out which internal organs may have been damaged, as we shall see when we take a look inside the abdomen.

Internal Anatomy of the Abdomen

Viewed from the inside, the superior border of the abdominal cavity is formed by the *diaphragm,* which arches high into the chest. An imaginary plane from the sacrum to the pubis forms the inferior abdominal border (Fig. 18-2). The muscle of the anterior abdominal wall forms the anterior boundary of the abdomen, while the thoracic and lumbar spine make up the posterior boundary. Lining the abdominal cavity is a smooth, thin layer of tissue, called the **peritoneum** (hence, the abdominal cavity is also sometimes referred to as the "peritoneal cavity").

FIGURE 18-2. **BOUNDARIES OF THE ABDOMINAL CAVITY.**

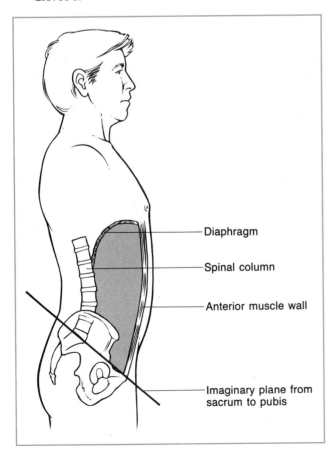

- Diaphragm
- Spinal column
- Anterior muscle wall
- Imaginary plane from sacrum to pubis

Divisions of the Abdominal Cavity

It is customary to divide the abdomen into three regions:

- The **intrathoracic abdomen** (Fig. 18-3A) is the portion of the abdomen protected by the rib cage. The intrathoracic abdomen contains the SPLEEN, STOMACH, LIVER, and DIAPHRAGM, which are most likely to be injured in association with fractures of the ribs or sternum. A direct blow, however, may also rupture the liver or spleen. And a powerful blow to the lower abdomen may squeeze the lower abdominal contents upward to cause rupture of the diaphragm. That mechanism is typical of *seat belt injuries*.
- The **true abdomen** (Fig. 18-3B) contains the LARGE AND SMALL BOWEL and the BLADDER; in women, it also contains the uterus, ovaries, and fallopian tubes. The bladder and female reproductive organs lie within the pelvic ring. The bladder, in fact, is outside the peritoneal cavity, between the peritoneum and the pubic bone. Its location makes it particularly vulnerable to injury when the pelvis is fractured.
- The **retroperitoneal abdomen** (Fig. 18-3C) is located behind the peritoneal membrane (*retro* = "behind"), that is, behind the true abdominal cavity. It contains the KIDNEYS, PANCREAS, DUODENUM, AORTA, and INFERIOR VENA CAVA. Injuries to structures within the retroperitoneum may be very difficult to detect, for bleeding into the retroperitoneum does not produce the kind of distention that may be seen with bleeding into the true abdomen.

Nearly all the organs of the abdomen are loosely suspended from the body walls by a delicate membrane called **mesentery,** which carries blood vessels and nerves to the abdominal organs. The mesentery is easily torn and, because it is so vascular, can bleed profusely when lacerated.

Body Systems Within the Abdominal Cavity

The abdominal cavity contains major portions of the digestive, lymphoid, and genitourinary systems.

The function of the DIGESTIVE SYSTEM (Fig. 18-4) is to convert the double burger, cole slaw, and fries you had for lunch into simple sugars, amino acids, fatty acids, and wastes. That is accomplished by breaking down the food you ingested, mechanically and chemically, into smaller and smaller components until it is in a form suitable for metabolism. The portions of the digestive system outside the ab-

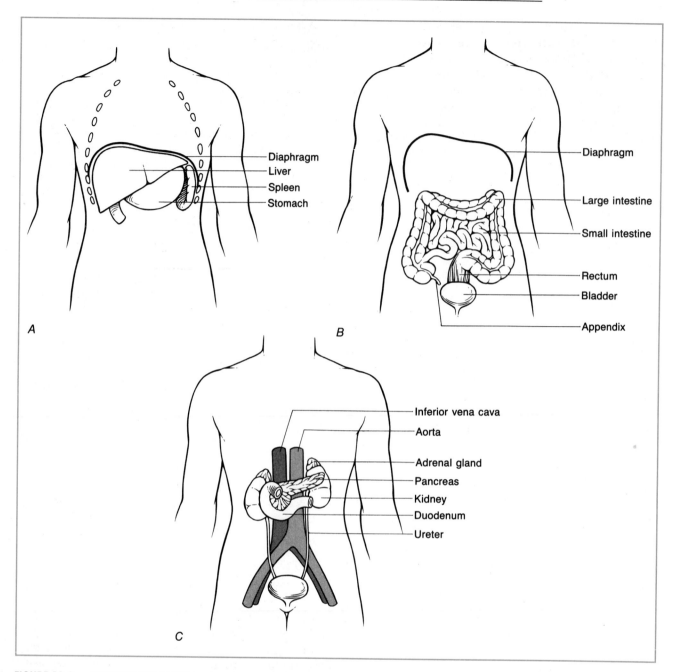

FIGURE 18-3. ANATOMIC REGIONS OF THE ABDOMEN. (A) Intrathoracic abdomen. (B) True abdomen. (C) Retroperitoneum.

dominal cavity include the *mouth* (which contains teeth and salivary glands to begin both mechanical and enzymatic breakdown of food), the *pharynx,* and the *esophagus.* **Peristalsis,** propulsive waves produced by sequential muscular contractions, drives the food down the esophagus (or even *up* the esophagus if you are swallowing upside down; consider how difficult it would be for a giraffe to drink if mammals had to rely on gravity in order to swallow!). Peristalsis operates throughout the hollow organs of the digestive system and can be detected by the gur-

gles and plops normally heard on auscultation over the abdomen. When there is injury or inflammation in the abdomen, however, peristalsis may stop altogether, and the belly becomes silent.

At the point where the esophagus joins the stomach, food enters the abdominal cavity proper. The **stomach** is a J-shaped organ that lies mostly in the left upper quadrant. Within the stomach, your lunch is churned up together with acid and pepsin, a digestive enzyme that begins the breakdown of the hamburger (protein). Normally, food will be emptied

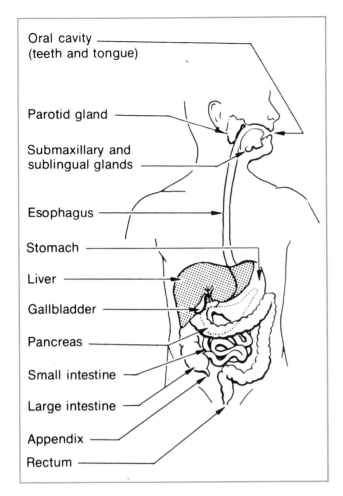

FIGURE 18-4. **COMPONENTS OF THE DIGESTIVE SYSTEM.**

from the stomach within 1 to 3 hours after it is ingested, but pain or injury can significantly delay gastric emptying. Although it is customary to inquire of an injured patient when he ate his last meal, it is safest to assume that

> ## EVERY INJURED PATIENT HAS A FULL STOMACH.

In emulsified form, then, the double burger, cole slaw, and fries depart the stomach and enter the first portion of the small intestine, the **duodenum**, which is about a foot long. Food passing into the duodenum is mixed with secretions from the pancreas and liver. The **pancreas** is a rather flat organ located, as we recall, in the retroperitoneal space. It contains two sorts of glands: one type secretes powerful digestive enzymes that are pumped into the duodenum; the second type of gland manufactures the hormone **insulin,** which is released into the bloodstream to regulate the concentration of sugar in the blood.

Bile, produced by the **liver** and concentrated in the **gallbladder** also enters the duodenum, to participate in the digestion of fat. The liver in fact has a number of crucial roles in the body, besides its role in digestion: It produces proteins essential for blood clotting; it detoxifies the blood by metabolizing many drugs and other poisons; and it stores sugar for emergency energy supply. To carry out such tasks, the liver needs, and has, a very generous blood supply. So when it is injured, the liver bleeds profusely.

After leaving the duodenum, your partially digested lunch now enters the second and third segments of the small intestine, the **jejunum** and **ileum,** respectively. Together, the jejunum and ileum are about 20 feet long, and within them the double burger, fries, and cole slaw undergo the final stages of digestion, being broken down into carbohydrate, protein, and fat subunits for absorption into the circulation. The part that is not absorbed, such as all the fiber from the cole slaw, continues on into the large intestine, or **colon,** where more of the fluid is absorbed and stool (feces) is formed. The colon consists of three sections: The first part (ascending colon) sweeps upward from the connection with the ileum (**ileocecal valve**) on the right side of the abdomen; the colon then crosses the abdomen (transverse colon) from right to left, and finally makes a right turn to sweep downward (descending colon) along the left side of the abdomen. Peristalsis drives the stool through the colon, into the **rectum,** and out of the body through the **anus.**

Near the junction of the ileum and the colon is a short, dead-end tube, the **appendix.** It has no role in digestion but may play a role in the development of normal immunity in children.

The main representative of the LYMPHORETICULAR SYSTEM in the abdomen is the **spleen,** which sits tucked up under the ribs in the (intrathoracic) abdomen. The major function of the spleen is to clear the blood of old, tired red blood cells and to replace them with new ones. Like the liver, the spleen is filled with thousands of small channels for blood flow, so it may bleed profusely if ruptured. Splenic rupture is most likely to occur with injuries to the *left lower ribs.*

A third organ system represented within the abdomen is the GENITOURINARY SYSTEM, which includes, as the name implies, the organs of urine formation and the organs of reproduction. The *urinary system* (Fig. 18-5) filters wastes from the blood, assists in the control of acid-base balance, and regulates the concentration of various electrolytes in the blood. The real work of the urinary system is carried out by the **kidneys,** paired organs that sit against the pos-

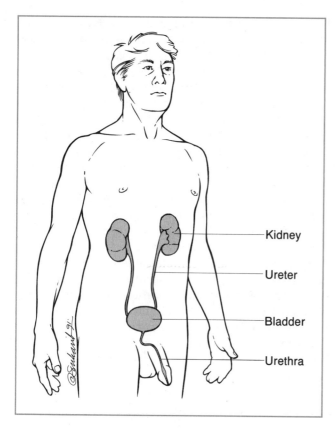

FIGURE 18-5.   COMPONENTS OF THE URINARY SYSTEM.

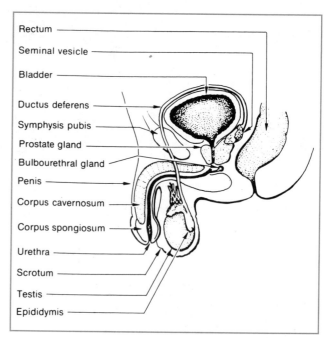

FIGURE 18-6.   MALE REPRODUCTIVE ORGANS.

terior abdominal wall at about the level of the twelfth thoracic to second lumbar vertebrae (T12–L2). A rich vascular supply brings blood to the kidneys, which filter out waste products and form urine. The urine is then collected through a system of tubules, which unite to empty into the **ureters,** the tubes leading to the bladder. The urinary **bladder** in turn empties to the outside of the body through another excretory passage, called the **urethra.** In the male the urethra passes through the penis, and in the female it opens in front of the vagina.

If the kidneys are damaged, waste products such as urea can no longer be efficiently removed from the bloodstream and instead accumulate, sometimes to toxic levels, within the body. Normal kidney function depends critically on blood flow; if blood flow is disrupted for any period of time, the kidneys may cease functioning altogether. Thus anything that produces inadequate perfusion (shock) may also produce renal failure.

The MALE REPRODUCTIVE SYSTEM (Fig. 18-6) is mostly *extra*-abdominal. It consists of the testes, a duct system, accessory glands, and the penile urethra. The **testes** (singular: *testis*) are the primary organs of reproduction in the male. They lie outside the

body cavity in a sac called the **scrotum.** Each testicle contains specialized cells that produce male hormones, seminal fluid, and sperm cells. The sperm, suspended in seminal fluid, are carried up the seminal ducts into the abdominal cavity, where they enter the **seminal vesicles** for storage. Seminal fluid, or **semen,** is ejaculated through the urethra during sexual intercourse. As semen passes through the urethra, it is joined by fluids from the **prostate gland** surrounding the urethral orifice. Special mechanisms prevent the passage of urine through the urethra during sexual intercourse. The **penis,** through which the urethra passes, is made up of specialized tissue rich in blood vessels. During sexual excitement, reflexes cause dilatation of the arteries supplying this *erectile tissue;* the resultant engorgement of the penile tissue with blood causes the penis to become rigid and assume an erect position.

The FEMALE REPRODUCTIVE SYSTEM (Fig. 18-7) consists of the ovaries, fallopian tubes, uterus, vagina, and external genitalia. Like the testes, the **ovaries,** which lie in the lateral portions of the lower abdomen, produce sex hormones and specialized reproductive cells—in this case *ova* (eggs). During a woman's reproductive years, her ovaries release an ovum at approximately monthly intervals. As we shall learn in more detail in Chapter 35, the mature ovum is released into the **fallopian tube,** through which it travels to the **uterus.** The latter is a hollow, muscular organ that opens through a narrow passage, called the **cervix,** into the **vagina.**

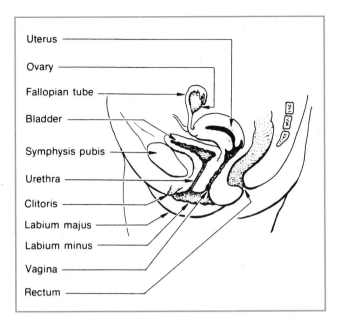

Uterus
Ovary
Fallopian tube
Bladder
Symphysis pubis
Urethra
Clitoris
Labium majus
Labium minus
Vagina
Rectum

FIGURE 18-7. **FEMALE REPRODUCTIVE ORGANS.**

Hollow Versus Solid Organs

The organs within the abdominal cavity are sometimes also classified according to whether they are hollow or solid, for the types of injury to which an organ is susceptible are not the same for hollow organs as for solid organs. Hollow organs are more liable to rupture and spill their contents into the peritoneal cavity, while solid organs are likely to bleed profusely if disrupted.

TYPES OF ABDOMINAL ORGANS

Hollow Organs	Solid Organs
Stomach	Liver
Small intestine	Spleen
Large intestine	Pancreas
Gallbladder	Kidneys
Ureters	Adrenal glands
Urinary bladder	

ASSESSMENT OF THE PATIENT WITH ABDOMINAL INJURY

Assessment begins, as always, with the ABCs. Abdominal injury is particularly likely to produce *vomiting*, which may jeopardize the **airway**. So have suction immediately available, and place the pa-

tient—other injuries permitting—in the stable side position, to enable vomitus to drain out of the mouth rather than back down the throat. Impairment of **breathing** suggests associated chest or spinal injury. Remember, severe compression injuries to the abdomen may drive abdominal contents upward and cause tears in the diaphragm. Assess the **circulation** in the usual fashion, by checking the pulse, skin condition, and capillary refill. A restless, anxious patient with cold, clammy skin and poor capillary refill may very likely be bleeding into his abdomen, *even if his pulse is normal or slow*. For reasons not well understood, severe intra-abdominal hemorrhage sometimes occurs *without* the tachycardic response that we usually associate with significant blood loss.

Once you have completed the primary survey, take a few moments to observe the scene and question those present to learn as much as you can about the MECHANISMS OF INJURY. If the patient was injured in a road accident, take a quick look at any *damage to the vehicle*. Note whether the patient is wearing a *seat belt* and, if so, what kind (lap belt only? shoulder harness?) and how it is being worn. Lap belts worn incorrectly across the belly, rather than across the hips, can cause laceration of the small intestine or rupture of the diaphragm. If the patient has been stabbed, try to get a look at the knife. How long is the blade? Was the assailant a man or a woman? (That is not a sexist consideration! Most men will wield a knife underhand and thrust upward into the abdomen; the average woman will thrust downward with an overhand motion, which causes considerably less damage.) If the patient was shot, what kind of firearm was used? At what range?

In taking a brief HISTORY from the patient, find out his chief complaint, which may help identify his injuries. If he has *pain*, what is it like? Blood or spilled digestive juices within the peritoneum produce peritoneal inflammation, which causes the patient severe pain that is made worse by any movement, even a cough. Pain radiating into the left shoulder (**Kehr's sign**) suggests blood beneath the left diaphragm and may be associated with a ruptured spleen.

Find out whether the patient has *vomited* since the accident. If so, was there blood in the vomitus (**hematemesis**)? When did he last urinate? A full bladder is much more likely to be ruptured than an empty one.

Record the VITAL SIGNS, and proceed to the HEAD-TO-TOE SURVEY. As you examine the *chest*, again keep in mind that

---

AN INJURY TO THE CHEST ANYWHERE BELOW THE NIPPLES IS ALSO AN INJURY TO THE ABDOMEN.

To examine the abdomen, expose the abdomen fully and

- LOOK. Inspect the anterior and posterior abdominal walls as well as the lower chest, the flanks, and the buttocks. Look for bruises, abrasions, lacerations, penetrating wounds, and eviscerations. Immediately after an accident, compression marks, such as those made by seat belts, may also be visible.
- FEEL for tenderness or rigidity. Muscular *guarding* represents voluntary spasm of the abdominal wall muscles in an attempt to prevent the pain of peritoneal irritation. Guarding may be caused by injury to the abdominal wall itself or to the structures within the abdomen. When the abdominal wall is truly rigid ("boardlike"), peritoneal irritation is almost certainly present. Do *not* test for rebound tenderness. If you want to verify peritoneal irritation, ask the patient to cough, and observe his face for a grimace of pain when he does so.

> **A DISTENDED, TENDER ABDOMEN AFTER INJURY MEANS INTERNAL BLEEDING. TREAT FOR SHOCK, AND TRANSPORT IMMEDIATELY.**

In the field, it is usually not worth the time it takes to listen for bowel sounds. To hear bowel sounds at all requires relatively quiet conditions, which are rarely to be found at the scene of a road accident, a shooting, a stabbing, or similar event. Furthermore, one must listen for at least a full minute to be able to state that "bowel sounds are absent," and a full minute is too much time to devote to such a low-yield procedure.

PENETRATING TRAUMA TO THE ABDOMEN

Penetrating injuries to the abdomen may result from knives, bullets, and a variety of other instruments that man has devised to harm his fellows. Penetrating injuries may be much more serious than they appear from the outside; beneath the clean little bullet hole, for example, may lie a disaster area of torn vessels, chewed up intestines, and so forth. Penetrating injuries most usually result in HEMORRHAGE, from laceration of a major blood vessel or solid organ and PERFORATION of a hollow organ, usually a segment of the bowel.

The TREATMENT of a patient with penetrating trauma to the abdomen includes the following:

- Attend first to the ABCs.
- COVER OPEN WOUNDS with dry, sterile dressings.
- If there is an IMPALED OBJECT in the abdomen, LEAVE IT THERE. Stabilize the impaled object in place with bulky dressings, and tape the dressings securely.
- If viscera are protruding through a large, open wound in the abdominal wall, DO NOT ATTEMPT TO REPLACE THE PROTRUDING ORGANS INTO THE ABDOMEN. Leave the viscera on the surface of the abdomen, and cover them gently with sterile aluminum foil or with sterile dressings that have been soaked in sterile saline. Do not use dry dressings in direct contact with protruding viscera, for dry dressings will stick and be difficult to remove later. Cover the foil or wet dressing with a clean towel or several additional layers of universal dressings to minimize heat loss across the wound.
- Start an IV (preferably TWO IVs) with large-bore catheters and lactated Ringer's. If the patient is already showing signs of shock when you first encounter him, start the IVs while en route to the hospital.
- Give NOTHING BY MOUTH.

BLUNT TRAUMA TO THE ABDOMEN

Blunt abdominal trauma may have few outward signs. Even bruises, the usual indication of blunt impact, may take several hours to develop in a person who has sustained a blow to the abdomen. Thus you will need to pay close attention to the mechanisms of injury and the patient's overall condition in order not to miss a blunt abdominal injury. Mechanisms of injury suggestive of blunt abdominal trauma include

- *Compression* of the abdominal contents against the spine
- *Direct blows* (e.g., a kick in the belly)
- Rapid *deceleration,* especially when the patient is restrained by an improperly applied lap seat belt

Be particularly alert for blunt abdominal trauma in the scenario of a *pedestrian struck by a moving vehicle.*

The organs most commonly injured by blunt trauma to the abdomen (including the part of the abdomen that is within the chest) are the liver, spleen, pancreas, duodenum, and mesentery of the small bowel. The LIVER, in the right upper quadrant, is easily torn by blunt injury, such as steering wheel trauma, and because of its rich blood supply can bleed massively. Similarly, severe hemorrhage may occur from rupture of the SPLEEN, located in the LUQ and also vulnerable to steering wheel trauma. The spleen is the most commonly injured organ in blunt abdominal trauma. Stashed up inside the ribs, the spleen is susceptible to rupture whenever there is a fracture of the left ninth and tenth ribs. It can also be compressed against the vertebral column or against other organs.

Damage to the PANCREAS, tucked away behind the stomach and liver, will result in spillage of digestive enzymes and consequent peritonitis, although the signs of peritonitis may take some time to develop.

Injuries caused by lap seat belts are apt to involve the INTESTINES and the LUMBAR SPINE.

TREATMENT of blunt abdominal trauma is principally aimed at anticipating shock and supporting the circulation:

- Attend first to the ABCs. Anticipate vomiting. If the patient is unconscious and has been intubated, consider inserting a nasogastric tube en route to hospital.
- If significant forces were involved in producing the injury, or if you see a seat belt mark on the abdomen, IMMOBILIZE THE SPINE.
- Use of the MAST in abdominal trauma is now somewhat controversial (see Chap. 9). Be guided by local protocols.
- Start TRANSPORT.
- Start one and preferably TWO LARGE-BORE IV LINES, and infuse lactated Ringer's solution.

Remember:

> **BLUNT ABDOMINAL INJURY MAY BE MUCH MORE SERIOUS THAN IT LOOKS. DON'T DAWDLE AT THE SCENE!**

GENITOURINARY INJURIES

Genitourinary injuries may be produced by either blunt or penetrating trauma. The KIDNEYS are relatively well protected from injury by the ribs and heavy muscles of the back; therefore any force powerful enough to damage the kidneys will usually produce other injuries as well, such as fractured ribs or vertebrae and damage to other abdominal organs. As always, consider the *mechanisms of injury.* Any blow to the flank or to the lower rib cage in the back should arouse suspicion of renal injury. In the secondary survey, finding a *hematoma over a rib fracture* involving the tenth, eleventh, or twelfth rib posteriorly should alert you to the possibility that the kidney has sustained significant injury; any *discoloration, penetrating wound, or mass in the flank* has the same potential significance.

The urinary BLADDER, located as it is just behind the pubic bone, is vulnerable to injury whenever there is *fracture of the pelvis.* Sudden *deceleration forces,* such as those experienced in a head-on collision, may also produce bladder injury, shearing the bladder off at the urethra. The drunk driver is especially prone to such injuries, since he is more likely to be driving with a full bladder. Deceleration forces may also result in avulsion of the URETER where it crosses the pelvic brim, especially in children. Examination of the patient with bladder injury may reveal a *lower abdominal mass* or tenderness, or there may be signs of peritonitis.

In most patients who have suffered injury to a kidney, the bladder, or both, the urinary tract injuries will not be their only injuries and often will not be their most serious injuries. Thus priorities of TREATMENT for such patients will usually be governed by their other injuries and their overall condition. Tenderness over the vertebrae, for example, requires that the patient be immobilized on a backboard; a fractured pelvis is best immobilized with the MAST; signs of shock mandate the placement of at least one intravenous line.

Injuries to the EXTERNAL GENITALIA are discussed in detail in most basic EMT texts (see, for example, *Emergency Medical Treatment,* Chap. 16). Such injuries are rarely life-threatening, even if often highly distressing to the owner of the genitals as well as to the rescuers. Genital injuries are treated according to the same principles that govern treatment of soft tissue injuries anywhere else in the body.

GLOSSARY

anus The outlet of the *rectum,* lying in the fold between the buttocks.

appendix Wormlike structure attached to the *cecum,* in the right lower quadrant of the abdomen.

cecum The first portion of the large intestine, into which the small intestine empties.

colon The large intestine.

costal arch The arch formed by the lowest ribs as they curve upward toward the sternum.

duodenum   The name given to the first 11 inches of the small intestine.

epigastrium   The upper middle region of the abdomen, within the sternal angle.

evisceration   Disembowelment; the protrusion of abdominal viscera outside the abdominal cavity.

fallopian tube   A tube extending from an *ovary* to the *uterus*.

hematemesis   Vomiting blood.

ileocecal valve   The point at which the distal end of the small intestine (the ileum) is joined to the first portion of the large intestine (cecum).

ileum   The third portion of the small intestine.

insulin   Hormone secreted by the pancreatic islets that promotes utilization of sugar by the body.

Kehr's sign   Pain in the left shoulder after rupture of the spleen.

mesentery   Tissues carrying blood vessels, lymphatics, and nerves, by which the intestines are connected to the back surface of the abdominal cavity.

ovary   The female sex organ in which eggs (ova) and female hormones are produced.

peristalsis   Successive waves of muscular contraction and relaxation proceeding uniformly along a hollow tube, such as the esophagus or intestines, which propel the contents of the tube forward.

peritoneum   The membrane that lines the abdominal cavity.

prostate   Gland at the base of the male bladder that surrounds the urethra.

quadrant   Term used to designate one-quarter of the abdomen.

rectum   Distal portion of the large intestine.

renal   Pertaining to the kidney.

testis   Male gonad.

ureter   Tube leading from the kidney to the bladder.

urethra   Passage from the bladder to the outside of the body.

uterus   Muscular organ of the female pelvis designed to house the developing fetus; womb.

FURTHER READING

Al Saleh BMS et al. Fractures of the penis seen in Abu Dhabi. *J Urol* 134:274, 1985.

Asbun HJ et al. Intra-abdominal seatbelt injury. *J Trauma* 30:189, 1990.

Baxt WG, Moody P. The impact of a physician as part of the aeromedical prehospital team in patients with blunt trauma. *JAMA* 257:3246, 1987.

Bietz DS. Abdominal injuries. *Emergency* 10(12):30, 1978.

Cwinn AA et al. Prehospital advanced trauma life support for critical blunt trauma victims. *Ann Emerg Med* 16:399, 1987.

Denis R et al. Changing trends with abdominal injury in seatbelt wearers. *J Trauma* 23:1007, 1983.

Edwards FJ. Liver trauma. *Emerg Med Serv* 19(3):28, 1990.

Fiedler MD et al. A correlation of response time and results of abdominal gunshot wounds. *Arch Surg* 12:902, 1986.

Freeark RJ. Penetrating wounds of the abdomen. *N Engl J Med* 291:186, 1974.

Frentz GD, Lang EK. Problem: Bladder injury. *Emerg Med* 15(12):111, 1983.

Knudson M et al. Hematuria as a predictor of abdominal injury after blunt trauma. *Am J Surg* 164:482, 1992.

Mackersie RC et al. Intra-abdominal injury following blunt trauma: Identifying the high-risk patient using objective risk factors. *Arch Surg* 124:809, 1989.

Majernick TG et al. Intestinal evisceration resulting from a motor vehicle accident. *Ann Emerg Med* 13:633, 1984.

Moore JB, Moore EE, Thompson JS. Abdominal injuries associated with penetrating trauma in the lower chest. *Am J Surg* 140:724, 1980.

Murr PC et al. Abdominal trauma associated with pelvic fracture. *J Trauma* 20:919, 1980.

Palomar JM, Halikiopoulos H, Polanco E. Primary repair of the fractured penis. *Ann Emerg Med* 9:260, 1980.

Pennell TC. Hepatic trauma: An overview. *Emerg Med Serv* 6(5):68, 1977.

Pons PT et al. Prehospital advanced trauma life support for critical penetrating wounds to the thorax and abdomen. *J Trauma* 25:828, 1985.

Stubbs AJ, Harrison LH. Injuries to the lower genitourinary tract and their management. *Emerg Med Serv* 5(5):25, 1976.

Stubbs AJ, Resnick MI. Emergency department evaluation and treatment of acute scrotal swelling. *Emerg Med Serv* 7(2):68, 1978.

Thompson D, Adams SL, Barrett J. Relative bradycardia in patients with isolated penetrating abdominal trauma and isolated extremity trauma. *Ann Emerg Med* 19:268, 1990.

Vayer JS et al. Absence of a tachycardic response to shock in penetrating intraperitoneal injury. *Ann Emerg Med* 17:227, 1988.

Ward KR, Sullivan RJ, Zelenak RR. Isolated blunt splenic trauma. *Emerg Med* 21(1):73, 1989.

Whitehurst AW, Resnick M. The kidney and trauma: Diagnosis and treatment. *Emerg Med Serv* 5(6):30, 1976.

19
Fractures, Dislocations, and Sprains

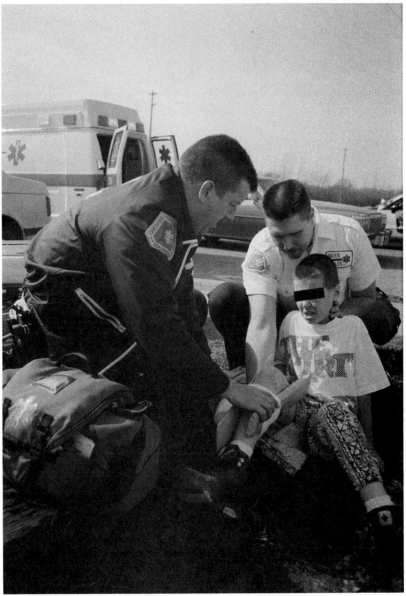

Fagen-Miller Ambulance Service, Highland, Indiana. Photo by Michael S. Kowal.

OBJECTIVES

Musculoskeletal injuries are common injuries. Usually they are obvious injuries, and sometimes they are very dramatic injuries. Only very rarely, however, are they life-threatening injuries, which is the reason we are considering them last. In this chapter, we shall review the anatomy of the musculoskeletal system and the ways in which bones and joints can be injured. We shall then consider the assessment and management of patients with injuries involving the musculoskeletal system. By the conclusion of the chapter, the student should be able to

1. Identify the major bones of the body, given a drawing of the skeleton or a description of the bones
2. List the bones that make up the major joints of the body
3. List five mechanisms of musculoskeletal injury, and give an example of an injury produced by each mechanism
4. List another injury likely to be present given a description of a musculoskeletal injury already detected in a patient
5. List six symptoms and signs of fracture
6. Given a description of the mechanisms of injury and clinical findings of several patients, identify a patient with a probable
   • Fracture
   • Dislocation
   • Sprain
   and describe the correct management of each
7. List six symptoms and signs of limb ischemia
8. Identify a patient with impending compartment syndrome, given a description of the patient's clinical findings, and describe the management of the patient
9. Describe the correct management of a patient who has suffered traumatic amputation of a limb, given a description of the patient's clinical findings
10. List in correct sequence the steps in treating a multitrauma victim who has sustained musculoskeletal injury
11. List the steps in assessing an injured extremity, given a description of the patient's overall condition
12. List three purposes of splinting an injured extremity
13. Identify correct and incorrect splinting procedures, given a description of various procedures
14. List the specific danger(s) associated with
    • Posterior sternoclavicular dislocation
    • Scapular fracture

• Supracondylar fracture of the humerus
• Pelvic fracture
• Posterior dislocation of the hip
• Dislocation of the knee
• Fracture of the tibia
and describe the correct management of each

REVIEW OF MUSCULOSKELETAL ANATOMY

The Body Scaffolding: The Skeleton

The skeletal system, comprising 206 bones, provides a framework for the body. It gives the body form and protects vital organs, like the brain, heart, and lungs, that are enclosed within it. The skeletal system consists of (1) *bones*, which form the hard framework of the body; (2) *tendons* and *ligaments*, which hold things together; and (3) *cartilage*, which provides connecting and supporting structures.

BONES consist of both organic and inorganic materials. The *organic* materials, including living cells and an interstitial protein matrix, give bone its limited pliability and its capacity to repair and remodel itself. *Inorganic* salts of calcium and phosphorus give bone its strength and hardness. When calcium is deficient, as in rickets, the bones are easily bent and distorted.

Bones are classified according to shape and structure. On the basis of *shape*, bones may be categorized as long (bones of the extremities), short (bones of the wrist, ankle), flat (ribs, scapulae), or irregular (vertebrae). On the basis of *structure*, bones are classified as compact (hard, dense outer layer of bones) or spongy (containing many marrow-filled cavities). The femur (Fig. 19-1), for example, is a long bone, with a main, central shaft (**diaphysis**) composed principally of compact bone; an **epiphysis**, or portion of spongy bone covered with compact bone, at each end; and a **marrow cavity** within the shaft, containing principally fat cells. The bone is covered with a membrane called **periosteum.**

Bones come together, or **articulate** at JOINTS of various types. Joints may be *fused*, such as those between the bones of the skull, allowing little or no motion between the component bones. Or they may permit motion in one or more planes. A **synovial joint** is one in which the articular surfaces are covered with cartilage and separated by an articular cavity filled with lubricating fluid (synovial fluid). The bone ends of a joint are held together by tough ligamentous bands that form the **joint capsule.** The thickness of the capsule is not uniform. At certain points the ligament is thinner and looser, allowing motion to oc-

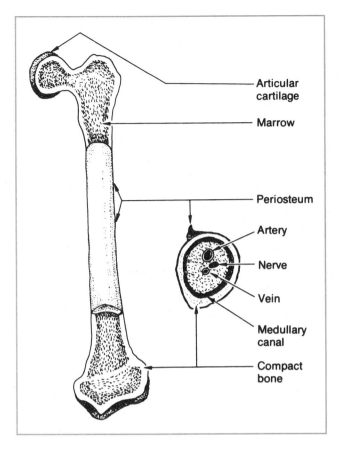

FIGURE 19-1.   **THE STRUCTURE OF A LONG BONE.**

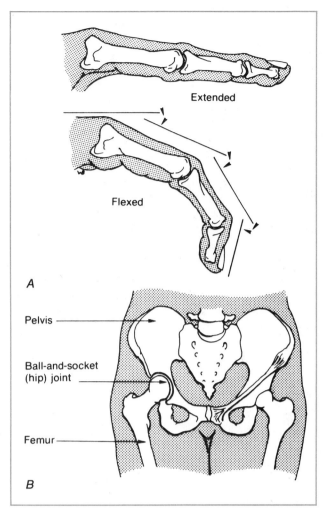

FIGURE 19-2.   **TYPES OF JOINTS.**   (A) Hinge joints permit flexion and extension. (B) Ball-and-socket joints allow motion in several planes.

cur; at other points, the ligament is thick and resistant to any stretch. The more range of motion allowed by the ligaments of the joint capsule, the greater the vulnerability of a joint to dislocation.

The type and degree of motion at any given joint are determined not only by the surrounding ligaments but also by the design of the joint itself. The structural types of joints include

- *Hinge joints,* such as those of the fingers (Fig. 19-2A), which permit flexion and extension
- *Ball-and-socket joints,* like those in the shoulders or hips (Fig. 19-2B), which permit a wide range of motions (and therefore have a greater vulnerability to dislocation)
- *Pivot joints,* like that between the radius and the ulna, which enable pronation and supination at the wrist (see below)
- *Gliding joints,* such as those between the bones of the hand, which allow very subtle and delicate movements

Motion at joints is made possible by the actions of attached muscles, which act as levers to produce movement as they contract and relax (see next section).

The connecting and supporting structures of the skeletal system include tendons, ligaments, and cartilage. **Tendons** are flat or cordlike bands of connective tissue that *attach muscle to bone.* **Ligaments** are similar in structure to tendons and *attach bones to one another.* **Cartilage** is another form of connective tissue that is widespread throughout the body. It forms the smooth surface over bone ends where they articulate, provides cushioning between the vertebrae, gives structure to the nose and external ear, and forms the framework of the larynx and trachea.

The skeleton as a whole (Fig. 19-3) permits an erect posture and gives the body its characteristic form. In previous chapters we have already considered the **axial skeleton**—that is, the skull, vertebral column, and thorax—and the injuries to which it is

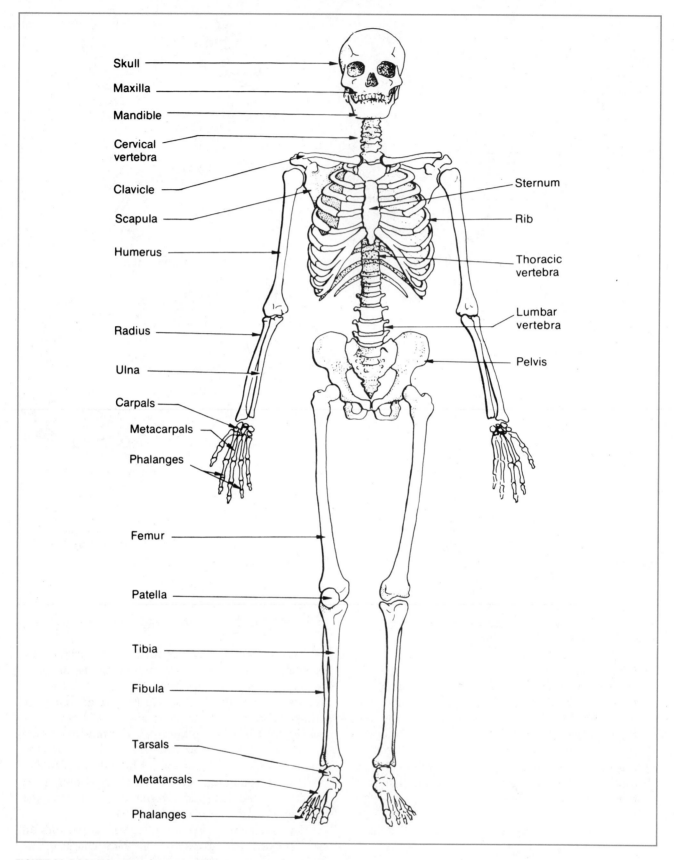

FIGURE 19-3. THE HUMAN SKELETON. The skull, vertebral column, and rib cage form the axial skeleton. The bones of the upper and lower extremities make up the appendicular skeleton.

susceptible. In this chapter we shall concentrate on the **appendicular skeleton,** the part of the skeleton that comprises the upper and lower extremities.

The Upper Extremities

The upper extremities consist of the bones of the shoulder girdle, arms, forearms, and hands.

The SHOULDER GIRDLE (Fig. 19-4) comprises the two scapulae and two clavicles. The shoulder blade, or **scapula,** is a flat, triangular bone held to the rib cage posteriorly by powerful muscles, which buffer the scapula against injury. The superior and lateral portion of the scapula forms the socket of the arm joint (the **glenoid fossa**), where motion is very free in all planes. The collar bone, or **clavicle,** is a slender, somewhat S-shaped bone attached by ligaments at the medial end to the sternum and at the lateral end to the raised tip of the scapula, called the **acromion.** The clavicle acts as a strut to keep the shoulder propped up; but being both very slender and very exposed, the clavicle is vulnerable to injury.

The ARM (Fig. 19-5) joins the shoulder girdle at the glenohumeral joint. The upper arm, or **humerus,** articulates proximally with the scapula and distally with bones of the forearm—the radius and ulna—to form the hinged elbow joint.

The radius and ulna make up the FOREARM. The **radius** is the larger of the two forearm bones, and it lies on the *thumb* side of the forearm. The proximal end of the **ulna,** called the **olecranon,** forms part of the elbow joint and can be palpated as the "funny bone." What makes it "funny" is the ulnar nerve passing along a groove on the outside of the ulna; when the elbow is bumped, the ulnar nerve is apt to be bruised, producing a "boing" sensation. Distally the ulna is narrow and is on the little-finger side of the forearm. It serves as the pivot around which the radius turns at the wrist to rotate the palm upward (**supination**) or downward (**pronation**). Because the radius and ulna are arranged in parallel, when one is broken the other is often broken as well.

The HAND (Fig. 19-5, inset) comprises three sets of bones: *wrist bones* (**carpals**), *hand bones* (**metacarpals**), and *finger bones* (**phalanges**). The carpals, especially the scaphoid (carpal navicular), are vulnerable to fracture when a person falls on an outstretched hand. Phalanges are more apt to come to grief in a slammed car door.

The back of the hand is referred to as the **dorsal** surface (or simply the *dorsum*) and the front as the palmar or **volar** surface. The thumb side of the hand and wrist is, as noted, called the **radial** side (after the radius), and the little finger side is called the **ulnar** side. (Question: Where do you take the radial pulse?) Thus if a doctor says "There is ecchymosis of the radial aspect of the dorsal surface of the right wrist," what he means is that there's a black-and-blue mark on the back of the right wrist at the base of the thumb.

FIGURE 19-4. **THE SHOULDER GIRDLE** is formed by the scapula and clavicle.

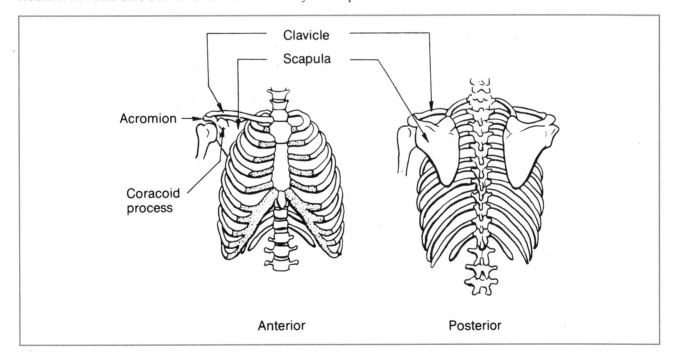

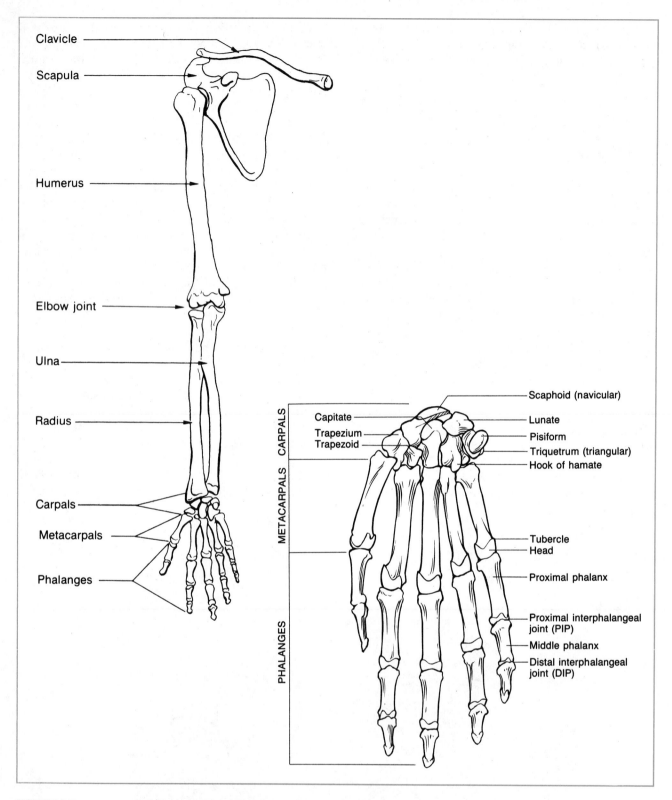

FIGURE 19-5.   THE BONES OF THE UPPER EXTREMITY.   At lower right are the bones of the hand and wrist.

The Lower Extremities

The lower extremities consist of the bones of the pelvis, upper legs, lower legs, and feet. The hip bone, or PELVIC GIRDLE (Fig. 19-6), is in reality three separate bones—the **ischium, ilium,** and **pubis**—fused together to form a bony ring. The two iliac bones are joined posteriorly by tough ligaments to the sacrum, at the **sacroiliac joints;** the two pubic bones are connected anteriorly, by equally tough ligaments, to one another at the **symphysis pubis.** Those joints allow very little motion, and therefore the pelvic ring is strong and stable. On each side, the three pelvic bones unite at a socketlike depression, the **acetabulum,** which accommodates the head of the long leg bone, the femur. The posterior portions of the ischium, called the **ischial tuberosities,** can be palpated as a hard bump in each buttock and are important landmarks for applying a traction splint.

The LEG (Fig. 19-7) joins the pelvic girdle at the acetabulum to form the hip. The thigh bone, or **femur,** is a long, powerful bone articulating proximally in the ball-and-socket joint of the pelvis and distally in a hinge joint at the knee. The femur consists of a *head,* the ball-shaped part that fits into the acetabulum, and a *neck* about 3 inches long, which is set at an angle to the *shaft.* The femoral neck is a common

site for fractures, especially in the elderly. The prominence of the **greater trochanter** is easily palpated in the lateral thigh and is sometimes called the "hip bone," so fractures of the proximal femur are sometimes referred to as hip fractures.

The LOWER LEG consists of two bones, the tibia and the fibula. The **tibia,** or shin bone, forms the inferior component of the knee joint, where it is shielded anteriorly by the knee cap, or **patella.** The tibia runs down the front of the leg, where it is very vulnerable to direct blows, and can be felt just beneath the skin of the lower leg. The much smaller **fibula** runs posteriorly and laterally. The fibula is not a component of the knee joint, but it does make up the lateral knob of the ankle joint (**lateral malleolus**) in its distal articulation. The **medial malleolus,** or bony knob on the inner side of the ankle, is the distal end of the tibia. (Question: On which side of the ankle—medial or lateral—do you find the posterior tibial pulse?)

The FOOT, like the hand, is composed of three classes of bones (Fig. 19-7, inset): *ankle bones* (**tarsals**), *foot bones* (**metatarsals**), and *toe bones* (**phalanges**). The largest of the tarsal bones is the heel bone, or **calcaneus,** which is subject to injury when a person jumps from a height and lands on his feet.

The same terminology for the surfaces of the hand and arm applies to those of the foot and leg (although, because most of us no longer walk on all fours, what we consider to be the *back* of the hand we consider as the *front* of the leg!). The *front* of the foot is its **dorsal** surface; the sole of the foot is its **plantar** surface. So when you *dorsiflex* the foot, you bend it upward, toes toward the sky. (Question: Which surface of the foot do you palpate for the *dorsalis* pedis pulse?)

The Moving Force: Muscles

Muscles are specialized tissues that contract when stimulated and, by their contraction and relaxation, produce motion—in themselves or in other body structures. Muscles are divided into three types on the basis of their structure and function: smooth muscle, cardiac muscle, and skeletal (striated) muscle.

SMOOTH or INVOLUNTARY MUSCLE mostly constitutes the muscles of the internal organs; it is found in the walls of the digestive tract, trachea and bronchi, urinary bladder, and blood vessels. Smooth muscles are innervated by nerves of the autonomic nervous system (see p. 500). The actions of smooth muscles are for the most part *not* under voluntary control; rather, smooth muscles contract slowly in re-

FIGURE 19-6. **THE PELVIC RING** consists of pelvic bones—ilium, ischium, and pubis—fused posteriorly with the sacral region of the spine.

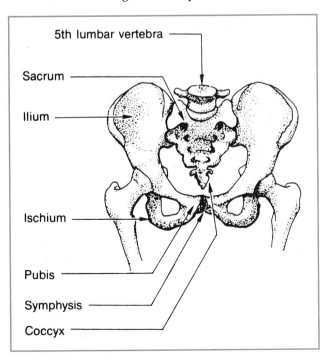

- 5th lumbar vertebra
- Sacrum
- Ilium
- Ischium
- Pubis
- Symphysis
- Coccyx

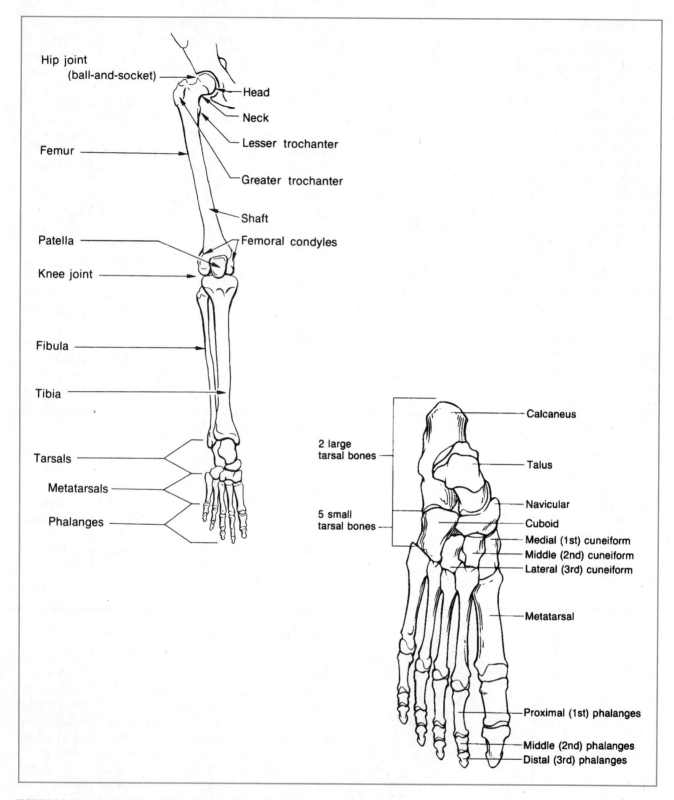

FIGURE 19-7. THE BONES OF THE LOWER EXTREMITY. At lower right are the bones of the foot and ankle.

sponse to signals from various visceral motor centers in the brain.

CARDIAC MUSCLE is a highly specialized form of muscle found only in the heart. Like smooth muscle, cardiac muscle receives innervation from the autonomic nervous system. But, in addition, cardiac muscle has the unique property of being able to initiate its own contractions—a property known as **automaticity.**

The kind of muscle with which we are concerned in this chapter is SKELETAL MUSCLE. As the name implies, skeletal muscle comprises all the muscles attached to the skeleton (Fig. 19-8). It also constitutes the muscles of the tongue, soft palate, scalp, pharynx, upper esophagus, and eye. Skeletal muscles are also called *voluntary* muscles, since their contractions are largely under voluntary control. Skeletal muscles are profoundly affected by the amount of training and work to which they are subjected. Muscles that remain unused tend to **atrophy** (grow smaller), while training increases the size and strength of muscles.

As noted earlier, skeletal muscles are attached to various parts of the bone structure by *tendons*. Tendons cross joints to create a pull between two bones when a muscle contracts. The biceps muscle (Fig. 19-9), for example, has its origins on the scapula; the biceps tendon passes over the head of the humerus, where it fuses with the body of the biceps muscle; at the distal end of the biceps, a tendon passes over the anterior surface of the elbow and inserts onto the radial bone. Thus when the biceps muscle contracts, the force exerted causes the elbow to bend (flex).

When any muscle contracts, it generates a small electric current that can be detected by electrodes on the surface of the skin. That is the basis for the electrocardiogram (ECG), which records the electric currents generated during *cardiac* muscle contraction.

Muscle contraction requires energy, which is derived from metabolism of glucose and results in the production of **lactic acid,** or lactate. Lactic acid, in turn, must be converted into carbon dioxide and water, a process requiring oxygen. For that reason,

FIGURE 19-8. **THE SKELETAL MUSCLES** are largely under voluntary control.

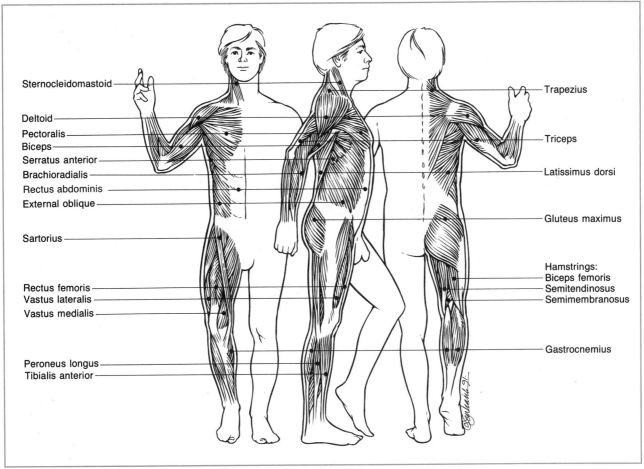

Sternocleidomastoid

Deltoid
Pectoralis
Biceps
Serratus anterior
Brachioradialis
Rectus abdominis
External oblique

Sartorius

Rectus femoris
Vastus lateralis
Vastus medialis

Peroneus longus
Tibialis anterior

Trapezius

Triceps

Latissimus dorsi

Gluteus maximus

Hamstrings:
Biceps femoris
Semitendinosus
Semimembranosus

Gastrocnemius

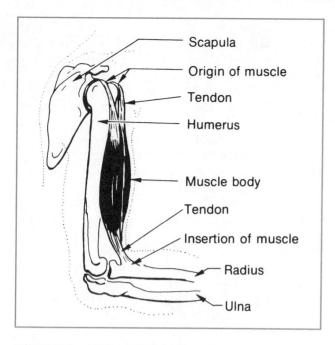

FIGURE 19-9. **THE BICEPS** tendon crosses the elbow joint to permit flexion of the arm.

vigorous muscular activity is often followed by an increased respiratory rate, which increases both oxygen delivery to the tissues and carbon dioxide removal from the tissues.

The sensation of muscle *fatigue* occurs when the energy supply to the muscle is inadequate to meet the energy demands. If muscle fatigue occurs as a result of excessive muscular activity, rest produces quick recovery. Muscle fatigue may also occur, however, from lack of essential nutrients, electrolytes (such as sodium or calcium), or oxygen. In anemia, for example, the oxygen-carrying capacity of the blood is reduced, so less oxygen reaches the muscles and they fatigue more easily.

Of the total energy used in muscle contraction, only about one-third is expended in the performance of work; the rest is liberated in the form of *heat*, which is used to maintain body temperature. When the body is exposed to cold environmental temperatures, it can augment the production of heat through voluntary activity, such as walking, or through involuntary muscular movements, such as shivering.

MECHANISMS OF MUSCULOSKELETAL INJURY

Orthopedic trauma may result from a variety of mechanisms and should be suspected whenever any of those mechanisms have been involved in producing the injury.

To begin with, musculoskeletal injury may be caused by a DIRECT BLOW, in which the bone is broken *at the point of impact* with a solid object, such as a dashboard or automobile bumper. INDIRECT INJURIES, on the other hand, involve a fracture or dislocation at some distance along the bone from the point of impact, as, for example, a hip fracture that occurs when a knee has been rammed against the car dashboard. Indirect forces may be transmitted along the entire length of a bone or several bones in series and may do their damage anywhere along the line. Thus a person falling on an outstretched hand may suffer any one or more of the following injuries as the result of forces transmitted proximally from the point of impact: (1) fracture of the scaphoid bone of the hand (direct blow); (2) fracture of the distal ulna and radius (Colles' fracture); (3) fracture/dislocation of the elbow; (4) fracture/dislocation of the shoulder; (5) fracture of the clavicle.

TWISTING INJURIES, such as commonly occur in football or skiing, result in fractures, sprains, and dislocations. Typically, the distal part of the limb remains fixed, as when cleats or a ski hold the foot to the ground, while torsion develops in the proximal section of the limb; the resulting forces cause shearing of tendons and ligaments and spiral fractures of bone. POWERFUL MUSCLE CONTRACTIONS, as occur in seizures or tetanus, may tear muscle from bone or actually break away a piece of bone. At least half of all posterior shoulder dislocations, for example, occur as a result of seizures. FATIGUE FRAC-

TABLE 19-1. MUSCULOSKELETAL INJURIES THAT COMMONLY OCCUR TOGETHER

IF YOU FIND:	LOOK FOR:
Scapular fracture	Rib fracture; pulmonary contusions
Carpal scaphoid fracture	Elbow fracture Shoulder fracture
Pelvic fracture	Lumbosacral spine fracture; bladder injury
Hip dislocation	Fracture of acetabulum or femoral head
Hip fracture	Dislocation of contralateral hip
Femoral fracture	Dislocation of ipsilateral hip
Patellar fracture	Fracture/dislocation of ipsilateral hip
Knee dislocation	Tibial fracture
Calcaneal fracture	Fracture of the other calcaneus Fracture of L1 or L2 of the spine

TURES, or march fractures, are caused by repeated stress and most commonly occur in the feet after prolonged walking. PATHOLOGIC FRACTURES are seen in patients with diseases that weaken areas of bone, such as metastatic cancer, and may occur with minimal force. The elderly also have weaker, more brittle bones and are thus more prone to fractures, especially hip fractures, than younger people.

When evaluating a patient who has sustained musculoskeletal injury, then, think like an engineer: Try to determine the nature of the force that produced the injury and the direction in which it was applied. Some injuries are commonly found together because of the way the causative forces are transmitted, so if you find one, start looking for the other(s) (Table 19-1). Pain and swelling over the scaphoid (navicular) bone of the wrist, for example, mean that the patient fell hard against an outstretched hand, so there may be other injuries anywhere along the axis from the hand to the shoulder, as described above.

TYPES OF MUSCULOSKELETAL INJURY

Musculoskeletal injuries fall into three general categories—fractures, dislocations, and sprains—any of which can occur by itself or in association with another type of injury.

Fractures

A fracture is a break in the continuity of bone. A fracture may be either **closed** (*simple*), in which the overlying skin is intact, or **open** (*compound*), in which there is a wound over the fracture site, with or without bone protruding through it. Open fractures have a far greater potential for complications than do closed fractures, for open fractures are more prone to infection and may also bleed more profusely.

Fractures are also classified according to their appearance on x-ray (Fig. 19-10). Although you will not have x-ray equipment available to you in the field, you should nonetheless become familiar with the terminology that derives from the x-ray appearance of the fracture; and you should be able, based on the mechanism of injury, to make an intelligent guess about what the x-ray will show.

A **transverse fracture** cuts across the bone at right angles to its long axis and is most usually produced by a direct blow. **Greenstick fracture** occurs in children, whose bones are still pliable (like green sticks), and is also a break straight across the bone—but it goes only part way through the bone. **Spiral fractures** usually result from twisting injuries, and the fracture line has the appearance of a spring. Twisting forces or other indirect forces may also produce **oblique fractures,** in which the fracture line crosses the bone at an oblique angle. In an **impacted fracture,**

FIGURE 19-10. **TYPES OF FRACTURE.** The x-ray appearance of a fracture reflects the mechanisms of injury.

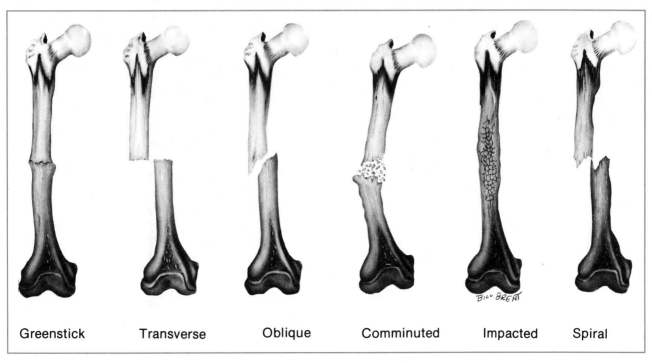

| Greenstick | Transverse | Oblique | Comminuted | Impacted | Spiral |

the broken ends of the bone are jammed together; impaction occurs from indirect forces, when a bone is trapped along its long axis between two unyielding objects. Finally, a **comminuted fracture** is one in which the bone is fragmented into more than two pieces and is the result of very powerful direct forces.

Signs and Symptoms of Fractures

The primary *symptom* of fracture is PAIN, usually well localized to the fracture site. In addition, the patient may report that he heard something snap or felt the bone break. Usually that information is quite accurate. The *signs* of fracture, detected on physical examination, include the following:

- DEFORMITY is one of the most reliable signs. The limb may be found in an unnatural position or show motion at a place where there is no joint.

> **THE BEST WAY TO DETECT DEFORMITY OR ANY OTHER ABNORMALITY IN AN EXTREMITY IS TO COMPARE IT TO THE EXTREMITY ON THE OTHER SIDE.**

- Comparing one limb to the other will also permit you to notice any SHORTENING in the injured limb. Shortening occurs in fractures when the broken ends of a bone override one another. Shortening is characteristic, for example, of hip fractures, because the broken femoral bone no longer serves as a strut to oppose spasm in the powerful thigh muscles.
- Visual inspection will usually also reveal SWELLING at the fracture site, due to both bleeding from the broken bone and the accumulation of edema fluid. As blood infiltrates the tissues around the broken bone ends, ECCHYMOSIS will become apparent as well.
- GUARDING and LOSS OF USE characterize most fractures. The patient will try to keep a fractured bone still and will avoid putting any stress on it. Sometimes the measures a patient takes to protect a fractured bone from movement are so characteristic that one can almost diagnose the fracture without examining the extremity. The patient who walks to the ambulance holding the dorsum of one wrist in his other hand, for example, almost certainly has a Colles' fracture (a type of fracture involving the distal radius and ulna). A patient standing with his head cocked

toward a "knocked-down shoulder" most probably has a fracture of the clavicle on the side to which the head is leaning.
- A fractured bone is almost invariably TENDER TO PALPATION over the fracture site.
- Palpation may also reveal GRATING or CREPITUS over the broken bone ends. Crepitus may be noted as an incidental finding during splinting attempts; do *not* try to elicit that sign, for you may cause further injury to the bone and surrounding soft tissue, not to mention severe pain to the patient.
- In an open fracture, EXPOSED BONE ENDS may be visible in the wound.

Potential Complications of Fractures

Fractures are ordinarily low-priority injuries, quite a way down the list after injuries that threaten the airway, breathing, and so forth. Nonetheless, fractures may have some serious consequences and should not, therefore, be treated carelessly.

BLEEDING from the broken ends of a fractured bone can be of significant volume. A fractured tibia can release a unit of blood into the lower leg; a fractured femur may pour 2 units of blood into the thigh; and a pelvic fracture can result in up to 6 units of blood loss, more than enough to produce profound hemorrhagic SHOCK. Quite aside from the danger of shock, however, bleeding into a closed space, such as the forearm or lower leg, is also dangerous because it increases the pressure within that closed space. As the pressure rises, vital structures, such as nerves and other blood vessels, are squeezed. If such compression—known as a **compartment syndrome**—is allowed to continue for more than a few hours, there will be permanent damage to the limb and lifelong disability. It is therefore essential to spot the signs of impending compartment syndrome early. Those signs can be summarized as the SIX Ps:

- PAIN is the earliest and most reliable sign, especially pain elicited by passively extending the fingers or toes of the affected limb; the pain will be localized to the region of the forearm or calf muscles. Although all fractures are painful, when there is a compartment syndrome, the patient will report the development of a qualitatively different kind of pain, or a return of pain after splinting had provided relief.
- PALLOR or a deterioration in capillary refill may be an early sign of compromised blood flow to the limb.
- When the blood supply to the distal limb is cut off altogether, by extreme pressure squeezing

down against the arterial walls, PULSELESS-NESS will occur, but that is already a late sign.

- PARESTHESIAS, that is, pins-and-needles sensations or frank numbness, occur as pressure on the sensory nerves increases.
- At the same time, pressure on the motor nerves will lead to PARESIS (weakness) and finally outright PARALYSIS. Paralysis occurs when there has been complete ischemia (absence of blood supply) of the peripheral nerve for more than 10 minutes.
- There is usually some degree of swelling, or PUFFINESS, both from the initial injury and from the obstruction to venous return as pressure within the compartment increases. As in the case of pulselessness and paresis, swelling is usually a *late* sign.

The finding of *any* sign of neurovascular compromise should prompt *immediate transport* of the patient to a hospital.

When the patient has an *open* fracture, EXTERNAL BLEEDING and bacterial CONTAMINATION of the wound are additional potential complications. Contamination of a fracture wound is very likely to lead to infection, which may delay healing of the fracture or even cause death from sepsis.

Dislocations

A dislocation is the displacement of a bone end from its articular surface, sometimes with associated tearing of the ligaments that normally hold the bone ends in place. The shoulder, elbow, fingers, hips, and ankles are the joints most frequently affected.

The principal *symptom* of dislocation is PAIN or a feeling of pressure over the involved joint, as well as LOSS OF MOTION of the joint. A patient with a posterior dislocation of the shoulder, for example, is unable to raise his arm but holds it tightly against his side instead. Sometimes the joint will seem "frozen" altogether. The principal *sign* of dislocation is DEFORMITY. When the shoulder pops out anteriorly, for instance, the acromion will suddenly seem very prominent, and the head of the humerus will be palpable in front of the shoulder joint.

In describing the position of a dislocated limb, we need to recall four special terms: **Abduction** is movement of a limb *away* from the body, whereas **adduction** is movement of a limb *toward* the body. When a limb is turned *outward* (laterally), it is said to be **externally rotated;** when turned *inward* (medially), it is **internally rotated.** (Question: When you *pronate* your arm, is it internally rotated or externally rotated?)

Thus, for example, when a patient suffers a posterior dislocation of the hip, the affected hip is usually found *flexed, adducted,* and *internally rotated.* (Picture that configuration. Is the knee pointing laterally or medially?)

What makes dislocations very urgent injuries is their potential to compromise the nerve supply or blood supply to the distal extremity. If the dislocated bone end is pressing on a *nerve,* there may be NUMBNESS or WEAKNESS distal to the dislocation; if an *artery* is being compressed, there may be ABSENCE OF THE DISTAL PULSE. That is yet another reason why it is important to

---

ALWAYS CHECK THE PULSES, STRENGTH, AND SENSATION DISTAL TO A MUSCULOSKELETAL INJURY.

The absence of pulses or any neurologic deficit distal to the injury means that the extremity is in grave danger, and transport to the hospital should not be delayed. In such cases, radio ahead so that the hospital will have time to alert an orthopedic surgeon to be standing by when the patient arrives.

Sprains

Sprains are injuries in which ligaments are partially torn, usually caused by the sudden twisting of a joint beyond its normal range of motion. The ankle and the knee are the joints most commonly affected. A sprain differs from a dislocation in that the continuity of the joint is *not* disrupted in a sprain, although the structures that support the joint are separated. Therefore deformity is less likely to be a significant feature in sprains, but PAIN, SWELLING, and DISCOLORATION may all be prominent parts of the picture. The common clinical features of fractures, dislocations, and sprains are summarized in Table 19-2. In actual practice, however, it is not always easy to differentiate among those three types of injury in the field. For that reason, it is best to err on the side of caution and

---

TREAT EVERY SEVERE SPRAIN AS IF IT WERE A FRACTURE.

TABLE 19-2. SIGNS OF COMMON ORTHOPEDIC INJURIES

FRACTURE	DISLOCATION	SPRAIN
Pain	Pain	Pain on motion
Tenderness		Tenderness
Deformity	Deformity	
Loss of use	Loss of motion	Painful motion
Swelling		Swelling
Ecchymosis		Redness
Grating		
Exposed bone ends (if compound)		

Strains

Strains are soft tissue injuries or muscle spasms around a joint and are characterized by pain on active movement. There is no deformity or swelling associated with a strain, and passive movement elicits little if any pain. If there is any doubt, however, as to the nature of the injury, treat it as a sprain pending evaluation in the emergency department.

Traumatic Amputations

The amputation of a limb or part of a limb is a dramatic and disabling injury. Amputation may also be a life-threatening injury if there is massive hemorrhage from the severed blood vessels. Usually, however, bleeding is self-limited because of spasm in the cut arteries, and direct pressure on the stump, using dressings that have been moistened in sterile saline, will usually control bleeding readily. DO NOT USE A TOURNIQUET EXCEPT AS A VERY LAST RESORT, when all other measures to control bleeding have failed; a tourniquet applied to an amputation stump will reduce the viability of the distal stump and thus lessen the chances of successfully reimplanting the amputated limb.

The care of an amputated part has already been described (see p. 307). We shall deal with the assessment and management of other musculoskeletal injuries in the sections that follow.

GENERAL PRINCIPLES OF ASSESSMENT AND MANAGEMENT

The most important principle in the treatment of musculoskeletal injuries has already been alluded to more than once:

> **MUSCULOSKELETAL INJURIES ARE RARELY IF EVER AN IMMEDIATE THREAT TO LIFE. A FRACTURE CAN WAIT. THE AIRWAY CANNOT.**

Often in the victim of multiple trauma, a mangled limb is the most dramatic and immediately obvious injury; it is unlikely, however, to be the most serious injury, and it should not distract the rescuer from the usual priorities of ABC.

The Primary Survey

As always, attention must be directed first to securing an airway, ensuring adequate breathing, and controlling external hemorrhage. If the patient is critically injured, starting the ABCs may be all you have time for in the field. When a multiply injured patient must be transported immediately, there will not be time to splint each fracture one by one. The best way to stabilize multiple fractures when the patient's overall condition is critical is to splint the axial skeleton, that is, *immobilize the whole patient* on a long backboard, a procedure that is called for anyway because of the likelihood of spinal injury in such circumstances.

> **WHEN A PATIENT WITH MULTIPLE FRACTURES REQUIRES IMMEDIATE TRANSPORT, IMMOBILIZE THE WHOLE PATIENT ON A LONG BACKBOARD.**

If the patient is otherwise stable, however, proceed to the secondary survey.

The Secondary Survey

As you begin the secondary survey, try to determine the MECHANISMS OF INJURY by examining the scene and questioning the patient, if he is conscious. Ask how the injury occurred and in what position the limb was at the time it occurred. For example, in the case of a twisted ankle, did the injury occur with the ankle bent outward or bent inward? Was the patient walking when it happened, or had he just jumped 6 feet from a stone wall? Has the bone or joint ever been injured before? Does the patient have any serious illnesses (e.g., cancer) that might help account for an otherwise unexplained fracture?

Don't forget to find out the patient's CHIEF COMPLAINT. Most patients with significant musculoskeletal injury will complain of PAIN, usually well localized to the area of the injury. But the patient may have sustained other injuries that are not so obvious as his orthopedic injury, and failure to elicit the chief complaint may mean failure to find injuries that are more serious than the fracture. The patient may, for instance, have obvious swelling over the sternoclavicular joint, leading you to suspect a posterior dislocation at the joint. But unless you ask him what is bothering him the most, you may not hear about his dyspnea and be alerted to the pneumothorax beneath the dislocated bone.

In the HEAD-TO-TOE survey, quickly assess the full length of each extremity. Besides looking for the injury itself, your most important task will be to assess neurovascular function distal to the injury. First LOOK at all four extremities, always comparing one extremity to its mate. Note the *position* of the extremity—is it unnatural in any way? Is there *deformity* in the extremity? *Unnatural motion? Swelling? Cyanosis?* FEEL each extremity for tenderness, swelling, and deformity. (One can also—strange as it seems—LISTEN for a fracture, using a stethoscope placed over the bone to detect changes in sound transmission, but such methods are rarely practical under field conditions.)

Assuming there are no other injuries, it is the status of the blood supply to the limb and the innervation of the limb that will determine the urgency of the patient's fracture or dislocation. It is therefore worthwhile to review in detail here the assessment of neurovascular status.

To ASSESS THE CIRCULATION TO AN EXTREMITY, first note the *skin condition* (color, warmth, moisture). Remember that *pallor* is one of the Six Ps. Test *capillary refill* by depressing the fingernail until it blanches and seeing how long it takes to "pink up" again (the nail bed should refill before you've had time to say, "Normal capillary refill"). Palpate the *pulse distal to the extremity* (the radial pulse for the upper extremity, the dorsalis pedis and posterior tibial pulses for the lower extremity—Fig. 19-11), comparing the pulse on the injured side to that on the uninjured side.

To ASSESS THE NERVE SUPPLY TO THE INJURED EXTREMITY, it is necessary to examine sensation and motor function of the specific areas innervated by the radial, ulnar, and median nerves in the upper extremity and the peroneal and tibial nerves (the two branches of the sciatic) in the lower extremity. The sensory and motor provinces of each of those nerves are summarized in Table 19-3. For practical purposes, however, all that is necessary to test sensation is to pinprick over the fingertips, dorsum of the hand, heel, and dorsum of the foot and to ask the patient to dorsiflex and palmar flex his hands and dorsiflex and plantar flex his feet.

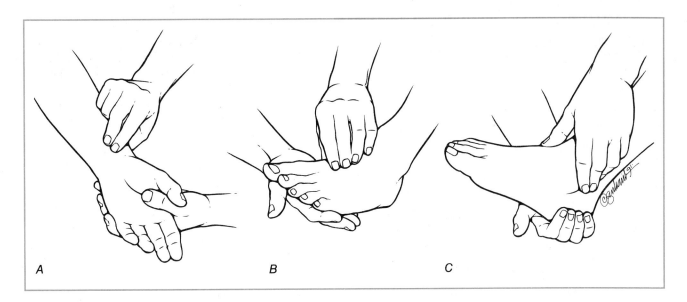

FIGURE 19-11.　CHECKING THE DISTAL PULSES. (A) The radial pulse. (B) The dorsalis pedis pulse. (C) The posterior tibial pulse.

TABLE 19-3. TESTING THE KEY PERIPHERAL NERVES

TO CHECK:	MODALITY	CARRY OUT THIS PROCEDURE
Upper extremity:		
Radial nerve	Motor	Ask patient to dorsiflex wrist.
	Sensory	Check pinprick over dorsal web space (between thumb and index finger).
Median nerve	Motor	Ask patient to touch his fingertips with the thumb of the same hand.
	Sensory	Check pinprick over the tips of the middle and index fingers.
Ulnar nerve	Motor	Ask patient to spread his fingers wide apart, then to make a cup with his hand.
	Sensory	Check pinprick over tip of little finger.
Lower extremity:		
Peroneal nerve	Motor	Ask patient to dorsiflex great toe.
	Sensory	Check pinprick on dorsum of foot.
Tibial nerve	Motor	Ask patient to plantar flex foot and toes.
	Sensory	Check pinprick over back of heel.

SUMMARY: ASSESSING NEUROVASCULAR STATUS IN AN INJURED LIMB

- Assessing CIRCULATION to the limb
  1. Warmth and color
  2. Capillary refill
  3. Peripheral pulse(s)
- Assessing NERVE SUPPLY to the limb
  1. Upper extremities
     a. Sensory: Pinprick over fingertips, dorsum of hand
     b. Motor: Dorsiflexion and palmar flexion of wrist
  2. Lower extremities
     a. Sensory: Pinprick over heel and dorsum of foot
     b. Motor: Dorsiflexion and plantar flexion of foot

SPLINTING INJURED EXTREMITIES

The mainstay of treatment for musculoskeletal injuries is immobilization of the injured extremity with an appropriate splint. As noted earlier, for the patient in critical condition, time may not permit more than securing the whole patient to a long backboard. But in cases of isolated musculoskeletal injury, when the patient is otherwise stable, it is worth taking the time to splint the injured extremity properly.

The Purpose of Splinting

Splinting an injured extremity accomplishes several nice things for the patient:

- Splinting ALLEVIATES PAIN. Providing relief of pain is not only a kind and humane thing in itself; it is also important to the patient's overall condition, for pain is stress, and stress can aggravate shock.
- By restricting movement of a fractured extremity, splinting can MINIMIZE FURTHER DAMAGE to muscles, nerves, and blood vessels that might otherwise occur if jagged bone ends were permitted to move freely. By the same token, a properly applied splint will PREVENT A CLOSED FRACTURE FROM BECOMING AN OPEN FRACTURE.
- By holding the injured extremity immobile, splinting also HELPS CONTROL BLEEDING. Motion of an extremity increases blood flow to the extremity and also disrupts the process of hemostasis. By keeping the extremity still, one gives the platelets a chance to seal off leaking blood vessels.

General Principles of Splinting

There are a number of general principles that apply to splinting irrespective of the location of the injury or the type of splint used to immobilize it.

- EXPOSE THE ENTIRE EXTREMITY to be splinted, so that you can properly assess the extent of the injury. Cut away clothing as necessary.
- DRESS WOUNDS BEFORE SPLINTING FRACTURES.
- Check the distal PULSE, SENSATION, and MOTOR FUNCTION before you splint the extremity, and record your findings.
- STRAIGHTEN SEVERELY ANGULATED FRACTURES before splinting. Explain to the patient that straightening the fracture may cause momentary pain, but that relief will be significant once the fracture is straightened and splinted. To straighten a fractured extremity, grasp the limb firmly with both hands—one hand below the fracture site and one above it—and exert *longitudinal traction*. If possible, have an assistant exert countertraction by holding the patient in place. Maintain traction until the splint has been applied and secured. If you encounter resistance to traction, however, DO NOT USE FORCE; splint the limb in the angulated position.
- DO NOT TRY TO STRAIGHTEN FRACTURES INVOLVING JOINTS, such as the shoulder, elbow, wrist, or knee. Splint such fractures in the position in which they are found.
- SPLINT DISLOCATED EXTREMITIES IN THE POSITION IN WHICH THEY ARE FOUND. Do not try to straighten or reduce a dislocation unless specifically ordered to do so (see discussion of knee dislocation, p. 418). Since it is often difficult to distinguish in the field between a fracture and a dislocation of a joint (and since the two may be present together), the simplest general rule to follow is

---

> **WHEN THERE IS INJURY TO A JOINT, SPLINT THE EXTREMITY IN THE POSITION IN WHICH IT IS FOUND.**

- When dealing with a *compound fracture*, DO NOT ATTEMPT TO PUSH EXPOSED BONE ENDS BACK BENEATH THE SKIN. Simply cover the wound with a sterile dressing, and moisten the dressing with sterile saline. Sometimes the process of straightening an angulated compound fracture will itself pull the exposed bone ends back into the wound; opinions differ regarding what to do in such a situation. It is the view of this author that it is better to straighten a severely

angulated fracture and risk infection than to leave it angulated and risk ischemia and loss of the limb. Consult your own medical director, however, for local guidelines.

- Make sure you use a long enough splint to IMMOBILIZE THE JOINTS ABOVE AND BELOW THE FRACTURE or, if the fracture is in a joint, immobilize the *bones* above and below it. Thus, for example, a Colles' fracture of the radius and ulna requires immobilization of both the wrist and elbow.
- Splint firmly, but not so tightly as to occlude the circulation. RECHECK THE PULSE, SENSATION, and MOTOR FUNCTION distal to the injury once the splint is in place, to be certain that the circulation is still adequate. If the pulse is weak or absent, loosen the splint until the pulse becomes palpable again. LEAVE FINGERS AND TOES OUT OF THE SPLINT, so that you can inspect them easily during FREQUENT RECHECKING OF THE DISTAL CIRCULATION. Similarly, check and recheck air splints to make certain they are not overinflated. Inspect the ankle hitch on a traction splint lest it be applied too tightly across the foot.
- PAD RIGID SPLINTS GENEROUSLY, especially where there are bony prominences. Be sure that the proximal end of a lower extremity splint is not pressing against the groin (a conscious patient will doubtless let you know if it is!).
- When time permits, IMMOBILIZE ALL FRACTURES BEFORE MOVING THE PATIENT.
- Whenever possible, ELEVATE THE INJURED EXTREMITY once it is splinted.
- WHEN IN DOUBT as to whether the patient has indeed suffered a serious musculoskeletal injury, treat the injury as a fracture and SPLINT.

Types of Splints

Any device used to immobilize a fracture or dislocation is a splint. It may be an improvised device, such as a rolled newspaper, cane, ironing board, or virtually any other object that can provide stability; it may be the patient's own body; or it may be one of the several commercially available splints, such as board splints, inflatable splints, and traction splints. It is with those latter devices that we shall be concerned in this section. However, the lack of a commercially made splint should never prevent a paramedic from properly immobilizing an injured patient; multiple casualties may tax the resources of even the best equipped ambulance, and in such circumstances, you will have to improvise.

Rigid Splints

A rigid splint is any inflexible device attached to a limb to maintain stability. It may be simply a padded board, a piece of heavy cardboard, or an aluminum "ladder" molded to fit the extremity. Whatever its construction, however, it must be generously padded and long enough to be secured well above and below the fracture site (beyond the proximal and distal joints).

To apply a rigid splint, grasp the extremity above and below the fracture site, and apply gentle traction (Fig. 19-12A). An assistant then places the splint, which should be adequately padded to ensure even pressure along the extremity, alongside the limb. While you maintain traction, your assistant wraps the limb and splint in self-adhering bandages, applying them tightly enough to hold the splint firmly to the extremity, but not so tightly as to occlude circulation (Fig. 19-12B). Be sure to leave the fingers or toes out of the bandage so that you can monitor capillary refill to check the adequacy of distal circulation.

Air Splints

Air splints, or inflatable splints, are useful primarily for immobilizing fractures involving the lower leg or forearm. Because they also provide circumferential pressure, air splints have the additional advantage that they can help slow bleeding and minimize swelling. Air splints should *not* be used on severely angulated fractures or fractures involving joints, since the pressure generated by the splint will place tension on the joint to straighten it.

How you apply an air splint depends on whether it is equipped with a zipper. If it is not, gather the splint on your own arm so that its proximal edge is just above your wrist. Grasp the patient's hand or foot while an assistant maintains proximal countertraction, and slide the air splint over your hand onto the patient's extremity (Fig. 19-13A). Position the air splint so that it is free of wrinkles. Then, while you continue to maintain traction, instruct your assistant to inflate the splint *by mouth* (Fig. 19-13B). Do *not* use a compressed air tank to inflate an air splint.

If the air splint has a zipper, apply it to the injured area while an assistant maintains traction proximally and distally; then zip it up and inflate. In either instance, inflate the splint just to the point at which finger pressure will make a slight dent in the splint's surface.

Air splints must be watched carefully to be certain that they do not lose pressure or become overinflated. *Overinflation* is particularly apt to occur when the splint is applied in a cold area and the patient is subsequently moved to a warmer area, for the

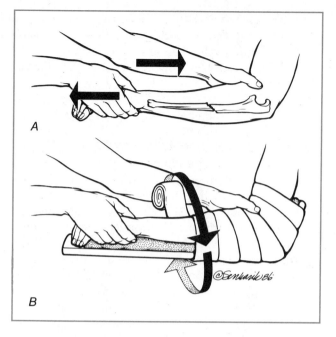

FIGURE 19-12.   APPLICATION OF A RIGID SPLINT.
(A) Apply traction along the long axis of the broken bone to keep the bone ends from overriding.
(B) Splint the joint above and the joint below the fracture.

air inside the splint will expand as it gets warmer. Air splints will also expand in going to higher altitude, a factor that must be taken into account when patients are transported by air ambulance.

Keep in mind that the MAST can be deployed as an air splint and is especially useful in that role for fractures of the pelvis.

Traction Splints

Traction splints are used to provide constant pull on a fractured femur and thereby prevent the broken bone ends from overriding as a result of unopposed muscle contraction. A traction splint is, in fact, simply a mechanical means of providing the traction that is always a part of immobilizing a fracture; the splint is not intended to reduce the fracture but simply to oppose spasm of the thigh muscles and prevent free motion of the broken bone ends. Keeping the leg under traction, furthermore, can significantly reduce bleeding into the thigh. Normally, the thigh is shaped like a cylinder. When there is a femoral fracture, and the thigh is shortened, it becomes spherical. The volume of a sphere is 50 percent greater than that of a cylinder, so a person with an untreated femoral fracture can accumulate 50 percent more blood in the thigh than a person whose thigh has not been deformed.

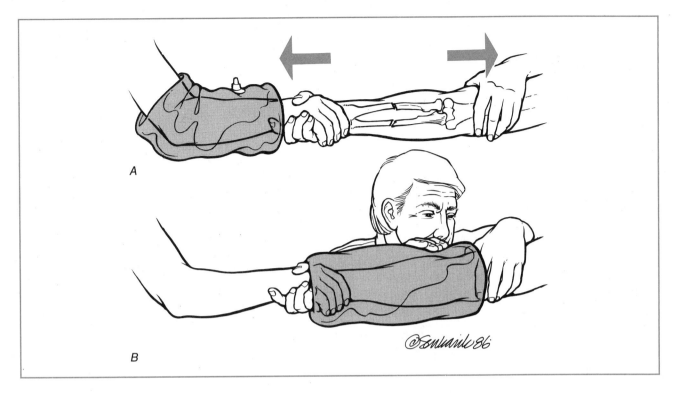

FIGURE 19-13. APPLICATION OF AN AIR SPLINT. (A) Apply traction along the long axis of the broken bone(s) to keep the bone ends from overriding. After sliding the air splint over the patient's arm, so that it includes the joint above and below the fracture, inflate the splint *by mouth* (B).

The most commonly used traction splints are the Thomas half-ring splint and the Hare traction splint. The basic principles of application are the same for both:

- Apply TRACTION to the injured extremity by grasping the ankle and calf and exerting a gentle pull in line with the long axis of the limb (Fig. 19-14A). An ankle hitch is then secured to the foot and thereafter used to maintain traction.
- While you continue holding the leg in longitudinal traction, an assistant slides the splint beneath the leg and secures the half-ring in position, pressing it firmly (but not too firmly!) against the ischial tuberosity (Fig. 19-14B).
- After securing the half-ring, your assistant then secures the ankle hitch to the distal end of the traction splint (you are still holding the leg in traction).
- Traction is developed by tightening the windlass until the patient experiences relief of pain (Fig. 19-14C). Once traction has been developed in the splint itself, you may release your hold on the ankle hitch.

- The patient's leg is then secured to the splint with cravats or Velcro fasteners, and the splint is elevated so that the patient's foot is clear of the ground or the stretcher (Fig. 19-14D).
- Check sensation and capillary refill in the foot every 5 to 10 minutes after the traction splint has been applied.

Sling

An arm sling may be fashioned from a triangular bandage or a kerchief and is useful as an adjunct to a rigid splint of the upper extremity; the sling immobilizes the injured part against the chest wall and also takes some of the weight off the injured area (Fig. 19-15).

To apply a sling, place the splinted extremity in a comfortable position across the chest. Then lay the long edge of a triangular bandage along the patient's side opposite the injury. Bring the bottom edge of the bandage up over the forearm and tie it *at the side* of the neck. The pointed end of the sling, at the elbow, is tied or pinned to form a cradle. Secure the sling so that the hand is carried higher than the elbow and

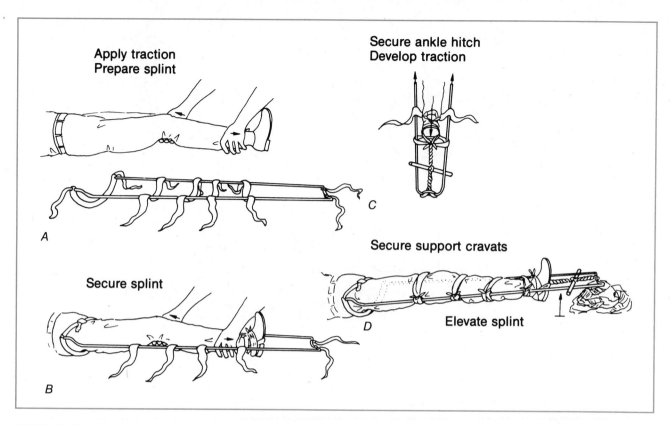

Apply traction
Prepare splint

A

Secure splint

B

Secure ankle hitch
Develop traction

C

Secure support cravats

D

Elevate splint

FIGURE 19-14.   APPLYING A TRACTION SPLINT.

the fingers are visible for checking peripheral circulation.

Sling and Swath

An arm suspended in a sling can be further immobilized by using another one or two triangular bandages to secure the arm firmly to the chest wall (Fig. 19-16). That type of immobilization is particularly useful for injuries to the clavicle and for anterior dislocations of the shoulder. (When a sling and swath are used for a shoulder dislocation, it is usually necessary to use a pillow or two to fill the gap between the arm and the chest wall.) The sling is applied in the manner already described, and then one or two wide cravats, which can be fashioned from folded triangular bandages, are applied around the chest and tied firmly in place.

Pillow Splint

A pillow is an effective means to immobilize an injured foot or ankle. To do so, simply mold an ordinary pillow around the foot in a position of comfort, and secure it in place with several cravats (Fig. 19-17). Pillows can also be molded around an injured knee or elbow and are invaluable for padding backboards

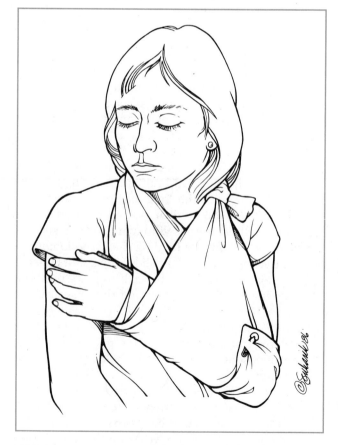

FIGURE 19-15.   A SLING is useful for immobilizing injuries of the scapula, clavicle, and humerus.

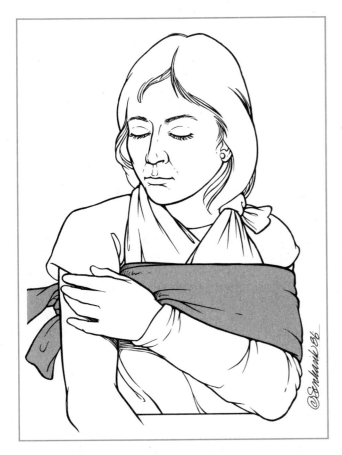

FIGURE 19-16. **A SLING AND SWATH** gives firmer immobilization than a sling by using the chest wall as a splint.

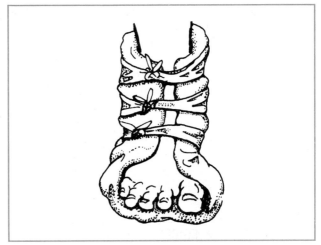

FIGURE 19-17. **A PILLOW SPLINT** is often the most comfortable way to immobilize the foot and ankle.

when used to immobilize patients with dislocated hips.

Vacuum Splints

The vacuum splint was developed in Europe and only recently has come into use in the United States. The prototype consists of a sealed mattress that is filled with air and thousands of small plastic beads. The mattress is laid out on the stretcher, and the patient is placed on top of it and allowed to settle into a comfortable position. Then a suction pump attached to the mattress is used to evacuate all of the air from inside the mattress. That creates a vacuum inside the mattress, which compresses the beads in such a way that the whole splint becomes rigid—like a plaster cast that has been molded to conform to the contour of the patient's entire posterior surface. Thus the vacuum mattress in effect provides a tailor-made posterior body cast for each patient.

The vacuum mattress is an excellent splint, but it has several significant drawbacks that limit its usefulness. To begin with, the mattress-type vacuum splint is quite bulky and thus not only takes up a lot of storage room in the vehicle but also can be difficult to work with in cramped quarters. Furthermore, it requires that one carry along a mechanical suction pump, yet another piece of equipment. Finally, the vacuum mattress is relatively expensive and may not be within the means of every ambulance company. Smaller vacuum splints, for upper and lower extremities, are also available, however, and can be a valuable addition to the trauma kit. Perhaps most useful of all is the *vacuum cervical collar*, which has recently been found to be superior to all other methods of immobilizing the cervical spine in the prehospital setting.

SOME SPECIFIC MUSCULOSKELETAL INJURIES

The treatment of specific orthopedic injuries is dealt with in considerable detail during basic EMT training, and we shall not review all of that detail here. Those who wish to refresh their knowledge of the subject are referred to *Emergency Medical Treatment*, Chapter 17, or the relevant chapter of any other textbook for EMT-As. We shall deal here only with those musculoskeletal injuries that may present a threat to life or limb.

Upper Extremity Injuries

Posterior Sternoclavicular Dislocation

Posterior dislocation at the junction of the clavicle with the sternum most often occurs as a result of a direct blow to the clavicle, but it is also sometimes seen after strong pressure is applied to the posterior shoulder, as may befall the football player who ends up at the bottom of a pileup. Usually the injury is not difficult to identify, for there is pain and swelling at the sternoclavicular joint. What makes this a potentially dangerous, and even potentially fatal, injury is not the dislocation itself but the possible damage to underlying structures—specifically, the trachea, esophagus, jugular vein, subclavian vein and artery, carotid artery, and other vascular structures. Any symptoms that suggest such underlying injury—such as *dyspnea, pain on swallowing,* a *sensation of choking, loss of pulses,* or a *sensory deficit* in the upper extremity on the same side—are DANGER SIGNALS and should prompt you to TRANSPORT THE PATIENT AS RAPIDLY AS POSSIBLE to the hospital. En route, position the patient supine, with the arm on the affected side abducted and a rolled towel under the shoulder blade, a position that may help take some of the pressure off the structures beneath the sternoclavicular joint.

Scapular Fractures

The importance of a scapular fracture lies in what it tells you about the *mechanisms of injury,* namely, that massive forces must have been applied directly to the upper back—for otherwise the heavy and well-buttressed shoulder blade could not be broken. A fractured scapula will present with swelling, tenderness, and ecchymosis over the shoulder blade, and occasionally deformity as well. Those signs are a tip-off to search for more serious injury involving underlying and adjacent structures—contusion of the lung, pneumothorax, spinal injury—whose treatment will have priority over that of the scapular fracture. A sling and swath are sufficient to immobilize the scapula itself, but most patients subjected to forces sufficient to fracture the scapula should have complete spinal immobilization on a backboard.

Fractures of the Distal Humerus (Elbow)

Supracondylar fractures of the humerus occur most often in children under the age of 11. The typical mechanism is a fall onto an outstretched hand with the elbow in extension, thereby breaking the distal humerus; as a result, the distal fragment of the humerus is pushed backward and the humeral shaft is pulled forward, where it can compress the brachial artery and the radial and median nerves (Fig. 19-18). If not handled properly, this type of fracture can lead to a dreaded complication called **Volkmann's ischemic contracture,** which leaves the fingers permanently contracted and useless.

The child with a supracondylar fracture of the humerus usually has a very swollen, painful elbow,

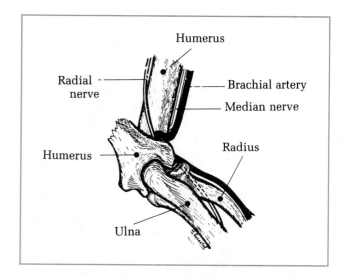

FIGURE 19-18. SUPRACONDYLAR FRACTURE OF THE HUMERUS. The broken bone ends impinge on the brachial artery, endangering circulation to the distal limb. Pressure on the radial nerve may, in addition, produce "wrist drop."

which he may hold splinted to his chest in order not to move it at all.

Splint the injured elbow IN THE POSITION IN WHICH YOU FIND IT. If any of the "Six Ps" is present and if you are more than about 20 minutes from the hospital, contact your base physician for instructions. He or she may advise you to try to apply straight traction to the humerus and extend the elbow *very slightly and very gently* until a radial pulse is detectable or the extremity pinks up, and then to splint the arm in that position.

The treatment of a variety of upper extremity injuries is summarized in Table 19-4.

Lower Extremity Injuries

Fracture of the Pelvis

Pelvic fractures, particularly in the young, bespeak powerful forces of injury and almost invariably occur in the context of other injuries as well. Pelvic fracture is most commonly caused by motor vehicle trauma but may also occur as a result of a crush injury or fall from a height. Usually, the pelvis is fractured by an *indirect* force transmitted upward along the femoral shaft; but direct compression may occur when a pedestrian is run over by a car or a motorcyclist is thrown from his bike, and the injuries from direct compression are likely to be much more serious than those produced by indirect forces.

TABLE 19-4. UPPER EXTREMITY INJURIES

REGION	INJURY	MECHANISMS OF INJURY	SYMPTOMS AND SIGNS	POSSIBLE COMPLICATIONS	PREHOSPITAL TREATMENT
Sternoclavicular joint	Anterior dislocation	Shoulder jammed back	Prominent proximal clavicle; tender sternoclavicular joint	None	None needed
	Posterior dislocation	Direct blow Football pileup with pressure to posterior clavicle	Pain, swelling over joint; depression of medial clavicle	Damage to trachea, esophagus, vascular structures behind the joint; pneumothorax	Rapid transport if there is dyspnea, difficulty swallowing, loss of pulses
Acromioclavicular joint	Dislocation	Direct pressure to point of shoulder	Knocked-down shoulder Cannot lift arm or bring arm across chest Skin stretched over lateral clavicle		Cold pack Sling & swath
Clavicle	Fracture	Direct blow or blow delivered through arm	Holds injured arm against chest with good arm Head cocked toward injured side	Permanent bump at fracture site Subclavian artery injury	Cold pack Sling & swath (*not* figure-of-eight)
Scapula	Fracture	Massive direct force	Can't move shoulder	Associated injuries to ribs, lungs	Other injuries take priority (shock, pneumothorax) Sling for scapular fracture
Shoulder	Anterior dislocation	Falling backward on outstretched hand	Supports arm with other hand Prominent acromion Palpable humeral head Arm abducted and externally rotated Can't touch elbow to side	Axillary artery and axillary nerve injury Associated fracture	Pad axilla (pillow) Sling & swath
	Posterior dislocation	Seizures; direct blow; landing on outstretched arm	Arm internally rotated and held tightly against body Severe pain; no motion	Associated fracture	Pad and strap arm to body
Humerus	Shaft fracture	Direct blow (motor vehicle accident) Gunshot wound Fall on outstretched arm	Swelling, deformity, ecchymosis	Radial nerve injury: wrist drop	Sling & swath or padded board splint
Elbow	Fracture	Fall on extended or flexed elbow (e.g., skateboard injury)	Massive swelling Often open fracture	Volkmann's ischemic contracture	Padded board or pillow splint Rapid transport for any of the "6 Ps"
	Dislocation	Fall on hyperextended arm	"Locked," painful elbow; extreme deformity Same as for fracture	Vascular injury	Splint as found with padded board or sling & swath
Forearm	Fracture	Direct or indirect Warding off a blow in isolated ulnar fracture ("nightstick fracture")	Swelling, deformity, ecchymosis		Air splint or padded board splint

TABLE 19-4.   UPPER EXTREMITY INJURIES (continued)

REGION	INJURY	MECHANISMS OF INJURY	SYMPTOMS AND SIGNS	POSSIBLE COMPLICATIONS	PREHOSPITAL TREATMENT
Wrist	Fracture	Colles': fall on outstretched hand Smith's: backward fall on extended wrist (motorcyclist)	Colles': dinner-fork deformity Smith's: garden spade deformity		Air splint
	Dislocation	Fall on outstretched arm Sports injury	Deformity	Associated wrist fracture	Air splint
Carpals/ metacarpals	Fracture	Scaphoid: fall on outstretched hand hyperextended 5th metacarpal: boxer's fracture	Swelling; pain on pronation and ulnar deviation; tenderness		Splint in intrinsic-plus position
Phalanges	Fracture	Hand slammed in car door Industrial accident	Pain, tenderness, ecchymosis		Foam-padded, flexible aluminum splint (*not* frog splint) No circumferential taping
	"Jammed finger"	Baseball finger	Tenderness	Tendon injury	Same as above

BLEEDING is the major cause of death in patients with pelvic fractures, in which up to 30 percent of the total blood volume may be lost into the surrounding soft tissues and pelvic cavity. Pelvic fractures are also frequently associated with injuries to the urinary and gastrointestinal tracts.

Pelvic fracture can usually be recognized by pain and instability of the pelvis when you try to compress the iliac wings. In the *treatment* of a patient with pelvic fracture, the ABCs have priority. The MAST may be used both to stabilize the pelvis and tamponade bleeding, and the whole patient should be immobilized on a LONG BACKBOARD. At least one, and preferably TWO LARGE-BORE IVs should be started en route to the hospital.

Posterior Dislocation of the Hip

Posterior dislocation of the hip is a true emergency because of the danger it presents to both the blood supply to the femur and the nerve supply to the leg. The head of the femur gets most of its blood supply from arteries that emerge from the acetabulum; when the hip is dislocated, therefore, the femoral head is torn away from its blood supply. If the dislocation is not reduced promptly, there is a high probability that the patient will develop AVASCULAR NECROSIS OF THE FEMORAL HEAD. The destroyed femoral head will subsequently disintegrate, and the patient will need an artificial hip.

Posterior dislocation of the hip also puts stress on the *sciatic nerve*, which controls flexion and extension at the ankle. A patient with permanent sciatic nerve damage will be unable to dorsiflex his foot ("foot drop") and will therefore develop an abnormal gait.

Most hip dislocations occur in motor vehicle accidents, when the knee hits the dashboard, forcing the femur backward and driving the femoral head out of the rather lax hip joint.

> **WHEN YOU FIND A KNEE INJURY IN THE VICTIM OF A CAR ACCIDENT, LOOK FOR POSTERIOR DISLOCATION OF THE HIP.**

When the hip is dislocated posteriorly, it will usually be found *flexed, adducted,* and *internally rotated* such that the knee is pointing medially. The buttock may be very prominent (from the head of the femur), and the injured leg usually looks *shorter* than the leg on the uninjured side.

In assessing the patient, be sure to CHECK DISTAL PULSES (the dorsalis pedis and posterior tibial) and CHECK SCIATIC NERVE FUNCTION. You will not be able to test the sciatic nerve itself, but you can

TABLE 19-5. LOWER EXTREMITY INJURIES

REGION	INJURY	MECHANISMS OF INJURY	SYMPTOMS AND SIGNS	POSSIBLE COMPLICATIONS	PREHOSPITAL TREATMENT
Pelvis	Fracture	Indirect force along shaft of femur Direct compression; fall from height; pedestrian hit by car; motorcyclist thrown from bike; straddle injury	Pain on compression of iliac wings Instability Hematoma of scrotum or perineum	Shock Bladder/urethra injury Associated spinal injury	Priority to ABCs MAST Backboard IV fluids
Hip	Posterior dislocation	Force applied to flexed knee (e.g., dashboard injury)	Hip flexed, adducted, internally rotated Knee crosses midline Prominent buttock Injured leg looks shorter	Associated fracture of acetabulum Femoral head necrosis Sciatic nerve injury with foot drop	Long backboard Pillows as padding
	Anterior dislocation (rare)	Forced abduction ("split") Fall from height	Hip flexed, abducted, *externally* rotated Knee points *away* from midline Injured leg looks longer		Long backboard Pillows as padding
	Fracture	Sudden twisting Fall Motor vehicle accident (younger patient)	Severe pain Leg externally rotated, shortened	Shock	MAST Traction splint, or padded board or body splint plus long backboard IV fluids
Femoral shaft	Fracture	Major trauma with direct blow Gunshot wound	Pain, deformity, shortening	Shock Damage to blood vessels	MAST Traction splint IV fluids
Knee	Sprain	Athletic injury	Pain, sometimes swelling, deformity		Cold packs Pillow splint
	Dislocation	Hyperextension	Severe pain Swelling, deformity Unable to move knee	Popliteal artery injury: ischemia Peroneal nerve damage	If no pedal pulse, try once to straighten Long padded board Immediate transport Notify hospital
	Patellar dislocation	Knee twisted while foot stayed planted Direct lateral blow	Pain Knee held in flexion Abnormal medial bulge		Pillow splint or long padded board
	Fracture	Direct blow	Same as dislocation	Associated hip dislocation Popliteal artery injury	Long padded board
Tibia/fibula	Fracture	Direct blow (motorcyclist's fracture) Twisting force (ski boot fracture)	May be severely angulated Often open	Compartment syndrome: damage to blood vessels Infection (if open)	Cover open wounds Long leg air splint Transport at once for any of 6 Ps
Ankle	Fracture Dislocation Sprain	Twisting forces Inversion	Swelling Deformity Limitation of motion		Pillow splint or air splint Elevate; cold packs
Heel	Fracture	Fall from height, landing on feet	Extreme pain Ecchymoses Extreme tenderness	Associated lumbar spine fracture Associated fracture of other heel	Pillow splint to feet Backboard
Metatarsals	Fracture	Marching (stress fracture) Object fell on foot	Pain on top of foot on weight-bearing Extreme tenderness		Pillow splint Elevation
Toe	Fracture	Stubbed toe Object fell on toe	Tenderness, swelling, Ecchymosis		Elevate foot Cold pack

test the function of its two main branches, the *tibial* and *peroneal* (review Table 19-3), basically by checking sensation over the foot and the ability to dorsiflex and plantar flex the foot. RECORD YOUR FINDINGS, and recheck often.

As noted, hip dislocation is a true emergency, and the patient should therefore be transported without delay to the hospital, where an orthopedic surgeon should be notified to stand by. If for some reason it will not be possible to reach a hospital promptly, and if you receive instructions to do so, try *once* to reduce the dislocation, as follows:

- Explain the procedure to the patient, and obtain consent.
- If the patient's condition is otherwise stable, allow him to self-administer nitrous oxide (Nitronox) for analgesia (see Drug Handbook at the end of this textbook).
- Have the patient's knee and hip each flexed 90 degrees.
- While an assistant holds the pelvis to keep it from moving, apply strong upward traction along the axis of the femur, and *gently* rotate the hip slightly back and forth—internally and externally. Traction should be slow and steady to overcome muscle spasm.
- Success in reducing the dislocation will be signalled by the femoral head "popping" back into the joint. The patient will experience immediate relief of pain, and the leg will assume its normal position.
- Immobilize the patient on a long backboard. If reduction has been successful, immobilize the leg lying straight (i.e., at 180 degrees). If reduction was not successful, immobilize the leg in 90 degrees of flexion, supported and padded by pillows.

Dislocation of the Knee

The most common form of knee dislocation is an anterior dislocation, which usually results from a hyperextension injury. Like dislocation of the hip, knee dislocation is a potentially catastrophic injury primarily because it may damage the *popliteal artery* and compromise circulation to the foot. Furthermore, the peroneal nerve is often badly damaged as well.

Usually a dislocation of the knee is not hard to spot, for the knee is apt to be bruised and swollen; it is not possible in the field, however, to know whether a fracture of the joint is also present. As always, check for distal pulses, sensation, and motion. A dislocated knee needs to be reduced very quickly, especially if there is any sign of vascular or neurologic deficit. If you are not within a few minutes of the hospital, try *once* to reduce the dislocation, as follows:

- Explain the procedure to the patient, and obtain consent.
- Have the patient self-administer nitrous oxide (Nitronox).
- Have an assistant apply longitudinal traction to the leg, either by hand or by traction splint.
- As traction is developed, keep one hand on the patient's tibia and one hand on his femur, in order to guide them back into position. DO NOT USE EXCESSIVE FORCE!

Tibial Shaft Fracture

Tibial fractures may be the result of either direct or indirect forces. A direct blow to the tibia tends to produce a comminuted fracture, often open, of the type seen most commonly among motorcyclists. Indirect fractures are usually the result of twisting injuries, typically seen in skiers, and thus tend to be spiral or oblique fractures. The principal danger associated with a tibial fracture is the development of a **compartment syndrome** as the result of bleeding and soft tissue swelling in the tight muscle compartments of the lower leg. As noted earlier, the *symptoms and signs* of impending compartment syndrome are those of limb ischemia in general—the **Six Ps.** The presence of any of those signs is a danger signal, and should prompt immediate transport of the patient. There is no definitive treatment for the compartment syndrome that can be undertaken in the field, since treatment requires making incisions into the muscle compartments to release the pressure within them. Whenever there is a tibial fracture, therefore, COOL AND ELEVATE THE LIMB, and TRANSPORT WITHOUT DELAY.

The treatment of a variety of upper extremity injuries is summarized in Table 19-5.

GLOSSARY

abduction Movement *away* from the midline of the body.

acetabulum The cup-shaped cavity in which the rounded head of the femur rotates.

acromion Lateral extension of the scapula that forms the highest point of the shoulder.

adduction Movement *toward* the midline of the body.

appendicular skeleton The part of the skeleton comprising the upper and lower extremities.

articulation Place of junction between two or more bones of the skeleton; a *joint*.

atrophy Wasting away of a tissue.

automaticity The property of cardiac muscle of being able to initiate its own contractions.

axial skeleton   The part of the skeleton comprising the skull, spinal column, and rib cage.

carpals   The eight small bones of the wrist.

cartilage   Tough, elastic substance that covers opposable surfaces of moveable joints and also forms part of the skeleton.

clavicle   Collar bone.

comminuted fracture   Fracture in which the bone is broken into three or more pieces.

compartment syndrome   *Ischemia* of a limb caused by increased pressure within muscular compartments of the limb that compromises circulation through the limb.

compound fracture   Open fracture; fracture beneath an open wound.

diaphysis   The shaft of a long bone.

dorsal   Referring to the back or posterior side of the body or an organ.

dorsiflexion   Backward bending of the hand or foot.

epiphysis   The end of a long bone.

external rotation   Rotation of an extremity in a lateral direction.

fibula   The smaller of the two bones of the lower leg.

glenoid fossa   Socket in the scapula in which the head of the humerus rotates.

greenstick fracture   Type of fracture occurring most frequently in children in which there is incomplete breakage of the bone.

humerus   The bone of the upper arm.

ilium   The broad, uppermost bone of the pelvis.

internal rotation   Rotation of an extremity in a medial direction.

ischemia   Tissue anoxia as a result of diminished blood flow.

ischial tuberosity   The protuberance on the inferior portion of the ischium (the part of the ischium we sit on).

ischium   The lowermost dorsal bone of the pelvis.

joint   Point at which two or more bones articulate, or come together.

joint capsule   Saclike envelope that encloses the cavity of a synovial joint.

lactic acid   Metabolic end product of the breakdown of glucose that accumulates when metabolism proceeds in the absence of oxygen.

ligament   Tough band of tissue that connects bone to bone around a joint or supports internal organs within the body.

malleolus   Large, rounded bony protuberance on either side of the ankle joint.

metacarpals   The five bones that form the palm and back of the hand.

metatarsals   The five long bones extending from the tarsus to the phalanges of the foot.

olecranon   Proximal bony projection of the *ulna* at the elbow; the part of the ulna that constitutes the "funny bone."

patella   Knee cap.

periosteum   Dense, fibrous tissue that covers bone.

phalanx   Any bone of the finger or toe.

plantar   Referring to the sole of the foot.

pronation   The act of turning the palm of the hand backward or downward, performed by internal rotation of the forearm.

pubis   One of two bones that form the anterior portion of the pelvic ring.

radius   The bone on the thumb side of the forearm.

sacroiliac joint   The point of attachment of the *ilium* to the sacrum.

scapula   Shoulder blade.

simple fracture   Closed fracture; fracture in which there is no break in the overlying skin.

supination   To turn the forearm laterally so that the palm faces forward (if standing) or upward (if lying supine).

symphysis pubis   The midline articulation of the pubic bones.

synovial joint   Joint that permits movement of its component bones.

tarsals   Ankle bones.

tendon   The fibrous portion of muscle that attaches to bone.

tibia   The shin bone.

trochanter   Either of the two processes below the neck of the femur.

ulna   The larger bone of the forearm, on the side opposite that of the thumb.

volar   Pertaining to the palm or sole; referring to the flexor surfaces of the forearm, wrist, or hand.

Volkmann's ischemic contracture   Contraction of the fingers and sometimes also the wrist, with loss of muscular power, that sets in rapidly after severe injury around the elbow joint.

FURTHER READING

Anast GT. Fractures and splinting. *Emergency* 10(11):42, 1978.

Bostian LC et al. Survey of common athletic injuries. *EMT J* 5(4):265, 1981.

Boswick JA, Phelps DB. Care of the injured hand: Part I. Basic principles of management of the injured hand. *Emerg Med Serv* 7(1):16, 1978.

Burtzloff HE. Splinting closed fractures of the extremities. *Emerg Med Serv* 10(3):70, 1981.

Canan S. Grasping objectives of long-bone splinting. *Rescue* 2(5):45, 1989.

Caroline NL. *Emergency Medical Treatment: A Text for EMT-As and EMT-Intermediates* (3rd ed.). Boston: Little, Brown, 1991. Chap. 17.

Connolly JF. Fracture pitfalls (series):
    The ankle. *Emerg Med* 16(7):49, 1984.
    The elbow. *Emerg Med* 15(11):163, 1983.
    The femur. *Emerg Med* 15(21):51, 1983.
    The forearm. *Emerg Med* 15(13):235, 1983.

General principles. *Emerg Med* 14(17):161, 1982.

The humerus. *Emerg Med* 15(9):170, 1983.

The knee: Bone and soft tissue. *Emerg Med* 16(1):205, 1984.

Metacarpals and phalanges. *Emerg Med* 15(15):201, 1983.

Pathologic fractures. *Emerg Med* 16(11):61, 1984.

Tibial fractures. *Emerg Med* 16(5):43, 1984.

The wrist. *Emerg Med* 15(14):195, 1983.

Connolly JF. Foot fractures: Catching the common troublemakers. *Emerg Med* 23(20):21, 1991.

Cote DJ et al. Comparison of three treatment procedures for minimizing ankle sprain swelling. *Phys Ther* 68:1072, 1988.

Evers BM, Cryer HM, Miller FB. Pelvic fracture hemorrhage: Priorities in management. *Arch Surg* 124:422, 1989.

Gordon L, Buncke HJ Jr, Alpert BS. From amputation to reimplantation. *Emerg Med* 15(10):61, 1983.

Gormley P. The dislocation dilemma. *Emerg Med Serv* 22(9):75, 1993.

Gustafson JE. Contraindications to the repositioning of fractured or dislocated limbs in the field. *JACEP* 5:184, 1976.

Haverson G, Iverson KV. Comparison of four ankle splint designs. *Ann Emerg Med* 16:1249, 1987.

Hedges JR, Anwar RAH. Management of ankle sprains. *Ann Emerg Med* 9:298, 1980.

Jupiter JB, Krushell RJ. Evaluating hand injuries. *Emerg Med* 21(3):79, 1989.

Kay DB. The sprained ankle: Current therapy. *Foot Ankle* 6:22, 1985.

Knight K. The effects of hypothermia on inflammation and swelling. *Athletic Training* 11:7, 1976.

Lhowe D. Basics of broken bones for the nonorthopedist: 2. Primary care for nondisplaced fractures. *Emerg Med* 19(16):89, 1987.

Martinez AJ, Lee MJ. A step-by-step look at lower extremity trauma. *JEMS* 17(4):42, 1992.

McGraw S. Pelvis problems. *Emerg Med Serv* 23(1):39, 1994.

McNamara RM. Reduction of anterior shoulder dislocations by scapular manipulation. *Ann Emerg Med* 22:1140, 1993.

Menkes JS. Pitfalls in orthopedic trauma:

Part I. The upper extremity. *Emerg Med* 21(5):64, 1989.

Part II. The lower extremity. *Emerg Med* 21(6):108, 1989.

Misurya RK et al. Use of tuning fork in diagnostic auscultation of fractures. *Injury* 18:63, 1987.

Murphy R, Boswick JA, Phelps DB. Care of the injured hand: Part V. Tendon injuries. *Emerg Med Serv* 7(5):48, 1978.

Phelps DB. Emergency care of the injured hand: Part IX. Mutilating hand injuries and reimplantation. *Emerg Med Serv* 8(4):33, 1979.

Powell JB, Lloyd GJ, Rintoul RF. New clinical test for fracture of the scaphoid. *Can J Surg* 31:237, 1988.

Rayburn BK. Prehospital care of fractures and dislocations of the extremities. *EMT J* 4(2):61, 1980.

Rector J, Phelps DB. Care of the injured hand: Part VI. Fractures and dislocations. *Emerg Med Serv* 8(1):16, 1979.

Sherman M. Hot or cold: Which treatment is recommended? *Am Pharm* 20:46, 1980.

Shirreffs TG. Compartment syndrome: An extremity at risk. *Emerg Med* 22(6):103, 1990.

Sloan JP et al. Effects of cold and compression on edema. *Phys Sports Med* 16:116, 1988.

Sonzogni JJ. Physical assessment of the injured ankle. *Emerg Med* 21(1):62, 1989.

Stanley D, Norris SH. Recovery following fractures of the clavicle treated conservatively. *Injury* 19:162, 1988.

Thompson DA et al. The significance of scapular fractures. *J Trauma* 25:974, 1985.

Thygerson AL. Finger injuries. *Emergency* 13(4):28, 13(5):82, 1981.

Thygerson AL. The sprained ankle. *Emergency* 13(2):20, 1981.

Tomford W. Basics of broken bones for the nonorthopedist: I. The fundamental principles. *Emerg Med* 19(15):25, 1987.

Wald DA, Ziemba TJ, Ferko JG. Upper extremity injuries. *Emergency* 21(3):25, 1989.

Winspur I, Phelps DB. Emergency care of the injured hand: Part XI. Hand dressings, splints, and casts. *Emerg Med Serv* 9(1):22, 1980.

Young MRA et al. Clinical carpal scaphoid injuries. *Br Med J* 296:825, 1988.

20
Multiple Injuries: Summary of Advanced Trauma Life Support

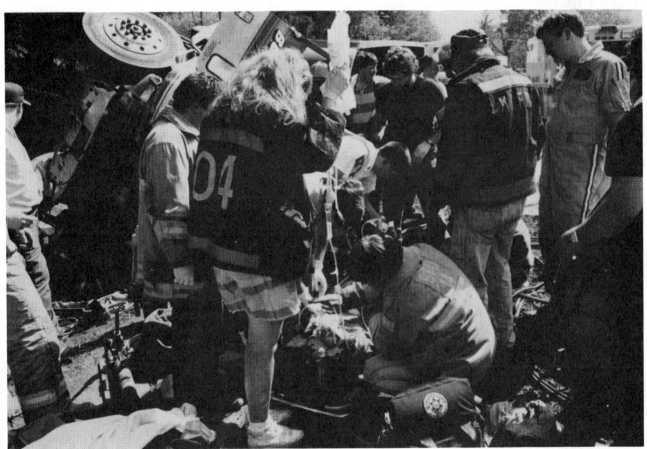

Smethport Volunteer Fire Department and Smethport Area Ambulance Service, Smethport, Pennsylvania; Paramedic Services, Bradford Regional Medical Center, Bradford, Pennsylvania; Kane Volunteer Fire Department, Kane, Pennsylvania; Port Allegany Volunteer Fire Department, Port Allegany, Pennsylvania; Star Flight Medical Helicopter, WCA Hospital, Jamestown, New York. Photo by Jay K. Bradish.

OBJECTIVES

We have covered a lot of material in the previous six chapters on trauma. Urgent messages in capital letters blare out from the printed page with important principles of managing head injuries, spine injuries, chest injuries, belly injuries. It is easy to become overwhelmed by so many bits of vital information; it is even easier to become overwhelmed by a patient who presents with a whole variety of serious injuries. What is needed in multitrauma is a road map, to guide us through the evaluation and care of the patient. In this chapter, we shall try to provide that road map and, in the process, bring together the principles we have learned in the six chapters that preceded. We shall start by considering the concept of the Golden Hour and some of the ways a paramedic can shave seconds and minutes off the time spent in the field. We shall then review the steps of the primary survey—the very special kind of primary survey that is conducted on seriously injured patients. We shall examine the factors that go into deciding at what point to transport the injured patient, and we shall review the components of the complete secondary survey in trauma. Finally, we shall consider some of the methods of record-keeping for the injured patient. By the end of this chapter, then, the student should be able to

1. List at least three ways of saving seconds or minutes of the "Golden Hour" without compromising the quality of patient care
2. List the equipment that should be carried in the first trip from the ambulance to a severely injured casualty
3. Describe precisely what should be checked during the primary survey of a severely injured patient in assessing
   - The airway
   - Breathing
   - Circulation
   - Neurologic status
4. Identify patients who are critically injured, given a description of the findings in the primary survey of a number of patients, and describe the correct management of each patient—both those who are critically injured and those who are not
   - At the scene
   - En route to the hospital
5. List the most important things to check in the secondary survey of the
   - Head
   - Neck
   - Chest
   - Abdomen
   - Extremities

6. List the information that should be obtained in taking the history of a trauma victim
7. Indicate at what point communications should be initiated with the receiving hospital, given a description of the injured patient, and list the information that should be transmitted

THE GOLDEN HOUR

It has become customary among trauma experts to speak of the "Golden Hour" for the victim of critical injury. The phrase derives from the observation that seriously injured patients who manage to reach the operating room within an hour of being injured have the highest rates of survival. So we refer to that hour—the hour after the moment of injury—as the Golden Hour, in which every minute is precious. Response times must therefore be prompt. Equipment must be assembled and organized *before* you reach the scene. And every action taken in the field must have a lifesaving purpose, for each procedure you undertake before starting transport eats up minutes of the Golden Hour.

> **TIME IS GOLDEN. WEIGH EVERY FIELD PROCEDURE AGAINST THE TIME IT WILL TAKE TO PERFORM. IS IT WORTH THE PRICE?**

Making an Efficient Response to the Scene

As noted, the clock starts ticking down the Golden Hour at the moment when the victim is injured, *not* the moment when you reach him. Thus, if it took 5 minutes for a bystander to get to a highway telephone, 1 minute for 911 to process the call, and 20 minutes for you to get to the scene, nearly half of the Golden Hour is already gone by the time you arrive on the scene. It is essential, therefore, to make the most efficient possible response to the scene. That does *not* mean driving like a competitor at the Indy 500; an efficient response is not one that endangers you and every other motorist on the road. It *does* mean getting on the road promptly as soon as you hear your unit called, even before you've been given all the details (and without delaying to finish that cup of coffee). It also means knowing the map, so that you can choose the shortest route or switch to an alternative route if your first choice is congested. Excessive speed will not make up for unfamiliarity with the map; you will just get lost faster!

Preparing the Necessary Equipment

Try to find out as much about the incident as you can from the dispatcher as you proceed toward the scene. What is the *nature of the call* (road accident, gunshot wound)? Are there any known *hazards* at the scene? *How many victims* are there? Will any *special equipment*, such as self-contained breathing apparatus, be needed?

ASSEMBLE YOUR EQUIPMENT EN ROUTE to the scene, so that you will be able to CARRY ALL ESSENTIAL EQUIPMENT TO THE PATIENT when you first approach him. Otherwise you will waste precious minutes running back and forth to the ambulance to fetch things you've left behind there. Haul out the long backboard (if it's in exterior storage, bring it inside the ambulance before you leave your base), and arrange the required equipment on top of it; then use the backboard straps to secure the equipment to the board, so it won't all tumble off as you are carrying the backboard from the ambulance to the patient. The equipment that you will need to take with you for initial management of the patient includes the following:

**EQUIPMENT TO CARRY
TO A TRAUMA VICTIM**

- Long BACKBOARD with at least three STRAPS, cervical COLLAR, and a device for immobilizing the head (e.g., blanket roll)
- Full OXYGEN cylinder assembled with reducing valve and flow meter
- Portable SUCTION unit, hooked up to tonsil suction catheter
- Oropharyngeal and nasopharyngeal AIRWAYS
- POCKET MASK with oxygen inlet and/or BAG-VALVE-MASK with oxygen reservoir
- WOUND KIT (Table 20-1)
- MAST, if used in your service
- STETHOSCOPE
- FLASHLIGHT

The equipment listed will be sufficient to carry out all of the lifesaving procedures of the primary survey and to package the patient for transport if you should

TABLE 20-1.   WOUND AND BURN KIT

QUANTITY	EQUIPMENT
24	4-by-4-inch sterile gauze pads
24	Bandaids
6	Medium dressings
4	Multitrauma (universal) dressings
4	Petrolatum gauze dressings
2	Sterile burn sheets
6	Water Jel dressings, various sizes
1	Roll sterilized aluminum foil
6	Rolls self-adhering roller bandage
12	Triangular bandages
1	Roll 1-inch adhesive tape
1	Roll 3-inch adhesive tape
12	Safety pins
1	Pair heavy-duty scissors

find that a "load-and-go" situation exists. If, on the other hand, it turns out that the patient is *not* in critical condition, and that you therefore have time to carry out a more painstaking survey and additional stabilizing measures (e.g., splinting individual fractures), you will also have time to return to the ambulance for whatever additional equipment is required.

When You Reach the Victim

Once you reach the scene of the incident, you will have to carry out five steps as expeditiously as possible:

1. SURVEY OF THE SCENE (see Chap. 6)—to determine:
   - Whether there are any *hazards* to the patient or rescuers.
   - Whether you will need *backup* (figure one ambulance for every critically injured patient).
   - Whether you will need any special *equipment to gain access* to the patient.
2. The PRIMARY SURVEY—to identify injuries that could kill the patient if not managed immediately.
3. TRANSPORT DECISION and CRITICAL INTERVENTIONS—deciding whether there is a "load-and-go" situation and, if so, whether there are any lifesaving actions—such as decompression of a pneumothorax—that you have to carry out before you start transport.
4. The SECONDARY SURVEY—to find injuries that were not considered life-threatening on the pri-

mary survey, along with life-threatening complications that may have developed since completion of the primary survey. In critically injured patients, the secondary survey must be carried out during transport.

5. COMMUNICATION WITH THE RECEIVING HOSPITAL, to enable them to prepare appropriately to receive this specific patient with his particular collection of injuries.

Some trauma experts specify a "platinum 10 minutes" as the maximum time that paramedics should spend carrying out the above five steps at the scene. That time limit may not always be reasonable or practical, but it is a good goal to shoot for.

THE EXTENDED PRIMARY SURVEY

The primary survey is the rapid, initial assessment to detect life-threatening conditions. For the victim of trauma, the alphabet of the primary survey is extended from three letters to five letters—ABCDE—but the survey should nonetheless be accomplished in *under 2 minutes*. You should be able to move through the steps of the primary survey like a robot, stopping for nothing except to perform immediately lifesaving procedures (e.g., airway opening, rescue breathing, venting a tension pneumothorax).

> **DO NOT INTERRUPT THE PRIMARY SURVEY FOR ANY REASON EXCEPT TO OPEN AN OBSTRUCTED AIRWAY OR PERFORM OTHER IMMEDIATELY LIFESAVING PROCEDURES.**

Finding the casualty in respiratory distress is *not* a reason to interrupt the primary survey, for you will only delay detection of the cause, which is likely to become evident during examination of the chest.

We shall deal here with the steps of the primary survey in sequence, for that is how you should store them in your brain. It is important to point out, however, that often more than one step is being carried out simultaneously, especially—as *should* be the case—if two or more rescuers are working as a team. Thus, for example, one rescuer should immediately move to stabilize the cervical spine of an unconscious casualty while a second rescuer checks the airway and proceeds down the rescue alphabet. Similarly, when a patient is bleeding briskly from a wound of

the lower extremities, there is no reason why one rescuer has to wait until his or her partner has reached step C of the primary survey before applying pressure to the bleeding site. TEAMWORK IS ESSENTIAL!

Start by setting down the backboard so that all the equipment loaded on it will be within immediate reach of the rescuer who will be positioned at the patient's airway. While one member of the team starts unbuckling equipment from the backboard, the second team member addresses the first letter of the rescue alphabet—A, for airway.

Airway and Cervical Spine

As always, first priority goes to the **airway.** Is the airway open now? Will it *stay* open? If the patient is unconscious, OPEN THE AIRWAY by *jaw thrust, chin lift,* or *jaw lift* (Fig. 20-1), that is, maneuvers that will not move the head out of neutral position. A little bit of extension of the head probably won't hurt, but flexion of the head may be catastrophic, so AVOID FLEXING THE HEAD at all costs.

> **REMEMBER: ANY PATIENT WITH INJURY ABOVE THE CLAVICLES OR ANY PATIENT UNCONSCIOUS AFTER TRAUMA HAS A CERVICAL SPINE INJURY UNTIL PROVED OTHERWISE.**

Inspect the patient's mouth quickly, and SUCTION out secretions, blood, or vomitus. If the patient is unconscious, use an OROPHARYNGEAL OR NASOPHARYNGEAL AIRWAY to help keep the airway patent. Do not attempt endotracheal intubation at this juncture, for the patient will not have been adequately preoxygenated yet.

Breathing

If the patient is *conscious,* listen to him TALK. Is he able to speak in full sentences without gasping for breath? Can he take a deep breath?

If the patient is *unconscious,* expose his chest, and place your cheek over his mouth in order to LOOK, LISTEN, AND FEEL FOR BREATHING. If the patient is *not* breathing, give two full breaths, check for a carotid pulse, and start CPR as required. If he *is* breathing, however, check the *adequacy* of breathing by noting:

- Respiratory RATE.
- DEPTH of respirations (tidal volume).
- The NECK (look and palpate): Is the *trachea in the midline?*
- The CHEST:
  1. *Look* for open wounds, bruises, deformity, and flail segments. (If you detect a *sucking chest wound,* place a gloved hand over it until your partner can cover it with an occlusive dressing. Do *not* interrupt your survey.)
  2. *Feel* for instability over the rib cage.
  3. *Listen* with a stethoscope in each axilla for presence and equality of breath sounds. If breath sounds are not equal, *percuss* over both sides of the chest for dullness or hyperresonance on one side.

As soon as you moved from the patient's airway to his chest, your partner should have whipped an OXYGEN mask onto the patient's face (preferably a nonrebreathing mask) or started ASSISTED VENTILATION by bag-valve-mask, as required. It is very difficult to maintain an airway, hold a mask against the face with one hand, squeeze a bag with the other hand, *and* avoid moving the patient's head or neck. One way to stabilize the patient's head and neck during bag-valve-mask ventilation—pending more definitive immobilization on a backboard—is for the rescuer to kneel and hold the patient's head steady between his or her knees (Fig. 20-2).

Circulation

In practice, you will be assessing the patient's circulation at the same time as you are assessing his breathing; for both examinations require you to examine the neck and the chest, and it makes no sense to do that twice. In fact, assessment of the circulation begins as soon as you encounter the patient and place a hand on his forearm. Establishing immediate physical contact provides the patient with reassurance (if he is conscious, and even, perhaps, if he isn't conscious) and provides you with important information about his skin condition; if it is pale, cold, and sweaty, the patient is in shock until proved otherwise.

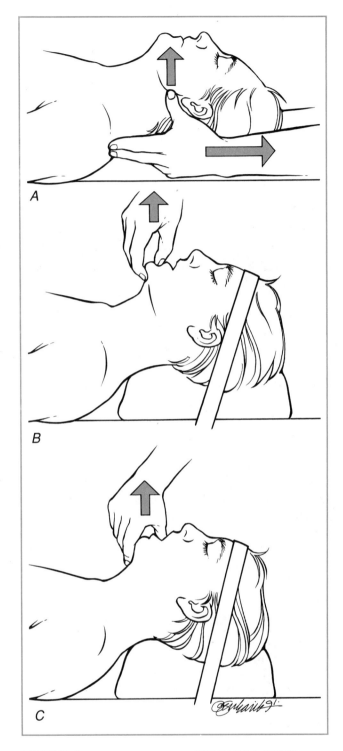

FIGURE 20-1. OPENING THE AIRWAY IN A SPINE-INJURED PATIENT. (A) Jaw thrust. (B) Chin lift. (C) Jaw lift. All maneuvers are performed with the head in neutral position.

> **ESTABLISH PHYSICAL CONTACT WITH THE INJURED PATIENT IMMEDIATELY WHEN YOU REACH HIM. IF HIS SKIN FEELS COLD AND SWEATY, HE IS IN SHOCK UNTIL PROVED OTHERWISE.**

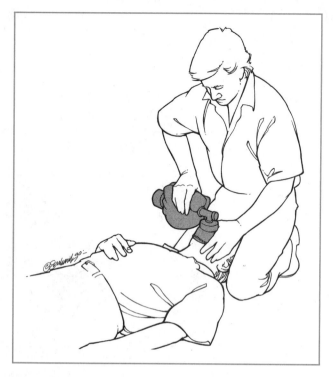

FIGURE 20-2. **VENTILATING A PATIENT WITH POSSIBLE CERVICAL SPINE INJURY.** Stabilize the patient's head in neutral position between your knees.

Other signs of shock may become evident as you continue your assessment of the circulation. While still at the patient's head, palpate the CAROTID PULSE, and note its rate and quality. As soon as you finish your examination of the chest, check for the presence of a FEMORAL PULSE in the groin and then a RADIAL PULSE in the wrist. Now you can make a rough estimate of the blood pressure:

If a pulse is present in:	The systolic pressure is at least:
The carotid artery	60 mm Hg
The femoral artery	70 mm Hg
The radial artery	80 mm Hg

If time and lighting permit, you may also check the fingernail or hypothenar eminence for CAPILLARY REFILL. Remember, peripheral perfusion is severely impaired if the nail does not pink up within the time it takes you to say, "Normal capillary refill."

When you've found signs of shock, you still have to determine what *kind* of shock: Is it cardiogenic shock, secondary to tension pneumothorax, cardiac tamponade, myocardial contusion, or air embolism?

Or is it hypovolemic shock, secondary to blood loss? Two things that can help you make the distinction are the patient's neck veins and his breath sounds. If the NECK VEINS are distended, look for a *cardiogenic* source of shock, such as tension pneumothorax or cardiac tamponade. If the neck veins are not distended, you have not ruled out diagnoses such as tension pneumothorax—for if there has been bleeding as well, the neck veins may remain flat. But the check you already made of the BREATH SOUNDS should help you zero in on the source of shock.

When the patient is in *hypovolemic* shock, the source may or may not be obvious. EXTERNAL BLEEDING must, of course, be controlled during the primary survey, initially by direct manual pressure on the wound. When the patient shows signs of hypovolemic shock and the source of bleeding is *not* obvious, consider the THREE AREAS OF HIDDEN BLOOD LOSS: the *chest*, the *abdomen*, and the *thigh*.

Disability (Brief Neurologic Examination)

For the primary survey, only the briefest neurologic evaluation is undertaken, specifically an assessment of PUPIL SIZE AND REACTION TO LIGHT and of the patient's LEVEL OF CONSCIOUSNESS, according to the AVPU scale. To review:

A   Alert (patient knows his name, where he is, what day it is)
V   Responds to **v**ocal stimuli
P   Responds only to **p**ainful stimuli
U   **U**nresponsive to any stimuli

A more detailed neurologic evaluation, such as the Glasgow Coma Scale, should be conducted and documented during the secondary survey.

A DECREASING LEVEL OF CONSCIOUSNESS MAY BE A SIGN OF HYPOXEMIA AND DEMANDS IMMEDIATE RE-ASSESSMENT OF THE PATIENT'S OXYGENATION.

Expose

The patient should now be completely undressed, to permit thorough assessment. Up to this point, you may have opened up the front of his shirt to see the anterior chest or perhaps cut open a trouser leg to get at a source of bleeding. But that is not sufficient for a complete examination. Cut through the front of shirts and trousers so that the sleeves and pant legs fold back from the extremities. (If the patient cannot be shielded from public view, defer this step until he is inside the ambulance.) As soon as you have completed the survey, COVER THE PATIENT with blankets to prevent heat loss.

SUMMARY: EXTENDED PRIMARY SURVEY

A AIRWAY, with cervical spine precautions
- Jaw thrust, with cervical spine stabilization
- Suction
- Oropharyngeal or nasopharyngeal airway

B BREATHING
- Present or absent? Look, listen, and feel
- Respiratory rate and depth
- Trachea deviated?
- Chest
  1. Look: Open wounds? Flail segment?
  2. Feel: Unstable ribs?
  3. Listen: Unequal breath sounds? One side dull or resonant with respect to the other?
- Oxygen
- Assisted ventilation (by Rescuer #2) as required

C CIRCULATION/BLEEDING
- External hemorrhage control: manual pressure (by Rescuer #2, while Rescuer #1 completes assessment)
- Skin condition
- Pulses (carotid, femoral, radial): rate, quality
- Neck veins

D DISABILILTY
- Pupils: Size and reaction to light
- Level of consciousness: AVPU rating

E EXPOSE

The steps of the primary survey, along with the steps that come immediately afterward, are summarized in flow-chart form in Figure 20-3.

It takes a lot longer to describe the steps of the primary survey than to perform them, and you should be able to carry out all of the steps listed above in less than 2 minutes. By the time you have done so, furthermore, you should have enough information to decide whether a "load-and-go" situation exists.

TRANSPORT DECISION AND CRITICAL INTERVENTIONS

Patients with critical injuries cannot be stabilized in the field. Those are the patients for whom the minutes of the Golden Hour are ticking down inexorably. You need to be able to recognize such patients, by means of the primary survey, and to get them promptly and safely to a trauma center.

CRITICALLY INJURED PATIENTS CANNOT BE STABILIZED IN THE FIELD. YOUR JOB IS TO KEEP THEM ALIVE AND PREVENT FURTHER INJURY DURING RAPID TRANSPORT TO A TRAUMA CENTER.

Load-and-Go Situations

Not surprisingly, the patients who fall into the category of critically injured are those in whom the ABCs (and D) are in immediate jeopardy:

- Patients whose AIRWAY is in jeopardy. These are patients in whom you **cannot establish a secure airway,** for whatever reason. A patient hurled against the steering wheel of a car, for example, may have suffered blunt laryngeal trauma that makes it inadvisable to try to intubate from above (through the mouth or nose); at the same time, massive swelling and ecchymoses of the neck may totally obscure the landmarks for cricothyrotomy. Such a patient will *urgently* need a tracheostomy carried out in the operating room, and the faster you can get him to the operating room, the better his chances of survival.
- Patients whose BREATHING is inadequate, including those with:
  1. **Respiratory arrest**
  2. **Open pneumothorax**
  3. **Tension pneumothorax**
  4. Large **flail chest**
- Patients with CIRCULATORY insufficiency (i.e., shock) including those with
  1. Full **cardiopulmonary arrest**
  2. **Shock**
     a. Hemorrhagic
     b. Cardiogenic (cardiac tamponade, myocardial injury)
     c. Spinal
  3. **Uncontrollable bleeding**

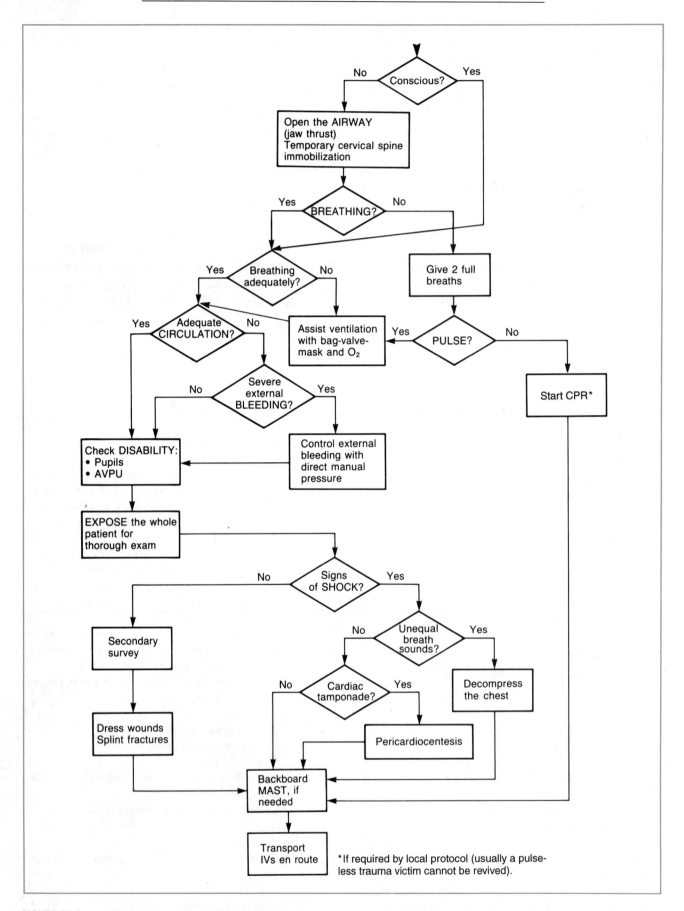

FIGURE 20-3. ASSESSMENT OF THE INJURED PATIENT.

- Patients with severe neurologic DISABILITY
  1. **Unconscious**
  2. **Deteriorating level of consciousness**
  3. Any other signs of **rising intracranial pressure** (see Chap. 16)

Only about 10 percent of all victims of trauma do in fact fall into the critical category, but for those 10 percent, every minute counts. If, therefore, a patient has any one or more of the critical conditions listed above, he should be immediately secured to a long backboard, loaded into the ambulance, and transported rapidly to the nearest trauma center. There are only a very few, lifesaving procedures that need to be done before you leave the scene.

Critical Interventions

Critical interventions are those that will make an immediate difference between life and death. They are the only interventions that should be permitted to delay transport of a patient judged to be critically injured according to the criteria just outlined. There are, in fact, very few procedures that qualify as critical interventions.

Establishing an Airway

The patient *must* have a patent airway. If you cannot ensure the airway manually, or with the help of an oropharyngeal airway, you will have to try other methods until you have established a reliable conduit between the patient's respiratory tract and the outside. When the patient's face is more or less intact, the safest method is ENDOTRACHEAL INTUBATION. The experts differ on whether it is preferable in trauma to intubate through the mouth or through the nose. This author personally favors orotracheal intubation—either visual or tactile—because it is usually faster and less traumatic. But the bottom line is: Use the method you do best. With either method, make sure an assistant is holding the patient's head steady, with the spine kept in alignment.

When there is massive maxillofacial trauma, endotracheal intubation is often unfeasible, and you may have no choice but to perform CRICO-THYROTOMY or PERCUTANEOUS TRANSLARYNGEAL VENTILATION (see Chaps. 7 and 8). Those are techniques that you are not apt to use very often, and you will not be able to perform them rapidly or correctly in an emergency if you don't practice, in the lab or the morgue, in between times.

External Hemorrhage Control

Major external hemorrhage was initially controlled, during the primary survey, by direct manual pressure on the bleeding sites. Clearly it is not practical to tie up one or two rescuers for any period of time holding manual pressure on wounds. The manual pressure must be supplanted by some sort of pressure dressing. When the wound is on an extremity, an AIR SPLINT is an excellent means of holding a dressing firmly against a bleeding wound. On the head or trunk, use triangular bandages or self-adhering roller gauze to secure bulky dressings against bleeding sites. Do *not* use clamps or other instruments to try to pinch off bleeding vessels; you are unlikely to succeed under field conditions, and meanwhile you may do irreparable damage to adjacent nerves and other structures.

Sealing Open Neck Wounds

Recall that bleeding from an open wound of the neck carries the particular danger of *air embolism*. On first encountering a patient with an open neck wound, you must cover the wound with whatever is immediately available—even your gloved hand if you do not have a dressing unwrapped and ready. Before transport, however, you need to cover the neck wound more securely, with an occlusive dressing and bulky dressings over that.

Sealing Open Chest Wounds

Holes in the chest must also be sealed properly, especially large holes through which you can hear air being sucked in with respiration. Use petrolatum gauze, aluminum foil, or plastic wrap as an occlusive dressing, and tape the dressing on *three sides only*, to permit air under pressure inside the chest to be vented out.

Stabilization of Flail Segments

When the chest is visibly flailing, each inhalation brings the ribs crashing down onto the underlying lung and thus bruises the lung further. Minimize movement of the flail segment by securing a pillow firmly against the segment or placing the patient flail-side down on the backboard.

Decompression of a Tension Pneumothorax

Tension pneumothorax presents as severe, progressive shock, and a patient in that condition may not make it alive to the hospital unless the pneumothorax is promptly decompressed. If the primary survey reveals a tension pneumothorax, therefore, you will need to put a needle in the patient's chest as quickly as possible (see Chap. 17).

Pericardiocentesis for Cardiac Tamponade

Cardiac tamponade is usually much harder to recognize than tension pneumothorax, especially when the classic signs, such as distended neck veins, are not present. You will need to have a high index of suspicion based on the mechanisms of injury, the presence of severe shock, and the very narrow pulse pressure. Sometimes you will not suspect tamponade until after an attempt to relieve a "tension pneumothorax" has failed. If the patient's condition is deteriorating rapidly, it is worth inserting a needle into the pericardium at that point and trying to draw off some blood. Removal of as little as 5 ml of blood may be lifesaving if there *is* cardiac tamponade.

SUMMARY: CRITICAL INTERVENTIONS

- AIRWAY management
- External HEMORRHAGE CONTROL
- SEALING OPEN WOUNDS
  1. Neck
  2. Chest
- Temporary stabilization of FLAIL chest
- CHEST DECOMPRESSION for tension pneumothorax
- PERICARDIOCENTESIS for cardiac tamponade

THE SECONDARY SURVEY

In patients who meet the criteria for critically injured, the secondary survey will have to be performed, often in abbreviated fashion, during transport to the hospital, along with various treatment measures such as starting intravenous therapy. In the 90 percent of trauma patients who are *not* found in critical condition, however, the secondary survey and stabilizing measures are carried out at the scene, in an orderly, systematic way.

General Principles

Table 20-2 reviews what you need to look for in performing the secondary survey of an injured patient. We shall not reiterate in this chapter all of the details concerning the assessment and treatment of specific injuries. Suffice it to recall a few important points from the past six chapters as we proceed through the head-to-toe survey:

- The most important clinical sign in *head injury* is a CHANGING STATE OF CONSCIOUSNESS.

TABLE 20-2. SECONDARY SURVEY OF THE MULTITRAUMA PATIENT

BODY REGION	WHAT TO LOOK FOR
HEAD	Depressed fracture; scalp laceration; cerebrospinal fluid leak from ears or nose; Battle's sign; maxillofacial injury (palpate bones of the face)
EYES	Penetrating injury: extraocular motions; pupils; visual acuity
MOUTH	Foreign bodies; loose or avulsed teeth; broken dentures; blood, vomitus, secretions; malocclusion
NECK	Open wounds; subcutaneous emphysema; tracheal deviation; jugular distention; tenderness or bruises over cervical spine (assume, in any case, that cervical injury is present)
CHEST	Bruises; open injuries; stability of clavicles and chest wall; equality of breath sounds; dullness or hyperresonance; audibility of heart sounds
ABDOMEN	Contusions and seat belt marks; open wounds; evisceration; distention; guarding; rigidity; cough "rebound" tenderness
PELVIS	Stability on compression of iliac wings
BACK	Open wounds
EXTREMITIES	Deformity, swelling, ecchymosis; color; temperature; pulses; sensation and motion (withdrawal from pain if unconscious)

Carefully document the patient's level of consciousness and other neurologic signs at frequent intervals in every head-injured patient.

- FALLING BLOOD PRESSURE IS ALMOST NEVER CAUSED BY A HEAD INJURY. Look for a source of major hemorrhage elsewhere in the body if a head-injured patient becomes hypotensive.
- DISTENDED NECK VEINS mean that blood is backing up behind the right side of the heart. Consider tension pneumothorax and cardiac tamponade as possible life-threatening causes.
- Whenever the mechanisms of injury suggest the *possibility* of spine injury, IMMOBILIZE THE SPINE. For practical purposes, that category in-

cludes *every* patient with MULTIPLE INJURIES, as well as any patient with serious HEAD INJURY, patients who have FALLEN FROM A HEIGHT, patients involved in significant DECELERATION INJURIES or DIVING ACCIDENTS—irrespective of whether clinical signs of spinal cord injury are present.

- A DISTENDED ABDOMEN in an injured patient is a danger signal.
- Check and recheck PULSES DISTAL TO AN INJURY.

Taking the History in Trauma

When dealing with the victim of serious trauma, the patient's history is usually obtained either simultaneously with the head-to-toe survey or en route to the hospital. Most courses in Advanced Trauma Life Support (ATLS) recommend an abbreviated format for obtaining the particular details of medical history that are important in managing trauma—a format that can be easily remembered by the mnemonic "Take an AMPLE history."

A ALLERGIES
M MEDICATIONS that the patient takes regularly or has taken today
P PAST MEDICAL HISTORY
  - Operations
  - Anesthetic complications during previous operations
  - Previous hospitalizations
  - Other serious illnesses
L LAST MEAL, that is, the last time the patient had any oral intake (which helps assess the risk of vomiting and aspiration during induction of anesthesia)
E EVENTS leading up to the incident (mechanisms of injury)

Trauma Scoring

Very nearly everyone agrees that it is useful to have some sort of scoring system to rate the severity of a patient's injuries and therefore help decide which patients ought to be referred directly to a trauma center and which can be transported to other, perhaps closer hospitals. The problem is that, as of this writing, there are more than 45 different systems for determining injury severity, of which at least 15 have been developed for prehospital use (see Further Reading at the end of this chapter).

Nearly all systems for scoring severity of trauma give numerical values to various physiologic and sometimes anatomic findings. The revised Trauma Score developed by Champion and his colleagues in Washington, D.C., for example, combines the Glasgow Coma Scale with an assessment of the systolic blood pressure and respiratory rate.

Whatever form of trauma scoring is employed in your EMS system, the important thing is to *know the system by heart* and to KEEP AN ACCURATE FLOW CHART OF REPEATED OBSERVATIONS. Whatever parameters are monitored—and usually they should include at least the level of consciousness and vital signs—should be *rechecked and recorded at least every 5 minutes* for the duration that the patient is in your care.

COMMUNICATIONS

As soon as you have a clear idea of the extent of the patient's injuries—which may be immediately after the primary survey in a critically injured casualty—MAKE CONTACT WITH MEDICAL COMMAND. It is absolutely critical that the receiving hospital be given as much time as possible to prepare for the arrival of your patient. A full-fledged trauma center may indeed have a team on standby at all times. But many hospitals will require lead time to summon the appropriate staff—for example, a neurosurgeon for the head-injured patient. The Golden Hour can be squandered in the hospital as well as in the field if the hospital is not adequately prepared to receive the patient you bring in. When you communicate by radio with medical command or with the receiving hospital, follow these guidelines:

- IDENTIFY YOUR UNIT CLEARLY with every transmission. Medical command may be dealing with more than one emergency, or even more than one unit at the accident scene with you, and it is important to keep the units and their patients sorted out.
- FOLLOW THE STANDARD REPORTING FORMAT:
  1. Patient's age, sex, and chief complaint or mechanism of injury.
  2. Abnormalities found on the primary survey.
  3. Vital signs.
  4. Secondary survey findings (in stable patient).
  5. Treatment you have given.
  6. Estimated time of arrival at hospital (ETA).
- BE BRIEF AND CONCISE.

STABILIZING MEASURES

Just how much you can do to stabilize the patient at the scene will depend, as we have observed, on how badly the patient is injured. A severely injured patient must be packaged as a single unit to a backboard and transported without delay, except for the few critical interventions necessary to prevent immediate death. In the majority of patients who are not critically injured, however, there will be time to carry out some basic stabilizing measures in the field.

Once again, we shall not review here all the details of the past six chapters but rather just highlight a few important points regarding stabilization of injuries:

- Dress all WOUNDS before splinting fractures.
- Cover EVISCERATED ABDOMINAL ORGANS with bulky, sterile dressings that have been soaked in sterile saline. Do not attempt to place eviscerated organs back into the abdomen.
- Stabilize IMPALED OBJECTS in place.
- Preserve AMPUTATED PARTS. Wrap them in sterile gauze that has been moistened in sterile saline, and seal them inside a plastic bag. Then place the plastic bag on ice or chemical cold packs.
- Splint FRACTURES before moving the patient.
- Unless a complicated extrication requires you to remain a long time at the scene, START IVs EN ROUTE. Get set up (assemble the administration set, tear the tape, apply the tourniquet, prep the skin) with the unit rolling. If necessary, have the driver stop while you insert the needle. Then get rolling again.
- KEEP THE PATIENT WARM!!! Turn up the heat in the ambulance, and cover the patient with blankets. Patients in shock are easily chilled, and hypothermia just worsens their situation.

A COLD GRAVE AWAITS A COLD PATIENT. KEEP THE TRAUMA VICTIM WARM!

FURTHER READING

American College of Emergency Physicians. Clinical policy for the initial approach to patients presenting with acute blunt trauma. *Ann Emerg Med* 22:1101, 1993.

Baxt WG et al. The failure of prehospital trauma prediction rules to classify trauma patients accurately. *Ann Emerg Med* 18:1, 1989.

Cales RH. Injury severity determination: Requirements, approaches, and applications. *Ann Emerg Med* 15:1427, 1986.

Cayten CG et al. Basic life support versus advanced life support for injured patients with an injury severity score of 10 or more. *J Trauma* 35:460, 1993.

Champion HR. Field triage of trauma patients (editorial). *Ann Emerg Med* 11:160, 1982.

Champion HR et al. Assessment of injury severity: The triage index. *Crit Care Med* 8:201, 1980.

Champion HR et al. Trauma score. *Crit Care Med* 9:672, 1981.

Champion HR et al. The effect of medical direction on trauma triage. *J Trauma* 28:235, 1988.

Champion HR et al. A revision of the trauma score. *J Trauma* 29:623, 1989.

Coats TJ, Wilson AW, Cross FW. On-scene medical decision making and overtriage. *Br J Surg* 80:1291, 1993.

Cox DM. Keeping score: Triage tools for organized patient care and evaluation. *Emergency* 25(5):42, 1993.

Ferko JG. The triage factor. *Emergency* 20(8):44, 1988.

Goodwin C. Rethinking triage. *Emergency* 26(3):41, 1993.

Gormican SP. CRAMS scale: Field triage of trauma victims. *Ann Emerg Med* 11:132, 1982.

Kane G et al. Empirical development and evaluation of prehospital trauma triage instruments. *J Trauma* 25:482, 1985.

Knopp R et al. Mechanism of injury and anatomic injury as criteria for prehospital trauma triage. *Ann Emerg Med* 17:895, 1988.

Knudson P, Frecceri CA, DeLateur SA. Improving the field triage of major trauma victims. *J Trauma* 28:602, 1988.

Koehler JJ et al. Prehospital index: A scoring system for field triage of trauma victims. *Ann Emerg Med* 15:178, 1986.

Koenig WJ. Management of severe multiple trauma. *Emergency* 11(2):27, 1979.

Larkin J, Moylan J. Priorities in the management of trauma victims. *Crit Care Med* 3:192, 1975.

Moreau M et al. Application of the trauma score in the prehospital setting. *Ann Emerg Med* 14:1049, 1985.

Morris JA et al. The trauma score as a triage tool in the prehospital setting. *JAMA* 256:1319, 1986.

Nixon RG. Assessment of the trauma patient. *Emerg Med Serv* 8(2):50, 1979.

Ornato J et al. Ineffectiveness of the trauma score and the CRAMS scale for accurately triaging patients to trauma centers. *Ann Emerg Med* 14:1061, 1985.

Phillips JA. Optimizing prehospital triage criteria for trauma team alerts. *J Trauma* 34:127, 1993.

Rogers LF. Common oversights in the evaluation of the patient with multiple injuries. *Skeletal Radiol* 12:103, 1984.

Rosemurgy AS. Prehospital traumatic cardiac arrest: The cost of futility. *J Trauma* 35:468, 1993.

Sampalis JS et al. Impact of on-site care, prehospital time, and level of in-hospital care on severely injured patients. *J Trauma* 34:252, 1993.

Spoor JE. Trauma responses: Beyond the ABCs. *Emergency* 12(2):33, 1980.

Spoor JE. Multiple trauma (from the scene to the surgeon). *Emerg Med Serv* 10(3):38, 1981.

Timberlake GA. Trauma in the golden hour. *Emerg Med* 19(20):79, 1987.

Trunkey DD. Is ALS necessary for pre-hospital trauma care? *J Trauma* 24:86, 1984.

Trunkey DD. Trauma: The first hour. *Emerg Med* 16(5):93, 1984.

21
The Multicasualty Incident

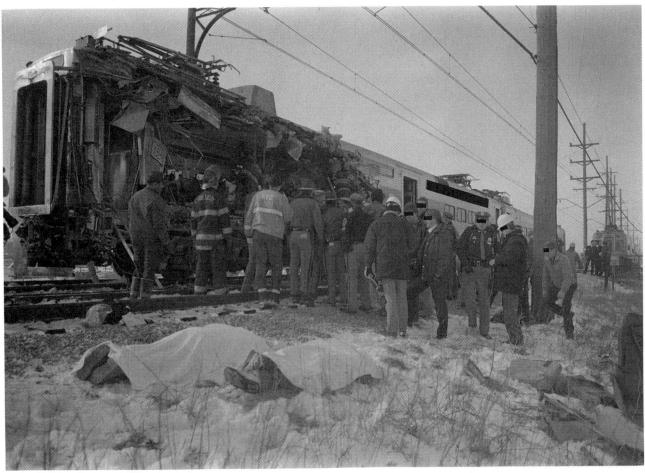

Gary, Indiana. Photo by Michael S. Kowal.

OBJECTIVES

The accident or disaster involving multiple casualties poses the ultimate challenge to the paramedic, for it requires the paramedic not only to deploy all of his or her skills—skills of judgment, organization, extrication, physical assessment, and treatment—but also to do so under the most difficult possible circumstances, which may involve mass panic along with other hazards to the safety of everyone at the scene. That is a tall order, and it will not be adequately filled unless the EMS system has a carefully developed disaster plan and stages periodic field exercises to drill all those involved in carrying out the plan. This chapter cannot substitute for such disaster drills. What we *can* do in this chapter is review the basic principles of responding to a multicasualty incident, organizing the work at the scene, sorting patients, and getting the patients bundled off safely to appropriate hospitals. By the end of this chapter, therefore, the student should be able to

1. List the information that the dispatcher should try to obtain regarding any multicasualty incident
2. Choose an appropriate place to position his or her ambulance, given a description of the incident scene
3. Choose an appropriate location for a triage area and for a staging area, given a description of an incident scene
4. List the equipment that is required in a triage area
5. Identify, given a description of several patients with different injuries,
   a. First-priority patients
   b. Second-priority patients
   c. Third-priority patients
6. Estimate how many ambulances will be needed, and what other services should be summoned, given a description of a multicasualty incident scene
7. List the information that should be recorded on the patient's triage tag or whatever other record accompanies him to the hospital
8. Indicate the order in which casualties should be evacuated from the scene, given a description of several casualties with different injuries and of the available transport resources
9. Identify common emotional reactions to mass casualty situations, and describe how to deal with people manifesting those reactions
10. List at least three ways in which bystanders can be usefully employed in mass casualty situations

The most common situation involving multiple casualties—and therefore the situation we shall use as our example in most of the following discussion—is the multivehicle highway accident. In 1988, there were approximately 42,000 serious motor vehicle accidents in the United States, in which more than 47,000 people lost their lives. Road traffic accidents also accounted for approximately 4 million injuries during the same year. In nearly half the cases, more than one vehicle was involved. Thus, nearly every rescue squad is likely to be faced with a multivehicle accident at some time. The principles of dealing with that situation are the same as for any other multicasualty incident.

RECEIVING THE CALL FOR HELP

The response to a multicasualty incident—whether it's a road accident or the crash of a jumbo jet—begins at the moment of notification, when the dispatcher receives the call for help. When the circumstances suggest that the incident may involve more than one or two casualties, the dispatcher should try to obtain as much of the following information as possible:

- The exact LOCATION of the accident or disaster:
  1. Specific directions, including helpful landmarks.
  2. The proper geographic designation (e.g., *East* Maple Street or *West* Maple Street?).
  3. The telephone number of the caller, which may help to pinpoint the caller's location and which will also enable the dispatcher to phone back if further directions are needed. (Obtaining the caller's telephone number also helps to discourage nuisance calls.)
- If the incident is a vehicular accident, the NUMBER AND TYPES OF VEHICLES involved:
  1. If there are trucks, what are they carrying? Are there hazardous cargoes?
  2. Are buses involved?
  3. In what condition are the vehicles? Is any vehicle on fire? If so, which vehicle?
- Number of VICTIMS and estimated extent of INJURIES.
- HAZARDS at the scene:
  1. *Fire.*
  2. Downed *electric wires.*
  3. *Hazardous materials* (see Chap. 34) carried by involved vehicles (e.g., explosives, chemicals, radioactive materials).
  4. *Traffic hazards* (Determine whether the road is fully or partially blocked by the accident and whether traffic is moving).
  5. Vehicles in unstable or *precarious positions* (e.g., vehicles under water).
  6. *Debris.*

Date _____   Log # _____

Times
Call received _____ A.M./P.M.
Car out _____
Arrived at scene _____
Left scene _____
Arrived at hospital _____
Back in service _____

Patient's name _____
Address _____
City/town _____

Patient status
Conscious?_____
Breathing?_____
Bleeding? _____
Other _____

If vehicular accident
Number and kinds of vehicles involved
_____cars _____trucks _____buses _____other
Number of persons injured _____
Extent of injuries _____
Are persons trapped? _____
Hazards
_____traffic _____wires down _____fire _____hazardous cargo
_____unstable vehicle _____debris _____submerged vehicle

Caller: Name _____ Phone no. _____

Vehicle dispatched _____
Crew _____   Other units called _____
_____   _____
_____   _____

FIGURE 21-1. A preprinted **DISPATCH FORM** helps remind the dispatcher of what information needs to be obtained.

A dispatch information form covering the above questions, like that shown in Figure 21-1, either printed or displayed on a computer terminal, can be of considerable help to the dispatcher in rapidly assembling all essential information. On the basis of that information, the dispatcher must then make the initial decision as to how many ambulances should be sent to the scene and what ancillary services (e.g., police, fire, utility company) need to be notified.

ARRIVING AT THE SCENE

On reaching the incident scene, the rescuer's first task is always to make a quick assessment of the overall situation. Studies have indicated that the first res-

cuers arriving at the scene of a multicasualty incident often tend to become overwhelmed by the magnitude of the situation or the severity of the injuries involved. Already en route to the scene, therefore, the most senior paramedic should be designated as team leader, whose job it will be on arrival to ensure that everyone gets straight down to business.

The very first, almost unconscious decision at the scene of a multicasualty incident will be WHERE TO POSITION THE AMBULANCE. From the point of view of safety, certain general principles apply:

• The ambulance should be parked OFF THE ROAD, out of the flow of traffic.
• If the ambulance is parked facing oncoming traffic, its HEADLIGHTS SHOULD BE TURNED

OFF. Flashing or revolving warning lights should remain on, however, to alert oncoming traffic of the hazard ahead.

- The ambulance should be parked BEYOND THE REACH OF DOWNED WIRES and AT LEAST 30 METERS FROM ANY BURNING VEHICLE. If there is spilled gasoline flowing along the road, the ambulance should not be parked where it will be downstream from the flow.
- The ambulance should be parked UPWIND FROM ACCIDENTS INVOLVING SPILLAGE OF DANGEROUS CHEMICALS.
- The ambulance should not be closer than 700 to 1,000 METERS FROM an accident involving EXPLOSIVE CARGOES.

The next decision that must be made on arrival at the incident scene is WHETHER THERE IS A HAZARD TO THE SAFETY OF THE RESCUERS. Multiple casualty incidents often involve multiple hazards—fire, downed wires, toxic chemicals. Those at the scene most skilled in hazard control, usually fire personnel, should be assigned to that responsibility, with paramedics maintaining close coordination. A paramedic can greatly assist hazard control personnel by first looking out for his or her own safety. The rescuer who rushes blindly into a hazardous environment is unlikely to be of much help and indeed may become part of the problem. It is therefore worthwhile to reiterate here:

> **ALWAYS LOOK FIRST TO YOUR OWN SAFETY.**
> **DEAD HEROES CAN'T SAVE LIVES.**

Finally, the initial, rapid survey of the scene should also enable you to decide whether the number of rescue personnel already present will be sufficient or whether ADDITIONAL HELP will be NEEDED. One ambulance and *at least* two rescuers will be required for every seriously injured victim. For the less seriously injured, two victims may be accommodated in a single ambulance. Ongoing triage will permit a more accurate determination of exactly how many and what types of rescue vehicles will be required, but the initial observation of the scene should enable the senior paramedic to decide if there is an *immediate* need for more help. Clearly, for example, a single ambulance with a crew of three will not be able to handle a multivehicle accident with 15 casualties, 5 of them critically injured. In such a situation, at least five

more ambulances should be summoned at once, and additional teams placed on standby. Furthermore, whenever possible, one or more doctors, preassigned to the task, should be requested to respond to the scene of a multicasualty incident, to take medical control on site.

Overall control of a disaster scene should be assumed as soon as possible by an Incident Commander. More and more jurisdictions throughout the United States are adopting an **Incident Command System** (ICS), based on fire service models, to provide unified command and clear lines of authority at incidents where several agencies must be involved in the response. The structure of the local Incident Command System should be known to all participants in the system, and chain of command procedures should be rehearsed at each disaster drill.

ESTABLISHING A TRIAGE AREA

In mass casualty situations—such as a train wreck, aircraft crash, large building collapse—one or two members of the rescue team should start immediately to establish a triage area while the rest of the team begins the initial sorting of patients. The **triage area** will be the place to which all casualties are brought as they are removed from the wreckage or the accident scene. It should be a large area with good lighting, well away from any hazards. Setting up the triage area will proceed much more efficiently if the local EMS system has at least one vehicle specially equipped for disasters—a mobile field hospital or, more accurately, a mobile medical storeroom—containing all of the medical and other supplies necessary for the initial treatment of large numbers of patients. That equipment should include individually packaged resuscitation kits, ventilation and suction equipment, high-power lights with their own generators, stretchers, and a variety of special-purpose kits (e.g., IV infusion kits), whose contents are clearly listed on the outside of the cartons. The deployment of all that equipment from the vehicle should be drilled in periodic field exercises.

The triage area should be arranged in such a way that the senior medical person can check the entire area at a glance. It should, furthermore, be located *between* the site from which the casualties are being removed and the place where the evacuation vehicles are parked (the **staging area**), to ensure an orderly sequence of triage, treatment, and evacuation (Fig. 21-2). Otherwise what inevitably happens is that casualties are loaded willy-nilly into ambulances and rushed off to hospitals, without regard to severity of

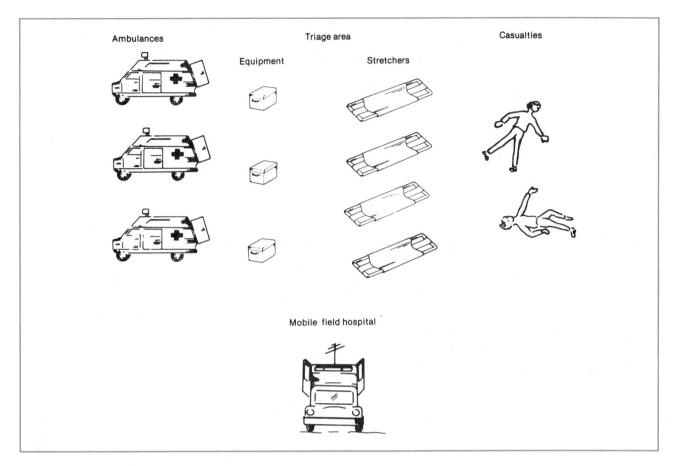

Ambulances   Triage area   Casualties

Equipment   Stretchers

Mobile field hospital

FIGURE 21-2. The **TRIAGE AREA** is interposed between the place where the casualties are found and the place where the ambulances are parked, to prevent evacuation of any casualty who has not been triaged.

injuries, capabilities of the receiving hospitals, or the necessity to account for each casualty.

Supplies and equipment centralized in the triage area should be immediately visible and accessible and should include

- Stretchers: Ideally, long backboards should be used from the outset at every stretcher position. Triage requires frequent movement of the casualty, and it is preferable that patients not have to be moved from one type of stretcher to another.
- At *every* stretcher position:
  1. IV equipment: catheters, infusion sets, intravenous fluid bags, devices for suspension of IV bags
  2. Stethoscope
  3. Sphygmomanometer
  4. Bag-valve-mask or pocket mask
  5. Oropharyngeal airways
  6. Portable oxygen and suction
  7. Wound care kit: dressings, self-adhering roller bandage, triangular bandages, heavy-duty scissors
- Conveniently and prominently located:
  1. Sterile, prepackaged sets for emergency procedures should be clearly labelled:
     a. Endotracheal intubation kit
     b. Cutdown set
     c. Cricothyrotomy and/or translaryngeal ventilation set
     d. Chest tube set with Heimlich valves
     e. Additional sterile dressings
     f. Urethral catheterization set
     g. Sterile syringes and needles
     h. Medication kits with prefilled syringes
  2. Military anti-shock trousers (MAST) kits
  3. Backboards, cervical collars, splints of all types
  4. At least one monitor/defibrillator unit

SORTING OF CASUALTIES

Triage refers to the *sorting* of problems or patients according to their degree of seriousness. The concept of triage had its origins in military medicine, where the goal was (and remains) to restore as many of the injured as possible to full combat duty and to save as many lives as the situation will allow. In civilian practice, the constraints of triage are a bit different. The numbers of seriously wounded are usually (but not always) fewer, and the tactical situation is rarely a major consideration. Nonetheless, the fundamental principles of triage are the same in both military and civilian practice, and apply equally to triage of the individual patient with multiple injuries and to triage of large numbers of separate casualties:

PRINCIPLES OF TRIAGE

- SALVAGE OF LIFE TAKES PRECEDENCE over salvage of limb.
- The principal immediate threats to life are AS-PHYXIA and HEMORRHAGE.

In the situation of mass casualties, the purpose of triage is to accomplish THE GREATEST GOOD FOR THE GREATEST NUMBER. For that very reason, triage decisions are very complicated and very difficult, sometimes requiring that critically injured patients are bypassed altogether. Responsibility for triage should therefore be assigned to the most highly trained and experienced person at the scene, preferably a senior surgeon or emergency physician.

Proper management of multiple casualties requires several *rounds* of triage. The initial round is carried out at the accident site, where the triage officer moves rapidly from one victim to another, deciding which victims require immediate treatment.

In the FIRST ROUND OF TRIAGE, priorities for treatment are founded on the familiar priorities of ABC: *Airway, Breathing,* and *Circulation.* Patients with AIRWAY OBSTRUCTION require immediate attention to relieve the obstruction by manual maneuvers. Artificial ventilation is begun on patients who are NOT BREATHING. Manual control of external bleeding is provided for patients with SEVERE BLEEDING. Whether anything will be done for patients found in CARDIAC ARREST depends on the number of rescuers available; if personnel are in short supply, *do not do CPR.* The chances of survival in trau-

matic cardiac arrest are very small—less than 1 in 1,000—and CPR takes a lot of time and resources that could be used to help more salvageable patients (the greatest good for the greatest number).

Besides victims of full cardiac arrest, it is also necessary in the first round of triage to BYPASS those who are HOPELESSLY INJURED (e.g., decapitated or suffering other devastating head trauma) and those with INJURIES THAT DO NOT POSE AN IMMEDIATE THREAT TO LIFE. (Which injuries *do* pose an immediate threat to life? If you don't remember, review Chap. 20!) During this first round of triage, which is basically the *primary survey of the scene,* the senior triage officer must keep moving from patient to patient, tagging patients and assigning assistants to begin immediate treatment as warranted. The person serving as senior triage officer should not stop to treat any one patient but should survey all of the patients first to obtain an overall evaluation of the scene.

It is important to bear in mind that victims may be scattered over a wide area, either by the accident itself or because they have wandered off, dazed, from the accident scene. Casualties may, therefore, be overlooked if a sufficient perimeter around the accident scene is not surveyed.

In the SECOND ROUND OF TRIAGE, which is best accomplished in the triage area, more definitive measures are taken to manage life-threatening problems—for example, endotracheal intubation to secure a jeopardized airway or chest decompression for tension pneumothorax. Only when conditions that pose an immediate threat to life are under control may efforts shift toward secondary injuries. In subsequent rounds of sorting, the critically injured victims undergo a methodical secondary survey—preferably while already en route to a trauma center—while the less seriously injured receive their initial evaluation at the scene (Table 21-1).

To summarize the triage process, let us look, as an example, at a mass casualty situation in which a school bus and a tractor-trailer have collided and there are upward of two dozen injured, ranging from minor to critical in severity. Let us also suppose that in the initial response, 10 rescuers arrived at the scene. Their initial deployment might be as follows:

- Two rescuers begin unloading equipment to establish a triage area.
- One or two rescuers attend to hazard control.
- The remaining rescuers move immediately to the wreckage to start triage and initial treatment:
  1. The most senior paramedic performs triage only, moving rapidly from one victim to another, to obtain an overview of the total situation.

TABLE 21-1. PRIORITIES OF TREATMENT IN TRIAGE

PRIORITY GROUP	PROBLEM	TREATMENT			
		1ST ROUND TRIAGE	**2ND ROUND TRIAGE**	**3RD ROUND TRIAGE**	**4TH ROUND TRIAGE**
First	Airway obstruction	Airway opened manually	Endotracheal intubation; cricothyrotomy		
	Sucking chest wound	Sealed manually	Sealed with occlusive dressing; O_2	Chest tube with Heimlich valve	
	Apnea	Mouth-to-mouth ventilation	Bag-valve-mask with O_2	Continue artificial ventilation	
	Cardiac arrest*	External cardiac compressions; try early defibrillation	Continue ECC; start IV; O_2	Drugs; defibrillation	
	Exsanguinating hemorrhage	Manual control of bleeding	MAST; IV infusions; O_2		
	Tension pneumothorax	O_2; needle decompression		Chest tube with Heimlich valve	
	Pericardial tamponade		O_2; ECC	Evacuate blood from pericardium	
	Impending shock		O_2; MAST	IV infusions	
	Massive hemothorax		O_2	Chest tube	
Second	Head injury		Secure airway; O_2		Stabilize cervical spine
	Evisceration			IV; cover viscera	
	Open fractures			Dress wounds	Splint
	Spinal injuries			Immobilize	
Third	Lesser fractures, wounds				Splint; dress wounds

*Treat only if cardiac arrest is not the consequence of trauma and there are more than enough rescuers at the scene; otherwise bypass.

2. The rest of the rescuers split off, one by one, to attend the first-priority patients as they are identified by the triage officer.

This process should be accomplished within the first minutes of arriving at the scene. As soon as the triage officer has completed his first round of triage, and therefore has a grasp of the magnitude of the situation, he or she should radio for whatever additional help is needed and also see that receiving hospitals are placed on standby alert. One rescuer should thereafter be assigned the job of communications officer, to maintain the flow of information from the scene to medical command or to receiving hospitals.

INFORMATION GATHERING AND RECORD KEEPING

One person at the scene should be assigned the task of collecting information from the victims. A record must be made of every casualty at the scene, and the record must be updated each time a casualty is evacuated from the scene, to indicate the patient's destination. It is also important to determine who is *not* at the scene; that is, are there any victims unaccounted for? People suffering injury may become dazed and wander off from an accident scene. Only by keeping track of who has already been treated will it be possible to determine whether it is necessary to start a search for missing casualties.

From conscious patients, it is important to obtain identifying information (name, age) along with an AMPLE medical history, as described in the previous chapter. That information, together with details of the physical assessment and treatment, is best recorded on a TRIAGE TAG affixed to the patient.

A triage tag should be made of a durable material than can withstand wet weather and dirt, and it should be big enough to be easily handled and readily seen. The tag should have a sturdy tie or wire to enable it to be attached to the patient's wrist or clothing, and it should have space for at least the following information:

TRIAGE TAG INFORMATION

- IDENTIFYING INFORMATION
  Name:
  Age:
  Address:
  Next of kin:
  Telephone:

- INFORMATION ABOUT THE SCENE
  Location in which patient was found:
  Position in which patient was found:
  Evidence relating to mechanism of injury:

- MEDICAL HISTORY
  A   Allergies:
  M   Medications:
  P   Past history of hospitalizations; blood type:
  L   Last meal:
  E   Events of the injury:

- PHYSICAL ASSESSMENT (name of examiner: _____)
  Vital and neurologic signs:
  Pertinent physical findings:

- TREATMENT
  Time, drug, dose, route:

- PRIORITY

The last-mentioned category of information, priority, is best indicated by using **color-coded tags** or affixing a color-coded sticker to the triage tag during the first round of triage. In some EMS systems, a priority *number* is simply written with blue felt-tip marker on each patient's forehead. Various other methods have been suggested for assigning priorities and tagging patients; in general, the simplest method is usually the best. The purpose of any labelling method—whether tags or stickers or numbers on the forehead—is to indicate to the rescuers which patients are most urgently in need of ongoing attention, according to the judgment of the triage team leader.

One way for an ambulance service to stay prepared for triage decisions in multicasualty incidents is to triage *every* patient seen during routine, day-to-day calls. If you get used to assigning a triage category as a matter of course in every call, it will not be so difficult to do so when the big call comes.

PRIORITIES FOR EVACUATION

It is necessary to assign priorities for evacuation only in instances where the number of casualties to be evacuated at any given moment vastly exceeds the immediate evacuation capability. That is usually *not* the case. In most mass casualty situations, in both peace- and wartime—at least in industrialized countries—there are a sufficient number of evacuation vehicles to maintain a steady flow of casualties from the scene, and the principle of evacuation under such circumstances is very simple:

THOSE WHO ARE STABILIZED FIRST ARE EVACUATED FIRST.

Thus, in a given situation, the first ambulance leaving the scene may be carrying a critically injured patient considered to be in the "load-and-go" category along with one of the "walking wounded" who requires little if any treatment at the scene.

In the situation in which there are insufficient numbers of evacuation vehicles, however, priorities must be assigned to decide who is evacuated first. There are various systems for determining those priorities, and opinions on the matter differ even among the experts. One widely used system is as follows:

PRIORITIES FOR EVACUATION

- **Priority I**: Patients in persisting danger of asphyxia or exsanguination, including patients with
  1. THORACIC INJURIES
     a. Massive hemothorax
     b. Cardiac tamponade
     c. Thoracoabdominal injuries
  2. Any INJURIES THAT THREATEN THE AIRWAY
  3. SHOCK
- **Priority II**:
  1. Stabilized PATIENTS IN DANGER OF SHOCK, such as those with
     a. Blunt abdominal trauma
     b. Widespread burns
  2. Patients with closed head injury and a DETERIORATING LEVEL OF CONSCIOUSNESS
- **Priority III**: Patients with
  1. SPINAL CORD injuries
  2. EYE injuries
  3. HAND injuries
  4. Major COMPOUND FRACTURES or injuries to large areas of muscle
- **Priority IV**: Patients with lesser fractures and soft tissue injuries
- **Priority V**: "Walking wounded"

Just as important as deciding who gets evacuated is deciding *where* they will be evacuated to. Close communications must be maintained with all hospitals within a reasonable distance of the incident to avoid overburdening any given hospital or sending patients with special needs to hospitals that cannot meet those needs. Just launching ambulances rapidly from the disaster scene, without regard to the situation at receiving hospitals, merely relocates the disaster from the street to the emergency room. One person at the scene must be in charge of "traffic control," to ensure a reasonable distribution of patients among regional hospitals. In general, it is a good idea to send patients with less serious injuries to the hospitals more distant from the disaster scene, since patients with minor injuries are more likely to be able to tolerate longer transport times. But one must also take into account the specialty capabilities of different hospitals (e.g., which hospital has a burn unit, which has a spinal cord unit) and their patient load at any given time.

As each evacuation vehicle leaves the scene, the communications officer or the driver of the vehicle should radio the receiving hospital with the following information:

INFORMATION FOR RECEIVING HOSPITAL

- Number of casualties en route
- For each casualty (starting with the most seriously injured):
  1. Age, sex, and chief complaint
  2. Level of consciousness
  3. Pulse, respirations, skin condition (blood pressure if taken)
  Do *not* waste time transmitting nonessential information!
- Estimated time of arrival (ETA)

GENERAL GUIDELINES FOR MASS CASUALTY INCIDENTS

Situations involving many casualties put everyone under stress—the victims, bystanders, and rescue personnel alike. Most people are not at their best under such circumstances, and it is important therefore to know what to expect from others and what to ask of oneself in a multicasualty situation.

Responses of Patients and Bystanders to Mass Casualties

As we learned in Chapter 4, it is possible to classify the most common responses to a disaster situation into five categories:

- The NORMAL REACTION is one of extreme *anxiety*, manifested by sweating, weakness, nausea, and sometimes even vomiting. EMS personnel are not immune to such reactions, but usually they or anyone else showing signs of severe anxiety can be quickly mobilized to provide useful assistance if given firm direction. Instructing an

EMT to "Get that leg splinted," for example, or telling a bystander, "Please hold this IV bag for me" may be all that is required to pull someone out of his initial emotional shock.

- A more worrisome reaction is BLIND PANIC, in which the person's judgment seems to disappear altogether. Blind panic is particularly dangerous because it can precipitate mass panic among others present. For that reason, a panicky bystander should be separated from others and placed under the supervision of a responsible person.
- Traumatic DEPRESSION is seen in the individual who sits or stands in a numbed, dazed state. Like the person experiencing a normal reaction to a disaster, the person who reacts with depression may also be capable of helping out if given firm guidance.
- The bystander displaying OVERREACTION, on the other hand—talking compulsively, joking inappropriately, running from one task to another without doing anything useful—cannot be of help. Such a person will only get in the way and impede the efforts of others, so he or she needs to be removed from the disaster scene, again in the company of a responsible person.
- Another not at all uncommon response to a disaster is a CONVERSION REACTION, in which the patient subconsciously converts his anxiety into a bodily dysfunction; he may be unable to see or hear or may become paralyzed in an extremity. Hysterical coma, sometimes called "shock" by lay persons, is in this category and may initially be difficult to distinguish from coma due to closed head injury. A person suffering a conversion reaction will not be able to assist the rescue effort in any way and, like the individuals showing signs of blind panic and overreaction, needs responsible supervision.

The rescuer who can quickly spot the characteristic reactions to disaster will be better able to organize those at the scene who are capable of helping out (and will be more tolerant of those who are not).

Guidelines for Behavior in Mass Casualties

By definition, multicasualty or mass casualty situations are exceedingly difficult situations. There is inevitably a lot of noise, confusion, blood, and gore. Working conditions are usually difficult and often downright hazardous. Victims are screaming for help. Rescue personnel are shouting orders to one another. Two-way radios are squawking on a dozen frequencies, and bullhorns are blaring. The equipment you need isn't where you put it because someone else has used it. Those things hardly ever happen during a disaster drill, but they almost always happen when the real thing comes along. So that is the first thing you need to remember about a mass casualty situation:

> **MASS CASUALTY INCIDENTS NEVER GO BY THE BOOK.**

Every multicasualty or mass casualty incident is different; each one will require a somewhat different response. But there *are* some general guidelines that apply across the board to all multicasualty incidents and that can help pilot you through a chaotic scene:

- TREATMENT OF SERIOUS PHYSICAL INJURIES HAS PRIORITY, but psychologic treatment should not be overlooked altogether. If you forget who belongs in which treatment category, use the ABCs as your guide to priorities.
- RESCUE PERSONNEL SHOULD IDENTIFY THEMSELVES and take command of the situation with self-assurance and a sympathetic but businesslike manner.
- ASSIGN TASKS TO RESPONSIBLE BYSTANDERS, both to keep them occupied (and thereby lessen their anxiety) and to relieve rescue personnel of nonmedical tasks. (Conduct a mental disaster drill and make a list for yourself of the tasks that bystanders can usefully carry out.)
- KEEP SPECTATORS AWAY. If bystanders are not usefully occupied, they should be kept out of the triage area. Ask public safety officers at the scene to help secure the area.
- ACCEPT EACH PERSON'S RIGHT TO HAVE HIS OWN FEELINGS. Let the patient know you are trying to understand his feelings in order to help him. Don't try to tell him how he *should* feel.
- ACCEPT EACH CASUALTY'S LIMITATIONS AS REAL, including emotional limitations; shattered feelings are just as disabling as shattered limbs. Do not try to force a casualty to overcome his handicaps. Rather, try to identify his remaining strengths that can be put to use.
- GIVE SEDATIVES ONLY AS A LAST RESORT. In most instances, they will only add to the victim's confusion and in the case of the physically injured may mask important symptoms. A calm, reassuring attitude on the part of the rescuer is the best sedative.

- ACCEPT YOUR OWN LIMITATIONS. Establish priorities, and do what is within your capabilities. If you try to do more than that, you will only decrease your potential effectiveness.

GLOSSARY

staging area Area at a mass casualty incident at which ambulances are stationed until they are needed for evacuation of patients.

triage System for categorizing and sorting patients according to the severity of their injuries.

triage area Area at a mass casualty incident in which casualties are assembled for more efficient sorting and treatment.

FURTHER READING

Auf der Heide E. *Disaster Response: Principles of Preparation and Coordination.* St. Louis: Mosby, 1989.

Beinin L. *Medical Consequences of Natural Disasters.* New York: Springer-Verlag, 1985.

Borden FW. Earthquake planning and preparedness. *Emerg Med Serv* 14(3):12, 1985.

Bowen TE, Bellamy RF (eds.). *Emergency War Surgery: Second United States Revision of the Emergency War Surgery NATO Handbook.* Washington, D.C.: U.S. Government Printing Office, 1988.

Butman AM. The challenge of casualties en masse. *Emerg Med* 15(7):110, 1983.

Caroline NL. *Emergency Medical Treatment: A Text for EMT-As and EMT-Intermediates* (3rd ed.). Boston: Little, Brown, 1991. Chap. 18.

Centers for Disease Control. Tornado disaster—Pennsylvania. *MMWR* 34(51), 1986.

Eisner ME et al. Evaluation of possible patient survival in a mock airplane disaster. *Am J Surg* 150:321, 1985.

Feldstein BD et al. Disaster training for emergency physicians in the United States: A systems approach. *Ann Emerg Med* 14:36, 1985.

Garcia B. Picking & choosing. *Rescue* 2(4):15, 1989.

Garvin JM et al. The logistics of a disaster drill: Medex 78. *Emerg Med Serv* 10(1):41, 1981.

Goodwin C. Rethinking triage. *Emergency* 26(3):41, 1993.

Griffiths RW. Management of multiple casualties with burns. *Br Med J* 291:917, 1985.

Halpin T. Who's on first? *Emergency* 22(8):34, 1990.

Hartman K, Allison J. Expected psychological reactions to disaster in medical rescue teams. *Milit Med* 146:323, 1981.

Haynes BE et al. A prehospital approach to multiple-victim incidents. *Ann Emerg Med* 15:458, 1986.

Kelly JT. Model for pre-hospital disaster response. *J World Assoc Emerg Disaster Med* 1:80, 1986.

Longmire AW, Ten Eyck RP. Morbidity of hurricane Frederic. *Ann Emerg Med* 13:334, 1984.

Mahoney LE, Reutershan T. Catastrophic disasters and the design of disaster medical care systems. *Ann Emerg Med* 16:1085, 1987.

Mathews TP. Triage 81. *J World Assoc Emerg Disaster Med* 1:153, 1985.

Orr SM, Robinson WA. The Hyatt Regency skywalk collapse: An EMS-based disaster response. *Ann Emerg Med* 12:601, 1983.

Rund DA, Rausch TS. *Triage.* St. Louis: Mosby, 1981.

Safar P. Resuscitation potentials in mass disasters. *J World Assoc Emerg Disaster Med* 2:34, 1986.

Sanner PH, Wolcott BW. Stress reactions among participants in mass casualty situations. *Ann Emerg Med* 12:426, 1983.

Schwartz TJ. Model for pre-hospital disaster response. *J World Assoc Emerg Disaster Med* 1:78, 1986.

Tornado disaster—North Carolina, South Carolina, March 28, 1984. *JAMA* 253:2637, 1985.

Villazon-Sahagun A. Mexico City earthquake: Medical response. *J World Assoc Emerg Disaster Med* 1:15, 1986.

When disaster strikes in Boston. *Emerg Med* 15(10):28, 1983.

Yates DW. Major disasters: Surgical triage. *Br J Hosp Med* 22:329, 1979.

V

MEDICAL EMERGENCIES

22
Respiratory Emergencies

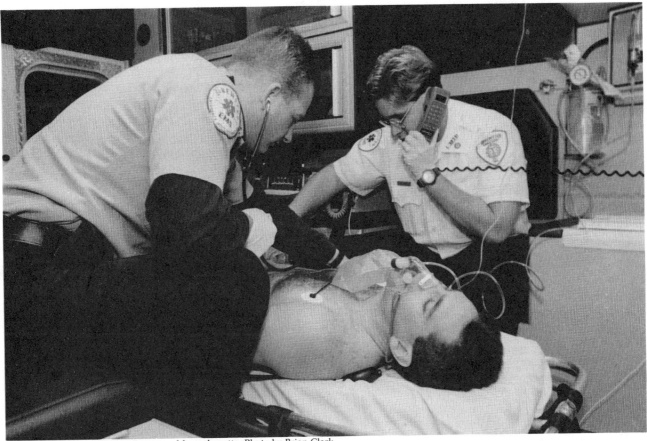

Brewster Ambulance Service, Brewster, Massachusetts. Photo by Brian Clark.

OBJECTIVES

There are few incentives to dial 911 more powerful than the feeling of being unable to breathe (dyspnea). In the majority of cases, that distressing feeling is caused by a problem in the respiratory system itself. In this chapter, we shall examine some of the respiratory problems that produce dyspnea. We shall begin by briefly reviewing the anatomy and function of the respiratory system. We shall next consider the assessment of a patient whose chief complaint is dyspnea—what aspects to emphasize in taking the history and carrying out the physical examination. Then we shall look at some of the problems that may beset each component of the respiratory system—from the respiratory control center in the brain to the smallest functional unit of respiration in the lung, the alveolus. In the process, we shall also consider what may happen to the lungs of a person who ascends very high into the mountains or descends into the watery deep. By the end of this chapter, the student should be able to

1. Describe the effects on arterial PCO_2 of
   • Increasing the minute volume
   • Decreasing the minute volume
2. List six conditions that can cause shunt
3. List six questions that should be asked in taking the history from a patient whose chief complaint is dyspnea
4. List four signs of respiratory distress
5. In the examination of a patient with respiratory complaints, explain the significance of
   • Various abnormal respiratory noises
   • Distended neck veins
   • An abnormal ratio of inhalation to exhalation
   • A silent chest
6. Given a description of several patients with different clinical findings, identify a patient with:
   • Chronic obstructive pulmonary disease (COPD)
   • Asthma
   • Pneumonia
   • Smoke or toxic gas inhalation
   • Pulmonary embolism
   • High-altitude pulmonary edema
   • Pickwickian syndrome
   • Hyperventilation syndrome
   • Pulmonary overpressurization syndrome
   • Dysbaric air embolism
   • Decompression sickness
   and describe the appropriate prehospital management of each
7. Explain in one word under what circumstances oxygen should be withheld from a dyspneic patient

8. List five clinical signs pointing to particular severity of an acute asthmatic attack
9. List four causes of wheezing other than asthma
10. List the steps that should be taken upon finding a swimmer
    • Struggling to stay afloat in deep water
    • Floating facedown in a swimming pool
11. List five symptoms or signs of acute mountain sickness, and specify which symptom or sign is the most reliable indicator of a potentially serious problem
12. List five symptoms or signs that a person rescued from a fire has probably suffered significant respiratory injury, and specify which symptom or sign indicates imminent airway obstruction
13. List the therapeutic effects, indications, contraindications, potential side effects, and correct dosages of
    • Oxygen
    • Terbutaline
    • Isoetharine or albuterol/salbutamol
    • Aminophylline
    • Magnesium sulfate
    • Sodium bicarbonate
    after studying the sections relevant to each of those drugs in the Drug Handbook at the end of this textbook.

REVIEW OF RESPIRATORY ANATOMY AND FUNCTION

In Chapter 8, we examined the structure and function of the respiratory system in some detail. Here we shall review that material only briefly, in order to appreciate what points in the system are vulnerable to illness or dysfunction.

Components of the Respiratory System

Take a moment to look at Figure 22-1 and to review the structures that make up the respiratory system. Recall that regulation of the whole system is carried out by centers in the medulla, part of the BRAINSTEM. There, information regarding the blood concentrations of oxygen, carbon dioxide, and hydrogen ions (pH), along with data on the degree of stretch in the lung at any given moment, is processed and orders are issued to the respiratory muscles. Impulses arising in those medullary control centers are then transmitted via the SPINAL CORD, then out through PERIPHERAL NERVES to the RESPIRATORY MUSCLES—specifically, the *diaphragm* and the *intercostal muscles*.

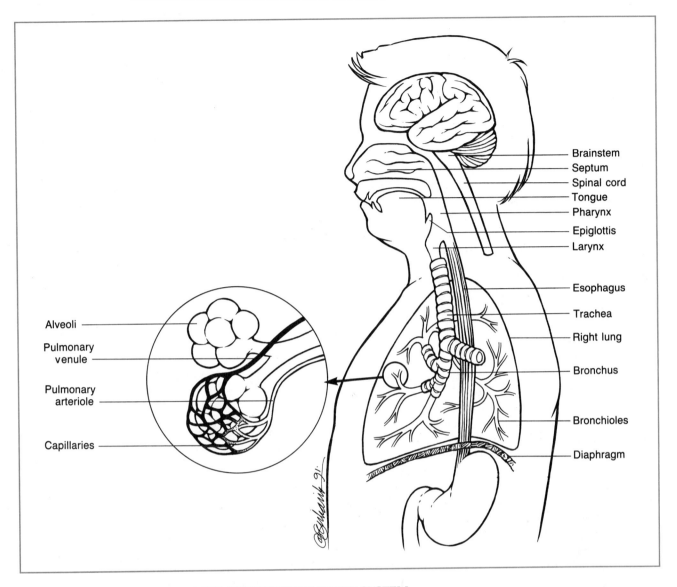

FIGURE 22-1. **MAIN COMPONENTS OF THE RESPIRATORY SYSTEM.**

The business end of the respiratory system resides in the lungs, which are made up primarily of air spaces and blood vessels. Air enters the body through the NOSE or MOUTH, which together with the PHARYNX and LARYNX constitute the *upper airway*. From the standpoint of emergency medicine, all the air passages south of the vocal cords—the TRACHEA, BRONCHI, and BRONCHIOLES—are considered the *lower airways*, terminating in the ALVEOLI, the tiny sacs in which the business of gas exchange actually takes place. (All the air passages from the mouth up *to* the alveoli are considered **dead space,** because the air in those passages does not participate in gas exchange with the blood.)

PULMONARY ARTERIES leaving the right side of the heart enter the lungs carrying blood that has been relatively depleted of oxygen in its transit through the body. Subdividing into smaller and smaller arterioles, the arteries at last become tiny CAPILLARIES that wrap around each alveolus. There, at the alveolar/capillary interface, venous blood gives up its excess carbon dioxide and takes on a fresh load of oxygen. It is then transported through a system of ever larger veins into the PULMONARY VEINS, which carry oxygenated blood back to the left side of the heart.

Breathing Revisited

Breathing, as we recall, is achieved through the rhythmic contraction and relaxation of the respiratory muscles, which leads to rhythmic changes in intrathoracic pressure. Contraction of the diaphragm and the intercostal muscles initiates *inhalation*. As the diaphragm contracts, it flattens and descends into the abdomen (thus the abdominal contents are pushed downward, and the wall of the abdomen bulges outward). At the same time, contraction of the intercostals moves the ribs upward and outward. The net effect is to increase both the vertical and horizontal dimensions of the chest cavity and thus to increase its volume. Since the air within the lungs now suddenly occupies a larger space, the pressure inside the chest falls below that of the atmosphere outside, and air flows from the outside of the body into the lungs until the pressures are equalized. Inhalation, therefore, is an *active* process, requiring muscle contraction, although ordinarily it is perceived as effortless.

Exhalation, on the other hand, is a passive process requiring only that the respiratory muscles relax and return to their resting state. As they do so, the chest wall recoils, intrathoracic pressure rises, and air is expelled from the lungs. Normally, the expiratory phase of breathing takes only about half as long as the inspiratory phase.

The movement of air in and out of the lungs (specifically, in and out of the alveoli) is called **ventilation,** and we can assess the efficiency of ventilation by measuring the amount of CARBON DIOXIDE in a person's blood. That, in fact, is precisely what the chemoreceptors in the brainstem are doing moment by moment to determine the optimal respiratory rate and depth, and under normal circumstances it is the CO_2 concentration in the blood that drives respiration. By definition, normal ventilation is that which maintains the arterial PCO_2 around 35 to 40 torr. Sometimes that may require breathing faster or more deeply than usual—as, for example, after you have run up six flights of stairs and your muscles have, in the process, generated an unusually large load of CO_2. So we cannot say that a person is "hyperventilating" or "hypoventilating" merely on the basis of his respiratory rate or depth. In the absence of arterial blood gas measurements (which are not usually available in the field!), we need to look for other clues to help us decide whether the patient is blowing off enough, too much (**hyperventilation**), or too little (**hypoventilation**) CO_2. We shall discuss some of those clues later on in the chapter.

The other job of the lungs, besides excreting carbon dioxide produced in metabolism, is of course to furnish the red blood cells with OXYGEN. To do so, the lungs need intact alveoli that are being regularly supplied with fresh air from outside the body. If some alveoli are collapsed or filled with anything other than fresh air (such as edema fluid, pus, toxic gases), the blood passing by those alveoli will not pick up oxygen; instead, it will return to the left side of the heart empty-handed, so to speak, as if it had never passed through the lungs at all. That situation—the return of deoxygenated blood from the lungs to the left heart—is what we call **shunt,** and its severity can be assessed by measuring the amount of oxygen in the patient's arterial blood. In a normal person breathing ambient air, the arterial PO_2 should be around 80 to 100 torr. When the arterial PO_2 falls significantly below that level, the patient is considered **hypoxemic.**

Sustained hypercarbia (i.e., failure to keep the arterial PCO_2 below 50 torr) or sustained hypoxemia (i.e., failure to maintain an arterial PO_2 above 60 torr) constitutes **respiratory failure.** The principal causes of carbon dioxide excess and oxygen deficiency were discussed in detail in Chapter 8 and are summarized here in Table 22-1.

A Systems Approach to Respiratory Emergencies

We have seen that the respiratory system consists of several components, not all of them in the chest:

COMPONENTS OF THE RESPIRATORY SYSTEM	
BRAIN	Seat of the respiratory center, thus the source of respiratory control.
SPINAL CORD, NERVES, and RESPIRATORY MUSCLES	The spinal cord and nerves transmit the orders of the respiratory center to the respiratory muscles, which carry them out.
AIRWAYS	The passages through which air travels to the lungs (pharynx, larynx, trachea, bronchi, and bronchioles).
ALVEOLI	The functional units of the lungs, where gas exchange with the blood is accomplished.
PULMONARY CIRCULATION	The vessels that carry blood to the alveoli for pickup of oxygen and elimination of carbon dioxide.

Each component of the respiratory system may suffer dysfunction, leading to respiratory insufficiency.

TABLE 22-1.   CAUSES OF BLOOD GAS ABNORMALITIES

Elevated PCO_2 (hypercarbia, hypercapnea)	• Increased CO_2 production
	  1. Fever
	  2. Muscular exertion
	  3. Anaerobic metabolism
	• Decreased CO_2 elimination (hypoventilation)
	  1. Decreased tidal volume
	    a. Pain (rib fractures, pleurisy)
	    b. Weakness (myasthenia gravis)
	    c. Paralysis (spinal cord injury, polio)
	  2. Decreased respiratory rate
	    a. Head injury
	    b. Depressant drugs
	    c. Cerebrovascular accident (stroke)

Decreased PO_2 (hypoxemia, shunt)	• Fluid in the alveoli
	  1. Pulmonary edema
	  2. Pneumonia
	  3. Near-drowning
	  4. Chest trauma
	• Collapsed alveoli (atelectasis)
	  1. Airway obstruction
	    a. By the tongue
	    b. By a foreign body
	  2. Failure to take deep breaths
	    a. Pain (rib fracture, pleurisy)
	    b. Paralysis of respiratory muscles (spinal cord injury, polio)
	    c. Depression of the respiratory center (head injury, drug overdose)
	  3. Collapse of the whole lung (pneumothorax)
	• Other gases in the alveoli
	  1. Smoke inhalation
	  2. Inhalation of toxic chemicals
	  3. Carbon monoxide poisoning
	• Respiratory arrest

Head trauma or anything else that disturbs the function of the BRAIN (Fig. 22-2A) may depress the respiratory control centers in the medulla. We have already seen, for example, how in closed head trauma increasing intracranial pressure may literally put the squeeze on the medulla to produce a variety of respiratory abnormalities including apnea. As we shall see in later chapters, a *stroke* may have a similar effect by depriving portions of the brain of circulation. *Overdose with drugs* such as heroin or barbiturates may also severely depress the activity of the respiratory center.

Looking at the next component of the respiratory system, we have already seen, in Chapter 16, how injury high in the SPINAL CORD may paralyze the intercostal muscles and even the diaphragm. *Polio*—thankfully now rare in developed countries—attacks the NERVES that supply the respiratory muscles, while certain chronic illness, such as *myasthenia gravis*, weaken the RESPIRATORY MUSCLES themselves. The net effect of any of those conditions is an inability of the respiratory muscles to contract normally in response to the respiratory drive. Thus, the tidal volume is shallow, and the minute volume is correspondingly decreased. (What happens to the arterial PCO_2?) Patients with such conditions often need assisted ventilations to increase the tidal volume.

The UPPER AIRWAY, as we learned in Chapter 7, may be jeopardized in a number of ways (Fig. 22-2B). Most commonly, the *tongue* is the culprit in upper airway obstruction, but a *foreign body, swelling* of structures within the airway, or *trauma* to the larynx or trachea may also compromise the upper airway. The LOWER AIRWAYS, that is, the subdivisions of the bronchi, are also subject to clogging, swelling, and muscular spasm in acute conditions like *asthma* and chronic conditions such as *chronic bronchitis*.

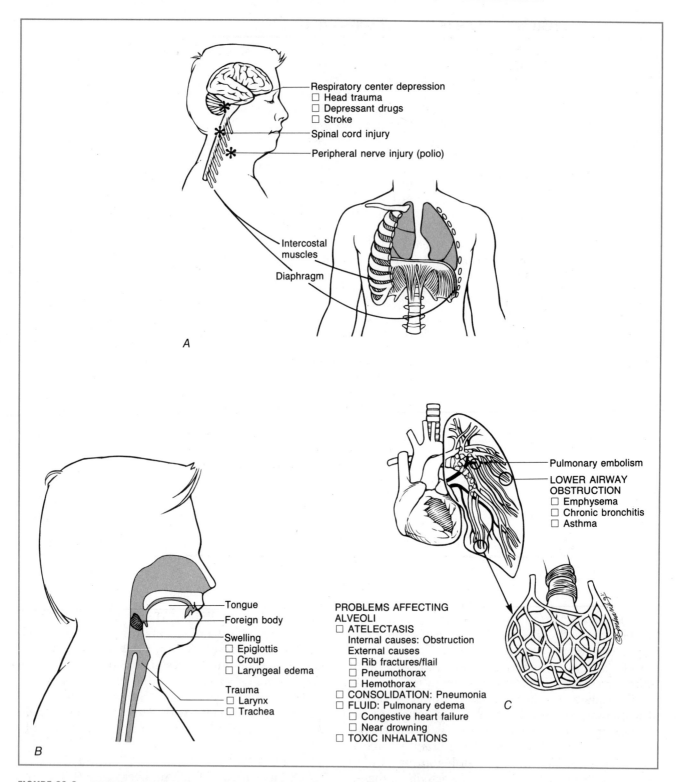

A

B

C

FIGURE 22-2. **LEVELS OF RESPIRATORY SYSTEM DYSFUNCTION.** (A) The respiratory center, spinal cord, peripheral nerves, and respiratory muscles. (B) The upper airway. (C) The lower airways, alveoli, and pulmonary arteries.

TABLE 22-2.　SYSTEMS APPROACH TO RESPIRATORY INSUFFICIENCY

RESPIRATORY SYSTEM COMPONENT AFFECTED	PATHOLOGIC CONDITION	FURTHER DISCUSSION
Brain: respiratory center	Head trauma	Chapter 16
	Overdose with depressant drugs	Chapter 27
	Cerebrovascular accident (stroke)	Chapter 24
Spinal cord, nerves, and respiratory muscles	Spinal cord injury	Chapter 16
	Nerve damage: poliomyelitis	
	Muscle weakness: myasthenia gravis	
Airway	Upper airway obstruction	Chapter 7
	Obstructive disease of the lower airways	Chapter 22
Alveoli	Atelectasis	
	• From airway obstruction	Chapter 7
	• From rib fracture, pneumothorax	Chapter 17
	Pneumonia	Chapter 22
	Drowning	Chapter 22
	Pulmonary edema	Chapter 23
	Toxic inhalations	
	• Toxic gases	Chapter 22
	• Carbon monoxide	Chapter 27
Pulmonary circulation	Pulmonary embolism	Chapter 22
	Air embolism	Chapters 9, 16
	Amniotic fluid embolism	Chapter 35
Other	Pickwickian syndrome	Chapter 22
	Hyperventilation syndrome	Chapter 22

Getting down to the business end of the lungs, the ALVEOLI are subject to any number of disorders (Fig. 22-2C). They may collapse (**atelectasis**) from *obstruction* somewhere in the proximal airways or from external pressures produced, for example, by *pneumothorax* or *hemothorax*. They may fill with pus in *pneumonia*, with blood in *pulmonary contusion*, or with fluid in *near drowning* or congestive *heart failure*. Or the nice fresh air that they are supposed to contain may be displaced by smoke or *toxic gases*.

Finally, the PULMONARY CIRCULATION may be compromised by a wandering blood clot (**embolism**), a globule of fat from a broken bone (fat embolism), a leakage of amniotic fluid from the amniotic sac of a pregnant woman (amniotic fluid embolism), or even an air bubble entering the circulation from a laceration of the neck or an improperly assembled IV administration set (air embolism). A large embolism, of whatever type, will lodge in a major branch of the pulmonary artery and act as a plug to prevent any blood flow through that branch.

The disorders affecting each component of the respiratory tract are summarized in Table 22-2, which also indicates in which chapter of this book the principal discussion of each respiratory disorder can be found.

ASSESSMENT OF PATIENTS WITH DYSPNEA

As noted earlier, *acute respiratory insufficiency* is defined, strictly speaking, as any situation in which the arterial PCO_2 rises above 50 torr or the arterial PO_2 falls below 60 torr or both. However, those measurements of arterial blood gases are not ordinarily available in the field—and certainly not when you need them the most! (If you doubt that assertion, try performing pulse oximetry on a 200-pound patient in heart failure who is frantic from hypoxemia. You won't try it a second time.) You must learn, therefore, to assess a patient's respiratory status from *clinical* observations, that is, from the patient's story and from the evidence of your senses.

As always, the assessment of the patient begins with the primary survey: ABC. Assuming that the patient is conscious and his airway is unobstructed, you may proceed straight to the secondary survey.

Taking the History

The Chief Complaint

The chief complaint of a patient with respiratory problems is almost invariably **dyspnea** or "air hunger," that is, the *sensation* of being short of breath. The patient with dyspnea *feels* that breathing is difficult. Ordinarily, as we mentioned earlier, breathing is nearly effortless, and we proceed with whatever we are doing without giving any thought to the contraction and relaxation of our respiratory muscles. When a person involuntarily becomes *aware* of his breathing, that is already a sign that something is not quite right; and when breathing requires conscious *effort*, there is definitely a problem.

Dyspnea, in fact, may arise from a number of different inputs to the brain—signals from chemoreceptors monitoring levels of CO_2, acid, and oxygen in the blood; from stretch receptors monitoring expansion and relaxation of the chest muscles; and from higher centers in the brain that interpret internal and external stimuli in light of past experience.

History of the Present Illness

Like any other chief complaint, the chief complaint of dyspnea requires elucidation. The same PQRST-A system we used to explore the chief complaint of pain can also be used, with a minor modification, to find out more about a patient's shortness of breath:

P   What PROVOKED the dyspnea? That is, what (if anything) brought it on? **Paroxysmal nocturnal dyspnea,** that is, dyspnea that comes on suddenly in the middle of the night, may signal heart failure or worsening of chronic obstructive pulmonary disease (COPD); it occurs because of accumulation of fluid in the alveoli or pooling of secretions in the bronchi during sleep. What PALLIATES the dyspnea (makes it better)? Is it provoked or palliated by any particular *position?* **Orthopnea** is dyspnea that gets worse in the recumbent position and is often related to congestive heart failure. (It should be noted, however, that *most* patients with dyspnea resist a recumbent

position and feel most comfortable sitting up straight, even leaning forward a bit.)

Q   What is the QUALITY of the dyspnea; that is, what precisely does it feel like? Ask the patient, "Do you feel as if you can't get air in, or do you feel as if you can't get air out—or both?"

R   When we were considering pain as a chief complaint, *R* stood for "radiation." With regard to dyspnea, *R* stands for RECURRENCE; that is, has this problem happened before? Dyspnea that has been present for a long time, or that has been coming and going over an extended period, has a very different significance from dyspnea that came on suddenly without any prior history of respiratory problems.

S   How SEVERE is the dyspnea? In taking the history, what you are interested in is the *patient's* assessment of the severity of his symptoms; when you perform the physical examination, you can form your own conclusions. If the patient suffers from a chronic problem, such as asthma or chronic bronchitis, ask him to compare this episode with others, or to compare the severity of his dyspnea today with that of a day ago. As a general rule, people with chronic illnesses do not call for help unless something has *changed*—usually for the worse—but it's worth inquiring precisely what the change has been. Ask in detail about any diminution of functioning (e.g., "How many stairs can you climb this week without stopping for breath? How many could you climb last week?").

T   What is the TIMING of the symptoms? When did the dyspnea start? Did it come on suddenly, from one moment to the next, or gradually over hours or days? The dyspnea associated with asthma or congestive heart failure may develop gradually, over several hours, while that associated with pulmonary embolism or spontaneous pneumothorax may come on with striking suddenness.

A   Are there any ASSOCIATED SYMPTOMS? Ask specifically whether the patient is a smoker and whether he has been *coughing.* If he has a cough, is he bringing up *sputum?* What does the sputum look like? Patients with COPD often "keep a cough" associated with thick, white sputum; when such patients decompensate, the volume of their sputum increases and it becomes **purulent**—yellow-green in color, sometimes with a bad smell. Purulent or rust-colored sputum may also be associated with pneumonia. The patient with pulmonary edema, on the other hand, often produces foamy, blood-tinged sputum—sometimes in alarming quantities. Coughing of frank blood may be associated with a variety of conditions, including heart disease, tuberculosis, and trauma to the lungs.

Ask also about *pain.* If there is pain associated with the dyspnea, what is it like? Dyspnea that comes on abruptly together with sudden, sharp chest pain may indicate a spontaneous pneumothorax; pulmonary pain, on the other hand, suggests heart failure secondary to myocardial infarction.

Other Medical Problems

After the inquiries into the patient's present illness are complete, it is still necessary, as we learned in Chapter 11, to obtain some further information about the patient's medical background, specifically:

- Does the patient have any MAJOR UNDERLYING MEDICAL PROBLEMS? Ask specifically about a history of lung diseases, heart disease, high blood pressure, and diabetes—any of which may be related to the episode of dyspnea. The patient in congestive heart failure, for example, may have a long history of cardiac problems or hypertensive disease. The patient with pneumonia may have an underlying illness, such as AIDS, that made him more susceptible to pneumonia.
- Find out what, if any, MEDICATIONS the patient takes regularly. "Breathing pills" and inhalants suggest obstructive airway disease; digitalis indicates that the patient is under treatment for an underlying cardiac problem. "Water pills" (diuretics) may be taken for high blood pressure or chronic heart failure. The patient taking "blood thinners" (anticoagulants) may have had a previous episode of pulmonary embolism. A list of medications commonly taken by patients with respiratory problems is provided in Appendix II at the end of this chapter.
- Does the patient have any known ALLERGIES? The patient who tells you that he is allergic to aspirin may well be an asthmatic, for the incidence of aspirin allergy is higher in asthmatics than in the general population.
- Who is the patient's DOCTOR, and at what HOSPITAL, if any, has he been treated in the past?

The Physical Examination

By the time you have elicited the history from a patient with respiratory complaints, you in fact already have some important information about the patient's physical signs, for you have already had a chance to observe his level of consciousness, his position, his degree of distress, and so forth. For didactic purposes, however, let us proceed through the steps of the physical assessment in sequence, noting at each step the points of particular relevance to the dyspneic patient.

General Appearance

Recall from Chapter 12 that the assessment of a patient's general appearance takes into account the following:

- The POSITION in which a dyspneic patient is found may be very revealing. As noted earlier, a patient who is truly in respiratory distress will almost invariably be sitting bolt upright, often leaning forward.
- Assessing the LEVEL OF CONSCIOUSNESS is enormously important in dyspneic patients. While we cannot ordinarily measure the patient's arterial blood gases in the field, the patient's brain is constantly doing precisely that. Any fall in arterial PO_2 (hypoxemia) will be registered as restlessness, confusion, and sometimes combative behavior. A rise in the PCO_2, on the other hand, usually has narcotic effects, making the patient sleepy and hard to rouse.
- The patient's DEGREE OF DISTRESS is usually not difficult to gauge. Is the patient struggling to breathe? Is he showing signs of stress, such as sweating? Did his dyspnea make it hard for him to answer your questions in full sentences, so that he could only gasp out a few words at a time? Or did questions easily distract him from his symptoms?
- The SKIN CONDITION can tell you about the patient's peripheral perfusion and perhaps something about his state of oxygenation. Cyanosis, if present, suggests hypoxemia—but its absence does not by any means rule out inadequate oxygenation.

Nearly all of the information just described in several paragraphs can, in fact, be taken in at a glance during the first moments of contact with the patient. That glance should tell you just how urgent the problem is and therefore what steps need to be taken right away. As a general rule, every patient whose chief complaint is dyspnea should be given oxygen within

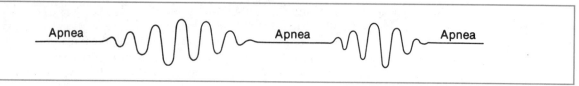

FIGURE 22-3.　CHEYNE-STOKES RESPIRATIONS.

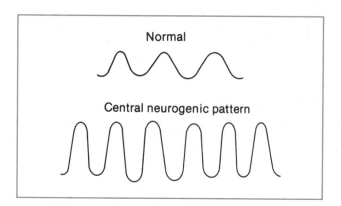

FIGURE 22-4.　CENTRAL NEUROGENIC HYPER-
VENTILATION.

the first minute of your contact with him. Whether
any further urgent measures are needed before you
complete the history and physical examination will
depend on the patient's overall condition.

Vital Signs

While all the vital signs must be measured in the dyspneic patient, clearly the vital sign with which we
shall be most concerned is *respiration:*

- First, count the respiratory RATE. Recall that in
  the healthy adult, the rate of breathing at rest is
  usually around **16 breaths per minute.** Very rapid
  breathing (**tachypnea**) may signal impending respiratory failure. Very slow breathing implies
  depression of the respiratory center and is more
  likely to be seen in unconscious patients than in
  those awake enough to report dyspnea.
- At the same time as you are counting the respirations, observe the respiratory RHYTHM. Normal breathing is fairly regular, but illness may
  produce an abnormal breathing pattern. Recall
  that in **Cheyne-Stokes** respirations (Fig. 22-3),
  periods of rapid, irregular breaths—in a cres-
  cendo-decrescendo pattern—alternate with periods of apnea. Cheyne-Stokes respirations may
  occur in a variety of neurologic or metabolic derangements, many of which are reversible. More
  worrisome is **central neurogenic hyperventila-**

tion (Fig. 22-4), characterized by very deep, very
rapid respirations (hyperpnea and tachypnea).
The **Kussmaul's breathing** of a diabetic in ketoacidosis is also very deep and rapid.

- Note the EASE OF RESPIRATIONS. Normal
  breathing, as we have noted, is relatively effortless. A patient in respiratory trouble, by contrast,
  will show signs of effort and distress:

**SIGNS OF
RESPIRATORY DISTRESS**

- NASAL FLARING—the nostrils open wide on
  inhalation.
- TRACHEAL TUGGING—the Adam's apple is
  pulled upward and the area just above the sternal notch is sucked inward with inhalation.
- RETRACTION OF THE INTERCOSTAL MUS-
  CLES on inhalation.
- Use of ACCESSORY MUSCLES in the neck and
  abdomen to assist breathing—PARADOXICAL
  RESPIRATORY MOVEMENT (the epigastrium
  is pulled in with inhalation, rather than bulging
  out).

- Try to evaluate the DEPTH of respiration (tidal
  volume). Bare the patient's chest, and *look* at the
  ventilatory excursions of the chest wall. Place the
  back of your hand near the patient's mouth and
  feel how much air is expelled during exhalation
  (for comparison, test your own exhalations the
  same way). A patient with an inflammation involving the pleura, and sometimes a patient with
  a pulmonary embolism, will breathe very shallowly because it hurts to take deeper breaths.
  Shallow breathing also characterizes patients
  who have overdosed with depressant drugs.
- Listen for ABNORMAL RESPIRATORY NOISES.
  As a general rule, *any* respiratory noises that you
  can hear without a stethoscope are abnormal
  noises, because normal breathing is quiet:

NOISY BREATHING IS OBSTRUCTED BREATHING.

Recall that **snoring** indicates partial obstruction of the upper airway by the *tongue*—a form of obstruction that is easily corrected by head tilt maneuvers; **gurgling** signals the presence of *fluid* in the upper airway; **stridor**, a harsh, high-pitched sound heard on inhalation, indicates *narrowing*, usually as a result of swelling (**laryngeal edema**).

- The last aspect of assessing the respirations at this point in the examination is to note any ABNORMAL ODORS ON THE BREATH. A fruity smell on the patient's breath, for example, may go a long way toward explaining why the patient has hyperpnea and tachypnea.

Head-to-Toe Survey

One of the principal purposes of the head-to-toe survey of the dyspneic patient is to try to establish whether the underlying problem comes from the lungs or from the heart. Pay particular attention, therefore, to the following:

- As you examine the *head*, check the MUCOUS MEMBRANES of the conjunctivae and lips for cyanosis.
- In the *neck*, look for JUGULAR VENOUS DISTENTION with the patient in a semisitting position, which provides a rough measure of the pressure in the right atrium of the heart; thus distended neck veins may implicate cardiac failure as the source of the patient's dyspnea. (In chest trauma, as we learned, neck vein distention may have other significance.)
- We now come to the more detailed examination of the *chest*.
  1. First *look* at the chest wall. Is its anterior-posterior diameter greater than normal (BARREL CHEST), suggesting chronic obstructive pulmonary disease? Is the SPINE ABNORMALLY CURVED (scoliosis), a condition that may lead to chronic respiratory difficulties? Does the chest appear HYPERINFLATED, as it sometimes does in severe cases of emphysema or asthma? If so, *percuss* over the chest to see whether it has an unusually hollow sound.
  2. Now, *listen* with a stethoscope. Listen for at least one respiratory cycle, first at each base, then at each apex, front and back. Note the RATIO OF INHALATION TO EXHALATION. As we mentioned earlier, inhalation normally occupies about two-thirds of the respiratory

cycle and exhalation one-third. A PROLONGED INSPIRATORY PHASE of respiration suggests obstruction of the *upper* airway (the patient will probably have stridor as well); a PROLONGED EXPIRATORY PHASE is most typically seen in conditions characterized by obstruction of the *lower* airways (e.g., asthma). Listen as well for ABNORMAL BREATH SOUNDS:

ABNORMAL BREATH SOUNDS

- **Crackles:** Any discontinuous noises heard on auscultation of the lungs, caused by the popping open of air spaces and usually associated with increased fluid in the lungs; formerly called *rales* and *rhonchi*.
- **Wheezes:** High-pitched, whistling sounds made by air flowing through narrowed airways. Wheezing may be diffuse in conditions like asthma and congestive heart failure or may be localized when due to a foreign body obstructing a bronchus.
- **Silence:** The most ominous breath sounds are no breath sounds at all! If you don't hear anything with your stethoscope, it means the patient is not moving enough air to ventilate his lungs. SILENCE MEANS DANGER!

---

3. *Feel* the chest for vibrations as the patient speaks (**vocal fremitus**). Normally those vibrations are felt equally on both sides of the chest. However, if air is not moving effectively into one side of the chest—as is the case, for example, when a bronchus is obstructed—vocal fremitus will be diminished or absent on the affected side.

- In examining the *abdomen*, pay particular attention to the LIVER in the right upper quadrant. A palpable, painful liver may signal the presence of congestive heart failure.
- Palpate the lower *back* for EDEMA, yet another tip-off to the presence of heart failure.
- Finally, in examining the *extremities*, look for CLUBBING of the fingers, a sign of chronic respiratory problems. The fingers may also reveal CIGARETTE STAINS, which speak for themselves. Check the lower extremities for PEDAL EDEMA (swelling of the feet), very often a sign of congestive heart failure.

By the time you have completed your assessment of the patient, which should not take more than 2 or 3 minutes, you should be able to form some impressions of the diagnostic possibilities, some of which we shall now proceed to consider.

OBSTRUCTIVE AIRWAY DISEASES

Obstructive airway diseases are those characterized by diffuse obstruction to air flow within the lungs. The most common obstructive airway diseases are emphysema, chronic bronchitis, and asthma, which as a group affect as many as 10 to 20 percent of adults in the United States. Emphysema and chronic bronchitis are together classified as *chronic obstructive pulmonary disease* (COPD), or chronic obstructive lung disease (COLD), for the changes in pulmonary structure and function are chronic, progressive, and irreversible. Asthma is considered a separate entity since—at least in its early stages—it is by definition a condition of *reversible* airway narrowing.

Chronic Obstructive Pulmonary Disease

Chronic obstructive pulmonary disease is a common disorder, affecting approximately 15 million Americans. In 1988, nearly 82,000 people in the United States died from COPD, and 82 percent of that mortality was attributable to CIGARETTE SMOKING. Mortality from COPD, furthermore, has been increasing steadily over the past 10 to 15 years. It is highly likely, therefore, that every ambulance service will see a considerable number of patients suffering from COPD. The condition is more common in men than in women, and more common in city dwellers than in rural populations; it is seen primarily in individuals between 45 and 65 years of age.

Clinical Features of COPD

Theoretically, COPD comprises at least two distinct clinical entities: emphysema and chronic bronchitis.

EMPHYSEMA is characterized by distention of the air spaces (groups of alveoli) beyond the bronchioles, with destructive changes in their walls. As the supporting structure of the air spaces is lost, the small airways are more prone to collapse under the negative pressure of inhalation. The patient with emphysema often reports *weight loss*, and the typical history is one of increasing *dyspnea on exertion*, with progressive limitation of activity. Coughing may *not* be a prominent feature of the illness; if the patient does

report a cough, it is usually productive of only small quantities of mucus. Patients with classic emphysema tend to maintain fairly normal arterial blood gases and are not usually cyanotic; for that reason, they are sometimes referred to as "pink puffers." On physical examination, the patient with emphysema appears *thin and wasted*, often with prominent neck muscles. The chest is *barrel-shaped* and *hyperresonant* to percussion, owing to air-trapping within the lungs. Breath sounds are distant and difficult to hear. The patient may appear obviously short of breath and often *purses his lips* during exhalation.

CHRONIC BRONCHITIS is officially defined as sputum production most days of the month for 3 or more months out of the year for more than 2 years. What the official definition makes clear is that a cardinal feature of chronic bronchitis is *excessive mucus production* in the bronchial tree, which is nearly always accompanied by a chronic or recurrent productive *cough*. The typical patient with chronic bronchitis is almost invariably a heavy cigarette smoker. He is usually somewhat obese, with a congested, sometimes bluish complexion—features that have inspired the term "blue bloater" to describe this type of patient. His blood gases tend to be abnormal, with an elevated PCO_2 (hypercarbia) and a decreased PO_2 (hypoxemia). Often he has associated heart disease and right heart failure (**cor pulmonale**).

It is important to point out that the "pink puffer" and "blue bloater" in fact represent two extremes of a whole spectrum of clinical pictures. In the real world, most patients with COPD fall somewhere between those two extremes, showing signs and symptoms of both.

Patients with COPD ordinarily come to some sort of *modus vivendi* with their disease. Over the years, they learn how much exertion they can tolerate, in what position sleep is possible, and so forth. So when a patient with COPD calls for an ambulance, it nearly always means that *something has changed*—changed for the worse. Patients with established COPD are extremely vulnerable to episodes of acute decompensation leading to respiratory failure. Such episodes are often triggered by respiratory infection, but they may be simply the result of exhaustion; for unlike a person with normal lungs, for whom breathing is a relatively effortless affair, the patient with COPD has to expend a great deal of effort to breathe; edema of the airways, secretions in the airways, bronchospasm—all of those add immensely to the mechanical load on the respiratory muscles.

The patient with an acute decompensation of COPD may report a *change in the character of his sputum*, usually an increase in volume along with a change in color from white to yellow or green. His dyspnea increases, often to the point that it disturbs his sleep. He may complain of headache, or others may report a change in his behavior.

On physical examination, the patient is likely to be in marked respiratory distress. Increasing degrees of hypoxemia lead to sweating, cyanosis, confusion, agitation, and sometimes twitching of the muscles, while hypercarbia is more likely to manifest itself as drowsiness. Vital signs will usually show tachypnea and tachycardia, often with an irregular heart beat. The blood pressure may be markedly elevated, in part because of the stress associated with hypoxemia. If right heart failure is part of the picture, there will be jugular venous distention. Patients with chronic bronchitis will usually have a very noisy chest, a veritable symphony of crackles and wheezes, while the chest of a patient who is more toward the emphysematous end of the spectrum may be ominously quiet.

SUMMARY: SYMPTOMS AND SIGNS OF DECOMPENSATION IN COPD

- Increasing dyspnea
- Sleep disturbance
- Change in color and volume of sputum
- Altered mental state:
  1. From hypoxemia: confusion, agitation, combativeness
  2. From hypercarbia: lethargy, drowsiness
- Marked respiratory distress
- Cyanosis
- Cardiac dysrhythmias

Treatment of COPD in Acute Decompensation

The prehospital management of a patient in acute decompensation of COPD is aimed primarily at *relieving hypoxemia*, for it is hypoxemia that will kill him fastest. OXYGEN, therefore, IS THE MAINSTAY OF TREATMENT IN COPD. Oxygen in itself improves respiratory muscle function, helps to correct right heart failure and pulmonary hypertension, and prevents complications of hypoxemia such as seizures and myocardial infarction. A great deal of nonsense has been promulgated on the subject of giving oxygen to patients with COPD, so it is worthwhile to take a moment here to consider the subject.

Even today, many textbooks carry dire warnings against giving supplemental oxygen to patients with COPD. The rationale is that patients with COPD pre-

sumably derive their drive to breathe from hypoxemia, so if you correct the hypoxemia, they will stop breathing. To begin with, there is *no convincing evidence* to support that view (see Aubier et al. and Sassoon et al. in the Further Reading list at the end of this chapter). To the contrary, the few careful studies done on the subject have demonstrated that, if anything, patients with COPD have a higher than normal drive to breathe and that giving oxygen does nothing to depress that drive. Even, however, if it *were* the case that oxygen therapy suppresses the drive to breathe in patients with decompensated COPD, that would *not* constitute sufficient grounds for withholding oxygen therapy—for the patient may die without oxygen. If there indeed exists a danger that oxygen administration will lead to apnea, the solution to the problem is to *keep an eye on the patient*, not to deny him the one drug that can save his life! If he stops breathing, ventilate him with a bag-valve-mask. This point cannot be overemphasized:

NEVER, NEVER, NEVER WITHHOLD OXYGEN THERAPY FROM ANY PATIENT IN RESPIRATORY DISTRESS, EVEN (OR ESPECIALLY) A PATIENT WITH COPD.

If the patient needs oxygen, provide it generously. Start with nasal cannula at about 4 to 5 liters per minute, because a frantic, combative patient may not tolerate a mask very well. If the patient develops respiratory depression—which is more likely to occur as a result of sheer exhaustion than of oxygen therapy—then assist him to breathe. But NEVER, NEVER hesitate to administer oxygen to any patient suspected of acute respiratory insufficiency. No patient with COPD ever died from respiratory depression secondary to supervised oxygen therapy; scores of patients with COPD die from hypoxemia. So once again, remember the golden rule:

NEVER WITHHOLD OXYGEN FROM ANY PATIENT WHO NEEDS IT. A PATIENT WITH COPD NEEDS IT.

As to *other measures* in the treatment of COPD, observe the following guidelines:

- The patient will probably be most comfortable in the SITTING position.
- Establish an IV LIFELINE with D5/W to a keep-open rate.
- Administer a selective **beta-2 sympathomimetic drug,** such as ALBUTEROL (salbutamol) *or* ISO-ETHARINE, by metered-dose inhaler (preferred) or nebulizer (see Appendix I of this chapter for the technique of giving drugs by metered-dose inhaler).
- While no longer considered a drug of choice, AMINOPHYLLINE is still used by some physicians in the treatment of COPD. If your supervising physician orders aminophylline, first confirm that the patient has not taken a similar drug himself during the past few hours (see Appendix II to this chapter). If he has not, add 250 mg of aminophylline to a 250-ml bag of D5/W, to run at a rate specified by the physician (usually about 0.5 mg/kg/hr).
- DO NOT GIVE SEDATIVES OR TRANQUILIZERS! If the patient is frantic, it's because he can't breathe and he's not getting enough oxygen. The treatment is to give him oxygen, not to depress his respirations further!
- Encourage the patient to cough up his secretions and to take deep breaths.
- MONITOR cardiac rhythm. Dysrhythmias are common in acute decompensations of COPD, and fatal dysrhythmias are not unlikely, especially if hypoxemia is not rapidly corrected.

Asthma

The word *asthma* is actually a Greek word that means "panting," and it was applied to the disease we know as asthma by the second century Greek physician Aretaeus, "because in the paroxysms, the patients also pant for breath."

Bronchial asthma is characterized by an increased reactivity of the trachea, bronchi, and bronchioles to a variety of stimuli. That hyperreactivity results in widespread, *reversible* narrowing of the airways (**bronchospasm**). The disease afflicts approximately 6 million Americans, of whom about 4,000 to 5,000 die from asthma each year. Asthma begins before age 10 in about half the cases and before age 30 in another third. Often the disease is present in more than one member of the same family. Asthma characteristically occurs in *acute attacks* of variable duration. Between attacks, the patient may be relatively symptom-free.

Three distinct pathologic processes produce the airway obstruction that leads to an ACUTE ASTHMATIC ATTACK:

- BRONCHOSPASM, that is, spasm of the smooth muscle that surrounds the bronchioles, causing a decrease in bronchiolar diameter; bronchospasm develops very rapidly and can be relieved very rapidly by giving medications that relax smooth muscles (see Table 22-3).
- SWELLING of mucous membranes in the bronchial walls. Mucosal edema develops relatively slowly, over hours to days, at least partly in response to chemical mediators of inflammation released from *mast cells.*
- PLUGGING of bronchi by thick, mucous secretions.

Clinical Features of the Acute Asthmatic Attack

The acute asthmatic attack may be brought on by an allergic reaction to inhaled irritants, by respiratory infection, or by emotional stress. Narrowing of the airway and increased amounts of tenacious sputum interfere with air flow, especially on exhalation, with the result that the chest becomes progressively *hyperinflated* and the patient is able to move less and less air in and out. If the attack has gone on for any period of time, *dehydration* is also often part of the picture and may contribute to the thickness of mucus in the airways.

In the typical attack, the patient is found sitting up, often leaning forward and fighting to breathe. He may be coughing spasmodically and unproductively. Use of accessory muscles of respiration is prominent, and the chest is relatively fixed in the inspiratory position. Hyperinflation makes the chest hyperresonant to percussion. Wheezing is usually quite audible, even without a stethoscope, *but* keep in mind that it takes two things to make a wheeze: narrowed airways *and* air flow. If the attack is very severe and there is scarcely any air moving in and out of the lungs, wheezes may be absent.

> **IN THE ACUTE ASTHMATIC ATTACK, SILENCE IS NOT GOLDEN—IT'S DEADLY!**

When you first encounter the patient, take a brief history to find out how long the attack has been going on and, very importantly, WHAT MEDICA-

TIONS HE HAS ALREADY TAKEN. The physician at medical command may be hesitant to order epinephrine in the field, for example, for a patient who has already taken a near overdose of related drugs from a pocket inhaler. As you question the patient, you can form an impression of his degree of distress and evidence of hypoxemia.

In examining the patient, be alert for the following signs that suggest a particularly severe attack:

SIGNS OF A SEVERE ASTHMATIC ATTACK

- Pulse rate > 130 per minute
- Respiratory rate > 30 per minute
- Pulsus paradoxus > 15 mm Hg*
- Retraction of the neck muscles on inhalation
- Restlessness, faintness, agitation
- Silent chest

Status asthmaticus is a severe, prolonged asthmatic attack that cannot be broken with conventional treatment. IT IS A DIRE MEDICAL EMERGENCY. Just as the patient with COPD ordinarily does not call for an ambulance unless there has been a marked change in his condition, so too the average asthmatic does not dial 911 unless the attack is much worse than those he usually has to deal with. So it is a reasonably safe assumption that

---

ANY ASTHMATIC WHO FEELS SICK ENOUGH TO CALL AN AMBULANCE IS IN STATUS ASTHMATICUS UNTIL PROVED OTHERWISE.

On examining the patient in status asthmaticus, you will find him fighting desperately to move air through his obstructed airways, with prominent use of accessory muscles of respiration. The chest is maximally hyperinflated. Breath sounds and wheezes may be entirely inaudible because air movement is negligible. The patient is usually exhausted, severely acidotic, and dehydrated.

---

*Recall from Chapter 17 that pulsus paradoxus is the decrease in systolic blood pressure with inhalation.

Treatment of the Acute Asthmatic Attack

The prehospital management of the acute asthmatic attack is aimed at relieving bronchospasm and thereby improving ventilation. Measures may also be taken to address the swelling and mucous plugging of the airways. Remember, however, that before administering any medications to an asthmatic, *find out what he has already taken!*

The types of medication used to treat bronchial asthma are summarized in Table 22–3. Of the medications listed in the table, clearly those of relevance to the prehospital phase of treatment are those with a rapid onset of action. Medications that require hours to days before they take effect can wait until the patient is thoroughly evaluated in the hospital.

The following, then, are the steps in treating the severe acute asthmatic attack:

- Ensure an open AIRWAY.
- Administer OXYGEN by nonrebreathing mask, if the patient will tolerate it, otherwise by nasal cannula at 4 to 6 liters per minute. Do *not* use the unmodified demand valve, since it delivers dry gases to the airway and thus tends to worsen the problem of thick secretions.
- Establish an IV LIFELINE with D5/W or normal saline.
- Give a beta-2 adrenergic drug by metered-dose inhaler (see Appendix I of this chapter for instructions on use of the inhaler). This author prefers ALBUTEROL (salbutamol) *or* ISOETHARINE, 1 to 2 inhalations. You may repeat the dosage after 15 minutes if there is no response.
- The patient with a *very severe asthmatic attack* may not be moving enough air to inhale medication from a metered-dose inhaler. If that is the case, you may be instructed instead to inject TERBUTALINE, 0.25 mg SQ (adult dosage). Repeated injections every 15 minutes may be needed in status asthmaticus.
- For patients in status asthmaticus, the physician may also order SODIUM BICARBONATE, 50 to 100 mEq IV, to counteract the metabolic component of the patient's acidosis.
- If you are a considerable distance from the hospital, it may also be worthwhile to start corticosteroids in the field, such as METHYLPREDNISOLONE, 60 to 100 mg IV.
- Recent research suggests that MAGNESIUM SULFATE is of considerable use in the treatment of acute asthmatic attacks. If ordered for asthma, the dosage is 1.2 gm of magnesium sulfate diluted in 50 ml of saline and infused IV over about 30 minutes.

TABLE 22-3. PHARMACOTHERAPY FOR BRONCHIAL ASTHMA

TYPE OF DRUG	COMMON EXAMPLES	MECHANISM OF ACTION	ONSET OF ACTION	MAXIMUM EFFECT	DURATION OF ACTION	SIDE EFFECTS
Beta agonist	Albuterol, metaproteronol, terbutaline, isoetharine	Bronchodilator	5 min (inhaled)	30 min	3–6 hr	Tremor, tachycardia, dysrhythmias, cramps
Methylxanthine	Theophylline	Bronchodilator Enhances contractility of the diaphragm Respiratory center stimulant	3–5 min (IV)	20 min	? hr	Tremor, tachycardia, dysrhythmias, seizures, gastrointestinal upsets
Anticholinergic	Ipratropium bromide	Smooth muscle relaxant	15 min (inhaled)	1–2 hr	3–6 hr	Minimal; can worsen glaucoma
Corticosteroids	Prednisone, prednisolone beclomethasone	Anti-inflammatory	8–12 hr (oral) Days (inhaled)	24 hr Not known	24 hr 4–6 hr	Multiple with long-term use Oral thrush
Mast cell inhibitors	Cromolyn sodium	Prevents release of chemical mediators of inflammation	Days to weeks	Days to weeks	Not known	Occasional allergic reaction

- DO NOT GIVE SEDATIVES, which may depress respirations, OR ANTIHISTAMINES, which may dry secretions. Do *not* give aspirin, since many asthmatics are allergic to aspirin.

The management of acute asthmatic attacks in children is discussed further in Chapter 30.

When dealing with any asthmatic patient, it is particularly important to maintain a calm, reassuring attitude. The asthmatic having an acute attack, particularly a severe attack, is invariably anxious and may indeed be panic-stricken, as would just about anyone who found themselves suddenly unable to breathe. If you allow yourself to be infected by the patient's panic, you will become part of the problem rather than part of the solution. Panic can also kill. What the asthmatic needs is to feel safe in competent hands.

Finally, a note of caution:

ALL THAT WHEEZES IS NOT ASTHMA.

Among the several other causes of diffuse wheezing are acute left heart failure ("cardiac asthma"), smoke inhalation, chronic bronchitis, and acute pulmonary embolism. Localized wheezing reflects an obstruction, by foreign body or tumor, in a specific area. Only a careful history and physical examination will enable you to reach the correct diagnosis. It is particularly important to distinguish the wheezing of asthma from that caused by left heart failure, since the treatment of the two conditions is markedly different. We shall discuss left heart failure in the next chapter, and the differentiation between it and asthma will be summarized in Table 23-6.

ALVEOLAR DYSFUNCTION

Up to now, we have considered illnesses that affect primarily the conducting airways. In this section, we shall consider a variety of conditions that interfere with alveolar function. Already in Chapter 17, we learned about some of those conditions—flail chest, pneumothorax, hemothorax—which interfere with alveolar function by causing alveolar collapse. Alveoli can also be rendered inoperative, however, if they become filled with any sort of fluid or any gas other than fresh air.

Pneumonia

One way that alveoli can become nonfunctional is if they fill up with pus, as occurs in pneumonia. Like the collapsed or fluid-filled alveolus, the alveolus consolidated with pus does not participate in gas exchange. Pus-filled alveoli thus contribute to *shunt,* and hypoxemia may be the result.

Pneumonia may be caused by a variety of bacterial, viral, and fungal agents. Bacterial pneumonia is responsible for about 10 percent of hospital admissions in the United States and, even in this era of antibiotics, still carries a mortality of between 5 and 10 percent. The elderly, patients with chronic illnesses, and smokers are at greater risk to contract the illness. The most common form of bacterial pneumonia is *pneumococcal pneumonia,* which strikes about 1 out of every 500 Americans annually, the peak incidence being in winter and early spring.

The patient with pneumonia usually reports several hours to days of *weakness,* productive *cough, fever,* and sometimes chest pain made worse by cough. The illness may have started abruptly with a shaking chill (**rigor**) or more gradually with progressive weakness.

On physical examination, the patient with pneumonia usually *appears very ill.* He may or may not be coughing. In classic pneumococcal pneumonia, cough may be absent early on, but when it does develop it is often productive of a rust-colored sputum. The skin of the patient with pneumonia feels hot. Depending on the degree of pulmonary consolidation, the patient may show minimal or marked respiratory distress, but vital signs usually reveal both *tachypnea* and *tachycardia. Crackles* may be heard on auscultation of the chest, and there may also be increased vocal fremitus. Sometimes the abdomen is distended.

Definitive treatment of pneumonia usually requires hospitalization. All that is necessary in the field is to administer OXYGEN (why?) and transport the patient in the position he or she finds most comfortable.

Near Drowning

Another possible source of alveolar dysfunction is *fluid* in the alveoli. When the fluid gets into the lungs from immersion in water, we are talking about drowning. About 1 out of every 9 or 10 submersion incidents in the United States results in death. When death does occur, we use the term **drowning;** when there is at least temporary survival after submersion, we call it **near drowning.**

Approximately 9,000 persons drown each year in the United States, making drowning the third leading cause of accidental death. At least another 70,000 people are *near*-drowning victims every year. Among adults, alcohol intoxication is a factor in about one-half of drownings. Among children, swimming pool drownings account for a third of the total, the vast majority of which occur at the child's own house or the house of a neighbor.

Pathophysiology of Drowning

Near drowning generally follows a predictable sequence, sometimes referred to as the "hypoxic march":

- As the victim goes under and water enters his mouth and nose, he begins to *cough* and *gasp,* and he *swallows* considerable amounts of water.
- At the same time, a very small amount of water is aspirated into the larynx and perhaps the trachea, setting off spasms of the laryngeal muscles (**laryngospasm**) that effectively seal off and protect the airway, at least temporarily, from further aspiration.
- Like any other form of airway obstruction, laryngospasm leads to **asphyxia,** that is, a combination of hypoxemia and hypercarbia, and the patient may *lose consciousness.* Hypoxemia, meanwhile, leads to a shift from aerobic to anaerobic metabolism, with the production of lactate and the development of *metabolic acidosis.* If the patient dies during this phase of laryngospasm, as occurs in about 10 to 15 percent of drowning cases, it is essentially a death from suffocation, for the lungs are still dry ("dry drowning"). More commonly, however, the drowning process progresses to the next phase.
- At a certain point, which varies from person to person, *water begins to enter the lungs.* That may occur because the hypercarbic and hypoxic drives stimulate inhalation or, if the patient has lost consciousness, because progressive asphyxia causes the laryngeal muscles to relax. In either case, the net effect is to permit water to gain access to the lungs ("wet drowning"). That triggers an increase in peripheral airway resistance along with constriction of pulmonary vessels, all of which decrease the compliance of the lungs. The lungs, that is, become stiff.
- The *decompensation stage* of drowning occurs next. The victim gasps for air, inhaling yet more water, which mixes with air and chemicals in the lung to form froth. *Apnea* recurs, and if he has not done so already, the patient loses consciousness. The process of hypoxic brain damage gets under way, and cardiac arrest also occurs.

Response to the Near-Drowning Incident

In general terms, the resuscitation of a victim of near drowning is the same as that for any other patient in respiratory or cardiac arrest, but clearly there are a few additional logistic problems.

First, of course, you must REACH THE VICTIM, with due concern for your own safety; it serves little purpose for an unqualified swimmer to enter the water in an attempt to rescue a drowning person, since the most likely outcome is two drowning persons. All water rescue courses teach the basic sequence of rescue procedures:

REACH AND PULL	When the victim is alert and close to shore, hold out something for him to grab—a rope, a stick, a ladder—and PULL him from the water.
THROW	If he is alert but too far to reach, THROW an object that will float (foam cushion, plastic cooler, inflatable splint, even the spare tire from the ambulance).
TOW	Once the victim is hanging on to a flotation device, find a way to TOW him to safety. Toss him a rope or wade out as far as waist deep to reach him with a stick.
GO	If the victim is too far out or unconscious, *and* if you know how to swim, GO to him by boat (you must wear a personal flotation device). Only as a *last resort,* when all of the other measures fail, may you GO into the water and swim to the patient—and then *only* if you are a qualified swimmer trained in lifesaving.

When you reach the victim, the steps of treatment follow the usual sequence of ABC. For purposes of treatment at the scene, it is of no importance whether the drowning occurred in fresh water or salt water. First priority, as always, goes to establishing the AIRWAY. If the near drowning occurred in a swimming pool or in other circumstances that may have produced neck injury, *support the victim's neck in neutral position* (without flexion or extension), and use chin lift or jaw lift alone to open the airway. When you suspect spine injury, furthermore, the victim should be floated supine onto some form of back support—a wooden backboard, a surfboard, even a door

removed from its hinges—before being removed from the water (see Fig. 16-24).

Rescue BREATHING should be started as soon as possible, *even before the victim is removed from the water.* Do not waste time trying to get water out of the victim's lungs. As noted, 10 percent of drowning victims do not aspirate any water at all; even among those who do aspirate water, the amount is usually modest and—if it is fresh water—it is rapidly absorbed from the lungs into the circulation. Do *not* perform manual thrusts (Heimlich maneuver) to remove water from the lungs. It will not remove water from the lungs, but may very effectively displace it from the stomach *into* the lungs. Reserve the Heimlich maneuver, therefore, for cases in which you find the airway completely obstructed by a foreign body.

As soon as the victim has been removed from the water, start supplementary OXYGEN at the same time as you quickly determine whether a pulse is present. If there is no pulse, begin CHEST COMPRESSIONS. SUCTION as needed. Early ENDOTRACHEAL INTUBATION is indicated in every unconscious near-drowning victim to permit POSITIVE PRESSURE VENTILATION and to protect the airway from aspiration during the vomiting that is almost inevitable in resuscitation from near drowning.

A word here about a technique called positive end-expiratory pressure or PEEP, which means maintaining some degree of positive pressure at the end of the expiratory phase of respiration. Recall that during normal, spontaneous breathing the pressure in the airways at the end of exhalation is effectively zero. As a result, a certain number of alveoli normally collapse during the expiratory phase of the respiratory cycle. When there is widespread atelectasis and shunt—as in near drowning—it is desirable to maintain some positive pressure at the end of exhalation, both to keep alveoli open and to drive any fluid that may have accumulated in the alveoli back into the interstitium or capillaries. In the field, PEEP is indicated for intubated patients who must be transported long distances to the hospital after near drowning or who have other conditions that produce significant shunt.

While there are several ways to create PEEP, the device most useful in the field is a Boehringer valve, which consists of a cylinder in which a metal ball is suspended. When connected to the expiratory port of a bag-valve unit, the valve creates PEEP by forcing the patient to exhale against the weight of the ball. Different valves are available to provide 5, 10, and 15 cm H_2O expiratory pressures. For the device to function properly, the bag-valve must be held so that the Boehringer valve is exactly vertical. In all other respects, ventilation with the bag-valve device is carried out in the usual fashion.

Once an endotracheal tube is in place (but not before!), insert a NASOGASTRIC TUBE to decompress the stomach (see Chap. 27 for technique of nasogastric tube insertion). If the pulse is absent, further advanced life support measures are similar to those in any other case of cardiopulmonary arrest (see Chap. 23): establishment of an IV lifeline, administration of epinephrine, cardiac monitoring, and electric conversion of ventricular fibrillation. In general, near-drowning victims, regardless of whether they suffer cardiac arrest, tend to develop *severe metabolic acidosis,* so—unlike the garden variety cardiac arrest—near-drowning victims may require SODIUM BICARBONATE early in resuscitation. If ordered to do so, give **1 mEq per kilogram** of bicarbonate by IV push as soon as the IV line has been initiated. The patient's acid-base status should be assessed by arterial blood gases at the earliest moment after his arrival at the hospital.

Patients rescued from near drowning are prone to develop bronchospasm from the irritation to their airways. If you hear wheezes, administer a BETA-2 ADRENERGIC AGENT, such as albuterol or isoetharine, by metered-dose inhaler, as you would for a patient having an acute asthmatic attack.

Even if a near-drowning victim seems to have recovered at the scene, he should be transported to a hospital for evaluation. Delayed deaths due to pulmonary edema ("secondary drowning") and aspiration pneumonia are not uncommon, and it is impossible to evaluate the state of the patient's lungs or the adequacy of arterial oxygenation at the scene. Thus, EVERY NEAR-DROWNING VICTIM MUST BE EVALUATED AT A HOSPITAL. While transporting the patient, continue to administer 100% oxygen, and continue resuscitation measures as needed.

One other point deserves emphasis: DO NOT GIVE UP ON A DROWNING VICTIM, especially if the victim is a child and if drowning occurred in cold water. Successful resuscitations with complete neurologic recovery have been reported even in cases in which the victim had been submerged for more than an *hour* in cold water. So even when the victim has been fished out of the water after a relatively long submersion (i.e., more than the "magic" 4 minutes), there is every possibility of restoring him to useful life.

SUMMARY: MANAGEMENT OF NEAR DROWNING

- Do not enter the water to save a drowning victim if you are not a qualified swimmer.
- Ensure an open AIRWAY and start rescue BREATHING even before the victim is removed from the water.
- Continue artificial ventilation, and remove the victim from the water.
- Determine whether the victim has a pulse. If not, start external CARDIAC COMPRESSIONS.
- INTUBATE the trachea of the unconscious victim, and administer OXYGEN under positive pressure.
- Establish an IV LIFELINE.
- Give a BETA-2 ADRENERGIC DRUG by metered-dose inhaler for wheezing.
- Provide advanced life support measures as required.
- Insert a NASOGASTRIC TUBE in intubated patients.
- TRANSPORT *every* near-drowning victim to the hospital, even those who seem to recover at the scene.
- Use BLANKETS to keep the patient warm en route to the hospital.

More and more studies are indicating that if a near-drowning victim is going to be saved at all, he will be saved in the prehospital setting, not in the emergency room or the intensive care unit. This means that prompt, good CPR and advanced life support by paramedics at the scene will make the difference between life and death for the near-drowning victim.

High-Altitude Pulmonary Edema

In drowning, the fluid that gains access to the alveoli comes mostly from *outside* the body. In other circumstances, however, fluid may cross into the alveoli from the pulmonary circulation, a situation referred to as **pulmonary edema.** By far the most common scenario of pulmonary edema is failure of the left side of the heart, causing blood to back up into the pulmonary circulation. We shall consider that condition, known as congestive heart failure, in some detail in the next chapter. There are, however, a number of other pathologic conditions that can produce pulmonary edema, including the aspiration of irritating substances, inhalation of certain toxic fumes, and even insults remote from the lungs such as head injury and heroin overdose. In this section, we shall consider yet another possible cause of pulmonary edema—ascent to high altitudes. Needless to say, this material will be of more relevance to paramedics working in the Rocky Mountain region than those in the plains states!

Precursors: Acute Mountain Sickness

Most people who ascend rapidly to elevations above 8,200 feet (2,500 meters) experience some unpleasant symptoms, at least for a while. And about 1 out of every 10 such people will develop a syndrome called **acute mountain sickness.** One study, for example, found a 12-percent incidence of acute mountain sickness among skiers visiting a Colorado resort at an altitude of between 7,900 and 9,200 feet.

Acute mountain sickness usually develops during the first 8 to 24 hours at altitude. The more rapidly a person makes the ascent, the more likely he is to experience symptoms. Being young and fit confers no particular protection and may even be a liability.

The *symptoms* of acute mountain sickness vary widely in severity among different persons but are all suggestive of a mild increase in intracranial pressure:

SYMPTOMS OF ACUTE MOUNTAIN SICKNESS

- Throbbing, bilateral frontal HEADACHE, worse in the morning and in the supine position, and exacerbated by strenuous exercise
- ANOREXIA (loss of appetite), and in severe cases NAUSEA and VOMITING
- LASSITUDE (fatigue and listlessness)
- SLEEP DISTURBANCE
- DYSPNEA ON EXERTION
- ATAXIA (staggering gait)

Mild forms of acute mountain sickness, which are often described as similar to those of a hangover, do not require any special treatment. The victim must simply stop his ascent and rest, and the symptoms will ordinarily clear up within a day or two.

The most useful sign of progression from mild to moderate mountain sickness is **ataxia,** and any patient complaining of any of the symptoms listed above should have his gait tested. If he cannot walk heel-to-toe, he should, if at all possible, be brought down at once 1,000 to 2,000 feet. If the circumstances make immediate descent impossible, the patient should be kept at rest and given oxygen (at low flows to preserve the oxygen supply) until rescue can be arranged. When you anticipate a long delay, administer *dexamethasone*, 4 mg by mouth every 6 hours.

It is very important to recognize moderate mountain sickness and deal with it promptly, because the majority of patients who develop life-threatening altitude syndromes, such as high-altitude cerebral edema (HACE) or high-altitude pulmonary edema (HAPE), pass through the stage of acute mountain sickness first.

High-Altitude Pulmonary Edema: Signs and Treatment

High-altitude pulmonary edema occurs in susceptible individuals within 24 to 72 hours of making a rapid ascent to altitudes greater than 7,500 feet (2,286 meters). Children and adolescents seem to be particularly vulnerable, as are residents of higher elevations who return home after a period at lower altitude. The onset of symptoms is usually preceded by strenuous exertion, but symptoms may worsen dramatically during sleep, perhaps as a consequence of gravitational effects in the recumbent position.

The earliest SYMPTOM of high-altitude pulmonary edema is usually *decreased exercise performance*, which the patient often shrugs off as fatigue. Other early symptoms, such as unproductive *cough, palpitations* (being aware of one's heart beat), and *dyspnea on exertion*, along with any of the *symptoms of acute mountain sickness* mentioned, also tend to be ignored by macho mountaineers (of both sexes!). Were the mountaineer to stop and rest at the point when such symptoms occur and to delay any further ascent, the symptoms would ordinarily disappear over the next day or two. But if the ascent continues, the full-blown picture of HAPE is very likely to appear.

SYMPTOMS AND SIGNS OF HIGH-ALTITUDE PULMONARY EDEMA

- Severe DYSPNEA
- Cheyne-Stokes respirations
- COUGH productive of pink, frothy sputum
- CYANOSIS
- CONFUSION and sometimes COMA
- Vital signs: TACHYPNEA and TACHYCARDIA
- Auscultation: CRACKLES (starting in the right middle lobe)
- Signs and symptoms of acute mountain sickness

Adequate TREATMENT of high-altitude pulmonary edema depends critically on prompt recognition, for once the victim has reached the stage of gurgling respirations and confusion, he may progress very quickly toward death. The mainstay of treatment is DESCENT to a lower altitude. The victim should be kept warm and assisted downhill so as to minimize his own exertions. If oxygen is available, it should be administered during descent, but descent should never be delayed to wait for someone to bring oxygen.

> **DESCENT TO LOWER ALTITUDE IS THE ONLY EFFECTIVE TREATMENT FOR HIGH-ALTITUDE PULMONARY EDEMA.**

If, for any reason, such as adverse weather conditions, it is impossible to begin the descent immediately, the patient should be kept warm and at rest, breathing supplemental OXYGEN. Ideally, 100% oxygen should be given by demand valve, but supplies of oxygen sufficient to permit sustained demand valve ventilation are rarely available in field situations. If evacuation of the patient is going to be significantly delayed, you may have to husband the oxygen, giving it at 2 to 3 liters per minute by nasal cannula. Delayed evacuation is also an indication for giving DEXAMETHASONE, 4 mg orally or intramuscularly every 6 hours. Other agents that are traditionally used for cardiogenic pulmonary edema—such as morphine and diuretics (see Chap. 23)—have *not* proved effective in HAPE.

Toxic Inhalations

The inhalation of smoke or toxic chemicals can interfere with alveolar function in two ways. To begin with, simply the presence in the alveoli of a gas other than fresh air means that blood passing through the pulmonary capillaries is going to find a reduced concentration of oxygen on the other side of the capillary/alveolar interface. The result will be shunt. Furthermore, in due time—which may be within minutes or, more commonly, hours—the irritant or toxic effects of the inhaled gases are likely to produce an inflammatory response within the lung, causing transudation of edema fluid into the alveolar spaces. The result: more shunt.

It is important to point out that in a fire, the inhalation of superheated *air* in itself rarely produces damage to the lung; dry air is a poor conductor of heat, and the mucous membranes of the upper respiratory tract provide an efficient cooling mechanism. Furthermore, a blast of hot air causes reflex closure of the vocal cords, reducing even further the probability of direct thermal injury to the lower respiratory tract; only inhalation of extremely hot, *wet* air (steam) is likely to cause *thermal injury* to the mucosa of the lungs. However, the *products of combustion* of a variety of common substances (Table 22-4) may produce significant *chemical* injury to the alveoli.

In fact, toxic gases may wreak havoc throughout the whole respiratory system, not just in the alveoli. Smoke inhalation, for example, can produce a broad pattern of respiratory injury, as detailed in Table 22-5.

The first danger that threatens the victim of

TABLE 22-4. TOXIC PRODUCTS OF COMBUSTION

SUBSTANCE	FOUND IN	PRODUCTS OF COMBUSTION	EFFECTS OF EXPOSURE
Polyvinyl chloride	Plastic bottles, electric insulation, car and aircraft upholstery, wall coverings, phonograph records	Hydrogen chloride, phosgene, chlorine, carbon monoxide	Pulmonary edema, mucosal irritation, chest tightness
Polyurethane	Thermal insulation, mattresses, carpets, seat cushions	Hydrogen cyanide, isocyanate, carbon monoxide	Asphyxia
Acrylics	Textiles, paints, aircraft windows	Acrolein, acetic acid, formic acid	Mucosal irritation, asphyxia
Nylon	Clothes, carpeting, upholstery	Ammonia, hydrogen cyanide	Pulmonary edema, asphyxia
Wood, paper, cotton	Furniture, structural materials, paper products, clothing	Acrolein, acetaldehyde, formaldehyde, acetic acid, formic acid	Mucosal irritation

TABLE 22-5. SMOKE INHALATION INJURIES

SITE OF DAMAGE	PATHOLOGIC PROCESS AND CONSEQUENCES*
Upper airway	Chemical mucosal burns by soluble gases (sulfur dioxide, ammonia, chlorine) → **laryngeal edema** and airway obstruction **Laryngospasm**
Trachea/ bronchi	Poisoning of cilia → inability to clear secretions **Bronchospasm** Necrosis of respiratory epithelium Hemorrhagic tracheobronchitis
Alveoli	Alveolar macrophages destroyed, allowing bacteria to proliferate → pneumonia Pulmonary surfactant destroyed → **atelectasis** Capillary leak → pulmonary edema

*Conditions in **boldface** are those that can develop within minutes of injury.

smoke inhalation is *hypoxemia*, for not only does the fire consume oxygen, it also produces other gases, such as methane or carbon monoxide, that can displace oxygen from the alveoli or from hemoglobin. As hypoxemia progresses, metabolism shifts to the anaerobic pathway, setting in motion a process that will lead to *metabolic acidosis*. Hypoxemia may be further aggravated by *bronchospasm*, and *laryngeal edema* may compromise the upper airway. With airway obstruction comes collapse of alveoli (atelectasis). Later on, transudation of fluid into the alveoli may produce chemical pulmonary edema, often complicated by bronchopneumonia. All of those changes add up to shunt.

Fire is the most common scenario of exposure to toxic gases, but certainly not the only scenario. *Chlorine gas exposure*, which may lead to both upper and lower respiratory tract injury, is most apt to take place in industrial settings, municipal swimming pools, or after transport accidents. Inhalation of *nitrogen dioxide*, producing the cough, dyspnea, and crackles characteristic of "silo-filler's disease," rarely occurs any more in silos but does result from exposure to diesel exhaust and from accidents in the transport of nitric acid. The "dung lung" syndrome of pulmonary edema, metabolic acidosis, and cardiovascular collapse, produced by *hydrogen sulfide* (H_2S), got its name because of the hydrogen sulfide hazards to individuals working in sewage systems. In general, gases with high water solubility, like ammonia, are quickly absorbed in the *upper* airway and so do their

principal damage there, causing runny nose, sore throat, and laryngeal edema. The intense upper airway irritation usually prompts the victim to leave the exposure environment as fast as possible, so the lower airway is relatively protected. Gases that are less soluble in water, on the other hand, such as phosgene, may reach the *lower* airway and even the alveoli in sufficient doses to cause injury before there is any symptomatology in the upper airway.

The ABCs of Toxic Inhalation

The ABCs of managing a victim of toxic inhalation in fact begin *before* the ABCs! Recall that the very first step of the primary survey is the survey of the *scene*, and the very first question the rescuer must ask is: "Is it safe for *me* to approach the scene?" Before you even reach the victim, therefore, carry out the following steps:

- ASSESS THE SCENE. Is there any evidence of a chemical agent that could endanger the rescue team? (We shall consider the approach to hazardous materials incidents in more detail in Chap. 34.)
- If you suspect the presence of a toxic or asphyxiating gas, SECURE THE AREA, and summon the appropriate agencies (e.g., police, fire department). Do not allow unauthorized persons to approach.
- Check and then don SELF-CONTAINED BREATHING APPARATUS before entering any suspect environment. When you do enter, use the BUDDY SYSTEM and safety lines.
- Do not under any circumstances remove your breathing mask at any time while you are in the suspect environment.
- Remove the victim to a place UPWIND from the exposure.

Once you and the victim have reached a safe place, it is possible to proceed with the primary and secondary surveys. Conduct the *primary survey* as you would for any other patient, with particular attention to symptoms or signs that foretell impending jeopardy to the AIRWAY. Recall that in patients removed from a fire, burns of the face, singed eyebrows or nasal hairs, blistering inside the mouth, and sooty sputum are all signs that significant smoke inhalation has probably occurred. If in addition you hear hoarseness, stridor, or a brassy cough, it means that *laryngeal edema* is already developing, and it may be only minutes before the airway closes off altogether. If you hear stridor, GET MOVING! And be prepared to perform a cricothyrotomy en route to the hospital.

Any patient who is not BREATHING adequately will need *assisted ventilation*, preferably by demand valve or bag-valve-mask with PEEP to help keep alveoli from collapsing. In any event, *oxygen* must be administered in high concentrations as early as possible.

Some toxic inhalants, such as hydrogen sulfide, are toxic to the heart as well as to the lungs (any toxic inhalation that produces significant hypoxemia will be indirectly toxic to the heart); until you can attach a cardiac monitor, therefore, keep a finger on the patient's pulse, and be prepared to deal with cardiac arrest.

The Secondary Survey and Management

In the course of the secondary survey, try to find out as much as you can about the exposure, particularly:

- The NATURE OF THE INHALANT or combusted material. Many irritant gases combine with water to form corrosive acids and alkalis that cause burns of the upper respiratory tract. Such gases include *ammonia* (which forms ammonium hydroxide), *nitrogen oxide* (nitric acid), *sulfur dioxide* (sulfurous acid), and *sulfur trioxide* (sulfuric acid). In addition, victims of fire may inhale *phosgene*, a gas that is formed by the decomposition of chlorinated hydrocarbons at high temperatures and is a powerful alveolar irritant. (*Poisoning* from smoke inhalation may be due to carbon monoxide or cyanide, discussed in Chap. 27.)
- The DURATION of the exposure.
- Whether the patient was in a CLOSED ENVIRONMENT when the exposure took place. As a general rule, victims trapped in a closed space with toxic fumes are more likely to sustain respiratory tract damage than those out in the open.
- Whether the patient LOST CONSCIOUSNESS in a smoky environment, in which case reflex mechanisms that ordinarily protect the lower respiratory tract may have been impaired.

At the scene of a fire or any other toxic gas exposure, victims may include those found at the scene and rescue personnel. Some victims may remain relatively asymptomatic for periods of a few minutes up to as long as 18 hours before showing signs of pulmonary edema and severe respiratory distress. For that reason, *any* person, including a member of the rescue services, exposed to smoke or toxic gases must be kept under surveillance for 24 hours. Hospitalization may not be necessary, but some form of supervision is. To repeat, NO VICTIM OF SMOKE INHALATION SHOULD BE LEFT ALONE DURING THE FIRST 18 HOURS FOLLOWING THE EXPOSURE, and those keeping an eye on the exposure victim—whether family or colleagues at work—should be aware of the signs of developing respiratory problems.

To summarize, then, the management of patients exposed to smoke or other toxic fumes:

SUMMARY: MANAGEMENT OF PATIENTS EXPOSED TO TOXIC FUMES

- Ensure your own SAFETY before entering a suspect environment.
- REMOVE THE PATIENT from the exposure environment.
- Establish and maintain an AIRWAY. Rapidly developing laryngeal edema may necessitate early endotracheal intubation or cricothyrotomy in the field. *Transport patients with stridor urgently.*
- Assist BREATHING, as required, with the demand valve or bag-valve-mask plus PEEP.
- Administer humidified OXYGEN in high concentrations to *all* patients removed from the area of a fire or from other toxic fumes, regardless of whether they do or do not appear to be in respiratory distress.
- MONITOR cardiac rhythm.
- Establish an IV LIFELINE with D5/W.
- All victims of smoke inhalation should be treated for carbon monoxide poisoning and evaluated for cyanide poisoning as well (see Chap. 27).
- All victims of intense exposure to smoke or toxic fumes should remain under supervision for 18 to 24 hours.

DISRUPTION OF THE PULMONARY CIRCULATION: PULMONARY EMBOLISM

As we have observed, adequate gas exchange in the lungs requires functional alveolar units to provide oxygen and take up carbon dioxide; but gas exchange also requires intact pulmonary vessels to convey oxygen-poor blood to the alveoli. In the preceding section, we looked at some of the pathologic conditions that can interfere with alveolar function. However, even normal alveoli will be of little use if the venous blood cannot reach them. That is the situation in pulmonary embolism.

A **pulmonary embolism** is the sudden blocking of a pulmonary artery or one of its branches by a clot or other obstructing material carried to the site by the blood current. Pulmonary emboli may arise from a variety of sources. Most commonly, BLOOD CLOTS forming in the veins of the legs or pelvis break loose and are swept downstream, through the venous circulation, through the right heart, until they are trapped in the progressively narrowing network of pulmonary vessels. Several factors favor the development of such clots, including:

- *Heart disease,* particularly chronic congestive heart failure.
- Chronic pulmonary diseases, especially *COPD.*
- *Advanced age.*
- *Prolonged immobilization,* as in bedridden patients (or even people sitting for a long time on an aircraft), which causes blood to stagnate in the lower extremities, thus favoring clot formation. Immobilization of the lower extremities in a cast similarly predisposes to the formation of blood clots.
- *Malignancy* (cancer), especially that involving the lungs, gastrointestinal tract, or prostate.
- *Thrombophlebitis,* that is, inflammation of veins, especially those in the legs and pelvis, increases the risk of clot formation and embolism. Patients with thrombophlebitis in the leg will sometimes complain of calf pain, and the calf may be tender to palpation. But thrombophlebitis in the deep pelvic veins may not produce any symptoms at all.
- Certain *drugs*—notably birth control pills—increase the risk of developing pulmonary emboli.

Pulmonary emboli may also form from materials other than blood clots. FAT PARTICLES released from disrupted ends of bone in massive trauma may be carried in the bloodstream and lodge in the pulmonary circulation. Similarly, AMNIOTIC FLUID may find its way into the maternal circulation during delivery and be swept into the mother's lungs. Finally, AIR entering the circulation from a wound in the neck or an improperly functioning IV may obstruct a pulmonary artery as fully as any blood clot.

The *symptoms and signs* of pulmonary embolism will depend on the size of the obstruction. If a large clot lodges in a major pulmonary vessel, gas exchange will be severely impaired, and the patient will experience severe respiratory distress. At the same time, the right heart will have to work much harder than usual to push blood into the clogged pulmonary arteries, so signs of right heart failure (such as distended jugular veins) may also develop.

The typical patient with pulmonary embolism presents with the SUDDEN ONSET of severe, unexplained DYSPNEA. There may be no other symptoms, or the patient may have sharp CHEST PAIN that is made worse by COUGHING or taking a deep breath. On physical examination, there is almost invariably TACHYCARDIA and TACHYPNEA, and the patient may be laboring to breathe. In very severe cases, the blood pressure falls, and the patient has all the symptoms of shock. The head-to-toe survey rarely reveals any abnormalities. If right heart failure accompanies the pulmonary embolism, there may be JUGULAR VENOUS DISTENTION. Examination of the chest is usually normal. Occasionally the source of the embolus is evident in a tender, swollen calf, but usually the source cannot be found.

Treatment of suspected pulmonary embolism in the field is supportive, for definitive therapy with anticoagulants requires hospitalization.

PREHOSPITAL MANAGEMENT OF SUSPECTED PULMONARY EMBOLISM

- Ensure an open AIRWAY.
- Administer 100% OXYGEN.
- Assist BREATHING as needed.
- Establish an IV LIFELINE with normal saline. Run it at a keep-open rate unless there is a drop in blood pressure, in which case open the IV wide.
- MONITOR cardiac rhythm.

DISORDERS OF VENTILATION

Ventilation, as we learned, is the movement of air in and out of the lungs. Under normal circumstances, the volume of ventilation (minute volume) is regulated by the need to maintain the arterial PCO_2 in the range of 35 to 40 torr. In a person at rest, that goal is usually accomplished by breathing a tidal volume of around 500 ml at a rate of about 12 to 16 breaths per minute, that is, with a minute volume in the range of 6 to 8 liters. In deep sleep, a smaller minute volume may suffice, while muscular exertion may require a larger minute volume. But so long as the arterial PCO_2 remains in the normal range, the ventilation is considered normal.

In this section, we shall look at two conditions in which ventilation is decidedly *ab*normal. In the first, the Pickwickian syndrome, ventilation is insufficient; in the second, the hyperventilation syndrome, ventilation is excessive.

The Pickwickian Syndrome

The pickwickian syndrome is the name given to the combination of extreme obesity (usually over 130 kg, or 286 lb) and sleepiness reminiscent of the fat boy, Joe, in Charles Dickens's *Pickwick Papers*. The syndrome is, in fact, probably a form of what is known as the *sleep apnea* syndrome, in which patients suffer periods of apnea, sometimes accompanied by cardiac dysrhythmias, during sleep. The cause of hypoventilation in the pickwickian syndrome is not entirely clear, but it may at least in part be related to the high energy cost of respiration in a very fat person. That hypothesis is supported by the fact that dramatic improvement in all symptoms of the pickwickian syndrome takes place when a pickwickian patient loses weight.

The typical patient with pickwickian syndrome isn't simply fat; he is VERY, VERY FAT, and often has been so for many years. The *patient's* chief complaint is apt to be HEADACHE, but those around him are more likely to complain about his **somnolence** (sleepiness), often in extremely inappropriate circumstances. The patient may doze off, for example, while eating, driving a car, or even in the middle of a sentence when you are taking the history. Typical findings on physical examination include *cyanosis*, periods of *apnea*, muscle *twitching*, and signs of right heart failure (*distended neck veins, ankle edema*).

The only *definitive* treatment for a pickwickian patient is a weight reduction diet, but secondary problems such as heart failure may need attention in the meanwhile. In the field, all that is necessary is to assist ventilations as needed, so that periods of apnea do not lead to dangerous cardiac dysrhythmias. Since Murphy's Law predicts that any 300-pound patient will live in a fourth floor apartment (no elevator), you will doubtless be sorely tempted to suggest that the patient proceed to the ambulance under his own steam. Resist that temptation. If the patient had any steam left, he probably would not have called for an ambulance.

Hyperventilation Syndrome

At the other end of the spectrum from the hypoventilating pickwickian patient is the patient who is *hyper*ventilating. The hyperventilating patient is usually relatively young—a teenager or young adult—and ordinarily doesn't know that he is hyperventilating. His chief complaint is often about something else altogether—fatigue, dizziness, nervousness. The patient may report a sensation of *tingling or numbness around the mouth* and in the *hands* and *feet. Sharp, stabbing chest pain* is also a frequent chief complaint and may lead the patient to the panicky conclusion that he or she is suffering a heart attack.

On physical examination, it may or may not be immediately apparent that the patient is hyperventilating. If the history is suggestive, try to assess the *depth* of respiration as you count the respiratory rate. Patients with marked hyperventilation will often develop **carpopedal spasm,** in which the hands contort in a flexed position, with the thumb curved toward the palm. Patients who are predisposed to seizures are especially likely to seize during an episode of hyperventilation.

Hyperventilation, by definition, leads to a fall in arterial PCO_2, which in turn can cause significant derangements of electrolytes. The *treatment* of hyperventilation, therefore, is aimed at restoring the PCO_2 toward normal. We used to recommend having the patient breathe into a paper bag for that purpose—the idea being that the patient would thereby rebreathe his own exhaled CO_2, which in turn would help bring the CO_2 levels in his blood back up to normal. Recently, however, "paper bag therapy" of hyperventilation has been called into question. When a person rebreathes his own exhaled air from a paper bag, the oxygen content of his inspired air progressively falls. After the patient has taken several breaths, the air in the paper bag will contain only a very low concentration of oxygen. Continuing to breathe that oxygen-poor air could be dangerous, especially if the patient is already suffering from some degree of hypoxemia (e.g., a patient with an unsuspected pulmonary embolism). The only way to be certain that the patient is *not* hypoxemic is to measure his arterial blood gases, which is not really practical in the field. For that reason, it is safest *not* to use paper bag therapy outside the hospital. Instead, try to calm the patient verbally, and help him to take conscious control of his breathing.

Once the acute episode is resolved, it is worthwhile to explain and demonstrate to the patient how his symptoms came about, for patients with hyperventilation syndrome tend to have repeated attacks. Have the patient intentionally hyperventilate under your supervision, to demonstrate that it is his "overbreathing" that produces the uncomfortable feelings experienced during the acute attack. Understanding the causes of his symptoms may not prevent the patient from hyperventilating again in the future, but it will certainly help keep him from panicking the next time it happens and may save you many more calls to the same address.

A reminder:

> **NOT EVERY PATIENT WHO IS BREATHING DEEPLY AND RAPIDLY IS HYPERVENTILATING.**

Remember, hyperventilation refers to the situation in which a person's minute volume is *in excess of his need to blow off CO₂*. A patient with diabetic ketoacidosis may be breathing very deeply and very rapidly, but he does NOT have hyperventilation syndrome because he needs to maintain that increased minute volume just to normalize his PCO_2. If you stick a paper bag over *his* face, you will simply worsen his already severe acidosis. So don't assume that every patient with tachypnea and hyperpnea is hyperventilating. Take a careful history and a close look at the patient first.

There is one more category of respiratory emergencies that we shall consider in this chapter and that is pulmonary barotrauma along with other injuries sustained in diving. Before we move on to that specialized topic, however, it is worthwhile to review Table 22-6, which summarizes the features of the more common conditions that present as dyspnea.

PULMONARY BAROTRAUMA AND OTHER DIVING INJURIES

There are 5 million recreational scuba divers in the United States, not to mention those who are engaged in diving for commercial and military purposes, and about 200,000 Americans receive scuba instruction every year. Paramedics who work in coastal or lake-

TABLE 22-6.　DIFFERENTIAL DIAGNOSIS OF DYSPNEA

	PULMONARY EDEMA	COPD	SPONTANEOUS PNEUMOTHORAX	PULMONARY EMBOLI	ASTHMA
Possible history	Symptoms of acute myocardial infarction "Water pills" Sudden weight gain Cough, watery sputum Orthopnea	Emphysema, bronchitis Heavy smoking Recent cold *Chronic* dyspnea "Breathing pills" or inhalers	Sudden, sharp chest pain *Sudden* dyspnea, brought on by strenuous exertion, coughing, air travel Patient often young, tall, thin	Sudden, sharp chest pain *Sudden* dyspnea Prolonged immobilization, recent surgery or trauma to lower extremities Thrombophlebitis Sickle cell anemia Birth control pills	Acute, episodic dyspnea Often younger patient Allergic history Relieved by shots in the past Cold or flu may have preceded attack
Possible physical findings	Distended neck veins Crackles S₃ gallop	↑ Anteroposterior diameter of chest Purse-lip breathing Wheezing, crackles Prolonged expiratory phase of respiration Use of accessory muscles to breathe	↓ Breath sounds and ↑ resonance on side of collapsed lung Tracheal deviation	Tachypnea Tachycardia Hypotension Pleural rub Phlebitis in legs	Wheezing Hyperresonance If bronchospasm severe, chest may be silent
Treatment in the field	OXYGEN Monitor IV: D5/W to KO M.D. may order morphine, furosemide, nitroglycerin	OXYGEN—but watch for depression of breathing; be prepared to ventilate Monitor IV: D5/W to KO M.D. may order aminophylline	OXYGEN Monitor IV at discretion of M.D.	OXYGEN Monitor IV: D5/W to KO	OXYGEN Monitor Epinephrine SQ M.D. may order aminophylline IV: D5/W for hydration

front areas are therefore sooner or later likely to encounter a diving casualty. It is also not improbable that the casualty—especially if he is a professional diver—will know a lot more about diving medicine than the paramedic; and if conscious, the casualty will often put forward his own ideas about the diagnosis. Nonetheless, it is not advisable for medical personnel, paramedics included, to depend on patients—scuba divers or any others—to diagnose and treat themselves in emergencies; and paramedics operating in areas where diving is popular should become at least as conversant with diving medicine as the enthusiasts of the sport.

There are, in fact, four different modes of diving:

- BREATH-HOLD DIVING, or free diving, does not require any equipment, except sometimes a snorkel.
- In SURFACE-TENDED DIVING, air is piped to the diver through a tube from the surface.
- The most popular form of diving is SCUBA DIVING, named for the **s**elf-contained **u**nderwater **b**reathing **a**pparatus that the diver carries on his back.
- In SATURATION DIVING the diver remains at depth for prolonged periods.

All divers, irrespective of the type of diving they do, are subject to the increased ambient pressures that occur under water. In order to understand the things that can go wrong in diving, we need to understand a little bit about pressure and its effects on gases.

Pressure Effects: Physical Principles

Pressure is defined as *force per unit area,* and it may be expressed in a number of different ways, depending on the units one chooses. Thus the weight of air at sea level, for example, can be expressed as 14.7 pounds per square inch (**psi**), as 760 **mm Hg** (torr), or as 1 atmosphere absolute (**ATA**). It is the last-mentioned system—measurement in atmospheres absolute—that is used most commonly in diving medicine. Because water is much denser than air, relatively small changes in depth produce large changes in ambient pressure. For every 33 feet of seawater (**fsw**), the pressure increases 1 ATA, so knowing the depth of the dive permits one to estimate the pressure to which the diver was exposed: At a depth of 33 fsw, the pressure is 2 ATA; at 66 fsw, it is 3 ATA, and so forth. The majority of scuba diving is done at depths between 60 and 120 fsw, that is, at pressures between about 2 and 4 ATA.

Most tissues of the body, being themselves composed primarily of water, are not compressible and therefore are not significantly affected by the pressure changes experienced in descent or ascent through water. Gas-filled organs are another matter, however, for gases *are* compressible. To understand the behavior of gases within the body during diving, we need to know a little bit of the physics that governs all gases. Three gas laws are relevant here:

- **Boyle's law** states that at any given temperature, the volume of a gas is inversely proportional to its pressure:

$$PV = K, \text{ or } P = \frac{K}{V}$$

where P = pressure, V = volume, and K = a constant

What this equation tells us is that if you double the pressure on a gas, you halve its volume. (Suppose you filled a balloon with 1 liter of air and brought the balloon down to 33 feet below the surface of the water. What would the volume be there? What would it be at 99 feet below the surface? See Figure 22-5 to check your answer.)

FIGURE 22-5. BOYLE'S LAW. As a bubble descends through water, its volume changes in inverse proportion to the ambient pressure.

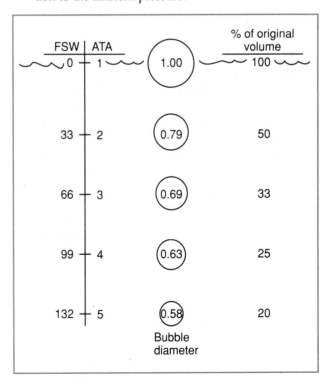

- **Dalton's law** has to do with the pressure exerted by mixtures of different gases. Dalton's law states that each gas in mixture exerts the same *partial pressure* that it would exert if it were alone in the same volume, and that the total pressure of a mixture of gases is the sum of the partial pressures of all the gases in the mixture. Thus for fresh air:

$$P_{total} = PO_2 + PCO_2 + PN_2$$

In fact, we learned Dalton's law already in Chapter 8, when we considered the partial pressures of gases in room air, although we did not mention the law by name. Dalton's law becomes important in understanding how decompression sickness develops.

- **Henry's law** states that the amount of gas dissolved in a liquid is directly proportional to the partial pressure of the gas above the liquid. As we shall see, Henry's law also helps explain how decompression sickness comes about.

With that brief background in physics, let us look at some of the injuries that can occur during diving.

Barotrauma

Barotrauma literally means injury caused by pressure; more precisely, it is injury that results from a pressure imbalance between gas-filled spaces inside the body and the external atmosphere. The various types of barotrauma, especially that involving the ears, comprise the most common injuries suffered by divers. In our discussion here, we shall focus on barotrauma involving the lungs. Other types of barotrauma are summarized in Table 22-7.

In fact, barotrauma can occur from two different mechanisms—from the compression of gases within body spaces during descent or from the expansion of gases within those spaces during ascent. We shall look at those mechanisms one at a time.

Barotrauma of Descent

Recall Boyle's law and the balloon filled with a liter of air at sea level. When we bring the balloon down 33 feet (2 ATA), it will contain only half a liter, so it will shrink to about 80 percent of its former diameter; if we descend to 99 feet (4 ATA), it will contain a quarter of a liter, so its diameter will be 60 percent of what it was at the surface (Fig. 22-5). The tendency of a sealed, gas-filled space, therefore, is to shrink and *im*plode as it descends. What, then, keeps all the gas-filled spaces in the body from imploding during descent through water?

The person who is scuba diving is theoretically protected, for he is breathing compressed air, which will be at the same pressure as the surrounding environment. So as long as the air-filled cavities of the body can equilibrate freely, they will not implode. When there is an obstruction somewhere in the system, however, the tendency is indeed toward implosion. Thus, for example, when there is blockage in the eustachian tube, which connects the middle ear with the nasopharynx, the pressure in the middle ear cannot be equalized with that of the outside and a characteristic "middle ear squeeze" syndrome develops.

The corresponding injury to the lung, called **lung squeeze,** in fact is quite rare and tends to occur only in breath-hold diving, for the scuba diver can constantly reequilibrate the pressure in his lungs simply by breathing. For lung squeeze to occur, the breath-hold diver must descend to a depth in which his total lung volume is significantly compressed, which usually means a depth of at least 100 fsw. (By what factor would total lung volume be reduced at that depth?) The negative pressure within the lung then pulls interstitial fluid and blood into the shrunken air spaces, so the CLINICAL MANIFESTATIONS of lung squeeze are, not surprisingly, *dyspnea, chest pain, cough, hemoptysis,* and *pulmonary edema.*

Prehospital TREATMENT of suspected lung squeeze is similar to that for pulmonary edema from any other cause *except* that positive pressure ventilation or PEEP should NOT be given—lest it induce gas embolism from the injured lung. Therefore, administer 100% oxygen by nonrebreathing mask, start an IV, keep the patient sitting up, and transport him to the hospital.

Barotrauma of Ascent

As the diver ascends, and the ambient pressure around him *decreases*, the gases within his body's air-filled spaces—so Boyle's law again tells us—will expand. For example, the lung volume of a scuba diver who has inhaled to his total lung capacity at a depth of 33 fsw would double by the time he reached the surface if he were to hold his breath during ascent. For that reason, all student divers are trained to exhale constantly as they are ascending, in order to vent air from their lungs. That training, however, may be forgotten in an emergency ascent—for instance, when the diver experiences some difficulty with his equipment and panics—and the diver may then follow his instinctive impulse to hold his breath under water. The result will be one of the worst forms of barotrauma of ascent, the **pulmonary overpressurization syndrome,** appropriately enough called "POPS" for short, and known to divers as "burst

TABLE 22-7. DIVING INJURIES

MECHANISMS AND PATHOPHYSIOLOGY	BODY REGION	CONDITION	CLINICAL FEATURES	TREATMENT
BAROTRAUMA During DESCENT: compression of gas in closed spaces	Ear	External ear squeeze (*barotitis externa*)	Otalgia, bloody otorrhea	Keep ear canal dry; no swimming or diving until healed
		Middle ear squeeze (*barotitis media*)	Severe ear pain, nausea, vertigo	Decongestants; no diving until healed
		Inner ear squeeze	Tinnitus, vertigo, hearing loss; pallor, diaphoresis	Bed rest; surgical repair
	Paranasal sinuses	Sinus squeeze	Pressure/pain over frontal and maxillary sinuses; painful upper teeth	Decongestants; antibiotics
	Face	Face mask squeeze	Erythema, ecchymoses, petechiae of skin beneath face mask; bulging eyes; scleral/ conjunctival hemorrhage	
	Lungs	Lung squeeze (in breath-hold dives)	Dyspnea, chest pain, cough, hemoptysis, pulmonary edema	100% oxygen (avoid demand valve, PEEP) IV fluids
During ASCENT: expansion of gas in closed spaces	Teeth	Tooth squeeze (*barodontalgia*)	Toothache; tooth may explode	Refer to dentist
	Gastrointestinal tract	"Gas in gut" (*aerogastralgia*)	Colicky belly pain, belching, flatulence	Usually none required
	Lungs	Pulmonary barotrauma (PBT), "burst lung," pulmonary overpressurization syndrome (POPS)	Dyspnea, dysphagia, hoarseness, substernal pain; subcutaneous emphysema around neck; pneumothorax, syncope	100% oxygen Decompress pneumothorax; rest
		Dysbaric air embolism (DAE)— complication of PBT	Like a cerebrovascular accident: hemi- or polyplegia; blindness, deafness, vertigo, dizziness, seizures, aphasia, sudden loss of consciousness on surfacing; sudden death	100% oxygen Left lateral head-down position Hyperbaric therapy Steroids
DECOMPRESSION SICKNESS	Skin		Pruritus, subcutaneous emphysema, swelling, rashes	Symptomatic; observe for complications
	Joints & muscles	Bends ("Pain-only bends")	Arthralgias, especially in elbows and shoulders, relieved by pressure	Analgesia; observe
	Cerebrum		Multiple sensory/motor disturbances	Hyperbaric therapy IV fluids
	Cerebellum	The "staggers"	Unsteadiness, incoordination, vertigo	Steroids for all patients with anything more than skin and musculoskeletal involvement
	Spinal cord		Paraplegia, paraparesis, bladder dysfunction (inability to void)	
	Lungs	Venous air embolism (the "chokes")	Chest pain, cough, dyspnea, signs of pulmonary embolism	
DISSOLVED NITROGEN	CNS	Nitrogen narcosis: "Rapture of the deep"	Symptoms like those of alcohol intoxication	Ascent to shallower water
HYPERVENTILATION BEFORE DIVE	CNS	Shallow water blackout (in breath-hold dives)	Loss of consciousness just before reaching surface	100% oxygen Assisted breathing

lung." Because the relative pressure and volume changes are greatest near the surface of the water, that is also the area of greatest danger for burst lung. It takes only a very small overpressurization—that which can be produced by breath-holding for only the last *6 feet* of ascent—to rupture alveoli.

When alveoli do rupture, the SYMPTOMS AND SIGNS produced will depend in part on where the air escaping from the lungs ends up. Most commonly, it leaks into the mediastinum and beneath the skin, causing *mediastinal and subcutaneous emphysema.* The patient may complain of a sensation of fullness in his throat, of pain on swallowing (**dysphagia**), of dyspnea, or of substernal chest pain. When he speaks, he may be hoarse or have a brassy quality to his voice. On physical examination, subcutaneous air may be palpable above the clavicles. Sometimes a crunching noise that is synchronous with the heart beat may be audible on auscultation. Theoretically, *pneumothorax* is also a possibility after alveolar rupture, so be sure to check for the characteristic signs: tracheal deviation, unequal breath sounds, and hyperresonance on the affected side of the chest.

By far the most dangerous possible consequence of "burst lung" is **dysbaric air embolism** (DAE), which is second only to drowning as the major cause of death among divers. Air bubbles from ruptured alveoli enter the pulmonary capillaries and coalesce into larger and larger bubbles as they travel through the pulmonary veins back to the left side of the heart. From the left ventricle the bubbles may enter the coronary arteries, producing all of the effects of acute myocardial infarction. The vast majority of air emboli, however, proceed to the cerebral circulation for the simple reason that the diver's head is usually the highest part of his body during ascent and bubbles rise.

The air does not, in fact, enter the circulation until the diver has reached the surface and taken his first breath. Up to that point, pulmonary blood flow was prevented by the overdistention of the lungs; but with the diver's first exhalation, the pressure on the pulmonary vessels is released and blood flow through them resumes. Thus it is customary to speak of a "lucid interval" in dysbaric air embolism—the time between surfacing and taking the first breath. The CLINICAL PICTURE OF AIR EMBOLISM tends to be very dramatic. Symptoms usually appear within seconds or minutes after surfacing and may involve just about any cerebral function. Most commonly, there is weakness or paralysis of one or more of the extremities, seizure activity, or unconsciousness; but a variety of other neurologic symptoms—including paresthesias, blindness, deafness, changes in mental status—are frequently reported.

> **ANY DIVER WHO LOSES CONSCIOUSNESS RIGHT AFTER A DIVE HAS SUFFERED AN AIR EMBOLISM UNTIL PROVED OTHERWISE.**

The prehospital TREATMENT of the patient with pulmonary barotrauma will depend, at least in its urgency, on whether there is associated air embolism. The patient who has suffered only pneumomediastinum and subcutaneous emphysema will probably be managed in the hospital with bed rest and oxygen therapy, and basically the same principles apply in the field: Give 100% oxygen (by nonrebreathing mask, *not* demand valve; that is, DON'T GIVE PEEP TO POPS!); keep the patient quiet; and transport him to the hospital. If, however, there is any reason to suspect he has suffered air embolism, he must reach a **hyperbaric chamber** facility as soon as possible for recompression (see next section).

TREATMENT OF SUSPECTED DYSBARIC AIR EMBOLISM

- Ensure an adequate AIRWAY. Intubate the unconscious patient.
- Administer 100% OXYGEN by nonrebreathing mask.
- Transport in LEFT LATERAL RECUMBENT position, with 10 degrees of HEAD-DOWN TILT. (Think about why.)
- IV LIFELINE with lactated Ringer's solution.
- MONITOR cardiac rhythm, and be prepared to treat dysrhythmias.
- Have the following drugs ready for immediate use if needed:
  1. Diazepam, 5 mg IV for SEIZURES.
  2. Dopamine infusion, 10 µg/kg/min for HYPOTENSION
- Notify medical command to make arrangements for reception at a HYPERBARIC CHAMBER facility.

Decompression Sickness

Various adverse effects on the body may be observed as a consequence of breathing gases—especially inert gases (i.e., gases that are not used up in metabolism, like nitrogen)—at higher than normal atmospheric pressure, both when the gases go into solution and when they come out of solution. Recall Henry's law: The amount of gas that will dissolve in a liquid is directly proportional to the partial pressure of the gas on the liquid. As the diver descends, the pressure increases, so the amount of any given gas that dissolves in the tissues increases as well. Oxygen that dissolves in the blood and tissues will be used in metabolism, but nitrogen, being inert, will simply accumulate, particularly in fatty tissues in which it is more soluble.

So long as the diver remains under pressure, the only effect he will experience of all the nitrogen dissolved in his tissues is an anesthetic effect, known as **nitrogen narcosis,** or "rapture of the deep." While not in itself dangerous, nitrogen narcosis may interfere with a diver's judgment and orientation and thus lead to serious diving accidents. It is said that every 50 fsw of descent has an effect equivalent to one martini, and that "martini rule" is often used to evaluate the relative narcotic effects of dives to different depths. At 100 fsw (= 2 martinis), many divers will feel lightheaded and euphoric. The treatment is simply to ascend to a depth in which the martini effect dissipates.

Much more serious than the effects of gases going into solution are the effects of gases *coming out of solution,* for those effects may result in the syndrome known as **decompression sickness.** As just pointed out, all the while that the diver is *descending,* increasing quantities of nitrogen and oxygen are, according to Henry's law, being dissolved in the blood and carried to the tissues.

As the diver *ascends* and ambient pressure decreases, essentially the reverse process occurs—nitrogen begins to diffuse out of the tissues. If the ascent is slow enough, the amount of nitrogen in the tissues will equilibrate with that in the alveoli. But if the ascent takes place more rapidly than nitrogen can be removed, the diver's tissues will literally begin to bubble, somewhat like the bubbling that occurs in a carbonated beverage when you remove the cap from the bottle. Bubbles do their damage both by interfering mechanically with tissue perfusion and by triggering chemical changes within the body. The result is a multisystem disorder that can potentially affect almost every organ in the body.

It has become customary to classify decompression sickness as type I or type II. Type I refers to mild forms of the syndrome that involve only the skin and the musculoskeletal system. Type II includes all the other manifestations and is regarded as more serious. That categorization system in fact is not very useful, and it is much more informative to specify the systems affected and the precise symptoms (see Table 22-7) when describing a particular patient with decompression sickness.

It may not always be possible to distinguish clinically between decompression sickness and air embolism, especially when the patient has neurologic symptoms. As a general rule, symptoms produced by air embolism usually reflect cerebral dysfunction, while in decompression sickness the spinal cord is more likely to be involved, but exceptions do occur. From the point of view of prehospital treatment, the distinction is somewhat academic, because the cornerstone management in either case will be to TRANSPORT THE PATIENT TO A HYPERBARIC FACILITY. At the hyperbaric center, however, it *will* be important to make the distinction, for treatment of air embolism requires recompression to significantly greater depth than treatment of decompression sickness. For that reason, it is very important to try to obtain as many details as you can about the dive and the onset of the patient's symptoms. It is helpful to keep a special form in the ambulance that has been specifically prepared for TAKING THE HISTORY OF THE DIVING ACCIDENT. The form should include the following:

WHAT TO FIND OUT ABOUT A DIVING ACCIDENT

- TYPE OF DIVING the patient was doing and the TYPE OF EQUIPMENT he was using.
- DIVING ACTIVITY (e.g., photographing, fishing).
- SITE OF DIVING and water temperature.
- NUMBER OF DIVES made during the past 72 hours, along with the DEPTH, BOTTOM TIME, and SURFACE INTERVAL for each.
- Details of the IN-WATER DECOMPRESSION.
- Whether the diver attempted IN-WATER RECOMPRESSION (a no-no!).
- DIVE COMPLICATIONS, if any.
- PRE-DIVE AND POST-DIVE ACTIVITIES.
- ONSET OF SYMPTOMS (e.g., when, what came first?). Decompression sickness will usually manifest itself within the first hour of surfacing, and certainly within the first 6 hours. Symptoms occurring within 10 minutes suggest air embolism.

The prehospital TREATMENT of a patient suffering from decompression sickness is basically supportive—to get him to a recompression facility in optimal condition:

TREATMENT OF DECOMPRESSION SICKNESS

- Ensure an adequate AIRWAY.
- Give 100% OXYGEN by nonrebreathing mask.
- Start an IV with lactated Ringer's, and give fluids at the rate ordered. (For long-range transport of a catheterized patient, adjust fluids to produce a urine output of 1–2 ml/kg/hr.)
- Give STEROIDS, preferably methylprednisolone, 125 mg IV.
- Do *not* use nitrous oxide/oxygen (Nitronox) for analgesia!
- Arrange for TRANSPORT TO THE NEAREST HYPERBARIC FACILITY. (If you don't know where that is, telephone the Divers Alert Network for assistance: (919) 684-8111.)

Shallow Water Blackout

It remains to mention one further condition that may be seen by paramedics in any part of the country, even in desert states, for it may occur as easily in the backyard swimming pool as in the ocean—and that is shallow water blackout. The blackout is most frequently seen among adolescent boys competing to see who can remain the longest under water. One way of extending one's underwater endurance, at least among swimmers who don't know any better, is to hyperventilate just before diving beneath the surface. Hyperventilation decreases arterial PCO_2 and also causes cerebral vasoconstriction. Meanwhile, as the swimmer descends, his arterial PO_2 increases (Henry's law, remember?). Because the PCO_2 is relatively low, the diver's respiratory drive is suppressed, so he tends to remain under water longer than he ordinarily would—and all the while oxygen is being removed from his alveoli. He remains conscious because his cerebral function is being maintained by the increased PO_2 at depth. As he surfaces, however, and ambient pressure rapidly decreases, the arterial PO_2 plummets, and hypoxemia combined with cerebral vasoconstriction cause him to black out just before he reaches the surface. If he doesn't drown in the process, he may learn a lesson. If he does drown, or nearly drown, that's when you will be summoned. Treatment is the same as for any other case of near drowning. But when the patient comes around, as one hopes he will, explain to him and his buddies that hyperventilation before a breath-hold dive can indeed help a swimmer remain under water a long time—as long as forever.

Getting Help for Diving Accidents

A valuable resource for emergency medical personnel dealing with underwater diving accidents is the Divers Alert Network (DAN), which provides a 24-hour emergency consultation service. Emergency calls to the DAN number, (919) 684-8111, are received at DAN headquarters at Duke University Medical Center in Durham, North Carolina, and the caller is immediately connected with a physician experienced in diving medicine. The physician can assist with diagnosis, provide advice for early management of the accident, and supervise referral to an appropriate recompression chamber when necessary. DAN also produces the excellent *Underwater Diving Accident Manual*, which can be obtained by writing to: Divers Alert Network, Box 3823 F.G. Hall Laboratory, Duke University Medical Center, Durham, NC 22710.

GLOSSARY

acute respiratory insufficiency Any condition in which breathing is inadequate to supply oxygen to or remove carbon dioxide from body tissues; more specifically, any condition that results in an arterial PO_2 below 60 torr or an arterial PCO_2 above 50 torr.

anorexia Lack of appetite.

asphyxia Suffocation; more accurately, hypercarbia plus hypoxemia.

asthma Obstructive airways disease characterized by periodic attacks of dyspnea, bronchospasm, cough, and wheezing.

ATA Abbreviation for atmospheres absolute, a measurement of ambient pressure.

ataxia Inability to cooordinate the muscles properly; often used to describe a staggering gait.

barotrauma Injury resulting from pressure disequilibrium across body surfaces.

bronchodilator Agent that relaxes bronchial muscles and thereby increases the diameter of the airways.

bronchospasm Severe constriction of the bronchial tree.

carpopedal spasm Contorted position of the hand in which the fingers flex in a clawlike attitude and the thumb curls toward the palm.

chronic bronchitis Chronic obstructive pulmonary disease characterized by cough and excessive mucus production.

COPD Abbreviation for chronic obstructive pulmonary disease.

cor pulmonale Heart disease that develops secondary to a chronic lung disease, usually affecting primarily the right side of the heart.

crackles Any discontinuous adventitious sounds in the lungs, caused by the popping open of air spaces.

dead space The portion of the tidal volume that does not reach the alveoli and thus does not participate in gas exchange.

drowning Death by submersion in water.

dysphagia Pain or difficulty in swallowing.

dyspnea The *sensation* of being short of breath.

embolism A mass (embolus, sing.; emboli, pl.) of solid, liquid, or gaseous material that is carried in the circulation and may lead to occlusion of blood vessels.

emphysema A chronic obstructive pulmonary disease characterized by distention of the alveoli and destructive changes in the lung parenchyma.

fsw Abbreviation for feet of seawater, an indirect measure of pressure under water.

HAPE Abbreviation for high-altitude pulmonary edema.

hyperventilation Increased rate and/or depth of breathing that results in abnormal lowering of the arterial PCO_2.

hypoventilation Breathing that is inadequate to remove the carbon dioxide produced by metabolism, resulting in an elevated arterial PCO_2.

laryngospasm Severe constriction of the larynx, in response to allergy, noxious stimuli, or illness.

lassitude Condition of listlessness and fatigue.

lung squeeze Injury to the lung caused by breath-holding during descent through water.

minute volume The volume of air inhaled or exhaled during one minute, calculated by multiplying the respiratory rate times the tidal volume.

nasal flaring Marked widening of the nostrils on inhalation—a sign of respiratory distress.

near drowning Submersion in water with temporary or long-term survival thereafter.

nitrogen narcosis State resembling alcohol intoxication produced by nitrogen gas dissolved in the blood at high ambient pressure; also called rapture of the deep.

orthopnea Severe dyspnea experienced when recumbent and relieved by sitting or standing up.

palpitation Abnormal awareness of one's heart beat or the sensation that the heart is "skipping a beat."

paroxysmal nocturnal dyspnea Severe shortness of breath occurring at night after several hours of recumbency, during which fluid pools in the lungs.

PEEP Abbreviation for positive end-expiratory pressure.

POPS Abbreviation for pulmonary overpressurization syndrome.

pulmonary arteries The arteries that carry blood poor in oxygen from the right ventricle of the heart to the lungs.

pulmonary veins The veins that carry oxygenated blood from the lungs to the left atrium of the heart.

purulent Full of pus; having the character of pus.

rigor A shaking chill.

scuba Abbreviation for self-contained underwater breathing apparatus.

shunt The portion of the output of the right heart that returns unoxygenated to the left heart after passage through the lungs.

somnolence Sleepiness.

status asthmaticus Severe, prolonged asthmatic attack that cannot be broken with epinephrine.

tidal volume The amount of air inhaled or exhaled during one breath.

ventilation The movement of air in and out of the lungs, or, more accurately, in and out of the alveoli.

vertigo Hallucination of movement; a sensation that the external world is spinning.

vocal fremitus The vibrations palpable on the chest wall when someone speaks.

wheezes High-pitched, whistling sounds associated with narrowing or partial obstruction of the lower airways.

APPENDIX I: HOW TO ADMINISTER MEDICATIONS WITH A METERED-DOSE INHALER OR NEBULIZER

Use of a Metered-Dose Inhaler

Adrenergic agents—such as albuterol, isoetharine, and metaproterenol—are most effectively administered in the field with a metered-dose inhaler (MDI). Previously, nebulizers were considered the preferred method of delivering beta-adrenergic drugs for the treatment of asthmatic attacks. But recent studies have shown that MDIs, especially when used with spacing devices (see below), are at least as effective as nebulizers and have several distinct advantages:

- MDIs are *more convenient* than nebulizers. They do not require any setup time or the drawing up of drugs in syringes. Nor do they require a source of compressed gas.

- MDIs are *more reliable* than nebulizers. With a nebulizer, one cannot be certain that the patient is getting the full dose of the drug. MDIs deliver a more consistent amount of drug aerosol.
- Since most asthmatics use MDIs at home, employing the MDI in an emergency provides an excellent opportunity to *educate the patient* in proper use of the device. Studies have shown that more than half of patients using MDIs at home employ incorrect and ineffective technique. Showing a patient the correct technique—and demonstrating its effectiveness — can improve the outcome of subsequent asthmatic attacks, so that next time there may not be a need to call for an ambulance.

Correct Metered-Dose Inhaler Technique

- Confirm the medication order with the physician.
- Explain and demonstrate the entire procedure to the patient.
- SHAKE the MDI cannister before use.
- Have the patient hold the MDI UPRIGHT 1–2 inches in front of his mouth.
- Instruct the patient to EXHALE COMPLETELY.
- Instruct the patient to BEGIN A SLOW DEEP BREATH. As he starts his inhalation, have him TRIGGER THE MDI and inhale.
- When he completes the inhalation, instruct him to HOLD HIS BREATH FOR 10 SECONDS, to give the medication time to deposit out in the lungs.
- After 1–5 minutes, REPEAT THE INHALATION if needed, according to the same procedure. Waiting a few minutes before taking the next puff permits the medication already delivered to dilate some airways and therefore improve penetration of the next dose.

The metered-dose inhalers that you carry on the ambulance should ideally be equipped with **spacers.** A spacer is a device that collects the medication as it is released from the cannister, allowing more to be delivered to the lungs and less lost to the environment. When a spacer is used, the patient does not have to worry about timing the inhalation to coincide with discharge of the inhaler. Spacers also reduce deposition of the drug into the mouth and oropharynx.

Use of a Nebulizer

Nebulizers provide another means of delivering medications directly to the patient's respiratory tract and are used in many ambulance services. Employing compressed air or oxygen as a power source, a nebulizer turns the liquid medication into an aerosol of tiny droplets that can be inhaled deep into the patient's lungs. (Because aerosols are deposited deep within the lung, care must be taken to maintain the sterility of medications and diluents. The best way to keep things sterile for prehospital care is to stock *unit-dose packages* that are used for one treatment only and then discarded. Multidose vials are much more apt to become contaminated.) To administer a medication by nebulizer, proceed as follows:

- Confirm the medication order with the physician.
- Explain the procedure to the patient.
- ASSEMBLE THE EQUIPMENT according to the instructions supplied with it. Be sure there is a 6-inch reservoir tube. If at all possible, give the treatment by mouthpiece rather than by mask.
- FILL THE NEBULIZER with the medication according to the dosage ordered (see dosage table below). If you are using a unit-dose drug, give it at full strength. Medications supplied in concentrated form, on the other hand, need to be diluted with 3 ml of normal saline.
- Have the patient SIT UP.
- Adjust the oxygen flow to 6 liters per minute.
- When you see a fine mist coming from the mouthpiece, have the patient place the mouthpiece in his mouth, INHALE DEEPLY, and THEN HOLD HIS BREATH for a few seconds.
- Instruct the patient to continue the same sequence: SLOW, DEEP BREATH—HOLD—EXHALE. Encourage him to cough if secretions are present.
- Continue until the medication has been completely nebulized (usually about 10 minutes).

DOSAGE OF DRUGS GIVEN BY NEBULIZER

Drug	Adult Dosage
Albuterol	0.5 mg (0.5 ml) in 3 ml of normal saline
Isoetharine	0.25–0.5 ml in 3 ml of normal saline
Metaproterenol	0.2–0.3 ml in 3 ml of normal saline
Racemic epinephrine	0.25–0.5 ml in 3 ml of normal saline

APPENDIX II: MEDICATIONS COMMONLY PRESCRIBED TO PATIENTS WITH RESPIRATORY PROBLEMS

The pill bottles on the patient's nightstand can tell you a great deal about the patient's underlying illnesses even when the patient himself cannot. It is useful, therefore, to become familiar with the names of some of the drugs prescribed to patients with chronic respiratory problems.

The majority of such drugs are various types of **bronchodilators,** used to prevent and treat the bronchospasm that is a prominent feature of both ASTHMA and CHRONIC BRONCHITIS. **Corticosteroids** may be prescribed to asthmatics to suppress an inflammatory component of their condition, while patients with COPD are often given **antibiotics** to deal with the intercurrent bacterial infections to which they are susceptible.

Although it's rare nowadays, at least in industrialized countries, to see tuberculosis, you should also know the names of the drugs used to treat that condition.

CATEGORY AND GENERIC NAME OF MAJOR COMPONENT	SOME TRADE NAMES	FORMS*
I. BRONCHODILATORS		
A. Beta agonists		
Albuterol	**Ventolin**	IH/Sy/T
	Proventil	IH
Epinephrine	**Medihaler-Epi**	IH
Isoetharine	**Bronkosol**	IH
	Bronkometer	IH
	Bronkotabs	T
Isoproterenol	**Isuprel**	IH
Metaproterenol	**Alupent**	IH/Sy/T
	Metaprel	T
Pseudoephedrine hydrochloride	**Actifed**	C/T/Sy
	Sudafed	C/T/Sy
Terbutaline	**Brethine**	T
	Bricanyl	T
B. Methylxanthines		
Theophylline	**Elixophyllin**	C/Sy
	Marax	T/Sy
	Quadrinal	T
	Quibron	T
	Slo-Phyllin	C/Sy
	Tedral	T/Sy
	Theo-Dur	T
Aminophylline		Su
C. Anticholinergics		
Ipratropium bromide	**Atrovent**	T
II. CORTICOSTEROIDS		
Beclomethasone	**Beconase**	IH
	Beclovent	IH
	Vancenase	IH
	Vanceril	IH
Prednisone		T
Triamcinolone	**Aristocort**	T/Sy
III. MAST CELL INHIBITORS		
Cromolyn	**Aarane**	IH
	Intal	IH

CATEGORY AND GENERIC NAME OF MAJOR COMPONENT		SOME TRADE NAMES	FORMS*
IV.	ANTIBIOTICS		
	Ampicillin	**Omnipen**	C/Sy
		Polycillin	C/Sy
	Erythromycin	**Ery-tab**	C
	Trimethoprim	**Bactrim**	C
		Cotrim	C
V.	ANTITUBERCULOUS		
	Isoniazid (INH)		T
	Capreomycin	**Capastat**	C
	Rifampin	**Rifamate/Rifadin**	C
	Streptomycin		
	Ethambutol	**Myambutol**	T
	Pyrazinamide		T

*C = capsule; T = tablet; Sy = syrup; Su = suppository; IH = inhaler.

FURTHER READING

RESPIRATORY ANATOMY, PHYSIOLOGY, AND ASSESSMENT

Fedullo AJ et al. Complaints of breathlessness in the emergency department: The experience at a community hospital. *NY State J Med* 86:4, 1986.

Kettel LJ. Acute respiratory acidosis. *Hosp Med* 12:31, 1976.

Miller WC. The ABCs of blood gases. *Emerg Med* 16(3):37, 1984.

Nixon RG. The respiratory system: An overview. *Emerg Med Serv* 19(1):18, 1990.

The Respiratory System. Bowie, Md: Brady, 1972.

Schecter AD, Kamholz SL. Assessing acute dyspnea. *Emerg Med* 22(9):19, 1990.

Stein JM. Interpreting arterial blood gases. *Emerg Med* 18(1):61, 1986.

COPD

Aubier M et al. Central respiratory drive in acute respiratory failure of patients with chronic obstructive pulmonary disease. *Am Rev Respir Dis* 122:191, 1980.

Aubier M et al. Effects of the administration of O_2 on ventilation and blood gases in patients with chronic obstructive pulmonary disease during acute respiratory failure. *Am Rev Respir Dis* 122:747, 1980.

Auerbach J. Expanding the choices in COPD cases. *JEMS* 16(3):67, 1991.

Baigelman W. Exacerbation of chronic obstructive pulmonary disease. *Emerg Med* 19(9):79, 1987.

Bates D. Chronic bronchitis and emphysema. *N Engl J Med* 278:546, 1968.

Campbell EJM. Management of acute respiratory failure in chronic bronchitis and emphysema. *Am Rev Respir Dis* 96:626, 1967.

Centers for Disease Control. State-specific smoking-attributable chronic obstructive pulmonary disease mortality—United States, 1986. *MMWR* 38:552, 1989.

Ersoz CJ. Prehospital support of the patient with chronic lung disease. *Emerg Med Serv* 8(3):63, 1979.

Farber SM, Wilson RHL. Chronic obstructive emphysema. *Clin Symp* 1968.

Ferguson GT, Cherniack RM. Management of chronic obstructive pulmonary disease. *N Engl J Med* 328:1017, 1993.

Hunt D. Common respiratory emergencies. *Emerg Med Serv* 19(1):19, 1990.

Marcus P. Pharmacotherapy for chronic obstructive lung disease. *Emerg Med* 24(3):35, 1992.

Murphy TF, Sethi S. Preventing or treating COPD flare-ups. *Emerg Med* 25(5):65, 1993.

Palevsky HI, Fishman AP. Chronic cor pulmonale. *JAMA* 263:2347, 1990.

Rice KL et al. Aminophylline for acute exacerbations of chronic obstructive pulmonary disease. *Ann Intern Med* 107:305, 1987.

Sassoon, CSH, Hassell KT, Mahutte CK. Hyperoxic-induced hypercapnia in stable chronic obstructive pulmonary disease. *Am Rev Respir Dis* 135:907, 1987.

Schmidt GA, Hall JB. Acute or chronic respiratory failure. *JAMA* 261:3444, 1989.

Seidenfeld JJ et al. Intravenous aminophylline in the treatment of acute bronchospastic exacerbations of chronic obstructive pulmonary disease. *Ann Emerg Med* 13:248, 1984.

Selinger SR et al. Effects of removing oxygen from patients with chronic obstructive pulmonary disease. *Am Rev Respir Dis* 136:85, 1987.

ASTHMA

Aberman A. A battle plan for acute asthma. *Emerg Med* 23(13):67, 1991.

Aspirin sensitivity in asthmatics (editorial). *Br Med J* 281:958, 1980.

Bailskus M, Niersbach C. Matters of life and breath. *Emergency* 21(4):12, 1989.

Battan FK. Inhalation therapy. *Emergency* 23(8):22, 1991.

Benatar SR. Fatal asthma. *N Engl J Med* 314:423, 1986.

Ben-Zvi Z et al. An evaluation of repeated injections of epinephrine for the initial treatment of acute asthma. *Am Rev Respir Dis* 127:101, 1983.

Bowler SD et al. Corticosteroids in acute severe asthma: Effectiveness of low doses. *Thorax* 47:584, 1992.

Brenner BE. Bronchial asthma in adults: Presentation to the emergency department. I. Pathogenesis, clinical manifestations, diagnostic evaluation, and differential diagnosis. *Am J Emerg Med* 1:50, 1983.

Carden DL et al. Vital signs including pulsus paradoxus in the assessment of acute bronchial asthma. *Ann Emerg Med* 12:80, 1983.

Cydulka R et al. The use of epinephrine in the treatment of older adult asthmatics. *Ann Emerg Med* 17:322, 1988.

DiGiulio GA et al. Hospital treatment of asthma: Lack of benefit from theophylline given in addition to nebulized albuterol and intravenously administered corticosteroids. *J Pediatr* 122:464, 1993.

Eitel DR et al. Prehospital administration of inhaled metaproterenol. *Ann Emerg Med* 19:1412, 1990.

Emerman CL et al. Ventricular arrhythmias during treatment for acute asthma. *Ann Emerg Med* 15:699, 1986.

Engel T et al. Glucocorticosteroid therapy in acute severe asthma: A critical review. *Eur Respir J* 4:881, 1991.

Fanta CH et al. Glucocorticoids in acute asthma: A critical controlled trial. *Am J Med* 74:845, 1983.

Gross NJ. Drug therapy: Ipratropium bromide. *N Engl J Med* 319:486, 1988.

Groth ML, Hurewitz AN. Diagnosing and managing bronchial asthma: Treatment. *Emerg Med* 24(12):19, 1992.

Idris AH et al. Emergency department treatment of severe asthma: Metered-dose inhaler plus holding chamber is equivalent in effectiveness to nebulizer. *Chest* 103:665, 1993.

Johnson AJ. Circumstances of death from asthma. *Br Med J* 288:1870, 1984.

Josephson GW et al. Cardiac dysrhythmias during the treatment of acute asthma. *Chest* 78:429, 1980.

Kampschulte S, Marcy J, Safar P. Simplified physiologic management of status asthmaticus in children. *Crit Care Med* 1:69, 1973.

Karetzky MS. Acute asthma: The use of subcutaneous epinephrine in therapy. *Ann Allergy* 44:12, 1980.

Kattan M et al. Corticosteroids in status asthmaticus. *J Pediatr* 96(Part 2):596, 1980.

Kavuru MS, Ahmad M. Ambulatory management of acute asthma. *Emerg Med* 20(21):111, 1988.

Kelly HW et al. Should we stop using theophylline for the treatment of the hospitalized patient with status asthmaticus? *Ann Pharmacother* 23:995, 1989.

Kerem E et al. Efficacy of albuterol administered by nebulizer versus spacer device in children with acute asthma. *J Pediatr* 123:313, 1993.

Kuitert L, Kletchko S. Intravenous magnesium sulfate in acute, life-threatening asthma. *Ann Emerg Med* 20:1243, 1991.

Lam A et al. Management of asthma and chronic airflow limitation: Are methylxanthines obsolete? *Chest* 98:44, 1990.

Leffert F. The management of acute severe asthma. *J Pediatr* 96:1, 1980.

Lewis M. Aerosol medication administration. *Emergency* 24(9):18, 1992.

Littenberg B. Aminophylline treatment in severe, acute asthma. *JAMA* 259:1678, 1988.

Martinez AJ. Nebulization, southwestern style. *JEMS* 16(8):86, 1991.

Matera P. Breathe easy: Diagnosing and treating asthma in the field. *JEMS* 18(11):40, 1993.

Mullen M, Mullen B, Carey M. The association between β-agonist use and death from asthma. *JAMA* 270:1842, 1993.

Nixon RG. A sigh of relief: Pharmacologic intervention for respiratory distress. *Emerg Med Serv* 22(6):39, 1993.

Noppen M et al. Bronchodilating effect of intravenous magnesium sulfate in acute severe bronchial asthma. *Chest* 97:373, 1990.

Okayama H et al. Treatment of status asthmaticus with intravenous magnesium sulfate. *J Asthma* 28:11, 1991.

Potter PC et al. Hydration in severe acute asthma. *Arch Dis Child* 66:216, 1991.

The proper use of aerosol bronchodilators (editorial). *Lancet* 1:23, 1981.

Ratto D et al. Are intravenous corticosteroids required in status asthmaticus? *JAMA* 260:527, 1988.

Richards W, Siegel S. Status asthmaticus. *Emerg Med* 9(2):294, 1974.

Rossing TH. Methylxanthines in 1989. *Ann Intern Med* 110:502, 1989.

Rothstein RJ. Intravenous theophylline therapy in asthma: A clinical update. *Ann Emerg Med* 9:327, 1980.

Rowe BH et al. Effectiveness of steroid therapy in acute exacerbations of asthma: A meta-analysis. *Am J Emerg Med* 10:301, 1992.

Schneider SM et al. High-dose methylprednisolone as initial therapy in patients with acute bronchospasm. *Asthma* 25:189, 1988.

Self TH et al. Inhaled albuterol and oral prednisone therapy in hospitalized adult asthmatics: Does aminophylline add any benefit? *Chest* 98:1317, 1990.

Skobeloff EM et al. Intravenous magnesium sulfate for the treatment of acute asthma in the emergency department. *JAMA* 262:1210, 1989.

Spevetz A et al. Inpatient management of status asthmaticus. *Chest* 102:1392, 1992.

Stadnyk AM, Grossman RF. Management of life-threatening asthma. *Emerg Med* 19(15):103, 1987.

Stewart MF et al. Risk of giving intravenous aminophylline to acutely ill patients receiving maintenance treatment with theophylline. *Br Med J* 288:450, 1984.

Young GP, Gilden DJ. Acute bronchospasm. *Emerg Med Serv* 21(1):28, 1992.

NEAR DROWNING

Allman FD et al. Outcome following cardiopulmonary resuscitation in severe pediatric near-drowning. *Am J Dis Child* 140:571, 1986.

Bierens JJLM et al. Submersion in the Netherlands: Prognostic indicators and results of resuscitation. *Ann Emerg Med* 19:1390, 1990.

Bolte RG et al. The use of extracorporeal rewarming in a child submerged for 66 minutes. *JAMA* 260:377, 1988.

Cairns FJ. Deaths from drowning. *NZ Med J* 97:65, 1984.

Colby PH. Plunging into water rescue. *JEMS* 15(7):31, 1990.

Conn AW et al. Cerebral resuscitation in near drowning. *Pediatr Clin North Am* 26:691, 1979.

Dean JM, Kaufman ND. Prognostic indicators in pediatric near-drowning: The Glasgow coma scale. *Crit Care Med* 9:536, 1981.

Dietz PE, Baker SP. Drowning: Epidemiology and prevention. *Am J Public Health* 64:303, 1974.

Drinking and drowning (editorial). *Lancet* 2:194, 1978.

Frewen TC et al. Cerebral resuscitation therapy in pediatric near-drowning. *J Pediatr* 106:615, 1985.

Harries MG. Drowning in man. *Crit Care Med* 9:407, 1981.

Harries MG. Clinical course of 61 serious immersion incidents. *Disaster Med* 1:263, 1983.

Hooper HA. Near drowning. *Emergency* 12(5):75, 1980.

Jacobson WK et al. Correlation of spontaneous respiration and neurologic damage in near-drowning. *Crit Care Med* 11:487, 1983.

Keating WR et al. Exceptional case of survival in cold water. *Br Med J* 292:171, 1986.

Knopp R. Near drowning. *JACEP* 7:249, 1978.

Martin TG. Near drowning and cold water immersion. *Ann Emerg Med* 13:263, 1984.

Modell JH. Near-drowning. *Int Anesthesiol Clin* 15:107, 1977.

Modell JH. Is the Heimlich maneuver appropriate as first treatment in drowning? *Emerg Med Serv* 10(6):63, 1981.

Modell JH. Drowning. *N Engl J Med* 328:253, 1993.

Munt PW, Fleetham JA. Corticosteroids and near-drowning. *Lancet* 1:665, 1978.

National Safety Council. *Accident Facts, 1984.* Chicago: National Safety Council, 1984.

Nemiroff MJ. Reprieve from drowning. *Sci Am* 237:57, 1977.

Nichter MA et al. Childhood near-drowning: Is cardiopulmonary resuscitation always indicated? *Crit Care Med* 17:993, 1989.

Nussbaum E. Prognostic variables in nearly drowned, comatose children. *Am J Dis Child* 139:1058, 1985.

Orlowski JP. Prognostic factors in pediatric cases of drowning and near drowning. *JACEP* 8:176, 1979.

Orlowski JP. Drowning, near-drowning, and ice-water drowning (editorial). *JAMA* 260:390, 1988.

Orlowski JP, Abulleil MM, Phillips JM. The hemodynamic and cardiovascular effects of near-drowning in hypotonic, isotonic, or hypertonic solutions. *Ann Emerg Med* 18:1044, 1989.

Ornato JP. The resuscitation of near-drowning victims. *JAMA* 256:75, 1986.

Pearn J. Secondary drowning in children. *Br Med J* 281:1103, 1980.

Pearn J. Drowning and alcohol. *Med J Aust* 141:6, 1984.

Pluekhahn V. Alcohol and accidental drowning. *Med J Aust* 141:22, 1984.

Pratt FD et al. Incidence of "secondary drowning" after saltwater submersion. *Ann Emerg Med* 15:1084, 1986.

Quan L, Kinder D. Pediatric submersions: Prehospital predictors of outcome. *Pediatrics* 90:909, 1992.

Redding JS. Drowning and near-drowning. *Postgrad Med* 74:85, 1983.

Redmond AD et al. Resuscitation from drowning. *Arch Emerg Med* 1:113, 1984.

Sarnaik AP et al. Near-drowning: Fresh, salt, and cold water immersion. *Clin Sports Med* 5:33, 1986.

Schuman SH et al. Risk of drowning: An iceberg phenomenon. *JACEP* 6:139, 1977.

Simcock AD. Hospital management of cold water drowning. *Disaster Med* 1:268, 1983.

Sladen A, Zauder HL. Methylprednisolone therapy for pulmonary edema following near-drowning. *JAMA* 215:1793, 1971.

Stanford TM. Near-drowning. *Emergency* 21(6):30, 1989.

Thygerson AL. Drowning. *Emergency* 12(7):29, 1980.

Wintemute GJ et al. Drowning in childhood and adolescence: A population-based study. *Am J Public Health* 77:830, 1987.

Young RSK et al. Neurologic outcome in cold water drowning. *JAMA* 244:1233, 1980.

HIGH-ALTITUDE PULMONARY EDEMA

Blumen IJ, Dunne MJ. Altitude and flight physiology. *Emergency* 24(7):36, 1992.

Bock J, Hultgren HN. Emergency maneuver in high-altitude pulmonary edema (letter). *JAMA* 255:3245, 1986.

Grissom CK et al. Acetazolamide in the treatment of acute mountain sickness: Clinical efficacy and effect on gas exchange. *Ann Intern Med* 116:461, 1992.

Hackett PH, Roach RC. Medical therapy of altitude illness. *Ann Emerg Med* 16:980, 1987.

Hackett PH et al. Dexamethasone for prevention and treatment of acute mountain sickness. *Aviat Space Environ Med* 59:950, 1988.

Honigman B et al. Acute mountain sickness in a general tourist population at moderate altitudes. *Ann Intern Med* 118:587, 1993.

Houston CS. High altitude illness: Disease with protean manifestations. *JAMA* 236:2193, 1976.

Johnson TS, Rock PB. Current concepts: Acute mountain sickness. *N Engl J Med* 319:841, 1988.

Kasic JF et al. Treatment of acute mountain sickness: Hyperbaric versus oxygen therapy. *Ann Emerg Med* 20:1109, 1991.

Kleiner JP, Nelson WP. High altitude pulmonary edema: A rare disease. *JAMA* 234:491, 1975.

Levine B et al. Dexamethasone in the treatment of acute mountain sickness. *N Engl J Med* 321:1707, 1989.

McNab AJ. Heightening awareness of acute mountain sickness. *JEMS* 16(11):43, 1991.

Montgomery BA, Mills J, Luce JM. Incidence of acute mountain sickness at intermediate altitude. *JAMA* 261:732, 1989.

Pollard AJ et al. Altitude induced illness. *Br Med J* 304:1324, 1992.

Rennie D. The great breathlessness mountains (editorial). *JAMA* 256:81, 1986.

Schoene RB. High-altitude pulmonary edema: Pathophysiology and clinical review. *Ann Emerg Med* 16:987, 1987.

Scoggin CH et al. High-altitude pulmonary edema in the children and young adults of Leadville, Colorado. *N Engl J Med* 297:1269, 1977.

Sophocles AM. High-altitude pulmonary edema in Vail, Colorado, 1975–1982. *West J Med* 144:569, 1986.

Wilson R. Acute high-altitude illness in mountaineers and problems of rescue. *Ann Intern Med* 78:421, 1973.

TOXIC INHALATIONS

Bascomb R, Kennedy T. Toxic gas inhalation. *Emerg Med Serv* 13(7):17, 1984.

Baud FJ et al. Elevated blood cyanide concentrations in victims of smoke inhalation. *N Engl J Med* 325:1761, 1991.

Beckerman B, Brody G. Smoke inhalation. *Emerg Med* 24(15):49, 1992.

Birky MM, Clark FB. Inhalation of toxic products from fires. *Bull NY Acad Med* 57:997, 1981.

Centers for Disease Control. Chlorine gas toxicity from mixture of bleach with other cleaning products—California. *MMWR* 40:619, 1991.

Cohen MA, Guzzardi LJ. Inhalation of products of combustion. *Ann Emerg Med* 12:628, 1983.

Dimick A, Wagner RG. A matter of burns and breath. *Emerg Med* 22(13):123, 1990.

DiVincenti FC, Pruitt BA Jr, Reckler JM. Inhalation injuries. *J Trauma* 11:109, 1971.

Done AK. It's a gas. *Emerg Med* 11(5):305, 1976.

Fein A. Toxic gas inhalation. *Emerg Med* 21(7):53, 1989.

Fein A, Leff A, Hopewell PC. Pathophysiology and management of the complications resulting from fire and the inhaled products of combustion. *Crit Care Med* 8:94, 1980.

Felegi WB. The silent killers: Part II. Methane. *Emerg Med Serv* 12(3):62, 1983.

Hedges JR. Acute noxious gas exposure. *Curr Top Emerg Med* 2(10), 1978.

Heimbach DM, Waeckerle JF. Inhalation injuries. *Ann Emerg Med* 17:1316, 1988.

Jelenko C, McKinley JC. Postburn respiratory injury. *JACEP* 5:455, 1976.

Kirk MA, Gerace R, Kulig KW. Cyanide and methemoglobin kinetics in smoke inhalation victims treated with the cyanide antidote kit. *Ann Emerg Med* 22:60, 1993.

Kulig K. Cyanide antidotes and fire toxicology (editorial). *N Engl J Med.* 325:1801, 1991.

Levy DB, Peppers MP. Poisoning with cyanide. *Emergency* 22(9):18, 1990.

Maslowski DE. H₂S emergency response. *Emergency* 11(4):17, 1979.

Moylan JA, Chan CK. Inhalation injury: An increasing problem. *Ann Surg* 188:24, 1978.

Mrvos R et al. Home exposures to chlorine/chloramine gas: Review of 216 cases. *South Med J* 86:654, 1993.

Robinson NB et al. Steroid therapy following isolated smoke inhalation. *J Trauma* 22:876, 1982.

Trunkey DD. Inhalation injury. *Surg Clin North Am* 8:1133, 1978.

Venus B et al. Prophylactic intubation and continuous positive airway pressure in the management of inhalation injury in burn victims. *Crit Care Med* 9:519, 1981.

Wroblewski DA, Bower GC. The significance of facial burns in acute smoke inhalation. *Crit Care Med* 7:335, 1979.

PULMONARY EMBOLISM

Bell WR, Simon TL, DeMets DL. The clinical features of submassive and massive pulmonary emboli. *Am J Med* 62:355, 1977.

Bone RC. Pulmonary embolism: New approaches to a complex problem. *Emerg Med* 25(14):144, 1992.

Cooke DH. Focusing in on pulmonary embolism. *Emerg Med* 17(9):86, 1985.

Dismuke SE, Wagner EH. Pulmonary embolism as a cause of death. *JAMA* 255:2039, 1986.

Goldhaber SZ. Recent advances in the diagnosis and lytic therapy of pulmonary embolism. *Chest* 99:173S, 1991.

Goodall RJR et al. Clinical correlations in the diagnosis of pulmonary embolism. *Ann Surg* 191:219, 1980.

Green RM et al. Pulmonary embolism in younger adults. *Chest* 101:1507, 1992.

Hoellerich VL et al. Diagnosing pulmonary embolism using clinical findings. *Arch Intern Med* 146:1699, 1986.

Huet Y et al. Hypoxemia in acute pulmonary embolism. *Chest* 88:829, 1985.

Langdon RW, Swicegood WR, Schwartz DA. Thrombolytic therapy of massive pulmonary embolism during prolonged cardiac arrest using recombinant tissue-type plasminogen activator. *Ann Emerg Med* 18:678, 1989.

McGlynn TJ, Hamilton RW, Moore R. Pulmonary embolism: 1979. *JACEP* 8:532, 1979.

Mohindra SK, Udeani GO. Treatment of massive pulmonary embolism with centrally-administered tissue-type plasminogen activator. *Ann Emerg Med* 22:1349, 1993.

Palmer LB, Schiff MJ. Pulmonary embolism and venous thrombosis. *Emerg Med* 20(15):37, 1988.

Stein PD et al. Clinical characteristics of patients with acute pulmonary embolism *Am J Cardiol* 68:1724, 1991.

Sutton GC, Honey M, Gibson RV. Clinical diagnosis of acute massive pulmonary embolism. *Lancet* 1:271, 1979.

Valenzuela TD. Pulmonary embolism. *Ann Emerg Med* 17:209, 1988.

Williams MH. Pulmonary embolism. *Emerg Med* 16(4):135, 1984.

PICKWICKIAN SYNDROME AND
HYPOVENTILATION DISORDERS

Chua W, Chediak A. Obstructive sleep apnea. *Postgrad Med* 95(2):123, 1994.

Feinsilver SH. Recognizing and treating the sleep apnea syndromes. *Emerg Med* 24(6):83, 1992.

Kuna ST, Sant'Ambrogio G. Pathophysiology of upper airway closure during sleep. *JAMA* 266:1384, 1991.

Orlowski JP, Herrell DW, Moodie DS. Narcotic antagonist therapy of the obesity hypoventilation syndrome. *Crit Care Med* 10:604, 1982.

Smith PL et al. The effects of oxygen in patients with sleep apnea. *Am Rev Respir Dis* 130:958, 1984.

Strohl KP, Cherniack NS, Gothe B. Physiologic basis of therapy for sleep apnea. *Am Rev Respir Dis* 134:791, 1986.

Strohl KP et al. Obstructive sleep apnea in family members. *N Engl J Med* 299:969, 1978.

Walsh RE et al. Upper airway obstruction in obese patients with sleep disturbance and somnolence. *Ann Intern Med* 76:185, 1972.

HYPERVENTILATION SYNDROME

Blau JN et al. Unilateral somatic symptoms due to hyperventilation. *Br Med J* 286:1108, 1983.

Callaham M. Hypoxic hazards of traditional paper bag rebreathing in hyperventilation syndrome. *Am J Med* 18:622, 1989.

Chelmowski MK, Keelan MH. Hyperventilation and myocardial infarction. *Chest* 93:1095, 1988.

Demeter SL et al. Hyperventilation syndrome and asthma. *Am J Med* 81:989, 1986.

Grossman JE. Paper bag treatment of acute hyperventilation syndrome (letter). *JAMA* 251:2014, 1984.

Pfefer JM. Hyperventilation and the hyperventilation syndrome. *Postgrad Med* 60(Suppl 2):47, 1984.

Rice RL. Symptom patterns of the hyperventilation syndrome. *Am J Med* 8:691, 1950.

Saltzman JA, Heyman A, Sieker HO. Correlation of clinical and physiological manifestations of sustained hyperventilation. *N Engl J Med* 268:1431, 1963.

Smith CW Jr. Hyperventilation syndrome: Bridging the behavioral-organic gap. *Postgrad Med* 78(2):73, 1985.

Smith M, Sealby N. A matter of life and breath: Prehospital treatment of hyperventilation. *JEMS* 16(6):83, 1991.

Stoop A et al. Hyperventilation syndrome: Measurement of objective symptoms and subjective complaints. *Respiration* 49:37, 1986.

Tavel ME. Hyperventilation syndrome with unilateral somatic symptoms. *JAMA* 187:301, 1964.

Tavel ME. Hyperventilation syndrome: Hiding behind pseudonyms? *Chest* 97:1285, 1990.

Wheatley CE. Hyperventilation syndrome: A frequent cause of chest pain. *Chest* 68:195, 1975.

Yu PN et al. Hyperventilation syndrome. *Arch Intern Med* 103:902, 1959.

PULMONARY BAROTRAUMA AND OTHER
DIVING INJURIES

Arthur DC, Margulies RA. A short course in diving medicine. *Ann Emerg Med* 16:689, 1987.

Balk M, Goldman JM. Alveolar hemorrhage as a manifestation of pulmonary barotrauma after scuba diving. *Ann Emerg Med* 19:930, 1990.

Bayne CG. Acute decompression sickness: 50 cases. *JACEP* 7:351, 1978.

Boettger ML. Scuba diving emergencies: Pulmonary overpressure accidents and decompression sickness. *Ann Emerg Med* 12:563, 1983.

Bove A, Davis JC. *Diving Medicine* (2nd ed.). Philadelphia: Saunders, 1989.

Cales RH et al. Cardiac arrest from gas embolism in scuba diving. *Ann Emerg Med* 10:589, 1981.

Dick APK, Massey W. Neurologic presentation of decompression sickness and air embolism in sport divers. *Neurology* 35:667, 1985.

Divers Alert Network. *1991 Underwater Diving Accident Manual*. Durham, N.C.: Duke University, 1990.

Hansen D, Hooker K. Barotrauma: Under pressure. *Emergency* 21(4):32, 1989.

Kizer KW. Corticosteroids in treatment of serious decompression sickness. *Ann Emerg Med* 10:485, 1981.

Kizer KW. Disorders of the deep. *Emerg Med* 16(17):18, 1984.

LaCombe DM. Under pressure: Recognizing and managing diving emergencies. *JEMS* 17(2):36, 1992.

Melamed Y, Shupak A, Bitterman H. Medical problems associated with underwater diving. *N Engl J Med* 326:30, 1992.

Whitcraft DD, Karas S. Air embolism and decompression sickness in scuba divers. *JACEP* 5:355, 1976.

23

Cardiovascular Emergencies

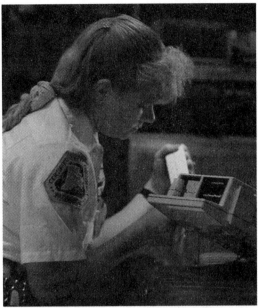

Fagen-Miller Ambulance Service, Highland, Indiana.
Photo by Michael S. Kowal.

OBJECTIVES

It was for the purpose of providing early, definitive treatment for patients with acute myocardial infarction that paramedics first came into being more than 20 years ago. Still today, approximately half a million Americans die every year of coronary artery disease, two-thirds of those deaths occurring outside the hospital, during the first minutes and hours after the onset of symptoms. For that reason, the recognition and management of cardiac emergencies continue to receive strong emphasis in paramedic training.

This chapter is intended to prepare the paramedic to assess and manage those cardiac emergencies that arise from coronary atherosclerosis as well as other conditions that involve pathology of the cardiovascular system. We shall begin by reviewing the anatomy and function of the cardiovascular system, with particular attention to the influence of the autonomic nervous system on cardiac function. We shall then look at some of the clinical manifestations of atherosclerotic and hypertensive cardiovascular disease. Considerable emphasis in this chapter is given to the interpretation of cardiac dysrhythmias and their management within the context of the patient's overall clinical condition. In the final sections of the chapter, we shall examine the pharmacologic and other treatment modalities that make up advanced cardiac life support. By the end of this chapter, then, the student should be able to

1. Identify the major structures of the heart, given a diagram of the heart or a description of its component structures
2. Trace the route taken by blood in one complete circuit through the body
3. Describe the circulatory effects of
   • Failure of the right side of the heart
   • Failure of the left side of the heart
4. Identify the main coronary arteries, and describe their distribution
5. Given a diagram of the cardiovascular system, identify the following arteries and veins:
   • Aorta
   • Pulmonary arteries
   • Common carotid artery
   • Subclavian artery
   • Axillary artery
   • Brachial artery
   • Radial artery
   • Femoral artery
   • Posterior tibial artery
   • Dorsalis pedis artery
   • Superior vena cava
   • Inferior vena cava
   • Pulmonary veins
   • Internal jugular vein
   • External jugular vein
6. Describe the effects of various changes in heart rate and stroke volume on the cardiac output
7. Explain the influence of
   • Preload
   • Afterload
   on the cardiac output and overall cardiac function
8. List the
   • Primary nerves
   • Chemical mediators
   • Effects of stimulation
   associated with the parasympathetic and sympathetic nervous systems
9. Given a list of drugs that act on the autonomic nervous system or a description of a drug's action, identify
   • Cholinergic drugs
   • Parasympathetic blocking agents
   • Alpha sympathetic drugs
   • Beta sympathetic drugs
   • Beta blocking agents
10. List the electrolytes that are most important in normal cardiac function, and describe the role of each
11. Outline the normal pathway of electric conduction through the heart
12. Identify on an ECG
    • The isoelectric line
    • The P wave
    • The P–R interval
    • The QRS complex
    • The S–T segment
    • The T wave
    • The R–R interval
    and describe the cardiac event associated with each
13. List three areas of the heart that can function as a pacemaker, and state the intrinsic rate of firing of each
14. List six questions that should be asked in taking the history of a patient with cardiac problems, given the patient's chief complaint
15. In the history of a patient with cardiac problems, state the possible significance of
    • Chest pain
    • Dyspnea
    • Dizziness or fainting
    • Palpitations
16. State the most likely underlying cardiac problems of a patient given a list of the cardiac medications he or she takes at home
17. In a patient with cardiac problems, state the possible significance of
    • An altered level of consciousness

- Cold, sweaty skin
- An irregular pulse
- Crackles or wheezes
- Right upper quadrant tenderness
- Pedal or sacral edema
- Poor capillary refill

18. List seven risk factors for coronary artery disease, and indicate which of those risk factors can be modified by changes in behavior

19. Given a description of several patients with different clinical findings, identify a patient with
    - Angina pectoris
    - Acute myocardial infarction
    - Left heart failure
    - Right heart failure
    - Cardiogenic shock
    - Aortic aneurysm
    - Hypertensive crisis

    and describe the correct prehospital management of each

20. Identify correct and incorrect techniques of applying monitoring electrodes, given a description of several techniques

21. List the steps in analyzing an electrocardiogram (ECG) rhythm strip

22. Given an ECG rhythm strip,
    - Describe the rhythm
    - Calculate the rate and the P–R interval
    - Describe the P waves and QRS complexes

23. Identify the following ECG rhythms and dysrhythmias, given a 6-second ECG strip, and describe the treatment for each in a symptomatic patient:
    - Normal sinus rhythm
    - Sinus arrhythmia
    - Sinus arrest
    - Sinus bradycardia
    - Sinus tachycardia
    - Wandering pacemaker
    - Premature atrial contractions
    - Premature junctional contractions
    - Paroxysmal supraventricular tachycardia
    - Atrial fibrillation
    - Atrial flutter
    - Junctional rhythm
    - First-degree atrioventricular (AV) block
    - Second-degree AV block, types I and II
    - Third-degree AV block
    - Bundle branch block
    - Premature ventricular contractions
    - Ventricular tachycardia (VT)
    - Ventricular fibrillation (VF)
    - Asystole
    - Artificial pacemaker rhythms
    - ECG artifacts

24. State which leads in a standard 12-lead ECG reflect the condition of
    - The inferior wall of the heart
    - The anterior wall of the heart
    - The lateral wall of the heart

25. Identify
    - A normal ECG
    - An ECG showing changes of ischemia, injury, or infarction given several 12-lead ECGs

26. List the steps of basic life support in the correct sequence

27. List the steps of advanced life support for
    - Ventricular fibrillation/pulseless ventricular tachycardia (VF/VT)
    - Pulseless electrical activity (PEA)
    - Asystole

28. State the indications for
    - Defibrillation
    - Electric cardioversion
    - Cough CPR and precordial thump
    - Carotid sinus massage*
    - Intracardiac injections*
    - Mechanical CPR devices

    and describe the correct utilization of each

29. State the therapeutic action, prehospital indications, contraindications, potential side effects, and adult dosage of
    - Oxygen
    - Morphine sulfate
    - Magnesium sulfate
    - Aminophylline
    - Sodium bicarbonate

    after reviewing the relevant material for each of those drugs in the Drug Handbook at the end of this textbook. (The student should have learned the pharmacology of these drugs already in previous chapters.)

30. State the therapeutic action, prehospital indications, contraindications, potential side effects, and adult dosage of
    - Adenosine
    - Atropine sulfate
    - Bretylium tosylate
    - Dopamine
    - Epinephrine
    - Furosemide
    - Labetolol
    - Lidocaine hydrochloride
    - Nifedipine
    - Nitroglycerin
    - Nitrous oxide
    - Norepinephrine
    - Propranolol

---

*Not required by USDOT for certification as a paramedic.

- Streptokinase
- Tissue plasminogen activator
- Verapamil

after studying the relevant material about each of those drugs in the Drug Handbook at the end of this textbook

31. Identify cases in which it is theoretically permissible (assuming there is local enabling legislation) to stop CPR in the field, given a description of several scenarios of resuscitation

CARDIOVASCULAR ANATOMY AND PHYSIOLOGY

Structure and Function

The cardiovascular system is composed of the heart and blood vessels. Its function is nothing more or less than to deliver oxygenated blood and nutrients to every cell in the body. At the same time, it is also responsible for delivering chemical messages (hormones) here and there and for transporting the waste products of metabolism from the cells to sites of recycling or waste disposal.

The Heart: Two Pumps in One

The moving force behind this extensive pickup and delivery service is the HEART (Fig. 23-1), a quite remarkable little pump that sits in the chest, right above the diaphragm, posterior to and slightly to the left of the lower sternum (**retrosternal**). The heart is not much larger than a man's fist and weighs only about 250 to 300 gm (about 9 ounces), but that is big and strong enough to move about 7,000 to 9,000 *liters* of blood around the body every single day of our lives.

Surrounding the heart, as we learned earlier, is a tough, fibrous sac, the **pericardium**. The pericardium normally contains about 30 ml of serous fluid, which serves as a lubricant, enabling the heart muscle, as it contracts and relaxes, to slide easily within the pericardial sac. The pericardium, being tough and fibrous, does not readily stretch, so it cannot accommodate any sudden accumulations of fluid. If more than about 100 ml of blood or other fluid accumulates rapidly within the pericardium, the pressure inside the tough bag rises to very high levels and literally puts the squeeze on the heart, preventing the ventricles from filling. We have already seen the conse-

FIGURE 23-1. ANATOMY OF THE HEART.   Cutaway view showing the cardiac chambers.

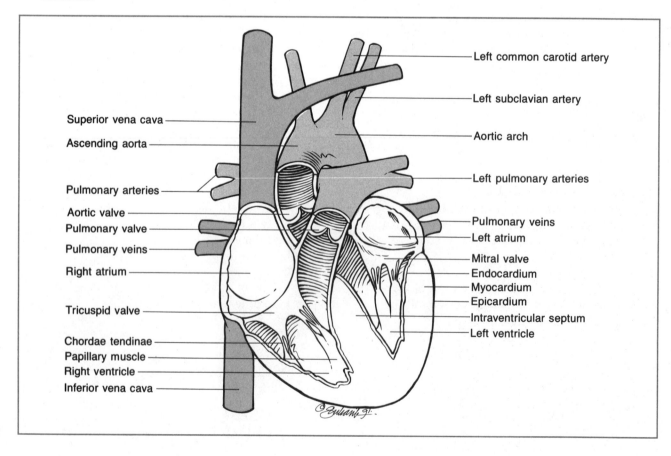

quences of that situation when we considered **cardiac tamponade** in an earlier chapter.

The wall of the heart is made up of three layers. Outermost is the surface layer, or **epicardium,** which is in fact a thin serous membrane; innermost is a smooth layer of connective tissue, the **endocardium;** and in between is the muscular layer of the cardiac wall, the **myocardium.** Like cells anywhere else in the body, myocardial cells require an uninterrupted supply of oxygen and nutrients; indeed, the cardiac demand for oxygen is particularly unremitting because the heart never stops to rest (or not without catastrophic consequences), so it is essential that the heart have an absolutely dependable blood supply. Oxygenated blood reaches the heart through the **coronary arteries** (Fig. 23-2), which branch off the *aorta* just above the leaflets of the aortic valve. There are two main coronary arteries—left and right. The **left main coronary artery** subdivides into the **left anterior descending** and **circumflex** arteries, both of which in turn branch widely to supply the more muscular left ventricle of the heart along with the interventricular septum and part of the right ventricle. The **right coronary artery** supplies the right atrium and ventricle and part of the left ventricle. There are a lot of connections (**anastomoses**) between the arterioles of the various coronary arteries, which allows for the development of alternative routes of blood flow (**collateral circulation**) in the event of blockage. As we shall see later on, the coronary arteries are subject to narrowing in atherosclerotic heart disease, and when the lumen (channel) of one of those arteries becomes so narrowed that blood flow through it is impeded, the symptoms of angina occur.

The arteries and the main **coronary vein** cross the heart in a groove that separates the atria from the ventricles, called the **coronary sulcus.** Venous blood empties into a large vessel in the posterior part of the coronary sulcus, the **coronary sinus,** which in turn ends in the right atrium of the heart.

Structurally, the heart consists of four separate chambers. Looking again at Figure 23-1, we can see that the upper chambers of the heart, or atria, are separated from their respective lower chambers, or ventricles, by **atrioventricular (AV) valves** whose job it is to prevent backflow during ventricular contraction. The **tricuspid valve** separates the right atrium from the right ventricle, and the **mitral valve** separates the left atrium from the left ventricle. Anatomic guy wires, called **chordae tendinae,** attached to **papillary muscles** within the heart, anchor those two valves and keep them from flipping inside out during ventricular contraction. Injury or disease, however, may disrupt the chordae tendinae and permit a valve leaflet to invert (**prolapse**), which in turn allows blood to regurgitate from the ventricle into the atrium.

Two other valves in the heart, collectively known as **semilunar valves** because of their shape, are found at the junction of the ventricles and the pulmonary circulation. The **pulmonic valve** separates the *right* ventricle from the pulmonary artery, preventing backflow from the artery into the ventricle; the **aortic valve** serves the same function for the *left* ventricle, preventing blood that has already entered the aorta from flowing back into the ventricle.

The **cardiac cycle** comprises one complete phase of atrial and ventricular relaxation (**diastole**) followed by one atrial and ventricular contraction (**systole**). During the relatively longer relaxation phase (normally 0.52 second), the left atrium fills passively with blood, under the influence of venous pressure; about 80 percent of ventricular filling occurs during this time as well. With atrial contraction (normally both atria contract at the same time), the contents of each atrium are squeezed into its respective ventricle to complete ventricular filling; the contribution to ventricular filling made by contraction of the atrium is referred to as **atrial kick,** for it is the amount of blood "kicked in" by the atrium. With completion of ventricular filling, the AV valves snap shut, the two ventricles contract (ventricular systole), and the semilunar valves are forced open. Blood squeezed out of the *right* ventricle moves forward, through the pulmonic valve, into the pulmonary arteries, while blood from the *left* ventricle is pushed through the aortic valve and out into the periphery. Systole is usually accomplished in a little over half the time it takes to fill the ventricles, that is, about 0.28 second. (When the heart rate speeds up, it is diastole that gets shorter. What, then, do you think happens to ventricular filling when the heart rate speeds up?)

We mentioned that the heart is a pump, but that is not quite accurate. In fact, functionally the heart is actually *two* pumps—a right pump and a left pump, separated by a thin wall (the **interventricular septum**)—that just happen, for purposes of efficiency, to be housed in one organ and to work in parallel (Fig. 23-3). The RIGHT HEART, composed of the right atrium and right ventricle, is a *low-pressure* system, for it pumps against the relatively low resistance of the pulmonary circulation. The **right atrium** collects oxygen-poor venous blood from the **venae cavae** and the coronary sinus and pumps it into the **right ventricle,** which in turns pumps the oxygen-poor blood into the **pulmonary artery** for distribution to the alveoli and oxygenation. The **pulmonary veins** then collect the oxygen-rich blood and return it to the LEFT HEART, specifically the **left atrium,** which pumps it into the powerful **left ventricle.** The left heart is a *high-pressure* pump, for it has to drive blood out of the heart against the relatively high resistance of the systemic arteries.

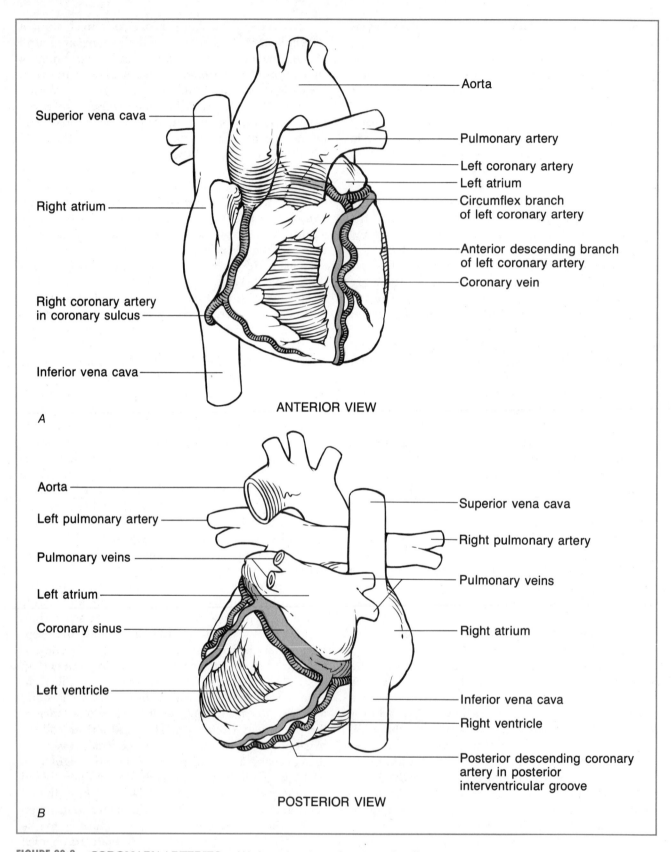

Superior vena cava

Right atrium

Right coronary artery
in coronary sulcus

Inferior vena cava

Aorta

Pulmonary artery

Left coronary artery
Left atrium
Circumflex branch
of left coronary artery

Anterior descending branch
of left coronary artery
Coronary vein

ANTERIOR VIEW

A

Aorta

Left pulmonary artery

Pulmonary veins

Left atrium

Coronary sinus

Left ventricle

Superior vena cava

Right pulmonary artery

Pulmonary veins

Right atrium

Inferior vena cava
Right ventricle

Posterior descending coronary
artery in posterior
interventricular groove

POSTERIOR VIEW

B

FIGURE 23-2.   CORONARY ARTERIES. (A) Anterior view, showing takeoff
point of left and right main coronary arteries from the aorta. (B) View from
below and behind, showing the coronary sinus.

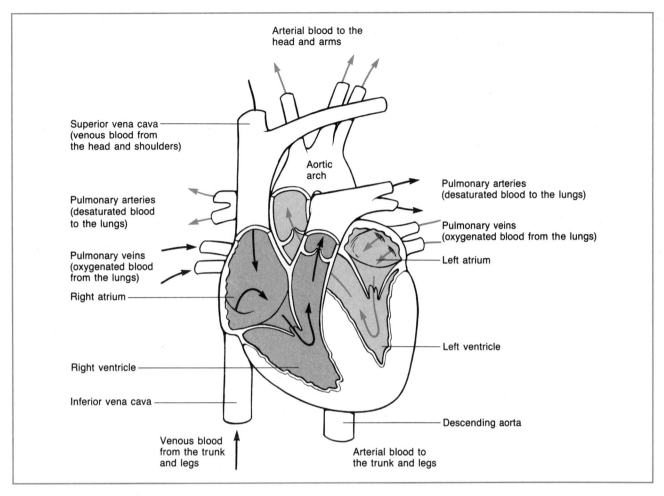

FIGURE 23-3. **BLOOD FLOW THROUGH THE HEART.** Desaturated blood enters the right atrium from the venae cavae, proceeds into the right ventricle and thence out the pulmonary arteries to the lungs. Oxygenated blood enters the left atrium from the pulmonary veins, proceeds to the left ventricle and thence to the body via the aorta.

If there are two pumps, there have to be two sets of tubing into which the pumps empty. And that is precisely the case in the human body, which has, in effect, two circulations. The first is the **systemic circulation** (Fig. 23-4A), that is, all of the blood vessels beyond the left ventricle up to the right atrium, which receive the output of the *left* side of the heart. The second circulation is the **pulmonary circulation** (Fig. 23-4B), comprising all of the blood vessels between the right ventricle and left atrium, which receive the output of the *right* side of the heart.

At any given time, a major proportion of the blood flow may be shunted into one or the other of these two circulations. If, for example, the *right* side of the pump fails and cannot squeeze out its contents efficiently, blood will back up behind the right atrium into the *systemic* veins. Those veins will, as a consequence, become engorged and distended. The most

visible of the systemic veins are the external jugular veins, which reflect the condition of *all* the other systemic veins. When the *external jugular veins* become *distended*, we know that there is considerable back pressure from the right heart throughout the whole systemic circulation. As pressure increases within the systemic veins, fluid starts to leak out into the surrounding tissues, causing those tissues to swell. When a large enough volume of fluid has leaked into the interstitial spaces, that swelling is visible as **edema** in the subcutaneous tissues; it is not so visible, but equally present, in the liver, the walls of the intestine, and other internal tissues.

If, on the other hand, it is the *left* side of the pump that fails, blood backs up behind the left atrium into the *pulmonary* circulation. As pressure builds up in the pulmonary veins, fluid is squeezed out into the alveoli, producing all the characteristic

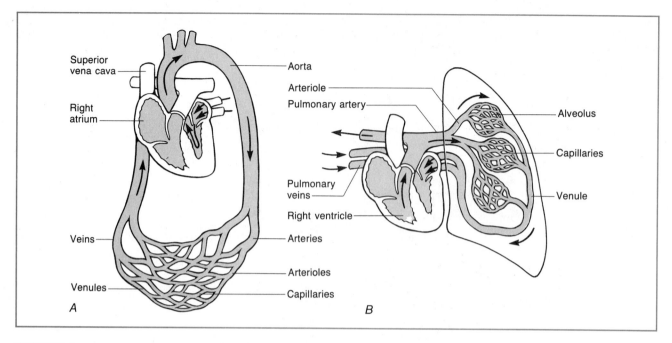

FIGURE 23-4.   DUAL HUMAN CIRCULATION.   (A) The *systemic circulation* consists of all the blood vessels distal to the left ventricle. (B) The *pulmonary circulation* consists of all the blood vessels between the right ventricle and the left atrium.

signs and symptoms of **pulmonary edema:** dyspnea, bubbling crackles, and frothy sputum.

As noted, the two pumps—right and left—in fact operate simultaneously, so that both atria contract first, then both ventricles.

The Blood Vessels

Besides the "cardio" component (the heart), there is, as the name of the system tells us, a second component to the cardiovascular system—the "vascular" component, that is, the blood vessels. There are two principal types of blood vessels in the human body: arteries and veins. Both types share a common structure (Fig. 23-5). There is, first of all, a protective fibrous tissue covering, the **tunica adventitia,** which gives the blood vessel the strength to withstand high pressure against its walls. A middle layer of elastic fibers and muscle, the **tunica media,** gives strength and contractility to the blood vessel. This medial layer is much thicker and more powerful in arteries than in veins. The innermost layer of the blood vessel, the **tunica intima,** is a smooth inner lining only one cell thick.

ARTERIES are thick-walled, muscular vessels—as befits pipes operating in a high-pressure system—that carry blood away from the heart. Usually, arteries carry *oxygenated* blood; the only exceptions are the

pulmonary arteries, which carry oxygen-depleted blood from the right ventricle to the lungs (again, they are carrying blood *away* from the heart). Arteries range in size from the largest artery in the body, the **aorta** to the tiniest arterial branch, or **arteriole.** The major arteries in the body are shown in Figure 23-6.

As we shall see shortly, arterial walls are highly sensitive to stimulation from the autonomic nervous system and, in response to that stimulation, can change their caliber considerably as they contract and relax. In that fashion, the arteries help to regulate **blood pressure,** that is, the pressure exerted by the blood against the arterial walls. Blood pressure is generated by repeated forceful contractions of the left ventricle, which keep blood flowing through the body. But as we shall see, the magnitude of the blood pressure is influenced not only by the output of the heart and the volume of blood present in the system but also by the relative constriction or dilatation of arteries.

VEINS, since they operate on the low-pressure side of the system, have much thinner walls than arteries and consequently less capacity to change their diameter. Veins carry blood *to* the heart—as a rule, *oxygen-poor blood.* Again, the only exceptions are the pulmonary veins, which carry oxygenated blood *to* the heart. The smallest veins, or **venules,** gradually coalesce into larger and larger veins, finally terminat-

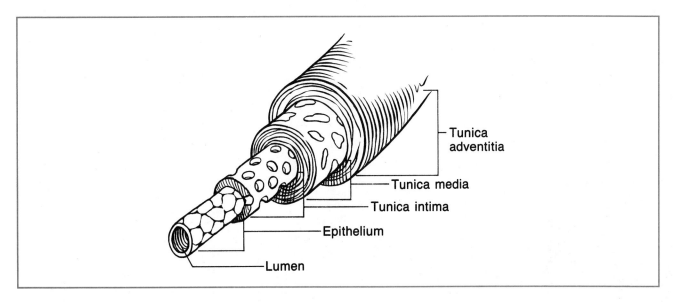

FIGURE 23-5. STRUCTURE OF A BLOOD VESSEL.

ing in the two largest veins of the body, the inferior and superior **venae cavae.**

Between the tiny arterioles and venules at the tissue level is a net of microscopic blood vessels called CAPILLARIES. The walls of capillaries are extremely thin—only one cell deep—enabling the exchange of gases and nutrients across them; the capillary *diameter* is so small that red blood cells must pass through them single file.

The Pump at Work

In order to understand how the heart functions as a pump, it is first necessary to learn some new technical terms:

cardiac output (CO)   The amount of blood that is pumped out by either ventricle, measured in liters per minute. Since the left and right ventricles are connected in series, the two ventricles have equivalent outputs.
stroke volume (SV)   The amount of blood pumped out by either ventricle in a single contraction (heart beat). Normally the stroke volume is between about 60 to 100 ml, but the healthy heart has considerable spare capacity and can easily increase stroke volume by at least 50 percent.
heart rate (HR)   The number of cardiac contractions (heart beats) per minute, in other words, the pulse rate.

Those three factors are related to one another in the following manner:

$$\text{CARDIAC OUTPUT} = \text{STROKE VOLUME} \times \text{HEART RATE}$$

That is, the volume of blood that either ventricle pumps out per minute equals the volume of blood it pumps out in a single contraction times the number of contractions per minute.

To meet changing demands, the heart must be able to increase its output several times over in response to increased oxygen needs in the body, as arise, for example, during exercise. The cardiac output equation tells us that the heart can increase its output either by increasing its stroke volume or increasing its rate or both.

In a mechanical piston pump, the stroke volume is a fixed quantity related to the distance travelled by the piston. The heart, by contrast, has several WAYS OF INCREASING STROKE VOLUME. To begin with, one of the characteristics of cardiac muscle is that when it is stretched, it contracts with greater force. That property is called the **Frank-Starling mechanism,** after the men who first described it. If for any reason an increased volume of blood is returned from the systemic veins to the right heart, or from the pulmonary veins to the left heart, the muscle surrounding the cardiac chambers will have to stretch to accommodate the larger volume; the more the cardiac muscle stretches, the greater will be the force of its contraction, the more completely it will empty, and

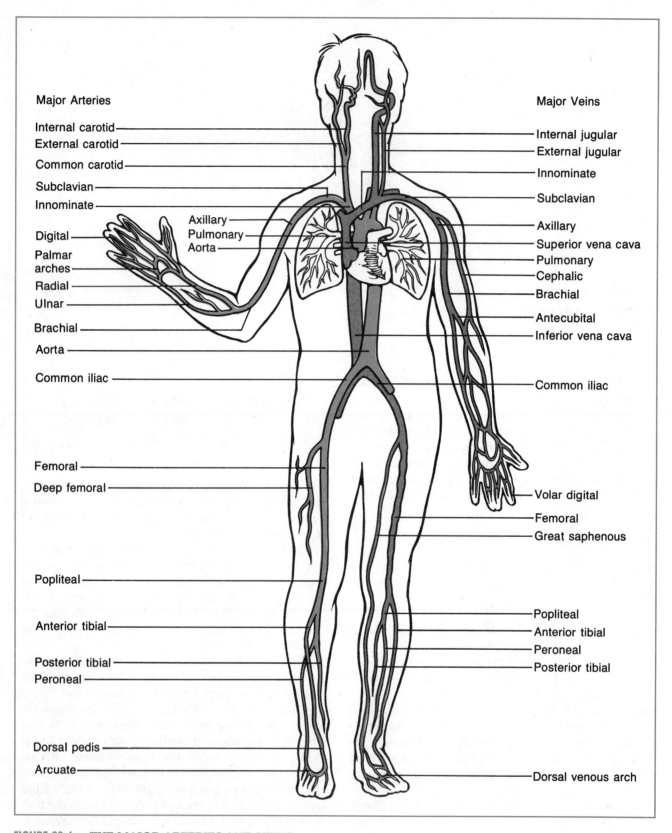

FIGURE 23-6. THE MAJOR ARTERIES AND VEINS.

therefore the greater will be the stroke volume. If we recall our equation:

$$\text{CARDIAC OUTPUT} = \text{STROKE VOLUME} \times \text{HEART RATE}$$

it is clear that any increase in stroke volume, with the heart rate held constant, will cause an increase in the overall cardiac output. The pressure under which a ventricle fills is called the **preload** and is influenced by the volume of blood returned by the veins to the heart. In situations of increased oxygen demand, the body returns more blood to the heart (preload increases), and cardiac output therefore increases through the Frank-Starling mechanism. In the diseased heart, the same mechanism is used to achieve a normal resting cardiac output (that is why some diseased hearts become enlarged).

The heart also has the capacity to vary the speed and degree of contraction of its muscle *without* varying the stretch on the muscle—a property called **contractility.** The ventricles are never completely emptied of blood with any single beat. However, if the heart squeezes into a tighter ball when it contracts, a larger percentage of the ventricular blood will be ejected, thereby increasing stroke volume and overall cardiac output. Nervous controls regulate the contractility of the heart from beat to beat. When the body requires an increase in cardiac output, nervous signals increase myocardial contractility and thereby augment stroke volume.

If we look once more at our equation:

$$\text{CARDIAC OUTPUT} = \text{STROKE VOLUME} \times \text{HEART RATE}$$

it is evident that the heart can also increase its output, given a constant stroke volume, by increasing the number of contractions per minute, that is, by INCREASING THE HEART RATE. Let us look, for example, at a heart that has a resting stroke volume of 70 ml per beat and a resting rate of 70 beats per minute:

$$\text{CARDIAC OUTPUT} = \frac{70 \text{ ml}}{\text{beat}} \times \frac{70 \text{ beats}}{\text{min}}$$
$$= \frac{4,900 \text{ ml}}{\text{min}}$$

Suppose that the owner of that heart now begins to exercise. His oxygen demand increases, and nervous mechanisms stimulate the heart to increase its rate. If, for example, the heart rate increases to 110 per minute, without any change in the stroke volume, the cardiac output would increase as follows:

$$\text{CARDIAC OUTPUT} = \frac{70 \text{ ml}}{\text{beat}} \times \frac{110 \text{ beats}}{\text{min}}$$
$$= \frac{7,700 \text{ ml}}{\text{min}}$$

(Beyond certain limits, further increases in heart rate will not increase cardiac output. Why do you think that is so? Hint: What is occurring between ventricular systoles?)

Of the mechanisms described, the Frank-Starling mechanism is an intrinsic property of heart muscle, that is, not under nervous control; contractility and changes in heart rate, on the other hand, are regulated by the nervous system.

The Electric Conduction System of the Heart

Heart muscle is unique among body tissues in that it has the ability to generate its own electric impulses without stimulation from nerves, a property known as **automaticity.** In addition, the heart is endowed with specialized conduction tissue that can propagate electric impulses with great speed to the muscular tissue of the heart. The area of conduction tissue in which the electric activity arises at any given time is called the **pacemaker,** because it sets the pace, or rate, for cardiac contraction.

Theoretically, any cell within the cardiac conduction system can act as pacemaker; but in the normal heart, the dominant pacemaker is the **sinoatrial (SA) node,** located in the right atrium, near the inlet of the superior vena cava (Fig. 23-7). The SA node is the fastest pacemaker in the heart, normally firing 60 to 100 times per minute. Electric impulses generated in the SA node spread across the two atria through specialized conduction pathways in the atrial wall in about 0.08 second, causing the atria to contract, and then reach the **atrioventricular (AV) node** in the region of the **AV junction.** The AV node serves as a sort of gatekeeper to the ventricles, delaying conduction of the impulse just a bit (normally around 0.12 second) so that ventricular contraction lags a bit behind atrial contraction and there is time for the "atrial kick" to occur. When the atrial rate becomes very rapid, as we shall discuss later on, not all the atrial impulses can get through the AV junction. Normally, though, impulses reaching the AV junction pass through it into the **bundle of His,** then move rapidly into the **right and left bundles** located on either side of the interventricular septum, and spread into

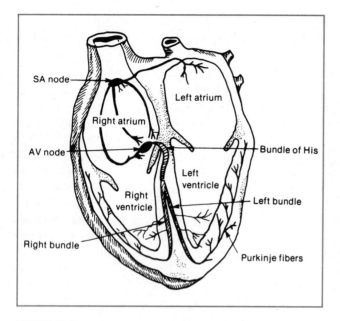

FIGURE 23-7.   ELECTRIC CONDUCTION SYSTEM OF THE HEART.   Impulses that originate in the SA node spread through the atria to the AV node and thence down the bundle of His and right and left bundles into the Purkinje network of the ventricles.

the **Purkinje fibers,** thousands of fibrils distributed through the ventricular muscle. It takes about 0.08 second for an electric impulse to spread across the ventricles, and as it does so, the ventricles contract.

The process by which muscle fibers are stimulated to contract is called **depolarization,** and it comes about through changes in the concentration of electrolytes across cell membranes (Fig. 23-8). Myocardial cells, like all other cells in the body, are bathed in electrolyte solution. Chemical pumps inside the cell maintain the concentrations of ions within the cell and in the process create an electric gradient across the cell wall. The result is that a resting (polarized) cell normally has a net charge of -90 millivolts (mV) with respect to the outside of the cell (Fig. 23-8A1). When the myocardial cell receives a stimulus from the conduction system (Fig. 23-8A2), the permeability of the cell wall changes in such a way that sodium (Na^+) rushes into the cell, causing the inside of the cell to become more positive. (Calcium [Ca^{++}] also enters the cell, although more slowly, with the same effect.) A reversal of electric charge—depolarization—starts at one spot in the cell and spreads in a wave along the cell until the cell is completely depolarized (Fig. 23-8A3). As the cell depolarizes, it contracts.

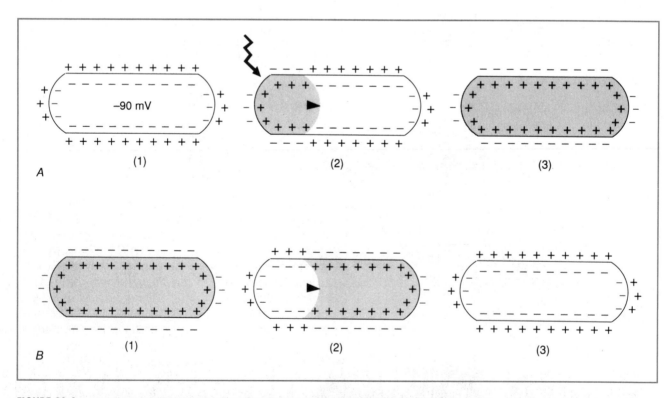

FIGURE 23-8.   MOVEMENT OF IONS TO PRODUCE NET CURRENT FLOW.
(A) Depolarization. (1) At rest, the cellular interior has a net charge of -90 mV. (2) The wave of depolarization begins as sodium ions pour into the cell. (3) The depolarized cell. (B) Repolarization. (1) Depolarized cell. (2) Wave of repolarization begins as potassium leaves the cell. (3) Repolarized cell.

If the cell were to remain depolarized, it could never contract again! Fortunately, the cell is able to recover from depolarization through a process called **repolarization** (Fig. 23-8B). Repolarization starts with the rapid escape of potassium (K^+) from the cell, to help restore the inside of the cell to its negative charge; then the proper electrolyte distribution is re-established by pumping sodium out of the cell and allowing the potassium to reenter. The roles of electrolytes in cardiac function are summarized in Table 23-1.

A myocardial cell cannot respond to an electric stimulus from the conduction system normally unless it is fully polarized. So the period when the cell is depolarized or in the process of repolarizing is called the **refractory period,** because the cell is refractory to further stimulation until it has fully repolarized.

As already noted, the SA node is normally the heart's dominant pacemaker because the SA node normally has the most rapid intrinsic rate of firing (60–100 times/min)—so it will literally "outpace" any slower conduction tissue. However, any component of the conduction system may act as a secondary pacemaker should the SA node be damaged or suppressed. The farther removed the conduction tissue is from the SA node, the slower will be its intrinsic rate of firing. Thus the *AV junction* (which includes the AV node and its surrounding tissue along with the bundle of His) will spontaneously fire 40 to 50 times per minute, while the ventricular *Purkinje sys-tem*, which is farther removed from the SA node, will spontaneously fire only 30 to 40 times per minute. Suppose, for example, that the SA node is damaged by ischemia (tissue injury caused by hypoxemia) and doesn't fire. The AV junction, failing to receive any impulses from the SA node, might then begin firing at its own rate (40–60 times/min), and the electrocardiogram (ECG) would show a "junctional rhythm" at a rate of 40 to 60 per minute.

The electric events in the heart can be recorded on an ECG as a series of waves and complexes (Fig. 23-9), each of which have been given a name. The *depolarization of the atria* produces the **P wave.** Then there is a brief pause as conduction is momentarily slowed through the AV junction, followed by the **QRS complex,** representing *depolarization of the ventricles.* Repolarization of the atria and ventricles produces **T waves;** however, the atrial T wave is small and usually buried in the QRS complex, so it isn't seen. The larger, ventricular T wave follows the QRS complex.

The intervals between waves and complexes also have names. The **P–R interval** is the distance from the beginning of the P wave to the beginning of the QRS complex. It represents the time required for an impulse to traverse the atria and AV junction, which is normally 0.12 to 0.20 second (3–5 little boxes on ECG paper). The **S–T segment** is the line from the end of the QRS complex to the begining of the T wave and should normally be at the same level as the baseline (**isoelectric line**). An S–T segment that is elevated above or depressed below the isoelectric line may indicate myocardial ischemia or damage. The **R–R interval** is the time between two successive QRS complexes, thus representing the interval between two ventricular depolarizations.

TABLE 23-1. ROLE OF ELECTROLYTES IN CARDIAC FUNCTION

ELECTROLYTE	ROLE IN CARDIAC FUNCTION
Sodium (Na^+)	Flows into cell to initiate depolarization
Potassium (K^+)	Flows out of cell to initiate repolarization *hypo*kalemia → increased myocardial irritability *hyper*kalemia → decreased automaticity/conduction
Calcium (Ca^{++})	Major role in depolarization of pacemaker cells and in myocardial contractility *hypo*calcemia → decreased contractility and increased myocardial irritability *hyper*calcemia → increased contractility
Magnesium (Mg^{++})	Stabilizes cell membrane; acts in concert with potassium and opposes actions of calcium

---

COMPONENTS OF THE ELECTROCARDIOGRAM

ECG Representation	*Cardiac Event*
P wave	Depolarization of the atria
P–R interval	Depolarization of the atria and delay at the AV junction
QRS complex	Depolarization of the ventricles
S–T segment	Period between ventricular depolarization and repolarization
T wave	Repolarization of the ventricles
R–R interval	Time between two ventricular depolarizations

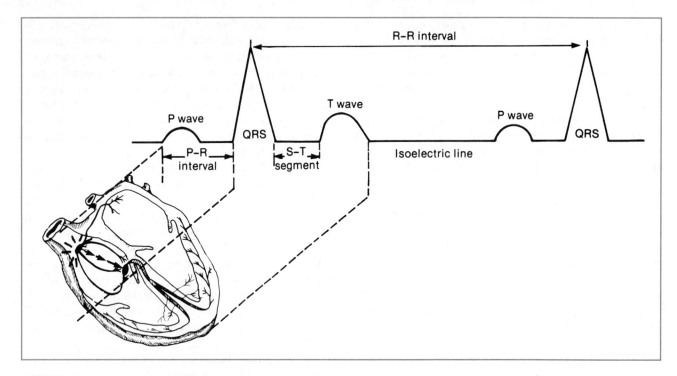

FIGURE 23-9. **THE ECG AND CARDIAC EVENTS.**   Progress of the depolarizing current through the heart produces characteristic waves and complexes on the ECG.

We shall return to the ECG later in this chapter, when we consider various disturbances in cardiac rhythm. We need first, however, to consider the factors that are most important in regulating normal cardiac rhythm and function.

The Autonomic Nervous System and the Heart

Throughout this textbook, in a variety of different contexts, we have made mention of the autonomic nervous system. It is time now to stop and take a closer look at that system, for it plays a key role in regulating the activity of the whole cardiovascular system; furthermore, the majority of pharmacologic agents we use in the field to manage cardiac disorders interact in one way or another with the autonomic nervous system.

The **autonomic nervous system** refers to that part of the human nervous system that controls *automatic*, or *involuntary* actions. Its importance can be gauged by considering the alternative: Suppose all bodily functions were solely under *voluntary* control. Sixty times a minute, 24 hours a day, you would have to remind your heart to beat. Twelve times a minute, 24 hours a day, you would be required to order your lungs to inflate and relax. You would be constrained

to warn your stomach that food was on the way, tell your pancreas and gallbladder to step up their activities, urge your gut to speed up or slow down according to the circumstances. Furthermore, any time you changed your level of activity, as for example in exercise, you would be forced to issue a complex series of orders to your cardiovascular system to ensure that cardiac output increased sufficiently to meet increased metabolic demands. Fortunately, all that administrative work is accomplished for us, without any conscious effort on our part. It happened more or less like this:

In the beginning, when God was working out the circuitry for man, Adam persuaded Him to include an autonomic nervous system. "Look," said Adam, "I don't want to spend all my time thinking about my cardiac output and my ventilation and my digestion. I want to think great philosophic thoughts, and maybe have a little fun on the side."

"We'll see what We can do," said God.

So after some debate, they worked out a compromise. "I tell you what I'll do for you, Adam. I'll give you *two* nervous systems: one that's fully automatic—an autonomic nervous system—so that your bodily functions can proceed without your having to bother yourself about them; the other voluntary, so that you can consciously control the movement of your muscles."

That seemed reasonable, and Adam agreed. So it came to pass that human beings have two nervous systems.

One day God noticed that Adam was looking very sad.

"What's the matter, Adam?" asked God.

"It's my autonomic nervous sytem," said Adam. "It's not quite right yet."

"What do you mean, it's not quite right? I designed it according to your specifications, didn't I?"

"I know. But I've noticed that my life is divided into two kinds of activity. I do a lot of rather vegetative things, like sleeping and digesting my food, during which my heart needs to slow down. But I also do really exciting things—especially since Eve arrived—during which my heart needs to speed up. What I really need are two autonomic nervous systems, one to take care of ordinary vegetative functions and another to equip me for things like fighting, running, and, uh, Eve."

"*Two* autonomic nervous systems! Adam, this is getting entirely out of hand."

"This is supposed to be Eden, isn't it? And everything's supposed to be perfect, isn't it? Well, if You were really concerned about my welfare, You'd give me two autonomic nervous systems like it says in the medical textbooks."

"All right, all right," said God. "I'll see what I can do."

So the next day, God said to Adam, "I've got everything fixed up. From now on, you'll have a voluntary nervous system and *two* autonomic nervous systems. One of them will be called parasympathetic, and it will regulate your vegetative functions; it will slow your heart rate, help you digest your food, and all that stuff. The other will be called the sympathetic nervous system, and that will speed up your heart, constrict your blood vessels, dilate your bronchi and pupils, and so forth."

"Why do they have to have such funny names?" asked Adam.

"Because *I* said so," said God, "and I'm still Boss around here, in case you've forgotten."

The Parasympathetic System

The parasympathetic system is concerned primarily with *vegetative* functions and sends its messages mainly through the **vagus nerve.** Suppose, for example, that the brain decided the heart should slow down a little; perhaps someone had applied a little pressure over the carotid or strained during a bowel movement (both of which are vagal stimuli). A message in the form of an electric impulse would then go barrelling down the vagus nerve to the place where the vagus abuts on the sinus node of the heart. At the end of the vagus, the electric impulse would cause the release of a naturally occurring chemical, **acetylcholine** (it is from this chemical that the parasympathetic nervous system derives its other name, the *cholinergic* nervous system). The acetylcholine (ACh, for short) would cross over to the sinus node of the heart and say, "Listen, sinus node, the brain says you ought to slow down; I just heard it from the vagus." Just to be on the safe side, another ACh molecule would wander down to talk to the AV node of the heart: "We've just instructed the sinus node to slow down; but just in case he didn't get the message, we want you to make sure that no extra impulses get through to the ventricles, understand?"

"Sure thing," says the AV node, which is more sensitive to criticism from the vagus nerve. "They shall not pass."

"Right on," says ACh.

The only drug with which we shall be concerned that interacts directly with the parasympathetic nervous system is **atropine.** Atropine is a parasympathetic *blocker;* that is, it opposes the action of acetylcholine on the heart and elsewhere.

Suppose the heart is plodding along at a rate of 50 beats per minute, and you administer 0.5 mg of atropine intravenously. The atropine will travel through the bloodstream until it reaches the sinus node.

"You're firing a little slowly today, aren't you?" says atropine.

"Just following orders," says the sinus node. "The vagus told me to take it easy."

"The vagus, the vagus. That's all I ever hear. What do you want to listen to that old stick-in-the-mud for? Listen, stick with me and you'll have a little excitement in your life."

"No kidding?"

"No kidding."

So the sinus node speeds up. Meanwhile, the atropine reaches the AV node. "How are you doing, AV?" asks the atropine.

"Oh, it's kind of slow lately. The vagus ordered me to close down two lanes southbound."

"The vagus again. Listen, AV node, if you keep paying attention to the vagus, before you know it he'll close down the whole highway to the ventricles, and they'll go off merrily on their own."

"Gee whiz," says the AV node. "What should I do?"

"Take my advice, sonny, and open the gates wide. Let all the impulses through."

"Are you sure that's a good idea? The vagus said. . . ."

"Forget about the vagus. He's just an old obstructionist."

"OK," says the AV node, always eager to please

when there's atropine around. And he opens all southbound lanes.

The Sympathetic System

The sympathetic nervous system is concerned with preparing the body to respond to various *stresses;* it is, in fact, the very same "fight or flight" system that we learned about in Chapter 4. As Adam properly noted, the parasympathetic system is fine for routine, everyday activities like keeping the heart plodding along during rest or coordinating digestion, but it provides no mechanism for the body to adapt to changing demands. It is the sympathetic nervous system that increases the heart rate, strengthens the force of cardiac muscle contractions, and provides a variety of other adaptive responses to ensure that increased oxygen demands of the tissues are met by increased cardiac output.

Suppose you start running to catch a bus. After a few seconds, your muscles will have used up all the oxygen and nutrients immediately on hand. "It's getting awfully stuffy down here," says one muscle to another.

"You said it!"

"I wish the heart would increase the delivery of oxygen."

So the muscles send a message through the sympathetic nervous system: "HELP! We can't breathe!"

The message travels through sympathetic nerves, originating in the thoracic and lumbar ganglia, and ultimately arrives at the heart. Whereas the vagus nerve releases acetylcholine, sympathetic nerves convey their commands through release of a different chemical, **norepinephrine** (NE). Norepinephrine travels to the sinus node, AV node, and ventricles, spreading the command from the sympathetic nerves: "Let's speed this operation up," says NE. "The muscles are suffocating and threatening to bomb the circulation with lactic acid if they don't get more oxygen." So the heart speeds up, increasing cardiac output and hence the delivery of oxygen and nutrients throughout the body.

When there is intense stimulation of the sympathetic nervous system, a special hormone—**epinephrine**—may also be mobilized to spread the alarm. Epinephrine is produced in the *adrenal gland* and thus is also sometimes called **Adrenalin,** from which the other name of the sympathetic system—the *adrenergic* system—is derived. Epinephrine, like norepinephrine, commands the heart to speed up.

DRUGS THAT INFLUENCE THE SYMPATHETIC NERVOUS SYSTEM are classified according to the *receptors* with which they interact. A drug receptor can be visualized as an ignition switch. When the proper key is fitted into the switch, a specified series of reactions is triggered. When the key is inserted into the ignition of a car, a predictable sequence of events follows: The battery sends a current to the spark plugs, which fire; a combustion of gasoline and air occurs; and the engine turns over. Not every key will fit a specific car's ignition, but every key that does fit will cause the same reaction. The organs of the body have a number of such ignition switches. In the sympathetic nervous system, those switches, or **receptors,** are labelled *alpha* and *beta*. Whenever one of those switches is activated by a key (a drug or hormone) that fits, a predictable sequence of responses will occur. In the heart, arteries, and lungs, those receptors are as follows:

EFFECTS OF SYMPATHETIC STIMULATION

Effect on	*Alpha*	*Beta*
Heart	None	Increased rate
		Increased force
		Increased automaticity
Arteries	Vasoconstriction	Vasodilation
Lungs	None, or mild bronchoconstriction	Bronchodilation

The heart has only one ignition switch, that for a beta agent. Any beta agent that comes along will have the same effect on the heart, that is, to increase its rate, force, and automaticity. The arteries, by contrast, have receptors for both alpha and beta agents. When an alpha drug is given, it will turn on the switch that causes vasoconstriction; when a beta agent is given, the switch causing vasodilation will be activated. Similarly, the lungs have both alpha and beta receptors. Alpha agents don't have much effect, actually; at most they cause a little bronchoconstriction. But beta agents trigger bronchodilation. (Think back to the previous chapter and the drugs used to treat asthma.) These concepts are represented schematically in Figure 23-10.

Drugs that have alpha or beta sympathetic properties are called **sympathomimetic drugs,** because they imitate (mime) the actions of naturally occurring sympathetic chemicals. By knowing whether a sympathomimetic drug is an alpha or beta agent, we can predict what it will do with respect to to the heart,

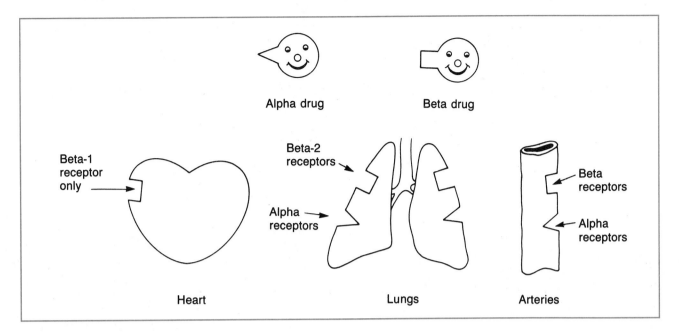

FIGURE 23-10. **RECEPTOR SITES** of the sympathetic nervous system in the heart, lungs, and arteries.

lungs, and arteries. Consider isoproterenol (Isuprel). It is a *pure beta* agent. Having carefully learned the properties of alpha and beta agents, we can immediately recognize that isoproterenol acts in the manner shown in Figure 23-11—to stimulate the heart, dilate the bronchi, and dilate the arteries.

Phenylephrine (Neo-Synephrine), on the other hand, is a *pure alpha* agent. By now, we all know what alpha agents do (Fig. 23-12).

Suppose a new drug called Peppynephrine appeared on the market, and the manufacturer stated the drug was a beta agent. Without being told anything further about the drug, we should now be able to describe the actions of Peppynephrine on the heart, lungs, and arteries.

Unfortunately, things are not always quite so simple as just described. While isoproterenol and phenylephrine are *pure* beta and alpha agents respectively, most other drugs have varying degrees of both alpha and beta activity. The drugs acting on the sympathetic nervous system can be pictured along a continuum from alpha to beta (Fig. 23-13). Norepinephrine (Levophed) is chiefly an alpha agent, and its alpha effects predominate; but because it does have some beta activity, it will—unlike a pure alpha agent—have effects on the heart. (What effects?) Conversely, epinephrine (Adrenalin) is chiefly a beta agent, and its beta effects predominate; but in high doses, epinephrine will produce some alpha effects, especially on the arteries.

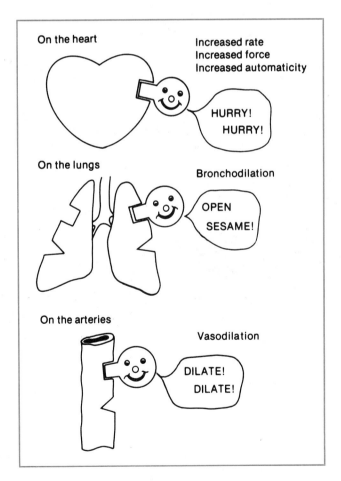

FIGURE 23-11. **BETA SYMPATHETIC AGENTS** increase the rate, force, and automaticity of the heart; dilate the bronchi; and dilate peripheral arteries.

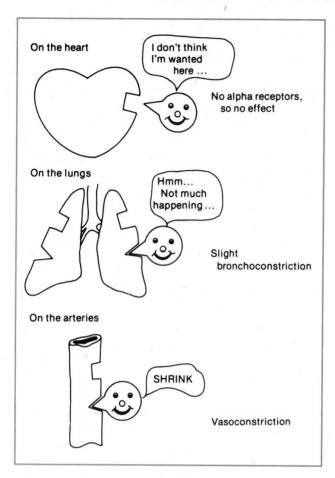

FIGURE 23-12.   **ALPHA AGENTS** have no direct effect on
the heart; they cause slight bronchoconstriction and
marked vasoconstriction.

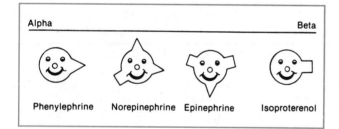

FIGURE 23-13. Many sympathomimetic agents have both
alpha and beta properties.

Among the drugs used in the field, there are
several commonly encountered sympathomimetic
agents:

• Isoproterenol (Isuprel)—pure BETA
• Albuterol (Ventolin), isoetharine (Bronkosol),
  and terbutaline (Bricanyl)—pure BETA
• Epinephrine (Adrenalin)—predominantly BETA
• Norepinephrine (Levophed)—predominantly
  ALPHA
• Dopamine (Intropin)—BETA at low doses;
  ALPHA at high doses
• Metaraminol (Aramine)—predominantly
  ALPHA

Two of those drugs, norepinephrine and epinephrine, are also naturally occurring chemicals of the
sympathetic nervous system. Their actions are the
same whether produced in the body and released
from the nervous system or manufactured in a factory and injected by a paramedic.

Based on what we have just learned about alpha
and beta effects, which of the above drugs would be
useful in treating an acute asthmatic attack? Which
would you use to raise the blood pressure by vasoconstriction?

It turns out that it is possible to subdivide *beta*
sympathetic agents into two groups, based on subtle
differences between the beta receptors in the heart
and those in the lungs. Drugs that act primarily on
cardiac beta receptors are called **beta-1** and those that
act chiefly on *pulmonary* beta receptors are called
beta-2. The newer bronchodilators, for example—
such as albuterol, isoetharine, and terbutaline—are
selective beta-2 agents, so they provide effective
bronchodilation with much fewer cardiac side effects.

There is another class of drugs that act on the
sympathetic nervous system—drugs known as sympathetic *blockers*. As their name implies, they block
the action of sympathetic agents by beating them to
the receptor site and preventing them from turning
on the ignition. The receptor sites, not being very
smart, cannot distinguish a blocker from a stimulator

FIGURE 23-14.   **A SYMPATHETIC BLOCKER** occupies the
receptor site for the stimulating drug, thus preventing
the stimulating drug from exerting its usual effect.

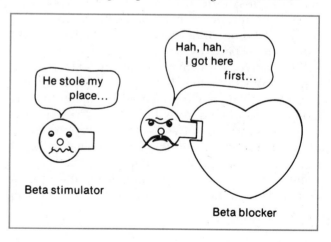

until it is too late. Sympathetic blockade is illustrated in Figure 23-14. With the blocker occupying the receptor site, the stimulating agent cannot get in to turn on the switch.

The only sympathetic blocking agents that may on occasion be used in the field, and that some patients may be taking at home, are **propranolol** (Inderal) and **labetalol** (Normodyne, Trandate), beta *blockers*. Propranolol may be considered a representative example of the group (Fig. 23-15). Propranolol occupies beta receptors in the heart, lungs, and arteries, as well as elsewhere in the body. Thus beta agents, whether released from sympathetic nerve endings or given intravenously, cannot have their full effect when propranolol has been administered previously (Fig. 23-16).

To sum up what we have learned so far: The human nervous system consists of a voluntary and involuntary system. The latter, also called the auto-

FIGURE 23-15. One of the principal sympathetic blocking agents is propranolol, a beta blocker.

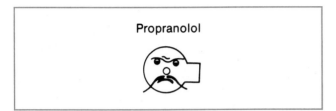

FIGURE 23-16. By occupying beta receptor sites, propranolol prevents epinephrine from having its usual effects on heart, lungs, and blood vessels.

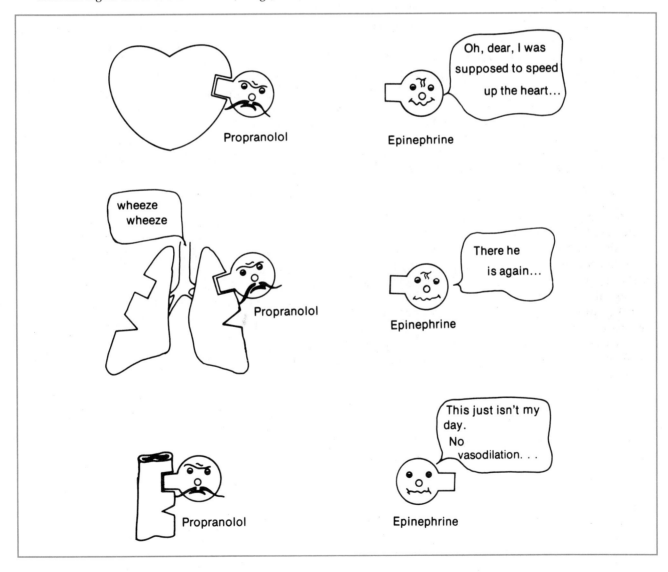

nomic nervous system, is further divided into the sympathetic and parasympathetic systems:

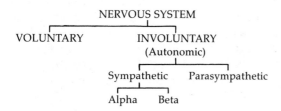

The *parasympathetic system* controls vegetative functions. It is mediated through the vagus nerve by release of a chemical called acetylcholine at nerve endings. The vagus can be stimulated in a number of ways, including pressure on the carotid sinus, straining against a closed glottis (**Valsalva maneuver**), and distention of a hollow organ (the bladder, the stomach). When the parasympathetic nervous system is stimulated, by whatever mechanism, the vagus *slows the heart* by depressing the activity of pacemaker sites. The influence of the vagus nerve can be opposed by the parasympathetic blocking agent, atropine.

The *sympathetic nervous system* enables the body to respond to stress. It is mediated through nerves arising in the thoracic and lumbar ganglia, via release of norepinephrine, and by the adrenal gland, via release of the hormone epinephrine. (Question: How does injury to the thoracic spinal cord produce spinal shock?) In addition to those naturally occurring chemicals, there are several synthetic agents, or drugs, that interact with the sympathetic nervous system. All sympathetic agents, whether naturally occurring or synthetic, are classified as alpha or beta. Alpha agents have no direct effect on the heart; they have minimal bronchoconstricting effects but significant vasoconstricting action. The alpha agent used most often in the field is norepinephrine (Levophed). Beta agents cause the heart to increase its rate and force of contraction, as well as increasing overall myocardial irritability. Beta agents dilate arteries and bronchi. Isoproterenol (Isuprel), epinephrine (Adrenalin), and the selective beta-2 adrenergics (like albuterol and isoetharine) are the beta agents used most often in the field.

Sympathetic *blockers* occupy receptor sites and prevent sympathetic stimulators from acting. Propranolol is a beta blocker and opposes beta effects; thus it slows the heart and prevents vasodilation and bronchodilation.

The properties of the autonomic nervous system are summarized in Table 23-2.

The *indications* for the major autonomic stimulating and blocking agents can be deduced easily now that we know the properties of those drugs and the manner in which they interact with the autonomic nervous system:

atropine   Parasympathetic blocker, opposing the vagus nerve. Hence, atropine is used to *speed up the heart* when excessive vagal firing has caused bradycardia.

norepinephrine   Sympathetic agent, primarily alpha, causing vasoconstriction. Norepinephrine is used to *increase the blood pressure* when hypotension is caused by vasodilation (e.g., neurogenic shock).

isoproterenol   Sympathetic agent, almost pure beta, causing an increase in heart rate and dilation of bronchi. Isoproterenol is used (1) to *increase cardiac output* and (2) to *dilate bronchi* in asthma.

epinephrine   Sympathetic agent, predominantly beta, with actions similar to isoproterenol, but having an additional, vasoconstrictor effect. Indications for epinephrine are similar to those for isoproterenol, but in addition epinephrine is indicated for (1) *asystole* or fine ventricular fibrillation (to increase the automaticity of the heart) and (2) *anaphylactic shock* (for *all* its effects: bronchodilation, vasoconstriction, increased cardiac output).

dopamine   Sympathetic agent, used at low (beta) doses to increase the force of cardiac contractions in *cardiogenic shock;* its beta effects on renal and mesenteric arteries are an added advantage, for by dilating those arteries, dopamine helps maintain urine flow and good perfusion to abdominal organs.

albuterol (salbutamol), **isoetharine, terbutaline**   Sympathetic beta-2 agents, used, because of their selective beta effects on the lungs, to induce bronchodilation in asthma, COPD, and other bronchospastic conditions.

metaraminol   Sympathetic agent, predominantly alpha, causing vasoconstriction. Metaraminol is thus used to *increase blood pressure* when hypotension is caused by vasodilation.

propranolol   Sympathetic beta blocker, opposing the actions of beta stimulating agents. Propranolol is used clinically (1) to *slow the heart rate* in certain tachyarrhythmias; (2) to *decrease the pain of chronic angina* (by decreasing the work of the heart); and (3) to *depress irritability in the heart* (by decreasing the tendency of the heart to fire automatically). Its use is contraindicated in asthmatics (Why?).

The Sympathetic Nervous System and Blood Pressure Regulation

Having learned something about the actions of the sympathetic nervous system on the heart and blood

TABLE 23-2. AUTONOMIC NERVOUS SYSTEM

FEATURES	PARASYMPATHETIC	SYMPATHETIC
Other name	Cholinergic	Adrenergic
Natural chemical mediator	Acetylcholine (ACh)	Norepinephrine Epinephrine
Primary nerve(s)	Vagus	Nerves from the thoracic and lumbar ganglia of the spinal cord
Effects of stimulation	Slows the heart Constricts pupils Increases salivation Increases gut motility	Speeds the heart Dilates pupils Constricts blood vessels Slows the gut
Stimulating drug	Neostigmine Reserpine	*Alpha*: phenylephrine *Beta*: isoproterenol *Beta-2*: albuterol Alpha + beta: Norepinephrine Epinephrine Metaraminol Dopamine
Blocking drugs	Atropine	Alpha: Chlorpromazine Phentolamine Beta: Propranolol Metoprolol Labetalol Atenolol

vessels, we are now in a position to consider how blood pressure is controlled. The body, as we learned in Chapter 9, attempts to maintain a fairly constant blood pressure to ensure perfusion of vital organs. At any given moment, the blood pressure is influenced by the cardiac output and the resistance (degree of constriction) of the arterioles:

> **BLOOD PRESSURE = CARDIAC OUTPUT ×**
> **PERIPHERAL RESISTANCE**

It is clear from the equation that the blood pressure can be increased by increasing either the cardiac output or the peripheral resistance or both. (How is cardiac output increased? How is peripheral resistance increased?) Under normal circumstances, the body balances flow and resistance to maintain a stable blood pressure. Alterations in one variable bring about compensatory changes in the other variable to restore blood pressure toward normal. Consider, for

example, the situation where cardiac ouput is suddenly decreased, as in hemorrhage. (Question: How does hemorrhage decrease cardiac output?) Since

$$\frac{\text{BLOOD}}{\text{PRESSURE}} = \frac{\text{CARDIAC}}{\text{OUTPUT}} \times \frac{\text{PERIPHERAL}}{\text{RESISTANCE}}$$

the fall in cardiac output will inevitably lead to a fall in blood pressure unless the peripheral resistance is altered. However, because the body attempts always to maintain a stable blood pressure, the falling cardiac output activates the sympathetic nervous system, which in turn causes the arterioles to constrict. (Question: Is that an alpha effect or a beta effect?) Vasoconstriction increases the peripheral resistance, thus tending to restore the blood pressure back toward normal.

Now let us look at the equation in a slightly different way. If we divide both sides of the equation by the peripheral resistance, we come up with a new equation that looks like this:

$$\frac{\text{CARDIAC}}{\text{OUTPUT}} = \frac{\text{BLOOD PRESSURE}}{\text{PERIPHERAL RESISTANCE}}$$

What that equation tells us is that, for any given blood pressure, the cardiac output will vary inversely with the peripheral resistance. In other words, the higher the peripheral resistance (i.e., the more constricted the arterioles), the lower the cardiac output. That makes intuitive sense, for clearly it is harder to push fluid through narrower pipes. There is, in fact, a special name given to the resistance against which the ventricle contracts, and that is **afterload.** The greater the afterload, the harder the ventricle has to work in order to pump out its blood. In conditions of chronically high afterload, such as high blood pressure, the left ventricle may eventually grow exhausted from the extra work and cease pumping efficiently.

PATIENT ASSESSMENT

The History in the Cardiac Patient

The most common chief complaints in patients suffering from cardiac problems are chest pain, dyspnea, fainting, and palpitations. Let us consider those chief complaints one at a time and see what we need to find out about each of them.

CHEST PAIN is often the presenting sign of acute myocardial infarction. The patient's description of the pain will be very important in assessing its significance. The PQRST-A format can help you remember the questions you need to ask about the patient's chest pain:

P What **provoked** the pain, that is, what if anything brought it on? What was the patient doing at the time? Just sitting in a chair? Changing a tire? Having an argument with his boss? What **palliates** the pain; that is, is there anything that makes it better? Patients with chronic coronary artery disease may take nitroglycerin for episodes of chest pain. Ask whether the patient did so and, if he did, whether it helped.

Q What is the **quality** of the pain, that is, what does it feel like? Dull? Sharp? Crushing? Heavy? Squeezing? Note the *exact words* the patient uses to describe his pain, and observe his body language as he does so.

R Does the pain **radiate?** From where to where? To the jaw? Down the left arm? Into the back?

S What is the **severity** of the pain; that is, how bad is it? If the patient suffers chronically from angina, ask him to compare the pain to his usual angina pain.

T What was the **timing** of the attack, that is, when did the pain come on? If there were other symptoms as well, which came first? Which came next?

A Is the patient experiencing any **associated symptoms,** such as nausea? Weakness? Dizziness? Palpitations?

Another common chief complaint among patients with cardiac problems is DYSPNEA, which we considered in some detail in the previous chapter. In the context of cardiac disease, dyspnea may be the first clue to failure of the left side of the heart. To explore that possibility, we need to know at least the following:

- **When** did the dyspnea start? Did it waken the patient from sleep? Recall that **paroxysmal nocturnal dyspnea (PND)** is an acute episode of shortness of breath in which the patient suddenly wakens from sleep with a feeling of suffocation. Often the patient will report going to a window to try to get "more air." PND is one of the classic signs of left heart failure, although it may occur as well in chronic lung diseases.
- Did the dyspnea come on **gradually or suddenly?**
- Does any **position** make the dyspnea better or worse? The dyspnea of pulmonary edema is usually worse when the patient is lying down (**orthopnea**), because blood pools in the lungs when the body is horizontal. Thus patients with significant orthopnea will often sleep with several pillows, or even sitting up in a chair, to maintain a semiupright position.
- Has the patient ever had dyspnea like this before? If so, under what circumstances?
- Again, we want to know if there were **associated symptoms** (e.g., coughing, chest pain, fever).

Recall that dyspnea may have a variety of causes. Not all of the causes are cardiac. So inquire also about other possible causes of dyspnea, such as chronic pulmonary problems, smoking history, and chronic cough.

FAINTING, or **syncope,** occurs when there is a reduction of cardiac output for any reason, leading to a reduction in cerebral perfusion. Among the *cardiac* causes of syncope are dysrhythmias, increased vagal tone, and various heart lesions. There are also numerous *non*cardiac causes of syncope, about which we shall learn in the next chapter. In taking a history from someone who has fainted, therefore, we are trying, among other things, to sort out whether the patient fainted from cardiac or noncardiac causes. Find out:

- Under what **circumstances** did the syncopal episode occur? What was the patient doing at the time it happened? A 20-year-old who faints at the sight of blood is unlikely to have significant underlying cardiac disease; a 60-year-old who faints after feeling some "fluttering" in the chest may be suffering a dangerous cardiac dysrhythmia.
- Were there any **warning feelings** before the faint, or did the fainting spell occur suddenly and without warning?
- In what **position** was the patient when he or she fainted? Standing? Sitting? Lying down? Losing consciousness while sitting or lying down has more ominous implications than fainting while standing up.
- Has the patient fainted before? If so, under what circumstances?
- Were there any **associated symptoms,** such as nausea, vomiting, urinary incontinence, or seizures?

Finally, the patient with cardiac problems may present with a chief complaint of PALPITATIONS. **Palpitations** refer to an abnormal awareness of one's heart beat—for except after extreme exertion, a person is normally quite *un*aware of his heart beat. The cause of palpitations is often a cardiac dysrhythmia, such as premature ventricular contractions (PVCs) or paroxysmal atrial tachycardia (PAT). The patient may not use the word *palpitations* but may report that he felt his heart "skip a beat" or words to that effect. As with the other chief complaints already mentioned, so too with palpitations it is necessary to inquire about the onset, frequency, and duration of this symptom as well as about previous episodes of palpitations. Again too, ask about the presence of associated symptoms (e.g., chest pain, dizziness, dyspnea).

After exploring the patient's chief complaint, inquire *briefly* about pertinent aspects of the patient's OTHER MEDICAL HISTORY, specifically:

- Is the patient taking any MEDICATIONS regularly? Take particular note of any of the following:
  Nitroglycerin, used by patients with coronary artery disease to relieve chest pain
  Digitalis (digoxin, digitoxin), often prescribed for heart failure and for certain chronic dysrhythmias (atrial fibrillation, atrial flutter)

Diuretics (such as hydrochlorothiazide, furosemide, ethacrynic acid), commonly prescribed to patients suffering from chronic heart failure or hypertension
  Procainamide (Pronestyl), **quinidine,** or **amiodarone** (Cordarone), prescribed to suppress chronic cardiac dysrhythmias
  Propranolol (Inderal), sometimes prescribed for chronic angina or hypertension
  (A more complete list of drugs commonly prescribed to patients with cardiac problems can be found in the Appendix at the end of this chapter.)
- Is the patient under treatment for any SERIOUS ILLNESSES? Ask specifically whether he has ever been known to have any of the following:
  Hypertension
  Diabetes
  Previous heart attack or heart failure
  Rheumatic fever
  Lung disease
- Does the patient have any known ALLERGIES? Ask specifically about Novocain or "numbing medicine used in the dentist's office." Novocain is related to lidocaine, a drug used to suppress certain cardiac dysrhythmias, and patients who have had a reaction to one may also react to the other.

Physical Examination of the Cardiac Patient

In the secondary survey, the fundamentals of physical assessment are similar in all patients. However, certain aspects of the physical examination bear particular emphasis in the patient whose chief complaint suggests a cardiac problem.

- In observing the patient's GENERAL APPEARANCE, pay particular attention to his *state of consciousness,* which is an excellent indication of the adequacy of cerebral perfusion. If a patient is alert and oriented, it means his brain is getting enough oxygen, and that in turn means that his heart is doing its job as a pump. Stupor or **confusion,** on the other hand, often indicates poor cardiac output, which may be the result of myocardial damage or dysfunction. *Skin color and temperature* are also valuable indicators of the state of the patient's circulation: The **cold, sweaty skin** of many patients with myocardial infarction reflects massive peripheral vasoconstriction.
- When you take the VITAL SIGNS, make a careful assessment of the patient's *pulse.* Is it regular or irregular? Is it abnormally fast or slow? Is it

strong or weak? An **irregular pulse** signals a disturbance in cardiac rhythm. A very rapid pulse (**tachycardia**) may simply indicate anxiety, but it can also be secondary to severe pain, congestive heart failure, or a cardiac dysrhythmia. A **weak, thready pulse** suggests a reduction in cardiac output. Measure the patient's *blood pressure*. A blood pressure over 140/90 is considered to signify hypertension, but in emergency situations an elevated blood pressure may be due to anxiety. A **systolic blood pressure lower than 90 mm Hg** suggests serious hypotension and shock. The *pulse pressure* (the difference between the systolic and diastolic pressures) may also provide useful information, for it gives a rough indication of the elasticity of the arterial walls and the stroke volume. In patients with arteriosclerosis, the arterial walls are stiffened, and the pulse pressure is increased. In cardiogenic shock, the stroke volume is reduced because the heart cannot pump effectively, so the pulse pressure is narrowed accordingly. Finally, note the rate and quality of the patient's *respirations*. Is the respiratory rate abnormally rapid (**tachypnea**)? Is the patient laboring to breathe? Respiratory distress in a cardiac patient suggests the presence of congestive heart failure, with fluid in the lungs.

- In the HEAD-TO-TOE SURVEY, pay particular attention to the patient's **jugular veins.** The external jugular veins reflect the pressure within the patient's *systemic* circulation. Normally the external jugular veins are collapsed when a person is sitting or standing; but if the function of the right heart is somehow compromised, blood will back up into the systemic veins behind the right heart and distend those veins. To estimate the patient's venous pressure, then, place the patient in a semisitting position (at about a 45-degree angle) with his head slightly rotated away from the jugular vein you are examining; then observe the height of the distended fluid column within the vein, and note how far up the distention extends above the sternal angle.
- *Look at* and *palpate* the chest. Is there a vertical scar over the sternum, suggesting previous cardiac surgery? Is there a nitroglycerin patch on the skin? Is there a bulge under the skin from an implanted pacemaker? Any such findings betoken a history of significant cardiac problems.
- Listen carefully to the *chest*. Listen for **crackles** or **wheezes** suggestive of left heart failure with pulmonary edema. Listen also for a **third heart sound** ("lub da-da" instead of "lub-dub"), known as an S_3 gallop, which again gives evidence of congestive heart failure.
- Examine the *extremities and back* for **edema,** a sign of failure of the right side of the heart.

PATHOPHYSIOLOGY AND MANAGEMENT OF CARDIOVASCULAR PROBLEMS

Coronary Artery Disease and Angina

It is estimated that 6.2 million Americans have coronary artery disease and that more than half a million Americans die each year from that cause.

The coronary arteries are the vessels that supply oxygen and nutrients to the myocardium. If a coronary artery becomes blocked, therefore, the area of muscle it supplies will be *deprived* of oxgyen (**ischemic**). If, furthermore, the oxygen supply is not quickly restored, the ischemic area of heart muscle will die (undergo **infarction**).

Arteriosclerosis is the disease that causes arteries in various parts of the body to become hardened and narrowed. A common type of arteriosclerosis, **atherosclerosis,** is of particular concern because it affects the inner lining of the aorta and cerebral and coronary blood vessels, leading to the narrowing of those vessels and reduction of blood flow through them.

The atherosclerotic process begins, probably in childhood, with small depositions of fatty material along the inner wall (intima) of arteries, usually at points of turbulent blood flow, such as where the arteries bifurcate or where there has been some sort of damage to the arterial wall. As the streak of fat enlarges, it eventually becomes a mass of fatty tissue, an **atheroma,** which gradually calcifies and hardens into a **plaque** (the word *atherosclerosis* literally means "hardening of an atheroma"). The atheromatous plaque infiltrates the arterial wall and decreases its elasticity. At the same time, it narrows the arterial lumen and interferes with blood flow through the lumen.

The narrowed, roughened area of the arterial intima provides a locus for the formation of a fixed blood clot, or **thrombus,** which may then obstruct the artery altogether (**coronary thrombosis**).

Who Is at Risk for Atherosclerosis

While atherosclerosis is widespread in industrialized countries, certain factors increase an individual's risk of developing atherosclerosis and coronary artery disease:

> **RISK FACTORS IN CORONARY ARTERY DISEASE**
>
> - Hypertension (high blood pressure)
> - Cigarette smoking

- Diabetes
- High serum cholesterol (which may be related to a high dietary intake of saturated fats and calories)
- Lack of exercise
- Obesity
- Family history of heart disease or stroke
- Male sex

Clearly, among those risk factors are things we can't do anything about; we cannot, for example, select our parents and grandparents or choose to be born female. But nearly half the risk factors for coronary artery disease *are* things that a person can do something about and for that reason are called **modifiable risk factors:**

- CIGARETTE SMOKING is the most important cause of preventable death in the United States, and a smoker's chances of sudden death are several times greater than those of a nonsmoker. The good news is that smokers who quit return very rapidly to the same risk level as nonsmokers.
- HYPERTENSION cannot be prevented or cured, but it *can* be controlled with changes in diet and with medications. A person with uncontrolled high blood pressure has double or triple the risk of coronary artery disease as compared to a person with normal blood pressure.
- The levels of SERUM CHOLESTEROL in the blood are at least in part a consequence of dietary intake of saturated fats. In populations with low fat intake, the incidence of coronary artery disease is also low. Furthermore, reduction in serum cholesterol levels has been shown to reduce the incidence of heart attacks and other dangerous cardiac events.
- One thing that may play a role in elevating serum cholesterol is LACK OF EXERCISE, which also has a variety of other untoward effects on the body. Exercise improves overall fitness, cardiac reserve, and probably collateral coronary circulation.
- OBESITY may go along with several of the other risk factors already mentioned (such as diabetes and hypertension). But obesity also probably itself contributes to an increased risk of coronary artery disease. Weight reduction, through a sensible diet and, more importantly, increased physical exeicse, can reap several benefits. Normalizing body weight will lower elevated blood pressure, serum cholesterol, elevated blood sugar, *and* the risk of coronary artery disease.

The data suggest that risk factor modification can make a significant difference. Between 1964 and 1984, there was a 39-percent decline in mortality from coronary artery disease in the United States. While it is impossible to know precisely what caused that decline (we would like to think that paramedic-staffed MICUs played a significant role!), there can be no doubt that reduction in smoking, better control of hypertension, changes in dietary habits, and an upsurge of interest in fitness all contributed substantially.

Angina Pectoris

The principal *symptom* of coronary artery disease is **angina pectoris,** which literally means "choking in the chest." Angina occurs when the supply of oxygen to the myocardium is insufficient to meet the demand. As a result, the cardiac muscle becomes ischemic, and a switch to anaerobic metabolism leads to the accumulation of lactic acid and carbon dioxide. The concept of *supply and demand* is critical here. The individual with heart disease who is at rest may have an adequate supply of oxygen to the heart for his sedentary needs, despite some narrowing of his coronary arteries. However, when the same individual exercises or experiences some other stress, the blood flow to his myocardium may not be able to keep up with the heart's increased demand for oxygen; in that case, angina will result. It is clear, then, that the patient who experiences angina at rest, when oxygen needs are minimal, has more severe coronary artery disease than the person who experiences angina only with vigorous exercise.

The experience of angina was described in 1768 by the physician William Heberdon:

> But there is a disorder of the breast marked with strong and peculiar symptoms, considerable for the kind of danger belonging to it, and not extremely rare, which deserves to be mentioned at more length. The seat of it, and sense of strangling and anxiety with which it is attended may make it not improperly be called angina pectoris. They who are inflicted with it are seized while they are walking . . . with a painful and most disagreeable sensation in the breast, which seems as if would extinguish life if it were to increase or continue. . . . The pain is sometimes situated in the upper part, sometimes in the middle, sometimes the bottom of the os sterni, and is more often inclined to the left than the right side. It likewise very frequently extends from the breast to the middle of the left arm. Males are more liable to that disease, especially such as have passed their fiftieth year. . . . Some have been seized while they were standing still or sitting; also upon first waking out of sleep; and the pain sometimes reaches to the right arm as well as the left, and even down to the hands . . . in a very few instances, the arm has at the same time been numbed and swelled.

Heberdon's description brings us to another concept that is important in taking the history from a patient with chest pain, and that is the distinction between stable angina and unstable angina. **Stable angina** follows a recurrent pattern: The person with stable angina experiences pain after a certain, predictable amount of exertion, such as climbing one flight of stairs or walking for three blocks. The pain also has a predictable location, intensity, and duration. The patient may report, for example, "Every time I walk up the hill to the bus stop, I get a squeezing pain under my breast bone, and I have to sit down for 2 or 3 minutes until it goes away."

Patients with chronic, stable angina often take a medication called **nitroglycerin** for relief of anginal pain. In its usual formulation, nitroglycerin is supplied as a little white tablet that is placed under the tongue and allowed to dissolve there; but it may also be given as sustained release capsules taken 2 or 3 times a day, as a cream rubbed into the skin, or as a patch worn on the skin. In whatever form it is used, nitroglycerin will have a predictable effect in stable angina, producing relief of symptoms within a few minutes.

Unstable angina (also called *preinfarction angina*) is much more serious than stable angina and indicates a greater degree of obstruction of the coronary arteries. It is characterized by noticeable *changes* in the frequency, severity, and duration of pain and often occurs without predictable stress. The patient may state that over the past several days or weeks, his anginal attacks have grown more frequent and severe, that they waken him from sleep or occur when he is otherwise at rest. Such attacks are often the warning signs of an impending myocardial infarction.

As a general rule, it is safe to assume that any patient who has called for an ambulance because of chest pain has, at the least, unstable angina and perhaps an evolving acute myocardial infarction (AMI)—for patients with chronic, stable angina rarely call for help unless something has changed, often dramatically, for the worse.

WHEN A PATIENT WITH CHEST PAIN CALLS FOR AN AMBULANCE IT IS BECAUSE HE NEVER HAD CHEST PAIN BEFORE OR BECAUSE HIS CHRONIC CHEST PAIN HAS CHANGED. EITHER WAY, IT'S SERIOUS.

For purposes of treatment outside the hospital, then, the patient with chest pain must be assumed to be suffering an acute myocardial infarction until proved otherwise and should therefore be treated as any other patient with a suspected AMI (see next section).

ANY MIDDLE-AGED OR OLDER PATIENT WITH CHEST PAIN SHOULD BE CONSIDERED TO BE SUFFERING AN ACUTE MYOCARDIAL INFARCTION AND TREATED ACCORDINGLY.

Acute Myocardial Infarction

An acute myocardial infarction (AMI), or "heart attack," occurs when a portion of the cardiac muscle is deprived of coronary blood flow long enough that the muscle dies (undergoes **necrosis,** or infarcts). Several things can diminish flow through coronary vessels, especially if those vessels are already narrowed by atherosclerotic disease: occlusion of a coronary artery by a blood clot (thrombus), spasm of a coronary artery, or reduction of overall blood flow from any cause (e.g., shock, dysrhythmias, pulmonary embolism).

The location and size of a myocardial infarct depend on which coronary has been blocked and where along its course the blockage occurred. The majority of infarcts involves the left ventricle. When the anterior, lateral, or septal walls of the left ventricle are infarcted, it is usually because of occlusion of the *left* coronary artery or one of its branches; inferior wall infarcts are usually the result of *right* coronary artery occlusion. When only the inner layer of muscle is affected by the ischemic process, the infarct is referred to as *subendocardial.* When the infarct extends through the entire wall of the ventricle, it is a **transmural** MI. Around the infarcted tissue there is invariably a ring of ischemic tissue—an area that is relatively deprived of oxygen but still viable. That ischemic tissue tends to be electrically very unstable and is therefore likely to be the source of cardiac dysrhythmias.

Acute myocardial infarction is the leading cause of death in the United States today, accounting for more than half a million deaths per year; of those deaths, 60 to 70 percent occur outside the hospital, during the first 2 to 3 hours after the onset of symptoms. Ninety percent of deaths from AMI are due to dysrhythmias, usually ventricular fibrillation, occurring most frequently during the early hours of the infarct. Dysrhythmias can be prevented or treated. What that means is that MOST DEATHS FROM AMI ARE PREVENTABLE, and the paramedic's knowledge and skills in emergency cardiac care can be of major significance in preventing the tragic, unnecessary waste of life associated with acute myocardial infarction.

Symptoms of Acute Myocardial Infarction

The typical patient with AMI is a middle-aged (45- to 65-year-old) man in his most productive years, although AMI can also occur in younger and older people, both men and women. The patient is often slightly overweight and may have recently overindulged at the dinner table or perhaps on the tennis court, but many heart attacks occur at rest or just after arising in the morning.

The most important symptom of AMI is CHEST PAIN, which occurs in 80 to 90 percent of patients with AMI. The pain is similar to that of angina but is much more severe and lasts much longer. If the patient suffers from chronic angina, he is aware that something very different from his previous anginal attacks is happening to him. The pain of AMI is typically felt just beneath the sternum and is variously described as *heavy, squeezing, crushing,* or *tight.* Often the patient unconsciously clenches his fist as he is describing the pain (Levine's sign), to convey in body language the squeezing nature of the pain. In about 25 percent of cases, the pain radiates to the arms, most often the left arm, and into the fingers; less commonly, and usually associated with blockage of the *right* coronary artery, the pain radiates to the neck, jaw, upper back, or epigastrium. The pain of AMI is not influenced by coughing, deep breathing, or other body movements. Occasionally, the patient mistakes the pain of AMI for indigestion, and he may take antacids in an attempt to relieve his discomfort.

In taking the history from a patient whose chief complaint is chest pain, be sure to ask—in addition to the usual PQRST-A questions outlined earlier in the chapter—whether he or she has taken anything for the pain and, if so, whether it helped. If the patient reports having taken nitroglycerin without relief, it is important to establish *why* the patient did not obtain relief. There are two possible reasons. One possibility is that the patient is indeed having an AMI, for which nitroglycerin would not provide pain relief. But another possibility is that the nitroglycerin had simply gone stale. In order to retain its potency, nitroglycerin must be stored in a dark, air-tight container; if it is out in the open for any period of time, it loses its therapeutic effectiveness. The way to distinguish between the two possibilities is to ask the patient whether he noticed the usual side effects when he took his nitroglycerin. Nitroglycerin that is therapeutically active causes a transient throbbing in the head with which any patient who has taken nitroglycerin is familiar. If the patient tells you that, yes, he did feel that throbbing, but his chest pain still wouldn't go away, then you know there was nothing wrong with the nitroglycerin and there may indeed be something very wrong with the patient.

Table 23-3 summarizes some of the differences between the pain of angina and the pain of AMI.

As soon as you have elicited a chief complaint of squeezing, pressing, crushing, heavy, or tight chest pain, you will need to start treatment of the patient; obtaining a detailed history and physical examination can wait.

> **START TREATMENT IMMEDIATELY IN ANY MIDDLE-AGED OR OLDER PATIENT WITH CHEST PAIN.**

TABLE 23-3. PAIN IN CORONARY ARTERY DISEASE

CHARACTERISTIC	ANGINA	AMI
Intensity	Mild to moderate	Very severe, intense, terrifying
Duration	Usually 3–5 min	May last hours
Precipitating factors	Exercise, stress, cold weather	May occur at rest
Relieving factors	Rest	Not relieved by rest
Effect of nitroglycerin	Often relieves	No effect
Associated symptoms	May be none	Often dyspnea, nausea, vomiting, diaphoresis, dizziness, feeling of impending death

For purposes of discussion, though, we shall continue here to proceed through the history and physical examination.

A word of caution: While it is true that *most* patients with AMI present with chest pain, keep in mind that 10 to 20 percent of patients with AMI *do not experience any chest pain at all.* A painless AMI is sometimes called a "silent AMI." The incidence of painless AMI rises sharply with age, and in the elderly patient, AMI may present instead as sudden *dyspnea,* progressing rapidly to pulmonary edema; sudden *loss of consciousness;* an unexplained *drop in blood pressure;* an apparent stroke; or simply *confusion.*

> **CONSIDER AMI IN ANY ELDERLY PATIENT WITH THE SUDDEN ONSET OF DYSPNEA, HYPOTENSION, OR CONFUSION.**

Besides pain (or, sometimes, in lieu of pain), there are a number of *other symptoms* commonly associated with AMI, including the following:

- DIAPHORESIS (sweating), often profuse, is principally the result of massive discharge by the autonomic nervous system. The patient may soak through his clothing and complain of a "cold sweat."
- DYSPNEA may be a warning of impending left heart failure.
- ANOREXIA (loss of appetite), NAUSEA, VOMITING, or BELCHING frequently accompanies myocardial infarction. HICCUPS may occasionally occur as well, due to irritation of the diaphragm by an inferior wall MI.
- WEAKNESS may be profound, and the patient may describe his feeling with phrases like "a limp rag."
- If cardiac output is significantly diminished, DIZZINESS may reflect the reduced circulation to the brain.
- PALPITATIONS are sometimes experienced by patients with cardiac dysrhythmias as a sensation that the heart has "skipped a beat."
- The patient may report a strong urge to move his bowels.
- Finally, a FEELING OF IMPENDING DEATH is very common among patients suffering myocardial infarction. The patient is frightened, looks frightened, and expresses his fear to those around him—all of which simply adds to a general atmosphere of panic and dread.

Signs of Acute Myocardial Infarction

While patients with AMI often show abnormalities in their physical examination, many have a relatively normal physical examination, and the diagnosis in the field (and, indeed, in the emergency room) depends chiefly on the history. Nonetheless, it is important to take note of a few specific things during the physical examination, in order to detect the development of complications to AMI, such as heart failure or cardiogenic shock. Pay attention, therefore, to the following:

- GENERAL APPEARANCE: Does the patient appear anxious? Frightened? In a lot of pain?
- What is his STATE OF CONSCIOUSNESS? Is he fully alert? Is he confused? Remember:

> **POOR PERFUSION CREATES CONFUSION.**

If the patient does not seem "all there," it may be because his heart is giving out and not enough oxygenated blood is reaching his brain.
- Is the SKIN pale, cold, and clammy?
- VITAL SIGNS: Is the *pulse* strong or weak? Regular or irregular? Is the *respiratory rate* abnormally rapid? Is the *blood pressure* abnormally high or low?
- Are there SIGNS OF LEFT HEART FAILURE (wheezes or crackles)?
- Are there SIGNS OF RIGHT HEART FAILURE (distended neck veins, pedal or presacral edema)?

The typical patient with AMI is very apprehensive, with an ashen-gray pallor and cold, wet skin. He *looks* scared. The pulse is usually rapid unless there is associated heart block. Blood pressure may be depressed, reflecting decreased cardiac output from the damaged heart, or it may be elevated from pain and anxiety.

Treatment of Uncomplicated Acute Myocardial Infarction

Treatment of AMI in fact begins as soon as the dispatcher receives a call indicating a "possible heart attack" or "chest pain." The ambulance must be dispatched at once, without any delay, and must move to the scene with *all possible safe speed,* full sirens, and flashing lights. Remember that more than half of the deaths from AMI occur within the first few hours, and patients often do not call for help until several hours after their pain has begun. Therefore, EVERY CARDIAC CALL MUST BE REGARDED AS AN EXTREME EMERGENCY. Early treatment may mean the difference between life and death for an otherwise healthy, productive, and relatively young man or woman.

On arrival at the scene, START TREATMENT AT ONCE for any middle-aged or older patient with chest pain, even before you complete the history and physical examination. The *goals* of treatment in AMI are threefold: (1) to alleviate the patient's fear and pain; (2) to prevent the development of serious cardiac dysrhythmias; and (3) to limit the size of the infarct. The following steps of management are designed to help accomplish those goals:

- PUT THE PATIENT MENTALLY AT EASE. It is quite literally a matter of life or death for the patient that you convey calm and confidence. Writing of his own experience of a heart attack, Norman Cousins observed, "One reason that so many heart attack victims never reach the hospital alive is that the heart, already in a precarious position, has had imposed upon it the additional burden of panic."

PATIENTS WHO DIE FROM AMI OFTEN DIE OF FRIGHT.

Panic literally kills. It causes the adrenals to squeeze out a surge of epinephrine, which in turn sends the damaged heart racing. At the same time, massive discharge throughout the "fight-flight" system puts the peripheral circulation in a state of severe vasoconstriction—so not only is the heart being flogged to go faster and faster, it also has to work harder and harder against the increased afterload. The heart's need for oxygen therefore soars precisely when it is already in a state of marked oxygen deprivation. That cycle can lead quickly to dysrhythmias and death. But the cycle can be interrupted by the arrival of a calm, steady person who puts a hand on the patient's shoulder and says, "OK, everything is under control now."

- PUT THE PATIENT PHYSICALLY AT EASE. Recall that one of our goals of treatment is to try to limit the size of the infarct, and one way to do that is to decrease the amount of work that the heart has to do. The position in which cardiac

work is minimal is the SEMIRECUMBENT POSITION, that is, reclining on the stretcher with the back of the stretcher raised about 30 degrees. The patient, of course, has to *get* to the stretcher, and he must *not* be permitted to do so on his own steam. From the time you arrive, the patient must not do *anything,* and certainly he must not be allowed to walk to the ambulance.

- Administer OXYGEN at the earliest opportunity. Oxygen is the mainstay of emergency cardiac care, for oxygen therapy has been proved to reduce the incidence of dysrhythmias following AMI. That is not surprising, really, for the underlying problem in AMI is, as we have seen, an imbalance between the heart's need for oxygen and the available supply of oxygen. By putting the patient at rest, we try to reduce the *need* for oxygen. By administering supplementary oxygen, we improve the *supply.* Oxygen should NEVER be withheld from a patient with chest pain for any reason.

Start oxygen therapy with 4 to 6 liters per minute by nasal cannula (the nasal cannula is usually more comfortable for the patient than a mask). When en route to the hospital, a 50 : 50 mixture of oxygen and nitrous oxide may be substituted (see below). But in any case, remember:

OXYGEN IS THE MOST IMPORTANT DRUG IN THE TREATMENT OF ACUTE MYOCARDIAL INFARCTION.

- Once the patient is breathing an enriched oxygen mixture, start an IV LIFELINE with D5/W, using a 250-ml bag and microdrip infusion set. Patients with AMI may have difficulty in handling salt loads or large volumes of fluid; for that reason, saline should not be used for the IV, and the infusion rate should be *just enough to keep the vein open*—no faster than about 10 microdrops per minute. The purpose of the IV is simply to have a line established just in case complications arise, so that medications can be administered through the line without any delay. Trying to start an IV in invisible, collapsed veins *after* the patient has had a cardiac arrest is much more difficult than getting the line in while there's still a good circulation.

- ATTACH ECG ELECTRODES, and run a strip to document the initial rhythm. Ideally, your monitor should have an audible tone that beeps with each QRS complex, so that you can keep track of the patient's cardiac rhythm even when you have to take your gaze from the monitor to do other things. The ear, in any case, is far more sensitive than the eye to slight irregularities in rhythm, so the chances are that you will *hear* the beginning of a cardiac dysrhythmia a lot sooner than you will see it on the monitor.

- RECORD THE VITAL SIGNS. Now that you have a way of keeping tabs on the patient's cardiac rhythm, move on to the vital signs. Measure the BLOOD PRESSURE, and repeat that measurement at least every 5 minutes. Measure the PULSE, and keep a finger on the pulse throughout transport. The ECG monitor provides information only about the *electric* activity of the heart; it gives no information whatsoever about the strength of the heart beat (*muscular* activity) or indeed about whether the heart is effectively beating at all! It is therefore necessary to monitor the patient's pulse to assess peripheral blood flow, especially during transport, when blood pressure measurements are difficult and unreliable.

- Some form of PAIN RELIEF must be provided, for the pain of AMI is very severe, and it places enormous stress on the patient's autonomic nervous system—stress that may itself contribute to complications. Start with **nitroglycerin**—a **0.4-mg** tablet placed under the patient's tongue. If the patient is indeed suffering from an AMI and not simply angina, the nitroglycerin is unlikely to relieve his pain, but it may in any case help to reduce the size of his infarction. Do *not* give nitroglycerin, however, if there is hypotension or bradycardia, and do *not* give it to patients having epigastric symptoms ("indigestion") or hiccups. If nitroglycerin brings no relief of pain within 2 to 3 minutes, then give **morphine sulfate** in titrated intravenous doses. To prepare the morphine, empty the contents of a 10-mg Tubex into a 10-ml syringe, and fill the remainder of the syringe (9 ml) with D5/W. Give 3 ml (=3 mg) IV at a time, checking the pulse and blood pressure after each dose, until the patient experiences relief of pain or there is a drop in pulse or blood pressure. If bradycardia occurs, notify the physician immediately. Remember that morphine should *not* be given to patients with low blood pressure (less than about 100 mm Hg systolic), patients suspected of having an AMI involving the inferior wall of the heart (which again means patients with prominent nausea, vomiting, or hiccups), or patients with severe chronic obstructive lung disease. In patients for whom morphine is contraindicated for any of those reasons, the preferred medication for treating the pain of AMI in the

field is **nitrous oxide** (N_2O), given as a 50 : 50 mixture with oxygen (Nitronox). Nitrous oxide should be *self-administered* by the patient, to minimize the risk of overdosage (the patient will get sleepy and drop the mask as the level of nitrous oxide in his system rises).

- Whenever you administer morphine to a patient with an AMI, you should have **atropine sulfate** drawn up and ready to inject in the event that the patient develops bradycardia from the morphine (or, for that matter, from the AMI itself). If indicated, the dosage of atropine is 0.5 mg by IV bolus. If the patient's heart rate does not pick up after the first dose of atropine, the physician may request that the dose be repeated once or twice.

- Keep the other ANTIARRHYTHMIC DRUGS that you stock close at hand so you can reach them quickly if the patient develops a cardiac dysrhythmia. (We shall deal with the specific drugs required for specific dysrhythmias in a later section of this chapter.)

- If it is part of the local protocol to do so, TAKE A 12-LEAD ECG, and report the results to Medical Command.

Only after you have completed all of the above steps (as appropriate) should you take time to OBTAIN A MORE DETAILED HISTORY AND PHYSICAL EXAMINATION. Find out if the patient has a history of cardiac disease; if he takes any heart medications such as digitalis, diuretics, or nitroglycerin; if he has had a heart attack before. Also obtain a more complete description of his present symptoms, as detailed earlier. Gathering that information should not, however, delay transport to the hospital. Once you have taken the necessary precautions to stabilize the patient (oxygen, IV lifeline, monitor, analgesia), there is no reason to remain any longer at the scene, unless there is a cardiac arrest or a dysrhythmia that requires immediate treatment. Take the rest of the history en route to the hospital.

Once the patient is stable, then, TRANSPORT him to the hospital in a SEMIRECUMBENT POSITION (unless he is in shock, in which case he should be supine). Do all you can to ensure that the patient is as relaxed and comfortable as possible. En route, some additional treatment measures may be worthwhile, especially when transport will take a long time:

- There is accumulating evidence that the administration of magnesium to patients with AMI decreases the incidence of dangerous cardiac dysrhythmias and lowers mortality for acute infarction. If you are some distance from the hospital, you may be asked, therefore, to start an infusion of **magnesium sulfate**. To do so, add **2.4 gm** of magnesium sulfate to 50 ml of D5/W and infuse over 20 to 60 minutes.

- You may also be instructed to administer **aspirin**, which is given for its anticlotting properties. The dosage is usually ½ tablet (165 mg) by mouth.

DO NOT RUSH and DO NOT USE SIRENS in transporting the patient to the hospital. High speed and sirens give the patient two clear messages: (1) There must be something terribly wrong; and (2) the personnel on the ambulance don't feel capable of dealing with the situation. Those are *not* the messages you want to convey to a frightened patient with a damaged heart! What that patient *needs* to feel is that things will be all right and those caring for him are fully in control of the situation.

If a serious dysrhythmia should occur in transport, STOP THE VEHICLE, institute treatment immediately, and notify medical command. Except under unusual circumstances, treatment of life-threatening situations should not be attempted in a moving ambulance. Whenever possible, the driver should pull over to the side of the road and then go to the back of the vehicle to help out.

Thrombolytic Therapy of Acute Myocardial Infarction

The majority of AMIs occur as a result of thrombus formation at the site of a preexisting atherosclerotic plaque. It is the thrombus, that is, fixed blood clot, that occludes the coronary artery and thereby prevents further blood flow through it. Therefore it seems reasonable to try to dissolve the occluding blood clot and thereby restore perfusion to the ischemic myocardium. That is what thrombolytic therapy is all about. In fact, the concept is not altogether new. Attempts to use thrombolytic agents in the treatment of AMI were reported at least 30 years ago, without success. In retrospect, we realize that one of the reasons the early attempts did not succeed was that thrombolytic therapy was started too late, after the damage to the myocardium was already irreversible. With that realization came the concept that "time is myocardium," that is, the longer a segment of myocardium remains unperfused, the smaller the chances of salvaging that tissue and restoring its normal function. The obvious corollary is that the sooner thrombolytic therapy can begin with respect to the onset of the blockage, the better the chances for saving the affected distal myocardium. Indeed, thrombolytic treatment given within 30 to 60 minutes of the onset of symptoms can sometimes prevent the infarct altogether. That is why we say:

> # TIME IS MYOCARDIUM.

There began, therefore, in the 1980s a trend to start thrombolytic treatment as soon as possible after the patient with an AMI reached the emergency room, rather than waiting until he was admitted to the coronary care unit; and, inevitably, applying the doctrine that "time is myocardium" led to the idea of starting thrombolytic treatment even earlier, in the *pre*hospital phase of care.

The administration of thrombolytic agents by paramedics is still, at the time of this writing, in its preliminary phases in the United States and is being carried out only in a small number of EMS systems on a trial basis. To date, despite theoretical advantages of starting thrombolytic therapy earlier, research has *not* shown any improvement in patient outcome from giving thrombolytic therapy in the prehospital phase of care. Nonetheless, some EMS systems may still opt to start thrombolytic treatment in the field, and in rural areas with very long transport times, prehospital initiation of thrombolytic therapy may make a lot of sense. Even in EMS systems where paramedics do not themselves give thrombolytic therapy, their ability to identify candidates for such therapy will play a decisive role in helping emergency room personnel administer thrombolytic therapy early enough to make a difference. It is therefore important for all paramedics to understand the principles of thrombolytic therapy for AMI.

The idea behind thrombolytic therapy is simple enough, and that is to administer, during the early hours of AMI, an agent that will activate the body's own internal system for dissolving clots, the *fibrinolytic system*. Once activated, that system can begin to dissolve the clot that has formed within the coronary artery, thereby reopening the artery (**recanalization**) and allowing the resumption of blood flow through it (**reperfusion**). The problem is that if an agent capable of promoting clot dissolution is given intravenously, its effects cannot be limited to the clot in the coronary artery; to the contrary, the thrombolytic agent can also act anywhere else in the body where clots are being formed, and may thus lead to bleeding. Thus the benefit of thrombolytic therapy—the possible salvage of myocardium—must always be weighed against its risks, principally the risk of bleeding. For that reason, various criteria have been developed, based on considerations of potential benefit versus potential risk, to determine who should be a candidate for thrombolytic therapy.

Since there *are* risks to giving thrombolytic agents, we need, first of all, to be as certain as possible that we are really dealing with a patient who is having an AMI; a patient having chest pain from another source would have *no* potential benefit from thrombolytic therapy—so he would be subjected to the risks for nothing. While it is very difficult in the early hours of an AMI to be certain of the diagnosis, "inclusion criteria" have been established to try to help us select those patients most likely to be suffering an AMI. At the same time, there are also "exclusion criteria" to identify those patients for whom the risk of thrombolytic therapy is unacceptably high, for example patients most likely to have hemorrhagic complications. The inclusion and exclusion criteria for thrombolytic therapy are summarized in Table 23-4.

Most treatment regimens for thrombolysis in AMI today use one of three agents: streptokinase (SK), recombinant tissue plasminogen activator (rt-PA), or anisoylated plasminogen streptokinase activator complex (APSAC). The properties of each are summarized in Table 23-5. All of them work by converting, in one way or another, the body's own clot-dissolving enzyme from its inactive form, plasminogen, to its active form, **plasmin.**

Paramedics working in EMS systems where thrombolytic therapy is initiated in the field will have to undergo special training in performing and interpreting 12-lead ECGs as well as in carrying out the particular protocol employed by their EMS system. (An introduction to 12-lead ECGs is provided later in this chapter.) All paramedics, however, should be alert for patients who are good candidates for thrombolysis, should know which hospitals in their area carry out thrombolytic therapy, and should provide early notification to the emergency room that a candidate for such therapy is en route.

TABLE 23-4.   CRITERIA FOR THROMBOLYTIC THERAPY

Inclusion criteria
- Alert and able to give informed consent
- Age > 30 years
- Chest pain for > 20 minutes and < 6 hours
- Pain not relieved by sublingual nitroglycerin
- Systolic BP > 80 and < 180 mm Hg
- Diastolic BP < 120 mm Hg
- Systolic pressure difference between the two arms < 20 mm Hg
- ECG: S–T elevation of > 1 mm in two adjacent leads*

Exclusion criteria
- Significant bleeding or known bleeding disorder
- Patient taking oral anticoagulant medications
- Stroke or transient ischemic attack
- History of gastrointestinal or genitourinary bleeding
- Major surgery or trauma within the past month
- Recent CPR with apparent chest wall trauma
- Insulin-dependent diabetes mellitus
- Severe hypertension (systolic BP > 180 mm Hg, diastolic > 120 mm Hg)
- Intravenous cannulas at noncompressible sites
- Terminal illness

*Requires 12-lead ECG.

AMI: SUMMARY

SYMPTOMS
- Chest pain: heavy, crushing, squeezing, tight
- Gastrointestinal symptoms: anorexia, nausea, belching, vomiting
- Sweating
- Weakness
- Light-headedness
- Feeling of impending doom

SIGNS
- Patient looks scared
- Skin: ashen-gray, wet, cold
- Often tachycardia

TREATMENT
- Calm, confident manner to put the patient at ease
- Semirecumbent position
- Oxygen
- Monitor
- IV lifeline
- Nitroglycerin
- Analgesia (nitrous oxide or morphine)
- 12-lead ECG
- Other medications as ordered:
  1. Magnesium sulfate
  2. Aspirin
- Transport—no panic, no sirens

Thus far, we have discussed chiefly the management of the uncomplicated AMI. And, indeed, proper initial treatment of the patient with AMI will do much to decrease the incidence of complications. However, even with the best prehospital management, complications will sometimes arise, and the

TABLE 23-5. COMPARISON OF THROMBOLYTIC DRUGS

	STREPTOKINASE	rt-PA	APSAC
Trade name(s)	Streptase, Kabikinase	Activase	Eminase
Dosage	1.5 million units over 1 hr	60 mg over first hour	30 units over at least 5 min
Half-life	18 min	4 min	95 min
Allergic potential	Yes	No	Yes
Cost per dose	$500–1,000	$2,500–4,000	$1,000

paramedic must be able to recognize those complications and begin the appropriate treatment promptly. In the following sections, we shall discuss two acute complications of AMI: congestive heart failure and cardiogenic shock. Two other acute complications, cardiac dysrhythmias and cardiac arrest, will be considered in later sections of this chapter.

Congestive Heart Failure

Congestive heart failure occurs when the heart is unable, for any reason, to pump powerfully enough or fast enough to empty its chambers; as a result, blood backs up into the systemic or pulmonary circuit or both. While congestive heart failure may develop in situations other than AMI—for example, in the patient with chronic high blood pressure—the basic principles of diagnosis and treatment are similar, whatever the precipitating factors.

Left Heart Failure

In AMI it is the left ventricle that is most commonly damaged. In chronic hypertension, it is also the left ventricle that suffers the long-term effects of having to pump against an increased afterload (constricted peripheral arteries). In both instances, the right side of the heart continues to pump relatively normally and to deliver normal volumes of blood to the pulmonary circulation. But the left side of the heart may no longer be able to pump out the blood being delivered from the pulmonary vessels. As a result, blood backs up behind the left ventricle, and the pressure in the left atrium and pulmonary veins increases. As the pulmonary veins become engorged with blood, serum is forced out of the capillaries into the alveoli. The serum mixes with air in the alveoli to produce foam (pulmonary edema).

As we learned earlier, when fluid occupies the alveoli, oxygenation is impaired. The patient experiences that impairment of oxygenation as shortness of breath, or DYSPNEA, particularly in the recumbent position (ORTHOPNEA). If left ventricular failure is the result of *chronic* overload (as opposed to AMI), the patient is likely to give a history of a week or two of PAROXYSMAL NOCTURNAL DYSPNEA. To compensate for the impairment in oxygenation, the patient increases his respiratory rate (TACHYPNEA); but even so, if his shunt is large enough, CYANOSIS may become evident. In some patients with pulmonary edema, especially the elderly, CHEYNE-STOKES RESPIRATIONS may be prominent. Fluid from the pulmonary vessels also leaks into the interstitial spaces in the lungs, and increasing interstitial pressure causes narrowing of the bronchioles. Air passing through those narrowed bronchioles creates WHEEZING noises, while that bubbling through the fluid-filled alveoli produces CRACKLES. Furthermore, the patient may cough up some of that edema fluid in the form of FOAMY, BLOOD-TINGED SPUTUM. Meanwhile, as the airways narrow and the lungs get heavier and heavier from the accumulation of fluid, the work of breathing increases, putting an even greater demand on the already floundering heart. Dyspnea and hypoxemia produce a state of panic, which induces the release of epinephrine from the adrenals. So the heart is pushed even harder, and its oxygen demand is increased precisely when fluid in the alveoli is reducing the amount of oxygen available. And to make matters even worse, the sympathetic nervous system response also produces peripheral vasoconstriction; so peripheral resistance (= afterload) goes up, and the weakened, hypoxic heart finds itself trying to push blood out into smaller and smaller pipes. Clinically, that peripheral vasoconstriction is apparent as PALLOR and ELEVATED BLOOD PRESSURE, and the massive sympathetic discharge also produces SWEATING of the pale, cold skin.

It is not unusual for a patient with left heart failure to become frantic from air hunger. He may pace or thrash about or may even be combative and struggle with the rescue team. Furthermore, hypoxemia results in an inadequate oxygen supply to the brain, often manifested as CONFUSION or DISORIENTATION. If hypoxemia is severe, CARDIAC ARREST may follow quickly.

Prehospital treatment of left heart failure is aimed at improving oxygenation and decreasing the workload of the heart, chiefly by reducing the volume of venous blood returned to the heart (the preload), so that the left ventricle is less overburdened.

- Administer 100% OXYGEN, preferably by demand valve or bag-valve-mask with PEEP, since positive pressure is helpful in driving fluid out of the alveoli. If the patient will not tolerate either of those two modalities, use the nonrebreathing mask. Monitor oxygenation with pulse oximetry.
- SIT THE PATIENT UP, WITH HIS FEET DANGLING. That position encourages venous pooling in the legs and thereby reduces venous return to the heart. The sitting position also makes breathing easier for the patient in respiratory distress.
- Start an IV LIFELINE with D5/W to a keep-open rate.
- Attach MONITORING ELECTRODES. Patients in congestive heart failure are prone to dysrhythmias.
- Pharmacologic therapy of left heart failure may vary slightly from place to place, but the mainstays of DRUG THERAPY include the drugs mentioned below (in order of the author's preference). Refer to your usual protocols and have the appropriate medications drawn up and ready, pending the physician's order to administer them:
  1. NITROGLYCERIN, 0.4 mg sublingually, may be ordered as a vasodilator to create venous pooling and thereby reduce the volume of blood returned from the periphery to the heart. Before ordering this medication, the physician will want to know how much, if any, nitroglycerin the patient has already taken. The initial 0.4-mg dose may be repeated at 5-minute intervals up to a total of 2.4 mg.
  2. FUROSEMIDE (Lasix) is a diuretic drug with two positive effects in left heart failure. Initially (within the first 5–10 minutes) it has a venodilating effect, to increase peripheral pooling of blood; subsequently, it removes excess fluid from the body by promoting its excretion by the kidneys. If ordered, furosemide is given in a dosage of 20 to 40 mg by IV bolus. Furosemide should *not* be given to elderly patients in the prehospital phase of management.

  3. MORPHINE SULFATE has long been part of the standard treatment of cardiogenic pulmonary edema and still has a useful role to play in many cases. Like nitroglycerin, morphine works as a vasodilator, to increase the pooling of blood in the periphery, but it also has a substantial calming effect on a frantic patient. To administer morphine sulfate, empty a Tubex (10 mg) into a 10-ml syringe and fill the remainder of the syringe with D5/W. That yields a concentration of 1 mg per milliliter. If morphine is ordered, first check the patient's blood pressure (do not give morphine if the patient is hypotensive). Then give approximately 3 ml (3 mg) of the diluted mixture slowly IV, and recheck the blood pressure. If the blood pressure remains stable, another 3 ml may be given. Proceed in that fashion until the total dose ordered by the physician has been administered.
  4. As we learned in the previous chapter, AMINOPHYLLINE is sometimes useful in circumstances where bronchoconstriction is a prominent part of the picture (i.e., when the patient has prominent wheezing), although the tendency now is to be much more cautious in the use of aminophylline. If aminophylline is ordered, attach an infusion set to a 250-ml bag of D5/W, and allow about 100 to 150 ml of the IV fluid to run out of the bag. To the remaining D5/W add 250 mg of aminophylline. Label the bag, and piggyback it into the IV; run in the contents over an hour.
  5. Under special circumstances, when transport will be prolonged, the physician may order DIGOXIN, a drug that strengthens the contractions of the heart, to be given in the field. The dosage is 0.5 mg slowly IV.
- TRANSPORT the patient to the hospital in a SITTING position, with his legs dangling down.

In some regions, rotating tourniquets are still used in the management of acute left heart failure. We do *not* recommend that technique, since there is no evidence to support its effectiveness. Furthermore, there are strong theoretical grounds for believing that rotating tourniquets may in fact worsen the condition of the patient in congestive heart failure by increasing an already significant burden of acidosis and by periodically reinfusing a volume load. Internal phlebotomy (removal of blood volume) accomplished by pharmacologic means (nitroglycerin, morphine) or even the actual phlebotomy of 1 unit of blood, drawn into a standard blood donor set, is a technique founded on a sounder theoretical basis and is to be preferred.

LEFT HEART FAILURE: SUMMARY

SIGNS AND SYMPTOMS
- Extreme restlessness and agitation
- Confusion
- Severe dyspnea and tachypnea
- Tachycardia
- Elevated blood pressure
- Crackles and often wheezes
- Frothy, pink sputum

TREATMENT
- 100% oxygen, preferably by demand valve
- Sit the patient up, with legs dangling
- IV lifeline (D5/W to kvo)
- ECG monitor
- Possible medications
  1. Nitroglycerin
  2. Furosemide
  3. Morphine sulfate
  4. Aminophylline
  5. Digoxin

In the last chapter, we noted that it may sometimes be difficult to distinguish the wheezing of asthma from that of left heart failure. Table 23-6 presents some of the features that can help you to differentiate the two conditions.

Right Heart Failure

Right heart failure most commonly occurs as a result of *left* heart failure. As blood backs up from the left heart into the lungs, the right side of the heart has to work harder and harder to pump blood into the engorged pulmonary vessels. Eventually the right heart is unable to keep up with the increased work load, and it too fails. Right heart failure may also occur as a result of pulmonary embolism or long-standing chronic obstructive pulmonary disease (COPD), especially chronic bronchitis.

When the right heart fails, blood backs up behind the *right* ventricle and increases the pressure in the *systemic* veins. The systemic veins as a consequence become engorged, and those veins visible on the surface of the body, such as the external JUGULAR VEINS, can be seen to be DISTENDED. Over time, as the pressure within the systemic veins increases, serum is forced out of the veins into the surrounding tissues, producing EDEMA. Edema is most likely to be visible in dependent parts of the body, such as the feet in a person who is sitting or standing, or the

lower back in a bedridden patient. Edema is also present, in right heart failure, in parts of the body that are *not* visible; a painful liver easily palpable in the right upper quadrant, for example, signals engorgement and swelling within that organ (**hepatomegaly**).

The development of right heart failure can actually improve *left* heart failure. That is because the failing right heart can no longer pump as much blood into the lungs. Thus the decrease in output from the right heart amounts to a decrease in preload for the left heart and may bring about a lessening of pulmonary congestion.

Right heart failure, by itself, is seldom a life-threatening emergency. Usually it develops gradually over days to weeks, and it likewise requires days to weeks to reverse the process by slowly ridding the body of its excess salt and water. Treatment in the field of the patient with right heart failure, therefore, is simply to make the patient comfortable, preferably in a semirecumbent position. Monitoring is always indicated in any patient with significant cardiac disease. If signs of associated left heart failure are present, treat as outlined in the previous section.

Cardiogenic Shock

Cardiogenic shock occurs when the heart is so severely damaged that it can no longer pump a volume of blood sufficient to maintain tissue perfusion. Acute myocardial infarction nearly always produces some impairment of left ventricular function. When about 25 percent of the left ventricular myocardium is involved in the AMI, left heart failure usually develops. When approximately 40 percent or more of the left ventricle has been infarcted, cardiogenic shock occurs. Cardiogenic shock therefore indicates that there has been extensive injury to the myocardium, and accordingly, it carries a very high mortality.

The *signs and symptoms* of cardiogenic shock are similar to those of any other kind of shock. Because of reduced cerebral perfusion, the patient is often CONFUSED or even COMATOSE; if awake, he is likely to be RESTLESS and anxious. Massive peripheral vasoconstriction (the body's attempt to maintain blood pressure) results in PALE, COLD SKIN, while poor renal perfusion is reflected in minimal or absent urine output. The RESPIRATIONS are RAPID AND SHALLOW, and the PULSE is RACING and THREADY. Finally, blood pressure is decreased, usually below 90 mm Hg systolic. The blood pressure may be deceptive however; in patients with preexisting hypertension, systolic pressures higher than 90 mm Hg may still be associated with shock.

Treatment of cardiogenic shock is aimed at im-

TABLE 23-6.   DIFFERENTIATION OF ASTHMA AND LEFT HEART FAILURE

	ASTHMA	LEFT HEART FAILURE
History	Often a younger patient	Often an older patient
	May have allergic history or family history of allergy	May have history of heart problems, hypertension
	Previous attacks of acute, episodic dyspnea	Dyspnea worse when lying down (orthopnea)
	May have had recent respiratory infection	Recent rapid weight gain
	MEDICATIONS may include INHALERS: Medihaler, Vaponefrin, microNEFRIN, Bronkosol, Isuprel PILLS: Tedrol, Sudafed, Quibron, Actifed, Marax	MEDICATIONS may include DIGITALIS: digoxin, Lanoxin, digitoxin DIURETICS: Diuril, Lasix, Esidrix, Edecrin, Naqua
	Unproductive cough	Cough with watery or foamy sputum
Possible physical findings	WHEEZING	WHEEZING
	Chest hyperinflated and hyperresonant	Crackles S_3 gallop
	Use of accessory muscles to breathe	Distended neck veins
	If bronchospasm severe, chest may be silent	Pedal/presacral edema
Treatment	OXYGEN (humidified)	OXYGEN
	IPPB	IPPB
	Monitor	Monitor
	IV: D5/W or D5/normal saline	IV: D5/W to keep open
	Selective beta-2 adrenergic	(Adrenergics usually contraindicated)
	Sometimes BICARBONATE	(Bicarbonate usually contraindicated)
	(Morphine contraindicated)	MORPHINE
	(Diuretics contraindicated)	DIURETICS (Lasix)
		NITROGLYCERIN

IPPB = intermittent positive pressure breathing.

proving oxygenation and peripheral perfusion without adding to the work of the heart. (Question: Why do we want to avoid increasing the cardiac work load?)

- Secure an AIRWAY, and administer 100% OXYGEN by mask. Endotracheal intubation will be necessary if the patient is comatose.
- Place the patient in a SUPINE position, unless pulmonary edema is present, in which case he should be semisitting.

- Start an IV LIFELINE with D5/W to a keep-open rate. The physician may order a trial of fluids to determine if there is a hypovolemic component to the shock. If so, rapidly infuse about 100 ml of D5/W and closely monitor the patient's pulse, blood pressure, and state of consciousness. Report those observations to the physician.
- Apply MONITORING ELECTRODES. Dysrhythmias may themselves bring about hypotension by causing severe disturbances in cardiac output; so until major dysrhythmias are corrected, one can-

not be certain that the patient's hypotension is indeed due to cardiogenic shock.

- Depending on the distance to the hospital and on local protocols, you may be asked to administer a VASOPRESSOR drug, such as one of those listed in Table 23-7. This author's preference is DOPAMINE because, at beta doses, it maintains renal perfusion better than the other agents listed. To prepare a dopamine infusion, add 1 ampule of dopamine (200 mg in 5 ml) to a 250-ml bag of D5/W, to yield a concentration of 800 µg per milliliter. The infusion rate will depend on the patient's weight and response, but it is usually *initiated* at **2 to 5 µg/kg/min.** (Problem: Calculate the initial infusion rate in microdrops per minute for 70-kg man. There are 60 microdrops in 1 ml.) The administration of dopamine or any other vasopressor drug requires *careful titration and frequent monitoring of the blood pressure.* Measure the blood pressure at least every 5 minutes. Slow the infusion if the systolic pressure rises above 90 to 100 mm Hg; speed up the infusion if the systolic pressure falls below 70 mm Hg. The effectiveness of dopamine may also be gauged by improvement in urine output. For that reason, it is helpful if the patient has a urinary catheter in place, especially if transport to the hospital will be prolonged.
- TRANSPORT the patient expeditiously to hospital. Except for the correction of life-threatening dysrhythmias, there are no measures that can stabilize the condition of a patient in cardiogenic shock in the field, so there is nothing to be gained by tarrying at the scene.

Aortic Aneurysm

The word **aneurysm** comes from a Greek word for a widening, and it refers to the dilatation or outpouching of a blood vessel. The aneurysms with which we are most concerned in emergency medicine are those that involve the aorta, particularly acute *dissecting* aneurysms of the thoracic aorta and expanding or *ruptured* aneurysms of the abdominal aorta.

Acute Dissecting Aneurysm of the Aorta

The proximal aorta is subject to enormous hemodynamic forces. Anywhere from 60 to 100 times a minute, 60 minutes an hour, 24 hours a day—that is, around 40 million times a year—pulsatile waves of blood come pounding out of the left ventricle against the aortic walls. Over the years, that pounding takes its toll, producing degenerative changes in the media (the middle layer) of the aorta, especially the *ascending* aorta (the part of the aorta that rises from the heart toward the aortic arch). Those degenerative changes are more pronounced with advancing age and in people with chronic high blood pressure, and their effect is to "unglue" the layers of the aortic wall from one another.

Eventually, the degenerative changes in the aortic media may lead to a disruption of the underlying intima (innermost layer of the artery). Tearing of the intima is most likely to occur in those portions of the thoracic aorta that are under the greatest stress, specifically in the ascending aorta just distal to the aortic valve (about 65 percent of cases) and the descending aorta just beyond the takeoff point of the left subclavian artery (Fig. 23-17A). Once the intima is torn, the process of **dissection,** or separation of the arterial wall, can begin. With each ventricular systole, a jet of blood is forced into the torn arterial wall, creating a false channel between the intimal and medial layers of the wall (Fig. 23-17B). As blood continues to be forced into the arterial wall, the channel is propagated distally and sometimes proximally along the length of the wall. If the dissection progresses back into the aortic valve, it may prevent the valve from closing, so that blood regurgitates back from the aorta into the left ventricle during systole. Recall, also, that the *coronary arteries* take off from the aorta just above

TABLE 23-7. VASOPRESSOR AGENTS*

DRUG	PREPARATION	CONCENTRATION	RATE
Dopamine HCl (Intropin)	5 ml (200 mg) dopamine in 250 ml D5/W	800 µg/ml	2–5 µg/kg/min (for 70-kg man: 150 µg/min, i.e., 12 microdrops/min)
Norepinephrine (Levophed)	1 ml (1 mg) norepinephrine in 250 ml D5/W	4 µg/ml	0.5–1.0 ml/min (30–60 microdrops/min)
Metaraminol (Aramine)	10 ml (100 mg) in 250 ml D5/W	0.4 mg/ml	20–30 microdrops/min

*The pharmacology of these agents is discussed in the Drug Handbook at the end of this book.

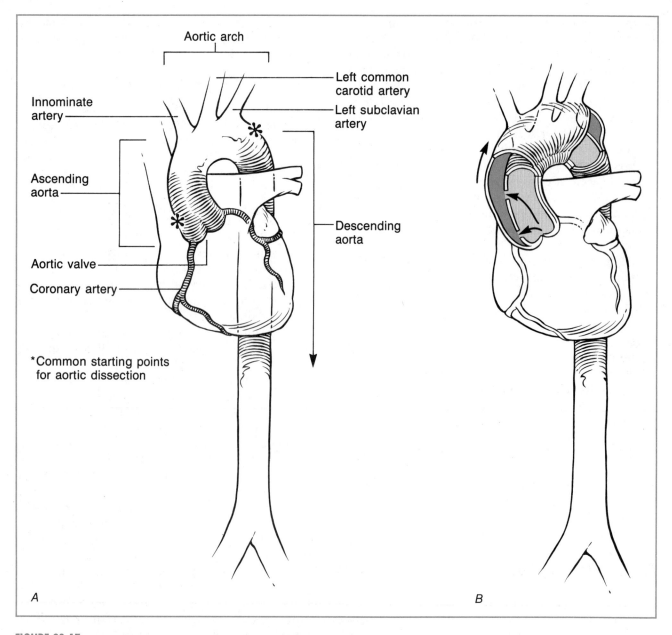

FIGURE 23-17.   DISSECTING AORTIC ANEURYSM.   (A) The most common
sites of intimal tears are just distal to the aortic valve and just beyond the
takeoff point of the left subclavian artery. (B) Blood may dissect down the
wall toward the aortic valve or distally, toward the arteries of the aortic arch.

the leaflets of the aortic valve; so if the valve is affected, chances are that coronary blood flow will be
affected as well. If the dissection involves the takeoff
point of the innominate, left common carotid, or left
subclavian artery, blood flow through the affected artery or arteries will be compromised.

The typical patient with a dissecting aneurysm is
a middle-aged or older man with chronic hypertension, although dissection may occur during pregnancy. By far the most common *chief complaint* is
CHEST PAIN, usually the worst pain the patient has

ever experienced. The patient may describe the pain
as "ripping," "tearing," "sharp," or "like a knife."
Usually the pain *comes on very suddenly* and is located
in the anterior chest or in the back between the shoulder blades. It may be very difficult, from the patient's
description, to differentiate the chest pain of a dissecting aneurysm from that of AMI, but there are a
number of distinctive features that may help. The
pain of AMI, to begin with, is often preceded by other
symptoms—nausea, "indigestion," weakness, sweating—and tends to come on gradually, getting more

and more severe with time. By contrast, the pain of a dissecting aneurysm usually comes on full force from one minute to the next, without any prodromal symptoms. Some of the differences in clinical presentation between AMI and dissecting aortic aneurysm are summarized in Table 23-8.

Other symptoms and signs of dissecting aneurysm will depend on the site of the intimal tear and the extent of the dissection. In dissections of the *ascending* aorta, which tend to occur in younger patients previously in good health, one or more of the vessels of the aortic arch are usually compromised. Thus, for example, disruption of flow through the innominate artery is likely to produce a DIFFERENCE IN BLOOD PRESSURE between the two arms (if you don't routinely *check* the blood pressure in both arms, you'll never pick up that sign!). Or you may find that one femoral or carotid pulse is missing. Disruption of blood flow into the left common carotid artery may produce SYMPTOMS AND SIGNS OF A STROKE. When the dissection extends proximally to the ostia of the coronary arteries, coronary blood flow is apt to be compromised, and ECG CHANGES of myocardial ischemia are likely. Death from dissection of the ascending aorta is nearly always a result of aortic rupture into the pericardium and resultant CARDIAC TAMPONADE. If that happens, you will see the characteristic signs of cardiac tamponade that we learned about in Chapter 17: distended neck veins, hypotension, narrow pulse pressure, pulsus paradoxus.

Dissection of the *descending* aorta occurs more commonly in older patients, especially those with a history of hypertension. The pain is apt to be somewhat less severe when the descending aorta is involved, and indeed the patient may wait a few days before seeking help. The dissection usually proceeds distally, so the aortic arch is spared, which means that blood pressure discrepancies between the two arms are *not* part of the picture; pulses in the *lower* extremities, however, may be affected.

The goal of prehospital management in a suspected dissecting aneurysm is primarily to provide adequate PAIN RELIEF. In the hospital, medications will be given to lower the patient's blood pressure and reduce myocardial contractility in order to take some of the hemodynamic load off the aorta. It would only be in very unusual circumstances, however, that such therapy would be started in the field, for it requires careful monitoring of intra-arterial pressure. The steps of prehospital management, then, in suspected dissecting aneurysm are as follows:

- Calm and reassure the patient.
- Administer 100% OXYGEN by nonrebreathing mask.
- Start an IV LIFELINE with crystalloid.
- Apply MONITORING ELECTRODES. Run a rhythm strip.
- If the patient is not hypotensive, administer MORPHINE sulfate, 3 mg IV at a time up to a total dose of 10 mg over 10 to 15 minutes.
- TRANSPORT WITHOUT DELAY. There is nothing that can be done to stabilize the patient in the field. He will need aggressive therapy in the intensive care unit and possibly surgery thereafter, so don't dawdle!

Expanding and Ruptured Abdominal Aortic Aneurysms

Abdominal aortic aneurysms affect about 2 percent of the American population over age 50 and account for about 15,000 deaths each year. Most commonly, the

TABLE 23-8. AMI VERSUS DISSECTING AORTIC ANEURYSM

	ACUTE MYOCARDIAL INFARCTION	DISSECTING ANEURYSM
Onset of pain	Gradual, with prodromal symptoms	Abrupt, without any prodromal symptoms
Severity of pain	Increases with time	Maximal from the outset
Timing of pain	May wax and wane	Does not abate once it has started
Location of pain	Substernal; back is rarely involved	Back is often involved, between shoulder blades
Clinical signs	Peripheral pulses equal	BP discrepancy between arms or decrease in a femoral or carotid pulse

aneurysm is located just distal to the renal arteries. An expanding aneurysm is, as the name implies, an aneurysm that is getting larger and producing symptoms by compressing on adjacent structures, although the aortic wall is still intact. When an aneurysm starts expanding and producing symptoms, one can assume that rupture of the aneurysm is imminent.

The typical patient with an abdominal aortic aneurysm is a man in his late 50s or 60s. So long as the aneurysm is stable, the patient will usually be entirely without symptoms. It is when the aneurysm starts to expand that the patient becomes symptomatic, with the sudden onset of ABDOMINAL OR BACK PAIN. When the pain is principally in the abdomen, it tends to be centered around the umbilicus. But in many cases, the pain may be located solely in the lower back, leading the patient to think he has "pulled a muscle" or otherwise injured his back. The pain is constant and moderate to severe; it cannot be relieved by changes in position. It tends to radiate into the thigh and groin. If the aneurysm is leaking blood into the retroperitoneal space, the patient may complain as well of an URGE TO DEFECATE. In some patients, an episode of SYNCOPE heralds the onset of symptoms.

The most characteristic physical finding in an abdominal aortic aneurysm is a PULSATILE MASS palpable in the abdomen. The patient is likely to be normotensive when first seen, but SIGNS OF SHOCK, with or without hypotension, may develop rapidly if the aneurysm has ruptured.

Prehospital *management* of an expanding or ruptured aortic aneurysm is aimed at getting the patient to the hospital as expeditiously as possible, since the definitive treatment requires urgent surgery. The key is to maintain a high index of suspicion whenever a middle-aged or older man presents with sudden back pain and a pulsatile abdominal mass.

- Administer OXYGEN.
- Apply (but do not inflate) the MAST.
- TRANSPORT without delay.
- Start an IV en route with normal saline or lactated Ringer's. If there are signs of shock, treat as for any other case of shock, with IV fluids, and consult the physician for orders to inflate the MAST.

Hypertensive Emergencies

It is estimated that **hypertension** (high blood pressure) afflicts nearly 60 million Americans and is directly responsible for more than 30,000 deaths per year. In addition, hypertension is a major contributing cause in many cases of myocardial infarction, congestive heart failure, and stroke.

Hypertension is present when the blood pressure *at rest* is *consistently* greater than about 140/90 mm Hg. Many conditions, such as anxiety or pain, can transiently elevate a person's blood pressure (especially the systolic blood pressure), so a single blood pressure measurement taken during an emergency scarcely constitutes adequate grounds for telling a patient that he or she is hypertensive.

> **ONE BLOOD PRESSURE MEASUREMENT DOTH NOT A HYPERTENSIVE MAKE.**

What one *may* tell a patient when a high blood pressure reading has been obtained is simply something like this: "Sir, your blood pressure is a little high right now. That may be simply because of the stress you are under and may not have any real significance; but to be absolutely sure, what you need to do is have your blood pressure rechecked a couple of times in the next few months under less stressful circumstances." Persistent elevation of the diastolic pressure *is* indicative of hypertensive disease. Untreated, hypertension significantly shortens the lifespan and predisposes to a variety of other medical problems.

In the majority of cases, hypertension is entirely ASYMPTOMATIC and is detected by chance in the course of routine examination. By the time symptoms do start to occur, hypertension is already in a more advanced stage and has probably started producing damage to the end organs most frequently affected, that is, the heart, the kidneys, and the brain. The symptoms that occur in advanced hypertensive disease may be related to the elevated blood pressure itself or to secondary complications. *Headache* is the most common symptom directly related to blood pressure elevation; hypertensive headache is usually localized to the occipital region of the head and occurs when the patient first wakens in the morning, then subsides gradually over the next few hours. Other common complaints in moderately severe hypertension include dizziness, weakness, epistaxis, and blurring of vision.

The most common complications of hypertension include renal damage, stroke, and heart failure—the last a result of the left ventricle having to pump for years against a markedly increased afterload.

Hypertensive *emergencies* occur in about 1 percent of all hypertensive patients. A hypertensive emergency is defined as an acute elevation of blood pressure with evidence of end-organ damage. That last phrase is important, for it is the evidence of end-organ dysfunction that determines the urgency of the situation, not the reading on the sphygmomanometer:

> ## TREAT THE PATIENT, NOT THE BLOOD PRESSURE.

We have already discussed two end-organ emergencies that may result from uncontrolled hypertension: left heart failure and dissecting aortic aneurysm. Less frequent but by far the most devastating complication of hypertension is **hypertensive encephalopathy.**

Hypertensive Encephalopathy

Hypertensive encephalopathy, or acute hypertensive crisis, may complicate any form of hypertension. Hypertensive crisis is usually signalled by a sudden, marked rise in blood pressure to levels greater than 200/130 mm Hg. Usually the first symptoms are SEVERE HEADACHE, NAUSEA, and VOMITING, followed by SEIZURES and ALTERATIONS IN MENTAL STATUS (lethargy, confusion, stupor, coma). Sometimes there may be focal neurologic signs, such as sudden BLINDNESS, APHASIA (disturbances in speech production or comprehension), or HEMIPARESIS. Widespread neuromuscular irritability may be signalled by MUSCLE TWITCHING.

The goal of *treatment* in hypertensive encephalopathy is to lower the blood pressure in a gradual, controlled fashion over 30 to 60 minutes so that cerebral blood flow is restored to normal. That is best accomplished under controlled conditions in a hospital, so if you are within 20 to 30 minutes of the nearest hospital, provide supportive treatment only:

- Secure the AIRWAY, and administer OXYGEN by nasal cannula.
- Establish an IV LIFELINE with D5/W to a keep-open rate.
- Apply MONITORING ELECTRODES and run a rhythm strip.
- TRANSPORT without delay. Be prepared to deal with seizures en route.

Paramedics working in rural areas or other circumstances where long transport times to the hospital are unavoidable may have to initiate DRUG THERAPY of hypertensive encephalopathy in the field. There used to be only one agent for rapidly lowering blood pressure that was at all suitable for prehospital use, and that was diazoxide (Hyperstat). There were problems with diazoxide, however, because it caused a precipitous drop in blood pressure that was very hard to control; diazoxide also increased myocardial oxygen demand, which made it undesirable for use in patients with possible cardiac disease. For those reasons, diazoxide has now been largely supplanted by other drugs, some better suited than others to prehospital care, and it will be necessary for the paramedic to learn and follow the protocols used in his or her own system. At the time of this writing, this author would recommend either of the following agents for prehospital use:

- NIFEDIPINE (Procardia) is a calcium channel blocker, that is, a drug that blocks the influx of calcium into smooth muscles, including those that make up the arterial walls. The result is to prevent vasoconstriction and thereby bring about arteriolar vasodilation. To administer nifedipine for a hypertensive emergency, take a 10-mg nifedipine capsule and puncture it a few times with a hypodermic needle, so that the fluid inside it can leak out. Then place it quickly *under the patient's tongue.* Given sublingually in that fashion, nifedipine is rapidly absorbed and has an onset of action within about 5 minutes. Alternatively, the patient may be given a 10-mg capsule and instructed to bite it and then swallow it.
- An alternative drug that is slightly more cumbersome to administer in the field is LABETALOL (Normodyne, Trandate), which has both alpha and beta blocking properties. As an alpha blocker, it prevents vasoconstriction and thereby decreases the overall peripheral vascular resistance. Meanwhile, its beta blocking actions prevent the reflex tachycardia that would otherwise occur in response to a drop in blood pressure. As a beta blocker, however, it is also relatively contraindicated in patients with asthma and COPD. To administer labetalol, add the contents of two 20-ml ampules (200 mg) to 160 ml of D5/W. That will yield a concentration of 1 mg per milliliter. Start the infusion at a rate of **2 mg per minute** (2 ml/min), and WATCH THE INFUSION LIKE A HAWK! A runaway IV could be disastrous. Monitor the patient's blood pressure every 2 to 3 minutes, and when the blood pressure has fallen to the target level specified by the physician, *stop the infusion.*

Whenever a drug to lower the blood pressure is being given, the patient should be kept SUPINE, and his blood pressure should be measured frequently, at least every 3 to 5 minutes. Each measurement should be recorded on a flow chart.

CARDIAC DYSRHYTHMIAS

Ninety percent of patients with acute myocardial infarction will experience some form of cardiac dysrhythmia sometime during the first week or two after their AMI. Of those episodes of dysrhythmia, 50 percent are life-threatening and will lead to cardiac arrest if not appropriately treated. Thus, in the majority of AMI patients who die before reaching the hospital, the cause of death is a dysrhythmia that was potentially treatable. Clearly, then, one of the most important tasks in the prehospital care of the AMI patient is to anticipate, recognize, and treat life-threatening dysrhythmias.

Dysrhythmias develop after AMI for two principal reasons. First, irritability of the ischemic heart muscle surrounding the infarct may cause the damaged muscle to generate abnormal currents of electricity that cause abnormal cardiac contractions. When the dysrhythmia arises from irritable spots in the myocardium (**ectopic foci**), it is usually a *rapid* dysrhythmia (tachyarrhythmia), such as ventricular tachycardia or premature atrial contractions (PACs) and premature ventricular contractions (PVCs). The second possible cause of dysrhythmias after AMI is damage by the infarct to the conduction tissues themselves. When that is the case, the abnormal rhythm is usually a block or *brady*arrhythmia.

Why do we worry about dysrhythmias at all? *Very slow heart rates* (less than 40–50/min) lead to inadequate cardiac output (why?) and often precede electric instability of the heart; furthermore, when the sinus rate becomes very slow, ectopic pacemakers in the ventricles are more likely to fire, leading to PVCs and ventricular dysrhythmias. *Very rapid heart rates* (over 120–140/min), on the other hand, increase the work of the heart, causing further myocardial ischemia and damage. Tachycardias may also be associated with decreased cardiac output secondary to decreased stroke volume, since the ventricles have less time to fill between beats. Electric instability of the ventricles, manifested by ectopic beats, is a serious warning that graver dysrhythmias, such as ventricular tachycardia or fibrillation, may be pending.

It must be mentioned that cardiac dysrhythmias may come about from a variety of causes, not solely because of AMI (Table 23-9). A cardiac dysrhythmia is simply a disturbance in the normal cardiac rhythm.

TABLE 23-9.   CAUSES OF CARDIAC DYSRHYTHMIAS

Myocardial ischemia or infarction

Other forms of heart disease
    Rheumatic heart disease
    Cor pulmonale

Generalized hypoxemia from any cause

Autonomic nervous system imbalance
    Increased vagal tone
    Increased sympathetic output

Distention of cardiac chambers (e.g., heart failure)

Electrolyte disturbances, especially those involving
    Potassium
    Calcium
    Magnesium

Drug toxicity

Certain poisons (e.g., organophosphate insecticides)

Central nervous system damage

Hypothermia

Normal variations

It may or may not be clinically significant. Thus it is always necessary to evaluate the dysrhythmia in the context of the patient's overall clinical condition, for it is the patient's clinical condition—not the lines and squiggles on a piece of paper—that should ultimately determine whether treatment is necessary:

> **TREAT THE PATIENT, NOT THE DYSRHYTHMIA.**

Application of Monitoring Electrodes

The first step in dysrhythmia recognition is the application of monitoring leads to the patient. The most commonly used electrodes for continuous monitoring are silver plate or clamp electrodes applied to the extremities or stick-on disc electrodes applied to the chest. Whichever type is used, there are certain basic principles that should be followed to minimize artifacts in the signal and to facilitate access to the patient.

- When electrodes are to be attached to the *extremities*, use the inner surfaces of the arms and legs, because they have relatively less hair.
- When the electrodes are to be placed on the chest, it may be necessary to shave the hair from

the chest to allow the discs to adhere properly. Leave the precordium adequately exposed to allow application of defibrillator paddles should the need arise.

- Rub the electrode site, wherever it is, briskly with an alcohol swab to remove oil and dead tissue from the surface of skin. Wait a moment for the skin to dry.
- Apply conductive electrode paste or gel to the electrodes, and attach the electrodes to the site you have prepped.
- Attach the electrodes to the ECG cables. Double-check that the appropriate electrode is attached to the appropriate cable (e.g., the right-arm electrode to the right-arm cable).
- Once the electrodes are hooked up, switch on the monitor and print out a sample rhythm strip. If there are a lot of extraneous lines on the strip, recheck to make sure that the electrodes are firmly applied to the skin.

Beware of artifacts. A straight-line ECG in an alert, communicative patient indicates a loose or disconnected lead, not asystole. Similarly, a wavy baseline resembling ventricular fibrillation may be caused by patient movement or muscle tremor. Before you lunge for the defibrillator paddles, LOOK AT THE PATIENT! If he is alert and in no obvious distress, recheck the leads.

In urgent situations, such as cardiac arrest, the paddles of most defibrillator/monitors can be used for immediate detection of dysrhythmias, as follows:

- Bare the patient's chest.
- Apply electrode gel or saline pads to the paddles. If you use saline pads, make sure they are not so waterlogged that saline oozes all over the chest.
- Apply the positive (red) paddle below the patient's left nipple and the negative (black) paddle on the upper right chest at the junction of the sternum and right clavicle.
- Press the paddles firmly on the chest, and read the rhythm off the monitor.

Reading an ECG Rhythm Strip

To analyze and correctly identify a dysrhythmia, you must have a SYSTEMATIC APPROACH to the ECG and examine each ECG in the same fashion. Using such an approach, you will find in most instances that even the most complex appearing dysrhythmias can be reduced to simple terms and correctly identified.

ECGs are recorded on standardized graph paper, which is moved past a stylus at a standardized speed.

Therefore a given distance on the graph paper represents a given time duration. Specifically, one small box is equivalent to 0.04 second, and one large box (which consists of five small boxes) is equivalent to 0.20 second.

Now, recall the components of the ECG (Fig. 23-18): the **P wave** representing atrial depolarization; the **QRS complex** reflecting ventricular depolarization; and the **T wave** occurring with ventricular repolarization. When examining the rhythm strip, proceed in the following, stepwise fashion:

- Is the RHYTHM **regular or irregular** (Figs. 23-19 and 23-20)? Another way of asking the same question would be: Are the distances between successive QRS complexes (i.e., the R–R intervals) equal? Often one can determine whether the rhythm is irregular at a casual glance, but sometimes it will be necessary to measure the R–R intervals and compare them (special ECG calipers are available for that purpose). Already in the first step of analysis, you have obtained a lot of information. An irregularly irregular rhythm is highly suggestive of atrial fibrillation; a rhythm with only occasional irregularities suggests an ectopic focus somewhere in the heart.
- What is the RATE? There are several ways to determine the cardiac rate from an ECG rhythm strip. The simplest and most accurate method is to count the number of QRS complexes in a *6-second strip* and multiply that number by 10 to obtain the rate per minute. Using that method, the rate in the strip shown in Figure 23-21 would be 50 per minute, since there are five QRS complexes in the 6-second strip. An alternative method to calculate the rate is to count the number of large boxes between any two QRS complexes (the R–R interval) and divide that number into 300. Thus in Figure 23-21, there are approximately 5.6 large boxes between two successive QRS complexes, and 300/5.6 = 54, so the rate would be about 54 per minute. The second method can be used only when the rhythm is absolutely regular.

  The normal heart rate is considered to be between 60 and 100 per minute. Rates *below* 60 per minute are called **bradycardia** (Fig. 23-22), and rates *above* 100 per minute are called **tachycardia** (Fig. 23-23).
- The P WAVE represents depolarization of the atria. In examining the ECG, determine:
  1. Are P waves *present* at all?
  2. Is there a P wave *before every QRS* complex?
  3. Conversely, is there a *QRS complex after every P* wave?

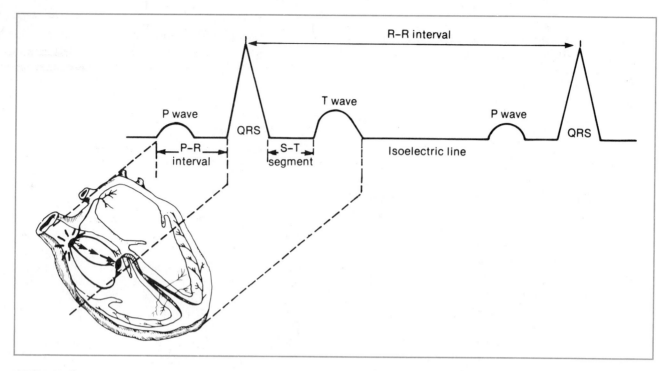

FIGURE 23-18. The P wave represents atrial depolarization, and the QRS complex reflects ventricular depolarization.

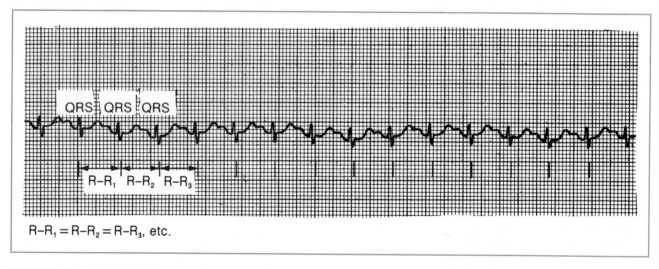

$$R-R_1 = R-R_2 = R-R_3, \text{ etc.}$$

FIGURE 23-19. **REGULAR RHYTHM.** When the rhythm is regular, the R–R intervals are the same.

4. Are all the P waves similar in size and configuration?

The answers to those questions tell us about the **pacemaker site** and the conduction system. If there are no P waves at all, the pacemaker for the heart is *not* in the SA node, and one must consider the possibility of atrial fibrillation or junctional rhythm. If a QRS complex is not preceded by a P wave, the pacemaker site for that beat is *not* in the SA node but rather in some ectopic focus. If a P wave is present but is not followed by a QRS complex, a block is present somewhere in the AV junction or below, preventing conduction from the atria to the ventricles. P waves that

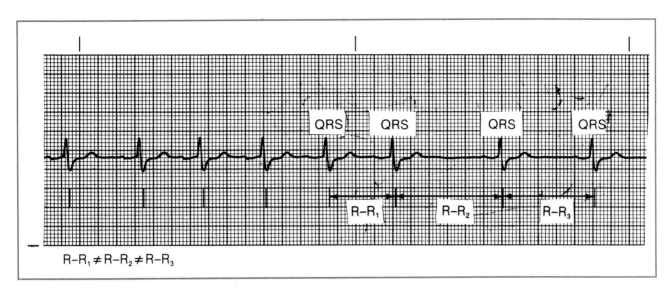

FIGURE 23-20. IRREGULAR RHYTHM. In an irregular rhythm, not all R–R intervals are the same.

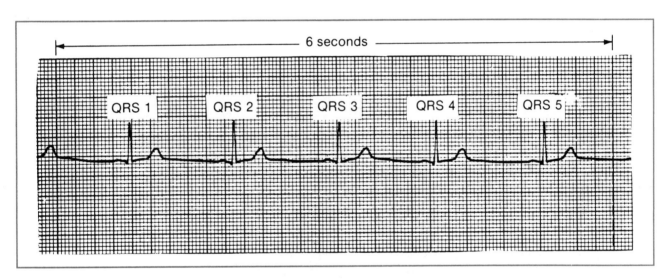

FIGURE 23-21. CALCULATION OF RATE. To calculate the rate, multiply the number of QRS complexes in a 6-second strip by 10.

vary in size and configuration mean that there are several pacemaker sites at different locations throughout the atria.

- The P–R INTERVAL represents the amount of time required for depolarization of the atria and conduction of the impulse through the AV junction. It is normally **0.12 to 0.20 second** (three to five little boxes), reflecting the slight delay that normally occurs in conduction through the AV junction (Fig. 23-24). When there is disease or damage in the AV node, as may occur in myocardial infarction, conduction through the junction may be slowed even more, and the P–R interval will therefore be lengthened (Fig. 23-25). A P–R interval exceeding 0.2 second (five little boxes) is called **first-degree AV block** and indicates injury (usually temporary) to the AV junction.

- The QRS COMPLEX represents depolarization of the ventricles. A normal QRS complex is narrow, with sharply pointed waves, and has a duration of less than 0.1 second (2.5 little boxes). It indicates that conduction of the impulse has proceeded normally from the AV junction, through the bundle of His, left and right bundles, and the Purkinje system. An abnormal QRS complex has a bizarre appearance and a duration longer than

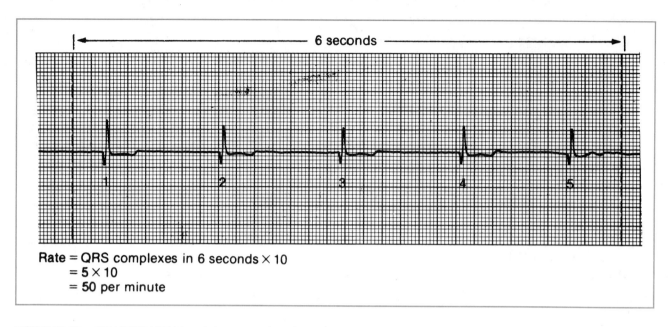

FIGURE 23-22.   **BRADYCARDIA.**   A heart rate less than 60 per minute is considered bradycardia.

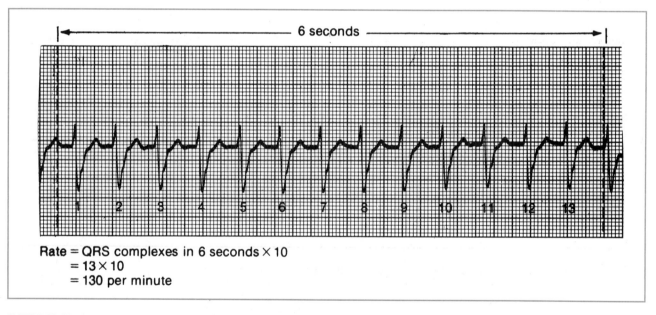

FIGURE 23-23.   **TACHYCARDIA.**   A heart rate greater than 100 per minute is considered tachycardia.

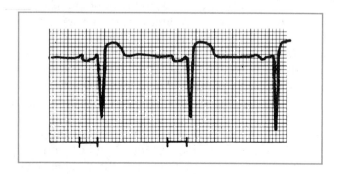

FIGURE 23-24.   **NORMAL P–R INTERVAL.**   The normal P–R interval is 0.12 to 0.20 second.

0.1 second. It signifies some abnormality in conduction through the ventricle (Fig. 23-26).

Again, note whether there is a P wave preceding every QRS. Do the P waves and QRS complexes have a constant relationship to each other, or do they seem to occur independently of one another?

• The S–T SEGMENT, or line between the QRS complex and the T wave, is normally at the same level as the baseline, that is, **isoelectric.** An S–T segment significantly above or below the isoelectric line is highly suggestive of myocardial is-

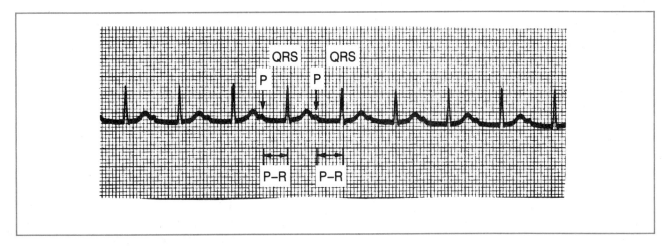

FIGURE 23-25. **PROLONGED P–R INTERVAL.** A P–R interval greater than 0.20 second is considered prolonged.

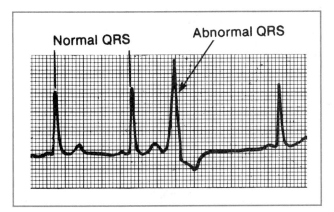

FIGURE 23-26. **QRS COMPLEXES.** An abnormal QRS complex is wider than the normal, and the T wave following it may be directed oppositely to the T wave that follows the normal QRS (e.g., a negative deflection instead of positive, as in this example).

SYSTEMATIC ANALYSIS OF THE ECG RHYTHM STRIP

- Is the RHYTHM regular or irregular?
- What is the RATE?
- Are there P WAVES? Is there a P wave before every QRS complex and a QRS complex after every P wave? Based on that, what is the pacemaker site?
- What is the P–R INTERVAL? Is it prolonged? Shortened?
- Are the QRS COMPLEXES normal or abnormal in shape, duration?
- Is the S–T SEGMENT isoelectric?
- Are the T WAVES of normal configuration?

---

chemia, although a full, 12-lead ECG is required to determine the precise significance of S–T elevation or depression.

- The T WAVE, representing ventricular repolarization, may also show abnormalities, especially in association with electrolyte disturbances. The T wave in hyperkalemia, for example, may be tall and sharply peaked. The T wave following a premature ventricular contraction (PVC) is usually directed opposite from the normal T wave. (Look at the T wave following the abnormal QRS in Fig. 23-26, and compare it to the T waves following the normal QRS complexes in the same rhythm strip.)

In summary, then, the analysis of every rhythm strip should proceed in order through the following steps:

By the time you have answered those questions, you should have a very good idea of the identity of the dysrhythmia in question.

Specific Cardiac Dysrhythmias

There are nearly as many systems for classifying cardiac dysrhythmias as there are cardiologists who have written books on the subject. Dysrhythmias may, for example, be categorized according to whether they are disturbances of automaticity versus disturbances of conduction, or whether they are tachyarrhythmias versus bradyarrhythmias, or whether they are life-threatening versus non-life-threatening. In this text, we shall study the cardiac dysrhythmias according to the *site from which they arise*. We shall start, therefore—after looking at a normal sinus rhythm for comparison—by examining the dysrhythmias that arise in the sinoatrial node. Then we'll examine the dysrhythmias that arise in the atrial tissue, then those that arise in the AV junction, and so on right down the conduction pathway. In each case, we shall learn how to identify the dysrhythmia and how to treat it, if indeed any treatment is necessary. In the pages that follow, then, we shall consider these specific cardiac dysrhythmias:

Dysrhythmias originating in the SA node
- Normal sinus rhythm (Fig. 23-27)
- Sinus arrhythmia (Fig. 23-28)
- Sinus arrest (Fig. 23-29)
- Sinus bradycardia (Fig. 23-30)
- Sinus tachycardia (Fig. 23-31)

Dysrhythmias originating in the atrium
- Wandering atrial pacemaker (Fig. 23-32)
- Premature atrial contractions (Fig. 23-33)
- Paroxysmal supraventricular tachycardia (Fig. 23-34)
- Atrial flutter (Fig. 23-35)
- Atrial fibrillation (Fig. 23-36)

Dysrhythmias originating in the AV node or AV junction
- Premature junctional contractions (Fig. 23-37)
- Junctional rhythm (Fig. 23-38)
- First-degree AV block (Fig. 23-39)
- Second-degree AV block
  1. Type I, Wenckebach (Fig. 23-40)
  2. Type II (Fig. 23-41)
- Third-degree (complete) AV block (Fig. 23-42)
- Bundle branch blocks (Fig. 23-43)

Dysrhythmias originating in the ventricles
- Premature ventricular contractions (Figs. 23-44 through 23-49)
- Ventricular tachycardia (Fig. 23-50)
- Ventricular fibrillation (Fig. 23-51)

Cardiac standstill
- Asystole (Fig. 23-52)

Rhythms originating outside the heart
- Pacemaker rhythms (Fig. 23-53)

For hotshots only
- Wolff-Parkinson-White (Fig. 23-54)

ECG artifacts
- Muscle tremor (Fig. 23-55)
- Patient cable movement (Fig. 23-56)

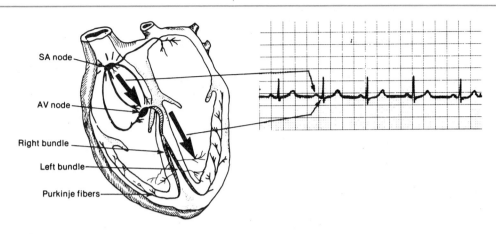

FIGURE 23-27. **NORMAL SINUS RHYTHM**

Rhythm: Regular.
Rate: 60 to 100 per minute.
P waves: Normal, preceding every QRS.
Pacemaker site: SA node.
P–R interval: Normal (0.12–0.20 sec).
QRS complexes: Normal, each preceded by a P wave.
Clinical significance: Normal rhythm.
Treatment: None.

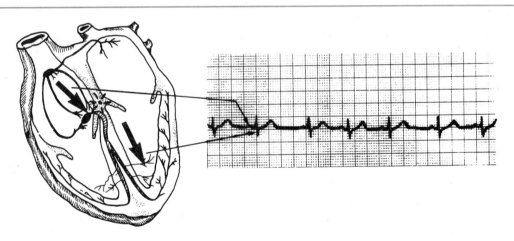

FIGURE 23-28. **SINUS ARRHYTHMIA**

Rhythm: Regularly irregular.
Rate: Normal.
P waves: Normal, preceding every QRS.
Pacemaker site: SA node.
P–R interval: Normal (0.12–0.20 sec).
QRS complexes: Normal, each QRS preceded by a P wave.
Clinical significance: Sinus arrhythmia is a normal phenomenon, caused by the effects of the parasympathetic nervous system of breathing.
Treatment: None.

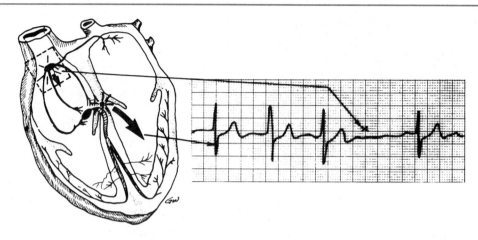

FIGURE 23-29.   SINUS ARREST

Rhythm: Irregular.

Rate: May be normal to slow.

P waves: Normal, where present, preceding each QRS. However, if the SA node does not discharge or is blocked, the entire P–QRS–T complex is absent.

Pacemaker site: SA node.

P–R interval: Normal (0.12–0.20 sec).

QRS complexes: Normal, each preceded by a P wave.

Clinical significance: Occasional episodes are not significant; however, if the heart rate is reduced below 30 to 50 per minute, cardiac output may fall and an ectopic focus in the ventricles may take over.

Treatment:

- None necessary if the patient is asymptomatic, blood pressure is well maintained, and there is no evidence of ventricular irritability.
- Treatment to increase the heart rate must be undertaken if there are signs of hypoperfusion or atrial or ventricular ectopic arrhythmias. In those instances, ATROPINE SULFATE, 0.5 mg, is given by IV bolus. The dose may be repeated at 5- to 10-minute intervals until the heart rate has increased to 70 or more per minute or until a maximum dose of 2.0 mg of atropine has been given.

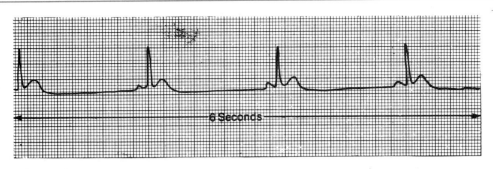

FIGURE 23-30.   SINUS BRADYCARDIA

Rhythm: Regular or very slightly irregular.

Rate: 35 to 60 per minute.

P waves: Normal, each preceding a QRS complex.

Pacemaker site: SA node.

P–R interval: Normal (0.12–0.20 sec).

QRS complexes: Normal, each preceded by a P wave.

Clinical significance: In young, healthy individuals, heart rates below 60 per minute may simply reflect good physical conditioning. However, in the context of AMI, sinus bradycardia implies (1) damage to the conduction system, (2) increased vagal (parasympathetic) tone, or (3) possible toxic levels of certain cardiac drugs (digitalis, quinidine). When the heart rate falls below about 50 per minute, cardiac output may be significantly reduced, leading to a decrease in perfusion of vital organs. Furthermore, bradycardia promotes electric instability of the ventricles and may thus lead to serious ventricular arrhythmias.

Treatment:

- No treatment is necessary if the blood pressure is normal, the patient is alert, and there is no ventricular ectopic activity.
- Treatment is indicated if either of the following circumstances is present: (1) HYPOTENSION (systolic pressure less than 80–90 mm Hg), especially with weak or absent pulse, cold and clammy skin, and confusion or coma; or (2) VENTRICULAR PREMATURE BEATS. In those instances, ATROPINE SULFATE, 0.5 mg, is given by IV bolus. The dose may be repeated at 5-minute intervals until the heart rate has increased to 70 or more per minute or until a maximum dose of 2.0 mg of atropine has been given.

   Remember: PREMATURE VENTRICULAR CONTRACTIONS IN THE CONTEXT OF BRADYCARDIA SHOULD BE TREATED FIRST WITH ATROPINE, *NOT* LIDOCAINE. Very often, merely speeding up the heart rate will abolish the PVCs, without the need for further medications. If atropine is ineffective in increasing the heart rate, the physician may order dopamine infusion starting at 5 to 20 μg/kg/min.

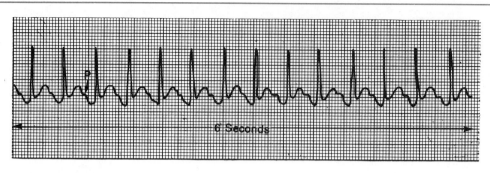

FIGURE 23-31.   SINUS TACHYCARDIA

Rhythm: Regular.

Rate: 100 to 160 per minute.

P waves: Normal, preceding each QRS complex. With very rapid rates, P waves may be buried in the previous T wave.

Pacemaker site: SA node.

P–R interval: Normal (0.12–0.20 sec).

QRS complexes: Normal, each preceded by a P wave.

Clinical significance: Sinus tachycardia may result from a variety of circumstances, including pain, fever, hypoxia, shock, and congestive heart failure, as well as from certain drugs (e.g., epinephrine, atropine, isoproterenol). Very rapid heart rates increase the work of the heart, leading in the AMI to further ischemia and infarction. In addition, cardiac output may be significantly reduced when the heart rate exceeds 120 to 140 per minute because there is inadequate time between contractions for the ventricles to fill completely with blood.

Treatment: Treat the *underlying cause* (e.g., hypoxia, congestive heart failure).

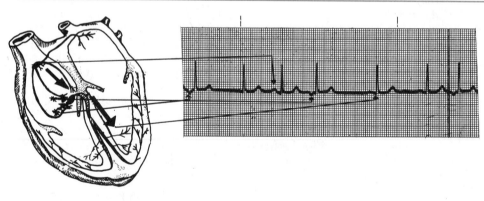

FIGURE 23-32.   WANDERING ATRIAL PACEMAKER

Rhythm: Slightly irregular.

Rate: Usually 60 to 100 per minute.

P waves: The size and shape of the P waves change from beat to beat; there are usually at least three P wave configurations visible in any given lead.

Pacemaker site: Multiple sites in the atria and AV junction (for that reason, the dysrhythmia is more properly called *multifocal atrial rhythm*).

P–R interval: Variable, depending on the distance between the atrial pacemaker site for a given beat and the AV node; may be less than 0.12 second with some beats.

QRS complexes: Normal.

Clinical significance: May occur in normal individuals or may reflect an increase in vagal tone, digitalis effect, or rheumatic fever.

Treatment: None required unless the rate exceeds about 120 per minute, in which case the underlying cause must be identified and treated.

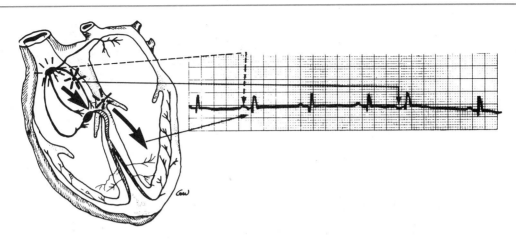

FIGURE 23-33. PREMATURE ATRIAL CONTRACTIONS (PACs)

Rhythm: Irregular.

Rate: Will be determined by the number of premature supraventricular beats.

P waves: The P waves of the premature atrial contractions are often different from the normal P waves in shape or size.

Pacemaker site: The pacemaker site of the premature supraventricular beat is an *ectopic focus* in some portion of the atria or AV junction other than the SA node.

P–R interval: Variable, depending on the distance between the ectopic pacemaker and the AV junction.

QRS complexes: Usually normal, but may be aberrantly conducted.

Clinical significance: Occasional PACs may occur in normal individuals, but frequent PACs suggest organic heart disease and may lead to atrial tachycardias. For purposes in the field, the chief importance of PACs is that they be correctly distinguished from PVCs.

Treatment: None.

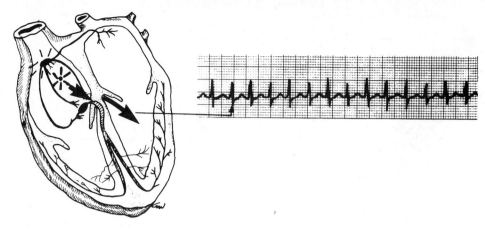

FIGURE 23-34. PAROXYSMAL SUPRAVENTRICULAR TACHYCARDIA (PSVT)

Rhythm: Usually regular, except at onset and termination.

Rate: About 140 to 220 per minute.

P waves: May be absent or abnormal.

Pacemaker site: A part of the atria or AV junction other than the SA node.

P–R interval: May be none; if a P wave precedes the QRS, the duration of the P–R interval will depend on the distance from the ectopic pacemaker site to the AV junction.

QRS complexes: Usually normal. **(If the QRS complexes are wide, treat the rhythm as ventricular tachycardia.)**

Clinical significance: Sometimes caused by structural damage to the SA or AV node or by digitalis overdose. One relatively common type of supraventricular tachycardia, however, occurs in otherwise healthy individuals and does not necessarily indicate cardiac disease: *paroxysmal atrial tachycardia* (PAT). In itself, PAT is a relatively benign dysrhythmia; but if it persists for any length of time, PAT may cause congestive heart failure. PAT can be precipitated in susceptible individuals by alcohol, heavy smoking, coffee, hyperventilation, and stress. It usually starts abruptly, and the heart rate in PAT is usually between 120 and 180 per minute, with 1 : 1 AV conduction (i.e., one P wave to every QRS).

Treatment: There are three approaches to treating PSVT—vagal stimulation, drug therapy, and electric cardioversion.

• *Vagal maneuvers* are indicated principally for patients who are hemodynamically stable, that is, who show no signs of shock or compromised cardiac function. Any maneuver that stimulates the vagus nerve will slow the heart and may therefore convert some PSVTs (notably PAT) back to normal sinus rhythm. Such maneuvers include the VALSALVA MANEUVER (straining against a closed glottis) and CAROTID SINUS MASSAGE (see p. 589 for technique). Immersion of the patient's face briefly in ICE WATER is also a potent and effective vagal stimulus, based on the mammalian diving reflex. Apply vagal maneuvers *only* if (1) you receive a physician's order to do so, (2) the patient is attached to a cardiac monitor, (3) an IV lifeline has already been established, and (4) atropine sulfate and lidocaine are immediately at hand.

• *Pharmacologic treatment.* If vagal maneuvers are unsuccessful in the stable patient, drug therapy should be tried. This is best carried out in the emergency department of the hospital. If transport to the hospital will take a long time, however, the physician may order you to administer ADENOSINE, 6 mg by rapid IV push (i.e., over 1–3 seconds). If the rhythm does not convert to sinus within about 2 minutes, you may give a *second dose of adenosine,* this time 12 mg given rapidly IV. If PSVT recurs after two doses of adenosine, it may be necessary to switch to another drug, VERAPAMIL. Since verapamil may produce serious side effects—including severe hypotension and even sudden death (if inadvertently given for ventricular tachycardia)—it is preferable to wait until the patient reaches the hospital before verapamil is administered.

• **Electric therapy (cardioversion)** of PSVTs is indicated in the field for
   1. Patients showing signs of severely compromised perfusion (shock, stupor, coma) or
   2. Patients with congestive heart failure or myocardial ischemia secondary to PSVT, when transport time to the hospital will be more than 5 to 10 minutes.

See p. 588 for technique of cardioversion.

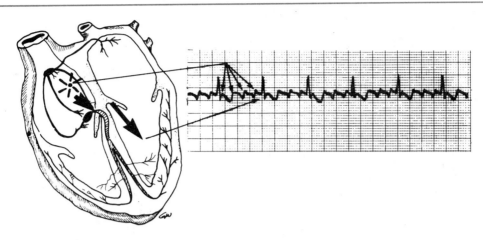

FIGURE 23-35.   ATRIAL FLUTTER

Rhythm: Atrial rhythm is regular; ventricular response is most often regular with 2 : 1 AV conduction, but it may be irregular.

Rate: Atrial rate is 240 to 360 per minute; ventricular rate is 140 to 160 per minute, but the ventricular rate may be slower, especially if the patient is taking digitalis.

P waves: No true P waves present. Instead, there are flutter waves (F waves), often in a jagged, "sawtooth" pattern.

Pacemaker site: An ectopic focus in the atrium.

P–R interval: Not measurable.

QRS complexes: Usually normal in configuration; a QRS may follow every second, third, or fourth flutter wave.

Clinical significance: Atrial flutter is usually caused by some underlying disease or damage to the heart. If the ventricular response is rapid, the work of the heart is increased, and cardiac output may be compromised.

Treatment:

- If the patient is clinically stable, without signs of hypoperfusion (e.g., falling blood pressure; cold, clammy skin; confusion or coma), no treatment is ordinarily indicated in the field. When transport time will be prolonged, however, as in some rural areas, the physician may order a drug to slow the ventricular rate. The drugs most commonly used in such circumstances are a beta blocker like PROPRANOLOL (1 mg IV over 5 minutes) OR a calcium channel blocker like VERAPAMIL (0.1 mg/kg over 1–2 minutes). Do *not* give both!

- If the ventricular rate (pulse) is in excess of 120 to 140 per minute, the patient evidences inadequate cardiac output (hypotension; cold, clammy skin; confusion or coma), and transport time to the hospital will be prolonged, *cardioversion* may be required in the field (see p. 588 for technique). In that event, it will be very important to inform the physician whether the patient has been taking digitalis at home, since cardioversion may be hazardous in the digitalized patient.

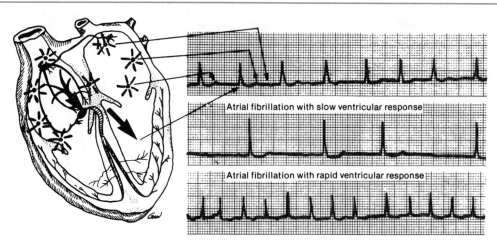

Atrial fibrillation with slow ventricular response

Atrial fibrillation with rapid ventricular response

FIGURE 23-36.   ATRIAL FIBRILLATION

Rhythm: *Irregularly irregular.*

Rate: Atrial rate is 350 to 600 per minute, not measurable on the rhythm strip; ventricular rate is 100 to 160 per minute if untreated, but may be slower if the patient is taking digitalis.

P waves: *Absent.* Instead there are fibrillatory waves (f waves), which may be very coarse or may be so fine that they resemble a straight line.

Pacemaker site: Multiple ectopic pacemaker sites throughout the atria.

P–R interval: Not measurable.

QRS complexes: Usually normal, but not preceded by demonstrable P waves.

Clinical significance: Atrial fibrillation is usually associated with underlying heart disease and, when it occurs in the setting of AMI, may indicate damage to the SA node or atria. Because in atrial fibrillation the atria and ventricles do not contract in sequence, the ventricles do not fill completely before contracting; thus the cardiac output may fall by as much as 25 percent. Furthermore, if the ventricular response in atrial fibrillation is in excess of 120 to 140 beats per minute, cardiac output is further compromised, and the work of the heart increased.

Treatment: Usually none in the field. Very rapid pulse associated with atrial fibrillation may require cardioversion or therapy with a drug such as propranolol, verapamil, or digoxin. Consult physician for orders, and indicate to him whether patient is taking any form of digitalis.

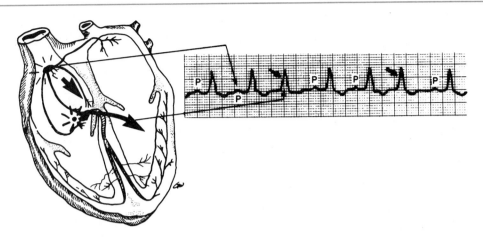

FIGURE 23-37.   PREMATURE JUNCTIONAL CONTRACTIONS (PJCs)

Rhythm: Irregular; the premature junctional beat is preceded by a shorter than normal R–R interval.

Rate: Will be determined by the number of PJCs.

P waves: May be present or absent in the PJCs; when present, they differ in shape from normal P waves and may occur before, during, or after the QRS.

Pacemaker site: An ectopic focus in the AV junction is the pacemaker site for the PJCs.

P–R interval: Less than 0.12 second for the PJC.

QRS complexes: Normal.

Clinical significance: Occasional PJCs are not significant; when multiple, they indicate irritability of the AV junction and may herald more serious dysrhythmias.

Treatment: None.

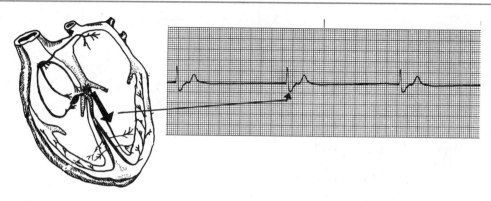

FIGURE 23-38. JUNCTIONAL RHYTHM

Rhythm: Regular.

Rate: The intrinsic rate of the AV junction, usually between 25 and 60 per minute.

P waves: If present at all, they are inverted in leads II, III, and aVF. P waves may occur *after* the QRS, depending on the pacemaker site in the AV junction.

Pacemaker site: AV junction.

P–R interval: Usually less than 0.12 second or nonexistent.

QRS complexes: Usually normal.

Clinical significance: Junctional rhythm can be caused by anything that *suppresses the SA node* and thereby allows the slower AV junctional tissue to "escape" from sinus control. Those causes include myocardial infarction (especially inferior wall AMI), congestive heart failure, anoxia, acidosis, hyperkalemia, and vagotonic drugs (e.g., morphine).

Treatment: Definitive treatment depends on identification and correction of the underlying cause. If the patient is stable, no treatment is required in the field. If the rate is very slow and the patient shows signs of inadequate cardiac output (cold, clammy skin; confusion; hypotension):

- Give 1 ampule (50 mEq) of SODIUM BICARBONATE IV and observe the monitor. If the ventricular rate increases or P waves begin to occur, the patient is probably suffering from acidosis or hyperkalemia or both, and additional bicarbonate may be needed en route.
- If there is no response to bicarbonate, give ATROPINE, 0.5 mg IV. That dose may be repeated twice, each time after waiting 5 minutes for a response.
- If there is no response to atropine and transport time will be prolonged, the physician may order a DOPAMINE drip to be started, at a rate of 5–20 µg/kg per minute.

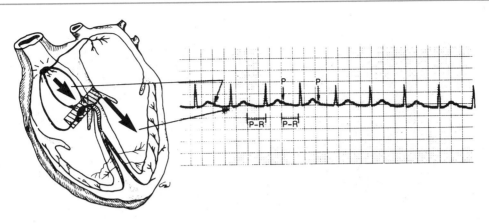

FIGURE 23-39.   **FIRST-DEGREE AV BLOCK**

Rhythm: Regular.
Rate: Normal.
P waves: Normal, preceding each QRS complex.
Pacemaker site: SA node.
P–R interval: Prolonged beyond 0.2 second (five little boxes).
QRS complexes: Normal, each preceded by a P wave.
Clinical significance: First-degree AV block may be caused by the following:
  • Damage to the AV junction
  • Increased vagal (parasympathetic) tone
  • Toxicity from certain cardiac drugs (e.g., digitalis, quinidine, procainamide)
    In the context of AMI, first-degree AV block may warn of impending, more advanced degrees of block.
Treatment: None indicated.

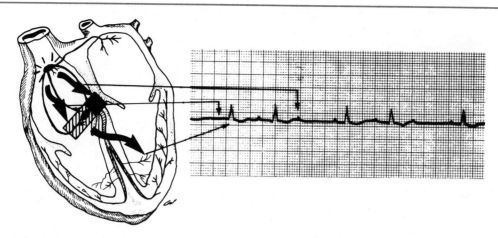

FIGURE 23-40.   SECOND-DEGREE AV BLOCK: TYPE I (WENCKEBACH)

Rhythm: Atrial (P wave) rhythm regular; ventricular (QRS) rhythm irregular.

Rate: Atrial rate normal; ventricular rate may be normal or slow depending on the degree of block.

P waves: Normal; a QRS complex is absent after every third, fourth, or fifth P wave. Hence P waves are more numerous than QRS complexes.

Pacemaker site: SA node.

P–R interval: Progressively widens until an atrial impulse is blocked altogether, and the P wave is not followed by a QRS.

QRS complexes: Normal, each preceded by a P wave.

Clinical significance: Wenckebach block is the less serious type of second-degree block, usually being transient and reversible. However, occasionally Wenckebach block will progress to complete heart block, and careful monitoring is therefore indicated.

Treatment: None if the heart rate is above 50 to 60 per minute and cardiac output is well maintained. However, if pulse is less than 50 to 60 per minute, accompanied by signs of inadequate cardiac output (hypotension; cold, clammy skin; confusion; or coma), ATROPINE SULFATE, 0.5 mg by IV bolus, may be ordered. The dose may be repeated at 5-minute intervals until the pulse reaches 70 or more per minute or until a maximum total dose of 2.0 mg has been given.

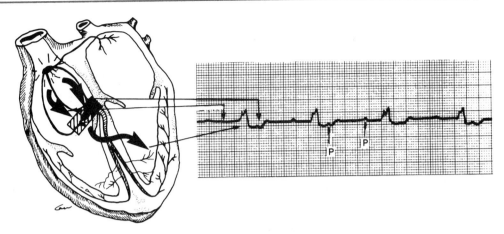

FIGURE 23-41. SECOND-DEGREE AV BLOCK: TYPE II

Rhythm: Atrial (P wave) rhythm regular; ventricular (QRS) rhythm may be regular or irregular.

Rate: Atrial rate normal; ventricular rate may be normal or slow depending on the degree of block.

P waves: Normal, but not every P wave is followed by a QRS. Hence the P waves are more numerous than the QRS complexes. The ratio of P waves to QRS complexes may be 2 : 1, 3 : 1, and so on.

Pacemaker site: SA node.

P–R interval: Normal or prolonged, but constant.

QRS complexes: Usually normal, each preceded by a P wave; may be widened.

Clinical significance: Second-degree AV block is a serious sign. It occurs in large anterior wall myocardial infarctions and may progress rapidly to complete AV block (third-degree heart block). Furthermore, if slow ventricular rates are associated with second-degree AV block, cardiac output may be substantially reduced.

Treatment: No treatment is necessary if the heart rate is above 50 to 60 per minute and the cardiac output is well maintained. In very slow heart rates accompanied by signs of inadequate cardiac output, the patient will need a pacemaker. Paramedics who are trained and equipped to do so should request orders to apply a TRANSCUTANEOUS PACEMAKER. Meanwhile, the receiving hospital should be notified to have a team standing by for immediate insertion of a transvenous pacemaker.

Atropine should *not* be given in type II second-degree heart block.

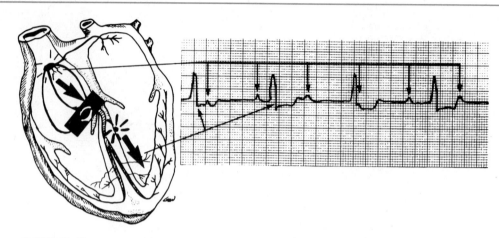

FIGURE 23-42. **THIRD-DEGREE AV BLOCK (COMPLETE HEART BLOCK)**

Rhythm: Regular.

Rate: Atrial (P wave) rate normal, *ventricular (QRS) rate is 30 to 40 per minute.*

P waves: Normal contour; *no consistent relationship to QRS complexes.*

Pacemaker site: The SA node is the pacemaker for the atria, but impulses from the SA node are blocked at the AV junction and cannot reach the ventricles; hence the ventricles are driven by a different pacemaker, in the AV junction or below. The lower the pacemaker lies in the ventricles, the slower the ventricular rate and the more bizarre the QRS complexes.

P–R interval: Strictly speaking, there is no P–R interval, since there is no consistent relationship between the P waves and the QRS complexes.

QRS complexes: May be normal if the ventricular pacemaker lies in the AV junction or bundle of His, but usually the QRS complexes are wide and bizarre.

Clinical significance: If the heart rate is below 35 to 50 beats per minute, cardiac output may be significantly reduced. In addition, because in third-degree heart block the atria and ventricles are no longer synchronized, the ventricles do not fill completely prior to each contraction, and cardiac output is further reduced.

Treatment: Initiated in the field if complete heart block is associated with signs of inadequate perfusion (e.g., hypotension, syncope, confusion).

- If trained and equipped to do so, obtain an order to apply a TRANSCUTANE-OUS PACEMAKER. Notify the receiving hospital to have a team standing by for immediate placement of a transvenous pacemaker.

- If a 12-lead ECG shows signs of an *inferior* wall infarction and QRS complexes are narrow, you may be asked instead to give either ATROPINE (0.5 mg IV, repeated up to 3 times) or a DOPAMINE infusion (5–20 μg/kg/min). Do *not* give atropine for third-degree block associated with *anterior* wall AMI or when QRS complexes are wide.

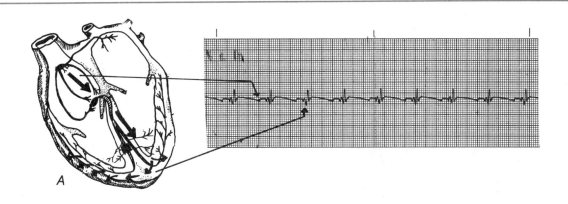

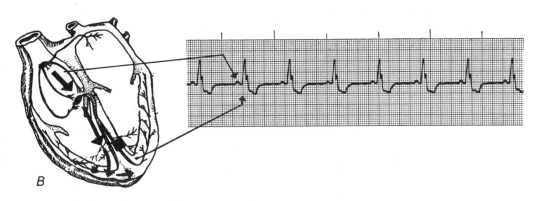

FIGURE 23-43.   BUNDLE BRANCH BLOCKS

Rhythm: Regular.

Rate: Usually normal, although sometimes a bundle branch block pattern becomes manifest only at rapid heart rates.

P waves: Normal.

Pacemaker site: SA node.

P–R interval: Normal.

QRS complexes: Prolonged and often bizarre in shape. In *right* bundle branch block (RBBB; Fig. 23-43A), the precordial leads usually show the "rabbit ear" pattern of RSR, reflecting the block of the excitation wave immediately after the septum; the wave must proceed down the (unblocked) left bundle and then pass back into the right ventricular myocardium. The QRS complexes in *left* bundle branch block (LBBB, Fig. 23-43B) often look like PVCs, with S–T depression and T wave inversion.

Clinical significance: In bundle branch blocks, conduction through one bundle is inhibited, so the ventricles are activated in series rather than in parallel. RBBB may be present in any type of heart disease; occasionally it is found in normal individuals. LBBB is a common finding in coronary artery disease or any condition that produces enlargement of the left ventricle (e.g., long-standing hypertension). Transient bundle branch block may occur in heart failure, AMI, acute infections, or as a consequence of digitalis or quinidine toxicity. Bundle branch blocks may, however, progress to complete heart block.

Treatment: In the field, watchful waiting: Be alert for slowing of the heart and the development of complete heart block. (Keep the beep tone of the monitor on, so you can *hear* the heart rate slow down.)

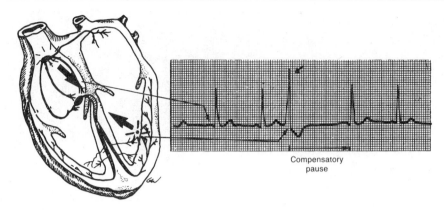

Compensatory
pause

FIGURE 23-44.   PREMATURE VENTRICULAR CONTRACTIONS (PVCs)

Rhythm: Irregular. A shorter than normal R–R interval separates the PVC from the preceding normal beat, hence the designation *premature*. Most PVCs are followed by a *compensatory pause*.

Rate: Determined by the number of PVCs.

P waves: Absent before PVCs.

Pacemaker site: The pacemaker site for the PVC is an ectopic focus in one of the ventricles.

P–R interval: None in the PVC, because it is not preceded by a P wave.

QRS complexes: *Distorted, wide* (greater than 0.12 sec, i.e., three little boxes), and *bizarre* in the PVCs. The T wave of the PVC is usually oppositely directed (i.e., if the QRS complex is upright, the T wave is inverted).

Clinical significance: Occasional PVCs may occur in normal persons. However, in the setting of AMI, PVCs indicate increased ventricular irritability and should be treated. Certain types of PVCs are of particular concern, because of their tendency to progress to ventricular tachycardia or fibrillation. These include the following:

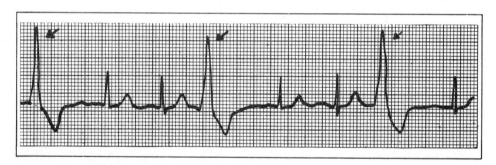

FIGURE 23-45.   FREQUENT PVCs (more than 6/min).

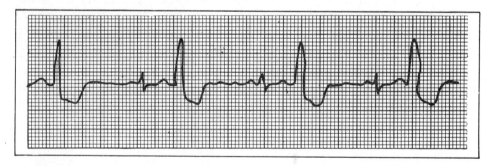

FIGURE 23-46.   BIGEMINY.   When PVCs occur every second beat, the rhythm is called *ventricular bigeminy*.

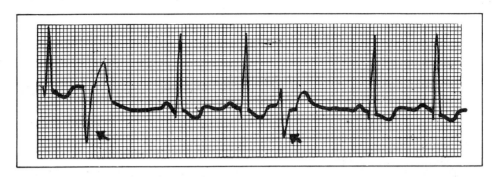

FIGURE 23-47.   **MULTIFOCAL PVCs** are of different sizes and shapes and indicate that there are multiple ectopic foci in the ventricle.

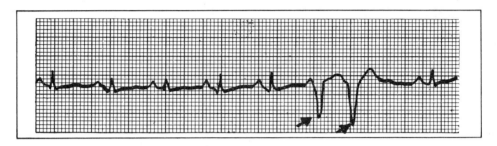

FIGURE 23-48.   **SALVOS.**   Bursts of TWO OR MORE PVCs IN A ROW (salvos) may progress rapidly to ventricular tachycardia.

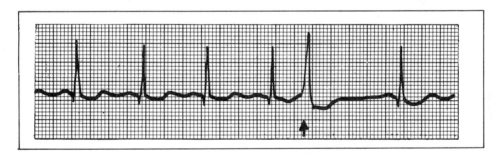

FIGURE 23-49.   **R–ON–T PATTERN.**   The T wave represents the vulnerable period of the cardiac cycle. A PVC falling on a T wave may thus precipitate ventricular fibrillation.

Treatment: In the setting of AMI, PVCs in the categories above should usually be treated:
- If you have not already done so, obtain permission to start an infusion of MAGNESIUM SULFATE (2.4 gm in 50 ml of D5/W infused over 20–60 minutes).
- Obtain orders to give LIDOCAINE, 75 to 100 mg by IV bolus, followed by a lidocaine infusion; the infusion is prepared by adding 0.5 gm of lidocaine to a 250-ml bag of D5/W and running the infusion at a rate of 60 to 90 microdrops per minute, to deliver a dosage of 2 to 3 mg per minute.

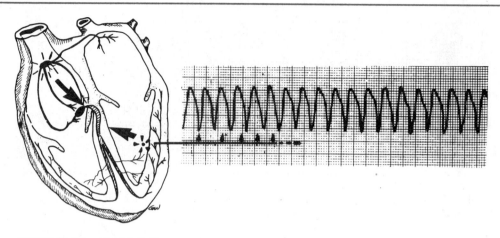

FIGURE 23-50. VENTRICULAR TACHYCARDIA

Rhythm: Regular or slightly irregular.

Rate: 100 to 250 per minute.

P waves: Often not seen because they are buried in the QRS complexes; when they are visible, they have no apparent relationship to the QRS complexes.

Pacemaker site: An ectopic focus in the ventricle.

P–R interval: None.

QRS complexes: Distorted, wide (greater than 0.12 sec), bizarre.

Clinical significance: This is a very serious and dangerous arrhythmia, which may lead to ventricular fibrillation and can itself cause marked reduction in cardiac output.

Treatment:

- *If the patient is alert* and has no signs of inadequate cardiac output, LIDO-CAINE, 75 to 100 mg, is given by IV bolus, followed by an infusion of lidocaine (0.5 gm added to a 250-ml bag of D5/W, run at 60–90 microdrops/min). If lidocaine is ineffective in converting the rhythm to sinus, the physician may order BRETYLIUM TOSYLATE as an infusion of 10 mg per kilogram given over 10 minutes (500 mg of bretylium is diluted in 50 ml of D5/W and given at a rate of 5 ml/min).

- In a *monitored* patient who suddenly becomes unconscious and whose rhythm is observed to be ventricular tachycardia, a sharp, quick PRECORDIAL THUMP may be delivered over the midsternum if a defibrillator is not immediately available. If the precordial thump is ineffective and there is continued evidence of inadequate cardiac output (hypotension; coma; cold, clammy skin), CARDIO-VERSION is indicated (see p. 588 for technique). Cardioversion is more likely to be successful if preceded by a bolus of lidocaine as described above.

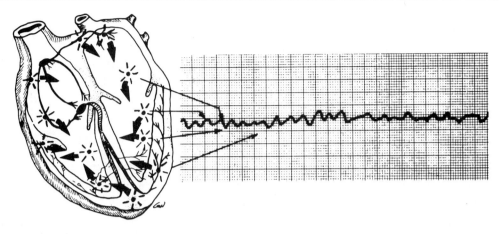

FIGURE 23-51.   VENTRICULAR FIBRILLATION

Rhythm: Totally irregular.
Rate: 150 to 300 entirely uncoordinated waves per minute.
P waves: Not seen.
Pacemaker site: Numerous ectopic foci scattered throughout the heart.
P–R interval: None.
QRS complexes: Absent. In place of QRS complexes there are fibrillatory waves of varying size, shape, and duration.

Clinical significance: In ventricular fibrillation, the ventricles fire in a totally disorganized fashion, and ventricular muscle simply quivers rather than beats. As a result, there is *no cardiac output,* and ventricular fibrillation is thus equivalent to *clinical death.* Biologic death inevitably follows unless CPR is initiated within a few minutes. It is obviously most important when a rhythm resembling ventricular fibrillation is seen on the monitor to check the patient rapidly to rule out muscle tremor, loose leads, or patient movement artifact as the source of the oscillating baseline.

Treatment:

- If ventricular fibrillation occurs in the rescuer's presence (*witnessed* cardiac arrest), GIVE AN IMMEDIATE COUNTERSHOCK of 200 joules (see p. 586 for technique). If a *monitored* patient is observed to go into ventricular fibrillation and a defibrillator is not immediately available, try a quick PRECORDIAL THUMP (see p. 589).

- If the patient has been in cardiac arrest for more than a few minutes or for an unknown period (*unwitnessed* cardiac arrest), INITIATE BASIC LIFE SUPPORT AT ONCE. Continue CPR until a defibrillator is available and charged. Then defibrillate as soon as possible. Further measures may be required to enable successful defibrillation. (For a more detailed discussion of the treatment of ventricular fibrillation, see the section on Advanced Cardiac Life Support later in this chapter.)

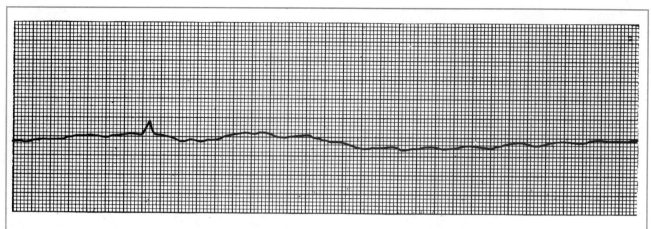

FIGURE 23-52. **CARDIAC STANDSTILL (ASYSTOLE)**

Rhythm: None—straight line.

Rate: Less than five ectopic beats per minute.

P waves: None.

Pacemaker site: None consistently.

P–R interval: None.

QRS complex: None or rare, bizarre.

Clinical significance: Asystole is total absence of electric activity in the heart and is thus a form of clinical death.

Treatment: CPR and drug therapy, including epinephrine (see pp. 581–584 for technique). If there is any doubt whether the rhythm is asystole or fine ventricular fibrillation, defibrillate at 200 joules. In refractory asystole, a pacemaker may be useful, and the hospital should be notified to have a pacemaker ready.

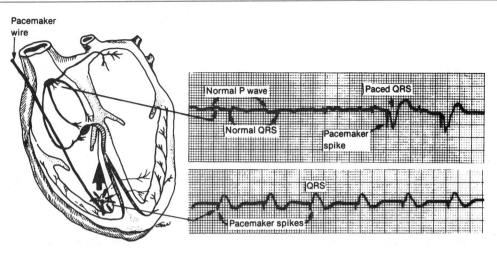

FIGURE 23-53.   PACEMAKER RHYTHMS

Rhythm: Regular or irregular.

Rate: Variable, depending on the pacemaker setting. The rate should not be below 60 per minute if the pacemaker is functioning properly.

P waves: Normal when present, and may or may not be followed by a QRS. Pacemaker spikes will precede those QRS complexes induced by the pacemaker.

Pacemaker site: Electronic pacemaker and sometimes SA node as well.

P–R interval: May be normal or prolonged when present.

QRS complexes: Those following a pacemaker spike are wide and bizarre, resembling PVCs.

Clinical significance: Pacemaker rhythms indicate that the patient has an electronic pacemaker in place. Most of the pacemakers used today are *demand pacemakers;* that is, they turn on when the patient's heart rate falls below a certain rate (usually about 60/min). Thus, a rhythm strip may show, as above, some normal sinus beats as well as beats originating from the electronic pacemaker.

Treatment: None. If the pacemaker is not "kicking in" when the patient's intrinsic heart rate falls below 60 to 70 per minute, or if the pacemaker is not sensing the patient's beats but rather is firing right after (or on top of) the normal QRS, the patient *must* be checked into the hospital for pacemaker malfunction.

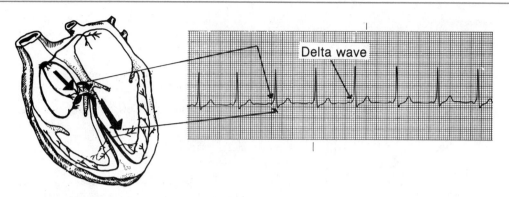

FIGURE 23-54.   WOLFF-PARKINSON-WHITE

Rhythm: Regular.

Rate: Can be normal, but often associated with rapid supraventricular tachycardias.

P waves: Normal.

Pacemaker site: SA node.

P–R interval: Less than 0.11 second. It is thought that the impulse travels through an accessory pathway, called the *bundle of Kent,* that bypasses the AV node—hence the normal delay at the AV node is not seen.

QRS complexes: Slurring of the upstroke of the QRS (*delta wave*) is diagnostic; QRS is longer than 0.11 second.

Clinical significance: May occur in young, otherwise healthy individuals (more commonly males); often diagnosed when an ECG is taken to investigate an episode of paroxysmal tachycardia. Rarely, Wolff-Parkinson-White is a sign of serious organic cardiac disease.

Treatment: None needed if the heart rate is normal. If the patient has a severe tachycardia that is producing clinical symptoms, treat for the specific dysrhythmia (e.g., vagal stimulation for PSVT, cardioversion for atrial fibrillation).

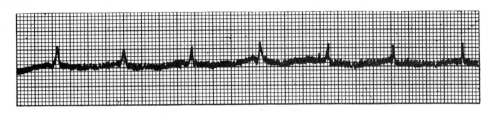

FIGURE 23-55. MUSCLE TREMOR.

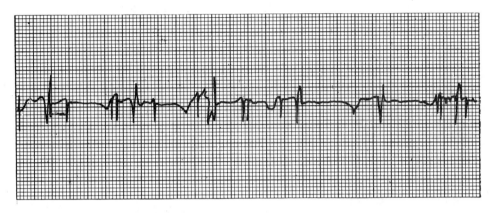

FIGURE 23-56. PATIENT CABLE MOVEMENT.

Improperly applied electrodes, loose or disconnected leads, inadequate electrode paste, oily skin, patient movement, muscle tremor, and a variety of other factors can produce artifacts in the ECG, some of which bear an alarming resemblance to life-threatening dysrhythmias. Thus, it is always necessary to correlate what is seen on the monitor with the patient's clinical status. A straight line on the monitored ECG of the patient who is conscious and alert should prompt a search for a disconnected lead, not initiation of CPR. Similarly, the ECG of a clinically stable patient that seems to show ventricular fibrillation may simply reflect muscle tremor, for which DC countershock is not a desirable treatment.

Two such tracings are illustrated here. Both are probably normal sinus rhythm.

Let us review for a few moments some of the concepts learned in the previous section.

Bedtime Stories: Tragic Tales of Dysrhythmias

CAST

SIDNEY SINUS: Sidney, the sinoatrial node, is boss of the heart. He ordinarily dispatches messengers 70 to 80 times a minute; those messengers are supposed to dash down the atria, slip through the AV junction, and depolarize the ventricles. Sidney is not terribly bright but is usually conscientious and reliable.

ALBERT AND ALICE ATRIA: Albert and Alice are the right and left atria, somewhat temperamental little pouches who normally contract in response to the messages sent by Sidney and squeeze their blood into the ventricles, providing the ventricles with an "atrial kick." Their contraction is represented on the ECG by the P wave.

AV ABE: Abe, the atrioventricular node, is a lower pacemaker who secretly yearns to be boss of the heart; but because of his lower intrinsic rate, he rarely gets the opportunity to run the show. Abe stands at the threshold of the ventricles and checks out every messenger sent by Sid Sinus. Normally Abe lets the messengers pass into the ventricles after a brief security check (P–R interval). However, as the node in charge of traffic control into the ventricles, Abe does regulate the flow of messengers and occasionally closes a few southbound lanes, especially when the traffic gets very heavy or when he's not feeling well.

VANCE AND VIRGINIA VENTRICLE: These are big, tough, muscular types, also not very bright, but charged with the enormous responsibility of pumping blood to the whole body. Normally, Vance and Virginia take their orders from the messengers sent by Sidney Sinus, but sometimes they grow irritable and contract without orders, especially when they run a little short on oxygen. They also tend to be impatient when they don't hear from Sidney on time, and under those circumstances, they will sometimes contract on their own.

MONTGOMERY, MIMI, MORTIMER, MILLICENT, ETC.: These are messengers, tiny electric impulses, earnest and dedicated; their job is to carry the orders for depolarization from Sidney's headquarters all the way to the ventricles.

First-Degree AV Block, or "The Little Messenger That Could"

One fine day, Sidney dispatched Mortimer Messenger with the usual order: "Depolarize the ventricles." Mortimer scampered down the atria without difficulty, but arrived at the AV node to find a huge pile of debris blocking the entrance to the ventricles. "Sorry," said Abe, "we're closed for repairs."

"But I *have* to get through," said Mortimer.

"Impossible," said Abe.

But Mortimer was brave and determined. "I think I can. I think I can. I KNOW I can," he said, gathering his few milliamps of strength. Finally, after a long struggle (prolonged P–R interval), Mortimer crashed through the AV junction into the ventricles and breathlessly issued the order to contract (Fig. 23-57). Thus, the ventricles were depolarized, and everyone lived happily ever after, until . . .

Type I (Wenckebach) Second-Degree AV Block

When Montgomery Messenger left for work that day, there was no sign there would be any trouble; he took his first set of orders from Sid Sinus, whistled down the atria, through the AV node, and smartly ordered the ventricles to depolarize. On the next trip down, however, he felt just a bit tired and slowed up slightly as he crossed the AV junction. "Why break my neck?" he thought. "So, the P–R interval will be a tiny bit prolonged. Who'll notice, anyway?" On his third trip, Montgomery encountered several roadblocks in the region of the AV junction and had to pick his way around them. Glancing at his watch as he reached the ventricles, he scowled. "Nuts," he said, "0.24 second. Boy, is Sidney going to be mad." Making his fourth trip from the SA node, Montgomery found the gates to the ventricles closed and locked. Frantically, he banged on the gates. "Come on, Abe, I know you're around somewhere. Let me through." To no avail. The gates remained shut. Defeated, Montgomery returned to the SA node, leaving a lonely P wave to chronicle his struggle (Fig. 23-58).

"What do you mean, you couldn't get through?" Sidney Sinus demanded.

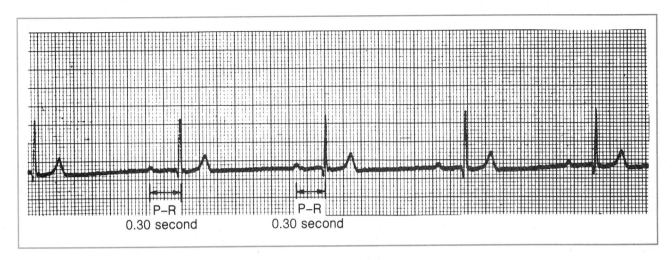

FIGURE 23-57. **FIRST-DEGREE AV BLOCK.** When there is trouble at the AV junction, it may take the messengers from the SA node longer to get through.

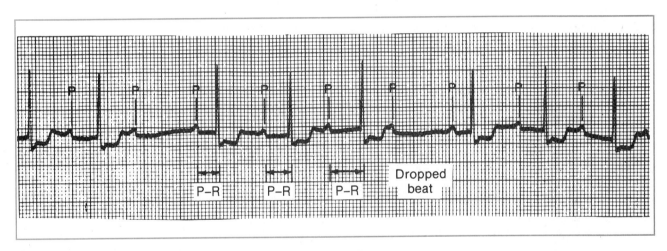

FIGURE 23-58. **TYPE I (WENCKEBACH) SECOND-DEGREE AV BLOCK.** Each transit through the AV junction is a bit slower, until finally the messenger cannot get through at all, and a beat is dropped.

"I couldn't get through," Montgomery said. "I'm telling you the gates were locked tight."

"OK," said Sid, "off to the showers. You've had it for the day." So Sidney called Mimi Messenger. "Now look," he told her, "I want you to go straight down to the ventricles and give them this message, and no fooling around at the AV junction, understand?"

"Oh, yes sir," said Mimi, always eager to please.

So off Mimi went, sailing down the atria, through the AV junction, and into the ventricles. "Hmm, 0.14 second," she noted to herself. "Sid can't complain about that." On her second run, however, she tripped over a shoelace and barely made it in under

0.2 second, and on the third trip some highway construction held her up for 0.24 second. But the fourth trip south was the worst, for she arrived at the AV junction to find that once again Abe had locked the gates. Mimi banged and banged on the gates. "Come on, Abe, open up. I'm going to lose my job." No response. Crestfallen, Mimi returned to the SA node.

"And what happened to you?" Sid demanded.

"I couldn't get through to the ventricles this time."

"Couldn't get through? Did you get lost, maybe?"

"But at least I made a nice P wave," Mimi ventured.

"A nice P wave! A nice P WAVE, she says. What good's a P wave without a QRS complex? Do you think the atria are going to supply blood to the whole body? They're strictly small time, sweetheart. The big guns are in the ventricles. That's why I sent you to depolarize them. Now you get to the showers."

And so it went. Messenger after messenger faltered at the AV junction, but the worst was yet to come.

Type II Second-Degree AV Block

It just wasn't Montgomery's week. Reporting for work the next day, he received the usual order from Sidney to depolarize the ventricles. Montgomery set out full of confidence and vigor, traversing the atria without difficulty. But when he arrived at the threshold of the ventricles, he found his path blocked by AV Abe.

"Let me through," Montgomery said. "I have an important message for the ventricles."

"Get lost," said Abe, who was feeling rather dyspeptic that day.

"But I have to get through. I've already used up 0.19 second."

"Beat it, sonny. I'm the boss around here."

Montgomery returned to Sidney Sinus disgraced. "What happened to you?" Sidney wanted to know. "You were supposed to order the ventricles to contract."

"I couldn't get past Abe," Montgomery replied.

"What do you mean, you couldn't get past Abe? I just sent your friend, Mimi Messenger down there, and she got through without any problem."

"But he wouldn't let me pass," whimpered Montgomery.

"I don't want to hear any excuses. You just go right back down there and deliver your message to the ventricles. I can't tolerate weaklings on my staff."

So Montgomery squared his shoulders, sailed down the atria again, and arrived once more at the gate of the ventricles.

"Are you here again?" said Abe. "I thought I told you to beat it."

"Please," said Montgomery, "I have to get through. You don't know what Sid is like when he gets upset."

"Sorry, sonny, I'm closed for lunch."

Montgomery returned to Sidney Sinus. "I couldn't make it," he said.

"Look, Montgomery," said Sidney, "Millicent Messenger just breezed by Abe right after you left. Now you march back down there and do your job."

"Yes, sir," said Montgomery.

Arriving again at the threshold of the ventricles, Montgomery once more found Abe blocking his path.

"Listen, Abe, I'm not kidding this time. If you don't let me through, I'm going to use some atropine and blast the gate open."

"Those are big words, sonny," said Abe, "but I'm not scared of a little atropine."

"The last time they used atropine, you were zonked for hours," Montgomery reminded him.

"I'll take my chances."

And so it went. Each time Montgomery reached the gate to the ventricle, AV Abe barred his path. Yet the messenger coming right after Montgomery kept getting through (2 : 1 block; Fig. 23-59).

"Montgomery," cautioned Sidney, "if this keeps up, they're going to put in a pacemaker, and we'll all be out of a job. Shape up."

But the worst was yet to come.

FIGURE 23-59. TYPE II SECOND-DEGREE AV BLOCK. Every second impulse from the SA node is blocked at the AV junction.

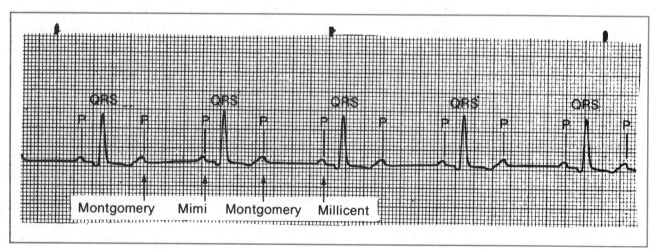

Complete Heart Block (Third-Degree AV Block)

The next day was even worse for Sidney's operation. It was bad enough, Montgomery not getting through. "Every second P wave not followed by a QRS," wailed Sidney. "My reputation is being ruined!" But then, suddenly, the situation became even worse. Sidney had just sent Mildred Messenger down to the ventricles, and she arrived at the AV junction to find the gate shut and bolted. A sign tacked to the gate read: "Closed until further notice."

"That's impossible," said Sidney when he heard the story. "Abe can't do that to me." So he sent another messenger, Marvin, to depolarize the ventricles. Marvin charged down the atria and ran smack into the closed gate. He banged and shouted, but there was no response.

"Impossible," said Sidney. "Abe must be sleeping." So he dispatched Melvin Messenger. Again the door was bolted tight.

"Oh, what I'd give for a bolus of atropine," sighed Sidney.

Meanwhile, the ventricles were starting to get nervous, and Vance, the right ventricle, said to Virginia, the left ventricle, "Have you heard anything from the atria lately?"

"Not a thing."

"Funny. Those messengers are usually pretty prompt."

"Must have run into some problems with Abe."

"Yeah. Every time that guy has a little too much digitalis, he gets delusions of grandeur and starts hassling the messengers."

"How long do you suppose we ought to wait?"

"I don't know. It's already been more than a second, and the brain is starting to complain about not getting enough oxygen."

"The brain is always complaining about something."

"Yeah, but the kidneys don't sound very happy either."

"OK, OK. Let's go ahead and contract. I hate to do it without authorization from above, though. The last time we decided to go ahead and fire on our own, some of that disgusting lidocaine came barrelling down the pipes. I was sick for a week."

So Vance and Virginia set off on their own, slowly (about 30 times a minute) so as not to attract much attention, little appreciating that back in the atria Sidney was frantically sending messenger after messenger, all in vain, to assault the closed gate (Fig. 23-60).

"What's happened to Sidney?" Virginia said to Vance, as they plodded along slowly.

"I wish I knew," said Vance.

Practice Session

Before moving on to the next subject, let's pause and practice some of the principles of ECG interpretation presented in the preceding sections. The following pages contain nine 6-second ECG strips (Fig. 23-61 through Fig. 23-69). Analyze each strip SYSTEMATICALLY, according to the questions listed under each. Then check your answers against those given at the end of the practice session. (Additional ECG exercises may be found in the *Study Guide for Emergency Care in the Streets, Fifth Edition*.)

FIGURE 23-60. THIRD-DEGREE AV BLOCK. The atria and the ventricles are marching to the beat of different drummers.

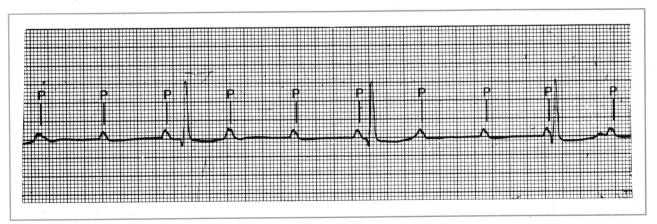

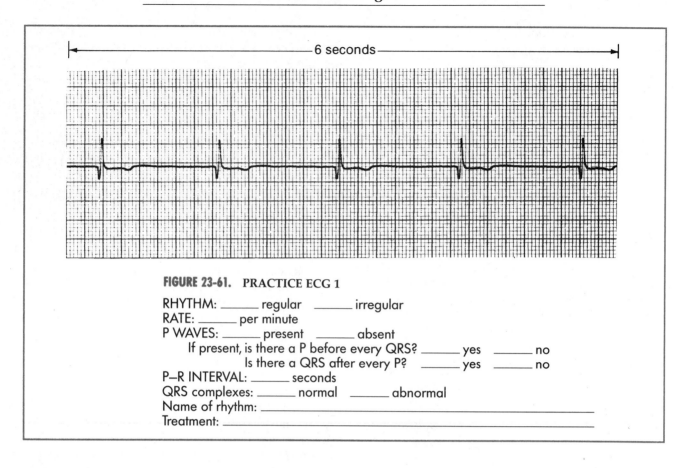

FIGURE 23-61. PRACTICE ECG 1

RHYTHM: _____ regular   _____ irregular
RATE: _____ per minute
P WAVES: _____ present   _____ absent
   If present, is there a P before every QRS? _____ yes   _____ no
      Is there a QRS after every P?   _____ yes   _____ no
P–R INTERVAL: _____ seconds
QRS complexes: _____ normal   _____ abnormal
Name of rhythm: _____
Treatment: _____

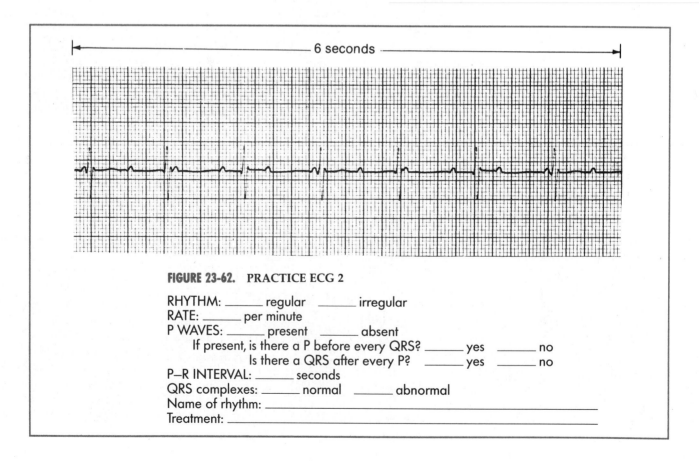

FIGURE 23-62. PRACTICE ECG 2

RHYTHM: _____ regular   _____ irregular
RATE: _____ per minute
P WAVES: _____ present   _____ absent
   If present, is there a P before every QRS? _____ yes   _____ no
      Is there a QRS after every P?   _____ yes   _____ no
P–R INTERVAL: _____ seconds
QRS complexes: _____ normal   _____ abnormal
Name of rhythm: _____
Treatment: _____

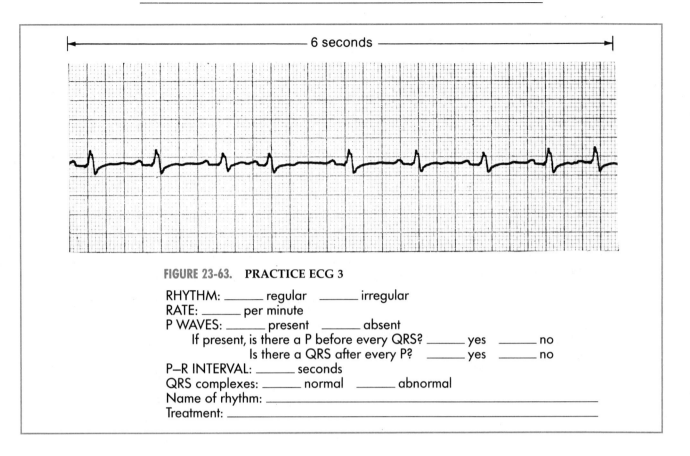

6 seconds

FIGURE 23-63. **PRACTICE ECG 3**

RHYTHM: _____ regular _____ irregular
RATE: _____ per minute
P WAVES: _____ present _____ absent
    If present, is there a P before every QRS? _____ yes _____ no
            Is there a QRS after every P? _____ yes _____ no
P–R INTERVAL: _____ seconds
QRS complexes: _____ normal _____ abnormal
Name of rhythm: _____
Treatment: _____

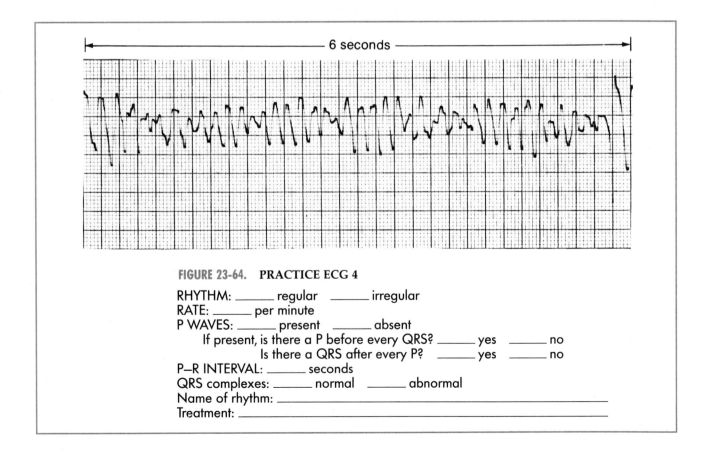

6 seconds

FIGURE 23-64. **PRACTICE ECG 4**

RHYTHM: _____ regular _____ irregular
RATE: _____ per minute
P WAVES: _____ present _____ absent
    If present, is there a P before every QRS? _____ yes _____ no
            Is there a QRS after every P? _____ yes _____ no
P–R INTERVAL: _____ seconds
QRS complexes: _____ normal _____ abnormal
Name of rhythm: _____
Treatment: _____

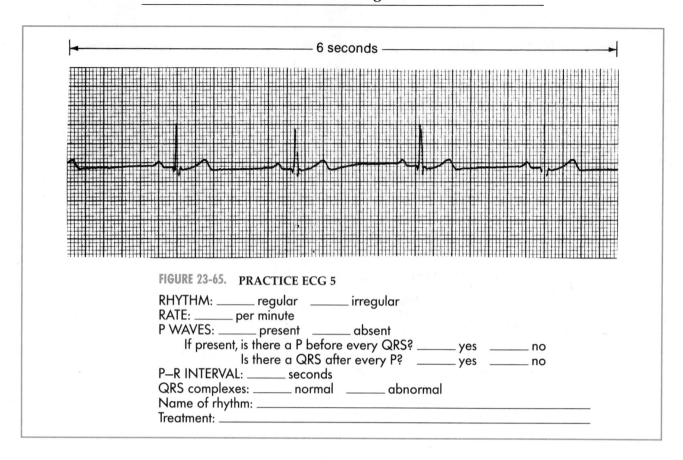

FIGURE 23-65. **PRACTICE ECG 5**

RHYTHM: _____ regular   _____ irregular
RATE: _____ per minute
P WAVES: _____ present   _____ absent
    If present, is there a P before every QRS? _____ yes _____ no
        Is there a QRS after every P? _____ yes _____ no
P–R INTERVAL: _____ seconds
QRS complexes: _____ normal   _____ abnormal
Name of rhythm: _____
Treatment: _____

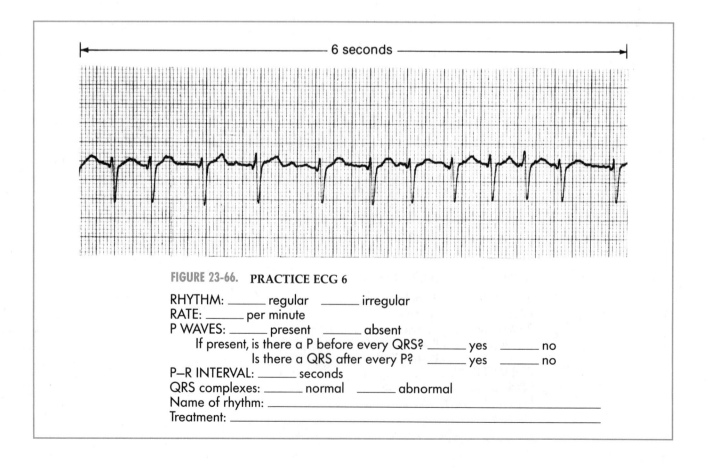

FIGURE 23-66. **PRACTICE ECG 6**

RHYTHM: _____ regular   _____ irregular
RATE: _____ per minute
P WAVES: _____ present   _____ absent
    If present, is there a P before every QRS? _____ yes _____ no
        Is there a QRS after every P? _____ yes _____ no
P–R INTERVAL: _____ seconds
QRS complexes: _____ normal   _____ abnormal
Name of rhythm: _____
Treatment: _____

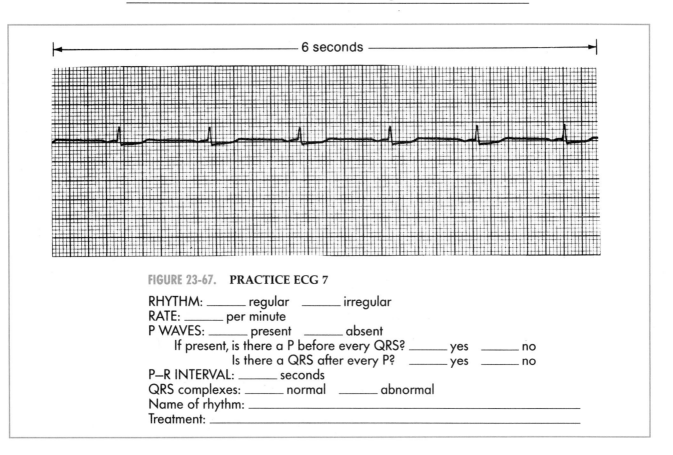

FIGURE 23-67. **PRACTICE ECG 7**

RHYTHM: _____ regular _____ irregular
RATE: _____ per minute
P WAVES: _____ present _____ absent
    If present, is there a P before every QRS? _____ yes _____ no
        Is there a QRS after every P? _____ yes _____ no
P–R INTERVAL: _____ seconds
QRS complexes: _____ normal _____ abnormal
Name of rhythm: _____
Treatment: _____

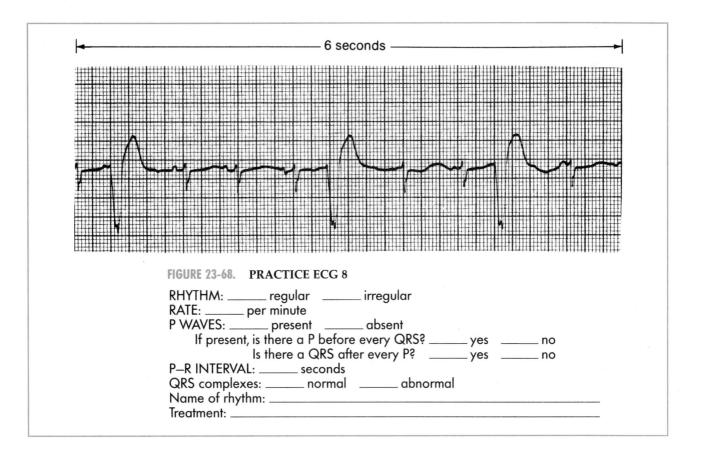

FIGURE 23-68. **PRACTICE ECG 8**

RHYTHM: _____ regular _____ irregular
RATE: _____ per minute
P WAVES: _____ present _____ absent
    If present, is there a P before every QRS? _____ yes _____ no
        Is there a QRS after every P? _____ yes _____ no
P–R INTERVAL: _____ seconds
QRS complexes: _____ normal _____ abnormal
Name of rhythm: _____
Treatment: _____

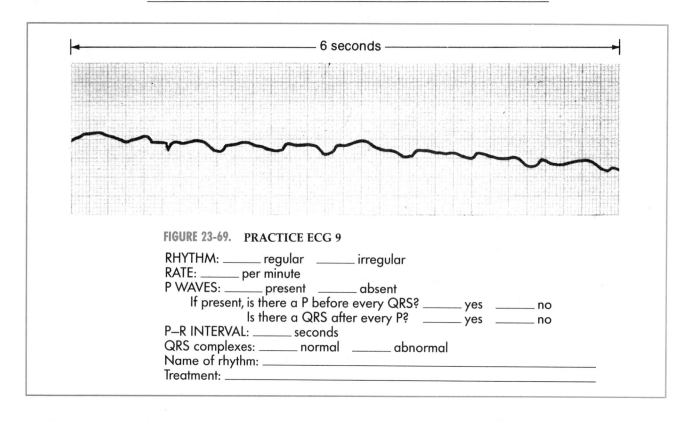

— 6 seconds —

FIGURE 23-69.   PRACTICE ECG 9

RHYTHM: _____ regular   _____ irregular
RATE: _____ per minute
P WAVES: _____ present   _____ absent
        If present, is there a P before every QRS? _____ yes _____ no
                    Is there a QRS after every P?   _____ yes _____ no
P–R INTERVAL: _____ seconds
QRS complexes: _____ normal   _____ abnormal
Name of rhythm: _____
Treatment: _____

Answers to Practice ECGs

Practice ECG 1

Rhythm: Regular.
Rate: 50 per minute (46/min using box-counting method).
P waves: Absent.
P–R interval: None.
QRS complexes: Normal.
Name of rhythm: **Junctional bradycardia.**
Treatment: If accompanied by signs of poor perfusion, give atropine, 0.5 mg IV.

Practice ECG 2

Rhythm: Regular.
Rate: 70 per minute.
P waves: Present, but without any consistent relation to the QRS complexes.
P–R interval: Not relevant.
QRS complexes: Normal.
Name of rhythm: **Third-degree AV block** (complete AV dissociation).
Treatment: None needed at this heart rate.

Practice ECG 3

Rhythm: Basic rhythm is regular, with two premature beats.

Rate: 90 per minute.
P waves: Present. There is QRS after every P; however, the last QRS complex is not *preceded* by a P wave.
P–R interval: 0.18 second.
QRS complexes: 0.12 second (upper limits of normal).
Name of rhythm: **Sinus, with PACs.**
Treatment: None.

Practice ECG 4

Rhythm: Chaotic.
Rate: Cannot be measured.
P waves: Not seen.
P–R interval: None.
QRS complexes: None; fibrillatory waves instead.
Name of rhythm: **Ventricular fibrillation** (VF).
Treatment: CPR and countershock.

Practice ECG 5

Rhythm: Regular.
Rate: 40 per minute (45/min by box-counting method).
P waves: Present before every QRS; QRS occurs after every P.
P–R interval: 0.2 second.
QRS complexes: Normal.

Name of rhythm: **Sinus bradycardia**

Treatment: None if the patient is asymptomatic; if there are signs of poor perfusion, give atropine, 0.5 mg IV, or a dopamine infusion.

Practice ECG 6

Rhythm: Irregularly irregular.
Rate: 120 per minute.
P waves: Absent.
P–R interval: None.
QRS complexes: Normal.
Name of rhythm: **Atrial fibrillation.**
Treatment: None necessary in the field at this heart rate.

Practice ECG 7

Rhythm: Regular.
Rate: 60 per minute.
P waves: Present (inverted).
P–R interval: 0.16 second.
QRS complexes: Normal.
Name of rhythm: Could be normal sinus if taken in lead aVR; in a standard monitoring lead (e.g., lead II), the inverted P wave is likely to signal an **atrial rhythm.**
Treatment: None.

Practice ECG 8

Rhythm: Irregular.
Rate: 90 per minute.
P waves: Present; there is a QRS after every P wave, *but* not every QRS complex is *preceded* by a P wave.
P–R interval: 0.12 second.
QRS complexes: There are three bizarre complexes and six normal complexes.
Name of rhythm: **Sinus rhythm with PVCs** (in this case, trigeminy, since there is a PVC occurring every third beat).
Treatment: Lidocaine, 75 to 100 mg IV bolus, followed by an infusion of 2 to 3 mg per minute.

Practice ECG 9

Rhythm: None.
Rate: None.
P waves: None.
P–R interval: None.
QRS complexes: None.
Name of rhythm: **Asystole** or **agonal rhythm.**
Treatment: CPR.

HOW TO INTERPRET 12-LEAD ECGs

Up to now, we have considered ECG rhythm strips obtained from monitoring a single lead. For purposes of rhythm interpretation, a single lead (usually lead II) is usually sufficient. But to localize the site of ischemia or injury to heart muscle, we need to be able to look at the heart from several different angles. That is precisely the purpose of a 12-lead ECG.

What Does a 12-Lead ECG Do?

Suppose you wanted to check out the condition of a used car you were thinking of buying. If all you needed to know was whether the motor was running, you could stand anywhere near the car and listen (just as you can use any one lead to monitor the cardiac rhythm). But if, on the other hand, you want to know what kind of shape the car body is in, you have to walk around the car and look at it from all sides. The driver's side may be in mint condition, but if you stroll around to the passenger's side, you may see that the whole door frame is staved in from a road accident. Similarly, each ECG lead looks at the heart from a different angle, and while one lead may see a normal myocardium, another may be looking at major damage.

The word *lead*, as it is used in electrocardiography, can be somewhat confusing. Sometimes the word is used to refer to one of the cables and monitoring electrodes that connect the ECG machine to the patient (e.g., the "right arm lead"). But more accurately, a **lead** is an electrical picture of the heart taken from a specified vantage point. Lead I, for instance, "looks" at the heart from the left, so it "sees" the left side of the heart. Lead aVF looks up at the heart from the feet (*F* stands for "foot"), so it "sees" the bottom of the heart. In the standard electrocardiogram, we record 12 leads, that is, 12 different pictures of the electrical activity of the heart.

Six of the leads—leads **I, II, III, aVR, aVL,** and **aVF**—are called **limb leads** because the pictures taken by those leads are derived from attaching cables to the patient's limbs. The limb leads look at the heart from the sides and from the feet, in the *vertical plane.* Figure 23-70 shows the viewpoint of each of the limb leads. So we can see, for example, that lead II has a direct view of the bottom of the heart (the *inferior* or diaphragmatic wall of the heart), while aVL (*L* stands for "left") is looking at the heart from the vantage point of the left shoulder. (Question: In which lead or leads do you think you'd be most likely to see indications of injury to the inferior wall of the heart?)

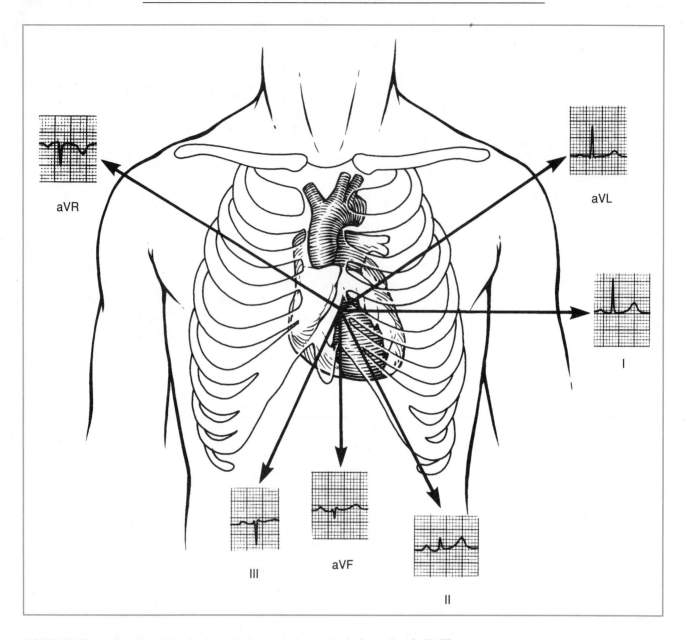

FIGURE 23-70. **LIMB LEADS** look at the heart in the vertical plane. Leads II, III, and aVF give us a picture of the wall of the heart that rests on the diaphragm, the *inferior* wall.

In addition to the limb leads, there are six **precordial leads** (**V₁ to V₆**), also called chest leads or V leads. The six precordial leads are placed on the anterior and lateral chest wall, usually with suction cups, in the positions shown in Figure 23-71. The chest leads look at the heart in the *horizontal plane,* as shown in the inset, so they provide a picture of the heart taken from the front (*anterior* wall of the heart) and from the left side (*anterolateral*). More specifically, leads V₁ and V₂ usually look at the *right ventricle*; V₃ and V₄ look at the intraventricular *septum,* as well

as the *anterior wall* of the left ventricle; and V₅ and V₆ look at the *anterior and lateral walls* of the left ventricle.

What Do ECG Leads Record?

What does a lead "see" when it looks at the heart? What the lead is looking at is the depolarizing or repolarizing current moving through the heart, from the inside of the heart to the outside of the heart.

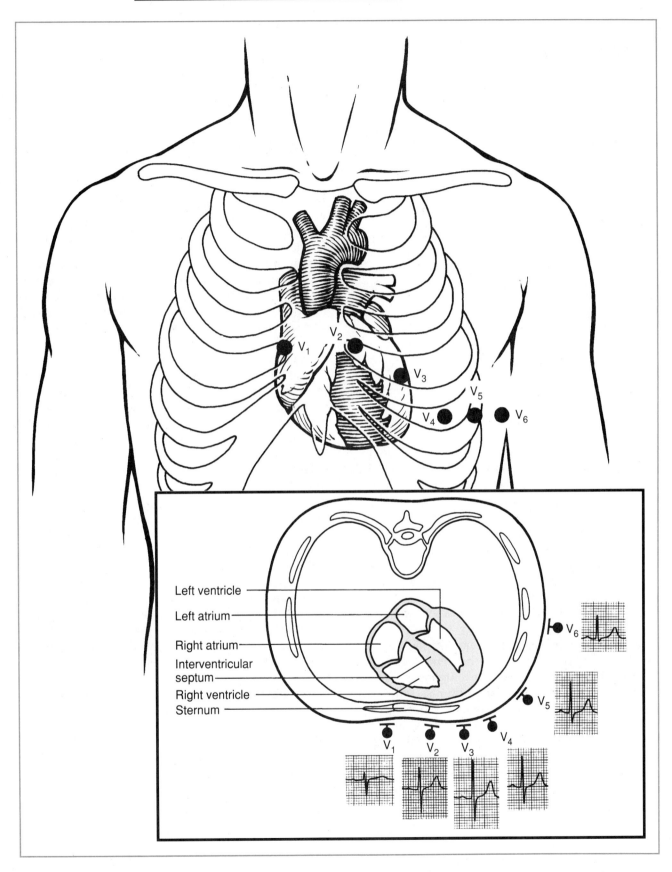

FIGURE 23-71. **PRECORDIAL LEADS** (chest leads) look at the heart in the horizontal plane. Inset: V_1 and V_2 look at the right ventricle. V_3 and V_4 "see" the interventricular septum. V_5 and V_6 see the anterior and lateral left ventricle.

WHAT THE LEADS ARE LOOKING AT	
Leads	*What They Are Looking at*
I and aVL	The left side of the heart in the vertical plane
II, III, and aVF	The inferior (diaphragmatic) wall of the heart
aVR	The right side of the heart in the vertical plane
V_1 and V_2	The right ventricle
V_3 and V_4	The intraventricular septum and anterior wall of the left ventricle
V_5 and V_6	The anterior and lateral walls of the left ventricle

When a current is moving *toward* a lead, it creates a *positive* (upright) deflection on the ECG tracing of that lead. Thus in Figure 23-72, the current depolarizing the ventricles is moving *toward* lead II, so what we see in lead II is an *upright* QRS complex (recall that the QRS complex is produced by depolarization of the ventricles). If the depolarizing current is moving toward lead II, then it must be moving *away* from lead aVR; so we would expect to see a *negative* deflection in aVR. And, indeed, the QRS complex in aVR is a *downward* deflection. That makes intuitive sense. If you and I are standing facing one another at opposite ends of a football field, a ball thrown *toward* me is going to look bigger and bigger to me as it approaches; the same ball will meanwhile look smaller and smaller to you as it travels the same course. Just so, leads II and aVR, being nearly opposite one another, will have nearly opposite pictures of the same wave of electrical depolarization. If a depolarizing wave is coming *toward* lead II, it will be going *away* from aVR. By reviewing the pictures received from each vantage point (each lead), we can determine the average direction in which the wave of depolarization spreads through the ventricle. We call that average direction the **cardiac axis,** and it is normally somewhere between −30 and +110 degrees. (In Fig. 23-72, for instance, the axis is around +3 degrees). Various conditions can shift the axis of a person's heart. For example, a person with long-standing hypertension may develop a very large left ventricle because the left ventricle has been working unusually hard to

pump out blood against the high resistance of constricted arteries. When the left ventricle enlarges (hypertrophies), the axis tends to swing to the left. An axis to the left of −30 degrees is called, logically enough, *left axis deviation.*

The 12-Lead ECG in a Damaged Heart

In addition to looking at the axis, we can also learn a great deal about the state of the heart by examining the shape of the P waves and QRS complexes in different leads. In the prehospital setting, however, we are not really interested in subtle indications of chronic processes. Generally we need to know only one thing in the field: Is there any ECG evidence that this patient is having an acute myocardial infarction? To answer *that* question, we must turn our attention to three particular parts of the ECG: the S–T segment, the Q wave, and the T wave.

Recall first the sequence of events in an acute myocardial infarction. As the blood supply to the affected area of heart muscle slows to a trickle, the muscle no longer receives sufficient oxygen; that is, the heart muscle becomes *ischemic* (deprived of blood). If ischemia persists more than a few minutes, it leads to actual *injury* to the heart muscle, which in turn will be followed by *infarction* (death of muscle) if the circulation to the area is not rapidly restored.

The ECG can give us a graphic record of that sequence of events. With the first decrease in blood supply through a coronary artery, the leads overlying the affected myocardium will reflect changes typical of myocardial **ischemia: T wave inversion** and often **depression of the S–T segment** below the isoelectric line. In Figure 23-73, for example, we see changes of ischemia most prominently in leads V_2 through V_5, where the T wave is inverted and the S–T segment is as much as 3 mm below the isoelectric line. (Question: What part of the heart is ischemic? That is, what part of the heart are leads V_2 through V_5 looking at?) Those S–T changes occur because the muscle, deprived of oxygen and nutrients, lacks energy for repolarization; thus there is a delay in the repolarization process.

As myocardial ischemia progresses to **injury,** the affected portion of the heart muscle can no longer depolarize completely; so at the end of depolarization, it is still more positively charged than normal muscle. That is reflected, in the ECG leads that look at the injured segment, in **S–T elevation.** In Figure 23-74, the anteroseptal leads show 2 to 3 mm of S–T elevation, typical of acute myocardial injury. (Question: Which leads are anteroseptal?)

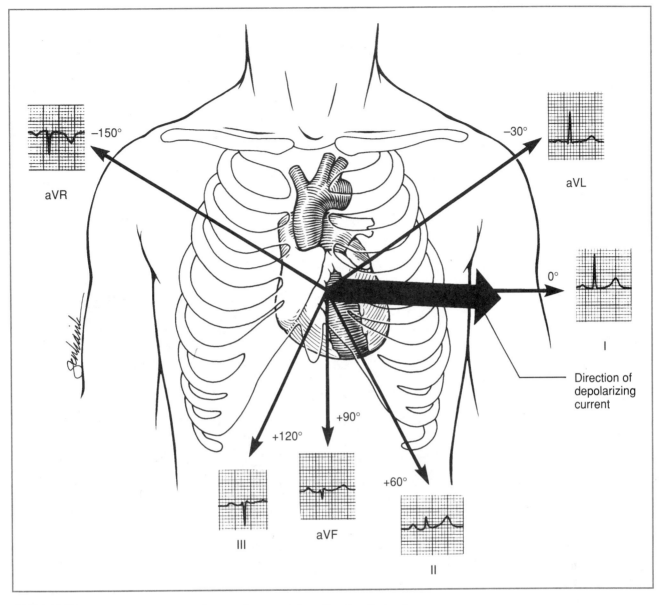

FIGURE 23-72. CARDIAC AXIS. The net direction of cardiac depolarization can be determined by looking to see which limb lead has the highest R wave.

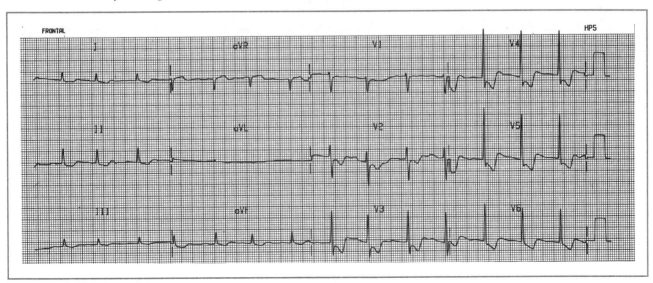

FIGURE 23-73. ISCHEMIA. S–T *depression* and *T wave inversion* in leads V_2 through V_5 indicate ischemia in the anterolateral wall of the left ventricle.

Finally comes the stage of tissue death, or **infarction.** No more will any waves of depolarization spread across the segment of muscle that is dead, for the dead are silent. Thus the infarcted area of muscle becomes electrically silent. So a lead that is looking at an infarcted wall of the heart will not see any wave of depolarization approaching across that wall. Instead, it will now be able to look straight through the infarcted wall to the opposite, healthy wall of the heart. And what the lead will see is the depolarizing

wave from that other wall travelling *away.* As we learned earlier, when an electric current (i.e., the wave of depolarization) moves *away* from a lead, what we see on the ECG tracing of that lead is a negative deflection. If the electric current in question represents the depolarization of the ventricles, that means what we will see is an initial **Q wave** in the QRS complex. Figure 23-75 shows Q waves in both the inferior (II, III, and aVF) and lateral (V_5 and V_6) leads. Small Q waves may occur normally in lead III

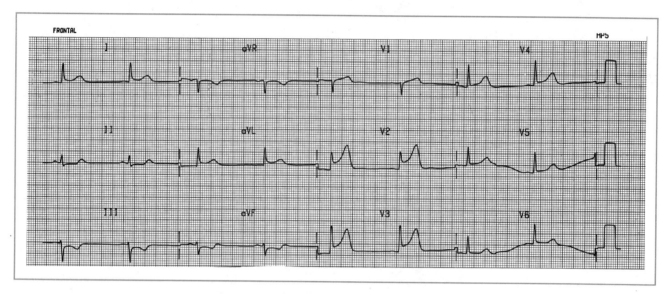

FIGURE 23-74.   **INJURY.**   S–T *elevation* in leads V_2 and V_3 signifies injury in the area of the interventricular septum. (What significance do the changes in leads II, III, and aVF have?)

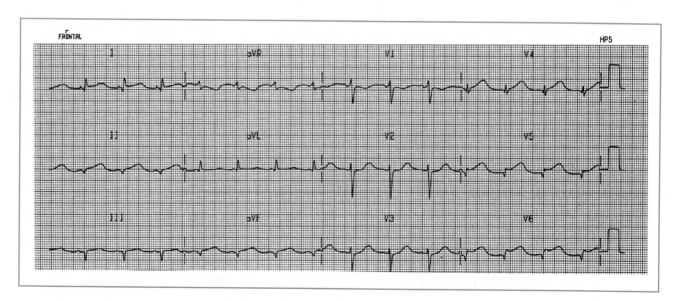

FIGURE 23-75.   **INFARCTION.**   Wide, deep Q *waves* in the inferior leads (II, III, and aVF) and in the lateral leads (V_5 and V_6) signify an inferolateral myocardial infarction.

and over the ventricular septum. But a Q wave wider than 0.04 second (one small box), deeper than 2 mm (two small boxes), or seen in more than two leads is likely to represent infarction.

If the infarcted portion of the heart can no longer undergo depolarization, it will not be repolarized either. So at some point one would also expect to see changes in the *T waves* after an AMI, since the T wave chronicles the repolarization of the ventricles. And indeed, within hours to days of the acute infarct, the T waves in the leads that look at the affected muscle flip upside down. So yet another ECG sign of myocardial ischemia or infarction is **T wave inversion.** The ECG changes of ischemia, injury, and infarction are summarized in Table 23-10.

The changes we have described—T wave inversion in ischemia, S–T elevation in injury, and Q waves with or without T wave inversion in infarct—are seen in the leads that "look at" the injured segment of myocardium. So if, for example, there is injury to the *inferior* wall of the heart, the wall that rests on the diaphragm, we would expect to see S–T elevation in the leads that look at the inferior wall, that is, leads II, III, and aVF, just as is shown in Figure 23-76.

There is another point of interest in Figure 23-76. Look at the S–T segment in leads aVR and aVL, the leads whose vantage point is opposite to that of leads II, III, and aVF. In leads aVR and aVL, the S–T segments are *depressed.* We call the changes in leads aVR and aVL **reciprocal changes.** Thus S–T segment elevation in one lead will be recorded by the opposite lead as S–T segment depression. Similarly, a Q wave (downward deflection) in one lead will be recorded as an R wave (upward deflection) by the opposite lead. That is because opposite leads, such as leads II and aVR, are looking at the electrical events from opposite vantage points. (Review Fig. 23-75. There is a Q wave in lead II, the lead that looks up at the heart from the bottom left. What would you expect to see in lead aVR, which is looking down at the heart from the direction of the right shoulder? Now examine aVR in the figure and see if you were correct.)

In Figure 23-77, on the other hand, we see injury

(S–T elevation) in the leads that look at the *anterior* wall of the heart, leads V₃ through V₅; while Figure 23-78 shows us signs of ischemia (T wave inversion) in the leads that look at the *anterolateral wall* of the heart, leads V₄ through V₆.

What we really need to know in the prehospital phase of care is simply the following: Does this patient have ECG evidence of ischemia, injury, or infarction? The answer to that question will help the receiving hospital to decide whether to mobilize their thrombolytic therapy team. Meanwhile, having taken the ECG, we have also obtained some information that can help *us* choose the most appropriate emergency management in the field. It is best, for example, *not* to give morphine to patients with *inferior* wall AMI, for morphine is more likely in those patients to cause undesirable side effects (vomiting, bradycardia). If we know which leads to check for signs of injury to the inferior wall of the heart, we will be able to identify patients who should have some other form of analgesia (such as nitrous oxide). The leads corresponding to different locations of myocardial injury are summarized in Table 23-11.

A Word of Caution

Studies have shown that performing a 12-lead ECG may add up to half an hour to the prehospital phase of patient care. There is only one reason for spending

TABLE 23-11.   LOCALIZATION OF AMI

SITE OF INFARCTION	PRIMARY ECG CHANGES SEEN IN:
Inferior (diaphragmatic) wall	Leads II, III, aVF
Anteroseptal	Leads V₁–V₃
Anterolateral	Leads V₄–V₆
Extensive anterior wall	Leads V₁–V₆, I, aVL
Posterior wall	Tall R waves in leads V₁–V₂ (reciprocal changes)

TABLE 23-10.   EVOLUTION OF AMI ON ECG

STAGE	ECG CHANGES IN OVERLYING LEADS*	TIMING
Ischemia	T wave inversion S–T depression	With the onset of ischemia
Injury	S–T elevation	Minutes to hours
Infarction	Q waves appear	Within several hours to several days

*Reciprocal changes will be seen in opposite leads.

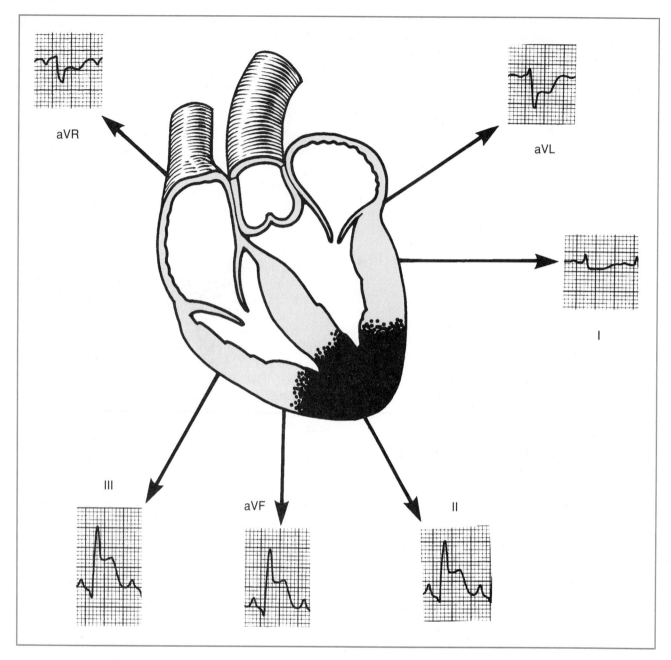

FIGURE 23-76.   INFERIOR WALL INJURY.   Note reciprocal changes in aVR and aVL.

the time to take a 12-lead ECG in the field, and that is to provide the receiving hospital with the information they need to mobilize (or not mobilize) their thrombolytic therapy team. Early notification from the field can save precious minutes and even hours once the patient reaches the emergency department; and in an AMI, as we have learned, "time is myocardium." Conversely, however, there is *no* justification for obtaining a 12-lead ECG on a patient who would not in any case be a candidate for thrombolytic therapy, for instance a patient with severe hypertension or one taking anticoagulant drugs. The decision to

perform an ECG should, therefore, be guided by a checklist of inclusion and exclusion criteria, such as that in Table 23-4.

It should be emphasized that the findings on the 12-lead ECG are *not* intended to determine whether the patient should be treated in the field for an acute myocardial infarction. That decision is made on clinical grounds alone! It may take hours for changes to appear in the ECG. Indeed, the patient may not live long enough to develop ECG changes if he does not receive appropriate treatment as soon as possible after the onset of his symptoms.

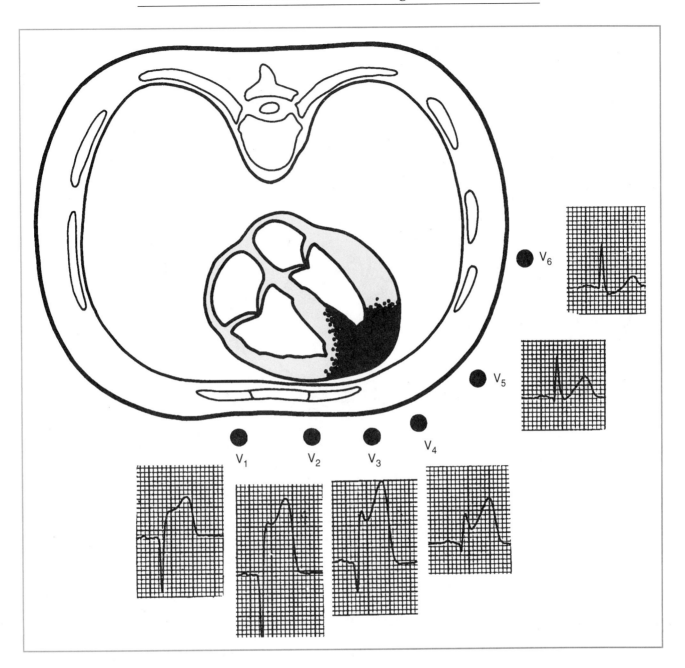

FIGURE 23-77. **ANTERIOR WALL INJURY.** (Question: What would *ischemia* in the anterior wall look like?)

EVERY PATIENT WITH A STORY OF HEAVY, CRUSHING, SQUEEZING, OR CHOKING CHEST PAIN MUST BE TREATED FOR AMI EVEN IF HIS ECG IS PERFECTLY NORMAL.

Paramedics who are authorized to perform 12-lead ECGs in the field should be equipped with por-table ECG machines that provide computerized ECG interpretation. Even if you are a whiz at reading 12-lead ECGs, computer ECG interpretations provide consistency and a high degree of accuracy. (They also provide on-the-job refresher training in ECG inter-pretation!) As soon as you have the ECG printout, contact the receiving hospital and read the computer ECG interpretation to the emergency physician there. If you have something to add to what the computer says, by all means do so (briefly!). And, of course, provide details of the patient's history and the find-ings on physical examination.

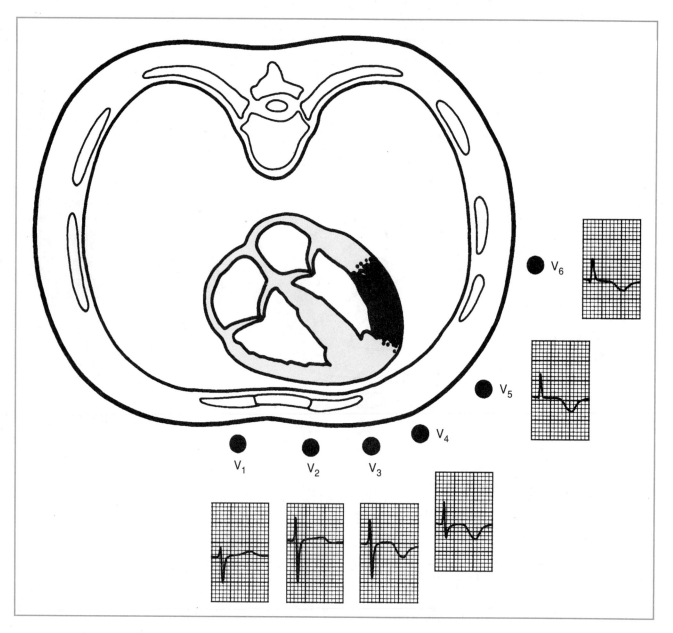

FIGURE 23-78.   ANTEROLATERAL WALL ISCHEMIA.

Taking a 12-Lead ECG: Guidelines

The only way to learn how to take a 12-lead ECG is to practice with the equipment itself. Here we can only present some guidelines to help ensure that the ECGs you obtain are of the highest quality possible.

- The patient should be *supine*. If he feels short of breath in that position, you may elevate the back of the stretcher about 30 degrees.
- Make sure the patient does not become chilled, because shivering will produce artifacts in the ECG tracing.
- Prepare the patient's skin as you would for placing monitoring electrodes (see p. 528).

- Connect the four limb electrodes. Double-check that the correct electrode is on each limb (the "LA" electrode on the left arm, the "RA" electrode on the right arm, etc.).
- Connect the six chest leads:

Lead	Placement
V$_1$	Fourth intercostal space at right sternal border
V$_2$	Fourth intercostal space at left sternal border
V$_3$	Equidistant between V$_2$ and V$_4$
V$_4$	Fifth intercostal space in left mid-clavicular line

V_5 Anterior axillary line (same horizontal plane as V_4)

V_6 Midaxillary line (same horizontal plane as V_4)

• Record the ECG.

MANAGEMENT OF CARDIAC ARREST

Nothing gets the adrenaline pumping more furiously—in the paramedic even if not in the patient—than a "code," a cardiopulmonary arrest. Management of cardiac arrest requires the paramedic to deploy a great many of the advanced life support skills that he or she has learned and to do so under very stressful circumstances, where minutes may make the difference between life and death. It is very difficult to think clearly in stressful circumstances, especially when there are likely to be other stressed and panicky people at the scene (the patient's family, for example). Therefore it is absolutely essential for paramedics to have *an orderly, systematic approach* to cardiac arrest emergencies. That approach needs to be rehearsed over and over again, in a team setting, until it is nearly automatic and must include the steps of both basic and advanced life support.

Basic Life Support: Review

The techniques and sequences of basic life support were covered in detail in Chapters 6 through 9, and by now any reader of this text should be able to rattle off the ABCs in his or her sleep. (If you cannot do so, meditate for a while on Fig. 23-79.) For our purposes in this section, we shall simply review the guidelines for ensuring maximally effective (and minimally damaging) CPR:

GUIDELINES FOR EFFECTIVE CPR

• Pay attention to the AIRWAY, to keep it fully open.
• AVOID EXCESSIVE INFLATION PRESSURES in artificial ventilation. Inflate just enough to make the chest rise.
• Maintain PROPER HAND POSITION:
  1. Fingers *off* the chest.
  2. Hands resting *lightly* on the sternum between compressions.
• Keep your compressions SMOOTH, REGULAR, AND UNINTERRUPTED.

---

1. Maintain each compression for at least half the compression-release cycle.
2. Avoid bouncing or jerky compressions.
• Keep your SHOULDERS DIRECTLY OVER THE victim's STERNUM, and keep your ELBOWS STRAIGHT.
• For adults, give 15 COMPRESSIONS to 2 VENTILATIONS at a rate of 80 to 100 per minute.
• DO NOT INTERRUPT CPR FOR MORE THAN 7 SECONDS AT A TIME except for
  1. Endotracheal intubation (20–30 seconds)
  2. Moving the victim (e.g., down stairs—may take 20–30 seconds).

We shall now consider how to integrate these well-rehearsed steps of basic life support into the sequences of advanced cardiac life support.

Advanced Cardiac Life Support

We defined *basic* life support as the maintenance of the airway, breathing, and circulation—the ABCs—*without adjunctive equipment*. Basic life support is a holding action only and is unlikely in itself to restore the heart to effective activity. Paramedics will be called on to deliver more definitive therapy as well, so the skills of *advanced* cardiac life support (ACLS) must also become second nature, to be deployed swiftly and systematically in the event of cardiac arrest.

What is Advanced Cardiac Life Support?

The American Heart Association has defined *advanced cardiac life support* for the patient in cardiac arrest (or the patient at immediate risk of cardiac arrest) to consist of the following elements:

• Use of ADJUNCTIVE EQUIPMENT for ventilation and circulation.
• Cardiac MONITORING for dysrhythmia recognition and control.
• Establishment and maintenance of an INTRAVENOUS INFUSION LINE.
• Employment of definitive therapy, including DEFIBRILLATION and DRUG ADMINISTRATION, to
  1. Prevent cardiac arrest.
  2. Aid in establishing an effective cardiac rhythm and circulation when cardiac arrest does occur.
  3. Stabilize the patient's condition.
• TRANSPORTATION with continuous monitoring.

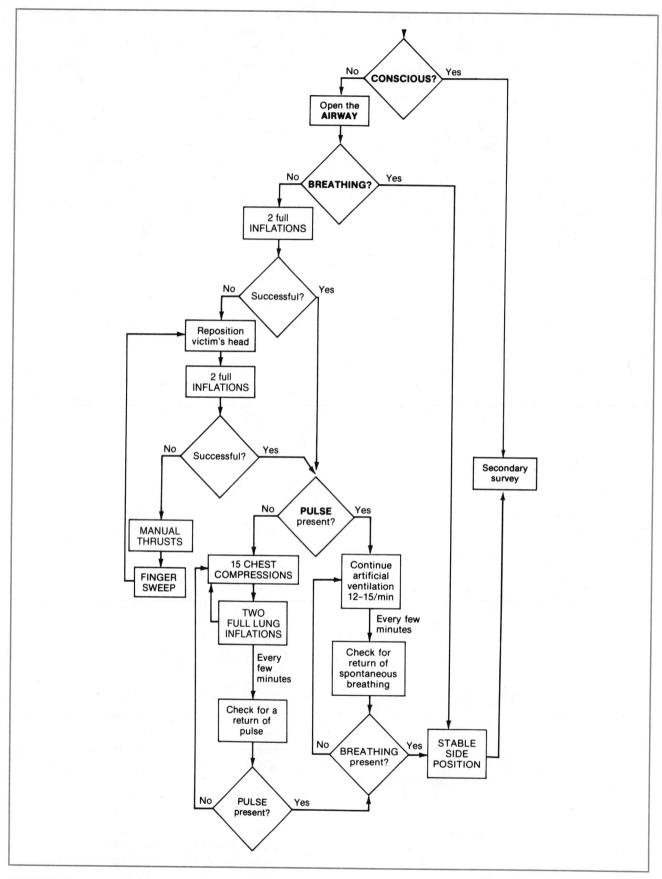

FIGURE 23-79. Sequence of steps in **BASIC LIFE SUPPORT.**

We have already discussed the use of airway adjuncts and equipment for artificial ventilation in Chapters 7 and 8. In this section, we shall deal with the *sequence of actions* in advanced cardiac life support. The last section of the chapter will describe some of the specific techniques—such as defibrillation—for restoring an effective cardiac rhythm.

The Universal Algorithm

The approach to *every* patient in cardiac arrest will start with the same steps. The American Heart Association calls those standard initial steps the *universal algorithm* because those steps are *always* deployed as soon as a person is found unresponsive and possibly in cardiac arrest. (An **algorithm** is a step-by-step procedure for solving a problem.) The universal algorithm includes measures that bystanders should take before your arrival (e.g., "Activate the EMS system"), so we need to modify the universal algorithm a bit to make it applicable to emergency medical services personnel. Here is the Universal Algorithm for Paramedics, which you will also find summarized in Figure 23-80:

- Whenever you are called for a case that *might* be a cardiac arrest ("man down," "unconscious patient," "choking," "stopped breathing," etc.), **carry the defibrillator with you** on your first trip from the ambulance to the patient. You should also carry a portable oxygen cylinder and a "jump kit" that contains equipment for managing the airway. If you have enough help—for instance, if you run with a three-person crew—by all means bring the intubation kit, the IV equipment, and the drug box as well. But if you're shorthanded, don't spend the time carting every piece of equipment from the ambulance to the patient. The two most vital things during the first minutes will be the defibrillator and the oxygen cylinder. You can send someone out to the ambulance for other equipment later. As soon as you reach the patient, one paramedic should ready the monitor/defibrillator while the other carries out the following steps:
- **Assess responsiveness.** If the patient is *not* responsive:
- **Open the airway** and **look, listen, and feel for breathing.** If the patient is *not* breathing:
- **Give two slow breaths.**
- **Assess the circulation: If no pulse, start CPR.** As soon as the monitor/defibrillator is ready, the second paramedic should:
- **Check the rhythm on the monitor.** At this point all you want to know is the answer to one question: *Is VF or VT present?*

- **If VF/VT is present** on the monitor/defibrillator, proceed as described in the algorithm for treating VF/VT (see next section).
- **If VF/VT is not present** on the monitor/defibrillator:
  1. **Intubate** the trachea.
  2. **Confirm** that the endotracheal tube is in the right place and that the chest rises adequately with each ventilation.
  3. **Determine the cardiac rhythm** and, if possible, the cause.

What you see on the monitor at this point will determine which algorithm you will now follow. If the patient is still in cardiac arrest, he may be in any one of the following three situations:

- Ventricular fibrillation or pulseless ventricular tachycardia
- Pulseless electrical activity (that is, you can see an organized rhythm on the monitor, but there is no detectable pulse)
- Asystole

Each of those situations requires a different, specific approach (a different *algorithm*). We shall deal with them one by one.

Ventricular Fibrillation/Pulseless Ventricular Tachycardia Treatment Algorithm

The algorithm for managing VF or pulseless VT is probably the most important for the paramedic to know because patients found in VF or VT are the most likely to be successfully resuscitated—*if* they receive timely and appropriate treatment. The steps, then, in managing VF/pulseless VT are as follows:

- **Check the ABCs,** as described in the universal algorithm.
- **Perform CPR until the defibrillator is attached.**
- **Confirm VF/VT on the monitor/defibrillator.**
- **Confirm absence of a pulse!** There are other things besides VF and VT that can make squiggly lines on a monitor, such as loose ECG leads or muscle tremor. Remember: Treat the *patient*, not the monitor:

YOU *MUST* VERIFY CARDIAC ARREST BY CLINICAL SIGNS. NEVER "DEFIBRILLATE" BEFORE YOU HAVE CHECKED FOR A PULSE.

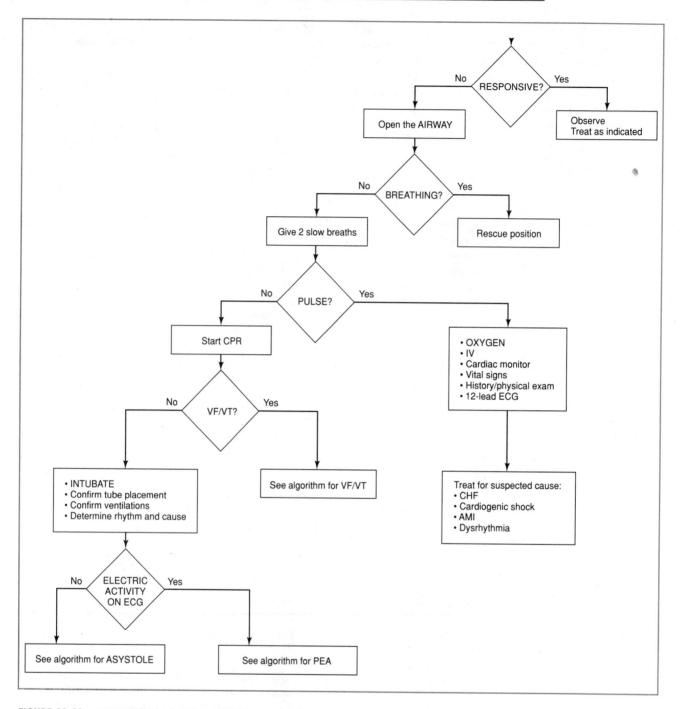

FIGURE 23-80.   UNIVERSAL ALGORITHM for adult emergency cardiac care. Adapted from Emergency Cardiac Care Committee and Subcommittees, American Heart Association. Guidelines for cardiopulmonary resuscitation and emergency cardiac care. *JAMA* 268:2172, 1992.

- **Defibrillate** up to three times, if needed, for persistent VF/VT:
  1. *First shock:* 200 joules. If not effective, or if VF/VT immediately recurs:
  2. *Second shock:* 200 to 300 joules. If not effective, or if VF/VT immediately recurs:
  3. *Third shock:* 360 joules. If not effective, resume CPR.

The three shocks are delivered one right after the other ("stacked"), taking time in between only to recharge the defibrillator and reassess the rhythm. Do *not* pause between shocks to perform CPR or (if the monitor shows persisting VF/VT) to check for a pulse. The sequence of actions, then, is as follows: SHOCK—Immediately RECHARGE the defibrillator while you look at the monitor screen—If VF/VT persists, SHOCK AGAIN as soon as the defibrillator is recharged.

- *If a rhythm other than VF/VT appears on the monitor screen:*
  1. Remove the paddles from the patient's chest.
  2. Disarm the defibrillator.
  3. Check for a pulse.
- *If the rhythm after three shocks is persistent VF/VT:*
- **Continue CPR.**
- **Intubate at once.**
- **Start an IV lifeline** with normal saline.
- As soon as the IV has been established, **administer epinephrine, 1 mg IV push,** and repeat every 3 to 5 minutes. Whenever you give a medication through a peripheral IV during CPR, follow it up immediately with a 20- to 30-ml bolus of intravenous fluid and then elevate the extremity, to facilitate delivery of the medication to the central circulation (which may take 1–2 minutes).
- **Recheck the monitor.**
- *If VF/VT is still present,* **defibrillate at 360 joules within 30 to 60 seconds** of giving the epinephrine dosage. You may deliver **up to three shocks in a row.**
- *If VF/VT is still present,* **administer lidocaine, 1.5 mg per kilogram IV push.**
- **Defibrillate** at 360 joules within 30 to 60 seconds.
- *If VF/VT is still present,* you may **administer a second bolus of lidocaine, 1.5 mg IV.**
- **Defibrillate** at 360 joules within 30 to 60 seconds.
- *If VF/VT is still present,* **administer bretylium, 5 mg per kilogram IV push.** Continue CPR for at least 1 to 2 minutes to circulate the drug. Consider giving **magnesium sulfate, 1 to 2 gm IV** as well. Then:
- **Defibrillate** at 360 joules.
- *If VF/VT is still present,* continue CPR for another 5 minutes, and then **administer a second dose of bretylium,** this time **10 mg per kilogram IV push.**
- **Defibrillate** at 360 joules.
- If at any point during this sequence, there is a *return of spontaneous circulation:*
  1. Assess the patient's vital signs.
  2. Support the airway and breathing, as required.
  3. Provide medications as indicated for maintaining the blood pressure, regulating the heart rate, and controlling cardiac dysrhythmias.

The steps of the VF/VT algorithm are presented schematically in Figure 23-81.

Pulseless Electrical Activity Treatment Algorithm

The term *pulseless electrical activity* (PEA) refers to an organized cardiac rhythm (other than VT) on the monitor that is not accompanied by any detectable pulse. This category includes what we used to call *electromechanical dissociation,* as well as a variety of conditions in which the heart is indeed beating, but beating so weakly that it cannot produce a palpable pulse. That may occur, for example, in cardiogenic or hypovolemic shock, in cardiac tamponade, in massive pulmonary embolism, in disturbances of electrolyte imbalance, or in drug overdoses. Clearly, when there are so many different potential causes of PEA, providing the appropriate treatment will depend significantly on identifying the cause of PEA in a specific case.

- **Continue CPR.**
- **Intubate at once.**
- Start an **IV lifeline** with normal saline.
- Treat for the cause, if known or suspected:

Possible Cause of PEA	Treatment
Hypovolemia	Trial of volume infusion
Hypoxemia	Ventilation with 100% oxygen
Tension pneumothorax	Needle decompression of chest
Others: Drug overdose, electrolyte disturbance, acidosis, massive AMI	Immediate transport

- Consider immediate transcutaneous pacing.
- Consider **epinephrine, 1 mg IV push,** repeated every 3 to 5 minutes.
- If PEA occurs in the context of *bradycardia,* give **atropine, 1 mg IV** (may be repeated every 3–5 minutes up to a total dosage of 0.04 mg/kg).

The steps in the algorithm for pulseless electrical activity are summarized in Figure 23-82.

Asystole Treatment Algorithm

A flat line on an ECG monitor may or may not be asystole, so one of the first things to do when you see a flat-line ECG is to rule out causes other than asystole.

- **Continue CPR.**
- **Intubate at once.**
- Start an **IV lifeline** with normal saline.
- **Confirm asystole.**

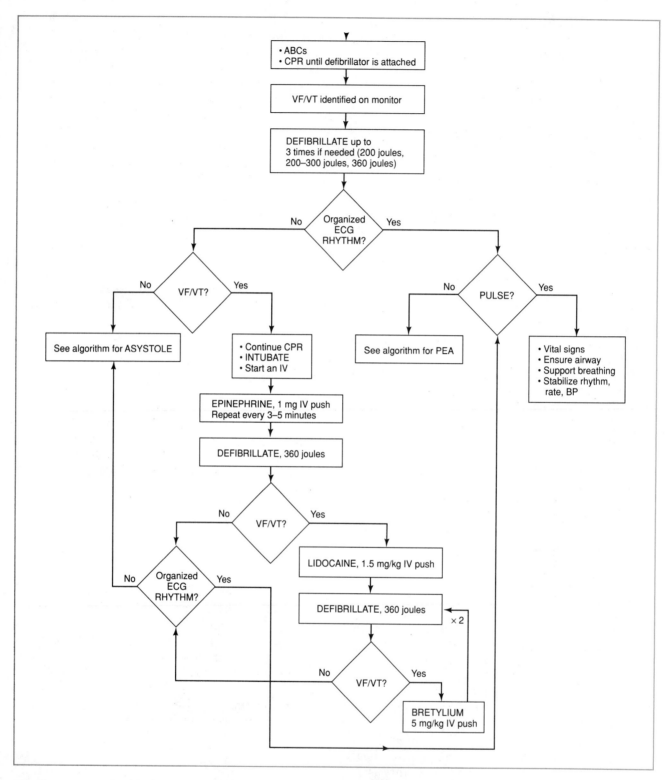

FIGURE 23-81. **ALGORITHM FOR VENTRICULAR FIBRILLATION AND PULSELESS VENTRICULAR TACHYCARDIA (VF/VT).** Adapted from Emergency Cardiac Care Committee and Subcommittees, American Heart Association. Guidelines for cardiopulmonary resuscitation and emergency cardiac care. *JAMA* 268:2172, 1992.

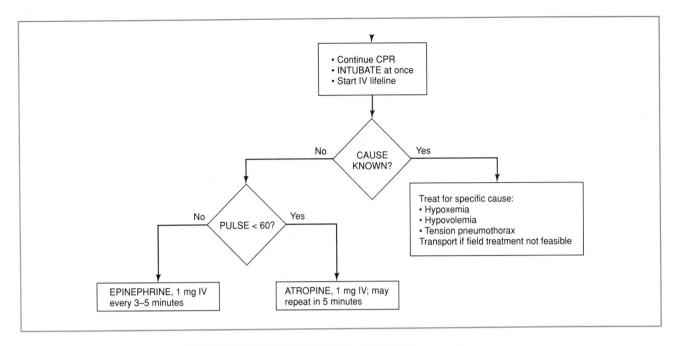

FIGURE 23-82. **ALGORITHM FOR PULSELESS ELECTRICAL ACTIVITY (PEA).** Adapted from Emergency Cardiac Care Committee and Subcommittees, American Heart Association. Guidelines for cardiopulmonary resuscitation and emergency cardiac care. *JAMA* 268:2172, 1992.

**POSSIBLE CAUSES
OF A FLAT-LINE ECG**

- Leads not connected to the patient
- Leads are loose
- Leads not connected to the monitor/defibrillator
- Very low–voltage ventricular fibrillation
- True asystole

Make sure that all the monitoring electrodes are firmly fastened to the patient and that the cables are hooked into the monitor. Switch to another lead (or move the quick-look paddles 90 degrees) to detect low-voltage VF. If the rhythm is indeed asystole, you need to be aware that the prognosis is very grim and the chances for successful resuscitation are poor.

- **Consider possible treatable causes.** The treatable causes of asystole include:
  1. Hypoxia
  2. Hyperkalemia or hypokalemia
  3. Preexisting acidosis
  4. Drug overdose
  5. Hypothermia

- Consider *immediate* **transcutaneous pacing.** To date, transcutaneous pacing of asystole in the field has been singularly *un*successful, but success rates might be higher if pacing is instituted immediately when asystole occurs, together with drug therapy.
- Give **epinephrine, 1 mg IV push,** and repeat every 3 to 5 minutes.
- Give **atropine, 1 mg IV.** The dosage may be repeated every 3 to 5 minutes up to a total dose of 0.04 mg per kilogram.
- **Consider termination of efforts.** We shall have more to say later in this chapter about stopping CPR in the field.

The steps in the asystole treatment algorithm are summarized schematically in Figure 23-83.

Postresuscitative Care

If an effective cardiac rhythm is restored in the field, the next task is to make sure that the rhythm *stays* restored and that optimal conditions are provided to promote recovery of the patient's brain from the hypoxic insult of cardiac arrest. To begin with, the *cardiac rhythm should be stabilized* to the degree possible. That means that if the arrest rhythm was ventricular fibrillation or ventricular tachycardia, a lidocaine bolus fol-

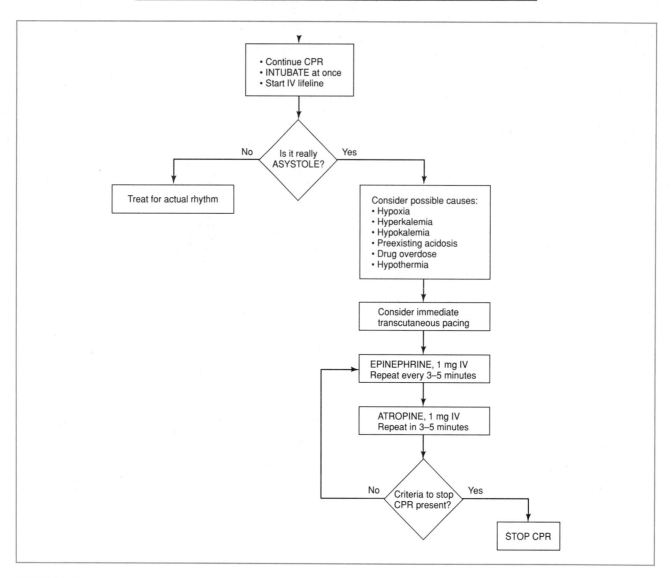

FIGURE 23-83.   ALGORITHM FOR ASYSTOLE.   Adapted from Emergency Cardiac Care Committee and Subcommittees, American Heart Association. Guidelines for cardiopulmonary resuscitation and emergency cardiac care. *JAMA* 268:2172, 1992.

lowed by an infusion of lidocaine is usually indicated. If severe bradycardia is present in the postarrest period, atropine or transcutaneous pacing may be required, and the receiving hospital should be alerted to prepare a transvenous pacemaker.

Once the cardiac rhythm is stable, attention turns to the brain itself and to ameliorating the effects of cardiac arrest on that vital organ. *Marked hypotension needs to be corrected rapidly,* for the brain will not be adequately perfused so long as the blood pressure is very low. If there is marked hypotension, then, and transport time to the hospital will be prolonged, the physician may order an infusion of dopamine or norepinephrine. The brain may also benefit from *moder-*

ate hyperventilation, to lower the PCO_2 to between 25 and 35 torr; that measure helps combat cerebral acidosis and also helps decrease intracranial pressure. In the intubated patient, *avoid tracheal suctioning* unless absolutely necessary, for suctioning provokes an increase in intracranial pressure. Finally, *elevate the patient's head* to about 30 degrees, to increase cerebral venous drainage.

It should be emphasized that postresuscitative care is complex and is best carried out in an intensive care unit, where careful monitoring and titrated therapy can most effectively be given. Thus, TRANSPORT TO THE HOSPITAL SHOULD NOT BE DELAYED FOR PATIENTS RESUSCITATED FROM

CARDIAC ARREST. If an effective cardiac rhythm is restored in the field, transport immediately. Only in situations where transport will be significantly prolonged (e.g., cardiac arrest occurring far from the hospital) should postresuscitative measures be started in the field, as directed by the physician.

POSTRESUSCITATIVE CARE: SUMMARY

- STABILIZE CARDIAC RHYTHM (lidocaine for post-VF/VT; atropine or a transcutaneous pacemaker for symptomatic bradycardia).
- NORMALIZE BLOOD PRESSURE (dopamine or norepinephrine infusion to raise systolic pressure to above 100 mm Hg).
- MODERATE HYPERVENTILATION (about 20 inflations/min by bag-valve-mask or bag-valve–endotracheal tube with oxygen).
- ELEVATE PATIENT'S HEAD to 30 degrees if blood pressure allows.

When to Stop CPR

Since the dawn of paramedic-staffed MICUs in the early 1970s, it has been the practice in most communities *not* to permit the termination of CPR in the field. That policy was established because, in most jurisdictions, only a physician is authorized to pronounce a person dead (and to stop CPR is considered equivalent to pronouncing a person dead). Cardiac arrest victims who were not successfully resuscitated at the scene, therefore, were invariably transported urgently to the hospital, with some semblance of CPR en route. However, with the accumulation of vast experience from EMS systems throughout the United States, it became clear that transport to the emergency room of adults who did not respond to an adequate trial of prehospital ACLS was an exercise in futility, for less than 1 percent of such patients survived. Furthermore, rapid transport of patients in cardiac arrest, with CPR en route, involves considerable *hazards to EMS personnel:* The risks of vehicular accidents or of injuries while working in a moving vehicle are greatly increased during urgent transport. Finally, the *costs* of continuing futile resuscitations in the emergency room are enormous. For all those reasons, the American Heart Association stated in their

most recent *Guidelines for Cardiopulmonary Resuscitation and Emergency Cardiac Care:*

> It is inappropriate, futile, and ethically unacceptable to routinely continue prehospital resuscitation efforts and require ambulance transport of all patients. . . . Cessation of efforts in the prehospital setting, following system-specific criteria and under direct medical control, should be standard practice in all EMS systems. . . .
> Resuscitation may be discontinued in the prehospital setting when the patient is nonresuscitable after an adequate trial of ACLS. . . . Physican ambulance medical directors remain ultimately responsible for determination of death, and pronouncement of death in the field should have the concurrence of on-line medical control.

Legislation will probably be required, at the state level, to permit pronouncement of death at the scene (such legislation already exists, for example, in New Jersey, where one-fourth of patients in cardiac arrest are now pronounced dead in the prehospital phase). Once such legislation is enacted, each EMS system will have to formulate criteria for the termination of CPR in the prehospital setting. A very good model is that proposed by Bonnin and co-workers in Houston (*JAMA* 270:1457, 1993):

CRITERIA FOR TERMINATION OF RESUSCITATION EFFORTS AT THE SCENE FOLLOWING UNMONITORED, OUT-OF-HOSPITAL, ADULT, PRIMARY CARDIAC ARREST

- Adult cardiopulmonary arrest (not associated with trauma, hypothermia, respiratory etiology, or drug overdose)
- Standard advanced cardiac life support for 25 minutes
- No restoration of spontaneous circulation (spontaneous pulse rate of faster than 60 beats per minute for at least one 5-minute period)
- Absence of persistently recurring or refractory VF/VT or any continued neurologic activity (e.g., spontaneous respiration, eye opening, or motor response)

It should be pointed out that gaining permission to stop CPR in the field will not necessarily make life easier for paramedics. There are delicate issues involved, such as the expectations of the patient's family or the disposition of the body. Paramedics may be under enormous pressure from bystanders to continue resuscitative efforts long after there is any medical justification for doing so. And it may also be very difficult for the paramedic to find himself or herself in the unaccustomed role of having to tell a family, "Your husband [father, etc.] is dead; there is nothing more that can be done." It is much easier to go careering off to the hospital with red lights and sirens and leave the emergency room staff with the unpleasant business of breaking bad news. So when it becomes legal in *your* EMS system to terminate CPR in the field, it's a good idea to meet with your medical director and "walk through" some of the scenes you may have to face. Role-play exercises can be particularly useful in helping you to pinpoint situations where you feel uncomfortable and to develop strategies in advance for dealing with those situations.

TECHNIQUES OF MANAGEMENT IN CARDIAC EMERGENCIES

In the sections that follow, we shall look at some of the devices and methods employed in the treatment of patients with cardiac emergencies. Not all of the techniques or devices described are used in every EMS system, and not all are required for certification as a paramedic. Direct your attention to the material that is relevant to local practice in your area.

Defibrillation

Defibrillation is the process by which a surge of electric energy is delivered to the heart. Recall that when the heart fibrillates, its individual muscle fibers get "out of synch" with one another and begin contracting individually. The result is that the heart as a whole ceases any useful movement; and if you were to look at a fibrillating heart, you would see movement resembling that of a bag of energetic worms. The idea behind *de*fibrillation is to deliver a current to the heart powerful enough to paralyze all of its component muscle cells, with the hope that when those cells recover from the shock—after a few seconds—they will all start up in unison and the heart as a whole will be restored to effective function.

Defibrillation needs to be carried out as soon as possible in VF or pulseless VT, for the likelihood of success declines rapidly with time. If a defibrillator is not immediately available, however, do not delay BLS. Start CPR at once, and defibrillate as soon as the equipment is on hand. Defibrillation is *not* useful in asystole. But if you are not sure whether the line you

see on the monitor is asystole or fine VF, try a countershock.

To perform defibrillation, turn the SYNCHRONIZE button on the machine to the OFF position, and turn the MAIN POWER switch ON. Set the ENERGY LEVEL to 200 joules, and CHARGE THE PADDLES.

It is then necessary to reduce the resistance of the patient's skin to passage of electric current by LUBRICATING THE PADDLES; otherwise the energy will be delivered largely to the skin itself, resulting in burns to the skin and ineffective energy delivery to the heart. Use either saline-soaked 4- by 4-inch pads or electrode paste to make good electric contact between the paddles and the skin. Saline pads have the advantage of not leaving a slippery residue on the chest to make subsequent cardiac compression difficult. The pads must be well soaked, but not so wet as to ooze saline over the chest. NEVER USE ALCOHOL-SOAKED PADS in defibrillation, as they will ignite into flames when electric current passes through them. If electrode paste is used, squeeze it generously onto the paddles and rub it into the skin with the paddles. Whichever method you choose—saline pads or electrode paste—take care to prevent contact (bridging) between the two conductive areas on the chest wall. If the saline or paste from one paddle comes in contact with that from the other paddle, the electric current will simply pass along the skin from one paddle to the other; effective current will thus bypass the heart, causing superficial burns of the skin instead. If there is a nitroglycerin patch on the patient's chest, remove it before you apply the defibrillator paddles. Although nitroglycerin does *not*—contrary to popular legend—explode, the backing used on some nitroglycerin patches can support electrical arcing during defibrillation, producing smoke, noise, and burns to the patient.

POSITION THE PADDLES so that the negative (black) paddle is just to the right of the upper sternum below the right clavicle and the positive (red) paddle is just below and to the left of the left nipple (Fig. 23-84). Exert firm pressure (20–25 lb) on each paddle to make good skin contact. Inadequate contact is another cause of burns and ineffective countershock.

When the paddles are in place, CLEAR THE AREA so that no one, including the operator, is in contact with the patient or stretcher; the operator should command, "Everyone off!" Then FIRE the DEFIBRILLATOR by pressing the button on each handle simultaneously. When using a machine for which a second operator must press a button on the panel rather than on the paddles, the rescuer wielding the paddles commands, "Hit it!" If current has reached the patient, contraction of his chest and other muscles will be evident. If you do not see contraction,

include the paddles, cables and connectors, power supply, monitor, ECG recorder, and any ancillary supplies (electrode gel, pads, spare battery, etc.). The U.S. Food and Drug Administration (FDA) has developed a very good Operator's Shift Checklist for inspecting both manual and automated defibrillators (see RD White, *Ann Emerg Med* 22:302, 1993). Conscientious use of that checklist should significantly reduce the incidence of defibrillator accidents and failures.

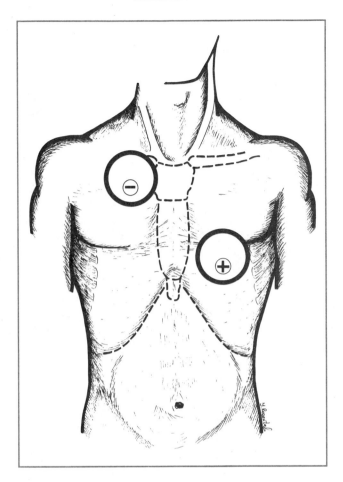

FIGURE 23-84. Position of the paddles for defibrillation.

PROCEDURES FOR DEFIBRILLATION: SUMMARY
• Turn the SYNCHRONIZE switch OFF, and turn the MAIN POWER ON. • Set the energy level at 200 JOULES. • CHARGE the paddles. • LUBRICATE the paddles, and POSITION them on the chest. • CLEAR the area. • FIRE the defibrillator. • Repeat at 200 to 300 joules and at 360 joules, as needed.

---

check the defibrillator to be certain the synchronizing switch is OFF and the battery is sufficiently charged.

Immediately after delivering the defibrillating current, RECHARGE THE DEFIBRILLATOR. Take the few seconds that the defibrillator is recharging to LOOK AT THE MONITOR. If VF/VT persists, SHOCK AGAIN AT 200–300 JOULES. Again, immediately recharge the defibrillator and look at the monitor. If you *still* see VF/VT, give a THIRD SHOCK at 360 JOULES. If at any point there is an organized rhythm on the monitor, check for a pulse.

If the patient requiring defibrillation has an implanted artificial *pacemaker*—which you may detect either from the spikes the pacemaker is producing on the ECG or the bulge it creates where its battery pack has been implanted under the patient's skin—that is *not* a contraindication to defibrillation. Just make certain that you do not place either of the electrode paddles directly over the pacemaker battery (the bulge beneath the skin).

The defibrillator should be *inspected* at the beginning of each shift, using a checklist to cover all aspects of the apparatus and its gear. Inspection should

The Automated External Defibrillator

The automated external defibrillator (AED) is a "smart defibrillator" that can—thanks to sophisticated computer chips—analyze the patient's ECG rhythm and determine whether a defibrillating shock is needed. AEDs may be either fully automatic or semiautomatic. The **fully automatic** versions assess the patient's rhythm and—if VF is present—charge the paddles and deliver countershocks, without any intervention by the rescuer. The **semiautomatic** AEDs, on the other hand, require decisions by the rescuer. That is, the semiautomatic AED identifies the rhythm and then instructs the rescuer what to do about it! If, for example, the AED detects ventricular fibrillation, a message may appear on the liquid crystal display (LCD) screen saying, "SHOCK ADVISED. PRESS TO SHOCK." The rescuer must then depress the "shock" button to defibrillate the patient.

Whether the AED is fully automatic or semiautomatic, the basic sequence of steps in using an AED are the same:

1. The patient's chest is exposed.
2. Two self-adhesive electrode pads are attached firmly to the patient's chest—one (the *sternal pad*)

at the junction of the right clavicle and upper border of the sternum; the other (the *apex pad*) along the left lower rib margin at the anterior axillary line.

3. The AED is turned on.
4. CPR is stopped, and everyone gets clear of the patient.
5. The AED assesses the rhythm (for about 6–20 seconds) and determines whether it is "shockable" (i.e., whether the rhythm is one that will respond to defibrillation).
6. If the AED does detect a "shockable" rhythm, it automatically starts charging up the paddles, which takes about 5 to 10 seconds.
7. Defibrillating shocks of 200 to 300 joules are then delivered, either automatically or by the rescuer, depending on the type of AED.

We shall not present here the details of operating the currently available automated external defibrillators. New AEDs are coming on the market all the time, and each model is furnished with its own operating manual. Paramedics who will be using an AED should train with the specific apparatus carried by their service, according to the manufacturer's instructions for that machine.

Cardioversion

Cardioversion is the use of the DC defibrillator to terminate dysrhythmias other than VF. In cardioversion, unlike defibrillation, the current is *synchronized* with the ECG so that it will not be delivered during the vulnerable period (i.e., on top of the T wave). Emergency cardioversion is indicated for rapid ventricular and supraventricular rhythms that are associated with severely compromised cardiac output—such as rapid ventricular tachycardia, or atrial flutter or atrial fibrillation with a rapid ventricular response. Emergency cardioversion should not, however, be used outside the hospital to convert rapid rhythms that may be due to digitalis toxicity (for practical purposes, that means any tachyarrhythmia in any patient taking digitalis).

In the field, cardioversion will be carried out *only* in patients whose cardiac output is so impaired that they are unconscious, so premedication need not be given. When cardioversion is performed electively on a conscious patient, the patient *must* first be anesthetized, preferably with a short-acting barbiturate such as methohexital, for cardioversion is a painful and terrifying experience for an awake patient.

NEVER PERFORM CARDIOVERSION IN AN AWAKE PATIENT.

Procedure for Cardioversion

- Turn the SYNCHRONIZE switch on the machine to the ON position (unlike for defibrillation), and turn the MAIN POWER ON.
- SET THE ENERGY LEVEL as ordered by the physician. Energy levels required for cardioversion vary depending on the type of dysrhythmia involved. Ventricular tachycardia, for example, can often be converted with energy levels as low as 25 to 50 joules. However, in emergencies, if an initial attempt to convert a rapid rhythm with low energy levels fails, immediately turn the setting up to 100 to 200 joules and repeat the shock.
- Prepare and APPLY THE PADDLES as described for defibrillation.
- CLEAR THE AREA by commanding, "Everyone off!"
- DEPRESS THE FIRING BUTTONS, AND KEEP THEM DEPRESSED until the synchronizer fires the machine. That may take a few moments, since the charge is synchronized to fire about 10 milliseconds after the peak of the R wave.
- If countershock produces VF, *immediately*
  1. Recharge the defibrillator to 200 to 300 joules.
  2. Turn the synchronizer circuit to the OFF position.
  3. Shock again.

Cough CPR and Precordial Thump

Two relatively simple techniques may be useful in special circumstances of cardiac arrest: cough CPR and the precordial thump. The paramedic should understand those maneuvers and know in which situations they are appropriate.

Research has shown that COUGHING can preserve consciousness during VF and can also sometimes convert ventricular tachycardia (VT) to normal sinus rhythm. That is probably because a cough produces changes in intrathoracic pressure that result in the forward flow of blood. Thus coughing and external chest compressions probably provide perfusion by similar mechanisms.

A sharp blow to the sternum (PRECORDIAL THUMP) has been documented to convert some episodes of VT and—rarely—VF to sinus rhythm. The mechanism of this effect is not known; but the blow to the chest may produce a low-energy electric current sufficient to "cardiovert" the heart when the myocardium is still well-oxygenated.

When are such measures appropriate? For the paramedic trained in ALS techniques, cough CPR or chest thumps are probably indicated only in the following situations:

- In a *monitored* patient seen to develop VT or VF when a defibrillator is not at hand, immediately coach the patient to COUGH forcibly several times. If the cough converts his rhythm to normal sinus, he may stop coughing. If VT or VF persists, coach him to continue coughing until a defibrillator is available. Then countershock at 100 to 200 joules (for the awake patient with VT, give an anesthetic first!).
- In *witnessed* cardiac arrest, when a defibrillator is not immediately available, deliver a sharp blow to the midsternum (PRECORDIAL THUMP), then recheck the pulse. If the pulse has returned, begin stabilizing procedures (oxygen, IV lifeline, lidocaine, and so forth). If the pulse is still absent, start CPR and call for a defibrillator.

Carotid Sinus Massage*

Carotid sinus massage is one of the most effective forms of vagal stimulation. It is sometimes used in an attempt to convert paroxysmal tachyarrhythmias associated with hypotension or a decreased level of consciousness. Carotid sinus massage works by increasing the output of the *para*sympathetic nervous system, which acts (remember?) to *slow* the heart. (Question: What other maneuver[s] increase the output of the parasympathetic nervous system?)

Procedure for Carotid Sinus Massage

- The patient must be closely monitored throughout the procedure. Therefore, APPLY MONITORING ELECTRODES, and place the oscilloscope where the screen can be viewed throughout the procedure. Make sure the beep tone is audible as well, for you can *hear* an irregularity in rhythm much sooner than you can see one. An IV LIFELINE should also have been established before you start this procedure.
- Assemble all the EQUIPMENT that may be necessary in the event of a cardiac arrest. Have a syringe of LIDOCAINE and a syringe of ATROPINE sulfate drawn up and ready.

---

*Not required by USDOT for certification as a paramedic.

- Gently palpate each carotid pulse *separately* to be certain there are equal pulses on each side; if one carotid pulse is absent or weak, ABORT THE PROCEDURE.
- POSITION THE PATIENT supine with his neck extended and his head turned slightly to the side opposite that on which you will be working (start on the right side—so the patient's head should be turned to the left).
- LOCATE THE CAROTID SINUS. It is found anterior to the sternomastoid muscle at the upper level of the Adam's apple or sometimes about one-half inch above it.
- Position yourself behind the patient.
- With two fingers, FIRMLY PRESS the carotid artery against the transverse process of the sixth cervical vertebra. You should be able to feel the pulsating artery beneath your fingertips. Maintain pressure NO LONGER THAN 15 TO 20 SECONDS while simultaneously massaging the area with the pressing fingers. KEEP AN EYE ON THE MONITOR THE ENTIRE TIME, and release pressure immediately if you see or hear the heart rate slowing.
- If massage of the right carotid sinus is unsuccessful, wait 2 to 3 minutes and then try the same procedure on the left side. Again, do not massage for more than 15 to 20 seconds, and cease immediately when the heart rate begins to slow down.
- NEVER, NEVER, NEVER MASSAGE BOTH CAROTID SINUSES SIMULTANEOUSLY!

Transcutaneous Cardiac Pacing*

Approximately 30 percent of patients suffering cardiac arrest outside the hospital are found to be in asystole or a pulseless bradycardia (bradyasystolic arrest) at the time the paramedics arrive. The prospects for resuscitating patients in bradyasystolic rhythms, even with the best advanced life support, are best described as dismal; salvage rates reported from various centers vary from 0 to 3 percent. Since pharmacologic therapy has been so unrewarding, several medical workers proposed using artificial pacemakers in the resuscitation of patients with bradyasystolic rhythms.

What artificial pacemakers do is deliver repetitive electric currents to the heart. Like the tiny electric currents generated by natural pacemakers, the current from an artificial pacemaker can cause the myocardial tissue to depolarize. So the artificial pacemaker can substitute for a natural pacemaker that has become blocked or nonfunctional.

The artificial pacemakers first developed for emergency use consisted of a small battery pack and a wire that had to be threaded through a vein into the right ventricle of the heart. Insertion of one of those *transvenous* pacemakers was a tricky and often time-consuming job, usually best undertaken in a coronary care unit. During the past 10 years or so, however, effective *transcutaneous* pacemakers—that is, pacemakers that deliver their current across the skin of the chest—have been developed and have come into widespread use. With the availability of equipment that made it possible to institute artificial pacing almost immediately, emergency physicians were eager to try the equipment out in bradyasystolic arrest.

The results were not very encouraging, but some researchers reasoned that they simply weren't getting to the patients quickly enough. It had already been demonstrated that the sooner a patient was paced following bradyasystolic arrest, the better the chances of success. So the logical next step was to try to institute pacing earlier in the course of cardiac arrest, and the most logical way to do *that* was to take the pacemaker out of the hospital and into the field.

Transcutaneous pacing has now been tested in several EMS systems. It has *not* proved useful in bradysystolic cardiac arrest—a fact that should not really be surprising. When asystole or bradycardia during cardiac arrest fails to respond to drugs, it is probably a sign of massive myocardial damage, so it is unlikely that *anything* will improve survival in such cases.

Nonetheless, asystolic cardiac arrest aside, transcutaneous cardiac pacing may have useful applications in prehospital care. Specifically, pacing may prove valuable for

- Interhospital transfer of patients needing pacemaker implantation (e.g., a patient with complete heart block admitted to a small community hospital that does not have the facilities to implant a permanent pacemaker)
- Symptomatic patients with artificial pacemaker failure
- Patients with bradyarrhythmias or blocks associated with severely reduced cardiac output and unresponsive to atropine, *prior* to cardiac arrest

In any of those circumstances, a transcutaneous pacemaker may buy time for the patient and enable him to reach the hospital in a state of optimal perfusion rather than in or near cardiac arrest.

There are currently about half a dozen different brands of transcutaneous external cardiac pacemakers on the market, and paramedics working with those devices will have to become familiar with the partic-

ular pacemaker used in their local EMS system. In general, though, the steps in initiating transcutaneous pacing are as follows:

- APPLY THE ELECTRODES—one anteriorly over the lower sternum, the other posteriorly just below the left scapula.
- Switch the POWER ON.
- Set the PACING RATE to 80 per minute.
- Set the CURRENT. Start at 50 milliamps (mA).
- CHECK FOR CAPTURE; that is, check whether every pacemaker spike is followed by a QRS complex. If not, it means that the pacemaker current is not depolarizing the ventricles. Increase the current gradually until there is consistent capture.

Transcutaneous pacemakers depolarize not only cardiac muscle but also muscles in the chest wall beneath the pacing electrode. As a result, patients who are conscious when transcutaneous pacing is initiated (or who regain consciousness during pacing) usually experience chest discomfort and sometimes severe pain from the procedure. Some form of ANALGESIA and sedation—such as nitrous oxide or morphine—should therefore be given to patients when transcutaneous pacemakers are used.

Intracardiac Injection*

When an intravenous route cannot be established readily during cardiac arrest, epinephrine is sometimes administered directly into the cardiac chambers by intracardiac injection. It should be emphasized that this technique has no advantages over instillation of epinephrine through an endotracheal tube. Furthermore, while endotracheal administration of drugs is a very safe procedure, intracardiac injection entails several serious *hazards:*

POTENTIAL HAZARDS OF INTRACARDIAC INJECTION

- Inadvertent laceration of a coronary artery
- Inadvertent injection into the heart muscle itself with resulting refractory ventricular fibrillation
- Pneumothorax
- Cardiac tamponade

---

*Not required by USDOT for certification as a paramedic.

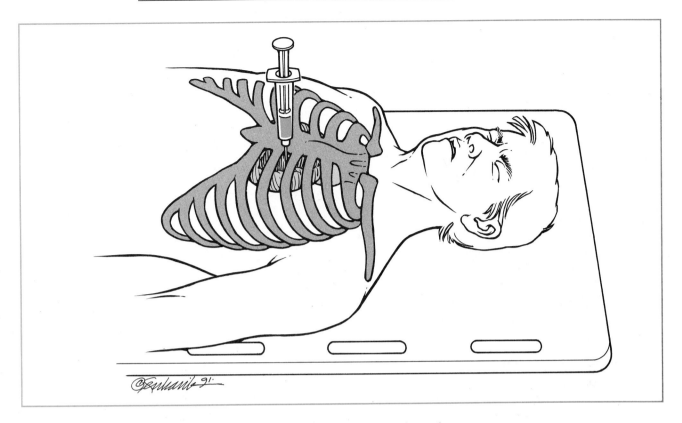

FIGURE 23-85. **INTRACARDIAC INJECTION.** Hold the syringe at right angles to the chest with the needle in the fourth left intercostal space at the left sternal border.

In addition, intracardiac injection requires interrupting ventilations and chest compressions. For all those reasons, many experts in resuscitation feel that the intravenous or endotracheal route is to be strongly preferred for administration of epinephrine during cardiac arrest.

If, nonetheless, intracardiac injection is ordered, it is performed as follows:

- Connect a long (spinal) needle of 20 to 22 gauge to the syringe of epinephrine. Many of the prefilled epinephrine syringes are supplied with such a needle already attached.
- Locate the fourth or fifth left intercostal space, approximately 1½ inches to the left of the sternal border (Fig. 23-85). Cleanse the area with an alcohol or povidone-iodine swab if readily available.
- Insert the needle at right angles to the chest wall, maintaining slight pull on the plunger of the syringe.
- When there is free aspiration of blood into the syringe, the tip of the needle has entered the ventricular lumen. At that point, inject the contents of the syringe as a bolus. Take care not to pull the needle out of the ventricle until you have fin-

ished injecting the contents of the syringe, lest the epinephrine be injected into the ventricular muscle itself.
- Rapidly withdraw the needle, and immediately resume external cardiac compressions.

Mechanical CPR Devices*

Various mechanical adjuncts are available to assist in delivering chest compressions to a patient in cardiac arrest. Such adjuncts are said to reduce or eliminate operator fatigue and to decrease the number of personnel required to perform CPR. Further, some authorities feel that mechanical CPR devices are especially suited for use in ambulances when extended transport with ongoing CPR is necessary. While the mechanical CPR devices differ considerably from one another, certain general observations apply to all of them:

- The safety and efficacy of mechanical CPR devices have not been clearly established.

---

*Not required by USDOT for certification as a paramedic.

- Use of these devices requires extensive training and frequent team drill to ensure correct application, coordination of team action, and efficient assembly time.
- MECHANICAL CPR DEVICES SHOULD *NOT* BE USED TO INITIATE CPR. Resuscitation should always be started manually, and the positioning of a mechanical CPR device should not be permitted to interrupt CPR for more than 15 to 20 seconds.
- Mechanical CPR devices should *not* be used in infants and children.

Mechanical CPR devices currently used in the field fall into three general categories: (1) active compression-decompression (ACD) units, (2) manually operated cardiac presses, and (3) automatic gas-powered compressors. The CPR vest, described in Chapter 9, has not yet come into widespread prehospital use.

The Active Compression-Decompression Unit

The ACD unit was developed by some California physicians after a letter to the *Journal of the American Medical Association* reported the successful resuscitation of a patient by his son using a toilet plunger applied to the chest to perform chest compressions. The commercially-produced ACD units now in use—such as the CardioPump pictured in Figure 23-86—are a bit more sophisticated than the household "plumber's helper," but the principle is the same: Pushing and pulling rhythmically on the plunger alternately compresses and reexpands the chest. The active rather than passive reexpansion of the chest seems to improve flow dynamics. The commerical version, furthermore, enables the rescuer to measure precisely how much pressure he or she is applying, so chest compressions can be delivered more effectively and consistently. The ACD device is indicated **only for adults** in cardiac arrest and may be deployed in either one- or two-rescuer CPR. Once applied, the ACD unit usually stays in place by suction, so there is no need for the single rescuer to keep reidentifying landmarks each time he returns to the chest to perform compressions. The procedure for use is as follows:

- Kneel close to the patient's side, as you would to perform standard CPR.
- Identify the COMPRESSION POINT, which is the same as that for manual CPR, on the lower third of the sternum.
- Place the center of the ACD unit on the sternum so that the lower edge of the vacuum cup lies just superior to the xiphoid.

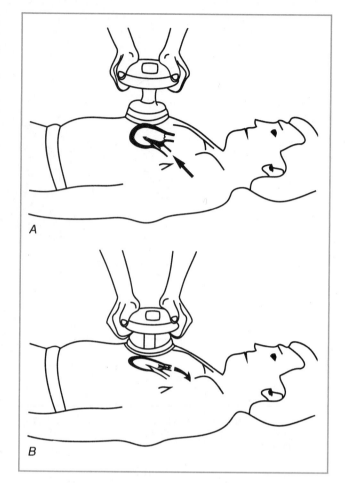

FIGURE 23-86. **ACTIVE COMPRESSION-DECOMPRESSION CPR** using the Ambu CardioPump. (A) As the handle of the ACD unit is depressed, blood is forced from the patient's heart. (B) As the ACD unit is lifted upward, the chest wall is pulled up, the thoracic cavity expands, and the heart refills with blood. Drawings courtesy of Testa-Laboratorium Export A/S, Denmark.

- Grip the rim of the ACD handle with both hands. The heels of your hands should rest on the surface of the handle.
- Straighten your arms and lock your elbows.
- COMPRESS straight down at a rate of 80 to 100 per minute. For an average adult, the compression force should be around 40 kg, but you will have to check in each case how much force it takes to depress the sternum 1½ to 2 inches (4–5 cm). Once you have determined how much pressure it requires, deliver that amount of pressure with every compression. Your compression should last for 50 percent of the compression-decompression cycle.
- DECOMPRESS by swinging your weight back up, as you would in standard CPR. But hold onto the ACD handle and *lift* the chest. Check the

gauge periodically to make sure you obtain an expansion force of at least 10 kg during active decompression.

The Cardiac Press

The cardiac press (Fig. 23-87) is a hinged, manually operated chest compressor, which usually provides an adjustable stroke of 1½ to 2 inches. It is relatively simple to assemble and, because of its simplicity, is unlikely to suffer mechanical breakdown. The procedure for its use is as follows:

- Start CPR with *manual methods*. The first rescuer continues CPR.
- The second rescuer slides the backboard of the press under the patient's back and places the frame into the position hole.
- The adjustment knob is loosened, and the plunger positioned centrally on the lower half of the sternum. The adjustment knob is then retightened.
- Cardiac compressions are now applied by the second rescuer pushing the handle of the press down with a brisk stroke; the handle is then released, allowing the press to return to its upward position. Compressions are continued at a rate of approximately 80 to 100 per minute.
- The first rescuer interposes a ventilation after every fifth compression.

The Automatic, Gas-Powered Compressor

The automatic, gas-powered compressor (Fig. 23-88) delivers compressions by a plunger mounted on a backboard and driven by compressed oxygen; the same oxygen source may be used to provide oxygen-

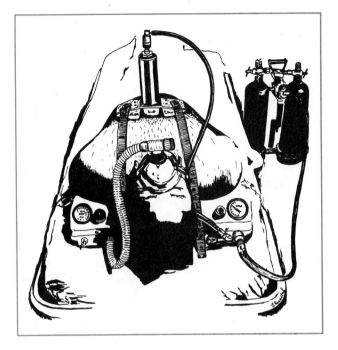

FIGURE 23-88. AUTOMATIC, GAS-POWERED CHEST COMPRESSOR.

enriched positive pressure ventilation with an inhaled oxygen concentration of up to 80 percent. When used in an ambulance, the device should be secured with a strap to the patient's chest to minimize shifts in plunger position due to vehicle motion. The procedure for applying a gas-powered compressor is as follows:

Rescuer 1	Rescuer 2
Initiate CPR by manual methods.	Secure equipment.
Roll patient onto his side (5 seconds).	Position base plate under patient so that lower part of patient's sternum is over center of plate.
Roll patient back to supine. Resume CPR.	Mount, position, and place in operation the automatic chest compressor.
Interpose a ventilation after every fifth compression. Switch to ventilation equipment.	Set up ventilation equipment.
Check to be sure chest rises with ventilations.	Check for carotid pulse with compressions.

FIGURE 23-87. CARDIAC PRESS.

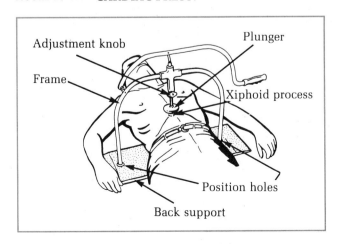

Adjustment knob
Plunger
Frame
Xiphoid process
Position holes
Back support

Catheterization of the Urinary Bladder*

Patients in severe left heart failure with pulmonary edema are usually given a strong diuretic, such as furosemide, to promote urinary excretion of their excess extracellular fluid. If the diuretic works as it should, the patient's bladder rapidly fills with urine—sometimes so rapidly that it obstructs outflow through the urethra, especially in older men with enlarged prostates. For that reason, older men treated in the hospital for congestive heart failure are often catheterized before they are given diuretics to ensure that they will be able to pass the increased volumes of urine they will shortly be producing. Catheterization of the bladder is also carried out in the hospital for any circumstance in which it is necessary to have a precise knowledge of the patient's urinary output and when the patient cannot, for one reason or another, void voluntarily at the appropriate intervals (e.g., an unconscious trauma victim).

In urban EMS systems, it will rarely if ever be necessary for a paramedic to carry out urinary catheterization in the field. In rural EMS systems, however, or in areas where paramedics are based in emergency departments, it may be necessary for paramedics to learn to insert a catheter into the bladder.

Catheterization of the bladder is *not* a pleasant experience for the patient. Your explanation of what is going to be done and why it is being done will be very important in establishing the patient's trust and gaining the patient's cooperation.

The EQUIPMENT for urinary catheterization should be sterilized and prepackaged as a set. Commercial catheterization kits are now widely available and quite suitable. If you make up your own kit, it should contain at least the following:

- Sterile gloves
- Sterile cleansing sponges
- Antiseptic solution (pHisoHex or Zephiran)
- Foley catheter with 5-ml balloon (usually No. 14 French for women, No. 16 French for men)
- Sterile towels
- 5-ml syringe of sterile saline, with needle
- 20-ml syringe
- Clamp
- Water-soluble, sterile lubricant
- Connecting tube and collecting bag
- Sterile basin
- Tape for securing the catheter

_____

*Not required by USDOT for certification as a paramedic.

Catheterization of a Male

- Place a towel beneath the patient's penis.
- Wash your hands, and don sterile gloves; arrange your equipment on a sterile towel where you can reach it easily. Test the balloon on the Foley catheter to make sure it doesn't leak.
- With your right hand (if you are positioned on the patient's left side), retract the patient's foreskin, if present, and hold the penis by the shaft.
- With your left hand, use the clamp to pick up a sterile sponge soaked in antiseptic solution; wash the glans.
- Touch nothing but the catheter and sterile equipment with your left hand. Lubricate the distal end of the Foley catheter and the urethral meatus, and introduce 10 to 15 ml of lubricant into the urethra via the large syringe (Fig. 23-89A).
- Raise the shaft of the penis straight up with your right hand (Fig. 23-89B), and rapidly introduce and advance the catheter. Advance it almost to its bifurcation before inflating the balloon with 5 ml of sterile saline.
- Pull back slightly on the catheter so that the balloon will be flush against the prostatic urethra.
- Connect the catheter to tubing of the drainage system.
- Tape the tubing, *not* the catheter, to the inner surface of the patient's thigh (Fig. 23-89C); avoid tension on the catheter.
- If the bladder is full, do not allow it to empty all at once, for very rapid decompression of the bladder may cause profound vagal stimulation and slow the heart. Allow only about 100 ml at a time to be evacuated, then clamp the connecting tubing for a few moments. Unclamp, allow another 100 ml to pass, and clamp again. Continue until the bladder has emptied, at which point the tubing may be left unclamped.

Catheterization of a Female

- If the paramedic is a male, a female chaperone should be present.
- Place the patient supine with knees bent and hips abducted.
- Observe the same sterile precautions as in catheterization of the male; cleanse the urethral meatus thoroughly with antiseptic solution.
- Lubricate the catheter tip, and advance it into the urethra.
- Subsequent steps are the same as for catheterization of the male.

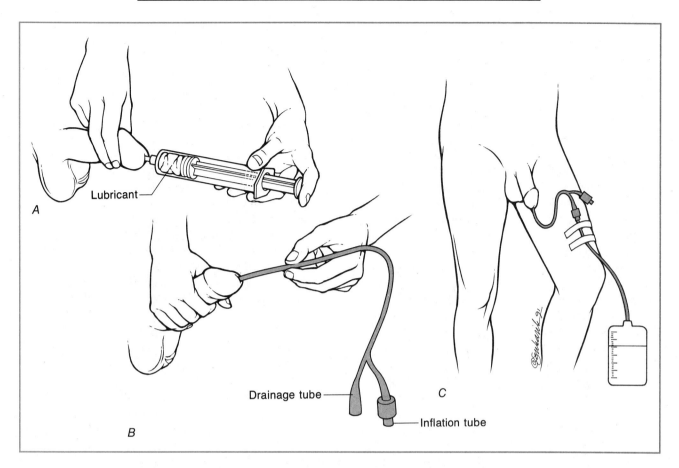

FIGURE 23-89. **CATHETERIZATION OF THE BLADDER.** (A) Lubricate the urethra. (B) Rapidly advance the catheter. (C) Tape the collection tubing (not the catheter) to the patient's inner thigh. Throughout the procedure, use one hand to touch the patient and the other to touch sterile equipment.

GLOSSARY

acetylcholine Chemical mediator of the *parasympathetic* nervous system.

afterload The resistance against which the ventricle contracts.

agonal rhythm Cardiac dysrhythmia seen just before the heart stops altogether; essentially asystole with occasional QRS complexes that are not associated with cardiac output.

algorithm Step-by-step procedure for solving a problem.

anastomosis Joining together of two tubelike structures, such as two blood vessels.

aneurysm Dilatation or outpouching of a blood vessel.

angina pectoris Sudden pain from myocardial ischemia, caused by relative insufficiency in the circulation to cardiac muscle.

anorexia Lack of appetite.

aortic valve Valve between the left ventricle and the aorta.

arteriole Small blood vessel that carries oxygenated blood.

arteriosclerosis Pathologic condition in which arterial walls become thickened and inelastic.

atheroma Mass of fatty tissue that develops in the intima of certain arteries.

atherosclerosis Common type of arteriosclerosis affecting the coronary and cerebral arteries.

atrial kick The addition to ventricular volume contributed by contraction of the atria.

atrioventricular (AV) junction Portion of the electric conduction system of the heart located in the upper part of the interventricular septum that conducts the excitation impulse from the atria to the bundle of His.

atrioventricular (AV) node Special structure located in the AV junction that slows conduction through the AV junction.

atrioventricular (AV) valves   Cardiac valves that separate the atria from their respective ventricles (the tricuspid and mitral valves).

automaticity   Spontaneous initiation of depolarizing electric impulses by pacemaker sites within the electric conduction system of the heart.

autonomic nervous system   Subdivision of the nervous system that controls largely involuntary bodily functions; it comprises the sympathetic and parasympathetic nervous systems.

bundle branches   Portion of the electric conduction system in the ventricles that conducts the depolarizing impulse from the bundle of His to the Purkinje network in the myocardium; subdivided into a right bundle branch and a left bundle branch.

bundle of His   Portion of the electric conduction system in the interventricular septum that conducts the depolarizing impulse from the AV junction to the right and left bundle branches.

cardiac axis   The average direction of current flow across the myocardium.

cardiac output   The amount of blood pumped by either ventricle per minute, calculated by multiplying the stroke volume by the heart rate.

chordae tendinae   Fibrous strands shaped like umbrella stays that attach the free edges of the AV valve leaflets to the papillary muscles.

collateral circulation   Network of arteries and capillaries that furnish blood to a segment of tissue whose original arterial supply has been obstructed.

contractility   Ability of a muscle to contract when depolarized by an electric impulse; the capacity of myocardial cells to vary their speed and degree of contraction without a change in their stretch.

coronary artery   Blood vessel that supplies the heart.

coronary sinus   Large vessel in the posterior part of the coronary sulcus into which the coronary veins empty.

coronary sulcus   Groove along the exterior surface of the heart that separates the atria from the ventricles.

depolarization   The process of discharging resting muscle fibers by an electric impulse that causes them to contract.

diaphoresis   Profuse sweating.

diastole   Period of ventricular *relaxation* during which the ventricles passively refill with blood.

dissecting aneurysm   Aneurysm formed by separation of the layers of the arterial wall.

diuretic   Drug used to promote elimination of excess extracellular fluid by increasing the renal secretion of urine.

ectopic focus   Pacemaker site located in some part of the electric conduction system other than the sinoatrial node.

electromechanical dissociation (EMD)   Condition in which ECG complexes are present without effective cardiac contractions.

endocardium   Thin membrane lining the inside of the heart.

epicardium   Thin membrane covering the outside of the heart; the visceral pericardium.

epinephrine   Hormone and drug with powerful beta stimulating properties.

hepatomegaly   Enlargement of the liver, seen, for example, in chronic right heart failure.

hypokalemia   Abnormally low concentration of potassium in the blood.

infarction   Death of a localized area of tissue caused by the cutting off of its blood supply; necrosis.

interventricular septum   Thin, muscular wall dividing the right and left ventricles.

ischemia   Tissue anoxia from diminished blood flow, usually caused by narrowing or occlusion of the artery to the tissue.

lead   Any one of the records of the ECG, depending on the direction of current flow.

mitral valve   Valve between the left atrium and left ventricle.

myocardium   Heart muscle.

necrosis   Death of tissue, usually caused by cessation of its blood supply.

norepinephrine   A naturally occurring neurotransmitter and a synthetically made drug with powerful alpha sympathetic properties.

orthopnea   Dyspnea produced or exacerbated by the recumbent position.

pacemaker   Specialized tissue within the heart that initiates excitation impulses; also, an electronic device used to stimulate cardiac contraction when the electric conduction system of the heart is malfunctioning.

palpitation   Sensation, usually perceived under the left breast, of the heart's "skipping a beat," most often caused by a premature ventricular contraction.

papillary muscles   Protrusions of the myocardium into the ventricular cavities to which the chordae tendinae are attached.

paroxysmal nocturnal dyspnea (PND)   Severe shortness of breath occurring at night after several hours of recumbency.

pericardium   Tough, fibrous sac containing the heart and the origins of the great vessels.

phlebotomy   The withdrawal of blood from a vein.

plaque   Calcified atheroma.

plasmin   Naturally occurring clot-dissolving enzyme,

usually present in the body in its inactive form, plasminogen.

preload   The pressure under which a ventricle fills.

pulmonic valve   Valve between the right ventricle and the pulmonary artery.

Purkinje network   System of fibers in the ventricles that conduct the excitation impulse from the bundle branches to the myocardium.

recanalization   Opening up of new channels through a blocked artery.

reperfusion   Resumption of blood flow through an artery.

repolarization   Electric process of recharging depolarized muscle fibers back to their resting state.

retrosternal   Behind the sternum.

semilunar valves   The aortic and pulmonic valves of the heart.

sinoatrial (SA) node   Dominant pacemaker of the heart, located at the junction of the superior vena cava and the right atrium.

stroke volume   Volume of blood pumped forward with each ventricular contraction.

sympathomimetic   Mimicking the properties of the sympathetic nervous system neurotransmitters.

syncope   Fainting; a brief loss of consciousness.

systole   Period during which the ventricles *contract.*

thrombolysis   The process of dissolving blood clots.

thrombus   A fixed blood clot that forms inside a blood vessel.

tricuspid valve   Valve between the right atrium and right ventricle.

tunica adventitia   Protective fibrous covering that gives a blood vessel the strength to withstand pressure against its walls.

tunica intima   Thin, innermost layer of a blood vessel.

tunica media   Middle, muscular layer of a blood vessel that gives the vessel its contractility.

vagotonic   Mimicking the action of the vagus nerve, hence stimulating parasympathetic effects.

Valsalva maneuver   Forced exhalation against a closed glottis, the effect of which is to stimulate the vagus nerve and thereby slow the heart rate.

venule   Very small vein.

to identify the patient's specific problem on the basis of a medication that he is taking. Beta blockers, for example, are prescribed for the relief of angina, to lower blood pressure in hypertension, and to prevent recurrence of AMI. Similarly, diuretic medications may be given simply to help rid the body of excess fluid in chronic heart failure or because of their effects in lowering blood pressure. Thus one needs to look at any given medication on the patient's bedside table or in his bathroom medicine cabinet in the context of his clinical history and the other medications he is taking.

Digitalis Preparations

Digitalis preparations are prescribed either for the treatment of chronic CONGESTIVE HEART FAILURE or for certain rapid ATRIAL DYSRHYTHMIAS (e.g., rapid atrial flutter, atrial fibrillation, supraventricular dysrhythmias). Digitalis acts by (1) increasing the strength of cardiac contractions, thereby improving cardiac output, and (2) slowing down conduction through the AV junction (thus, in atrial fibrillation or flutter, allowing fewer impulses to be conducted through to the ventricles—so the overall heart rate slows). At least 30 to 40 percent of patients taking digitalis develop some symptoms of *toxicity* from the drug. Those symptoms may include loss of appetite, nausea, vomiting, headache, blurred vision, yellow vision, and various cardiac dysrhythmias. VIRTUALLY ANY CARDIAC DYSRHYTHMIA MAY BE CAUSED BY DIGITALIS TOXICITY, so it is important to question all patients with disturbances in cardiac rhythm to determine whether they are taking digitalis.

Patients taking digitalis are very sensitive to *calcium* preparations. They are also very sensitive to a *fall in serum potassium*, so caution must be exercised in giving agents that might reduce the body's potassium stores, for instance, diuretics or large quantities of sodium bicarbonate.

APPENDIX: MEDICATIONS COMMONLY PRESCRIBED TO PATIENTS WITH CARDIOVASCULAR DISEASES

Patients with diseases affecting the cardiovascular system may be taking a wide variety of medications for a variety of reasons, and it is not always possible

---

COMMONLY USED DIGITALIS PREPARATIONS

Generic name	*Trade name*
Digoxin	**Lanoxin**
Digitoxin	**Crystodigin**

Antianginal Agents

Three main classes of drugs are used to relieve the pain of angina—nitrates, beta sympathetic blockers, and calcium channel blockers. All of them work exclusively or primarily on the demand side of the oxygen supply/demand equation; that is, all of them diminish, in one way or another, myocardial oxygen demand.

Nitrates

Nitrates were the first drugs to be used for the relief of angina. The prototype of the group is nitroglycerin, which comes as rapid-acting sublingual tablets, sustained release oral tablets, topically applied ointment, and patches that are stuck onto the skin. In its sublingual form, nitroglycerin is one of very few drugs that is taken by the sublingual route; so if a patient reports that he takes a medicine that he puts under his tongue, more likely than not that medicine is nitroglycerin.

Nitroglycerin is thought to exert its therapeutic effect by decreasing the work of the heart. Thus the heart's need for oxygen is decreased, as is the anginal pain that results from insufficient oxygenation. Nitroglycerin usually takes effect within 3 to 5 minutes of administration.

Nitroglycerin also causes significant *vasodilatation* and for that reason is sometimes used in the field as adjunctive therapy in the treatment of pulmonary edema secondary to left heart failure. Used in that circumstance, nitroglycerin produces an "internal phlebotomy," that is, a pooling of blood within the venous vessels that reduces the blood volume in the pulmonary vasculature just as if blood had been physically withdrawn from the body (**phlebotomy**).

When a patient reports that he has taken nitroglycerin for his chest pain, you need to find out: (1) HOW MANY nitroglycerin tablets did the patient take? and (2) Did the nitroglycerin relieve the pain? Failure of nitroglycerin to relieve anginal pain can occur for one of two reasons—either the pain is of extraordinary severity, such as that associated with acute myocardial infarction, or the nitroglycerin is stale and no longer effective. Nitroglycerin loses its potency very quickly after the bottle has been opened, and by 30 days after exposure to air, it may be entirely inactive. To distinguish between the two possibilities—very severe pain versus outdated nitroglycerin—you need to ask a few more questions. Fresh, potent nitroglycerin has certain distinct side effects, among them a transient, throbbing headache. It also has a rather bitter taste. If the patient did not find the pill bitter or did not experience a headache when he took the nitroglycerin, chances are the drug was outdated and ineffective. If, however, he did experience the throbbing in his head but still got no relief from his chest pain, one must suspect that the patient is having an AMI.

As noted, nitrates are also available in long-acting preparations that are swallowed rather than taken sublingually. The names of some of the more commonly prescribed nitrates are as follows:

COMMONLY PRESCRIBED NITRATES

Cardilate	**Nitrol**
Iso-Bid	**Nitrong**
Isordil	**Nitrostat**
NitrAnol	**Pentritol**
Nitro-Bid	**Peritrate**
Nitro-Dur	**Sorbide**
Nitroglycerin	**Sorbitrate**
Nitroglyn	**Tridil**

Beta Blockers

Drugs that block beta sympathetic receptors are also prescribed for the relief of angina. They work by decreasing the rate and strength of cardiac contractions and thereby decreasing the heart's demand for oxygen. Patients taking beta blocking drugs on a regular basis usually become resistant to the action of beta stimulating agents, such as epinephrine. When such patients suffer cardiac arrest, therefore, the administration of epinephrine during resuscitation attempts may not have the desired effect because the action of epinephrine may be blocked.

BETA BLOCKING AGENTS

Generic name	*Trade name*
Acebutolol	**Sectral**
Atenolol	**Tenormin**
Labetalol	**Normodyne**
	Trandate
Metoprolol	**Lopressor**
Nadolol	**Corgard**
	Corzide
Pindolol	**Visken**
Propranolol	**Inderal**
Timolol	**Blocadren**
	Timolide

Calcium Channel Blockers

Calcium channel blockers, as their name implies, block the influx of calcium ions into cardiac muscle. It is thought, therefore, that these agents relieve angina in two ways—first of all by preventing spasm of the coronary arteries, and secondly by weakening cardiac contraction and thereby decreasing myocardial oxygen demand. *Hypotension* may be a significant side effect.

CALCIUM CHANNEL BLOCKERS

Generic name	Trade name
Diltiazem	**Cardizem**
Nifedipine	**Aldalat**
	Procardia
Verapamil	**Calan**
	Isoptin

Antiarrhythmic Drugs

Antiarrhythmic drugs are used to control chronic disturbances in cardiac rhythm. Thus, when you encounter a patient taking one of these agents, you know the patient has had significant dysrhythmias in the past, which justifies particular surveillance for recurrent rhythm disturbances. PATIENTS TAKING ANTIARRHYTHMIC DRUGS SHOULD BE MONITORED while under the paramedic's care.

Some of the drugs that we've already encountered under other categories are also used for their antiarrhythmic activity. Digitalis preparations, as noted, are used to suppress atrial dysrhythmias. The beta blockers are sometimes prescribed for their suppressive effect on myocardial excitability, as are some of the calcium channel blockers. Finally, the seizure medication, phenytoin sodium (Dilantin), is occasionally used for cardiac dysrhythmias, particularly for those dysrhythmias due to digitalis toxicity.

COMMONLY USED ANTIARRHYTHMIC DRUGS

Generic name	Trade name	Indications
Amiodarone	**Cordarone**	Ventricular tachycardia and other life-threatening ventricular dysrhythmias
Bretylium tosylate	**Bretylol**	Ventricular tachycardia; ventricular fibrillation
Digoxin	**Lanoxin**	Atrial flutter/fibrillation
Disopyramide	**Norpace** **Persantine**	Ventricular dysrhythmias
Flecainide	**Tambocor**	Life-threatening ventricular dysrhythmias
Mexiletine	**Mexitil**	Ventricular dysrhythmias
Procainamide	**Procan** **Pronestyl**	Ventricular dysrhythmias
Quinidine	**Cardioquin** **Duraquin**	Ventricular dysrhythmias
	Quinidex **Quinaglute** **Quinora**	Some atrial dysrhythmias
Tocainide	**Tonocard**	Ventricular dysrhythmias
Verapamil	**Calan** **Isoptin**	Supraventricular tachycardias

---

Diuretics ("Water Pills")

Diuretics are prescribed to patients with chronic fluid overload, principally those in CHRONIC CONGESTIVE HEART FAILURE, but they are also used as primary or adjunctive therapy in the treatment of HYPERTENSION. Diuretics act by tricking the kidneys into excreting more sodium and water than usual (the desired effect). Not being very smart, however, the kidneys also tend to dump out potassium along with the sodium (an undesired effect). Thus patients taking diuretics often become depleted of potassium if they are not given potassium supplements. Those patients who do develop potassium deficits (**hypokalemia**) are prone to cardiac dysrhythmias—especially if they are also taking digitalis.

COMMONLY PRESCRIBED DIURETICS

Generic name	Trade name
Bumetanide	**Bumex**
Chlorthalidone	**Hygroton**
Ethacrynic acid	**Edecrin**
Furosemide	**Lasix**
Hydralazine	**Apresoline**

Indapamide	**Lozol**
Methyclothiazide	**Aquatensen**
Metolazone	**Diulo**
	Zaroxolyn
Quinethazone	**Hydromox**
Spironolactone	**Aldactone**
Thiazides	**Anhydron**
	Diuril
	Dyazide
	Esidrix
	HydroDIURIL
	Maxzide
	Metahydrin
	Naqua
	Saluron
Triamterene	**Dyrenium**
Combination	**Aldactadine**
drugs	**Corzide**
	Diucardin

Labetalol*	**Normodyne**
	Trandate
Lisinopril	**Prinivil**
	Zestril
Methyldopa	**Aldomet**
Prazosin	**Minipress**
Propranolol*	**Inderal**
Reserpine	**Sandril**
	Ser-Ap-Es
	Serpasil
Trimethophan	**Arfonad**

*beta blocker

Antihypertensive Drugs

As the term implies, antihypertensive agents are used to treat HYPERTENSION (high blood pressure). Many of the *diuretic agents* already listed are also used as antihypertensives or in combination with antihypertensives for a synergistic effect. Similarly, *beta blockers* are used in the treatment of hypertension.

It is often difficult to regulate the dosage of antihypertensives so that the patient's blood pressure is lowered enough but not too much. Thus, some patients taking these agents may suffer symptoms of *hypotension,* including weakness and dizziness. A feeling of giddiness when going from a recumbent to a sitting or standing position is particularly common; it is termed **orthostatic hypotension,** that is, hypotension that occurs with a change in posture. Every patient taking antihypertensive drugs, therefore, should have his or her blood pressure checked in both the recumbent and sitting position, to detect orthostatic hypotension.

Anticoagulant Drugs ("Blood Thinners")

Anticoagulant drugs diminish the ability of the blood to clot and are prescribed to patients who have had recurrent problems with blood clots (e.g., patients who have suffered pulmonary emboli) as well as to those who might be prone to develop clots (e.g., some patients who have had a myocardial infarction in the past; patients with artificial heart valves or valvular heart disease). Because these agents interfere with blood clotting, patients taking them are apt to bleed excessively from minor trauma or even venipuncture, and the paramedic should be alert to that possibility. The principal *oral* anticoagulant drug is warfarin (**Coumadin, Panwarfin**). Patients on home dialysis may be taking the intravenous anticoagulant, heparin, during their dialysis cycle.

FURTHER READING

ANATOMY, PHYSIOLOGY, AND PATIENT ASSESSMENT
Caroline NL. *Emergency Medical Treatment: A Text for EMT-As and EMT-Intermediates* (3rd ed.). Boston: Little, Brown, 1991. Chaps. 7 and 8.
Dennison DA Jr. Visual clues to cardiac diagnosis. *Emerg Med* 16(19):99, 1984.
Lampe B. Documenting cardiac emergencies. *Emergency* 25(2):44, 1993.
Maydayag TM. Emergency cardiac assessment. *Emerg Med Serv* 7(5):42, 1978.

ANGINA
Birdwell BG et al. Evaluating chest pain: The patient's presentation style alters the physician's diagnostic approach. *Arch Intern Med* 153:1991, 1993.
Chatterjee K, Rouleau JL, Parmley WW. Medical management of patients with angina. *JAMA* 252:1170, 1984.

COMMONLY PRESCRIBED ANTIHYPERTENSIVE AGENTS

Generic name	*Trade name*
Captopril	**Capoten**
Clonodine	**Catapres**
Enalapril	**Vasotec**
Guanethedine	**Ismelin**

Conti CR, Christie LG. Sorting out chest pain. *Emerg Med* 16(3):155, 1984.

Cooke DH. To stabilize unstable angina. *Emerg Med* 24(9):99, 1992.

Fein SA. Unstable angina: What should we do? *Emerg Med* 24(4):127, 1992.

Hultgren HN, Giacomini JC, Miller C. Treatment of unstable angina. *JAMA* 253:2555, 1985.

Rahimtoola SH. Unstable angina: Current status. *Mod Concepts Cardiovasc Dis* 54(4):19, 1985.

Rotche R, Sobotka PA, Wehrmacher WH. Is it unstable angina or acute MI? *Emerg Med* 21(15):59, 1989.

Wheatley CE. Hyperventilation syndrome: A frequent cause of chest pain. *Chest* 68:195, 1975.

Yusuf S, Wittes J, Friedman L. Overview of results of randomized clinical trials in heart disease: II. Unstable angina, heart failure, primary prevention with aspirin, and risk factor modification. *JAMA* 260:2259, 1988.

ACUTE MYOCARDIAL INFARCTION

American College of Cardiology/American Heart Association. Guidelines for the early management of patients with acute myocardial infarction. *J Am Coll Cardiol* 16:249, 1990.

Aronow WS. Prevalence of presenting symptoms of recognized acute myocardial infarction and of unrecognized healed myocardial infarction in elderly patients. *Am J Cardiol* 60:1182, 1987.

Assey ME. Ischemia without symptoms. *Emerg Med* 20(7):26, 1988.

Ayres SM. The prevention and treatment of shock in acute myocardial infarction. *Chest* 93(Suppl):17S, 1988.

Barsky AJ et al. Silent myocardial ischemia: Is the person or the event silent? *JAMA* 264:1132, 1990.

Bayer AJ et al. Changing presentation of myocardial infarction with increasing old age. *J Am Geriatr Soc* 34:263, 1986.

Case RB et al. Living alone after myocardial infarction: Impact on prognosis. *JAMA* 267:515, 1992.

Cousins N. *The Healing Heart: Antidotes to Panic and Helplessness.* New York: Norton, 1983.

Cummins RO. Interhospital transfer of acutely ill cardiac patients (editorial). *JAMA* 259:1707, 1988.

Deedwania PC, Carbajal EV. The dangers of silent ischemia. *Emerg Med* 24(3):165, 1992.

Flaker GC, Singh VN. Prevention of myocardial reinfarction. *Postgrad Med* 94(6):94, 1993.

Gibler WB et al. Prehospital diagnosis and treatment of acute myocardial infarction: A north-south perspective. *Am Heart J* 212:1, 1991.

Goldberg RJ et al. Recent changes in attack and survival rates of acute myocardial infarction (1975–1981). *JAMA* 255:2774, 1986.

Goldberg RJ et al. Time of onset of symptoms of acute myocardial infarction. *Am J Cardiol* 66:140, 1990.

Gore JM et al. Feasibility and safety of emergency interhospital transport of patients during early hours of acute myocardial infarction. *Arch Intern Med* 149:353, 1989.

Grace WJ, Chadbourne JA. The first hour in acute myocardial infarction. *Heart Lung* 3:737, 1974.

Hargarten KM et al. Limitations of prehospital predictors of acute myocardial infarction and unstable angina. *Ann Emerg Med* 16:1326, 1987.

Heriot AG, Brecker SJ, Coltart DJ. Delay in presentation after myocardial infarction. *J R Soc Med* 86:642, 1993.

Herlihy T et al. Nausea and vomiting during acute myocardial infarction and its relation to infarct size and location. *Am J Cardiol* 60:20, 1987.

Hine LK et al. Meta-analytic evidence against prophylactic use of lidocaine in acute myocardial infarction. *Arch Intern Med* 149:2694, 1989.

Hollander JE et al. Cocaine-induced myocardial infarction: An analysis and review of the literature. *J Emerg Med* 10:169, 1992.

Kahn JK et al. Aggressive treatment of acute myocardial infarction. *Postgrad Med* 94(8):51, 1993.

Kannel WB, Abbott RD. Incidence and prognosis of unrecognized myocardial infarction: An update on the Framingham Study. *N Engl J Med* 311:1144, 1984.

Kaplan L, Walsh D, Burney RE. Emergency aeromedical transport of patients with acute myocardial infarction. *Ann Emerg Med* 16:55, 1987.

Karlson BW et al. Clinical factors associated with delay time in suspected acute myocardial infarction. *Am Heart J* 120:1213, 1990.

Kereiakes DJ et al. Time delays in the diagnosis and treatment of acute myocardial infarction: A tale of eight cities. *Am Heart J* 120:773, 1990.

Ledwich JR et al. Chest pain during myocardial infarction. *JAMA* 244:2171, 1980.

Luria MH et al. Long-term follow-up after recovery from acute myocardial infarction: Observations on survival, ventricular arrhythmias, and sudden death. *Arch Intern Med* 145:1592, 1985.

Madden JF. Rapid diagnosis of acute MI. *Emerg Med* 23(16):107, 1991.

McCarthy BD et al. Missed diagnoses of acute myocardial infarction in the emergency department: Results from a multicenter study. *Ann Emerg Med* 22:579, 1993.

Mitchell JM. The golden hour of MI. *Emerg Med* 22(16):19, 1990.

Muller RT et al. Painless myocardial infarction in the elderly. *Am Heart J* 119:202, 1990.

National Heart Attack Alert Program Coordinating Committee. Emergency department: Rapid identification and treatment of patients with acute myocardial infarction. *Ann Emerg Med* 23:311, 1994.

O'Doherty M et al. Five hundred patients with myocardial infarction monitored within one hour of symptoms. *Br Med J* 286:1405, 1983.

Rubenstein DG et al. Transfer of acutely ill cardiac patients for definitive care: Demonstrated safety in 755 cases. *JAMA* 259:1695, 1988.

Smith HWB et al. Acute myocardial infarction temporally related to cocaine use. *Ann Intern Med* 107:13, 1987.

Subramaniam PN. Complications of acute myocardial infarction. *Postgrad Med* 95(2):143, 1994.

Teo KK et al. Effects of prophylactic antiarrhythmic drug therapy in acute myocardial infarction. *JAMA* 270:1589, 1993.

Topol EJ et al. Safety of helicopter transport and out-of-hospital fibrinolytic therapy in patients with evolving myocardial infarction. *Cathet Cardiovasc Diagn* 12:151, 1986.

Turi ZG et al. Implications for acute intervention related to time of hospital arrival in acute myocardial infarction. *Am J Cardiol* 58:203, 1986.

Willich SN et al. Physical exertion as a trigger of acute myocardial infarction. *N Engl J Med* 329:1684, 1993.

Winsor T. The electrocardiogram in acute myocardial infarction. *Clin Symp*, 1968.

Wroblewski M et al. Symptoms of myocardial infarction in

old age: Clinical case retrospective and prospective studies. *Age Aging* 15:99, 1986.

Yusuf S, Wittes J, Friedman L. Overview of results of randomized clinical trials in heart disease: I. Treatments following myocardial infarction. *JAMA* 260:2088, 1988.

THROMBOLYTIC THERAPY IN AMI

Adams J et al. Earliest electrocardiographic evidence of myocardial infarction: Implications for thrombolytic treatment. *Br Med J* 307:409, 1993.

Anderson HV, Willerson JT. Thrombolysis in acute myocardial infarction. *N Engl J Med* 329:703, 1993.

Applebaum D et al. Feasibility of pre-hospital fibrinolytic therapy in acute myocardial infarction. *Am J Emerg Med* 4:201, 1986.

Aufderheide TP et al. Feasibility of prehospital r-TPA therapy in chest pain patients. *Ann Emerg Med* 21:379, 1992.

Bossaert L et al. Prehospital thrombolytic treatment of acute myocardial infarction with anisoylated plasminogen streptokinase activator complex. *Crit Care Med* 16:823, 1988.

Bourn S. Clot busters or bust. *JEMS* 18(5):83, 1993.

Bresler MJ. Future role of thrombolytic therapy in emergency medicine. *Ann Emerg Med* 18:1331, 1989.

Burney RE, Walsh DG. Identification and transport of patients with acute myocardial infarction for thrombolytic therapy. *Ann Emerg Med* 17:1158, 1988.

Burney RE et al. Reperfusion arrhythmia: Myth or reality? *Ann Emerg Med* 18:240, 1989.

Califf RM et al. Experience with the use of tPA in the treatment of acute myocardial infarction. *Ann Emerg Med* 17:1176, 1988.

Castaigne A et al. Prehospital administration of anisoylated plasminogen streptokinase activator complex in acute myocardial infarction. *Drug* 33(Suppl 3):231, 1987.

Cross SJ et al. Safety of thrombolysis in association with cardiopulmonary resuscitation. *Br Med J* 303:1242, 1991.

Cummins RO, Eisenberg MS. From pain to reperfusion: What role for the prehospital 12-lead ECG? *Ann Emerg Med* 19:1343, 1990.

Doorey AJ et al. Thrombolytic therapy of acute myocardial infarction: Keeping the unfulfilled promises. *JAMA* 268:3108, 1992.

Eisenberg MS et al. Thrombolytic therapy. *Ann Emerg Med* 22:417, 1993.

European Myocardial Infarction Project Group. Prehospital thrombolytic therapy in patients with suspected acute myocardial infarction. *N Engl J Med* 329:383, 1993.

Grim PS, Feldman T, Childers RW. Evaluation of patients for the needs of thrombolytic therapy in the prehospital setting. *Ann Emerg Med* 18:483, 1989.

Handberg E, Keith T, Rucinski P. Clot busters: The future of EMS thrombolytics. *JEMS* 17(4):74, 1992.

Handlin LR, Vacek JL. Thrombolytic therapy for acute myocardial infarction: Are inclusion criteria too stringent? *Postgrad Med* 95(4):77, 1994.

Hartmann JR et al. Intravenous streptokinase in acute myocardial infarction: Experience in community hospitals served by paramedics. *Am Heart J* 11:1030, 1986.

Heras M et al. Emergency thrombolysis in acute myocardial infarction. *Ann Emerg Med* 17:1168, 1988.

Hillman DE et al. Reducing time delays in the administration of thrombolytic therapy to patients with acute myocardial infarction. *Ann Pharmacother* 25:1096, 1991.

Holmberg S et al. Very early thrombolytic therapy in suspected acute myocardial infarction. *Am J Cardiol* 65:401, 1990.

Karagounis L et al. Impact of field-transmitted electrocardiography on time to in-hospital thrombolytic therapy in acute myocardial infarction. *Am J Cardiol* 66:786, 1990.

Kennedy JW et al. Recent changes in management of acute myocardial infarction: Implications for emergency care physicians. *J Am Coll Cardiol* 11:446, 1988.

Krumholz HM et al. Cost effectiveness of thrombolytic therapy with streptokinase in elderly patients with suspected acute myocardial infarction. *N Engl J Med* 327:7, 1992.

Levy DB. rt-PA. . .A new era. *Emergency* 21(1):19, 1989.

Linderer T et al. Prehospital thrombolysis: Beneficial effects of very early treatment on infarct size. *J Am Coll Cardiol* 22:1304, 1993.

Linnik W, Tintinalli JE, Ramos R. Associated reactions during and immediately after rtPA infusion. *Ann Emerg Med* 18:234, 1989.

Mathey DG et al. Prehospital thrombolysis treatment of acute myocardial infarction: A randomized double-blind study. *Dtsch Med Wochenschr* 115:803, 1990.

Mercer S. Thrombolysis for the acute myocardial infarction. *Emergency* 24(2):29, 1992.

Peppers MP. Thrombolytics update. *Emergency* 25(2):24, 1993.

Rapaport E. Thrombolytic agents in acute myocardial infarction. *N Engl J Med* 320:861, 1989.

Reperfusion injury after thrombolytic therapy for acute myocardial infarction (editorial). *Lancet* 2(8664):655, 1989.

Ruffing M. New help for AMI. *Emergency* 22(6):43, 1990.

Schmidt SB et al. The prehospital phase of acute myocardial infarction in the era of thrombolysis. *Am J Cardiol* 65:1411, 1990.

Schofer J et al. Prehospital thrombolysis in acute myocardial infarction. *Am J Cardiol* 66:1492, 1990.

Schreiber TL. Review of clinical studies of thrombolytic agents in acute myocardial infarction. *Am J Med* 83 (Suppl 2A):20, 1987.

Schreiber TL. Aspirin and thrombolytic therapy for acute myocardial infarction: Should the combination now be a routine therapy? *Drugs* 38:180, 1989.

Sherrid M et al. A pilot study of paramedic-administered prehospital thrombolysis for acute myocardial infarction. *Clin Cardiol* 13:421, 1990.

Sherry S. Mistaken guidelines for thrombolytic therapy of acute myocardial infarction in the elderly. *J Am Coll Cardiol* 17:1237, 1991.

Stewart C. Prehospital thrombolysis. *Emerg Med Serv* 22 (11):47, 1993.

Tebbe U et al. Single-bolus injection of recombinant tissue-type plasminogen activator in acute myocardial infarction. *Am J Cardiol* 64:448, 1989.

Theroux P. Coronary thrombolysis: Prehospital use. *Can J Cardiol* 9:521, 1993.

Tisdale J et al. Steptokinase-induced anaphylaxis. *Ann Pharmacother* 23:984, 1989.

Weaver WD et al. Prehospital-initiated vs hospital-initiated thrombolytic therapy. *JAMA* 270:1211, 1993.

Weiss AT et al. Prehospital coronary thrombolysis: A new strategy in acute myocardial infarction. *Chest* 92:124, 1987.

HEART FAILURE

Abrams J. Vasodilator therapy for chronic congestive heart failure. *JAMA* 254:3070, 1985.

Barnett JC et al. Sublingual captopril in the treatment of acute heart failure. *Curr Ther Res* 49:274, 1991.

Bersten AD et al. Treatment of severe cardiogenic pulmonary edema with continuous positive airway pressure delivered by face mask. *N Engl J Med* 325:1825, 1991.

Bertel O, Steiner A. Rotating tourniquets do not work in acute congestive heart failure and pulmonary edema. *Lancet* 1:762, 1980.

Centers for Disease Control. Mortality from congestive heart failure—United States, 1980–1990. *MMWR* 43:77, 1994.

Cohn JN, Fanciosa JA. Vasodilator therapy of cardiac failure. *N Engl J Med* 279:27, 254, 1977.

Forrester JS, Staniloff HM. Heart failure. *Emerg Med* 16(4):121, 1984.

Francis GS et al. Acute vasoconstrictor response to intravenous furosemide in patients with chronic congestive heart failure. *Ann Intern Med* 103:1, 1985.

Genton R, Jaffe AS. Management of congestive heart failure in patients with acute myocardial infarction. *JAMA* 256:2556, 1986.

Hoffman JR, Reynolds S. Comparison of nitroglycerin, morphine and furosemide in treatment of presumed prehospital pulmonary edema. *Chest* 92:586, 1987.

Kraus PE. Acute preload effects of furosemide. *Chest* 98:124, 1990.

Levy DB, Pollard T. Failure of the heart. *Emergency* 20(12):22, 1988.

Marantz PR et al. Clinical diagnosis of congestive heart failure in patients with acute dyspnea. *Chest* 97:776, 1990.

Markiewicz W et al. Sublingual isosorbide dinitrate in severe congestive failure. *Cardiology* 67:172, 1981.

McKee PA et al. The natural history of congestive heart failure: The Framingham study. *N Engl J Med* 285:1441, 1971.

Melandri G et al. Comparative haemodynamic effects of transdermal vs intravenous nitroglycerin in acute myocardial infarction with elevated pulmonary artery wedge pressure. *Eur Heart J* 11:649, 1990.

Morgan MT. Rotating tourniquets: A critical evaluation. *STAT* 2(2):63, 1980.

Murphy PM, Borgio JP. Successfully treating congestive heart failure. *JEMS* 16(9):46, 1991.

Posner MD. Cardiac failure: Tourniquets vs. phlebotomy (letter). *N Engl J Med* 290:1485, 1974.

Ramirez A, Abelmann WH. Cardiac decompensation. *N Engl J Med* 290:499, 1974.

Rasanen J et al. Continuous positive airway pressure by face mask in acute cardiogenic pulmonary edema. *Am J Cardiol* 55:296, 1985.

Roberts R. Inotropic therapy for cardiac failure associated with acute myocardial infarction. *Chest* 93(Suppl 1):22S, 1988.

Robin ED, Carroll IC, Zelis R. Pulmonary edema. *N Engl J Med* 288:239, 292, 1972.

Roth A. Are rotating tourniquets useful for left ventricular preload reduction in patients with acute myocardial infarction and heart failure? *Ann Emerg Med* 16:764, 1987.

Tresch DD et al. Out-of-hospital pulmonary edema: Diagnosis and treatment. *Ann Emerg Med* 12:533, 1983.

Vaisanen IT, Rasanen J. Continuous positive airway pressure and supplemental oxygen in the treatment of cardiogenic pulmonary edema. *Chest* 92:481, 1987.

Wuerz RC, Meador SA. Effects of prehospital medications on mortality and length of stay in congestive heart failure. *Ann Emerg Med* 21:669, 1992.

Wulf-Dirk B, Schupp D. Effect of sublingual nitroglycerin in emergency treatment of severe pulmonary edema. *Am J Cardiol* 41:931, 1978.

CARDIOGENIC SHOCK

Abdulla AM. On vasoactive drugs in cardiogenic shock. *Emerg Med* 15(2):28, 1983.

Goldberg LI. Dopamine: Clinical uses of an endogenous catecholamine. *N Engl J Med* 291, 707, 1974.

Handler CE. Cardiogenic shock. *Postgrad Med* 61:705, 1985.

Holzer J et al. Effectiveness of dopamine in patients with cardiogenic shock. *Am J Cardiol* 32:79, 1973.

Sibbald WJ. The Trendelenburg position: Hemodynamic effects in hypotensive and normotensive patients. *Crit Care Med* 7:218, 1975.

AORTIC ANEURYSM

Bessen H. Averting aortic catastrophes. *Emerg Med* 25(10):57, 1993.

Czekaj PS, Athas DP, Grishkin B. Sudden onset of severe back pain in a 38-year-old man. *Ann Emerg Med* 15:58, 1986.

Ernst CB. Abdominal aortic aneurysm. *N Engl J Med* 328:1167, 1993.

Grubbs TC. The ultimate emergency: Managing aortic aneurysms. *JEMS* 16(10):56, 1991.

Jehle D. Aortic disasters: No time for delay. *Emerg Med* 23(3):59, 1991.

Mohindra SK, Udeani GO. Intravenous esmolol in acute aortic dissection. *Ann Pharmacother* 25:735, 1991.

Rigolin VH et al. Update on aortic dissection. *Emerg Med* 25(13):17, 1993.

Spittell PC et al. Clinical features and differential diagnosis of aortic dissection: Experience with 236 cases (1980 through 1990). *Mayo Clin Proc* 68:642, 1993.

Tintinalli JE. Ruptured aortic aneurysm. *JACEP* 4:440, 1975.

Wheat MW. Acute dissecting aneurysms of the aorta: Diagnosis and treatment—1979. *Am Heart J* 99:373, 1980.

HYPERTENSION AND HYPERTENSIVE EMERGENCIES

American Society of Hypertension. Recommendations for routine blood pressure measurement by indirect cuff sphygmomanometry. *Am J Hypertens* 5:207, 1992.

Angeli P et al. Comparison of sublingual captopril and nifedipine in immediate treatment of hypertensive emergencies: A randomized, single-blind clinical trial. *Arch Intern Med* 151:678, 1991.

Bannon LT et al. Single dose oral atenolol for urgent blood pressure reduction. *Drugs* 25(Suppl 2):84, 1983.

Bertel O et al. Nifedipine in hypertensive emergencies. *Br Med J* 286:19, 1983.

Bledsoe BE. Hypertensive emergencies. *JEMS* 15(4):67, 1990.

Cressman MD et al. Intravenous labetalol in the management of severe hypertension and hypertensive emergencies. *Am Heart J* 107:980, 1984.

Ferguson RK, Vlasses PH. Hypertensive emergencies and urgencies. *JAMA* 255:1607, 1986.

Garrett BN, Kaplan NM. Efficacy of slow infusion of diazoxide in the treatment of severe hypertension without organ hypoperfusion. *Am Heart J* 103:390, 1982.

Gifford RW. Management of hypertensive crisis. *JAMA* 266:829, 1991.

Gonzalez ER et al. Dose-response evaluation of oral labetalol in patients presenting to the emergency department with accelerated hypertension. *Ann Emerg Med* 20:333, 1991.

Haft JI. Use of the calcium-channel blocker nifedipine in the management of hypertensive emergency. *Am J Emerg Med* Suppl 3(6):25, 1985.

Haft JI, Litterer WE. Chewing nifedipine to rapidly treat hypertension. *Arch Intern Med* 144:2357, 1984.

Huey J et al. Clinical evaluation of intravenous labetalol for the treatment of hypertensive urgency. *Am J Hypertens* 1(3, Part 3):284S, 1988.

Huysmans FTM, Thien T. Koene RA. Acute treatment of hypertension with slow infusion of diazoxide. *Arch Intern Med* 143:882, 1983.

Kannel WB et al. Role of blood pressure in the development of congestive heart failure. *N Engl J Med* 287:781, 1972.

Lebel M et al. Labetalol infusion in hypertensive emergencies. *Clin Pharmacol Ther* 37:615, 1985.

Maharaj B et al. A comparison of the acute hypotensive effects of two different doses of nifedipine. *Am Heart J* 124:720, 1992.

Maxwell MH et al. Error in blood pressure measurement due to incorrect cuff size in obese patients. *Lancet* 2:33, 1982.

O'Mailia JJ et al. Nifedipine-associated myocardial ischemia or infarction in the treatment of hypertensive urgencies. *Ann Intern Med* 107:185, 1987.

Phillips RA. Nifedipine and hypertensive urgencies. *Emerg Med* 22(15):91, 1990.

Rahn KG. How should we treat a hypertensive emergency? *Am J Cardiol* 63:48C, 1989.

Segal JL. A primer on hypertensive emergencies. *Emerg Med* 10(8):23, 1975.

Wright S. Use of nifedipine in hypertensive emergencies. *J Emerg Med* 6:584, 1988.

ECG INTERPRETATION AND SPECIFIC DYSRHYTHMIAS

Adgey AAJ et al. Initiation of ventricular fibrillation outside hospital in patients with acute ischaemic heart disease. *Br Heart J* 47:55, 1982.

Aufderheide TP et al. The diagnostic impact of prehospital 12-lead electrocardiography. *Ann Emerg Med* 19:1280, 1990.

Baerman JM et al. Differentiation of ventricular tachycardia from supraventricular tachycardia with aberration: Value of the clinical history. *Ann Emerg Med* 16:40, 1987.

Bilitch M. *A Manual of Cardiac Arrhythmias*. Boston: Little, Brown, 1971.

Bissett GS et al. The ice bag: A new technique for interruption of supraventricular tachycardia. *J Pediatr* 97:593, 1980.

Bluxhas J et al. Ventricular tachycardia in myocardial infarction: Relation to heart rate and premature ventricular contractions. *Eur Heart J* 6:745, 1985.

Caroline NL. *Ambulance Calls: Review Problems in Emergency Care* (3rd ed.). Boston: Little, Brown, 1991.

Cranefield PF. Ventricular fibrillation. *N Engl J Med* 289:732, 1973.

DeSouza N et al. Evaluation of warning arrhythmias before paroxysmal ventricular tachycardia during acute myocardial infarction in man. *Circulation* 60:814, 1979.

Dubin D. *Rapid Interpretation of EKGs* (3rd ed.). Tampa: Cover, 1974.

Hoffman JR et al. Postdefibrillation idioventricular rhythm: A salvageable condition. *West J Med* 146:188, 1987.

Levitt MA. Supraventricular tachycardia with aberrant conduction versus ventricular tachycardia: Differentiation and diagnosis. *Am J Emerg Med* 6:273, 1988.

Liberthson RB et al. Pathophysiologic observations on prehospital ventricular fibrillation and sudden cardiac death. *Circulation* 49:790, 1974.

McDonald JL. Coarse ventricular fibrillation presenting as asystole or very low amplitude ventricular fibrillation. *Crit Care Med* 10:790, 1982.

Mehta D et al. Relative efficacy of various physical manoeuvres in the termination of junctional tachycardia. *Lancet* 1(8596):1181, 1988.

Mercer S. 12-lead ECGs: Ready to hit the streets. *Emergency* 25(11):46, 1993.

Morady F et al. Clinical symptoms in patients with sustained ventricular tachycardia. *West J Med* 142:341, 1985.

Northover BJ. Ventricular tachycardia during the first 72 hours after acute myocardial infarction. *Cardiology* 69:149, 1982.

Otto LA, Aufderheide TP. Evaluation of ST segment elevation criteria for the prehospital electrocardiographic diagnosis of acute myocardial infarction. *Ann Emerg Med* 23:17, 1994.

Schaeffer WA, Cobb LA. Recurrent ventricular fibrillation and modes of death in out-of-hospital ventricular fibrillation. *N Engl J Med* 293:259, 1975.

Spokick DH et al. Normal sinus heart rate: Sinus tachycardia and sinus bradycardia redefined. *Am Heart J* 124:1119, 1992.

Taigman M, Canan S. The push for 12-lead ECGs. *JEMS* 17(4):65, 1992.

Tye K et al. R on T or R on P phenomenon? Relation to the genesis of ventricular tachycardia. *Am J Cardiol* 44:632, 1979.

Waxman MB et al. Vagal techniques for termination of paroxysmal supraventricular tachycardia. *Am J Cardiol* 46:655, 1980.

Wayne MA. Conversion of paroxysmal atrial tachycardia by facial immersion in ice water. *JACEP* 5:434, 1976.

Wertz EM. The art of ECG analysis *Emergency* 25(2):56, 1993.

Younger M. The top 10 misconceptions in electrocardiography. *Emergency* 26(2):33, 1994.

CARDIAC ARREST: CAUSES AND MECHANISMS

Adelson L, Hoffman W. Sudden death from coronary disease. *JAMA* 176:129, 1961.

Bass E. Cardiopulmonary arrest: Pathophysiology and neurologic complications. *Ann Intern Med* 103(Part 1):920, 1985.

Becker LB et al. Racial differences in the incidence of cardiac arrest and subsequent survival. *N Engl J Med* 3329:600, 1993.

Clinton JE et al. Cardiac arrest under age 40: Etiology and prognosis. *Ann Emerg Med* 13:1011, 1984.

Cobb LA. Cardiac arrest during sleep. *N Engl J Med* 311:1044, 1984.

Crozier I et al. Sudden death due to painless spasm in near normal coronary arteries. *Aust NZ J Med* 16:64, 1986.

Cummins RO. Cardiopulmonary resuscitation and sudden cardiac death: An annotated bibliography of the 1984 literature. *Am J Emerg Med* 3:485, 1985.

Eisenberg MS et al. Out-of-hospital cardiac arrest: Significance of symptoms in patients collapsing before and after arrival of paramedics. *Am J Emerg Med* 4:116, 1986.

Goldberg AH. Cardiopulmonary arrest. *N Engl J Med* 290:381, 1974.

Goldstein S et al. Analysis of cardiac symptoms preceding cardiac arrest. *Am J Cardiol* 58:1195, 1986.

James TN. Mysterious sudden death. *Chest* 62:454, 1972.

Kirschner RH, Eckner FAO, Baron RC. The cardiac pathology of sudden, unexplained nocturnal death in southeast Asian refugees. *JAMA* 256:2700, 1986.

Lynch P. Soldiers, sport and sudden death. *Lancet* 7:1235, 1980.

McCabe WC et al. Sudden death revisited. *Cardiovasc Med* 10(9):10, 1985.

Medendorp GS et al. Analysis of cardiac symptoms preceding cardiac arrest. *Am J Cardiol* 58:1195, 1986.

Muller JE et al. Circadian variation in the frequency of sudden cardiac death. *Circulation* 75:131, 1987.

Neuspiel DR, Kuller LH. Sudden and unexpected natural death in childhood and adolescence. *JAMA* 254:1321, 1985.

Pfeiffer RJ. Cardiac arrest and jogging. *Ann Emerg Med* 11:678, 1982.

Phillips M et al. Sudden cardiac death in air force recruits: A 20-year review. *JAMA* 256:2696, 1986.

Raymond JR, Berg EK, Knapp MJ. Nontraumatic prehospital sudden death in young adults. *Arch Intern Med* 148:303, 1988.

Safranek DJ, Eisenberg MS, Larsen MP. The epidemiology of cardiac arrest in young adults. *Ann Emerg Med* 21:1102, 1992.

Sarvesvaran R. Sudden natural deaths associated with commercial air travel. *Med Sci Law* 26:35, 1986.

Siscovick DS et al. The incidence of primary cardiac arrest during vigorous exercise. *N Engl J Med* 311:874, 1984.

Van Hoeyweghen RF et al. Survival after out-of-hospital cardiac arrest in elderly patients. *Ann Emerg Med* 21:1179, 1992.

Warren JV. Recurrent sudden death (editorial). *N Engl J Med* 293:298, 1975.

CPR: INDICATIONS

Blackhall LJ. Must we always use CPR? *N Engl J Med* 317:1281, 1987.

Council on Ethical and Judicial Affairs, American Medical Association. Guidelines for the appropriate use of do-not-resuscitate orders. *JAMA* 265:1868, 1991.

Crimmins TJ. The need for a prehospital DNR system. *Prehosp Disaster Med* 5(1):47, 1990.

Crimmins TJ. Ethical issues in adult resuscitation. *Ann Emerg Med* 22:495, 1993.

Forgues M. In the best interests of the patient. *Emergency* 23(12):34, 1991.

Haynes BE et al. Letting go: DNR orders in prehospital care. *JAMA* 254:532, 1985.

Henry GL. Legal rounds. Problem: Deciding not to resuscitate. *Emerg Med* 18(5):142, 1986.

Iserson KV. Foregoing prehospital care: Should ambulance staff always resuscitate? *J Med Ethics* 17:19, 1991.

Miles SH, Crimmins TJ. Orders to limit emergency treatment for an ambulance service in a large metropolitan area. *JAMA* 254:525, 1985.

Murphy DJ et al. The influence of the probability of survival on patients' preferences regarding cardiopulmonary resuscitation. *N Engl J Med* 330:545, 1994.

Ramos T, Reagan JE. "No" when the family says "go": Resisting families' requests for futile CPR. *Ann Emerg Med* 18:898, 1989.

Schiedermayer DL. The decision to forego CPR in the elderly patient. *JAMA* 260:2096, 1988.

Stephens RL. "Do not resuscitate" orders: Ensuring the patient's participation. *JAMA* 255:240, 1986.

Stratton SJ. Withholding CPR in the prehospital setting. *Prehosp Disaster Med* 5(1):45, 1990.

Tomlinson T, Brody H. Futility and the ethics of resuscitation. *JAMA* 264:1276, 1990.

Tresch DD et al. Should the elderly be resuscitated following out-of-hospital cardiac arrest? *Am J Med* 86:145, 1989.

Veatch RM. Deciding against resuscitation: Encouraging signs and potential dangers (editorial). *JAMA* 253:77, 1985.

Youngner S. Who defines futility? *JAMA* 260:2094, 1988.

Youngner S. Futility in context. *JAMA* 264:1295, 1990.

CPR: HAZARDS AND COMPLICATIONS

Achong MR. Infectious hazards of mouth-to-mouth resuscitation. *Am Heart J* 100:759, 1980.

Bedell SE et al. Unexpected findings and complications at autopsy after cardiopulmonary resuscitation (CPR). *Arch Intern Med* 146:1725, 1986.

Emergency Care Committee, American Heart Association. Risk of infection during CPR training and rescue: Supplemental guidelines. *JAMA* 262:2714, 1989.

Kern KB. CPR injuries: The effect of three different external chest compression techniques. *Emerg Med Serv* 18(4):53, 1989.

Krischer JP et al. Complications of cardiac resuscitation. *Chest* 92:287, 1987.

Lawes EG et al. Pulmonary aspiration during unsuccessful cardiopulmonary resuscitation. *Intensive Care Med* 13:379, 1987.

Lonergan JH, Youngberg JZ, Kaplan JA. Cardiopulmonary resuscitation: Physical stress on the rescuer. *Crit Care Med* 9:793, 1981.

Longstreth WT. The neurologic sequelae of cardiac arrest. *West J Med* 147:175, 1987.

Ornato JP. Providing CPR and emergency care during the AIDS epidemic. *Emerg Med Serv* 18(4):45, 1989.

Nagel EL et al. Complications of CPR. *Crit Care Med* 9:424, 1981.

Raviglione MC, Battan R, Taranta A. Cardiopulmonary resuscitation in patients with the acquired immunodeficiency syndrome. *Arch Intern Med* 148:2602, 1988.

BASIC LIFE SUPPORT

Brody GM, Beckerman B. CPR: A review of "new" techniques. *Emerg Med* 22(17):119, 1990.

Chandra N. Mechanisms of blood flow during CPR. *Ann Emerg Med* 22:281, 1993.

Emergency Cardiac Care Committee and Subcommittees, American Heart Association. Guidelines for cardiopulmonary resuscitation and emergency cardiac care. *JAMA* 268:2171, 1992.

Fisher JM. ABC of resuscitation: Recognising a cardiac arrest and providing basic life support. *Br Med J* 292:1002, 1986.

Johnson LM. Giving a CPR form new life. *Am J Nurs* 86:60, 1986.

Knopp RK. CPR: Separating the wheat from the chaff (editorial). *Ann Emerg Med* 12:547, 1983.

Kouwenhoven WB, Knickerbocker GG. Closed-chest cardiac massage. *JAMA* 173:1064, 1960.

Lee RV et al. Cardiopulmonary resuscitation of pregnant women. *Am J Med* 81:311, 1986.

Liss HP. A history of resuscitation. *Ann Emerg Med* 15:65, 1986.

Little K, Auchincloss JM, Reaves CS. A mechanical cardiopulmonary life-support system. *Resuscitation* 3:63, 1974.

Mahoney BD et al. Efficacy of pneumatic trousers in refractory prehospital cardiopulmonary arrest. *Ann Emerg Med* 12:8, 1983.

Maier GW et al. The physiology of external cardiac massage: High-impulse cardiopulmonary resuscitation. *Circulation* 70:86, 1984.

Marsden AK. Basic life support. *Br Med J* 299:442, 1989.

McDonald JL. Systolic and mean arterial pressures during

manual and mechanical CPR in humans. *Crit Care Med* 9:382, 1981.

McIntyre KM. CPR: Old problems, new techniques. *Cardiovasc Med* 10(9):16, 1985.

Melker RJ. Recommendation for ventilation during cardiopulmonary resuscitation: Time for a change? *Crit Care Med* 13:882, 1985.

Melker RJ, Banner MJ. Ventilation during CPR: Two-rescuer standards reappraised. *Ann Emerg Med* 14:397, 1985.

Newton JR et al. A physiologic comparison of external cardiac massage techniques. *J Thorac Cardiovasc Surg* 95:892, 1989.

Niemann JT. Cardiopulmonary resuscitation. *N Engl J Med* 327:1075, 1992.

Ornato JP et al. Measurement of ventilation during cardiopulmonary resuscitation. *Crit Care Med* 11:79, 1983.

Rudikoff MJ et al. Mechanisms of blood flow during cardiopulmonary resuscitation. *Circulation* 61:345, 1980.

Safar P, Bircher N. *Cardiopulmonary Cerebral Resuscitation* (3rd ed.) Philadelphia: Saunders, 1988.

Sanders AB, Meislin HW, Ewy GA. The physiology of cardiopulmonary resuscitation. *JAMA* 252:3283, 1984.

Smith JP et al. Guidelines for discontinuing cardiopulmonary resuscitation in the emergency department after prehospital nonparamedic-directed cardiac arrest. *West J Med* 143:402, 1985.

Stapleton ER. Comparing CPR during ambulance transport: Manual vs mechanical methods. *JEMS* 16(4):63, 1991.

Steen-Hansen JE et al. Pupil size and light reactivity during cardiopulmonary resuscitation: A clinical study. *Crit Care Med* 16:69, 1988.

Swanson RW. Psychological issues in CPR. *Ann Emerg Med* 22:350, 1993.

Swenson RD et al. Hemodynamics in humans during conventional and experimental methods of cardiopulmonary resuscitation. *Circulation* 78:630, 1988.

Taylor GJ et al. Importance of prolonged compression during cardiopulmonary resuscitation in man. *N Engl J Med* 296:1515, 1977.

Warren ET et al. External cardiopulmonary resuscitation augmented by the military antishock trousers. *Am Surg* 49:651, 1983.

Yatsu FM. Cardiopulmonary-cerebral resuscitation. *N Engl J Med* 314:440, 1986.

ADVANCED CARDIAC LIFE SUPPORT

American College of Emergency Physicians. Prehospital advanced life support skills, medications, and equipment. *Ann Emerg Med* 17:1109, 1988.

Brooks R et al. Current treatment of patients surviving out-of-hospital cardiac arrest. *JAMA* 265:762, 1991.

Emergency Cardiac Care Committee and Subcommittees, American Heart Association. Guidelines for cardiopulmonary resuscitation and emergency cardiac care. *JAMA* 268:2171, 1992.

Jespersen HF et al. Feasibility of intracardiac injection of drugs during cardiac arrest. *Eur Heart J* 11:269, 1990.

Koscove EM, Paradis N. Successful resuscitation from cardiac arrest using high-dose epinephrine therapy: Report of two cases. *JAMA* 259:3031, 1988.

Longstreth WT et al. Intravenous glucose after out-of-hospital cardiopulmonary arrest: A community-based, randomized trial. *Neurology* 43:2534, 1993.

Perkins KC. ALS: The figures are in. *Emergency* 22:(4):52, 1990.

Rothrock SG et al. Successful resuscitation from cardiac ar-

rest using sublingual injection for medication delivery. *Ann Emerg Med* 22:751, 1993.

Schleien CL et al. Controversial issues in cardiopulmonary resuscitation. *Anesthesiology* 71:133, 1989.

Stavrakis P. Central vein cannulation during CPR. *Emerg Med* 20(21):80, 1988.

*For references on drug therapy in ACLS, see under the specific drug in the Drug Handbook at the end of this text.

WHEN TO STOP CPR

Bonnin M et al. Distinct criteria for termination of resuscitation in the out-of-hospital setting. *JAMA* 270:1457, 1993.

Chipman C et al. Criteria for cessation of CPR in the emergency department. *Ann Emerg Med* 10:11, 1981.

Eisenberg MS, Cummin RO. Termination of CPR in the prehospital arena (editorial). *Ann Emerg Med* 14:1106, 1985.

Frank M. Should we terminate futile resuscitations in the field? Can we afford not to? *Ann Emerg Med* 18:594, 1989.

Gray WA. Prehospital resuscitation: The good, the bad, and the futile (editorial). *JAMA* 270:1471, 1993.

Gray WA et al. Unsuccessful emergency medical resuscitation: Are continuing efforts in the emergency department justified? *N Engl J Med* 325:1393, 1991.

Kellerman AL. Criteria for dead-on-arrivals, prehospital termination of CPR, and do-not-resuscitate orders. *Ann Emerg Med* 22:47, 1993.

Kellerman AL, Hackman BB, Somes G. Predicting the outcome of unsuccessful prehospital advanced cardiac life support. *JAMA* 270:1433, 1993.

Kellerman A, Staves DR, Hackman BB. In-hospital resuscitation following unsuccessful prehospital advanced cardiac life support: "Heroic efforts" or an exercise in futility? *Ann Emerg Med* 17:589, 1988.

Newman J. Prehospital termination of cardiac care. *Emergency* 26(2):28, 1994.

Reigel M, Barnes D. A sensitive solution. *Emergency* 26(2):44, 1994.

Smith JP. Guidelines for discontinuing prehospital CPR in the emergency department: A review. *Ann Emerg Med* 14:1093, 1985.

Van Hoeyweghen R et al. Decision making to cease or to continue cardiopulmonary resuscitation (CPR). *Resuscitation* 17(Suppl):S137, 1989.

Van der Hoeven JG. Prolonged resuscitation efforts for cardiac arrest patients who cannot be resuscitated at the scene: Who is likely to benefit? *Ann Emerg Med* 22:1659, 1993.

DEFIBRILLATION AND CARDIOVERSION

Bocka J. Automatic external defibrillators. *Ann Emerg Med* 18:1264, 1989.

Cooke DH. Ventricular fibrillation: The state of the art. *Emerg Med* 18(5):115, 1986.

Copass M, Eisenberg MS, Damon SK. *EMT Defibrillation* (3rd ed.). Westport, Ct.: Emergency Training, 1989.

Cummins RO. Defibrillation. *Emerg Med Clin North Am* 6(2):217, 1988.

Cummins RO. From concept to standard-of-care? Review of the clinical experience with automated external defibrillators. *Ann Emerg Med* 18:1269, 1989.

Cummins RO et al. Sensitivity, accuracy, and safety of an automatic external defibrillator. *Lancet* 2:318, 1984.

Cummins RO et al. Automatic external defibrillation: Clinical issues for cardiology. *Circulation* 73:381, 1986.

Cummins RO et al. Automatic external defibrillators used by emergency medical technicians: A controlled clinical trial. *JAMA* 257:1605, 1987.

Cummins RO et al. Training lay persons to use automatic external defibrillators: Success of initial training and one-year retention of skills. *Am J Emerg Med* 7(2):143, 1989.

Cummins RO et al. Defibrillator failures: Causes of problems and recommendations for improvement. *JAMA* 264:1019, 1990.

Defibrillator/monitor/pacemakers. *Health Devices* 22:211, 1993.

DeSilva RA et al. Cardioversion and defibrillation. *Am Heart J* 100:881, 1980.

Ditchey RV et al. Safety of electrical cardioversion in patients without digitalis toxicity. *Ann Intern Med* 95:676, 1981.

Eisenberg MS et al. Treatment of ventricular fibrillation: Emergency medical technician defibrillation and paramedic services. *JAMA* 251:1723, 1984.

Eisenberg MS et al. Defibrillation by emergency medical technicians. *Crit Care Med* 13:921, 1985.

Ewy GA. Optimal technique for electrical cardioversion of atrial fibrillation. *Circulation* 85:1645, 1992.

Fotre TV. Automated defibrillators: Their history and utilization. *Emerg Med Serv* 18(4):33, 1989.

Gibbs W, Eisenberg M, Damon SK. Dangers of defibrillation: Injuries to emergency personnel during patient resuscitation. *Am J Emerg Med* 8(2):101, 1990.

Gonzales ER, Ornato JP. Electrical countershock for prehospital bradyasystolic cardiac arrest. *Emerg Med Serv* 17(6):42, 1988.

Graves JR, Austin D, Cummins RO. *Rapid Zap: Automated Defibrillation.* Englewood Cliffs, N.J.: Brady, 1989.

Hargarten KM et al. Prehospital experience with defibrillation of coarse ventricular fibrillation: A ten-year review. *Ann Emerg Med* 19:157, 1990.

Hoekstra JW et al. Effect of first-responder automated defibrillation on time to therapeutic interventions during out-of-hospital cardiac arrest. *Ann Emerg Med* 22:1247, 1993.

Hummel RS et al. Spark-generating properties of electrode gels used during defibrillation: A potential fire hazard. *JAMA* 260:3021, 1988.

Hunt RC et al. Influence of emergency medical services systems and prehospital defibrillation on survival of sudden cardiac death victims. *Am J Emerg Med* 7(1):68, 1989.

Iverson WR et al. AICDs spark hope for cardiac cure. *JEMS* 14(9):37, 1989.

Kellerman AL et al. Impact of first-responder defibrillation in an urban emergency medical services system. *JAMA* 270:1708, 1993.

Kerber RE. Electrical treatment of cardiac arrhythmias: Defibrillation and cardioversion. *Ann Emerg Med* 22:296, 1993.

Kowey PR. The calamity of cardioversion of conscious patients (editorial). *Am J Cardiol* 61:1106, 1988.

Lown B, Amarasingham R, Neuman J. New method for terminating cardiac arrhythmias: Use of synchronized capacitor discharge. *JAMA* 182:548, 1962.

Lown B et al. The energy for ventricular defibrillation: Too little or too much? *N Engl J Med* 288:1252, 1978.

Meade DM, Matoba RD. Current affairs. *Emerg Med Serv* 22(7):33, 1993.

Mercer S. Automated external defibrillation. *Emergency* 25(2):36, 1993.

Moore JE et al. Lay person use of automatic external defibrillation. *Ann Emerg Med* 16:669, 1987.

Ornato JP et al. Treatment of presumed asystole during prehospital cardiac arrest: Superiority of electrical countershock. *Am J Emerg Med* 5:395, 1985.

Ruffy R et al. Out-of-hospital automatic cardioversion of ventricular tachycardia. *J Am Coll Cardiol* 62:482, 1985.

Sedgwick ML et al. Performance of an established system of first responder out-of-hospital defbrillation. The results of the second year of the Heartstart Scotland project in the "Utstein style." *Resuscitation* 26:75, 1993.

Smith M. Rules for joules. *JEMS* 17(2):13, 1992.

Stults K. *EMT-D Prehospital Defibrillation.* Englewood Cliffs, N.J.: Brady, 1986.

Stults K et al. Efficacy of an automated external defibrillator in the management of out-of-hospital cardiac arrest: Validation of the diagnostic algorithm and initial clinical experience in a rural environment. *Circulation* 73:701, 1986.

Stults K et al. Self-adhesive monitor/defibrillation pads improve prehospital defibrillation success. *Ann Emerg Med* 16:872, 1987.

Ten-Eyck RP. Automated external defibrillator training and skills maintenance in Air Force emergency medical service systems. *Milit Med* 158:579, 1993.

Vukov LF et al. New perspectives on rural EMT defibrillation. *Ann Emerg Med* 17:318, 1988.

Weaver WD et al. Use of the automatic external defibrillator in the management of out-of-hospital cardiac arrest. *N Engl J Med* 219:661, 1988.

Weigel A, Atkins JM, Taylor J. *Automated Defibrillation.* Englewood, Colo.: Morton, 1988.

White RD. Maintenance of defibrillators in a state of readiness. *Ann Emerg Med* 22:302, 1993.

White RD, Feldman RA. The automatic internal cardioverter defibrillator (AICD): Description and guidelines for interaction during cardiac arrest. *Ann Emerg Med* 18:586, 1989.

COUGH CPR AND PRECORDIAL THUMP

Bircher N et al. Cerebral and hemodynamic variables during cough-induced CPR in dogs. *Crit Care Med* 10:104, 1982.

Caldwell G et al. Simple mechanical methods for cardioversion: Defence of the precordial thump and cough version. *Br Med J* 291:627, 1985.

Cary JM. Cough causes systemic blood flow. *Thorax* 39:192, 1984.

Chest thump in ventricular tachycardia (editorial). *Lancet* 1:488, 1971.

Niemann JT et al. Cough CPR. *Crit Care Med* 8:141, 1980.

Pennington JE, Taylor J, Lown B. Chest thump for reverting ventricular tachycardia. *N Engl J Med* 283:1192, 1970.

Rosborough JP et al. Cough supported circulation. *Crit Care Med* 9:371, 1981.

Scherf D, Bornemann C. Thumping of the precordium in ventricular standstill. *Am J Cardiol* 5:30, 1960.

Wei JY et al. Cough-facilitated conversion of ventricular tachycardia. *Am J Cardiol* 45:174, 1980.

Yakaitis RW, Redding JS. Precordial thumping during cardiac resuscitation. *Crit Care Med* 1:22, 1973.

TRANSCUTANEOUS CARDIAC PACING

Altamura G et al. Treatment of ventricular and supraventricular tachyarrhythmias by transcutaneous cardiac pacing. *PACE* 12:331, 1989.

Barthell E et al. Prehospital external cardiac pacing: A prospective, controlled clinical trial. *Ann Emerg Med* 17:1221, 1988.

Bocka JJ. External transcutaneous pacemakers. *Ann Emerg Med* 18:1280, 1989.

Cummins RO et al. Out-of-hospital transcutaneous pacing by emergency medical technicians in patients with asystolic cardiac arrest. *N Engl J Med* 328:1377, 1993.

Dalsey WC, Syverud SA, Hedges JR. Emergency department use of transcutaneous pacing for cardiac arrests. *Crit Care Med* 13:399, 1985.

Eitel DR et al. Noninvasive transcutaneous cardiac pacing in prehospital cardiac arrest. *Ann Emerg Med* 16:531, 1987.

Falk RH et al. External noninvasive cardiac pacing in out-of-hospital cardiac arrest. *Crit Care Med* 11:779, 1983.

Grubb BP et al. The use of external, noninvasive pacing for the termination of supraventricular tachycardia in the emergency department setting. *Ann Emerg Med* 22:714, 1993.

Hedges JR et al. Prehospital trial of emergency transcutaneous cardiac pacing. *Circulation* 76:1337, 1987.

Heller MB et al. A comparative study of five transcutaneous pacing devices on unanesthetized human volunteers. *Prehosp Disaster Med* 4(1):15, 1989.

O'Toole KS et al. Emergency transcutaneous pacing in the management of patients with bradyasystolic rhythms. *J Emerg Med* 5:267, 1987.

Paris PM et al. Transcutaneous pacing for bradyasystolic cardiac arrests in prehospital care. *Ann Emerg Med* 14:320, 1985.

Quan L et al. Transcutaneous cardiac pacing in the treatment of out-of-hospital pediatric cardiac arrests. *Ann Emerg Med* 21:905, 1992.

Roberts JR, Greenberg MI. Emergency transthoracic pacemaker. *Ann Emerg Med* 10:600, 1981.

Rosenthal E et al. Transcutaneous pacing for cardiac emergencies. *PACE* 11:2160, 1988.

Syverud SA, Dalsey WC, Hedges JR. Transcutaneous and transvenous cardiac pacing for early bradyasystolic cardiac arrest. *Ann Emerg Med* 15:121, 1986.

Vukov LF, Johnson DQ. External transcutaneous pacemakers in interhospital transport of cardiac patients. *Ann Emerg Med* 18:738, 1989.

Wertz EM. External cardiac pacing. *Emergency* 26(2):53, 1994.

Zoll PM et al. External noninvasive electric stimulation of the heart. *Crit Care Med* 9:393, 1981.

Zoll PM et al. External noninvasive temporary cardiac pacing: Clinical trials. *Circulation* 71:937, 1985.

MECHANICAL CPR DEVICES

Cohen TJ et al. Active compression-decompression: A new method of cardiopulmonary resuscitation. *JAMA* 267:2916, 1992.

Cohen TJ et al. A comparison of active compression-decompression cardiopulmonary resuscitation with standard cardiopulmonary resuscitation for cardiac arrests occurring in the hospital. *N Engl J Med* 329:1918, 1993.

Halperin H, Weisfeldt M. New approaches to CPR: Four hands, a plunger, or a vest (editorial). *JAMA* 267:2940, 1992.

Halperin H et al. A preliminary study of cardiopulmonary resuscitation by circumferential compression of the chest with the use of a pneumatic vest. *N Engl J Med* 329:762, 1993.

Little K, Auchincloss JM, Reaves CS. A mechanical cardiopulmonary life-support system. *Resuscitation* 3:63, 1974.

Stapleton ER. Comparing CPR during ambulance transport: Manual vs. mechanical methods. *JEMS* 16(9):63, 1991.

Ward KR et al. A comparison of chest compressions between mechanical and manual CPR by monitoring end-tidal PCO_2 during human cardiac arrest. *Ann Emerg Med* 22:669, 1993.

CPR: OUTCOME AND EVALUATION

Aprahamian C et al. Decision making in prehospital sudden cardiac arrest. *Ann Emerg Med* 15:445, 1986.

Backman J, McDonald GS, O'Brien PC. A study of out-of-hospital cardiac arrests in northeastern Minnesota. *JAMA* 256:447, 1986.

Becker LB et al. Outcome of CPR in a large metropolitan area: Where are the survivors? *Ann Emerg Med* 20:355, 1991.

Bergner L et al. Health status of survivors of out-of-hospital cardiac arrest six months later. *Am J Public Health* 74:505, 1984.

Bonnin MJ, Swor RA. Outcomes in unsuccessful field resuscitation attempts. *Ann Emerg Med* 18:507, 1989.

Cummins RO, Eisenberg MS. Prehospital cardiopulmonary resuscitation: Is it effective? *JAMA* 253:2408, 1985.

Curry L, Gass D. Effects of training in cardiopulmonary resuscitation on competence and patient outcome. *Can Med Assoc J* 137:481, 1987.

Dean NC, Haug PJ, Hawker PJ. Effect of mobile paramedic units on outcome in patients with myocardial infarction. *Ann Emerg Med* 17:1034, 1988.

Diamond NJ, Schofferman J. Factors in successful resuscitation by paramedics. *JACEP* 6:42, 1977.

Eisenberg MS, Bergner L, Hallstrom A. Out-of-hospital cardiac arrest: Improved survival with paramedic services. *Lancet* 1:812, 1980.

Eisenberg MS et al. Evaluation of paramedic programs using outcomes of prehospital resuscitation for cardiac arrest. *JACEP* 8:458, 1979.

Eisenberg MS et al. Long-term survival after out-of-hospital cardiac arrest. *N Engl J Med* 306:1340, 1982.

Eisenberg MS et al. Cardiac arrest and resuscitation: A tale of 29 cities. *Ann Emerg Med* 19:179, 1990.

Eitel D et al. Out-of-hospital cardiac arrest: A six-year experience in a suburban-rural system. *Ann Emerg Med* 17:808, 1988.

Ewy GA. Improving survival with CPR. *Cardiovasc Med* 10(10):10, 1985.

Guzy PM, Pearce ML, Greenfield S. The survival benefit of bystander cardiopulmonary resuscitation in a paramedic served metropolitan area. *Am J Public Health* 73:766, 1983.

Hearne TR, Cummins RO. Improved survival from cardiac arrest in the community. *PACE* 11:1968, 1988.

Hunt RC et al. Influence of emergency medical services systems and prehospital defibrillation on survival of sudden cardiac death victims. *Am J Emerg Med* 7:68, 1989.

Jakobsson J et al. Effects of early defibrillation of out-of-hospital cardiac arrest patients by ambulance personnel. *Eur Heart J* 8:1189, 1987.

Kaye W et al. Can better basic and advanced cardiac life support improve outcome from cardiac arrest? *Crit Care Med* 13:916, 1985.

Kowalski R et al. Bystander CPR in prehospital coarse ventricular fibrillation. *Ann Emerg Med* 13:1016, 1984.

Lauterbach SA, Padafora M, Levy R. Evaluation of cardiac arrests managed by paramedics. *JACEP* 7:355, 1978.

Lemire JG, Johnson AL. Is cardiac resuscitation worthwhile? A decade of experience. *N Engl J Med* 286:970, 1972.

Lombardi G, Gallagher J, Gennis P. Outcome of out-of-hospital cardiac arrest in New York City. *JAMA* 271:678, 1994.

Longstreth WT, Diehr P, Inui TS. Prediction of awakening after out-of-hospital cardiac arrest. *N Engl J Med* 308:1378, 1983.

Longstreth WT et al. Neurologic recovery after out-of-hospital cardiac arrest. *Ann Intern Med* 98:588, 1983.

Mayer JD. Emergency medical services: Delays, response time and survival. *Med Care* 17:818, 1979.

McSwain GR, Garrison WB, Artz CP. Evaluation of resuscitation from cardiopulmonary arrest by paramedics. *Ann Emerg Med* 9:341, 1980.

Murphy DJ et al. Outcomes of cardiopulmonary resuscitation in the elderly. *Ann Intern Med* 111:199, 1989.

Peacock JB, Blackwell VH, Wainscott M. Medical reliability of advanced prehospital cardiac life support. *Ann Emerg Med* 14:407, 1985.

Pionowski RS et al. Resuscitation time in ventricular fibrillation: A prognostic indicator. *Ann Emerg Med* 12:733, 1983.

Pressley JC et al. A comparison of paramedic versus basic emergency medical care of patients at high and low risk during acute myocardial infarction. *J Am Coll Cardiol* 12:1555, 1988.

Ritter G et al. The effect of bystander CPR on survival of out-of-hospital cardiac arrest victims. *Am Heart J* 110:932, 1985.

Roth R et al. Out-of-hospital cardiac arrest: Factors associated with survival. *Ann Emerg Med* 13:237, 1984.

Rowley JM et al. Advanced training for ambulance crews: Implications from 403 consecutive patients with cardiac arrest managed by crews with simple training. *Br Med J* 295:1387, 1987.

Solomon NA. What are representative survival rates for out-of-hospital cardiac arrest? *Arch Intern Med* 153:1218, 1993.

Spaite DW et al. Analysis of prehospital scene time and survival from out-of-hospital, non-traumatic, cardiac arrest. *Prehosp Disaster Med* 6(1):21, 1991.

Steuven H et al. Bystander/first responder CPR: Ten years experience in a paramedic system. *Ann Emerg Med* 15:707, 1986.

Tresch DD et al. Long-term survival after prehospital sudden cardiac death. *Am Heart J* 108:1, 1984.

Warner LL et al. Prognostic significance of field response in out-of-hospital ventricular fibrillation. *Chest* 87:22, 1985.

Weaver WD et al. Improved neurologic recovery and survival after early defibrillation. *Circulation* 69:943, 1984.

Weaver WD et al. Considerations for improving survival from out-of-hospital cardiac arrest. *Ann Emerg Med* 15:1181, 1986.

Weaver WD et al. Factors influencing survival after out-of-hospital cardiac arrest. *J Am Coll Cardiol* 7:752, 1986.

Weil MH et al. Acid-base determinants of survival after cardiopulmonary resuscitation. *Crit Care Med* 13:888, 1985.

CPR TRAINING

Abrams JI et al. Guidelines for rescue training of the lay public. *Prehosp Disaster Med* 8(2):151, 1993.

Angus DC et al. Recommendations for life-supporting first-aid training of the lay public for disaster preparedness. *Prehosp Disaster Med* 8(2):157, 1993.

Atkins JM. Training in resuscitation: Is it worthwhile? *Chest* 89:474, 1986.

Bernhard WN et al. Impact of cardiopulmonary resuscitation training on resuscitation. *Crit Care Med* 7:257, 1979.

Carter WB et al. Development and implementation of emergency CPR instruction via telephone. *Ann Emerg Med* 13:695, 1984.

Cummins RO et al. Ventilation skills of emergency medical technicians: A teaching challenge for emergency medicine. *Ann Emerg Med* 15:1187, 1986.

Curry L, Gass D. Effects of training in cardiopulmonary resuscitation on competence and patient outcome. *Can Med Assoc J* 137:491, 1987.

Eisenberg MS et al. Emergency CPR instruction via telephone. *Am J Public Health* 75:47, 1985.

Gass DA et al. Physicians' and nurses' retention of knowledge and skills after training in cardiopulmonary resuscitation. *Can Med Assoc J* 128:550, 1983.

Gombeski WR et al. Impact on retention: Comparison of two CPR training programs. *Am J Public Health* 72:849, 1982.

Hudson AD. Herpes simplex virus and CPR training manikins: Reducing the risk of cross-infection. *Ann Emerg Med* 13:1108, 1984.

Kaye W et al. The problem of poor retention of cardiopulmonary resuscitation skills may lie with the instructor, not the learner or the curriculum. *Resuscitation* 21:67, 1991.

Mandel LP, Cobb LA. CPR training in the community. *Ann Emerg Med* 14:669, 1985.

Mandel LP, Cobb LA. Reinforcing CPR skills without mannequin practice. *Ann Emerg Med* 16:1117, 1987.

Marchette L et al. The effect of an advanced cardiac life support course on advanced cardiac life support ability. *Heart Lung* 14:594, 1985.

Martin WJ, Loomis JH, Lloyd CW. CPR skills: Achievement and retention under stringent and relaxed criteria. *Am J Public Health* 73:1310, 1983.

Martin WJ, Loomis JH, Lloyd CW. Cardiopulmonary resuscitation skills: Do we expect too much? (editorial). *Arch Intern Med* 144:699, 1984.

Messick WJ, Rutledge R, Meyer AA. The association of advanced life support training and decreased per capita trauma death rates: An analysis of 12,417 trauma deaths. *J Trauma* 33:850, 1992.

Montgomery WH et al. Citizen response to cardiopulmonary emergencies. *Ann Emerg Med* 22:428, 1993.

Naughton MJ et al. Community trends in CPR training and use: The Minnesota heart survey. *Ann Emerg Med* 21:698, 1992.

Recommendations for decontaminating mannikins used in cardiopulmonary resuscitation training—1983 update. *Infect Control* 5:399, 1984.

Rowley JM et al. Simple training program for ambulance personnel in the management of cardiac arrest in the community. *Br Med J* 291:1099, 1985.

Stross JK. Maintaining competency in advanced cardiac life support skills. *JAMA* 249:3339, 1983.

Tweed WA et al. Retention of cardiopulmonary resuscitation skills after initial overtraining. *Crit Care Med* 8:651, 1980.

Van Kalmthout PM et al. Evaluation of lay skills in cardiopulmonary resuscitation. *Br Heart J* 53:562, 1985.

Wilson E, Brook B, Tweed WA. CPR skills retention of lay basic rescuers. *Ann Emerg Med* 12:482, 1983.

24
Unconscious States

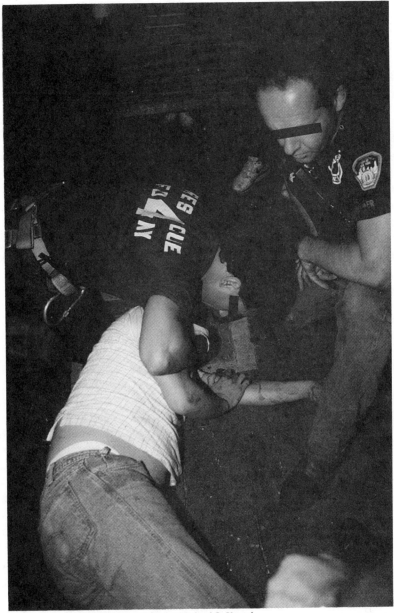

Rescue 4, Queens, New York. Photo by Michael S. Kowal.

OBJECTIVES

An unconscious patient is a patient in danger. Many of the reflexes that protect a waking person are in abeyance when consciousness is depressed by any cause. The eyelids do not blink away dust and irritants. The larynx does not gag and cough in reaction to secretions oozing down the airway. The body does not seek a more comfortable position in response to compression of a limb in an awkward position. The tongue goes slack. The airway is at risk. The patient is helpless and vulnerable.

In this chapter, we shall consider the plight of the unconscious patient. We shall first survey the various causes of unconsciousness and the clues to their detection. We shall also review the general principles of management that apply to *all* unconscious patients. Then we shall examine four specific causes of unconsciousness in some detail—diabetic states, syncope, seizures, and stroke. Other conditions that may produce unconsciousness, such as head injury or drug overdose, are dealt with elsewhere in this text, but by the end of *this* chapter, the student should be able to

1. List at least three dangers facing the comatose patient
2. List
   - The questions to be asked of bystanders
   - The points of emphasis in the physical examination

   when a patient is found unconscious and the cause is not known
3. Describe a patient's level of consciousness, given a list of findings from his neurologic examination
4. Identify the possible diagnostic significance of various physical findings in a comatose patient, given a list of findings
5. Identify the possible diagnostic significance of various medications found in the home or on the person of a patient in coma of unknown cause, given a list of medications
6. List nine causes of coma
7. List in the correct sequence the steps in managing a patient in coma from any cause
8. Given a description of several patients with different clinical findings, identify a patient suffering from
   - Diabetic ketoacidosis
   - Insulin overdose (hypoglycemia)

   and describe the correct treatment of each
9. Describe two mechanisms that can bring about syncope
10. List the questions that should be asked in taking the history of a patient who has fainted, and de-

scribe the correct prehospital treatment for fainting
11. List six causes of seizures, and describe the points of emphasis in examining a patient who has had a seizure
12. Given a description of several patients with different clinical findings, identify a patient suffering from
    - Syncope
    - Status epilepticus
    - Thrombotic stroke
    - Embolic stroke
    - Hemorrhagic stroke

    and describe the correct treatment of each
13. List the therapeutic effects, indications, contraindications, possible side effects, and correct dosages of
    - 50% glucose (D50)
    - Thiamine
    - Diazepam

    after studying the information about those agents in the Drug Handbook at the end of this textbook

THE COMATOSE PATIENT

Unconsciousness, or **coma,** is a state of unreponsiveness from which the patient cannot be roused. As noted, the patient in coma, from *any* cause, is a patient in danger. Coma depresses the reflexes that normally protect the airway from aspiration and obstruction; thus the comatose patient may very quickly be a dead patient if steps are not taken immediately to substitute for the patient's lost reflexes. For that reason, basic life support measures must be instituted *at once* for every comatose patient, before any attempt is made to gather a history or perform a detailed physical assessment.

> **A PATIENT IN COMA IS A PATIENT IN DANGER. INSTITUTE THE ABCs IMMEDIATELY.**

As always, the primary survey starts with the ABCs, so first priority goes to the AIRWAY. When a patient has simply been found unconscious and you don't know what might have happened to produce his coma, you have to assume there has been a head injury—and thus an associated cervical spine injury—until proved otherwise. So take care in opening the airway not to cause undue motion of the head or neck (use the jaw thrust, jaw lift, or chin lift maneuver *without* backward tilt of the head). Insert an *oropharyngeal airway* and see if the patient gags. If he does, he has some reflex activity left and can probably be managed with manual maneuvers to keep the airway open. If he does *not* gag, his airway is in jeopardy from aspiration, and he should be intubated.

Check for BREATHING. A detailed assessment of the patient's respiratory patterns can wait until the secondary survey. What you need to determine at this point is whether the patient is breathing adequately. (Is his respiratory rate greater than about 12 per minute? Is he moving a sufficient volume of air with each breath?) If the patient's minute volume does not seem adequate to you (or, needless to say, if he is not breathing at all!), *assist ventilations* with a bag-valve-mask, at a rate of about 20 to 25 breaths per minute (i.e., slight hyperventilation). And in any case, administer *oxygen.*

Evaluate the CIRCULATION by checking for a pulse. If the pulse is absent, start external chest compressions. If it is present, note its quality. A rapid, thready pulse should prompt a search for external BLEEDING.

Only when the ABCs are under control is the patient out of immediate danger. At that point, you may turn your attention to the secondary survey, whose purpose will be to try to narrow down the source of the patient's coma.

Assessment of the Comatose Patient

Taking the History

Taking a history from a comatose patient is obviously not a straightforward matter. The patient himself can't talk, so you will have to rely on bystanders who can and on your own powers of observation to learn as much as possible about the background of what happened. If family members, friends, or bystanders are present, try first to find out as much as you can from them. It's extraordinary how many mysterious cases of coma can be illuminated just by asking a few simple questions such as, "Do you have any idea what might have caused this?" ("Gee, I'm no doctor, but maybe it was all those sleeping pills he took. . . ."). Ask about the circumstances preceding the onset of coma: Did the coma come on gradually or suddenly? When did it start? Did the patient complain of anything in particular before he lost consciousness, such as a headache, stiff neck, dizziness? Was there a seizure? Had the patient suffered any recent trauma, especially head trauma, even if it seemed trivial at the time? Is there a background of

drug or alcohol abuse? Friends or family members may not want to divulge that the patient has been using illegal drugs, so it's helpful—when you ask about the possibility of drug use—to add a disclaimer like this: "Ma'am, I'm a paramedic, not a police officer, and the only thing I'm interested in is making sure your friend gets the right treatment. That's why I need to know whether he might have taken any particular drug."

Try as well to find out whatever you can about the patient's *medical history.* Is he under a doctor's care for any particular disorder? If so, what disorder (and what is the name of the doctor)? Is the patient known to suffer from diabetes? Heart disease? High blood pressure? Renal disease? Does he take any prescription medications regularly? Has he been sick lately?

As we learned in Chapter 11, *observations of the scene* in which the patient is found can also furnish valuable information regarding what might have happened to him. Check bureau tops, bedside tables, and medicine cabinets for medications that might give a clue to the patient's underlying illnesses. Check out the refrigerator for insulin. Look around as well for empty liquor bottles or drug paraphernalia (e.g., hypodermic syringes, crack pipes). If you do find medication bottles, bring them along with the patient to the hospital. They can help both to pinpoint the patient's underlying medical problems and to identify his physician, who may be able to provide a lot more information.

Physical Assessment

The goals of the physical examination in the comatose patient are twofold: (1) to determine the patient's level of consciousness with precision, so that other examiners who assess him later can readily determine whether his condition is improving or deteriorating; and (2) to look for signs that might provide clues to the source of coma (Table 24-1).

We start the physical assessment, as usual, by observing the patient's GENERAL APPEARANCE, and the first thing we will notice is the POSITION in which he is found. That is of some importance. Patients found in awkward, uncomfortable-looking positions often have brainstem damage, while a natural posture tends to be a good sign. Decorticate or decerebrate posturing should also be noted, if present; both are *bad* signs.

In appraising the LEVEL OF CONSCIOUSNESS, there are only three descriptive words that are universally understood:

- **Drowsiness** is a state in which the patient seems to be asleep but can be easily roused by verbal

TABLE 24-1. CLUES IN THE PHYSICAL ASSESSMENT OF THE COMATOSE PATIENT

ASSESSMENT	SIGN	SUGGESTIVE OF
VITAL SIGNS		
Pulse	Severe bradycardia	Heart block causing syncope; increased intracranial pressure
Blood pressure	Hypertension	Increased intracranial pressure; hypertensive encephalopathy; stroke; intracranial bleeding
	Hypotension	Blood loss; septic shock; myocardial infarction; pulmonary emboli
Respirations	Slow, regular	Narcotics or barbiturate overdose
	Cheyne-Stokes	Increased intracranial pressure; some overdoses
	Hyperpnea/tachypnea	Metabolic acidosis; midbrain lesions
Temperature	Elevated	Infection (e.g., meningitis); heat stroke
	Subnormal	Dehydration; alcohol or barbiturate overdose
HEAD	Battle's sign, CSF leak from nose or ears, coon's eyes	Skull fracture
PUPILS	Pinpoint	Narcotics overdose
	Fixed and dilated	Cerebral anoxia; barbiturate overdose; local agents (e.g., atropine eyedrops)
	Unequal	Increased intracranial pressure
MOUTH	Bleeding tongue	Recent seizure
	Fruity odor to breath	Diabetic ketoacidosis
NECK	Rigidity	Meningitis; intracranial hemorrhage
EXTREMITIES	Needle tracks	Narcotics overdose
	Flaccidity	
	Hemiplegia	Cerebral stroke
	Quadriplegia	Damage to the brainstem; associated cervical spine injury
	Decorticate posture	Cerebral damage
	Decerebrate posture	Brainstem damage

stimuli. Drowsiness is typified by the paramedic student sitting beside you in class, who nods off during an after-lunch lecture. You lean over and whisper, "Come on, wake up." His head jerks up; he says, "I'm wide awake. What do you want from me?" and he nods off again.

- **Stupor** is the stage beyond drowsiness (it takes a *really* boring lecturer to produce stupor!). The stuporous person does *not* respond to verbal stimuli but only to some sort of painful stimulus, like a pinch. Then he'll wake up briefly, but quickly revert to sleep.
- **Coma** is the state in which the patient does not respond to *any* stimulus—verbal or painful. If he reacts at all to a painful stimulus, it is with a reflex movement (e.g., a decorticate response), not a purposeful one.

Those three terms are the *only* terms that should ever be used in describing a patient's state of consciousness; any other terms—such as lethargic, obtunded, "zonked"—mean too many things to different people and therefore have no clinical utility. Best of all is to describe a patient's state of consciousness in terms of specific responses to specific stimuli. The **Glasgow Coma Scale** (Table 24-2) is a good guide so long as you keep a record of how you calculated the score. Simply saying that the patient has a Glasgow coma score of, say, 7, is not very informative, for the next person to examine the patient does not know specifically whether the patient did or did not open his eyes, had a decerebrate or a decorticate response, made garbled sounds or no sounds at all. So if you use the Glasgow Coma Scale, be sure to record the results in each category (eye opening, best motor response, verbal response), not just the total.

The CONDITION OF THE SKIN may be very informative. Cold, clammy skin is classically a sign of shock but may also signal severe hypoglycemia, as from an insulin reaction. Hot, dry skin suggests fever or, if the circumstances are appropriate, heat stroke. Cold, dry skin may indicate overdose of sedative drugs or alcohol.

In checking the VITAL SIGNS, look for the combination of *hypertension and bradycardia,* suggesting increased intracranial pressure. Be alert for *abnormal respiratory patterns.* Cheyne-Stokes breathing usually points to a *non*-neurologic source of the coma. More

TABLE 24-2. GLASGOW COMA SCALE

		TEST	PATIENT'S RESPONSE	SCORE
Eye opening		Spontaneous speech	Opens eyes on own	4
			Opens eyes when asked to in a loud voice	3
		Pain	Opens eyes when pinched	2
		Pain	Does not open eyes	1
Best motor response		Commands	Follows simple commands	6
		Pain	Pulls hand away when pinched	5
		Pain	Pulls a part of body away when examiner pinches him	4
		Pain	Flexes body inappropriately to pain (decorticate posturing)	3
		Pain	Body becomes rigid in an extended position when examiner pinches victim (decerebrate posturing)	2
		Pain	No motor response to pain	1
Verbal response (talking)		Speech	Carries on a conversation correctly and tells examiner where he is, who he is, month, and year	5
		Speech	Confused and disoriented	4
		Speech	Speech is clear but makes no sense	3
		Speech	Makes garbled sounds that examiner cannot understand	2
		Speech	Makes no sounds	1

- Assess the patient's score in each category, and total the scores of the three categories. A total score of 7 or less indicates coma.
- Assess the patient's score in each category frequently, and record each observation and the time it was made. Keep a parallel record of vital signs.

worrisome are other abnormal breathing patterns, such as central neurogenic ventilation or any sort of huffing and puffing that does not seem to be moving much air. Look for "para-respiratory" motions, such as sneezing and yawning. It takes an intact brainstem to produce a sneeze or a yawn, so both of those actions have positive prognostic significance. Hiccuping and coughing, on the other hand, may indicate brainstem damage.

Once trauma has been ruled out, the first thing we come to in the HEAD-TO-TOE SURVEY are the PUPILS. Are they pinpoint, suggesting narcotics overdose? Are they fixed and dilated, as in severe cerebral hypoxia or some barbiturate overdoses? Is one pupil widely dilated and unreactive to light, suggesting cerebral edema and herniation? Describe your findings precisely, for example, "The pupils are 5 mm in diameter and react to light directly and consensually." (*Don't* try to look smart by writing PERRLA—the abbreviation for "pupils equal, round, and reactive to light and accommodation"—on the trip sheet, because it will just be obvious you're faking it; it's impossible to check accommodation in an unconscious patient.)

If you have any reason to suspect that the coma might be psychogenic in origin ("hysterical coma"), place a fingertip very lightly on the patient's EYE-LASH on either side. In a patient whose coma does not have an organic source, the response will usually be vigorous bilaterally blinking, while a patient in coma from organic causes will not respond at all. An-

other atraumatic way of checking for hysterical coma is to insert a wisp of cotton into the patient's nose; again, the patient in hysterical coma will usually react. There is *no* excuse for applying painful or potentially dangerous stimuli—such as dropping the patient's hand on his face—to test for hysterical coma.

Examine the MOUTH for *bleeding* that might have occurred if the patient bit his tongue during a seizure. At the same time, notice whether there are any *unusual odors* on the patient's breath, such as the fruity odor of diabetic ketoacidosis, the almond odor of cyanide poisoning, or the odor of alcohol.

If there is no evidence of trauma, attempt to flex the patient's NECK; rigidity of the neck indicates that blood or pus has entered the cerebrospinal fluid (CSF) and is irritating the meningeal membranes.

In examining the EXTREMITIES, check for a bracelet or anklet that may identify the patient as a diabetic or epileptic, for example. Look for needle tracks on the arms that will identify a user of intravenous drugs. Try to evaluate the muscle tone in the extremities to determine whether one side seems flaccid compared to the other—a finding that would be suggestive of stroke.

Causes of Coma

Having gathered all that information, you can start to narrow down the list of possible causes of coma. One

TABLE 24-3.   MNEMONIC FOR THE CAUSES OF COMA

A	Alcohol, acidosis (hyperglycemic coma)
E	Epilepsy (also electrolyte abnormality, endocrine problem)
I	Insulin (hypoglycemic shock)
O	Overdose (or poisoning)
U	Uremia and other renal problems
T	Trauma; temperature abnormalities (hypothermia, heat stroke)
I	Infection (e.g., meningitis)
P	Psychogenic ("hysterical coma")
S	Stroke or space-occupying lesions in the cranium

widely used mnemonic for the causes of coma is AEIOU/TIPS (Table 24-3). For reasons that will become evident, this author prefers to put "A" for "alcohol" at the end of the list. But however you remember them, the possible causes of coma, and the clues to their presence, include

- TRAUMA: Trauma may or may not be evident from examination of the patient. Pay attention to the surroundings and possible mechanisms of injury; and when in doubt, immobilize the spine.
- DIABETES: The patient may be in coma from either excessive or inadequate levels of sugar in the blood (see next section). Does he have a Medic Alert tag? Is he carrying any medication such as Orinase or Diabinese in his pockets? Are there insulin syringes in the house or insulin in the refrigerator? Does his breath have a fruity odor?
- OTHER MEDICAL PROBLEMS: Again, look for a medical identification bracelet, anklet, or necklace that might tell of thyroid, adrenal, renal, or other problems. Check the surroundings for medications such as Synthroid or cortisone.
- DRUG OVERDOSE: Are there needle tracks on the patient's arms? Are the pupils pinpoint (suggesting narcotics overdose) or widely dilated (suggesting barbiturate overdose)? Is the patient carrying any sedative drugs on his person? Are the respirations very slow and deep or unusual in any other way? (We shall cover drug overdose in detail in Chapter 27.)
- HYPERTENSIVE EMERGENCIES AND STROKE: What is the blood pressure? Are the pupils equal? Is there paralysis on either side of the body? Is the patient carrying antihypertensive medications on his person?

- MENINGITIS: Had the patient complained of a severe headache before he lost consciousness? Had he had a fever or been confused prior to going into coma? Does he have a rash? Is his neck rigid?
- POSTICTAL PHASE OF A SEIZURE: Does the patient have a known history of seizures? Did anyone see him seize? Is there evidence that he bit his tongue? That he lost bladder or bowel control? Is he carrying Dilantin, phenobarbital, or Mysoline?
- ALCOHOL INTOXICATION: Is there alcohol on the patient's breath? Are there bottles lying about? Does the patient have a history of drinking to excess? Even so, we put alcohol intoxication at the end of the list because it is a diagnosis of exclusion:

> **JUST BECAUSE A PATIENT IS A KNOWN ALCOHOLIC OR BECAUSE HIS BREATH SMELLS OF ALCOHOL DOES NOT MEAN THAT HE CANNOT BE IN COMA FROM OTHER CAUSES.**

It's all too easy to assume that a comatose patient smelling of alcohol is "just another wino sleeping it off." The patient may or may not be an alcoholic. And even if he is an alcoholic, his coma may be from a different source altogether—indeed any one of the causes of coma mentioned previously.

In many cases, it will not be possible in the field to identify the precise reason for the patient's unconscious state. *Treatment* is therefore aimed at supporting the patient's vital functions, preventing any further deterioration in the patient's condition, and giving trial therapy for the immediately reversible causes of coma.

General Principles of Managing the Comatose Patient

We have already mentioned the ABCs, which were carried out during the primary survey. To reiterate the key points:

- A patient whose gag reflex is absent cannot protect his own AIRWAY from aspiration and should therefore be intubated at the earliest opportunity.

- If BREATHING is abnormally slow or shallow, assist ventilations by bag-valve-mask. If in doubt, err on the side of *hyper*ventilating the patient (i.e., about 20 to 25 breaths per minute).
- Give OXYGEN whether the patient is breathing spontaneously or being ventilated.

Further steps of treatment for coma of unknown cause include the following:

- Establish an IV LIFELINE with D5/W. Draw at least one red-top Vacutainer tube for blood tests. If you carry a glucometer or reagent strips for measuring blood sugar, make an immediate determination of the blood glucose level, and treat if the reading is less than 60 mg per deciliter. If you do not have the means to measure blood sugar, assume the patient is hypoglycemic and treat as follows: First, give **100 mg of thiamine** slowly IV, followed by **50 ml of 50% dextrose (D50);** i.e., 25 gm of dextrose. If the patient wakes up, you've got both a diagnosis and a cure! A dosage of 25 gm of dextrose will reverse most cases of hypoglycemic coma. (The thiamine is given just in case the patient is an alcoholic with nutritional deficiencies; for giving dextrose alone in such a situation can bring on a very serious neurologic disorder called **Wernicke's encephalopathy.** Thiamine prevents dextrose from precipitating Wernicke's encephalopathy.) If the patient *doesn't* come around after a dose of D50 or if you have any other reason to suspect narcotics overdosage (pinpoint pupils, needle tracks on the arms, depressed respirations):
- Give **naloxone, 0.8 mg, slowly IV.** If *that* wakes the patient up, you have good evidence that he has overdosed on a narcotic (see Chap. 27). If there is no response, you may repeat the dose twice.
- MONITOR the cardiac rhythm of every comatose patient.
- Recheck vital and neurologic signs frequently, and KEEP A FLOW SHEET of your findings (such as that in Fig. 16-11). Remember, the most important aspect of neurologic assessment is not a single measurement at a single point in time but rather the *trend* shown by several measurements. So recheck vital signs, pupils, and level of consciousness at least every 5 to 10 minutes and *record your findings* immediately.
- PROTECT THE PATIENT'S EYES by taping them shut or by closing them gently and covering them with moist gauze pads. A patient in coma may have lost his blinking reflex as well as his gag reflex, and the corneal surfaces may become dried out or coated with foreign materials if the eyes are not shielded.
- TRANSPORT the comatose patient *supine* if he is intubated, otherwise in the stable side position (unless injuries preclude that position). If the patient must be supine (e.g., because of suspected spine injury) and cannot be intubated, keep his mouth and pharynx suctioned free of secretions, vomitus, and blood.

It has become fashionable in some paramedic services to use noxious inhalants, such as spirits of ammonia, to rouse unconscious patients and send them on their way, instead of transporting the patients to the hospital for evaluation. This practice usually occurs in the setting of police pressure to remove a "vagrant" from a public place and "get him moving along." Whatever the priorities of the police may be, the priority of a *paramedic* MUST be the welfare of the patient. This author does not minimize the difficulties paramedics face in dealing with their "regular customers" or in bringing those patients to an unwelcoming emergency room staff. But the practice of medicine does not give us the luxury of treating only nice, well-behaved, well-groomed people. A doctor, nurse, paramedic, or other health professional undertakes an obligation to treat every patient who is in need of care, and the decision *how* to treat each patient must be a *medical* decision, not one based on the financial or social circumstances of the patient. So before you thrust a vial of ammonia under the nose of an unconscious person to "wake him up and send him on his way," think about whether that is how you would treat one of your parents or friends if they were found unconscious.

MANAGEMENT OF THE COMATOSE PATIENT: SUMMARY

- Ensure an open AIRWAY; intubate if there is no gag reflex.
- ASSIST VENTILATIONS as needed.
- Start an IV LIFELINE with D5/W.
- Administer THIAMINE followed by 50% DEXTROSE. If there is no response, try
- NALOXONE.
- MONITOR cardiac rhythm.
- Protect the patient's eyes.
- Recheck and record VITAL AND NEUROLOGIC SIGNS frequently.
- Transport without delay.

DIABETIC EMERGENCIES

Diabetes mellitus is a systemic disease affecting many organs, among them the pancreas, which becomes incapable of producing **insulin.** Insulin is a critical hormone in the body's metabolism, for it promotes the utilization of glucose by cells. In the absence of insulin, glucose accumulates in the blood to very high levels, causing a variety of untoward reactions. Many diabetics take a synthetic form of insulin by injection to compensate for their body's insulin deficiency. However, there is a very delicate balance involved in glucose regulation, and the insulin dose taken on any given occasion may be too much or too little. Diabetics get into trouble when, for whatever reason, their blood sugar becomes too high (**hyperglycemia**) or too low (**hypoglycemia**).

Hyperglycemia and Diabetic Ketoacidosis

Diabetic ketoacidosis occurs when the blood sugar becomes too high, either because the insulin dose was too small or because it was neglected altogether. Patients who suffer diabetic ketoacidosis tend to be young—teenagers and young adults. Often episodes of ketoacidosis are precipitated by some stress, such as a recent infection, emotional upset, or pancreatitis.

In diabetic ketoacidosis, the body faces the prospect of starvation in the midst of plenty; for while the blood sugar is high—so theoretically there is lots for the cells to metabolize—the deficiency of insulin prevents that sugar from being taken up into the cells. From the viewpoint of the cells, therefore, famine is at hand, and a distress signal goes out over the sympathetic nervous system, causing the release of various "stress hormones." Since the body cannot utilize glucose, it turns instead to other sources of energy, principally fat. The metabolism of fat generates *acids* and *ketones* as waste products. (It is the ketones that give the characteristic fruity odor to the breath of a patient in diabetic ketoacidosis.)

Meanwhile, since glucose cannot be taken up by the cells, it continues to accumulate in the blood. As the blood sugar rises, the patient undergoes massive **osmotic diuresis** (passing large amounts of urine because of the high solute concentration of the blood), which, together with vomiting, causes *dehydration* and even *shock*.

The processes described usually progress slowly, over a period of 12 to 48 hours, with the patient's level of consciousness deteriorating only gradually. (Patients in diabetic ketoacidosis are seldom deeply comatose; so if the patient is totally unresponsive,

start looking for another source of the coma, such as head injury, stroke, or drug overdose).

The signs and symptoms of diabetic ketoacidosis are mostly predictable from the underlying pathophysiology:

SIGNS AND SYMPTOMS OF DIABETIC KETOACIDOSIS

- POLYURIA (excessive urine output), because of osmotic diuresis.
- POLYDIPSIA (excessive thirst), because of dehydration.
- POLYPHAGIA (excessive eating), probably related to inefficient utilization of nutrients.
- NAUSEA and VOMITING, the latter worsening dehydration.
- TACHYCARDIA as a consequence of dehydration.
- Deep, rapid respirations (KUSSMAUL'S BREATHING), the body's attempt to compensate for acidosis by blowing off carbon dioxide.
- WARM, DRY SKIN and dry mucous membranes, also reflecting dehydration.
- FRUITY ODOR of ketones on the breath.
- Sometimes fever, abdominal pain, and hypotension. (Indeed, the presentation with nausea, vomiting, and abdominal pain may lead to a mistaken diagnosis of an "acute abdomen.")

The *treatment* of diabetic ketoacidosis in the field depends on making the correct diagnosis. *If you are unsure* whether the diabetic in coma is suffering from hyperglycemia or hypoglycemia, it is always safer to assume it is *hypo*glycemia. If, however, the patient's history and physical examination are consistent with ketoacidosis and—better still—if you have been able to measure the patient's glucose level in the field and have found it markedly elevated (over 300 mg/dl), the physician will probably order treatment for ketoacidosis. The goals of prehospital treatment in diabetic ketoacidosis are to begin rehydration of the patient and correction of his electrolyte and acid-base abnormalities. In most instances, specific treatment with insulin should await the patient's arrival at the hospital, where therapy can be closely monitored with laboratory determinations of blood sugar, ketones, and so forth.

TREATMENT OF DIABETIC KETOACIDOSIS

- Follow the procedure for any comatose patient with regard to AIRWAY maintenance and oxygen. Be particularly alert for *vomiting*, and have suction ready.
- Start an IV LIFELINE, draw blood for laboratory tests, and INFUSE A LITER OF NORMAL SALINE over the first half hour or at the rate ordered by the physician. Remember, a patient in ketoacidosis is severely dehydrated, often to the point of shock, and needs volume, usually at a rate of about 1 liter per hour for at least the first few hours.
- MONITOR cardiac rhythm. Changes in serum potassium caused by acidosis can lead to marked myocardial instability. Note the contour of the *T waves* on the rhythm strip; if they are sharply peaked (Fig. 24-1), the patient's potassium level may be dangerously high, and the physician may want you to administer sodium bicarbonate.

Hypoglycemia

Hypoglycemia in the insulin-dependent diabetic is often the result of having taken too much insulin, too little food, or both. Unlike other tissues, which can metabolize fat or protein in addition to sugar, the tissues of the central nervous system (most importantly, the brain) depend entirely on glucose as their sole source of energy. If the level of glucose in the blood suddenly drops very low, the brain is literally starved. The resulting symptoms reflect both the disordered function of hungry brain cells and the alarm reaction (sympathetic nervous system discharge) set off by the brain's distress. If hypoglycemia persists, cerebral dysfunction progresses very quickly to permanent brain damage.

Hypoglycemia, in contrast to ketoacidosis, develops *very rapidly*, over minutes to a few hours. It should be suspected in any diabetic presenting with bizarre behavior, neurologic signs, or coma. Often the hypoglycemic patient appears intoxicated, because of slurred speech and incoordination, and may be paranoid, hostile, and aggressive as well.

It should be pointed out that diabetics are not the only patients who are prone to episodes of hypoglycemia. Alcoholics; patients who have ingested certain poisons or overdosed with certain drugs (notably aspirin); and patients with certain cancers, liver disease, kidney disease, and a variety of other conditions may all suffer hypoglycemic episodes. Do not, therefore, discount the possibility of hypoglycemia in a comatose patient just because he is not known to be a diabetic. On the other hand, don't let the fact that a patient *is* a known diabetic prevent you from considering other causes of coma. Diabetics are not immune to head injury, stroke, seizures, meningitis, and so forth. So even if a Medic Alert tag informs you that the comatose patient is a diabetic, KEEP AN OPEN MIND, and assess the patient thoroughly.

As noted, the signs and symptoms of hypoglycemia reflect both cerebral dysfunction and the sympathetic nervous system response:

FIGURE 24-1. **TALL, PEAKED T WAVES** on the ECG are often a sign of hyperkalemia.

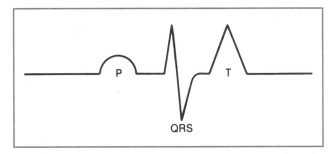

SIGNS AND SYMPTOMS OF HYPOGLYCEMIA

SIGNS OF A STARVING BRAIN
- Weakness and light-headedness
- Headache
- Mental confusion
- Fatigue
- Memory loss
- Incoordination; ataxic gait
- Slurred speech
- Irritable, nervous, belligerent, or bizarre behavior
- Seizures and coma in severe cases

SIGNS OF INCREASED SYMPATHETIC OUTPUT
- Weak, rapid pulse
- Cold, clammy skin
- Muscle tremors
- Dilated pupils

Whenever you *suspect* hypoglycemia, you must treat it *immediately,* for a hungry brain is a very unhappy brain, and permanent cerebral damage may ensue if blood sugar levels are not rapidly restored. If at all possible, first measure the patient's blood sugar, especially if his age or clinical history suggests that the cause of his coma might be stroke and not hypoglycemia—for administration of concentrated glucose solutions in that situation may exacerbate cerebral damage. So when the comatose patient is over about 55 years old or his family gives a history of recent transient ischemic attacks (see p. 626), a field glucose test (Dextrostix, Chemstrip BG) is strongly recommended before giving D50.

TREATMENT OF HYPOGLYCEMIA

- If the patient is still alert, is able to swallow, and has an intact gag reflex, give him sugar by mouth—a candy bar, a glass of orange juice to which a few teaspoons of sugar have been added, a cola drink—any of those should do the trick. Do *not,* however, give anything by mouth to a patient whose level of consciousness is depressed!
- If the patient is in coma, treat him as any other comatose patient, with attention to his AIRWAY and supplementary oxygen. Hold off endotracheal intubation, though, until you've tried giving D50; if the D50 works, the patient will simply pull out the endotracheal tube as soon as he wakes up!
- Start an IV LIFELINE with a *large-bore catheter* (no smaller than 18 gauge) in a *big vein,* draw blood for laboratory tests, and hook up a D5/W infusion.
- CHECK THE IV carefully to make sure it is patent and flowing freely. Inject a test bolus of 10 to 20 ml of your D5/W infusion fluid, to make sure the IV is not prone to infiltrate. Recheck by lowering the IV bag and looking for backflow of blood into the infusion set. The reason for all those precautions is that D50 is both hypertonic and acidic, and it can do a lot of damage if it infiltrates out of the vein into the surrounding tissue.
- If you are certain the IV is reliable, open the IV wide (do not pinch it shut) and administer 50 ML OF D50 *SLOWLY* IV, over at least 3 minutes. If the cause of coma is indeed hypoglycemia, the patient will often waken with dramatic

rapidity—although in cases of very severe hypoglycemia, another 50 ml of D50 may be required to restore a normal level of consciousness.

General Principles of Treating Diabetic Emergencies

Some of the features that distinguish diabetic ketoacidosis from hypoglycemic reactions are summarized in Table 24-4. While the distinctions look rather clearcut when presented in a table, the reality is sometimes less obvious, and in many cases it may be difficult to determine whether a comatose diabetic (or any other comatose patient) is *hyper*glycemic, *hypo*glycemic, or neither of the two. It is useful, therefore, to remember two general rules about the emergency treatment of diabetics (or others) in coma:

- ANY PATIENT IN COMA OF UNKNOWN CAUSE SHOULD RECEIVE GLUCOSE unless there is good reason to suspect stroke.
- Diabetics get into trouble from hyperglycemia and hypoglycemia. WHEN IN DOUBT, ASSUME THE DIABETIC IS *HYPO*GLYCEMIC AND GIVE GLUCOSE. You will not harm a hyperglycemic patient by giving glucose (the amount you administer is trivial compared to what he already has in his blood), but you could very seriously harm, and even kill, a hypoglycemic patient by withholding glucose.

WHEN IN DOUBT, GIVE GLUCOSE.

SYNCOPE

Syncope, or fainting, is a sudden, temporary loss of consciousness usually lasting less than 5 minutes. Syncope usually occurs because of one of three pathophysiologic processes:

- Seizure activity
- Inadequate glucose supply to the brain
- Inadequate oxygen supply to the brain

We have already discussed the symptoms and consequences of hypoglycemia, and we shall shortly

TABLE 24-4. DIFFERENTIATING DIABETIC EMERGENCIES

CHARACTERISTIC	DIABETIC KETOACIDOSIS	HYPOGLYCEMIC REACTION
Blood sugar	Excessively high (*hyper*glycemia)	Too low (*hypo*glycemia)
History		
Onset of symptoms	Gradual (12–48 hr)	Rapid (minutes to hours)
Food intake	Excessive	Inadequate; may have skipped a meal
Insulin intake	Inadequate	Excessive
Other precipitating factors	Infection, illness, stress	Strenuous exercise, alcohol ingestion
Symptoms	Polyuria, polydipsia, polyphagia, nausea, vomiting, abdominal pain	Headache, dizziness, irritability, hostile or bizarre behavior, confusion, weakness, diplopia
Physical findings		
Skin	Warm, dry, flushed	Cold, clammy, pale
Pulse	Rapid, thready	Rapid, may be weak
Blood pressure	Hypotension	Usually normal
Respirations	Kussmaul's (hyperpnea, tachypnea)	Normal or shallow
Temperature	May have slight fever	Normal or subnormal
Head-to-toe	Fruity odor to breath Soft eyeballs Tenting of the skin	Dilated pupils
Neurologic	Restlessness	Ataxia, tremors, sometimes hemiplegia or seizures; hyperactive reflexes; Babinski's sign present
Urine test		
Sugar	Present	Absent
Acetone	Present	Absent
Treatment	Rehydration: IV infusion of large volumes of normal saline; insulin at the hospital	Sugar: By mouth if alert; 50 ml of D50 IV if unconscious

come to the subject of seizures. By far the majority of cases of syncope, however, are a result of temporary interruptions in cerebral perfusion, which may come about because of changes in *vascular* tone that lead to pooling of blood in the periphery or because of disturbances in *cardiac* rhythm.

SIMPLE SYNCOPE, or **vasovagal syncope,** is the most common type of fainting and may occur in perfectly healthy individuals. It is usually precipitated by some stress (e.g., pain, fright, the sight of blood), which induces reflex dilation of blood vessels and consequent pooling of blood in the extremities. Simple syncope is more apt to occur when the person is sitting or standing, and consciousness rapidly returns when the patient becomes—intentionally or otherwise—horizontal. The simple faint may come on without warning or may be preceded by a brief period of symptoms, including weakness, cold sweat, nausea, abdominal discomfort, dimming of vision, and a roaring sound in the ears. While those symptoms are occurring, the patient usually grows quite

pale and may have a rapid pulse; but during the faint itself, the pulse usually slows to 50 or less per minute. The patient with simple syncope quickly regains consciousness after falling to the ground but may faint again if he tries to sit or stand up too quickly.

POSTURAL SYNCOPE (orthostatic syncope) is fainting that occurs when the patient sits or stands from a recumbent position. Usually either underlying disease (e.g., diabetes) or drugs that interfere with reflex vasoconstriction (e.g., antihypertensives, nitroglycerin, phenothiazines) are responsible. Prolonged standing in hot weather, as among soldiers on parade, may also produce this type of syncope, and athletes who suddenly stand still after vigorous exercise are also vulnerable. However, whenever a patient reports dizziness or fainting on sitting or standing up, the very first concern is to rule out *internal bleeding* and hypovolemia.

SYNCOPE OF CARDIAC ORIGIN may occur in any position. Syncope occurring when the patient is recumbent is almost always of cardiac origin and indicates a transient decrease in cardiac output. Recall the determinants of cardiac output:

$$\text{CARDIAC OUTPUT} = \text{HEART RATE} \times \text{STROKE VOLUME}$$

Thus, cardiac output can be decreased, first of all, by a marked decrease in *heart rate* (bradycardia)—usually to less than 40 beats per minute. As the equation shows, anything that decreases stroke volume can also decrease cardiac output. A very *rapid* heart rate (tachycardia)—over 150 beats per minute—is one thing that can decrease stroke volume, for it does not allow time for adequate ventricular filling in between systoles. Certain valvular diseases of the heart (aortic stenosis, mitral stenosis) may also diminish stroke volume or prevent outflow from the heart. Syncope of cardiac origin usually comes on abruptly and resolves quickly (in 1 or 2 minutes).

VAGAL CAUSES OF SYNCOPE are those that produce syncope by stimulating the vagus nerve and thereby causing profound bradycardia. (What does profound bradycardia do to cardiac output?) The person with a *hypersensitive carotid sinus*, for example, may faint while shaving or when buttoning a tight collar—actions that put pressure on the carotid sinus. Similarly, some patients may faint following other maneuvers that produce a vagal discharge, including laughter, urination ("micturition syncope"), or violent coughing.

Assessment of the Patient Who Has Fainted

In obtaining the HISTORY from a patient who has fainted, and from those who saw it happen, consider the episode in terms of three phases: what led up to the syncopal attack, the faint itself, and what happened immediately afterward.

- Before the patient fainted (history from the patient):
  1. What was he doing immediately before he fainted? Was there a stressful event preceding the faint?
  2. What *position* was he in?
  3. Did he have any *warning symptoms,* or did the faint come on "out of the blue"?

- About the faint itself (history from bystanders):
  1. What exactly did they see happen?
  2. Did the patient have any convulsive movements?
  3. How long was the patient unconscious?

- After the faint (history from bystanders and the patient):
  1. How long did it take before the patient recovered consciousness?
  2. Did he "come around" rapidly, or was he groggy for a while?
  3. Does the patient have any pain anywhere (that might suggest an injury sustained during the fall)?

Inquire as well into the patient's medical background, specifically whether he has any known *underlying disease* (particularly cardiovascular disease) and whether he is taking any *medications*.

In performing the PHYSICAL ASSESSMENT of the patient who has had a syncopal episode, pay particular attention to the following:

- Note the *position* in which the patient is found.
- Check the pulse and blood pressure in both arms. (Later, in the emergency room, the patient's blood pressure will be checked with the patient supine, sitting, and standing—but in the field, immediately after the faint, it is not a good idea to subject the patient to those changes in posture.)
- Make a careful survey for *injuries* that may have been sustained in a fall.

Treatment of a Syncopal Episode

While many if not a majority of syncopal episodes are of no clinical significance, that is a judgment that is best made in the emergency room and not in the field; so even if the patient seems to have recovered completely at the scene, it is still a good idea to transport him or her for further evaluation. Certainly any syncopal episode in a patient over 40 years old must receive further evaluation.

The basic principles of emergency treatment are the same for all syncopal episodes, regardless of the cause:

- Keep the patient in a *recumbent position* where he has fallen.

NEVER LIFT A PATIENT WHO HAS FAINTED INTO A SITTING POSITION. LEAVE HIM RECUMBENT.

It was the body's wisdom that caused the patient to fall in the first place, for perfusion of the brain is facilitated by the horizontal position, wherein the heart doesn't have to pump against gravity. So don't try to outsmart Mother Nature; she knows best. A sudden change in position to an upright posture may compromise cerebral blood flow so severely as to cause a stroke. Repeat: KEEP THE PATIENT FLAT.

- Ensure an open AIRWAY, and administer OXYGEN.
- Loosen any tight clothing on the patient.
- Elevate the patient's lower extremities for 10 to 20 seconds to facilitate venous return to the heart.
- Apply MONITORING electrodes, and check for dysrhythmias.
- If dysrhythmias are present, or if the patient is older than about 35, start an IV LIFELINE with D5/W to keep a vein open.
- Measure VITAL SIGNS frequently.
- Treat any injuries detected during the secondary survey.
- When the patient regains consciousness, discourage him from sitting up. Move him to a stretcher in a recumbent position, and transport him recumbent to the hospital.

SEIZURES

Seizures, or convulsions (or fits), occur when there is a massive discharge of a group or groups of neurons in the brain. Any person may suffer a seizure given the appropriate circumstances, but some people have a lower seizure threshold than others—either because they were born that way or because they suffered some insult that increased the irritability of part of the brain.

Seizures may be caused by a variety of conditions that lead to cerebral irritability.

CAUSES OF SEIZURES IN ADULTS

- Intracranial pathology
  1. Stroke, recent or remote
  2. Head trauma, recent or remote
  3. Space-occupying lesion (brain tumor, subdural hematoma)
- Hypoxemia
- Hypoglycemia
- Toxins, drugs, or withdrawal from drugs
- Withdrawal from alcohol
- Meningitis
- Eclampsia of pregnancy
- Idiopathic (cause unknown)—most epileptics are in this category

---

Among those several causes of seizures, probably the most common is failure of a known epileptic to take his or her prescribed medications. Seizures generally do not occur immediately after an epileptic stops taking seizure medications, but more usually several days or even 1 to 2 weeks afterward. Similarly, in seizures due to withdrawal from other drugs or alcohol, the seizures usually do not come on for about 24 to 72 hours after drug intake has been stopped. It is therefore necessary to make a careful inquiry as to when the last dose of a given drug, or the last drink of alcohol, was taken.

Seizures are of several types, classified according to the way they manifest themselves:

- GENERALIZED MOTOR SEIZURES (**grand mal seizures**) are characterized by loss of consciousness, tonic-clonic movement, and sometimes tongue-biting, incontinence, and mental confusion. The period of intense motor activity is usually followed by a period of coma or drowsiness, known as the **postictal state.** It is for the grand mal type of seizures (or behaviors that resemble grand mal seizures) that you are most likely to be summoned.
- FOCAL MOTOR SEIZURES usually involve only one part of the body, such as the face or an arm, in tonic-clonic twitching. Focal seizures may progress rapidly to generalized convulsions. If you witness the seizure, it is important to note *where it started* (e.g., the left side of the face), for that observation gives the physician useful information regarding the location of the irritable focus in the brain. For the same reason, pay attention to the direction toward which the patient's eyes deviate.
- PSYCHOMOTOR SEIZURES (temporal lobe seizures) usually don't look like seizures at all, and in most patients it takes a long time before a diagnosis is made. Temporal lobe seizures are often characterized by a sudden alteration in personality, which may be preceded by dizziness or a sensation of a peculiar, metallic taste in the mouth. In some patients, temporal lobe seizures will be manifested as sudden, unexplained attacks of

rage. In others, there will be stereotyped motor behavior. Or patients may experience hallucinations of vision, sound, taste, or smell.

- PETIT MAL SEIZURES are seen chiefly in children and rarely constitute an emergency. They are characterized by a very brief loss of consciousness—usually no longer than a few seconds—without loss of motor tone. The child will suddenly stare off into space for a few seconds and become entirely unresponsive. Then, just as suddenly, he will resume whatever he was doing, often quite unaware that anything unusual has happened.

All the types of seizures listed represent some sort of temporary cerebral dysfunction and must be distinguished from **pseudoseizures,** or hysterical seizures, which represent a psychologic disturbance. In the hysterical seizure, the movements tend to be bizarre and can often be interrupted by a sharp command. The patient having an hysterical seizure rarely if ever injures himself, bites his tongue, or becomes incontinent of urine and feces. Hysterical seizures, furthermore, almost invariably occur in front of an audience. In trying to differentiate the hysterical seizure from the genuine grand mal seizure, it is well to keep in mind the usual sequence of events in a generalized motor seizure:

- Many patients will first experience an **aura,** that is, a peculiar sensation that precedes and sometimes warns of an impending epileptic attack. The aura usually lasts a few seconds and may consist of visual or auditory hallucinations, a peculiar taste in the mouth, a painful feeling in the abdomen, or a sensation of movement in some part of the body when no movement is occurring.
- The patient then abruptly LOSES CONSCIOUSNESS.
- Immediately, a TONIC PHASE begins, characterized by continuous motor tension. The tonic phase may be heralded by a high-pitched cry, and it lasts about 15 to 20 seconds.
- Next comes a HYPERTONIC PHASE, lasting 5 to 15 seconds, during which the patient falls to the ground with his muscles held absolutely rigid in hyperextension. The patient is apneic during this phase and loses sphincter control, so urination or defecation may occur.
- The hypertonic phase is quickly followed by a CLONIC PHASE, or spasm in which rigidity and relaxation alternate in rapid succession. The clonic phase is accompanied by massive AUTONOMIC DISCHARGE, with hyperventilation, salivation, and tachycardia.

- Ordinarily the clonic phase lasts less than 5 minutes (although when you're watching it, it seems to last forever!). It is followed by a variable period of POSTICTAL COMA OR STUPOR, during which the patient's muscles are flaccid.
- Finally, CONSCIOUSNESS SLOWLY RETURNS, often with postictal symptoms of confusion, headache, and extreme fatigue.

Assessing the Seizure Patient

When you first reach the scene of a patient who is having, or has just had, a seizure, you will have to attend at once to the primary survey and to protecting the patient from injury. Only later will you be able to ask some questions of the patient and bystanders and to conduct a more thorough physical assessment.

In obtaining the HISTORY from the seizure patient and from those who witnessed the episode, try to find out the following:

- Does the patient have a *history of seizures?* If so, how frequently do they occur? Does he take medications for seizures? Has he been taking those medications regularly? Has he skipped any doses?
- While still on the subject of the patient's medical history, ask about a history of
  1. Head injury.
  2. Alcohol or drug use (if the patient is a substance abuser, find out when he or she last indulged).
  3. Diabetes (which might predispose to hypoglycemia).
  4. Heart disease (which may have caused a dysrhythmia and consequent cerebral hypoxia).
  5. Stroke (scars from an old stroke can act as irritable foci in the brain).
- Has the patient had a recent *fever, headache,* or *stiff neck* (suggesting the possibility of meningitis)?
- Get a *description of the seizure* if you did not see it yourself. Ask the patient whether he had any strange feelings before the seizure. Ask bystanders whether the spasmodic movements began in one area of the body and progressed or seemed to start all over the body at once. Ask also in which direction the patient's eyes deviated—left or right?

In carrying out the PHYSICAL EXAMINATION on a patient who has had a seizure, pay particular attention to the following:

- Assess the regularity of the *pulse*. (If it is at all irregular, monitor the patient from the outset.)
- Examine the *head* for evidence of trauma sustained during the seizure.
- Check the *pupils* for equality and reaction to light.
- Examine the *mouth* for injuries to the tongue and for swelling of the gums (**gingival hypertrophy**), the latter a sign of chronic therapy with the anticonvulsant drug phenytoin. If the patient is not yet conscious, determine whether he has a gag reflex.
- Check the *neck* for rigidity, suggesting meningeal irritation.
- Check for *injury elsewhere* in the body. Be especially alert for signs of POSTERIOR SHOULDER DISLOCATION after a major motor seizure.
- Examine the *extremities* for medical identification jewelry, needle tracks, and symmetry of deep tendon reflexes.
- Check the patient's pockets for medication containers.

Treatment of Seizures

The treatment necessary for seizures will depend on whether the patient has a single seizure or is having repetitive seizures, one after the other.

TREATMENT OF AN ISOLATED SEIZURE lasting less than 10 minutes is aimed at maintaining an airway and preventing the patient from injuring himself during the clonic phase of thrashing about. Clear all furniture and other objects away from the patient. DO NOT TRY TO RESTRAIN HIM during the tonic-clonic phase of the seizure—you will just risk injury to both the patient and yourself. Simply protect him from falling or banging into surrounding objects.

Bite-blocks and padded tongue blades are often brandished at patients having seizures, but such devices are rarely useful and can do a lot of damage. If the teeth are not already clenched, it is reasonable to place a tongue depressor that has been well padded with gauze between the upper and lower molars to minimize tongue biting. However, NEVER TRY TO JAM ANY OBJECT INTO THE MOUTH ONCE THE TEETH ARE CLENCHED; you will do more damage to the mouth than the patient will if just left in peace to bite his tongue. If possible, remove dentures before the teeth are clenched. Maintain an AIRWAY as best you can, and administer OXYGEN. As soon as the tonic-clonic phase of the seizure has abated, turn the patient onto his side, if he is not already in that position, and continue maintaining the airway. Have SUCTION nearby. Keep the patient in a quiet, calm atmosphere to minimize agitation and combativeness when he begins to wake up. Avoid tight restraints,

which may be frightening to the patient and cause him to struggle more vigorously, thus increasing the possibility of injury to himself. Transport the patient lying *on his side*, and continue giving oxygen en route.

Status epilepticus is defined as more than 30 minutes of continuous seizures or two or more seizures without a period of consciousness in between; it is a *dire medical emergency*. Repeated seizures, if not controlled, may lead to aspiration, anoxia, brain damage, fracture of the long bones and spine, cardiac muscle necrosis, and severe dehydration. The patient becomes metabolically and physically exhausted, and the body temperature may soar to dangerous levels. The most common *cause* of status epilepticus in adults is failure to take prescribed antiseizure medications. (Seizures and status epilepticus in children are discussed in Chap. 30.) As in the case of an isolated seizure, treatment of status epilepticus is aimed at maintaining the airway and preventing injury—but in status epilepticus, treatment has the additional objective of trying to stop the seizures.

TREATMENT OF STATUS EPILEPTICUS

- Place the patient on a wide bed or on the floor, away from furniture or other objects. Loosen any restrictive clothing. DO NOT TRY TO RESTRAIN HIM.
- Clear and maintain the AIRWAY. A soft nasopharyngeal airway may be helpful. If the patient has any period of flaccidity between seizures, take that opportunity to whip in an endotracheal tube, but don't attempt intubation during the tonic-clonic phase of a seizure.
- Administer OXYGEN in high concentration. Assist ventilations with a bag-valve-mask if there are long periods of hypoventilation or apnea. Hypoxia secondary to impaired breathing during seizure activity is the most serious threat to life. DEATHS FROM SEIZURES ARE HYPOXIC DEATHS. Therefore, they are preventable deaths.
- Start an IV LIFELINE with D5/W. Use a large-bore catheter in a big vein. Draw blood for laboratory studies. SECURE THE IV WELL, with lots of tape and self-adhering roller gauze, because the IV will be subjected to pulling, yanking, banging, and thrashing during the tonic-clonic phase of the seizure.
- If there is no reason to suspect a stroke, open the IV wide, and administer 100 mg of thiamine

followed by 25 gm of glucose (50 ml of D50) *slowly* IV.

- If the seizures do not stop within 10 minutes, the physician may order DIAZEPAM (Valium). Before administering diazepam, *record the blood pressure* accurately. Draw up **10 mg** (2 ml) into a syringe, and start injecting it into the IV line VERY SLOWLY. After each 0.5 ml (2.5 mg), stop and recheck the blood pressure. If the blood pressure begins to fall, discontinue the diazepam injection and notify medical command at once. If 10 mg of diazepam does not abort the seizures, do not attempt to give any more medication in the field, but transport the patient immediately to the hospital. If there are only two rescuers, you may wish to ask a bystander to accompany you in the back of the ambulance and assist in preventing the patient from injury while the paramedic maintains the airway.

STROKE

Stroke is the common term for a sudden vascular catastrophe—usually a clot or a hemorrhage—in the brain, leading to weakness, paralysis, speech disorders, confusion, coma, or some other neurologic deficit. Stroke is also referred to as a **cerebrovascular accident (CVA),** a less accurate and less descriptive term (we don't, after all, call the analogous event in the heart a "coronary artery accident"). The word *stroke* much more vividly describes the way a person is literally "struck down" from one moment to the next, as if by a stroke of lightning. Stroke, by definition, involves a neurologic deficit that lasts more than 24 hours and that corresponds to the distribution of a particular cerebral artery.

Strokes kill over 150,000 people in the United States each year and disable two to three times that number. They occur when the blood supply to a part of the brain is compromised in any way. Basically that can happen either because a cerebral artery becomes blocked (**ischemic stroke**) or because it ruptures and bleeds (**hemorrhagic stroke**). Those mechanisms are illustrated in Figure 24-2. The onset and symptomatology of the stroke will depend on which of those mechanisms has caused the stroke and which blood vessels are involved.

Ischemic Stroke

As the term implies, an ischemic stroke is caused by interruption of the blood supply to an area of the brain—in much the same way that myocardial ischemia is caused by interruption of the blood supply to a segment of the cardiac muscle. There are, in fact, two ways that a cerebral artery can become blocked—by the development of a clot in situ (thrombosis), again analogous to the process that occurs in coronary arteries, or by the impaction of a wandering blood clot (embolism) that reaches the cerebral circulation from another part of the body.

Thrombotic Stroke

About 60 percent of all strokes are the result of thrombosis in a cerebral artery, and in the vast majority of cases, the underlying disease is *atherosclerosis.* Atherosclerosis can affect cerebral vessels just as it does coronary vessels, to produce hardening, narrowing, and eventual thrombus formation.

Since atherosclerosis is a chronic, slowly evolving process, it is not surprising that patients who suffer thrombotic strokes tend to be older, with a peak incidence around age 70. Hypertension is present in about 60 percent of patients suffering thrombotic stroke, about 50 percent have evidence of atherosclerotic disease elsewhere (e.g., angina pectoris, absent peripheral pulses), and diabetes mellitus is present in 25 percent.

The vast majority—nearly 80 percent—of patients who suffer thrombotic strokes will have a series of "little strokes," or **transient ischemic attacks (TIAs)** in the months preceding their CVA. Transient ischemic attacks are recurrent neurologic deficits of any type (e.g., weakness, paralysis, speech disturbance) that correspond to the distribution of a particular cerebral artery and last anywhere from a few seconds to 12 hours; most commonly, they last up to 5 to 10 minutes, and it is unusual for a TIA to persist longer than 30 minutes. Between attacks, the neurologic examination may be entirely normal. In some patients, the onset of attacks is clearly related to standing up after lying or sitting, or it occurs in relation to exertion, emotional stress, or a bout of coughing. The patient who wakens in the morning with a TIA is especially likely to have a full-blown stroke in the near future.

Most commonly, thrombotic strokes come on during sleep or shortly after getting up in the morning. The *signs and symptoms* will depend on which cerebral artery has been blocked. The blood supply to the brain comes from four major vessels in the neck (Fig. 24-3): Two **carotid arteries** furnish about 80 percent of the blood flow (the so-called *anterior supply*), and two **vertebral arteries** furnish the remaining 20 percent (the *posterior circulation*). It is the carotids and their branches that are most commonly affected by thrombotic disease.

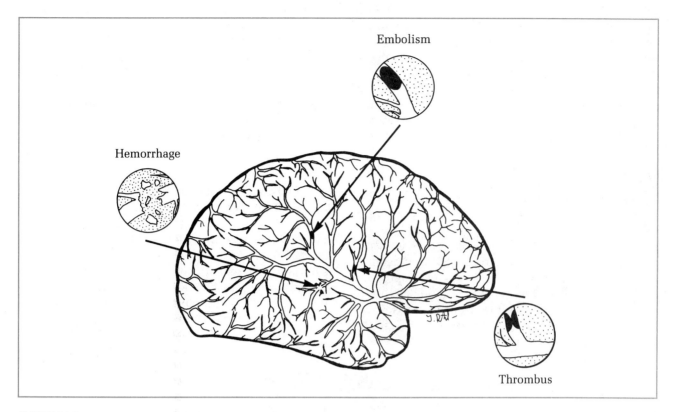

FIGURE 24-2. **MECHANISMS OF STROKE.**

FIGURE 24-3. **THE BLOOD SUPPLY TO THE BRAIN** comes from the two carotid and two vertebral arteries.

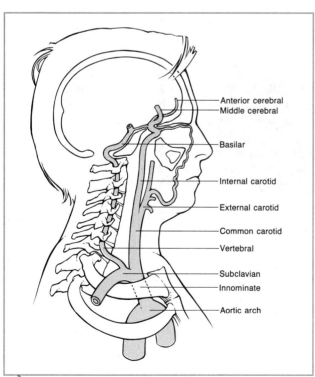

- Anterior cerebral
- Middle cerebral
- Basilar
- Internal carotid
- External carotid
- Common carotid
- Vertebral
- Subclavian
- Innominate
- Aortic arch

SIGNS AND SYMPTOMS OF THROMBOTIC STROKE

Carotid System Blockage	*Vertebrobasilar System Blockage*
Hemiparesis or hemiplegia*	Double vision
Unilateral numbness*	Numbness of the face
Aphasia†	Slurred speech (dysarthria)
Confusion or coma	Difficulty swallowing
Convulsions	Posterior headache
Sometimes incontinence	Dizziness or vertigo

*On the side of the body opposite the lesion

†If the stroke affects the dominant hemisphere (e.g., the left hemisphere of a right-handed person)

It is not necessary in the field to try to determine which cerebral vessel has been blocked, but it is useful to be aware of the various signs that may be produced by stroke syndromes and to make a careful record of the presence of those signs, even if you can't remember precisely what they mean. The doctor (one hopes) will know what the signs mean, and your trip sheet can thus be enormously helpful, especially if the patient's clinical picture is changing, as often occurs in a thrombotic stroke. Indeed, in thrombotic stroke it is difficult, if not impossible, to predict the eventual extent of disability on the basis of the patient's findings when first seen; for over the next 2 to 3 days, the patient's neurologic deficit may disappear altogether or it may extend and even lead to death.

Embolic Stroke

In contrast to thrombotic stroke, embolic stroke tends to *come on abruptly* at any time of the day or night, often when the patient is up and moving around. Furthermore, the embolic stroke *evolves very rapidly*, with the neurologic deficit reaching its maximum within seconds to minutes, rather than progressing gradually over several days in the fashion of a thrombotic stroke. In a significant percentage of cases, the embolic stroke begins with a *seizure*. About a quarter of patients will have a headache (although not a severe headache), and a third will have a transient *loss of consciousness*.

Embolic strokes most commonly occur in patients with rheumatic heart disease, atrial fibrillation, myocardial infarction, or any combination thereof. Women taking oral contraceptives and patients with sickle cell disease are also at increased risk.

Hemorrhagic Stroke

Hemorrhagic strokes can also be classified into two general types: intracerebral hemorrhage and subarachnoid hemorrhage.

Intracerebral Hemorrhage

Intracerebral hemorrhage is nearly always the result of hypertensive disease. After years of sustaining the increased stress of high blood pressure, small vessels in the brain start to develop areas of aneurysm. If one of those aneurysms finally gives way and ruptures, blood leaks out into the surrounding brain, disrupting brain tissue around it and, in addition, producing an almost instantaneous rise in intracranial pressure.

The average patient suffering an intracerebral hemorrhage is younger than the victim of thrombotic stroke—usually in his 50s or early 60s. The symptoms usually come on very abruptly when the patient is up and about (a frequent story is that the patient was straining to have a bowel movement and collapsed). The patient may be awake and fully alert when first seen, but usually his mental status deteriorates rapidly, and one sees all the symptoms and signs of increased intracranial pressure. (What *are* the symp-

toms and signs of increased intracranial pressure? If you don't remember, review Chap. 16!)

The prognosis for intracerebral hemorrhage is very bad—mortality is anywhere from 50 to 80 percent. But those who manage to make it through the first 12 to 24 hours may recover completely.

Subarachnoid Hemorrhage

Subarachnoid hemorrhage, as the term implies, means bleeding into the space around the brain, rather than into the brain tissue itself. The usual cause of subarachnoid hemorrhage is rupture of a slowly developing aneurysm, usually at the branch point of a vessel near the base of the brain. When the aneurysm blows out, there is a very sudden onset of symptoms, the most common of which is excruciating headache. The headache may be rapidly followed by nausea, vomiting, neck and back pain, confusion, or coma.

Assessment of the Patient Who May Have Suffered a Stroke

For purposes of discussion, we shall consider the patient who is conscious, for clearly any patient found unconscious—whether from a stroke or any other cause—requires primary attention to the ABCs and prompt transport.

In taking the HISTORY of a patient with a suspected stroke—from the patient himself or from members of his family—inquire about "little strokes" during the preceding weeks and months. Find out if the patient has a history of hypertension, cardiac disease, diabetes, or sickle cell disease. What *medications* does the patient take (if the patient is a woman under about 45 years of age, be sure to ask about birth control pills)? What *symptoms* did the patient notice first? Under what circumstances did they occur? Did anything seem to bring the symptoms on? Did the patient experience dizziness or palpitations? Does he have a headache? If so, in what part of his head? How bad is it? Is he having any problems with his vision? Is the patient right-handed or left-handed? (Why is that important?)

The signs of stroke elicited in the PHYSICAL EXAMINATION may be grossly obvious or quite subtle. Maintain a high index of suspicion in any older patient who presents with sudden confusion. Some of the more classic signs of stroke, any (or none) of which may be present in a given patient, include

- CONFUSION or other disturbances of mental status.
- In severe cases, SEIZURES or COMA.

- INAPPROPRIATE AFFECT, with excessive laughing or crying. Please note, however, that crying in itself is *not in the least* inappropriate under the circumstances. Imagine your own feelings if you woke up one morning unable to speak and unable to move your right arm and right leg.
- SPEECH DISTURBANCES, which may present as slurred speech (**dysarthria**), inability to speak at all (motor **aphasia**), inability to understand (sensory aphasia), or difficulty in naming objects. In the patient who is unable to speak, it is important to find out whether he is also unable to understand. Give the patient a simple command, such as "Squeeze my hand," and see if he can carry it out.
- IRREGULAR PULSE. Cardiac dysrhythmias occur in at least 50 percent of patients in the acute phase of a stroke, and potentially life-threatening dysrhythmias occur in as many as 20 percent of stroke victims.
- HYPERTENSION. (Remember, the combination of hypertension plus bradycardia suggests increasing intracranial pressure.)
- STIFF NECK (in patients with subarachnoid hemorrhage).
- HEMIPARESIS or HEMIPLEGIA (on the side of the body opposite the side of the cerebral lesion).
- Staggering gait or INCOORDINATION.

Treatment of Suspected Stroke

Treatment of stroke in the field is aimed at improving oxygenation of the brain and protecting the patient from possible complications secondary to his disabilities.

- Ensure an open AIRWAY. Even in a conscious patient, check the gag reflex to be certain that the patient can protect his airway; if the gag reflex is absent, the airway is in jeopardy. Since it is preferable to avoid performing an awake intubation under these circumstances (the process may precipitate an increase in intracranial pressure), try to keep the airway patent by suctioning as necessary and positioning the patient to facilitate drainage from his mouth.
- Therefore, place the patient who does not have a gag reflex in the STABLE SIDE POSITION. Other patients may be transported semisitting.
- Administer OXYGEN by nasal cannula.
- Record VITAL SIGNS frequently. Blood pressure is apt to be quite high, but it will usually come down by itself, without treatment—so don't lunge for the nifedipine. Indeed, treatment of el-

evated blood pressure in the setting of an acute ischemic stroke may be quite dangerous and should not be undertaken outside the hospital.
- MONITOR cardiac rhythm. Keep the beep tone on so that you can detect the onset of bradycardia or ventricular premature beats.
- Start an IV LIFELINE with normal saline and a microdrip infusion set; run the IV at a keep-open rate, and watch it closely to make sure it doesn't "run away," for patients with stroke should not receive a lot of fluids.
- PROTECT PARALYZED EXTREMITIES. The patient may not be able to feel or express discomfort when a paralyzed limb is, for instance, jammed against the side rail of the stretcher. So be extra careful.
- Provide comfort and HONEST REASSURANCE.

Keep in mind that to an alert patient, a stroke is a terrifying experience, especially when the patient has lost his speech and, with it, the ability to communicate his distress.

> **ALWAYS ASSUME THAT THE PATIENT CAN UNDERSTAND WHAT YOU ARE SAYING, EVEN IF HE OR SHE CANNOT TALK.**

Indicate to the patient that you understand the anxiety this condition is causing and that you know this is a frightening experience. Keep up a running conversation. Explain what you are doing as you go along (e.g., "Now I want to give you a little extra oxygen to breathe—I'll just put this elastic band around the back of your head, like this. . . ."), and reassure the patient, maintaining a hopeful attitude about improvement in symptoms. Do *not* use platitudes such as, "Everything will be all right," for the patient will simply feel that you don't understand the seriousness of the situation. But it *is* possible to tell the patient honestly that in many cases there is considerable and even complete recovery of neurologic function after a stroke, so there is every reason to hope for the best.

A word of warning: The lay person often interprets any sudden collapse as a stroke, so the call that comes in to the dispatcher as a "possible stroke" is often in reality a cardiac arrest. Proceed to the scene, therefore, with appropriate speed.

GLOSSARY

anticonvulsant Medication used to suppress seizures.

aphasia Defect in speaking or in understanding speech, caused by injury or disease affecting the speech centers of the brain.

aura Premonitory sensation of an impending epileptic seizure.

cerebrovascular accident (CVA) A stroke; the sudden cessation of effective circulation to a region of the brain.

coma State of unconsciousness from which a person cannot be roused by vocal or painful stimuli.

drowsiness State in which a person appears to be asleep but can be roused by vocal stimuli.

dysarthria Interference with proper articulation of words; slurring of speech.

gingival hypertrophy Overgrowth of the gums, seen in patients who have been taking phenytoin (Dilantin) for long periods.

grand mal seizure Generalized motor seizure.

hemiparesis Weakness on one side of the body.

hemiplegia Paralysis on one side of the body.

hyperglycemia Abnormally high concentration of sugar in the blood.

hypoglycemia Abnormally low concentration of sugar in the blood.

insulin Hormone secreted by the pancreatic islet cells that promotes the utilization of sugar by the body.

ketoacidosis Condition resulting from insufficient insulin, wherein the alternative metabolism of fat produces ketones and acids.

Kussmaul's breathing Respiratory pattern characteristic of the diabetic in ketoacidosis, with marked hyperpnea and tachypnea.

micturition syncope Fainting during urination.

orthostatic syncope Fainting on going from a recumbent or sitting position to an erect position.

osmotic diuresis Passage of large volumes of urine as a consequence of a high solute concentration in the blood.

petit mal seizure Type of epileptic attack seen in children, characterized by momentary loss of awareness without loss of motor tone.

polydipsia Excessive thirst and/or excessive intake of fluids.

polyphagia Excessive hunger and eating.

polyuria Excessive urination.

postictal Referring to the period after the convulsive stage of a seizure.

pseudoseizure Hysterical seizure; seizure occurring without there being an irritable focus in the brain.

seizure Convulsion; fit; attack of epilepsy.

status epilepticus The occurrence of two or more seizures without a full return to consciousness in between them.

stroke Relatively sudden onset of a neurologic deficit that corresponds to the distribution of a cerebral artery and lasts more than 24 hours.

stupor State in which a patient cannot be roused by vocal stimuli but can be roused by a painful stimulus.

subarachnoid hemorrhage Bleeding into the space around the brain, usually caused by rupture of an aneurysm.

syncope Fainting; a brief loss of consciousness usually caused by a transient inadequacy of blood flow to the brain.

transient ischemic attack (TIA) A "little stroke"; temporary neurologic deficit resulting from a transitory decrease in circulation to part of the brain, often warning of an impending stroke.

Wernicke's encephalopathy Nutritional deficiency syndrome involving mental disturbance, paralysis of eye movements, and ataxia of gait that can be precipitated by administering 50% glucose to susceptible individuals (e.g., chronic alcoholics); prevented by giving vitamin B_1 (thiamine).

APPENDIX: **MEDICATIONS COMMONLY PRESCRIBED TO PATIENTS WITH DIABETES OR SEIZURE DISORDERS**

In patients with underlying diseases that are liable to render them unconscious, it is particularly important to be able to identify the types of drugs they are taking—for the pill bottles on the bedside table may be your *only* clue to what caused the patient's coma.

Medications Prescribed to Diabetics

Insulin

Insulin is prescribed to diabetics to replace the hormone that their bodies lack. It is self-administered by subcutaneous injection in a wide range of formulations and dosages. Different insulin formulations—such as NPH, Lente, Ultralente, Protamine Zinc—vary in their speed of onset and duration of action. Most diabetics learn the dosage schedule that is best suited to their individual needs. But diabetics may get into trouble with *hyper*glycemia when they neglect to take their insulin or when the insulin dose they do take is too small; they develop *hypo*glycemia when they take too much insulin or skip meals.

Insulin must be kept cool, so the place to look for it is in the refrigerator. The bathroom medicine cabinet may, meanwhile, reveal a supply of special insulin syringes, marked off in "units" rather than in milliliters.

Trade names for different insulin formulations include the following:

INSULIN FORMULATIONS

Humulin
Iletin
Insulatard
Mixtard
Novolin
Velosulin

Oral Hypoglycemic Agents

Diabetics who still have some pancreatic function left may be prescribed oral hypoglycemic agents rather than insulin. Oral hypoglycemic agents act, in one way or another, to stimulate pancreatic release of insulin. The agents most commonly used today are as follows:

ORAL HYPOGLYCEMIC AGENTS

Generic Name	*Trade Name*
Acetohexamide	**Dymelor**
Chlorpropamide	**Diabinese**
Glipizide	**Glucotrol**
Glyburide	**DiaBeta, Micronase**
Tolazamide	**Tolinase**
Tolbutamide	**Orinase**

In some parts of the world, another oral hypoglycemic, phenformin (**DBI**) is still being used. There have been some fatal complications of phenformin use, notably refractory lactic acidosis.

Medications Prescribed to Patients with Seizures

Patients with chronic seizures are usually placed on long-term therapy with one or more drugs that suppress seizure activity (**anticonvulsant** drugs). One of the most common causes of recurrent seizures is failure to take those prescribed medications. For that reason, any patient presenting with seizures should be asked not only whether he takes medications for seizures but also whether he took his medications TODAY!

ANTICONVULSANT MEDICATIONS

Generic Name	*Trade Name*
Phenytoin	**Dilantin**
Mephenytoin	**Mesantoin**
Ethotoin	**Peganone**
Phenobarbital	**Luminal**
Mephobarbital	**Mebaral**
Metharbital	**Gemonil**
Primidone	**Mysoline**
Trimethadione	**Tridione**
Paramethadione	**Paradione**
Phensuximide	**Milontin**
Methsuximide	**Celontin**
Ethosuximide	**Zarontin**
Phenacemide	**Phenurone**
Carbamazepine	**Tegretol**
Clonazepam	**Clonopin**
Valproic acid	**Depakene**

FURTHER READING

THE COMATOSE PATIENT
Baehren D, Werman HA. Altered mental states. *JEMS* 11(7):67, 1989.
Bourn S. Treating the unconscious patient: Who's in the coma? *JEMS* 17(11):27, 1992.
Darmody WR. *Management of the Unconscious Patient.* St. Louis: Mosby, 1976.
Edwards FJ. Cases of coma. *Emergency* 23(11):38, 1991.
Garvin JM. Neurologic emergencies. *Emerg Med Serv* 17(7):40, 1988.
Haerer AF. Coma: Some differential considerations in the diagnosis and management. *Hosp Med* 12(4):68, 1976.
Henry GL. Neurologic emergencies: 1. The basic assessment. *Emerg Med* 20(3):29, 1988.

Hitchins J, Gullo R. Identifying types of coma in the elderly. *Emerg Med Serv* 14(2):33, 1985.

Jones C. Glasgow coma scale. *Am J Nurs* 79:1551, 1979.

Lipowski ZJ. Delirium (acute confusional states). *JAMA* 258:1789, 1987.

Posner J. The comatose patient. *Emerg Med* 11:107, 1977.

Redding JS, Tabeling BB, Parham AM. Airway management in patients with central nervous system depression. *JACEP* 7:401, 1978.

Samuels MA. A systematic approach to the comatose patient. *Emerg Med* 22(8):17, 1990.

Whitlow GD. The nervous system: A review of the physiology and common emergencies. *Emergency* 11(9):50, 1979.

Wilkinson HA. Evaluation and management of the unconscious patient. *Emerg Med Serv* 7(5):24, 1978.

DIABETIC EMERGENCIES

Adler PM. Serum glucose changes after administration of 50% dextrose solution: Pre- and in-hospital calculations. *Am J Emerg Med* 4:504, 1986.

Adrogue HJ, Barrero J, Eknoyan G. Salutary effects of modest fluid replacement in the treatment of adults with diabetic ketoacidosis: Use in patients without extreme volume deficit. *JAMA* 262:2108, 1989.

Andrade A et al. Hypoglycemic hemiplegic syndrome. *Ann Emerg Med* 13:529, 1984.

Auf der Heide E. Prehospital management of diabetic emergencies. *Emerg Med Serv* 9(5):9, 1980.

Baker FJ et al. Diabetic emergencies: Hypoglycemia and ketoacidosis. *JACEP* 5:119, 1976.

Bledsoe B. Dealing with diabetic emergencies. *JEMS* 16(12):40, 1991.

Bourn S. When sugar's not sweet. *JEMS* 14(12):81, 1989.

Browning RG et al. 50% dextrose: Antidote or toxin? *Ann Emerg Med* 21:20, 1992.

Carter WP. Hypothermia: A sign of hypoglycemia. *JACEP* 5:594, 1976.

Chisholm CD, Chisholm RL. Hypoglycemia: A metabolic disorder of many faces. *JEMS* 14(6):29, 1989.

Cotton EK, Fahlberg VI. Hypoglycemia with salicylate poisoning. *AM J Dis Child* 108:171, 1964.

deCourtern-Myers G, Myers RE, Schoolfield L. Hyperglycemia enlarges infarct size in cerebrovascular occlusion in cats. *Stroke* 19:623, 1988.

Dorin RI, Crapo LM. Hypokalemic respiratory arrest in diabetic ketoacidosis. *JAMA* 257:1517, 1987.

Felig P. Diabetic ketoacidosis. *N Engl J Med* 290:1360, 1974.

Hillman K. Fluid resuscitation in diabetic emergencies: A reappraisal. *Intensive Care Med* 13:4, 1987.

Hoffman JR et al. The empiric use of hypertonic dextrose in patients with altered mental status: A reappraisal. *Ann Emerg Med* 21:20, 1992.

Hogya PT et al. The rapid prehospital estimation of blood glucose using Chemstrip bG. *Prehosp Disaster Med* 4:109, 1989.

Iscovith AL. Sudden cardiac death due to hypoglycemia. *Am J Emerg Med* 1:28, 1983.

Jones JL et al. Determination of prehospital blood glucose: A prospective, controlled study. *J Emerg Med* 10:679, 1992.

Kunian L, Wasco J, Hulefeld L. Sweets for the alcoholic. *Emerg Med* 5(1):45, 1973.

Levine SN et al. Treatment of diabetic ketoacidosis. *Arch Intern Med* 141:713, 1981.

Morris LR et al. Bicarbonate therapy in severe diabetic ketoacidosis. *Ann Intern Med* 105:836, 1986.

Moss MH. Alcohol-induced hypoglycemia and coma caused by alcohol sponging. *Pediatrics* 46:445, 1970.

Rosenbloom AL. Intracerebral crises during treatment of diabetic ketoacidosis. *Diabetes Care* 13:22, 1990.

Slovis CM. Early recognition of diabetic ketoacidosis. *Emerg Med* 21(8):20, 1989.

Stapczynski JS, Haskell RJ. Duration of hypoglycemia and need for intravenous glucose following intentional overdoses of insulin. *Ann Emerg Med* 13:505, 1984.

Taigman M. Just a little sugar: Serious talk about D-50. *JEMS* 13(10):33, 1988.

Vukmir RB, Paris PM, Yealy DM. Glucagon: Prehospital therapy for hypoglycemia. *Ann Emerg Med* 20:375, 1991.

SYNCOPE

Day SC et al. Evaluation and outcome of emergency room patients with transient loss of consciousness. *Am J Med* 73:15, 1982.

Georgeson S et al. Acute cardiac ischemia in patients with syncope: Importance of the initial electrocardiogram. *J Gen Intern Med* 7:379, 1992.

Gibson TC et al. Diagnostic efficacy of 24-hour electrocardiographic monitoring for syncope. *Am J Cardiol* 53:1013, 1984.

Kapoor WN, Peterson PA, Karpf M. Micturition syncope: A reappraisal. *JAMA* 253:796, 1985.

Kapoor WN et al. Syncope in the elderly. *Am J Med* 80:419, 1986.

Martin GJ et al. Prospective evaluation of syncope. *Ann Emerg Med* 13:499, 1984.

SEIZURES

American College of Emergency Physicians. Clinical policy for the initial approach to patients presenting with a chief complaint of seizure, who are not in status epilepticus. *Ann Emerg Med* 22:875, 1993.

Bader T. Telling pseudoseizures from true. *Emerg Med* 17(13):41, 1985.

Bell HE, Bertino JS. Constant diazepam infusion in the treatment of continuous seizure activity. *Drug Intell Clin Pharm* 18:965, 1984.

Bernat JL. Getting a handle on an adult's first seizure. *Emerg Med* 21(1):20, 1989.

Camfield PR. Treatment of status epilepticus in children. *Can Med Assoc J* 128:671, 1983.

Cloyd JC, Gumnit RJ, McLain W Jr. Status epilepticus: The role of intravenous phenytoin. *JAMA* 244:1479, 1980.

Cox D. Diazepam use for seizures. *Emergency* 25(9):20, 1993.

Curry HB. Fits and faints: Causes and cures. *Emerg Med* 14(3):70, 1982.

Delgado-Escueta AV et al. Management of status epilepticus. *N Engl J Med* 306:1337, 1982.

Drawbaugh RE, Deibler CG, Eitel DR. Prehospital administration of rectal diazepam in pediatric status epilepticus. *Prehosp Disaster Med* 5(2):155, 1990.

Finelli PF, Cardi JK. Seizures as a cause of fracture. *Neurology* 39:858, 1989.

Gress D. Stopping seizures. *Emerg Med* 22(1):22, 1990.

Jagoda A, Riggio S. Refractory status epilepticus in adults. *Ann Emerg Med* 22:1337, 1993.

Klepser M, Levy DB. Status epilepticus. *Emergency* 25(7):59, 1993.

Leppik IE. Status epilepticus. *Clin Ther* 7:272, 1985.

Parrish GA, Skiendzielewski JJ. Bilateral posterior fracture-dislocations of the shoulder after convulsive status epilepticus. *Ann Emerg Med* 14:264, 1985.

Phillips SA, Shanahan RJ. Etiology and mortality of status epilepticus in children. *Arch Neurol* 46:74, 1989.

Riley TL. Epilepsy—or merely hyperventilation? *Emerg Med* 14(14):162, 1982.

Shaner DM et al. Treatment of status epilepticus. *Neurology* 38:202, 1988.

Sonander H et al. Effects of the rectal administration of diazepam. *Br J Anaesth* 57:578, 1985.

Working Group on Status Epilepticus. Treatment of convulsive status epilepticus. *JAMA* 270:854, 1993.

Wyler AR. Modern management of epilepsy. *Postgrad Med* 94(3):97, 1993.

See also references at the end of Chapter 30, Pediatric Emergencies.

STROKE

Alberts MJ, Bertels C, Dawson D. An analysis of time of presentation after stroke. *JAMA* 263:65, 1990.

Badui E et al. Coincidence of cerebrovascular accident and silent myocardial infarction. *Angiology* 33:702, 1982.

Baskin DS et al. Naloxone reversal of ischaemic neurological deficits in man. *Lancet* 2:272, 1981.

Berger JR. Differentiating stroke: A case study primer. *Emerg Med* 23(11):115, 1991.

Broderick J et al. Blood pressure during the first minutes of focal cerebral ischemia. *Ann Emerg Med* 22:1433, 1993.

Brott TG et al. Urgent therapy for stroke: Part I. Pilot study of tissue plasminogen activator administered within 90 minutes. *Stroke* 25:632, 1992.

Caplan LR. Diagnosis and treatment of ischemic stroke. *JAMA* 266:2413, 1991.

Caroline NL. *Emergency Medical Treatment: A Text for the EMT-A and EMT-Intermediate* (3rd ed.). Boston: Little, Brown, 1991. Chap. 22.

Edmeads J. Strategies in stroke. *Emerg Med* 15(4):163, 1983.

Elizabeth J et al. Arterial oxygen saturation and posture in acute stroke. *Age Ageing* 22:269, 1993.

Fallis RJ et al. A double blind trial of naloxone in the treatment of acute stroke. *Stroke* 15:627, 1984.

Fontanarosa PB. Recognition of subarachnoid hemorrhage. *Ann Emerg Med* 18:1199, 1989.

Jacobs FL. Stroke: Emergency assessment and management. *Emerg Med Serv* 14(2):41, 1985.

Klag MJ et al. Decline in US stroke mortality: Demographic trends and antihypertensive treatment. *Stroke* 20:14, 1989.

Komrad MS et al. Myocardial infarction and stroke. *Neurology* 34:1403, 1984.

Lavin P. Management of hypertension in patients with acute stroke. *Arch Intern Med* 146:66, 1986.

Marler JR et al. Morning increase in onset of ischemic stroke. *Stroke* 20:473, 1989.

Mikolich JR et al. Cardiac arrhythmias in patients with acute cerebrovascular accidents. *JAMA* 246:1314, 1981.

Myers MG et al. Cardiac sequelae of acute stroke. *Stroke* 13:838, 1982.

Parsons-Smith BG. First aid for acute cerebral stroke. *Practitioner* 223:553, 1979.

Powers WJ. Acute hypertension after stroke: The scientific basis for treatment decisions. *Neurology* 43:461, 1993.

Salzman B. Cerebrovascular accidents. *JEMS* 17(10):52, 1992.

Samuels MA. All about stroke. *Emerg Med* 18(6):94, 1986.

Tracey DF et al. Hyperglycaemia and mortality from acute stroke. *Q J Med* 86:439, 1993.

Walshaw MJ, Pearson MG. Hypoxia in patients with acute hemiplegia. *Br Med J* 288:15, 1984.

25
Acute Abdomen

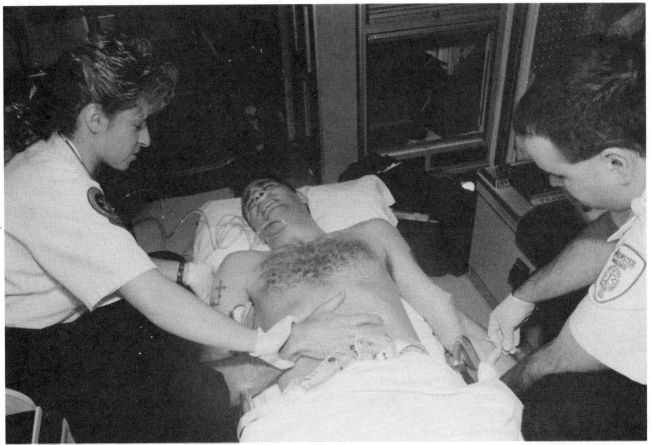

Brewster Ambulance Service, Brewster, Massachusetts. Photo by Brian Clark.

OBJECTIVES

Just about everyone suffers a bellyache at one time or another, and abdominal pain is, in fact, one of the most common presenting complaints in every emergency room. When we talk about the "acute abdomen," however, we are generally talking about something more serious than the garden variety abdominal pain. Although the term "acute abdomen" is not very precise, it usually refers to a condition that produces peritoneal irritation and, in many cases, requires surgical intervention. So it is important to be able to sort out those patients who may have an acute abdomen from those with a "deli belly" or other such relatively benign conditions. In this chapter, we shall, first of all, review what's inside the abdomen in order to appreciate the multitude of things that can go wrong there. We shall then consider the assessment of a patient whose chief complaint is abdominal pain and look at a few specific causes—nonhemorrhagic and hemorrhagic—of the acute abdomen. Finally, moving away from the acute abdomen to more chronic problems involving intra-abdominal organs, we shall examine the special considerations in dealing with a renal dialysis patient. By the end of this chapter, the student should be able to

1. List the abdominal organs or structures that belong to
   • The gastrointestinal system
   • The urinary system
   • The female reproductive system
   • The vascular system
2. Differentiate between visceral and somatic abdominal pain, given a description of several patients with qualitatively different abdominal pain
3. Give two examples of referred pain
4. List three mechanisms of abdominal pain
5. List four extra-abdominal conditions that can cause abdominal pain
6. List six questions that should be asked in taking the history of a patient whose chief complaint is abdominal pain
7. In a patient whose chief complaint is abdominal pain, describe the significance of
   • Coffee-ground vomitus
   • Melena
   • Tenting of the skin
   • Patient lying very still
   • Rigid abdomen
   • Pulsatile abdominal mass
8. List six symptoms and signs of hypovolemic shock

9. Given a description of several patients with different symptoms and signs, identify a patient with probable
   • Peptic ulcer disease
   • Diverticulitis
   • Mesenteric ischemia
   • Abdominal aortic aneurysm
   • Ureteral colic
   and describe the correct prehospital management of a patient with an acute abdomen
10. List eight medical problems to which renal dialysis patients are particularly susceptible
11. Identify the problem from which a dialysis patient is suffering, given a description of the clinical situation, and describe the prehospital management of that problem

REVIEW OF ABDOMINAL ANATOMY

Recall that the abdominal cavity is bounded by the diaphragm above, the pelvis below, the spine in back, and the muscular abdominal wall in front. As we learned in Chapter 18, the abdominal cavity can be viewed as consisting of three parts (Fig. 25-1): an *intrathoracic abdomen,* containing the liver, spleen and stomach; the *true abdomen,* containing the small and large bowel and the bladder; and the *retroperitoneum,* containing the pancreas, duodenum, kidneys and ureters, the abdominal aorta, and inferior vena cava. The abdominal cavity as a whole is lined by a smooth, membranous layer called the **peritoneum,** from which the abdominal cavity derives its other name—the **peritoneal cavity.**

The organs of the abdominal cavity can be classified in several ways. When we were dealing with abdominal *trauma,* it was very useful to classify abdominal organs according to whether they were solid organs or hollow organs (Table 25-1), for the type of injury to which an organ is vulnerable is influenced by its structure. In considering *non*traumatic problems affecting the abdomen, it is more useful to classify the abdominal organs according to the *organ system* to which they belong, for the patient's signs and symptoms will very often be referable to a particular organ system (Table 25-2). In general, the organs, or **viscera** (singular is **viscus**) of the abdomen belong to one of four organ systems. The bulk of the abdomen is occupied by viscera of the GASTROINTESTINAL SYSTEM, including the stomach, small and large bowel, liver, gallbladder, and pancreas. Most of the viscera of the URINARY SYSTEM lie in the retroperitoneal space—the kidneys and ureters—with the bladder alone more anteriorly placed in the pelvis. The female REPRODUCTIVE ORGANS are almost

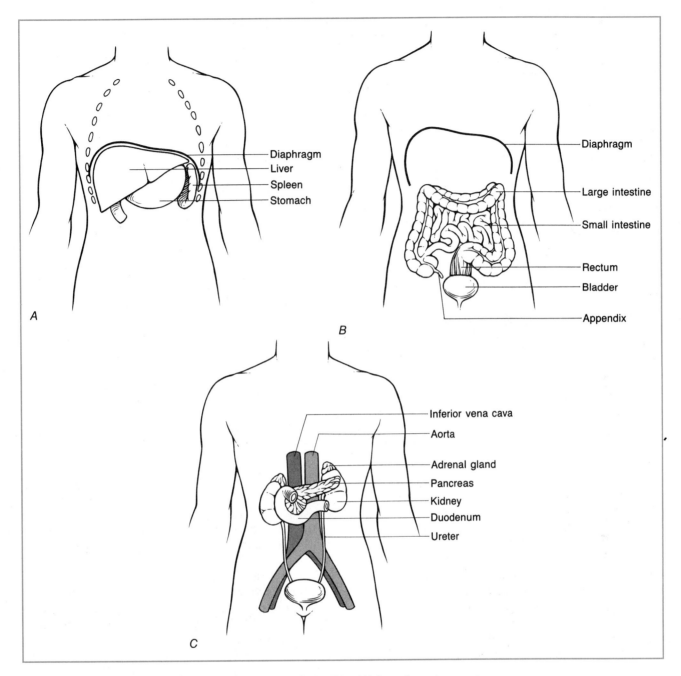

A

Diaphragm
Liver
Spleen
Stomach

B

Diaphragm
Large intestine
Small intestine
Rectum
Bladder
Appendix

C

Inferior vena cava
Aorta
Adrenal gland
Pancreas
Kidney
Duodenum
Ureter

FIGURE 25-1. **CONTENTS OF THE ABDOMINAL CAVITY.** (A) Intrathoracic abdomen. (B) True abdomen. (C) Retroperitoneum.

TABLE 25-1. **HOLLOW AND SOLID ORGANS OF THE ABDOMEN**

HOLLOW ABDOMINAL ORGANS	SOLID ABDOMINAL ORGANS
Stomach	Liver
Small and large bowel	Spleen
Gallbladder	Pancreas
Bladder	Kidneys
Uterus (females)	Ovaries (females)

entirely intra-abdominal—the ovaries, fallopian tubes and uterus being in the lower abdominal quadrants. Of the male reproductive organs, only the prostate and seminal ducts can really be considered abdominal structures, although pain from extra-abdominal structures, such as the testes, is often perceived as abdominal pain. Finally, the VASCULAR SYSTEM is well represented in the abdomen with the abdominal aorta and its branches along with the inferior vena cava and the veins that empty into it.

TABLE 25-2. ORGAN SYSTEMS OF THE ABDOMEN AND CLINICAL FINDINGS

ORGAN SYSTEM	COMPONENT ORGANS	SIGNS AND SYMPTOMS
Gastrointestinal	Stomach Small bowel (duodenum, jejunum, ileum) Large bowel (colon) Gallbladder Liver Pancreas	Anorexia Nausea Vomiting Hematemesis Diarrhea Constipation Bloody stools Tarry stools (melena)
Urinary	Kidneys Ureters Bladder	Flank pain Painful urination (dysuria) Frequent urination Blood in urine (hematuria)
Female reproductive	Ovaries Fallopian tubes Uterus	Menstrual irregularities Vaginal discharge/bleeding Pain during intercourse Signs of pregnancy
Male reproductive	Prostate Seminal ducts	Changes in urinary stream
Vascular	Aorta and all its branches Inferior vena cava and its sources	Tearing pain of a leaking aortic aneurysm Abdominal angina (mesenteric ischemia)

With so many different structures and systems represented in the abdomen, it is small wonder that so many things can go wrong and that most medical textbooks list at least 100 possible causes of an acute abdomen. It will usually not be possible, nor will it be necessary or useful, for the paramedic to identify the precise cause of a patient's abdominal pain. What *is* important, however, is to be able to rapidly identify conditions that have life-threatening potential and to assess the overall clinical status of the patient. To do so, one must take a relevant history and perform a brief but pertinent physical examination.

ASSESSING THE PATIENT WITH ABDOMINAL PAIN

It is useful, in questioning a patient about his belly pain, to understand the different mechanisms by which abdominal pain can come about. Three quite distinct types of pain response may be involved in producing pain in the abdomen: visceral pain, somatic pain, and referred pain.

- **Visceral pain** results from putting stretch on the autonomic nerve fibers that surround abdominal viscera. The distention of a hollow organ, for ex-

ample, as may occur in obstruction, increases the tension in its wall and thus the stretch on autonomic fibers there. Similarly, swelling inside a solid organ stretches the organ's capsule, with the same net effect. Visceral pain is classically described as being *colicky, crampy, dull,* or *gassy,* and typically it comes and goes. It tends to be diffuse and *poorly localized;* indeed, the patient may be surprised to find that the place where he is feeling pain is *not* the place that's tender when you palpate. Because it involves autonomic nerve stimulation, visceral pain is also likely to be accompanied by *other autonomic symptoms,* such as nausea, vomiting, tachycardia, and sweating.

- **Somatic pain** occurs when nerve fibers in the *peritoneum* are irritated by chemical or bacterial inflammation. Somatic pain is more localized than visceral pain. It is often described by the patient as *sharp* or knifelike, and it tends to be *constant* and to be exacerbated by coughing or any other jarring motion.

- **Referred pain** is any pain that is felt at a location removed from the diseased organ that is causing the pain. Knowing the classic patterns of referred pain (Fig. 25-2) can be helpful in narrowing down the cause of abdominal pain. When, for example, there is irritation of the diaphragm, by collections

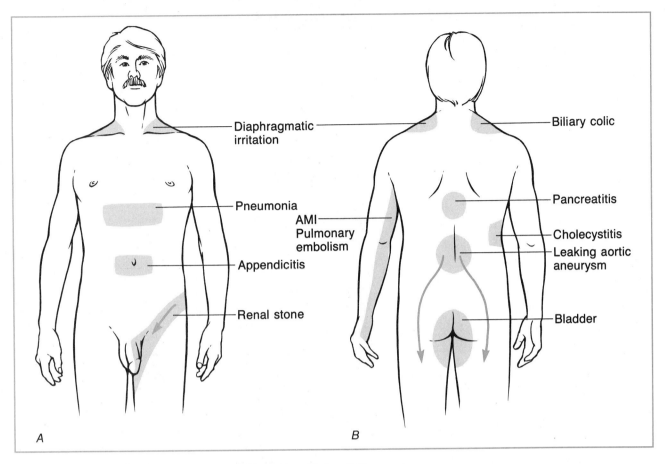

FIGURE 25-2. **CLASSIC PATTERNS OF REFERRED PAIN.** AMI = acute myocardial infarction.

of blood or pus beneath it, the pain often radiates to the side of the neck and shoulder. The pain of a stone passing through a ureter (**ureteral colic**) typically radiates down into the genitalia and inner thigh. A leaking aortic aneurysm is often experienced as pain in the lower back or buttocks.

The very existence of referred pain brings us to an important point:

NOT ALL ABDOMINAL PAIN IS FROM ABDOMINAL CAUSES.

We shall, in this chapter, be primarily concerned with the intra-abdominal causes of abdominal pain, which generally come about from one of three processes: obstruction of a hollow organ, peritoneal inflammation, or ischemia. But it is well to keep in

mind that other processes, outside the abdomen, may produce abdominal pain as well (Table 25-3).

With those considerations in mind, we can begin to ask the patient some questions about his or her abdominal pain.

Taking the History

In trying to learn more about a chief complaint of abdominal pain, the PQRST-A format is once again a useful guide:

P What, if anything, PROVOKED the pain, and what, if anything, PALLIATES IT? Try to establish in particular whether there was any relationship between the onset of pain and the consumption of food or drink. The pain of gallbladder disease, for example, can be provoked by a meal. Peptic ulcer pain is often made better by eating or by taking antacids.

TABLE 25-3.   CAUSES OF ABDOMINAL PAIN CLASSIFIED BY MECHANISM

MECHANISM	EXAMPLES
Intra-abdominal causes	
Obstruction of a hollow organ	Small bowel obstruction by adhesions
	Ureteral obstruction by kidney stones
	Common bile duct obstruction by gallstones
Peritoneal inflammation	Perforated duodenal ulcer
	Pancreatitis
Ischemia	Strangulated hernia
	Mesenteric thrombosis
Extra-abdominal causes	
Chest disorders	Pneumonia
	Acute myocardial infarction
	Pulmonary embolism
Genitalia	Testicular torsion
Nerve roots	Shingles (herpes zoster)
Metabolic and toxic	Diabetic ketoacidosis
	Sickle cell crisis
	Black widow spider bite
	Heavy metal poisoning (e.g., lead)

Q   What is the QUALITY of the pain; that is, what does it feel like? Constant abdominal pain is suggestive of inflammatory or destructive organ involvement, while cramping, intermittent ("colicky") pain suggests obstruction of a hollow organ. Pay attention to the adjectives the patient uses to describe his pain, for those adjectives are often a very sensitive diagnostic tool. The patient who describes his pain as "tearing" or "ripping" is likely to be bleeding from an aortic aneurysm, while the patient with "burning" epigastric pain may have a peptic ulcer that has eaten through the duodenal wall into the pancreas.

R   What is the REGION (location) of the pain, and where does it RADIATE? As noted earlier, visceral pain tends to be poorly localized, so the location of the pain may or may not correspond to the location of the diseased structure. Nonetheless, experience teaches that pain in certain areas is more likely to be associated with certain conditions. Figure 25-3 shows some of the causes of the acute abdomen in terms of the abdominal quadrant in which the pain is experienced.

S   How SEVERE is the pain? A stone lodged in the ureter, for example, generally produces pain that can make even a teamster cry. It should be mentioned, though, that the patient's description of the severity of his pain does not always correlate well with the severity of the problem, particularly in the elderly. Patients over about 65 to 70 years old usually have a higher pain threshold than younger patients and may therefore suffer only minor abdominal pain despite a major abdominal catastrophe.

T   What was the TIMING of the pain? Ask first about the *onset*: Did the pain come on suddenly, reaching its peak within minutes, or gradually, over hours or days? Sudden and explosive abdominal pain suggests the rupture of an abdominal structure (e.g., a ruptured aortic aneurysm, a ruptured ectopic pregnancy, a perforated duodenal ulcer) or sometimes intestinal ischemia ("intestinal angina"). The onset of pain in other conditions, on the other hand, such as appendicitis or **diverticulitis** (inflammation of an outpouching of the colon), may be much less dramatic. Find out also about the *duration* of the pain. As a general rule:

ANY SEVERE ABDOMINAL PAIN THAT COMES ON SUDDENLY AND LASTS MORE THAN SIX HOURS MUST BE CONSIDERED SERIOUS AND WILL PROBABLY REQUIRE SURGERY.

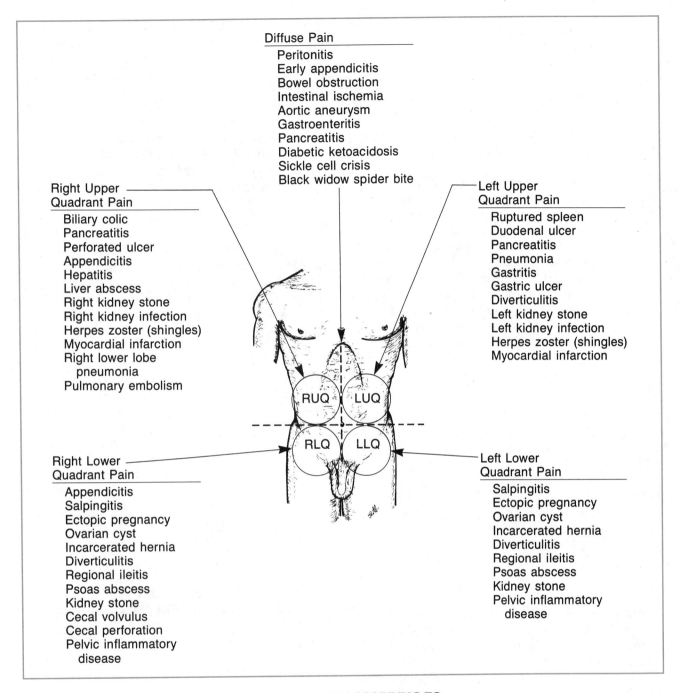

Diffuse Pain
Peritonitis
Early appendicitis
Bowel obstruction
Intestinal ischemia
Aortic aneurysm
Gastroenteritis
Pancreatitis
Diabetic ketoacidosis
Sickle cell crisis
Black widow spider bite

Right Upper Quadrant Pain
Biliary colic
Pancreatitis
Perforated ulcer
Appendicitis
Hepatitis
Liver abscess
Right kidney stone
Right kidney infection
Herpes zoster (shingles)
Myocardial infarction
Right lower lobe pneumonia
Pulmonary embolism

Left Upper Quadrant Pain
Ruptured spleen
Duodenal ulcer
Pancreatitis
Pneumonia
Gastritis
Gastric ulcer
Diverticulitis
Left kidney stone
Left kidney infection
Herpes zoster (shingles)
Myocardial infarction

Right Lower Quadrant Pain
Appendicitis
Salpingitis
Ectopic pregnancy
Ovarian cyst
Incarcerated hernia
Diverticulitis
Regional ileitis
Psoas abscess
Kidney stone
Cecal volvulus
Cecal perforation
Pelvic inflammatory disease

Left Lower Quadrant Pain
Salpingitis
Ectopic pregnancy
Ovarian cyst
Incarcerated hernia
Diverticulitis
Regional ileitis
Psoas abscess
Kidney stone
Pelvic inflammatory disease

FIGURE 25-3. **POSSIBLE CAUSES OF ABDOMINAL PAIN ACCORDING TO LOCATION.**

A Inquire about ASSOCIATED SYMPTOMS referable to the organ systems contained within the abdominal cavity. Specifically, ask about:
  • NAUSEA and VOMITING. While nausea and vomiting occur very frequently with abdominal pain and therefore do not provide much diagnostic information, it is important to know the following:

1. *How much* has the patient vomited? Once? Repeatedly for 2 days? (If the latter, look for signs of dehydration!)
2. What did the vomitus look like and taste like? Was it bitter, like bile? Did it smell like feces? Did the patient vomit blood (**hematemesis**) or material that looked like *coffee grounds* (which is blood that has remained for a while in the stomach)?

3. Which came first, the pain or the vomiting?

- Has there been any CHANGE IN THE PATIENT'S BOWEL HABITS? Constipation? Diarrhea? Change in the color of the stools? Has there been bright red blood in the stools? Have they been a tarry, black color (**melena**; which signals the presence of blood from the upper gastrointestinal tract)?
- Inquire about URINARY TRACT SYMPTOMS—painful urination (**dysuria**), frequency of urination, blood in the urine (**hematuria**).
- In women of child-bearing age, it is essential to obtain a recent MENSTRUAL HISTORY. At the least, find out the *date of the last menstrual period* to rule out the possibility of ectopic pregnancy (see Chap. 37).
- Ask about CHEST PAIN and DYSPNEA. As mentioned earlier, not all abdominal pain comes from the abdomen.

Finally, it is necessary to find out a few details about the patient's *medical history*—specifically whether he has any major UNDERLYING ILLNESSES, whether he has ever undergone ABDOMINAL SURGERY, and what MEDICATIONS he takes on a regular basis. Ask specifically about aspirin, antacids, and steroids.

Physical Assessment

The prehospital physical examination of a patient with abdominal pain should be brief, aimed at establishing the patient's general condition and the urgency of the problem.

In observing the patient's *general appearance*, note first his POSITION and DEGREE OF DISTRESS. A patient with peritoneal pain will usually lie very, very still, avoiding even the slightest movement, for even the shifting of abdominal viscera within the inflamed peritoneal cavity causes severe pain. The patient with an obstructed hollow organ, by contrast, will often be doubled over or thrashing about restlessly, searching for a position that brings relief from the pain. The patient with pancreatitis often lies on his side with his knees and hips flexed, to take tension off the inflamed abdominal musculature. The patient with appendicitis typically lies with the right hip and right knee flexed, again to minimize tension in the muscles overlying the inflamed structure.

Check the SKIN for sweating and pallor, which tend to be signs of serious illness. Pinch the skin over the back of the hand and see if it stays pinched or returns quickly to its normal form. Skin that stays pinched ("tents") signals dehydration.

Measure the VITAL SIGNS. *Tachycardia, hypotension*, or both suggest serious volume depletion and should serve as a reminder not to dawdle.

The ABDOMINAL EXAMINATION necessary in the field can be accomplished in less than a minute. Expose the abdomen, and first *inspect* it for distention, scars of previous surgery, and any obvious masses. Note as well whether the abdominal wall moves normally during respiration (a patient with peritoneal irritation will try to splint his abdominal muscles and prevent their movement). Then, with a warmed hand, palpate very gently to determine two things: (1) the *consistency* of the abdomen (soft? boardlike?) and (2) whether there is a *pulsatile mass*. Forget about listening for bowel sounds, because to do so properly requires several minutes in a quiet setting—conditions that cannot be met in the field, especially if the patient is in serious condition. Similarly, extensive palpation of a painful abdomen in the field serves no useful purpose; it will only increase the patient's discomfort and delay transport. Do not, therefore, spend a lot of time poking at the patient's belly. Decide whether it is soft or rigid and whether there is a pulsating mass, and leave it at that. The patient will be subjected to more than enough pushing and prodding in the emergency room; there is no need to add further to his pain in the field.

DO NOT SPEND A LOT OF TIME POKING AT THE BELLY OF A PATIENT WITH ABDOMINAL PAIN.

IMPORTANT CAUSES OF ABDOMINAL PAIN

Clearly we cannot, in the space of a short chapter, deal with all the causes of abdominal pain, nor would it be useful to do so. In this section, therefore, we shall merely mention some of the more serious conditions that may produce an acute abdomen. Once again, the purpose is *not* so that the paramedic can make an etiologic diagnosis in the field. The purpose of becoming familiar with some of the causes of abdominal pain is to be able to recognize when a serious condition exists, so that appropriate life support measures are undertaken.

One of the most important things to try to figure out is WHETHER THE PATIENT IS BLEEDING IN-

TERNALLY. Clues in the *history* include the vomiting of blood or coffee-ground material, bloody or tarry stools, or (in women) profuse vaginal bleeding. The physical examination, meanwhile, should provide confirmatory evidence with *signs of shock*. (What *are* the signs of shock? If you can't by now rattle them off in your sleep, go back and review Chap. 9.)

Among the most common causes of an acute abdomen with internal bleeding is PEPTIC ULCER DISEASE. The typical patient is a man between the ages of 35 and 45 who gives a history of chronic, vague pain or discomfort in the epigastrium, often just to the right of the midline. The chronic pain may be described as steady, dull, or burning. It is made worse by going for any period on an empty stomach, and it is usually relieved by the intake of food, liquids, or antacids.

Another quite common cause of the acute abdomen is DIVERTICULITIS. A **diverticulum** (plural: diverticula) is an outpouching in the wall of the colon. Diverticula become more common with advancing age and often are entirely asymptomatic. However, about 25 percent of patients who have colonic diverticula will experience an inflammatory complication (**diverticulitis**) at some time. What happens is that fecal material seeps through the thin-walled diverticula and causes inflammation and sometimes abscess formation in the colonic wall. The most characteristic symptom is steady, severe *left lower quadrant pain* that may have been present for several days (although sometimes the patient will report cramping pain that is relieved by a bowel movement). If perforation of the colon has occurred, the patient may also have signs of peritonitis.

A far less common but more dangerous cause of the acute abdomen is MESENTERIC ISCHEMIA, that is, compromise of the circulation to the intestines. Mesenteric ischemia, like cerebral ischemia, may occur in a number of ways. Most commonly, it is the result of *emboli* from the heart finding their way into the superior mesenteric artery, and patients most at risk are those who are most likely to be forming arterial emboli, namely those with atrial fibrillation, recent myocardial infarction, or rheumatic heart disease. As with emboli elsewhere (pulmonary, cerebral), the onset of symptoms in superior mesenteric artery embolism is usually abrupt, with severe, generalized abdominal pain that is all out of proportion to the findings on physical examination. Thus you are apt to find the patient in marked distress, but his abdomen may still be soft, and pushing on it doesn't increase the pain. A second possible mechanism for mesenteric ischemia is superior mesenteric artery *thrombosis*, which nearly always occurs in patients who have signs of atherosclerotic disease elsewhere (e.g., chronic angina pectoris). The onset of symp-toms in thrombosis is slower than with an embolus, with the pain getting slowly worse and worse over a period of several hours. Typically, the pain comes on after a heavy meal, because a heavy meal increases the bowel's oxygen demand in the same way that exertion increases the oxygen demand of the heart. For that reason, the pain of thrombotic disease in the bowel is sometimes referred to as "abdominal angina." Other signs of superior mesenteric artery thrombosis include *diarrhea* and *abdominal distention*.

Whatever the underlying cause, mesenteric ischemia is a *dire medical emergency* that carries a dismal mortality rate of between 70 and 90 percent. If the patient does not reach surgery within about 4 to 6 hours after the onset of pain, the part of the bowel that has been deprived of circulation will undergo necrosis and gangrene and will perforate. So if you have any reason to suspect mesenteric ischemia—for instance, when you get a history of abdominal pain that came on after a heavy meal or you find unexplained abdominal distention in an elderly person—you need to get moving quickly and to notify the receiving hospital of the possible diagnosis.

We have already discussed, in a previous chapter, the signs of an expanding or leaking ABDOMINAL AORTIC ANEURYSM. To review briefly, an aneurysm is an area of weakening and dilatation in the wall of an artery. When an abdominal aortic aneurysm begins leaking or ruptures, it classically produces a sudden onset of severe, constant pain that often radiates to the lower back, flanks, or buttocks. Palpation of the abdomen will usually reveal a *pulsatile mass*, and the femoral pulses may be decreased. Sometimes the skin over the abdomen appears mottled and the legs look paler than the rest of the body.

The patient with a KIDNEY STONE will usually be in extreme distress. In fact, so long as the stone sits in the kidney, it does not usually cause much trouble; symptoms occur when the stone starts migrating down the ureter, stretching the ureteral wall in the process. As it does so, the patient experiences the classic visceral pain associated with distention of a hollow organ. The pain of ureteral colic is usually located in the flank, radiating into the scrotum or labia. It is often associated with nausea and vomiting, and the patient may be markedly dehydrated. Given the location and radiation of the pain, one must also consider the possibility of an abdominal aortic aneurysm under such circumstances.

Finally, acute abdominal pain in a woman of child-bearing age, especially if accompanied by signs of shock, should be assumed to be an ECTOPIC PREGNANCY (a pregnancy developing in the abdomen, outside the uterus) until proved otherwise. We shall discuss ectopic pregnancy in more detail in Chapter 37.

MANAGEMENT OF THE PATIENT WITH ABDOMINAL PAIN

The prehospital treatment will be more or less the same for any patient with an acute abdomen and must be carried out with an appropriate *sense of urgency*.

> **IT IS NOT NECESSARY TO DIAGNOSE THE SPECIFIC CAUSE OF A PATIENT'S ABDOMINAL PAIN IN ORDER TO APPRECIATE THAT THE PATIENT IS IN SERIOUS CONDITION.**

When a patient is clearly in distress, his skin is cold and sweaty, and his pulse is rapid and weak, it is safe to assume that he has a potentially life-threatening problem and to act accordingly.

PREHOSPITAL CARE OF THE ACUTE ABDOMEN

- Ensure an adequate AIRWAY. If the patient is vomiting, position him on his side.
- Administer OXYGEN by nasal cannula.
- If you suspect an abdominal aortic aneurysm, apply (but do not inflate) the military anti-shock trousers (MAST), according to local protocols. Consult medical command regarding inflation.
- Start at least one LARGE-BORE IV en route. If the patient is tachycardic or has other signs of dehydration or shock, give large volumes of lactated Ringer's. Be particularly generous with fluids if you suspect a kidney stone. Consult medical command for fluid orders in elderly patients.
- MONITOR cardiac rhythm.
- TRANSPORT WITHOUT DELAY. When there is reason to suspect an acute surgical emergency (e.g., mesenteric ischemia), notify the receiving hospital to alert their surgical staff.

One item is conspicuously absent from the preceding list, and that is pain relief. There is no doubt that analgesia is a very important aspect of treatment for *any* patient suffering severe pain—not only for humani-

tarian reasons but also because pain is itself potentially harmful. Pain activates the body's fight/flight response, prompting an outpouring of adrenaline in an already overtaxed system. So it is highly desirable from every point of view to relieve the patient's pain. The problem is *how*. If you give a relatively long-acting analgesic, like morphine, the surgeons at the receiving hospital are going to be very upset; for you may relieve the patient's pain so effectively that the surgeons can no longer evaluate the findings on abdominal examination. On the other hand, what would otherwise be the ideal *short*-acting analgesic— nitrous oxide—is contraindicated in undiagnosed acute abdomen, for nitrogen tends to accumulate in closed spaces within the body (such as in an obstructed bowel) and worsen distention. So you are apt to be stuck in a situation where you may not give anything to relieve the pain of a patient in severe distress—a situation bound to cause any compassionate medical worker his or her own severe distress. What you *can* give, however, is the reassurance that comes from being cared for by a calm, well-organized professional. A large component of pain derives from fear, and fear is something you ought to be able to treat without drugs. Meanwhile, contact medical command and find out if it's OK to give at least a small dose of morphine. (If necessary, the surgeons can reverse the effects of morphine with naloxone when they come to assess the patient.) Every case is different, and in some cases analgesia may be permissible.

MANAGING THE RENAL DIALYSIS PATIENT

Approximately 40,000 people in the United States are receiving long-term dialysis for chronic renal failure, and those people are particularly subject to a number of medical emergencies.

Recall that the kidneys normally serve as the body's accountants, keeping careful track of the electrolytes, acids, and metabolic waste materials in the blood that pass through them. By sitting there counting passing ions and metabolites, the kidneys regulate the body's internal composition within narrow limits. If a few too many sodium ions (Na^+) pass by, the kidneys nab the next few and send them packing (by excreting them in the urine). If the hydrogen ion (H^-) count gets too high, the kidneys either excrete some of the excess hydrogen ions or hang onto some bicarbonate to buffer the extra acid. Similarly waste products of protein metabolism, principally **urea,** are monitored and banished with the urine when their levels get too high.

In view of that critical role that the kidneys play in maintaining chemical homeostasis in the body, it is not surprising that when the kidneys fail, for any reason, the body's internal chemical milieu goes completely haywire. Because he can no longer excrete the waste products of protein metabolism, the patient develops **uremia** (an excessive level of urea in the blood). But that is only part of his problem. Fluid and electrolyte balance cannot be maintained, so the patient retains fluid and the concentration of electrolytes in his blood becomes severely deranged. Particularly hazardous is *hyperkalemia*, which may cause dangerous and even lethal cardiac dysrhythmias. Fluid retention makes the patient vulnerable to *heart failure* and also increases a tendency to dangerously *high blood pressure*. Acids accumulate in the blood, along with all the uncollected metabolic wastes. Furthermore, the nonfunctional kidneys can no longer play their role in excreting various medications, so drugs taken by the patient in normal doses may build up to toxic levels in the blood. All told, the events following failure of the kidneys would inevitably be fatal within a matter of weeks if there were not some means to replace at least some of the functions previously carried out by the now-defunct kidneys.

Fortunately, there *is* a means to do so, and that means is renal dialysis, a technique for "filtering" the blood of its toxic wastes, removing excess fluids, and restoring the normal balance of electrolytes. Dialysis can be performed on an emergency basis simply by infusing large volumes of specially formulated dialysis fluid into (and back out of) the abdominal cavity (**peritoneal dialysis**). Patients on long-term treatment, however, are maintained on another form of dialysis, called **hemodialysis,** in which the patient's blood is circulated through a dialysis machine that functions in very much the same way (although not nearly as elegantly) as normal kidneys.

In order to facilitate their being hooked up to a dialysis machine, most patients undergoing chronic renal dialysis have some sort of a **shunt,** that is, a surgically created connection between a vein and an artery. When the patient undergoes dialysis, he is connected to the dialysis machine through that shunt, so that blood can flow from the body into the dialysis machine and then back into the body. In the Scribner shunt, for example, two plastic tubes, one fastened in the radial artery, the other in the cephalic vein, are joined together near the wrist with a Teflon connector. A Thomas shunt is a similar device but usually placed in the groin. Other patients will have a small, button-shaped device, a Hemasite, with a rubber septum that can be punctured with dialysis needles during treatment. Hemasites are usually placed in the upper arm or proximal anterior thigh. Finally, some patients have an *internal shunt* (an *arteriovenous [AV] fistula*), that is, an artificial anastomosis between a vein and an artery—usually in the forearm or upper arm.

Patients requiring chronic dialysis usually go "on the machine" every 2 or 3 days for a period of 3 to 5 hours. Many patients have their dialysis in the hospital or in community dialysis facilities, but a significant number have home dialysis units. Patients undergoing dialysis at home have usually had extensive training in the procedures, and often someone else in the home has also been trained—so if there's a problem with the machine, the patient may know a lot more about it than you do! It's a good idea, though, to keep the telephone number of the nearest dialysis facility at medical command, so that the local kidney center can be consulted for advice in an emergency.

Clearly a patient undergoing chronic dialysis can suffer the same spectrum of illnesses and injuries as any other patient. But dialysis patients are particularly vulnerable to certain problems, either because of the dialysis itself or because of their underlying renal failure. Some of those problems are described in the following section and are summarized in Table 25-4.

Problems Related to Dialysis

Problems associated with dialysis may come about because of too rapid shifts in fluids or electrolytes, accidental disconnection from the machine, or malfunction of the machine.

Hypotension and Shock

A sudden drop in blood pressure is not at all uncommon during or immediately after dialysis, and it can lead to cardiac arrest if not promptly detected and treated. The patient may feel light-headed or even become confused, and often he is yawning more than usual.

> **NOTE: WHEN YOU MEASURE THE BLOOD PRESSURE IN A DIALYSIS PATIENT, USE THE ARM THAT DOESN'T HAVE THE SHUNT!**

The emergency *treatment* of hypotension due to excess fluid removal is to put the stretcher into about 15 degrees of Trendelenburg (head-down tilt) or, if that is not possible, elevate the patient's legs on pillows. Then give **50 ml of normal saline IV,** and transport at once. Be sure to MONITOR cardiac rhythm, for dysrhythmias are always a possibility in dialysis patients.

A dialysis patient may also develop shock secondary to *bleeding*, from any number of causes. Pa-

TABLE 25-4. MEDICAL EMERGENCIES IN DIALYSIS PATIENTS

PROBLEM	PREHOSPITAL MANAGEMENT
Problems related to dialysis itself	
Hypotension	Give 50 ml of normal saline IV
Hemorrhage from the shunt	If the shunt cannot be reconnected, clamp it off; check for signs of shock
Potassium imbalance	For hypokalemia: Treat bradycardia with atropine
	For hyperkalemia: Calcium and bicarbonate
Disequilibrium syndrome	Supportive treatment only
Air embolism	Left lateral recumbent position in about 10 degrees of head-down tilt
Machine dysfunction	Turn off machine; clamp ends of shunt; disconnect patient from machine; transport
Problems to which dialysis patients are more vulnerable	
Congestive heart failure	Oxygen; sitting position; rapid transport to dialysis facility
Myocardial infarction and cardiac dysrhythmias	Treat as any other patient, but caution in administering any medications
Hypertension	Transport only; the treatment is dialysis
Pericardial tamponade	Emergency transport as soon as detected
Uremic pericarditis	Oxygen; position of comfort; transport
Subdural hematoma	Oxygen; urgent transport

tients with chronic renal failure are, for example, very prone to duodenal ulcers, and bleeding from those ulcers is not unusual. Bleeding may also occur from the dialysis cannula, in a variety of circumstances. Not by any means the least common scenario is a suicide attempt, in which the patient opens up the cannula and allows himself to exsanguinate. If you encounter that situation, immediately CLAMP OFF THE CANNULA and apply direct pressure. If that does not control the bleeding, use a tourniquet above the site of the shunt.

When you find a shunt *leaking* during a dialysis cycle, see if you can tighten up the connection. If it has become disconnected at the vein, clamp the cannula and disconnect the patient from the machine.

Potassium Imbalance

One of the consequences of renal impairment is the inability to excrete ingested potassium, so patients in chronic renal failure are prone to develop hyperkalemia, especially in circumstances of increased potassium intake or catabolic stress. This author witnessed a patient with chronic renal failure suffer a cardiac arrest 30 minutes after he had stealthily eaten a forbidden avocado (a very rich potassium source)! Usually, however, the signs of hyperkalemia come on somewhat less dramatically. The patient may present with profound muscular weakness. On the electrocardiogram (ECG), which should be monitored as soon as possible in *every* dialysis patient, the classic signs of hyperkalemia are **peaked T waves,** a prolonged QRS complex, and sometimes disappearance of the P waves. Complete heart block or asystole may occur. If you see those ECG signs, treatment is urgently required and will have to be undertaken in the field if you are any distance from the hospital:

EMERGENCY TREATMENT OF HYPERKALEMIA

- MONITOR the patient's cardiac rhythm throughout.
- If the patient has bradycardia (pulse less than about 46/minute), give **atropine 0.5 mg IV** (if

you don't have an IV line established, use the patient's shunt or AV fistula).

- Administer **10 ml of 10% calcium chloride IV.** Calcium antagonizes the effects of potassium on the heart.
- After the calcium has been well flushed out of the IV or shunt, give **sodium bicarbonate, 50 mEq IV.**
- The patient will need emergency dialysis, so ALERT THE HOSPITAL to get set up while you are en route.
- TRANSPORT without delay.

A much less common complication than hyperkalemia is *hypo*kalemia, which can occur as a consequence of overaggressive dialysis. For that reason, hypokalemia—if it is seen at all—is most likely to be seen during or immediately after a dialysis cycle. The patient may be hypotensive, and cardiac dysrhythmias are almost invariably present—usually bradycardias. Treat for the dysrhythmia you find if it is hemodynamically significant (e.g., atropine for severe bradycardia with hypotension).

Disequilibrium Syndrome

During dialysis, the concentration of urea in the blood is rapidly lowered while that in the cerebrospinal fluid (CSF) remains high. As we learned in an earlier chapter, water moves by osmosis from a solution of lower concentration into a solution of higher concentration. So as a consequence of dialysis, water initially shifts from the bloodstream into the CSF, producing an increase in intracranial pressure. The patient may, therefore, experience typical symptoms of mildly increased intracranial pressure, including nausea, vomiting, headache, and confusion. After a few hours, the fluid will reequilibrate between blood and CSF, and the patient's symptoms will get better on their own.

At the time you are called to see the patient, however, it may be impossible to distinguish between a disequilibrium syndrome and the development of a *subdural hematoma*, to which dialysis patients are particularly prone. The patient must, therefore, be transported expeditiously to the hospital for a full neurologic evaluation.

Air Embolism

If any of the fittings and connections in the dialysis system are not tight, air may enter the system and produce an air embolism. Recall the symptoms of air embolism: sudden dyspnea, hypotension, cyanosis.

If there is any reason to suspect air embolism, treat the patient as any other case of air embolism. Disconnect him from the dialysis machine, place him in the LEFT LATERAL RECUMBENT POSITION in about 10 degrees of HEAD-DOWN TILT, and transport immediately.

Machine Malfunction

If there is any question that a home dialysis machine is not functioning properly, follow these steps in disconnecting the patient from the machine (if the patient is alert, he will be able to instruct you himself):

- Turn the machine off.
- Clamp the ends of the shunt.
- Disconnect the shunt from the machine.

Problems to Which Dialysis Patients Are More Vulnerable

In addition to problems specifically related to dialysis itself, patients with chronic renal failure are at higher risk than the rest of the population from certain other medical problems, and it is important for the paramedic to be alert for those problems. They include the following:

MEDICAL PROBLEMS MORE LIKELY IN DIALYSIS PATIENTS

- Congestive heart failure (from fluid retention)
- Severe hypertension
- Myocardial infarction
- Cardiac dysrhythmias
- Pericardial tamponade (from uremic pericarditis)
- Peptic ulcer disease with gastrointestinal bleeding
- Subdural hematoma
- Septicemia
- Bleeding disorders (from failure to reverse anticoagulant therapy after dialysis)

As a general rule, the treatment of any of those problems is the same in dialysis patients as for any other patient with the same diagnosis. However, pharmacologic treatment in dialysis patients is usually best postponed until the patient reaches the hospital. For one thing, it will very often be ineffective. In congestive heart failure, for instance, diuretics and vasodilators are unlikely to work in dialysis patients; the only thing that *will* work is dialysis. Furthermore, even drugs that might be effective are very difficult to administer in appropriate dosages; what would be a therapeutic dosage in patient with normal kidneys may be a toxic dosage for a patient who lacks renal function. So a good rule of thumb is:

DON'T GIVE MEDICATIONS TO PATIENTS WITH CHRONIC RENAL FAILURE UNLESS SPECIFICALLY INSTRUCTED TO DO SO BY MEDICAL COMMAND.

GLOSSARY

arteriovenous (AV) fistula Surgically-created anastomosis between an artery and a vein, for purposes of facilitating *hemodialysis.*

cholecystitis Inflammation of the gallbladder.

colic Crampy pain associated with obstruction of a hollow organ.

diverticulitis Inflammation of *diverticula,* which may produce an acute abdomen.

diverticulosis Condition characterized by the presence of *diverticula,* sometimes a cause of painless lower gastrointestinal bleeding.

diverticulum (pl. **diverticula**) Pocket formed by a weakened area of the wall of the colon.

dysuria Pain or difficulty in urination.

hematemesis Vomiting blood.

hematuria The passage of blood in the urine.

hemodialysis Process of removing noxious agents and excess fluids from the blood by diffusion through a semipermeable membrane.

melena The passage of dark, tarry stools, signifying blood in the gastrointestinal tract.

peritoneal dialysis Process of removing noxious agents from the body by infusing balanced electrolyte solutions into the abdominal cavity and then withdrawing the solutions after they have equilibrated with the blood.

peritoneum The membrane that lines the abdominal cavity.

retroperitoneal The area of the abdomen behind the peritoneum, which contains the kidneys, ureters, and great vessels.

shunt In the context of renal dialysis, a shunt refers to the artificial connection created between a peripheral vein and a peripheral artery.

urea An end product of protein metabolism.

uremia The accumulation in the blood of urea and, by implication, other toxic wastes, as a consequence of the kidney's inability to remove those wastes.

viscus (pl **viscera**) Any large internal organ of the abdomen, pelvis, or thorax.

APPENDIX: MEDICATIONS COMMONLY PRESCRIBED TO PATIENTS WITH GASTROINTESTINAL PROBLEMS

There are literally thousands of medications taken for the relief of various gastrointestinal symptoms (just watch television for an evening and see how many such products are being advertised!). The medications that are of particular concern in emergency medicine are those that suggest the patient may be suffering from ulcer disease. Most prominent among those are ANTACIDS, which come as tablets (to be chewed) or solutions and which are taken to relieve the gastric acidity that is partially responsible for ulcer pain. Antacids are available "over the counter" (i.e., without a prescription), and many patients take antacids for relief without having had their symptoms investigated by a doctor. When, on the other hand, you find that a patient is taking cimetidine (**Tagamet**) or rantidine (**Zantac**), both of which are prescription drugs, you can be reasonably certain that a doctor is either treating an ulcer or trying to prevent an ulcer in a susceptible person.

COMMMONLY USED ANTACIDS

Alka-Seltzer
Aludrox
Amphojel
Delcid
Gaviscon
Gelusil
Maalox
Pepto-Bismol
Mylanta
Riopan
Rolaids
Romach
Silain-Gel
Titralac
Tums
WinGel

Bear in mind that simply because a person takes antacids, there is no guarantee that he or she indeed suffers from a gastrointestinal disorder. The pain of a myocardial infarction is commonly mistaken for "indigestion," and the patient who has taken Rolaids for that kind of indigestion is unlikely to obtain relief, no matter how you spell it. So always find out exactly what the pain is like and whether the antacids helped to relieve it.

FURTHER READING

Burns RP et al. Appendicitis in the mature patient. *Ann Surg* 201:695, 1985.

Fontanarosa PB. Acute abdominal pain. *JEMS* 14(11):28, 1989.

Kingsley AN et al. Colorectal foreign bodies—management update. *Dis Colon Rectum* 28:941, 1985.

Kraft J. The acute abdomen. *Emerg Med* 5:145, 1973.

Kraut JA. Emergency care of the dialysis patient. *Emerg Med Serv* 8(6):103, 1979.

McAllister CJ, Gibson R. Emergencies in dialysis patients. *JACEP* 7:96, 1978.

Meeroff JC. Algorithm for managing patients with severe GI hemorrhage. *Hosp Pract* 19(3):186, 1984.

Ozar MB. Urologic emergencies. *Emerg Med* 5:154, 1973.

Sacchetti A et al. ED management of acute congestive heart failure in renal dialysis patients. *Am J Emerg Med* 11:644, 1993.

Sheets CA. The urgency of mesenteric ischemia. *Emerg Med* 22(3):93, 1990.

Weiss JS et al. Abdominal pain in the emergency room: A study of 176 consecutive cases. *Mt Sinai J Med* 46:63, 1979.

26
Anaphylaxis

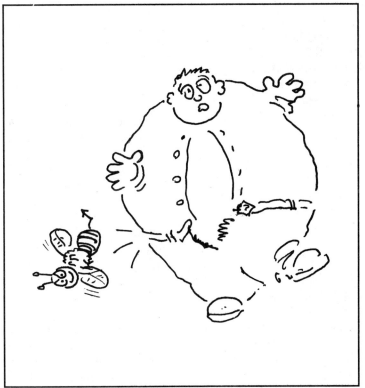

Peter Caroline

OBJECTIVES

Writing at the end of the seventeenth century, the clergyman Increase Mather observed:

> Some men also have strange antipathies in their natures against that sort of food which others love and live upon. I have read of one that could not endure to eat either bread or flesh; of another that fell into a swoonding fit at the smell of a rose. . . . There are some who, if a cat accidentally come into the room, though they neither see it, nor are told of it, will presently be in a sweat, and ready to die away.

Although one can't be certain without more information, it is highly likely that at least some of the individuals Increase Mather observed and read about were suffering from an exaggerated form of allergic reaction called anaphylaxis. In this chapter, we shall examine how such reactions come about and what agents most commonly cause susceptible people to fall into a "swoonding fit." We shall also look at the typical signs and symptoms of anaphylaxis and the emergency measures that are required to treat a patient suffering an anaphylactic reaction. By the end of this chapter, the student should be able to

1. Identify the correct definition of
   * Antigen
   * Antibody
   * Allergy
   * Anaphylaxis
   given a list of definitions
2. List six effects produced by the release from mast cells of histamine and other chemical mediators
3. List the symptoms and signs of an anaphylactic reaction referable to
   * The respiratory system
   * The cardiovascular system
   * The gastrointestinal system
   * The nervous system
   * The skin
   and explain the mechanism that produces each of those signs or symptoms
4. Identify a patient suffering an anaphylactic reaction, given a description of several patients with different clinical findings, and describe the correct management of an anaphylactic reaction
5. Describe the modifications in management of anaphylactic shock necessary when the patient is older than about 35 years of age
6. List four agents commonly implicated in causing anaphylactic reactions
7. List the therapeutic actions, indications, contraindications, and correct dosage for adults of
   * Epinephrine
   * Diphenhydramine
   * Aminophylline
   * Hydrocortisone
   after studying the information about those agents in the Drug Handbook at the end of this textbook

MECHANISMS AND CAUSES OF ANAPHYLAXIS

The word **anaphylaxis** comes from Greek root words meaning "without protection" (contrast the word *prophylaxis*, which means "for protection"). The term *anaphylaxis* is not, therefore, really accurate; for in fact the fundamental problem in an anaphylactic reaction is not lack of "protection" but *over*protection. That is, anaphylaxis is a form of allergy—a very extreme and devastating form—and allergy represents the body's protective, immune system gone overboard.

The Normal Immune Response

All normal people are endowed with an immune system to protect them from substances and microorganisms that do not belong in the body. Without such a protective system, normal life would be entirely impossible—as in the case of the "boy in the bubble"—for a person would be felled by the first bacteria that came along and decided to set up shop in the body. Fortunately, the vast majority of us are furnished with a quite wonderful immune system that is constantly on patrol to detect the incursion into the body of any unauthorized substances.

The moment a foreign substance does gain access to the body, especially through the skin or respiratory tract, alarms sound and a whole series of responses are triggered. Cells from the immune system quickly surround the foreign material and, as it were, check its identity papers. If those papers are not in order, the immune cells in effect open a file on the substance. Just as the police would record the fingerprints of a suspect for later identification, so the immune cells record the salient features of the foreign substance—usually one or two *proteins* on the surface of the substance—and design specific proteins of their own that will combine with the foreign proteins and inactivate them. Those specific *protective* proteins are given the name **antibodies,** while the *foreign* materials (usually proteins) capable of inducing antibody formation are called **antigens.**

The first time that an antigen gains access to the body, the response (called the *primary response*) is a bit slow, since it takes the cells of the immune system a while to ascertain that the substance is not "one of us," to take down all the details that will aid in future identification and to manufacture antibodies with a perfect "fit" to the antigen in question. Then the information about the potential saboteur has to be distributed to the whole body, for it won't do a punctured toe much good, for example, if only the deltoid muscle of the arm (which got a shot of the antigen) knows how to recognize the tetanus toxin. So just as the FBI distributes wanted posters to post offices throughout the country, the immune system distributes descriptions of known foreign invaders throughout the body. It does so by sticking the specific antibodies onto two related types of cells: **basophils** stationed in fixed guard posts within the tissues, and wandering **mast cells** that patrol through the connective tissues, bronchi, gastrointestinal mucosa, and other border areas vulnerable to foreign invasion.

Those two cell types are, in fact, the body's chemical weapons manufacturers and distributors. Within the tissue basophils and the mast cells are little granules containing a whole host of powerful substances ready to be released in the event of war with an invading foreign antigen. So long as everything stays quiet, the granules remain encapsulated and inactive within the mast cells. But should an antigen come along and combine with one of the antibodies on the surface of the mast cell, the granules will be expelled from the mast cell and detonated, releasing their chemical weapons into the surrounding tissue and the bloodstream (Fig. 26-1).

We know the identity of about a dozen of those chemical weapons (one of the most prominent is an agent called **histamine**); probably there are a lot more. Those agents are very important in carrying forward the immune response; they act, for example, to summon more white blood cells to the scene of battle—both by sending out chemical calls for help and by facilitating blood flow to the embattled area (dilating blood vessels, increasing capillary permeability). Those are all very useful effects when confined to the tiny area of the body under attack, such as an area of skin that has suffered a scratch. The effects of chemical immune mediators are not so useful if they are widespread throughout the body. Table 26-1 summarizes some of the physiologic effects of the chemical mediators released by mast cells.

As noted, the immune system is designed to serve a protective function in the body. Indeed, we exploit the body's natural immune mechanisms when we administer vaccines to *immunize* a person against a disease. When we give polio vaccine, for example, what we are doing is introducing the immune system to antigens of the polioviruses in a controlled fashion. Immune cells check out those antigens, identify them as alien, and set up the machinery to produce antibodies specifically designed to neutralize poliovirus. Now suppose that one fine day a few months or years later, an immunized person happens to drink some water contaminated with live, virulent poliovirus. The virus enters the body and, finding itself in

an apparently hospitable environment, cheerfully begins to replicate. But meanwhile, the cop on the beat—a wandering immune cell—spots the poliovirus. "Where have I seen that face before?" the immune cell asks himself. Then he remembers the wanted poster in the immune-cell locker room. Blowing his whistle, he activates the immune system. Lymphocytes, already fully tooled up from their earlier exposure to the antigen, go into full production of specific anti-poliovirus antibody. Before the viruses can multiply any further, they are swamped in gluey antibodies and then surrounded by a clean-up squad of hungry macrophages, which eat them all up. And the person who imbibed the contaminated water? He plods on, blissfully unaware of the drama that has been unfolding in an outpost of his gastrointestinal tract. That is the immune system at its best.

Abnormal Immune Reactions

Clearly, a vigilant immune system is essential to life and health. An *overzealous* immune system, however, can cause a lot of problems, ranging from the annoyance and misery of hay fever to the possibly fatal consequences of anaphylaxis. In **allergy,** the immune system is, for reasons we don't really understand, hypersensitive to one or more substances—very often substances, like ragweed pollen or penicillin, that in themselves would be harmless to the body. But the immune cells of an allergic person are jumpier than normal, a bit more trigger-happy. They react not only to the incursion of dangerous invaders, such as viruses or bacteria, but even to perfectly harmless substances. They are, in effect, like border guards gone berserk, who shoot not only enemy saboteurs but also tourists!

The allergic individual, then, suffers symptoms produced by localized mast cell bombing missions whenever a sensitized tissue comes in contact with the antigen (or **allergen**) to which it is sensitive. Generally, allergic reactions are, as implied, *localized* to a specific tissue. Thus in the person who suffers from **allergic rhinitis** (hay fever), the allergic reaction takes place primarily in the nasal mucosa and surrounding tissues. An inhaled allergen, such as ragweed pollen, triggers mast cell degranulation in the nasal mucosa. That in turn produces a local increase in capillary permeability, leading to nasal congestion. Other histamine effects produce red, itchy eyes, and so forth. In a person with a *food* allergy, on the other hand, it is the mucosa of the gastrointestinal tract that has been abnormally sensitized. When a food to which the person has been sensitized—typically a peanut or some kind of fish—reaches the gastrointestinal tract mucosa, resident mast cells detonate *their* chemical

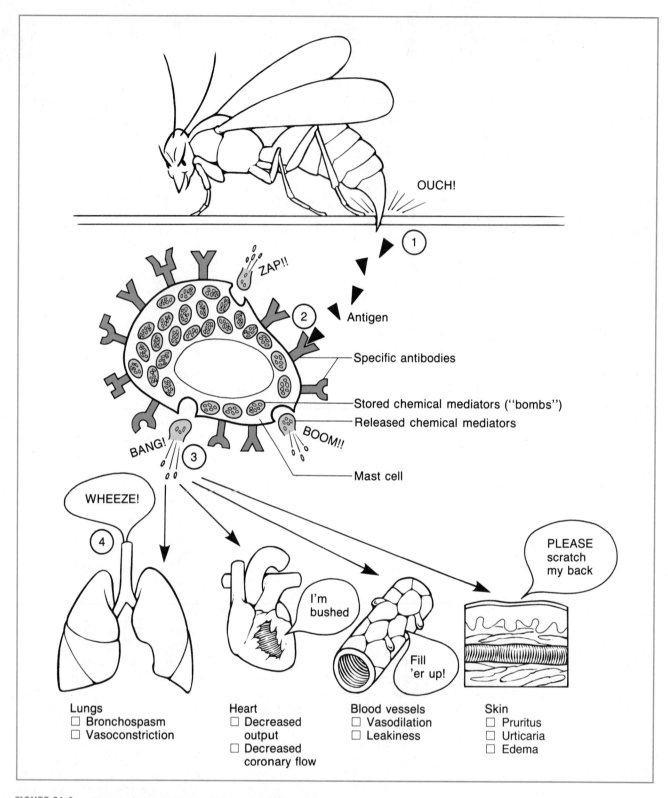

FIGURE 26-1. SEQUENCE OF EVENTS IN ANAPHYLAXIS. (1) Antigen introduced into the body. (2) Antigen-antibody reaction at the surface of a mast cell. (3) Release of mast cell chemical mediators. (4) Chemical mediators exert their effects on end organs.

TABLE 26-1.   EFFECTS OF SOME MAST CELL MEDIATORS

MEDIATOR	PHYSIOLOGIC EFFECTS
Histamine	Systemic vasodilation
	Increased permeability (leakiness) of blood vessels
	Decreased myocardial contractility
	Decreased coronary blood flow
	Dysrhythmias
	Bronchoconstriction
	Pulmonary vasoconstriction
Slow-reacting substance	Increased leakiness of blood vessels
	Decreased force of cardiac contraction
	Decreased coronary blood flow
	Bronchoconstriction
	Dysrhythmias
Serotonin	Pulmonary vasoconstriction
	Bronchoconstriction

TABLE 26-2.   AGENTS COMMONLY RESPONSIBLE FOR ANAPHYLAXIS

PHARMACEUTICAL PRODUCTS
  Penicillin and other antibiotics
  Sulfa drugs (sulfonamide, sulfisoxazole)
  Mismatched blood transfusion
  Animal serum products (horse serum, gamma globulins)
  Salicylates (aspirin)
  Vaccines
  Enzymes (chymotrypsin, penicillinase)
  Local anesthetics (procaine)
  Iodinated radiocontrast dyes used in taking x-rays
  Biologic extracts and hormones (insulin, heparin)
FOODS
  Shellfish and other seafoods
  Peanuts, pecans
  Milk and milk products
  Egg whites
  Chocolate
  Some fruits (mango, strawberries)
VENOM OF STINGING INSECTS
  Hymenoptera: Hornets, bees, wasps, yellow jackets
  Fire ants

bombs. There is swelling of the gut mucosa, with resultant cramps and diarrhea.

An **anaphylactic reaction** is the most extreme form of allergic reaction, usually affecting not just a localized tissue but the entire body. In an anaphylactic response, cells patrolling the body are in a state of red alert, highly sensitized to some particular antigen. Then along comes the allergen in question—say, penicillin or wasp venom—a substance to which the person has been previously exposed (whether he knows it or not). The mast cells take one look, and instead of simply dropping a few histamine bombs to create a little itch, they scream, "Geronimo! Nuke 'em!" and let loose a barrage of bombs and missiles all over the body. In so doing, they are very likely to kill the very organism they were designed to defend. That, in fact, happens to about 2,000 people in the United States each year who die from anaphylactic shock.

Virtually any foreign substances may serve as an allergen for an anaphylactic response, but some substances are implicated more commonly than others (Table 26-2). By far the most common culprits are drugs, especially penicillin. The stings of bees and their relatives also dispatch about 200 people every year. Finally foods—notably peanuts and fish—are responsible for several dozen fatal anaphylactic reactions each year, usually in restaurants or other places outside the home (at home, the sensitive individual can monitor what goes into his stomach; in a restaurant he has no way of knowing all the ingredients that are used to prepare the meal).

As is evident from the different types of agents that can elicit an anaphylactic response, the offending allergen can gain access to the body in different ways. Usually, the most rapid anaphylactic reactions occur after *injection* of an allergen—either by a six-legged creature with a venom pouch or a two-legged creature with a hypodermic needle. *Ingestion*, of course, is the route by which food allergens gain access to the body. Yet other allergens, such as antibiotic ointments, are *absorbed across the skin*. Finally allergens may be *inhaled*, although that is a very unusual route for producing an anaphylactic reaction.

THE CLINICAL PICTURE OF ANAPHYLAXIS

The signs and symptoms of anaphylaxis are readily predictable from the actions of mast cell mediators. When the mast cells start letting loose their chemical bombs, SKIN SYMPTOMS are usually the first to occur. Peripheral vasodilation produces *flushing*; fluid oozing from leaky capillaries produces *edema*; other histamine effects are responsible for **pruritus** (itching) and **urticaria** (hives). Swelling is apt to be most prominent in the face, especially around the eyes (**periorbital edema**).

RESPIRATORY SYMPTOMS are also often prominent. Bronchoconstriction produces a feeling of *dyspnea* and *tightness in the chest,* and breathing may be *wheezy.* As in the subcutaneous tissues, fluid leaking from capillaries in the area of the larynx creates localized swelling and produces a sensation of a *lump in the throat*. Itching in the throat may cause a dry, nonproductive *cough*. As laryngeal edema increases, the patient's voice may grow *hoarse* or *stridorous*.

A HOARSE VOICE IN A PATIENT HAVING AN ALLERGIC REACTION IS A DANGER SIGNAL! YOU MAY HAVE ONLY MINUTES TO SALVAGE THE AIRWAY.

CARDIOVASCULAR SYMPTOMS occur for a variety of reasons. The direct effects of histamine and other mediators on the heart, to begin with, weaken cardiac contractions, so cardiac output falls. A concomitant fall in coronary blood flow leads to myocardial ischemia and therefore makes the heart prone to *dysrhythmias*. Meanwhile, there is widespread peripheral vasodilatation. Part of the intravascular volume has already leaked out into the tissues; now, the volume that is left is suddenly in the much larger container produced by widened blood vessels. The net effect is hypotension and *shock*—in part hypovolemic (from plasma escaping into the tissues); in part cardiogenic (from decreased cardiac output); in part neurogenic (from loss of vasoconstrictive mechanisms). In response to the fall in blood pressure, the heart reflexly speeds up, so *tachycardia* is inevitably part of the picture. Indeed, flushing (from vasodilatation) and tachycardia are so characteristic of anaphylactic shock that it is very questionable to make the diagnosis without those two signs being present.

Plasma leaking into the wall of the gut to produce edema there is responsible for most of the GASTROINTESTINAL SYMPTOMS of anaphylactic shock. Those symptoms and signs may include *nausea, bloating, vomiting, cramps, abdominal distention,* and profuse, watery *diarrhea*.

Most of the CENTRAL NERVOUS SYSTEM MANIFESTATIONS of anaphylactic shock are secondary to stress and to inadequate cerebral perfusion: *headache, dizziness,* sometimes *confusion*. A characteristic symptom is the *feeling of impending doom*. Almost all patients with anaphylactic shock think that they are going to die (often with good reason).

The symptoms and signs of anaphylaxis, and the mechanisms that produce them, are summarized in Table 26-3.

TABLE 26-3.   SYMPTOMS AND SIGNS OF ANAPHYLAXIS

PATHOLOGIC PROCESS	RESULTING SYMPTOMS AND SIGNS
Constriction of bronchial smooth muscle (bronchospasm)	Dyspnea Chest tightness Wheezes (or silent chest in severe cases)
Peripheral vasodilation	Flushing of the skin Feeling of warmth Hypotension (neurogenic-type shock) Reflex tachycardia
Leakage of plasma into tissues → edema	
Edema of subcutaneous tissues	Swelling of eyelids, tongue, lips Relative hypovolemia, contributing to hypotension
Laryngeal and glottic edema	Feeling of a lump in the throat Hoarseness or stridor
Edema of gastrointestinal tract	Nausea, vomiting, cramps, diarrhea
Decreased myocardial contractility	Decreased cardiac output (cardiogenic component to shock)
Decreased coronary blood flow	Dysrhythmias Possible acute myocardial infarction
Other histamine effects	Pruritus Urticaria

MANAGEMENT OF ANAPHYLACTIC REACTIONS

An anaphylactic reaction is a dire medical emergency, and the patient will very likely die if lifesaving measures are not instituted within a few minutes. Thus, when a patient gives a history of becoming flushed and tachycardic after an injection, an insect sting, or a meal, you need to act very quickly:

- As always, first priority goes to the AIRWAY, which is likely to be in immediate jeopardy. If the patient is already hoarse or stridorous, he will need to be intubated as soon as possible; otherwise he's going to require an emergency cricothyrotomy in very short order. If you don't think you can handle an awake intubation on a panicky patient, you may be able to buy some time—enough time to get the patient to the hospital— by having the patient inhale 4 to 10 sprays of **1 : 1,000 racemic epinephrine by metered dose inhaler.** Then start OXYGEN administration by nasal cannula and get moving.
- Start at least one LARGE-BORE IV LIFELINE with lactated Ringer's solution and run it wide open. (If the anaphylactic reaction was caused by an injection or insect sting on an extremity, start the IV in the *other* extremity. Meanwhile apply a constricting band proximal to the injection or sting site, to retard further absorption of the antigen from the site.)
- MONITOR cardiac rhythm throughout.
- The drug of choice for anaphylactic reactions is EPINEPHRINE. Epinephrine does several very nice things in anaphylaxis. It stops the process of mast cell degranulation (the bombers go back to their bases!). Its *alpha*-adrenergic properties produce vasoconstriction, elevate the diastolic blood pressure, and improve coronary blood flow. Meanwhile, its powerful *beta*-adrenergic actions relieve bronchospasm in the lungs and increase the strength of cardiac contractions. However, those very same alpha and beta effects can be dangerous, especially in older patients. Excessive alpha activity can lead to hypertensive crisis, while too much beta stimulation can increase myocardial oxygen consumption to the point of producing a myocardial infarction. The trick, therefore, is to give *enough* epinephrine to accomplish all the good things we want to accomplish but not so much that we harm the patient. The following guidelines should help in choosing the right epinephrine dosage:
  1. For *mild reactions*, in which there are not yet signs of shock or respiratory compromise, give **0.3 to 0.5 ml of 1 : 1,000 aqueous epinephrine subcutaneously.** If the reaction is due to an injection or an insect sting, also inject 0.1 to 0.2 ml of the same solution at the injection site, to retard absorption of the antigen. (If it's a bee sting, first remove the stinger! Otherwise it will keep injecting venom. Take care not to squeeze the stinger as you remove it; use a scalpel blade or even a piece of paper to flick the stinger out of the skin.)
  2. For a *severe reaction in a young person* (under 35), give **5 to 10 ml (0.1 ml/kg) of 1 : 10,000 epinephrine slowly IV.** If you haven't been able to get an IV started but you do have an endotracheal tube in, spray the epinephrine down the tube and "bag it in" (i.e., immediately ventilate the patient with a bag-valve device). If you have neither intravenous nor endotracheal access, inject 0.5 ml of 1 : 1,000 aqueous epinephrine into the vascular plexus at the base of the tongue (inferior surface), from where it will be absorbed nearly as rapidly as if given IV.
  3. For a *severe reaction in an older person* (35 or over), a slow, continuous infusion of epinephrine is the safest option, for you can simply slow or stop the infusion if the blood pressure starts to climb too high or if the patient develops angina. Start by diluting **0.1 mg (0.1 ml) of a 1 : 1,000 solution of aqueous epinephrine in 10 ml of normal saline** and infuse that mixture **over 5 to 10 minutes.** Once that dose is in, you may start a continuous epinephrine infusion if the initial dose did not produce sufficient improvement. To prepare the infusion, add **1 mg (1 ml) of 1 : 1,000 aqueous epinephrine** to a **250-ml bag of D5/W,** which will yield a concentration of 4 µg per milliliter. The infusion should then be started at a rate of **1 µg per minute** (i.e., 0.25 ml/min, or 15 gtt/min with a microdrip infusion set), increasing slowly to a maximum 4 µg per minute if the initial dosage does not produce an effect. The patient *must* be carefully monitored—by electrocardiogram and with frequent blood pressure determinations—throughout the infusion.
- Most patients who have had an anaphylactic reaction are given an antihistamine, such as **diphenhydramine** (Benadryl). To a certain extent, giving antihistamines is a case of locking the barn door after the horses got away, but antihistamines may help counter some of the deleterious effects of the mast cell bombardment. If administered, the dosage of diphenhydramine is **25 to 50 mg IM.** If the patient is in shock, the intramuscular route won't be much good, so con-

sult medical command regarding whether to go ahead with the diphenhydramine IV. If given intravenously, diphenhydramine must be administered *slowly*—the total dosage should be delivered in no less than 3 to 5 minutes.

- In younger patients with prominent respiratory symptoms, the doctor may order **aminophylline.** The therapeutic effects of aminophylline in anaphylaxis include bronchodilation, stimulation of the respiratory drive, dilation of constricted pulmonary arteries, and strengthening the force of cardiac contractions. However, the combination of aminophylline and beta adrenergic agents like epinephrine may produce cardiac dysrhythmias. So think twice before you give the two drugs together, and monitor the patient's cardiac rhythm constantly if you do. The loading dose of aminophylline is **5 mg per kilogram** over about 20 minutes, followed by an infusion of 0.5 mg/kg/hr.

- Most patients suffering an anaphylactic reaction will be given corticosteroids somewhere along the line. If you are a considerable distance from the hospital, you may be asked to administer a steroid medication in the field, although there's no particular hurry. A dosage of **hydrocortisone, 100 to 200 mg** or the equivalent should be sufficient.

- TRANSPORT the patient without delay.

A CAUTIONARY TALE

Consider the following brief case history:

> Little Miss Muffit
> Sat on her tuffit
> Eating her curds and whey.
> She felt her face flush
> And her pulse start to rush.
> The funeral was held the next day.

The story might have ended differently. The chances are that Miss Muffit had already previously experienced some sort of allergic reaction to curds and whey. Perhaps she'd even been to an emergency room after a previous episode. But the care she got was not adequate if it did not include patient education. She should, of course, have been cautioned to avoid curds and whey. But that is not sufficient, because when dining out, one can't always know what ingredients were used in preparing the meal. So Little Miss Muffit should have been provided with an epinephrine auto-injector, such as the EpiPen, and instructed to take it with her to her tuffit or anyplace else where she might be apt to have a meal. Had Miss Muffit been carrying an EpiPen when she experi-

enced her allergic reaction, and had she been taught to use it at the onset of such a reaction, she might still be with us today.

GLOSSARY

allergen   Substance that produces an allergic reaction in a sensitive individual.

allergy   An abnormal susceptibility on reexposure to a substance that does not ordinarily cause adverse symptoms in the average person.

anaphylaxis   An exaggerated allergic reaction, characterized by bronchospasm and vascular collapse.

antibody   A protein produced in response to a specific foreign substance (antigen) that destroys or inactivates the foreign substance.

antigen   An agent that, when taken into the body, stimulates the formation of specific protective proteins called antibodies.

basophil   A white blood cell that contains chemical mediators of the immune/inflammatory process.

mast cell   A mobile chemical-mediator factory that releases histamine and related substances in response to an antigen/antibody reaction.

pruritus   Itching.

urticaria   Hives.

FURTHER READING

Austen KF. Systemic anaphylaxis in the human being. *N Engl J Med* 291:661, 1974.

Barach EM et al. Epinephrine for treatment of anaphylactic shock. *JAMA* 251:2118, 1984.

Casale TB, Keahey TM, Kaliner M. Exercise-induced anaphylactic syndromes. *JAMA* 255:2049, 1986.

Corey EC. Treatment for anaphylaxis. *Emergency* 25(10):48, 1993.

Fischer M et al. Volume replacement in acute anaphylactoid reactions. *Intensive Care* 7:375, 1979.

Frazier CA. Food allergy emergencies. *Emerg Med Serv* 12(2):71, 1983.

Fries JH. Peanuts: Allergic and other untoward reactions. *Ann Allergy* 48:220, 1982.

Goldberg M. Systemic reactions to intravascular contrast media. *Anesthesiology* 60:46, 1984.

Hollingsworth HM, Giansiracusa DF. Anaphylaxis. *Emerg Med* 24(12):142, 1992.

Hooper HA. Allergic reactions. *Emergency* 11(4):32, 1979.

Kaliner MA. Calling a halt to anaphylaxis. *Emerg Med* 21(6): 51, 1989.

Kelly JF, Patterson R. Anaphylaxis: Cause, mechanisms, and treatment. *JAMA* 227:1431, 1974.

Levy DB. Anaphylaxis. *Emergency* 21(4):42, 1989.

Lucke WC, Thomas H. Anaphylaxis: Pathophysiology,

clinical presentations and treatment. *J Emerg Med* 1:83, 1983.

Morrow DH, Luther RR. Anaphylaxis: Etiology and guidelines for management. *Anesth Analg* 55:493, 1976.

Perkin RM, Anas NG. Mechanisms and management of anaphylactic shock not responding to traditional therapy. *Ann Allergy* 54:202, 1985.

Raebel M. Potentiated anaphylaxis during chronic beta-blocker therapy. *Drug Intell Clin Pharm* 22:720, 1988.

Roth R. Allergic response. *Emergency* 22(6):28, 1990.

Runge JW et al. Histamine antagonists in the treatment of acute allergic reactions. *Ann Emerg Med* 21:237, 1992.

Sampson HA, Mendelson L, Rosen JP. Fatal and near-fatal anaphylactic reactions to food in children and adolescents. *N Engl J Med* 327:380, 1992.

Scheffer AL. Anaphylaxis. *J Allergy Clin Immunol* 75:227, 1985.

Schwartz HJ, Sher TH. Anaphylaxis to penicillin in a frozen dinner. *Ann Allergy* 52:342, 1984.

Stark BJ, Sullivan TJ. Biphasic and protracted anaphylaxis. *J Allergy Clin Immunol* 78:76, 1986.

Thompson T et al. Drug-induced, life-threatening angioedema revisited. *Laryngoscope* 103:10, 1993.

Vaneslow NA. Minutes to counter anaphylaxis. *Emerg Med* 20(15):121, 1988.

Wise SL, Stafford CT. Anaphylaxis from exercise. *Emerg Med* 23(11):141, 1991.

Yuninger JW et al. Fatal food-induced anaphylaxis. *JAMA* 260:1450, 1988.

27

Poisons, Drugs, and Alcohol

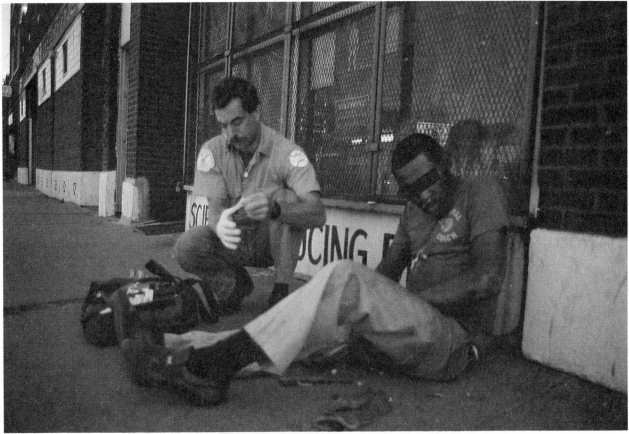

Chicago Fire Department, Chicago. Photo by Michael S. Kowal.

OBJECTIVES

"Why not just call the chapter, 'Poisons, Poisons, and More Poisons'?" inquired a colleague who saw the current title of this chapter when it was still in preparation. There is something to be said for that idea, for the unifying theme in this chapter is the idea of **toxicity**—the harmful effects of various substances on the body. Nonetheless, there *are* useful distinctions to be made among the three categories of toxic agents listed in the title of this chapter. A **poison** is a substance that is toxic *by its very nature*, no matter how it gets into the body or in what quantities it is taken. A **drug,** on the other hand, is a substance that is presumed to have some therapeutic effect when given under the appropriate circumstances and in the appropriate dosage. Drugs are toxic mainly when they are taken under *in*appropriate circumstances and in *in*appropriate amounts. One such drug, **alcohol,** is singled out for special attention because it is one of the most commonly abused drugs in our society.

In this chapter, then, we shall survey the spectrum of toxicologic emergencies that may arise from poisons, drugs, and alcohol. By the end of this chapter, the student should be able to

1. List five questions that should be asked in taking the history of a patient who may have been poisoned
2. List five points of emphasis in performing a physical examination on a patient who may have been poisoned
3. List six contraindications to the induction of vomiting in a poisoned patient
4. Identify patients for whom induction of vomiting is indicated and for whom it is contraindicated, given a description of several patients who have ingested various poisonous substances, and describe the correct method for induction of vomiting
5. List in the correct order the steps in treating
   • An alert patient
   • A comatose patient
   who has ingested an unknown poison
6. Given a description of several patients with different clinical findings, identify a patient who has ingested
   • A caustic substance
   • A hydrocarbon
   • Methyl alcohol
   • Ethylene glycol
   • Cyanide
   • A poisonous plant
   and describe the correct treatment of each

7. Give two examples each of commonly encountered
   • Strong acids
   • Strong alkalis
   • Hydrocarbons
   • Poisonous plants
8. Given a description of several patients with different clinical findings, identify a patient suffering from
   • Carbon monoxide poisoning
   • Hydrocarbon inhalation
   • Organophosphate poisoning
   and describe the correct treatment of each
9. Describe the treatment of an uncomplicated
   • Bee sting
   • Tick bite
10. Given a description of several patients with different clinical findings, identify a patient who has suffered a
    • Black widow spider bite
    • Brown recluse spider bite
    and describe the correct treatment of each
11. Describe how to determine whether a snakebite is envenomed, and list the steps in treating an envenomed snakebite
12. List the steps in treating
    • A coelenterate sting
    • The sting of an echinoderm or stinging vertebrate
13. Describe the dangers associated with
    • A dog bite
    • A human bite
    and list the steps of treatment of each
14. List five questions that should be asked in taking the history of a patient who has overdosed on drugs or appears to be suffering a toxic drug reaction
15. List five points of emphasis in the physical examination of a patient who has overdosed on drugs or appears to be suffering a toxic drug reaction
16. List in the correct sequence the steps in treating a patient found comatose and presumed to have taken an overdose of an unknown drug
17. Given a description of several patients with different clinical findings, identify a patient who has overdosed with
    • A narcotic drug
    • A barbiturate
    • Amphetamines or cocaine
    • An hallucinogen
    and describe the correct treatment of each
18. List five signs, behaviors, or features of the clinical history that should arouse suspicion that a patient has a problem with alcohol

19. List seven medical problems to which alcoholics are more prone than the general population

20. Given a description of several patients with different clinical findings, identify a patient suffering from
    - Acute alcohol intoxication
    - Alcohol withdrawal seizures
    - Delirium tremens

    and describe the correct treatment of each

21. List the therapeutic actions, indications, contraindications, and correct dosage of
    - Syrup of ipecac
    - Activated charcoal
    - Amyl nitrite
    - Atropine sulfate
    - Calcium gluconate
    - Naloxone (Narcan)
    - Thiamine
    - 50% dextrose
    - Diazepam

    after studying the relevant information about each in the Drug Handbook at the end of this textbook

POISONING: INTRODUCTION

Approximately 1 million poisonings are reported in the United States each year, and perhaps a similar number go unreported. The vast majority, approximately 75 percent, occur in children under 5 years of age, and most are caused by household products. What those data tell us is that approximately 75 percent of poisonings ought to be preventable. We shall deal with some of the more common causes of poisoning in children in Chapter 30.

Poisoning in adults is usually intentional, although accidents do occur both at home and in the workplace. While adult poisonings account for only about 10 to 20 percent of calls to Poison Control Centers, they account for nearly 90 percent of hospital admissions for poisoning. Poisoning in adults, that is, is apt to be a very serious matter.

Poisons gain access to the body in a variety of ways. By far the most common is by **ingestion** of a poisonous substance. Poisons in the form of gases, like carbon monoxide, or toxic vapors, like those of solvents, reach the body through **inhalation.** Yet other poisons, particularly the venoms of poisonous insects, snakes, and marine animals, enter the body by **injection.** Finally, some poisons—notably some of the widely used insecticides—can pass into the body by **absorption across the skin.** In the sections that follow, we shall look at some common examples of each of those modes of poisoning.

It is *not* the purpose of this chapter to provide an encyclopedia of poisons, nor can the human brain store all that information. That is the function of a **Poison Control Center,** staffed by experienced personnel who have immediate access to information on the more than 350,000 toxic substances to which the public may be exposed. There are more than 120 Poison Control Centers in the United States, serving every region; and if the paramedic remembers nothing else about poisoning, the one thing he or she *must* remember is how to get in touch with the regional Poison Control Center, which should be promptly notified of *every* poisoning call the ambulance service handles.

What can Poison Control do for you, as a paramedic? A lot! Suppose, for instance, you get called to a nice suburban home where you find a frantic mother hovering over a toddler who sits placidly beside the remains of a potted philodendron, most of which he apparently just had for lunch. Is the plant poisonous? How poisonous? Should you make the little tyke vomit? Is there an antidote? You can try to remember whether you once read something about philodendrons. You can guess. *Or,* you can call Poison Control and get a fast rundown on the ingestion, its potential toxicity, and what do do about it. Then, while you get started on treatment—treatment in which you can be confident—Poison Control will be faxing detailed information on the specific poison to the emergency department you name as your destination.

At the same time, your call to Poison Control helps *them* collect data on poisonings in the region. With your assistance and that of other EMS providers, Poison Control Centers can detect trends, spot developing public health problems, and also evaluate current treatment protocols for different poisonings.

INGESTED POISONS

Ingested poisons may produce immediate damage to tissues that they traverse, or their toxic effects may be delayed for several hours. Immediate injury is seen when the product ingested is some sort of caustic substance, like a strong acid or alkali. More often, however, the poison must be absorbed into the bloodstream before it can produce its toxic effects. Very little absorption occurs from the stomach, where the poison will sit for a variable period of time; the vast majority of absorption takes place in the small intestine. Thus a great deal of the management of poisoning by ingestion is aimed at trying to rid the body of the poison before the poison gains access to the intestinal tract.

General Principles of Assessment and Management

Taking the History

In order to choose an appropriate course of action in any given poisoning, one first needs to obtain some specific information about the poisoning. Find out at least the following:

- WHAT was ingested? If the substance was a commercial product, bring the container and all its remaining contents with the patient to the emergency department. If a plant was ingested, find out *what part of the plant* (roots, leaves, stem, flower, fruit), and bring a sample of the plant to the emergency room for identification. If vomiting has occurred, save a sample of the vomitus in a clean, closed container, and bring that along as well. The object of all those exercises is to enable a precise, specific identification of the poison or poisons ingested.
- WHEN was the poison ingested? The decision whether it is worthwhile to induce vomiting or to flush out (**lavage**) the stomach will be strongly influenced by the amount of time that has elapsed since the ingestion, for the likelihood of retrieving significant quantities of poison from the stomach decreases rapidly after the first 30 to 60 minutes.
- HOW MUCH was taken? A teaspoonful? A quart? In most poisonings, there is a direct relationship between the dosage and the toxic effects.
- WHAT ELSE was taken? A majority of intentional self-poisonings involve more than one substance. Or the patient may have tried to take something

as an **antidote** (something to counteract the effect of the poison).
- Has the patient VOMITED? If so, how soon after the ingestion? How much?
- It is also worthwhile to ask WHY the substance was taken. You may or may not get a reliable answer, but asking the question at least gives the patient an opening to talk about suicidal feelings if he or she wants to talk about them.

Physical Assessment

In addition to the standard procedures for the primary and secondary surveys, there are certain signs for which you need to be particularly alert in poisoned patients. ODORS are very important, for example. A garlicky smell may be the tip-off to an arsenic or organophosphate exposure, while patients poisoned with cyanide sometimes smell of almonds. Make careful note of the STATE OF CONSCIOUSNESS. A patient who has ingested certain mushrooms may be hallucinating, while other poisons may produce stupor or coma. The CONDITION OF THE SKIN can provide a great deal of information. Patients poisoned with atropine-like substances typically have red, hot, dry skin (some of the features mentioned in the old mnemonic for the signs of atropine poisoning: mad as a hatter; red as a beet; dry as a bone; blind as a bat; hot as hell!). Patients poisoned with organophosphate insecticides, on the other hand, are usually sweating profusely. The patient's VITAL SIGNS will tell you the extent to which the poison is already exerting systemic effects and may help identify the type of poison involved. Arsenic, for instance, generally increases the pulse, while gasoline may slow it down. Central nervous system (CNS) depressants slow respirations; poisons like methanol that cause metabolic acidosis lead to deep and rapid breathing. Some of the signs and symptoms that may help narrow down the cause of a poisoning are summarized in Table 27-1. It is not necessary to clutter up your head with all that information

TABLE 27-1. COMMON SIGNS AND SYMPTOMS OF POISONING

SIGN OR SYMPTOM	POSSIBLE CAUSATIVE AGENTS
Odor	
Bitter almonds	Cyanide
Garlic	Arsenic, organophosphates, phosphorus
Acetone	Methyl alcohol, isopropyl alcohol, aspirin, acetone
Wintergreen	Methyl salicylate
Pears	Chloral hydrate
Violets	Turpentine
Camphor	Camphor
Alcohol	Alcohol

TABLE 27-1 (continued)

SIGN OR SYMPTOM	POSSIBLE CAUSATIVE AGENTS
Pupils	
Constricted	Narcotics, organophosphates, jimson weed, nutmeg, Darvon
Dilated	Barbiturates, atropine, amphetamines, Doriden, LSD, cyanide, carbon monoxide
Mouth	
Salivation	Organophosphates, arsenic, strychnine, mercury, salicylates
Dry mouth	Atropine (belladonna), amphetamines, Benadryl, narcotics
Burns in mouth	Formaldehyde, iodine, lye, toxic plants, phenols, phosphorus, pine oil, silver nitrate, acids
Skin	
Pruritus	Jimson weed, belladonna, boric acid
Dry, hot skin	Atropine (belladonna), botulism, nutmeg
Sweating	Organophosphates, arsenic, aspirin, amphetamines, barbiturates, mushrooms, naphthalene
Respiratory	
Depressed respirations	Narcotics, alcohol, Darvon, carbon monoxide, barbiturates
Increased respirations	Aspirin, amphetamines, boric acid, cyanide, kerosene, methyl alcohol, nicotine
Pulmonary edema	Organophosphates, petroleum products, narcotics, carbon monoxide
Cardiovascular	
Tachycardia	Alcohol, amphetamines, arsenic, atropine, aspirin, cocaine, some antiasthma drugs
Bradycardia	Digitalis, gasoline, nicotine, mushrooms, narcotics, cyanide, mistletoe, rhododendron
Hypertension	Amphetamines, lead, nicotine, antiasthma drugs
Hypotension	Barbiturates, narcotics, tranquilizers, house plants, mistletoe, nitroglycerin, antifreeze
Central nervous system	
Seizures	Amphetamines, camphor, cocaine, strychnine, arsenic, carbon monoxide, petroleum products, scorpion sting
Coma	All depressant drugs (e.g., narcotics, barbiturates, tranquilizers, alcohol), carbon monoxide, cyanide
Hallucinations	Atropine, LSD, mushrooms, organic solvents, PCP, nutmeg
Headache	Carbon monoxide, alcohol, Antabuse
Tremors	Organophosphates, carbon monoxide, amphetamines, tranquilizers, poisonous marine animals
Weakness or paralysis	Organophosphates, botulism, eel, hemlock, puffer fish, pine oil, rhododendron
Gastrointestinal	
Cramps, nausea, vomiting, and/or diarrhea	Many if not most ingested poisons

or to try to remember which poison smells like bitter almonds and which smells like pears. It is always possible to look up the significance of an observation *if* you are alert enough to make the observation in the first place and then methodical enough to *write it down* on the patient's trip sheet.

> **RECORD ALL YOUR FINDINGS ABOUT A POISONED PATIENT, EVEN IF YOU DON'T KNOW THEIR SIGNIFICANCE. SOMEONE AT POISON CONTROL WILL KNOW.**

To Empty the Stomach or Not

As noted earlier, the objective in treating very nearly all toxic ingestions is to prevent poisonous material from reaching the small intestine, from where it can be most readily absorbed into the bloodstream. Basically, there are two ways of doing that: One can empty the patient's stomach—either by making the patient vomit or by putting a tube in the stomach and withdrawing the gastric contents—and thereby remove the poison before it has a chance to proceed into the small bowel; or one can try to inactivate the poison that is sitting in the stomach and perhaps also some of the poison that has already passed out of the stomach into the intestines. Which of those methods is best has become a matter of some controversy, and the paramedic should be guided by local protocols. We can, however, provide some general guidelines on the subject.

There is no doubt that vomiting is the most effective means of emptying the stomach, which is precisely what Nature designed vomiting to accomplish. The question is whether there is anything in the stomach worth emptying. The INDUCTION OF VOMITING is most likely to be useful if carried out very soon after the ingestion, that is, *within the first 15 to 20 minutes* after the poisonous substance was swallowed. Thereafter, making the patient vomit becomes literally a matter of progressively diminishing returns.

In certain cases, vomiting is contraindicated altogether, no matter how soon you reach the patient:

> **NEVER INDUCE VOMITING IN:**
>
> • A drowsy or STUPOROUS patient
> • A patient having SEIZURES

> • A PREGNANT patient
> • A patient with a possible ACUTE MYOCARDIAL INFARCTION
> • A patient who has ingested any of the following:
>   1. CORROSIVES (strong acids or alkalis)
>   2. HYDROCARBONS (kerosene, gasoline, lighter fluid, furniture products, solvents)
>   3. IODIDES
>   4. SILVER NITRATE (as in a styptic pencil)
>   5. STRYCHNINE (contained in some rat poisons)
>
> WHEN IN DOUBT, CALL FOR ADVICE.

When local protocol calls for the induction of vomiting, and there are no contraindications, the usual method is to administer **syrup of ipecac, 30 ml** (2 tablespoons) by mouth (adult dosage), followed by one or two glasses of water. Then encourage the patient to move around until he feels a need to vomit. At that point, support him in a head-down position, with his head lower than his hips, to minimize the possibility of aspiration. Save a sample of the vomitus. Then, if you have not already done so, administer **activated charcoal,** at least 5 tablespoons mixed in tap water to make a slurry. The stuff *looks* terrible, so it may take some coaxing to get the patient to swallow it, but it's absolutely essential that he do so.

If vomiting does not occur and your orders are to empty the stomach, the patient may require GASTRIC LAVAGE. Bear in mind that the same contraindications that apply to the induction of vomiting also apply to lavage. Furthermore, to be effective, gastric lavage should really be performed through a *very* large-bore (36 to 40 French) *oro*gastric tube that looks a lot like a garden hose and is no picnic to push down the esophagus of a conscious patient. So as a general rule, it's best to leave gastric lavage for the emergency department unless you are very far from the hospital. Even then, probably all you can aspire to in the prehospital phase is to slip down a more modestly proportioned *naso*gastric tube and remove as much as you can of the gastric contents.

The technique of passing a nasogastric tube is described in the Appendix at the end of this chapter. Once the tube is in, position the patient on his left side, head and face down to increase drainage and minimize the chances of aspiration. Aspirate the tube before you start the lavage, and save the contents. Then use a bulb syringe to instill about 50 ml of saline (for adults), draw it back out, and save it as well for laboratory analysis. Instill another 50 ml of saline, draw it back out, and discard it. Keep lavaging in that fashion until the aspirate is clear. Then instill a slurry of activated charcoal (at least 5 tablespoons in a small amount of tap water) down the nasogastric tube and clamp off the tube.

A reminder:

> **NEVER PASS A NASOGASTRIC TUBE IN A STUPOROUS OR COMATOSE PATIENT UNLESS YOU HAVE FIRST SECURED THE AIRWAY WITH A CUFFED ENDOTRACHEAL TUBE.**

Most paramedics will be very happy to hear that the trend nowadays is *not* to empty the stomach at all, by vomiting *or* gastric lavage, but simply to give activated charcoal by itself—which makes for much less mess at the scene and in the ambulance (unless the patient happens to vomit spontaneously). Newer forms of "superactivated" charcoal have a much increased adsorptive surface and can reduce the gastrointestinal absorption of toxic substances by as much as 50 percent. Activated charcoal has also been shown to increase the effectiveness of gastric-emptying methods when administered *before* or together with syrup of ipecac, or *before* gastric lavage. It is likely, therefore, that Poison Control Centers will soon be recommending that parents keep a supply of activated charcoal at home and administer *it*, rather than syrup of ipecac, as soon as possible after a toxic ingestion.

Treatment of Poisoning by Ingestion: General Principles

Putting the whole matter of gastric emptying into the context of overall treatment, the steps in managing a toxic ingestion are as follows:

- Maintain an open AIRWAY. This cannot be overstressed. The sleepy or comatose patient is in constant danger of aspiration. It is the paramedic's primary task to prevent that—usually by timely endotracheal intubation.
- Administer OXYGEN.
- If the patient is alert and has an intact gag reflex, and if not contraindicated, give ACTIVATED CHARCOAL, at least 5 tablespoons mixed into a slurry in tap water.
- Induce vomiting if called for by local protocols and if not contraindicated.
- If the patient is stuporous or comatose, insert a NASOGASTRIC TUBE *after* the patient's trachea

has been intubated, withdraw (and save) the gastric contents, and instill activated charcoal as described.
- BE PREPARED to manage *shock, coma, seizures,* and *dysrhythmias* as detailed in other sections of this book.
- TRANSPORT, preferably *left side down* to reduce absorption of the poison and minimize the risk of aspiration.

In the sections that follow, we shall look at some of the more common toxic ingestions and the specific measures required to treat them.

Caustic Ingestions

Caustic substances are those that cause direct chemical injury to tissues. The caustic substances most commonly ingested are either strong acids or strong alkalis (Table 27-2). Accidental ingestion of acids and alkalis (most commonly lye) occurs mostly among small children—some 5,000 to 8,000 annually—who

TABLE 27-2.   COMMON CAUSTIC SUBSTANCES

SUBSTANCE	FOUND IN
ACIDS	
Hydrochloric acid	Toilet bowl cleaners
	Swimming pool cleaners
Sulfuric acid	Battery acid
	Toilet bowl cleaners (as bisulfate)
Others	Bleach disinfectants
	Slate cleaners
ALKALIS	
Lye (sodium or potassium hydroxide)	Paint removers
	Washing powders
	Drain cleaners (e.g., Drano, Liquid Plumr, Plunge)
	Button batteries
	Clinitest tablets
Sodium hypochlorite	Clorox bleach
Sodium carbonate	Purex bleach
	Nonphosphate detergents
Ammonia	Hair dyes
	Jewelry cleaners
	Metal cleaners or polishes
	Antirust agents
Potassium permanganate	Electric dishwasher detergents

find the substances readily accessible in kitchen, bathroom, and garage cabinets. The rather strange but widespread practice of storing such substances in beverage containers (e.g., soft drink or beer bottles) only increases the likelihood that a child will regard the substance as something good to drink and try it out. Among adults, suicide attempts account for the majority of caustic ingestions.

Most patients who have swallowed caustic substances present with severe pain in the throat or chest. Usually the airway is *not* a problem, nor is the patient in shock. Although strong acids and strong alkalis probably produce their damage by different mechanisms, the initial management is similar for both types of ingestion, and the basic principle is to try to *dilute* the caustic substance.

- If, by chance, there *is* respiratory distress, it is most probably due to soft tissue swelling in the larynx, epiglottis, or vocal cords, which means that the patient is in immediate danger of complete airway obstruction. Therefore:

IF A PATIENT WHO SWALLOWED A CAUSTIC AGENT IS IN RESPIRATORY DISTRESS, GET MOVING WITHOUT FURTHER DELAY TO THE HOSPITAL. HAVE YOUR CRICOTHYROTOMY KIT READY.

- In the alert patient, give MILK—at least 6 to 8 ounces for a child, 8 to 12 ounces for an adult. If the patient ingested alkali *crystals*, such as Drano, have him first swish some milk around his mouth and spit it out, to get rid of any crystals that may still be sticking to the oral mucosa.
- Do NOT give any "neutralizing substances." Some product labels incorrectly advise neutralization of the caustic agent, for instance by giving lemon juice or dilute vinegar (weak acids) to a patient who has swallowed an alkali. When you mix an acid with an alkali, what you get is *heat*! So you are just adding thermal injury on top of the chemical injury.
- DO NOT INDUCE VOMITING. Do not perform gastric lavage.
- Do NOT give activated charcoal. It is not effective in acid or alkali ingestions, and it will just interfere with the patient's subsequent care—by blackening the field of vision for the endoscopist trying to inspect the esophagus and stomach for damage.

- Start an IV en route.
- TRANSPORT without delay.

Hydrocarbons

Hydrocarbons, as the name implies, are compounds made up principally of hydrogen and carbon atoms; most, but not all, are obtained from the distillation of petroleum. Hydrocarbons are found in a wide variety of products around the home—cleaning and polishing agents, paints and paint removers, lighter fluids and other fuels, pesticides, glues, spot removers. These products, like caustic agents, also tend to be stored in discarded soft drink bottles. Given the wide accessibility of hydrocarbons, then, and the likelihood of their being mistaken for potable beverages, it is not surprising that hydrocarbon ingestions account for nearly 5 percent of all accidental poisonings in children under 5. In adults, the incidence of hydrocarbon poisoning seems to follow the price of gasoline; when gasoline prices rise, there is an upsurge in ingestions that occur accidently during attempts to siphon fuel from vehicular gas tanks.

The potential hazards of swallowing a given hydrocarbon are directly related to the viscosity of the agent: The lower the viscosity, the higher the risk of aspiration and of other complications. The vast majority of hydrocarbon ingestions do *not* produce any lasting damage. But patients who develop symptoms within a few minutes of hydrocarbon ingestion are likely to have aspirated and are in need of immediate attention.

Hydrocarbons of low viscosity—such as kerosene, naphthas, toluene—can enter the lungs during the process of being swallowed. If the patient reports COUGHING, CHOKING, or VOMITING SPONTANEOUSLY immediately on swallowing the substance, he should be assumed to have aspirated. Similarly any signs of RESPIRATORY DISTRESS—air hunger, intercostal retractions, tachypnea, cyanosis—must be considered danger signals.

The same low viscosity that makes a hydrocarbon likely to get into the lungs also facilitates its uptake by tissues of the central nervous system and therefore its ANESTHETIC EFFECTS. There may, at first, be a period of excitement and euphoria, followed by weakness, incoordination, drowsiness, confusion, coma. Some petroleum products, notably gasoline, can also produce HYPOGLYCEMIA and CARDIAC DYSRHYTHMIAS.

Many hydrocarbon products also cause gastric irritation, producing ABDOMINAL PAIN, DIARRHEA, and BELCHING, sometimes for hours after the ingestion.

Treatment of Hydrocarbon Ingestion

If the patient who has swallowed a hydrocarbon product is asymptomatic at the time you arrive, the chances of his experiencing significant complications from the ingestion are very small. Most such patients can be safely observed at home, with instructions to call the regional Poison Control Center or a local emergency department if any symptoms develop. Consult medical command, though, before making any decision not to transport.

When, on the other hand, a patient who ingested a hydrocarbon has any of the signs or symptoms mentioned, emergency treatment and transport are required:

- Ensure an adequate AIRWAY. Anticipate a lot of secretions, and have suction ready. If the gag reflex is absent, endotracheal intubation will be needed as soon as possible, preferably carried out with the patient semisitting and with cricoid pressure to reduce the possibility of aspiration during the procedure.
- Administer OXYGEN.
- DO NOT INDUCE VOMITING.
- If and *only* if the patient has been intubated, pass a NASOGASTRIC TUBE and withdraw the contents of the stomach; then rinse a few times with saline.
- Do NOT give activated charcoal.
- Start an IV LIFELINE with D5/W. If coma or seizures are present, give 50 ml of 50% dextrose (D50).
- MONITOR cardiac rhythm; treat dysrhythmias as required.

Poisonous Alcohols

The form of alcohol consumed by humans in alcoholic beverages is *ethyl alcohol,* or **ethanol,** and it is not conventionally regarded as a poison—even though, when taken in sufficient quantities, it does have many properties of a poison. When we speak of poisonous alcohols, however, we are generally referring to types of alcohol manufactured for industrial or other nongastronomic purposes. Two such products that are most commonly implicated in poisonings are methyl alcohol and ethylene glycol.

Methyl Alcohol Poisoning

Methyl alcohol (wood alcohol, or **methanol**) is an alcohol present in paints, paint removers, varnishes, antifreeze, and canned fuels like Sterno. It is a popular substitute for ethanol among some of the more desperate and unenlightened alcoholics when they don't have the means to obtain a more conventional brew.

It is not methanol itself that is harmful but rather its metabolic breakdown products, formaldehyde and formic acid. Those products are responsible for the characteristic signs and symptoms of methanol poisoning. It does not take a lot of methanol to produce toxicity and even death: A dose of as little as 30 ml (1 ounce, or 2 tablespoons) should be regarded as potentially lethal in an adult.

The *symptoms* of methanol poisoning do not usually come on right away but rather begin anywhere from 8 to 72 hours after the ingestion, so the patient may or may not connect his symptoms to the fact that he took a swig of antifreeze a day or so earlier. The patient may complain of NAUSEA, VOMITING, and ABDOMINAL PAIN, usually the consequence of pancreatitis. VISUAL DISTURBANCES are also common, because of damage caused by formic acid to the optic disc. So the patient may report blurring of vision or tell you that everything "looks like in a snowstorm." Blindness may develop very quickly.

On physical examination, there may be an ODOR OF ALCOHOL on the patient's breath. ALTERATIONS IN THE STATE OF CONSCIOUSNESS are very common, ranging from what appears to be drunken behavior to seizures and coma. Vital signs are likely to reveal HYPERPNEA and TACHYPNEA in response to the severe metabolic acidosis that is characteristic of methanol ingestion. (Why is there hyperpnea and tachypnea in response to metabolic acidosis?) The PUPILS tend to be DILATED and to react sluggishly to light.

The *treatment* of a patient known to have ingested methanol must start as quickly as possible:

- *If the patient is still alert,* and if the ingestion took place within the previous 30 minutes, INDUCE VOMITING.
- If the patient is not alert, or if the gag reflex is absent, INTUBATE THE TRACHEA with a cuffed endotracheal tube. Once that is accomplished, pass a NASOGASTRIC TUBE, and aspirate the contents of the stomach. Save the aspirate in a closed container.
- Give 30 to 60 ml (1–2 ounces) of 80-PROOF WHISKEY. If the patient is alert, give the whiskey by mouth (the patient will probably be only too happy to accept that medicine!). If he is stuporous, give the whiskey down the nasogastric tube after endotracheal intubation. The reason for giving whiskey is that the alcohol contained therein, ethanol, is metabolized by the same en-

zymes that convert methanol to formic acid. By competing for those enzymes, ethanol inhibits the metabolism of methanol to formic acid and thus promotes the excretion of unaltered methanol from the body.

- Start an IV LIFELINE with D5/W.
- Give 50 mEq of SODIUM BICARBONATE IV to combat the metabolic acidosis.
- If the patient is in coma, treat as any other comatose patient.
- Most patients with serious methanol toxicity will require hemodialysis as soon as possible. Therefore NOTIFY the receiving hospital to tool up for a possible emergency dialysis.
- TRANSPORT without delay.

Ethylene Glycol Poisoning

Ethylene glycol is a colorless, odorless, but pleasant-tasting liquid that is present in a variety of antifreezes, deicers, coolants, polishes, and paints. Its relatively pleasant taste has made it a favorite substitute for ethanol among down-at-the-heel alcoholics, and its widespread availability has led to its use in suicide attempts as well. The lethal dosage of ethylene glycol is about 100 ml in adults.

Toxicity from ethylene glycol occurs in three stages, so the signs and symptoms you may see will depend on when you encounter the patient with respect to the time of his ingestion. During *stage 1,* which occurs anywhere from 20 minutes to 12 hours after the ingestion, the patient may simply APPEAR DRUNK, although the odor of ethanol on the breath is notably absent. There may also be nausea, vomiting, seizures, or coma. In *stage 2,* which occurs between 12 and 24 hours after the ingestion, PULMONARY EDEMA produces tachypnea, tachycardia, and crackles. Finally, during *stage 3,* 24 to 72 hours after the ingestion, the renal damage produced by ethylene glycol becomes evident in FLANK PAIN and ANURIA.

Treatment of ethylene glycol ingestion must be started as soon as the diagnosis is suspected. The treatment has three overall objectives: (1) to remove whatever is left of the ethylene glycol from the body (by emesis or gastric lavage in the field, and by hemodialysis in the hospital); (2) as in methanol poisoning, to block the metabolism of ethylene glycol to its toxic products; and (3) to prevent the formation of calcium oxalate crystals in the kidney, by keeping the kidneys well flushed.

- Administer OXYGEN by nasal cannula.
- *If the patient is alert and capable of protecting his airway,* INDUCE VOMITING with syrup of ipecac. Administer ACTIVATED CHARCOAL, at least 5 tablespoons mixed with tap water into a slurry.
- If the patient is not alert, or if his gag reflex is absent, INTUBATE THE TRACHEA. Only after the endotracheal tube is in place, pass a NASOGASTRIC TUBE into the stomach. Aspirate the contents of the stomach. Save the aspirate. Administer activated charcoal as above.
- Administer 60 ml (2 ounces) of WHISKEY—by mouth (as a chaser to the activated charcoal) to the alert patient, by nasogastric tube to the intubated, less-than-alert patient.
- Start an IV LIFELINE with lactated Ringer's, and run it at a rate of at least 200 ml per hour.
- Administer 50 mEq of SODIUM BICARBONATE IV.
- Consult medical command regarding other medications that may be required. Anticipate orders for any of the following:
  1. FUROSEMIDE, 40 mg IV, or MANNITOL, 35 gm IV, to promote renal clearance of ethylene glycol and oxalic acid.
  2. THIAMINE, 50 mg IV plus 50 mg IM, which acts as an enzyme cofactor in the detoxification of ethylene glycol.
  3. CALCIUM GLUCONATE, 10 ml of a 10% solution slowly IV, to treat the hypocalcemia that often accompanies ethylene glycol toxicity (should be given only after good urine flow is established, and after the IV line is flushed clear of sodium bicarbonate).
- BE PREPARED to deal with seizures.
- The patient will probably require hemodialysis, so NOTIFY the receiving hospital of the situation.
- TRANSPORT without delay.

Poisonous Plants

Of the many thousands of plant varieties, only a very small number are poisonous. But, strangely, a considerable proportion of those that *are* poisonous number among the most common ornamental garden shrubs and houseplants. Perhaps for that reason, plants are now the leading cause of poisoning in children under 5 years old, accounting for about 11 percent of all toxic ingestions in that age group. Fortunately, few of the affected children reported to Poison Control Centers required hospitalization, and none died. But the potential for very serious poisoning is there. A few examples:

For starters, there is the ubiquitous DIEFFENBACHIA, a lovely green plant with broad, variegated leaves. It is not by coincidence that dieffenbachia is nicknamed "dumbcane," for eating dieffenbachia can literally strike a person dumb. All parts of the dieffenbachia plant—leaves, stems, roots—contain sharp caladium oxalate crystals. When ingested, those crystals cause burns of the mouth and tongue and sometimes paralysis of the vocal cords. In severe cases, there may be edema of the tongue and larynx, leading to airway compromise.

CALADIUM, with its stunning multicolored leaves, is another hazard lurking in the flowerpot. Like dieffenbachia, it contains caladium oxalate crystals, so it can cause the same burning and swelling of the mouth and throat in anyone rash enough to chew on it. Nausea, vomiting, and diarrhea also commonly occur after ingestion.

LANTANA, also known as red sage or wild sage, is a perennial flowering shrub with clusters of little red berries, and it is the berries—particularly when they are ripe—that can lead to serious and even fatal poisoning. The green berries contain a poison, lantadene A, that causes stomach upsets, muscle weakness, shock, and sometimes death.

Then there's the real killer in the flowerpot: CASTOR BEAN. Indeed, the castor bean plant is so toxic that probably there should be a law forbidding its presence in any home with young children. It's the seed itself that is poisonous in castor bean, and chewing just a few or even one seed from this attractive shrub can kill a child. The poison in the castor bean seeds is called ricin, and it causes a variety of toxic effects: burning of the mouth and throat; nausea, vomiting, diarrhea, and severe stomach pains; prostration; failing vision; and kidney failure, which is usually the cause of death.

Those are just a few examples. More examples are contained in Table 27-3, mainly as a guide to plants that should not be kept around small children. When you encounter an actual case, get all the information you can from the parent, and then consult your regional Poison Control Center for advice. The information you need to collect is similar to that required in any other ingestion. Find out:

- WHEN was the plant ingested? If it was more than 12 hours ago and Junior still has no symptoms, chances are he will come out unscathed; most plant poisonings, if they are going to produce symptoms at all, do so within about 4 hours of ingestion. The possible exception to that rule, as applied to houseplants, is ingestion of the notorious castor bean, mentioned previously, where symptoms may be delayed from 1 to 3 *days* after ingestion.
- WHAT did the child eat? Find out not just what type of plant, but also WHAT PART(S) OF THE PLANT (leaves, root, stem, flower, fruit?). If

the child is transported to the hospital, take along the offending plant (or whatever is left of it).
- WHAT SYMPTOMS, if any, has the child shown?

Treatment of Plant Ingestions

As a general rule, the best approach to plant ingestion is to contact the regional Poison Control Center with the information described and ask for advice. There are, however, some general guidelines to keep in mind.

- *If* the child ate the plant within the past 4 hours, and *if* you don't know what the plant was, and *if* he is fully conscious, INDUCE VOMITING with 1 tablespoon of syrup of ipecac. If there is a responsible adult who can keep a close eye on the child over the next 12 hours or so, there is no real need to transport him to the hospital.
- If, on the other hand, the child is showing any symptoms following ingestion of any part of a plant, he will need to be evaluated in the emergency department. Follow the instructions of the Poison Control Center regarding the prehospital management.

INHALED POISONS

A person can suffer poisoning by inhalation only if the poison is present in the atmosphere around him. That fact, obvious as it seems, has at least two important implications. First of all, so long as the patient remains in the toxic environment, he will keep inhaling the poison—and so will you, if you enter that environment without protective breathing apparatus. The second implication is that when poisoning occurs because of a toxic environment, there is likely to be more than one victim. The other side of the coin is that when you are called to care for several people suffering from different symptoms, and they were all together in the same closed space, you need to think about an inhaled poison as the cause of the problem.

There are, then, two general guidelines that apply to all cases of poisoning by inhalation:

- THE MOST IMPORTANT ASPECT OF TREATMENT IN TOXIC INHALATIONS IS TO REMOVE THE PATIENT FROM THE TOXIC ENVIRONMENT, *but*:
- DO NOT ENTER A KNOWN TOXIC ENVIRONMENT WITHOUT PROTECTIVE BREATHING APPARATUS.

TABLE 27-3. POISONS IN SOME COMMON PLANTS

PLANT	POISONOUS PART	POISON	SIGNS AND SYMPTOMS OF POISONING
Apricot	Seeds	Cyanide	Headache, dizziness, weakness, nausea, vomiting, coma, seizures
Autumn crocus	Entire plant	Colchicine	Cramps, nausea, hematuria, diarrhea, coma, shock
Bird of paradise	Pod	Multiple	Vomiting, diarrhea
Bloodroot	Root	Sanguinarine	Cramps, diarrhea, dizziness, paralysis, coma
Buttercup	Entire plant	Protanemonin	Gastroenteritis, seizures
Caladium	Leaves and roots	Calcium oxalate	Burning of mucous membranes, swelling of tongue and throat, salivation, gastroenteritis
Cherry	Bark, leaves, seed	Amygdalin	Stupor, vocal cord paralysis, seizures, coma
Dieffenbachia	Leaves and roots	Calcium oxalate	Same as for caladium
Daffodil	Bulb	Multiple	Gastroenteritis
Deadly nightshade	Berry, leaf, root	Atropine	Fever; tachycardia; dilated pupils; hot, red, dry skin
Elderberry	Leaf, shoot, bark	Sambunigran	Gastroenteritis
Holly	Berries	Ilicin	Gastroenteritis, coma
Hyacinth	Bulb	Multiple	Severe gastroenteritis
Jack-in-the-pulpit	All parts	Calcium oxalate	Severe gastroenteritis, burning of oral mucosa
Jimson weed	All parts	Atropine	Dry mouth; hot, red skin; headache; hallucinations; tachycardia; hypertension; delirium; seizures
Laurel	All parts	Andromedotoxin	Salivation, lacrimation, rhinorrhea, vomiting, seizures, bradycardia, hypotension, paralysis
Lily of the valley	Leaf, flowers	Glycosides	Cardiac dysrhythmias, nausea
Mistletoe	All parts	Tyramine	Bradycardia, gastroenteritis, hypertension, dyspnea, delirium, sweating, shock
Morning glory	Seeds	LSD	Hallucinations
Narcissus	Bulb	Multiple	Gastroenteritis
Oleander	Entire plant	Oleanin	Cramps, bradycardia, dilated pupils, bloody diarrhea, coma, apnea (one leaf is lethal)
Philodendron	Entire plant	Calcium oxalate	Edema of tongue, throat
Poinsettia	Leaves, stem, sap	Multiple	Contact dermatitis, gastroenteritis
Potato	Green tubers, new sprouts	Solanine	Severe gastroenteritis, headache, apnea, shock
Rhododendron	Entire plant	Andromedotoxin	Salivation
Rhubarb	Leaves only	Oxalic acid	Cramps, nausea, vomiting, anuria
Wisteria	Pods	Glycoside	Severe gastroenteritis, shock

Cyanide Poisoning

Cyanide may gain access to the body through any of several routes. Poisoning can occur through the *ingestion* of cyanide-containing commercial products, such as silver polish, or the seeds of cherries, apples, pears, and possibly apricots. Cyanide poisoning can occur through *inhalation* of cyanide gas produced in household fires, from the combustion of materials that contain nitrogen (plastic furnishings, wool, silk, carpeting, synthetic rubber). Firefighters who neglect to wear self-contained breathing apparatus during the extinguishing and cleanup phases of a fire are particularly at risk of inhaling cyanide.

EVERY VICTIM OF SMOKE INHALATION SHOULD BE ASSUMED TO HAVE SUFFERED CYANIDE POISONING.

Regardless of the route of entry, cyanide is one of the most rapidly acting and most deadly poisons, and perhaps for that reason it is a great favorite among writers of murder mysteries.

Cyanide does its damage by combining with a crucial cellular enzyme, cytochrome oxidase, and thereby blocking the utilization of oxygen at the cellular level. The result is cellular suffocation, and death of the whole organism may follow within seconds if the cyanide was inhaled or within minutes to a few hours if it was ingested.

On physical examination, the patient who has been poisoned with cyanide may be confused or stuporous. If awake enough to answer questions, he may complain of HEADACHE, PALPITATIONS, or DYSPNEA. The classic ODOR OF BITTER ALMONDS on the patient's breath is highly suggestive but not diagnostic, and few people know what bitter almonds smell like anyway. RESPIRATIONS are usually RAPID AND LABORED early on, but later become slow and gasping. The PULSE is usually RAPID and THREADY. Vomiting, seizures, and coma are frequent. The patient's venous blood (and sometimes the patient himself) may be bright red because oxygen is not being taken up by the tissues. Cyanosis is rare; if the patient *is* cyanotic, either he has not been poisoned with cyanide or he's very near the end of the line.

Cyanide poisoning is a dire medical emergency, so *treatment* must be instituted as fast as possible. The aim of treatment is to displace cyanide from cytochrome oxidase by introducing another chemical (in the field, amyl nitrite is the easiest to use) that will "attract" the cyanide. The treatment is extremely effective if given in time.

- If the cyanide poisoning occurred as the result of a toxic inhalation, REMOVE THE PATIENT FROM THE CYANIDE SOURCE!
- Establish an AIRWAY.
- Administer 100% OXYGEN. Assist ventilations as necessary.
- If you carry the commercially available cyanide antidote kit (Eli Lilly), follow the instructions supplied with the kit, which include administration of 50 ml of 25% SODIUM THIOSULFATE solution IV. If you do not stock those kits, break a perle of AMYL NITRITE into a gauze pad or handkerchief and hold it over the patient's nose

for about *20 seconds* out of every minute; then have him breathe 100% oxygen for the rest of the minute. Keep alternating amyl nitrite and 100% oxygen in that fashion.
- While you are administering amyl nitrite, have your partner start an IV LIFELINE as quickly as possible.
- ANTICIPATE HYPOTENSION as a consequence of amyl nitrite therapy, and keep the patient supine with his legs elevated. If the systolic blood pressure falls below about 80 mm Hg, consult medical command regarding whether to hang a norepinephrine drip.
- MONITOR cardiac rhythm.
- NOTIFY the receiving hospital of the probable diagnosis, so that they can ready an infusion of sodium thiosulfate.
- TRANSPORT without delay.

Carbon Monoxide Poisoning

Carbon monoxide (CO) causes more poisoning fatalities than any other toxic substance—about 3,500 accidental and suicidal deaths in the United States each year. Carbon monoxide is produced during the incomplete combustion of organic fuels, most commonly in the automobile engine or home-heating devices. The latter make CO poisoning predominantly a winter phenomenon; problems commonly occur when a flue or ventilating system becomes blocked. However, at least half of successful adult suicide attempts are caused by CO, and obviously those may occur at any time of the year. An automobile in a small, closed garage can generate a lethal concentration of CO in 15 to 30 minutes. Carbon monoxide is also a major contributor to mortality from fires.

Carbon monoxide is a *colorless, odorless, tasteless gas,* and it is largely for that reason that CO is so dangerous. Usually the exposed victim of accidental CO inhalation has no idea he is inhaling a toxic material until it is too late. The toxicity of carbon monoxide is primarily due to its affinity for hemoglobin in red blood cells, where it displaces oxygen and thus prevents the red cells from carrying oxygen to the tissues. The atmospheric level of CO need not be high for poisoning to occur, for the affinity of hemoglobin for CO is more than 200 times that for oxygen. So even relatively small concentrations of carbon monoxide in the atmosphere can convert a significant proportion of normal hemoglobin into **carboxyhemoglobin** (hemoglobin combined with carbon dioxide), rendering it ineffective as an oxygen carrier. The result is suffocation at the cellular level.

Because the ability of the blood to transport oxygen is reduced in carbon monoxide poisoning, anything that increases the body's oxygen *requirements,* such as fever or physical exertion, will increase the severity of the poisoning. Similarly, children, whose metabolic rate is intrinsically higher than that of adults, tend to develop more severe symptoms at any given level of exposure, for their higher oxygen demand makes them feel the oxygen deficiency earlier.

The *symptoms* of CO poisoning are highly variable and often quite vague, leading in many cases to delays in diagnosis. Symptoms like headache, nausea, and vomiting sometimes cause CO poisoning to be misdiagnosed as "the flu." Other symptoms of CO poisoning may include a sensation of pressure in the head and roaring in the ears. With acute poisoning, the patient shows confusion and inability to think clearly. He may appear drunk. In more severe exposures, there is often vomiting and incontinence, followed by convulsions and coma. The physical examination reveals bounding pulses, dilated pupils, and pallor or cyanosis. The cherry red color of the skin that is mentioned in most textbooks is rarely seen. In the comatose patient, you may hear crackles indicative of pulmonary edema. There tends to be great variability in symptoms among different individuals having had the same exposure. Thus, consider the possibility of CO poisoning whenever you are confronted with an epidemic of varying symptoms among people who have shared the same accommodations for any period of time, especially if they have been quartered together in a closed area (e.g., a classroom) during winter. (When the family dog and cat are also acting funny, you can be nearly certain of the diagnosis.)

> WHENEVER YOU ENCOUNTER A BUNCH OF PEOPLE WITH A BUNCH OF DIFFERENT SYMPTOMS AND THEY WERE ALL TOGETHER IN THE SAME PLACE, THINK OF CARBON MONOXIDE.

Treatment of Carbon Monoxide Poisoning

The treatment of carbon monoxide poisoning is aimed at providing the highest concentration of oxygen possible, in an attempt to displace CO molecules from hemoglobin. The elimination half-time of carboxyhemoglobin in the serum of a person breathing room air is 520 minutes. When a person is breathing 100% oxygen, that half-time can be reduced to 80 minutes.

- REMOVE THE PATIENT FROM THE EXPOSURE ENVIRONMENT.
- Administer 100% OXYGEN by tight-fitting, non-rebreathing mask.
- If there is respiratory depression, assist ventilations with a bag-valve-mask (equipped with an oxygen reservoir).
- Keep the patient QUIET AND AT REST, to minimize his oxygen demand.
- If the patient has been removed from a structural or vehicular fire, consider the possibility of combined carbon monoxide and cyanide poisoning, especially if there are signs of shock, and consult medical command regarding the administration of amyl nitrite. If you carry a cyanide antidote kit, the definitive treatment is to give sodium thiosulfate, 12.5 gm IV.
- MONITOR cardiac rhythm and state of consciousness.
- Treat coma, if present, as outlined elsewhere. If the patient *is* comatose, or has any other signs of serious CO poisoning, he should ideally be treated in a HYPERBARIC OXYGEN chamber, where the elimination half-time of CO can be reduced to around 25 minutes. Notify medical command of the patient's condition, so that the process of arranging transfer to the nearest hyperbaric facility can be started.

Chlorine Gas Exposure

Accidents involving chlorine gas are relatively common because of the widespread use of chlorine compounds both in the home and in industry. Household exposures usually occur when someone mixes a cleaning agent containing sodium hypochlorite (such as bleach) with some strong acid in an overzealous attempt to "really clean" a toilet bowl. The resulting chemical reaction releases chlorine gas, often in high concentrations. Most cases of chlorine gas exposure occur outside the home, however, in situations of mass exposure. The chlorination of large swimming pools (where the gas rather than the liquid or solid forms of chlorine tends to be used) has led to numerous cases of mass exposure at hotels and community recreation centers. Leakage from industrial storage tanks or from trucks or trains carrying chlorine has also resulted in virtual epidemics of chlorine gas exposure. Thus, in the majority of instances in which the paramedic has to deal with chlorine gas inhalation, there will be a LARGE NUMBER OF VICTIMS, and the usual principles of triage must be applied.

The SYMPTOMS AND SIGNS of chlorine gas inhalation depend on the concentration of the inhaled gas and the duration of exposure. Chlorine gas is extremely irritating to all mucous membranes, and when it comes in contact with the moisture on those surfaces, it can form hydrochloric and other acids that are very damaging to tissue. With minor exposures, the patient will experience BURNING SENSATIONS in the eyes, nose, and throat and perhaps a slight cough. More intense exposure to chlorine gas causes CHEST TIGHTNESS, CHOKING, PAROXYSMAL COUGH, HEADACHE, NAUSEA, and sometimes WHEEZING. Patients with the most severe exposure are apt to present, in addition, with CYANOSIS, CRACKLES in the chest, SHOCK, CONVULSIONS, and COMA.

In treating the victims of chlorine gas inhalation, once again the first priority is to REMOVE THE VICTIMS FROM EXPOSURE TO THE GAS! To do so, the paramedic must take proper precautions to prevent his or her own exposure, which ideally means the use of a self-contained breathing apparatus. A makeshift gas mask for victims may be fashioned from a piece of cloth soaked in water and held over the victim's face until he is out of the exposure zone.

As soon as the victims have been removed to a safe environment, upwind from the gas spill, they must be rapidly TRIAGED. Oxygen cylinders and demand valves will usually be in short supply, so the most seriously affected must have priority for oxygen therapy. Those with dyspnea, wheezing, severe cough, or other signs of respiratory distress should receive humidified oxygen by mask; the demand valve should be reserved for victims with crackles or other indications of pulmonary edema. Once those patients have been treated and their evacuation to the hospital is under way, less serious problems may be addressed. Burning or itching eyes should be irrigated with tap water, as should any areas of the skin that may have come in contact with the chlorine.

Hydrocarbon Inhalation

The vast majority of hydrocarbon inhalations are "recreational" in nature. The rich alveolar capillary network makes the lungs a highly efficient mechanism for providing a quick drug "fix," as any smoker can attest. Indeed, it is this very property of the lungs that makes inhalation anesthesia possible. But it also makes possible the inhalation of a variety of toxic substances by those in search of the ever higher "high."

The modern epidemic of inhalation abuse began in the early 1960s, when sporadic reports of glue sniffing and its consequences started to appear. Within a very short time, the number of agents being inhaled to reach the ephemeral "high" had increased exponentially, as had the techniques for inhalation. Simple **sniffing** over the opening of a glue bottle did not provide an intense enough exposure for the serious abuser; so it was soon discovered that pouring the volatile material into a plastic bag, and then holding the bag over one's face to breathe in the fumes (a practice not surprisingly called **bagging**) provided a much better high. It also led to suffocation in a significant number of cases. Refining the techniques still further, users learned to pour the material onto a cloth, and then roll up the cloth into a tube through which the user breathes—a practice called **huffing.**

Sniffing, bagging, and huffing are most prevalent among very young abusers (peak incidence is between the ages of 13 and 15), as well as among the very poor, who can't afford designer drugs. The most commonly abused inhalants are volatile hydrocarbons, such as toluene, and persons habituated to such substances may use up to 4 pints of glue a day to sustain their habit.

Some of the substances most commonly abused by inhalation are summarized in Table 27-4. The acute effects of inhalation are similar in nearly all of them. The onset of action is very rapid, usually within seconds, with feelings of disorientation, dizziness, and euphoria. Often there are hallucinations, which may be frightening in character. The huffer may also experience a feeling that he is capable of anything—leaping tall buildings at a single bound, flying from a second story window, and so forth. Needless to say, if the "huffer" attempts one of those feats, he is apt to be disappointed in the outcome.

You are most likely to be called when something goes very wrong during a huffing or bagging session. Most often it will be because the abuser developed seizures or some major alteration in consciousness. It may or may not be possible to obtain a reliable history from bystanders, so you have to be alert to the clues that the youngster is an inhalant abuser.

CLUES TO INHALANT ABUSE

- Drunken behavior that resolves fairly rapidly
- Smell of a chemical solvent on the patient's breath
- Glue or paint on the face, hands, or clothes
- "Glue sniffer's rash" on the face of a chronic abuser
- Huffing or bagging paraphernalia at the scene (e.g., rags soaked with solvent)
- Product containers at the scene

TABLE 27-4.   COMPOUNDS COMMONLY ABUSED BY "SNIFFERS" AND "BAGGERS"

SUBSTANCE	FOUND IN	SIGNS AND SYMPTOMS OF TOXICITY
HALOGENATED HYDROCARBONS		
1,1,1-Trichloroethane (methylchloroform)	Cleaning solvents Typewriter correction fluid Aerosol propellant	Eye irritation, light-headedness, incoordination, CNS depression, respiratory failure, cardiac dysrhythmias, sudden death
Trichloroethylene	Degreasing solvent Aerosol propellant Rubber cement Plastic cement	Euphoria, anesthesia, weakness, vomiting, abdominal cramps, loss of coordination, neuropathy, blindness, cardiac dysrhythmias, "degreaser's flush" (flushed face, neck, and shoulders when taken along with alcohol)
Tetrachloroethylene (perchloroethylene)	Solvent Dry cleaning agent	Drunken behavior, dizziness, light-headedness, difficulty walking, numbness, sleepiness, visual disturbances, memory impairment, eye irritation, cutaneous flushing, sudden death
Methylene chloride (dichloromethane)	Refrigerant Paint remover Aerosol propellant	Fatigue, weakness, chills, sleepiness, nausea, dizziness, incoordination, pulmonary edema
Carbon tetrachloride	Cleaning fluid	Narcosis, sudden death
PETROLEUM HYDROCARBONS		
Benzene	Cable cleaner Industrial solvents Rubber cement	Delirium, agitation, convulsions, sudden death
Toluene	Spray paint Model/plastic cements Lacquer thinner	Narcosis, hallucinations, mania; impulsive, destructive, accident-prone behavior; sudden death
Gasoline		Sudden death

The most serious possible consequence of inhalant abuse is cardiac arrest, known as *sudden sniffing death*, or SSD. Sudden sniffing death has been reported most frequently in association with inhalation of typewriter correction fluid (trichloroethane), aerosol propellants (especially freons), and gasoline. If the patient is already in cardiac arrest when you reach the scene, you will have to treat the case as any other cardiac arrest. But the point to remember is that sniffers, huffers, and baggers who are still up and kicking are at significant *risk* of cardiac dysrhythmias and should be managed accordingly.

Treatment of Hydrocarbon Inhalation

The treatment of a patient experiencing toxic effects of hydrocarbon inhalation follows one simple principle:

> **TREAT THE PATIENT, NOT THE POISON.**

That is, tailor your management according to the patient's clinical situation, not according to what the book says about a particular inhalant. The patient may or may not experience any given toxic effect of an inhaled substance. A few general guidelines:

- Ensure a patent AIRWAY. Have suction handy in case of vomiting.
- Administer OXYGEN.
- MONITOR cardiac rhythm. Keep the beep tone audible so you can *hear* any premature beats or other rhythm disturbances as soon as they occur.
- Start an IV LIFELINE with D5/W.
- BE PREPARED to deal with seizures or coma.
- Use verbal reassurance for frightening hallucinations.

ABSORBED POISONS

Some poisons gain access to the body by absorption through the skin. We have already mentioned that cyanide can cause toxicity by that route. Of the poisonings that occur by absorption, those caused by organophosphates are the most common and the most serious.

Organophosphates

Organophosphates are a major component in many insecticides used both for agriculture and in the home. The very widespread use of those products has led to an increasing incidence of poisoning—in the range of 35,000 cases a year in the United States, of which about 10 percent require hospitalization. Among those hospitalized, the fatality rate is around 10 percent for adults and nearly 50 percent for children. Exposures to organophosphates occur in a number of ways. Suicide attempts account for a considerable proportion of organophosphate poisonings (in those cases, the poison is usually taken by mouth). Accidental agricultural exposure is another common source, and persons involved in the manufacture of organophosphates are also at increased risk. Children are often poisoned by handling equipment used to apply pesticides or by playing in areas that have been recently sprayed with organophosphates. Finally, American soldiers serving in the Persian Gulf, along with civilian populations within range of Iraqi missiles, were put at risk of mass organophosphate poisoning during the Gulf War. The nerve gases used in chemical weapons are in the same family of compounds as agricultural pesticides; nerve gases differ chiefly in their greater potency.

The symptoms of organophosphate poisoning are fundamentally the same whether the agent enters the body by mouth, by inhalation, or through the skin.

Organophosphates exert their toxic effects at the **synapses** (junctions) between nerve cells of the autonomic nervous system. Normally, conduction of an impulse from one nerve to another occurs by the release of a chemical, acetylcholine (remember?), at the junction between two nerve cells. Acetylcholine functions as a sort of chemical messenger, crossing the synapse to depolarize the nerve on the other side. Once it has delivered its message, the acetylcholine molecule must be inactivated. Otherwise it would continue stimulating the target nerve cell indefinitely, and the nerve could never receive another message from the brain. It would become like a telephone whose receiver was left off the hook. So nerve cells contain a special enzyme, called **cholinesterase,** whose job it is to inactivate acetylcholine after it has crossed the synapse from one nerve cell to another, so that the nerve can "take another call."

What organophosphates do is to combine with cholinesterase enzymes and prevent them from inactivating acetylcholine. The result is that acetylcholine accumulates at the synapses, causing overstimulation and eventually a breakdown in transmission in both the central and peripheral nervous systems.

Some of the most striking manifestations of organophosphate poisoning are those caused by stimulation of the *parasympathetic* nervous system, such as profuse salivation, bradycardia, and muscle twitching.

Organophosphate poisoning is apt to be missed in its early stages because the most common early SYMPTOMS—*headache, weakness, dizziness, nausea*—are nonspecific and may be brushed off as "the flu" or "something I ate." With more serious exposures, the patient develops *abdominal cramps, vomiting, diarrhea,* and—in very severe cases—*incontinence.* Patients with organophosphate poisoning often complain as well of *blurring of vision, tightness in the chest,* and *dyspnea.*

On PHYSICAL EXAMINATION, the patient with organophosphate poisoning may at first appear drunk because of a *staggering gait* and changes in mental status. The skin is apt to be very wet from *profuse sweating,* and vital signs may be notable for severe *bradycardia.* On head-to-toe survey, the pupils will usually be found to be very constricted (**miosis**), and there is *excessive salivation.* Sometimes a garlicky smell of the poison may be detectable on the patient's breath. The patient may be coughing up large amounts of watery fluid. *Wheezes* and *crackles* may lead the examiner to confuse the patient's condition with asthma or congestive heart failure (CHF). The tip-offs that the patient is *not* suffering from CHF, the flu, or food poisoning are the combination of bradycardia, miosis, and hypersalivation.

WHEN YOU SEE A PATIENT WITH BRADYCARDIA, CONSTRICTED PUPILS, AND HYPERSALIVATION, THINK OF ORGANOPHOSPHATES.

Treatment of Organophosphate Poisoning

The treatment of a patient showing signs of organophosphate poisoning is aimed at terminating his exposure to the poison and trying to reverse its effects on the autonomic nervous system (and, of course, keeping the patient alive in the meanwhile). The parasympathetic blocking agent **atropine** is used as the antidote to organophosphates because it prevents the acetylcholine that has accumulated in the synapses from working. Atropine thereby halts the parasympathetic overstimulation responsible for the toxic effects of organophosphate poisoning, but it takes very high doses of atropine to do so.

- If the patient is not fully alert, pay close attention to the AIRWAY. Copious secretions should be suctioned out thoroughly. If the patient does not have a gag reflex, intubate the trachea.
- Administer 100% OXYGEN, preferably with positive pressure (demand valve or bag-valve-mask plus positive end-expiratory pressure [PEEP]).
- If the poison was absorbed across the skin, DECONTAMINATE the patient. Wear protective clothing (gown and rubber gloves) to do so. Remove the patient's clothing, and stash it in a plastic bag. If he is at home or in an industrial workplace, have him take a shower and wash thoroughly with lots of soap and water; if out in the fields, try to find a hose or other water source that you can use to wash him down.
- If the organophosphate was taken by mouth, and the patient is still alert, administer activated charcoal and give syrup of ipecac to induce vomiting.
- Apply MONITORING electrodes.
- Start an IV LIFELINE with D5/W.
- Administer ATROPINE. Start with 2 mg IM and 1 mg IV as soon as possible, even before you've finished decontamination procedures. (The pediatric dosage is 0.05 mg/kg.) Repeat the IV dose at 5- to 10-minute intervals until signs of atropinization—dry mouth, increased pulse rate, widening of the pupils—are apparent. As noted, it may take truly massive doses of atropine to counter the effects of organophosphate poisoning, and the most common cause of treatment failure is inadequate atropinization.
- In rural areas, where agricultural exposures are common and transport times may be long, you may also be asked to give PRALIDOXIME (also called 2-PAM chloride or Protopam Chloride), which relieves the muscle weakness associated with organophosphate poisoning. One may give 600 mg IM by autoinjector right away, even before decontamination is complete. Thereafter, the recommended dosage is 1 to 2 gm diluted in 250 ml of normal saline and infused over 15 to 20 minutes. For children, the dosage is 10 to 25 mg per kilogram.
- Do NOT give morphine or aminophylline, even if there are signs of pulmonary edema.
- BE PREPARED to deal with *seizures* and *ventricular dysrhythmias*.

INJECTED POISONS AND OTHER BITE INJURIES

Injected poisons usually gain access to the body as the result of stings or bites from a variety of unpleasant little creatures (or sometimes not so little crea-

tures). In this section, we shall consider the ill effects that may come about from unfriendly encounters with creatures of the land, air, and sea—including some that look remarkably like ourselves.

Arthropod Bites and Stings

If sheer numbers were the sole criterion determining such things, arthropods would rule the world. The phylum Arthropoda includes at least a million and a half known species of "joint-footed" animals, ranging from the lobster to the mite. The classes of arthropods of medical importance—because of their ability to inject venom of one sort or another—are the *arachnids* (including spiders, scorpions, and ticks), the *chilopods* (centipedes), and the *insects* (including the hymenoptera).

Hymenoptera Stings

The Hymenoptera family of insects includes bees, wasps, hornets, yellow jackets, and ants. Among them, they kill more people each year than any other venomous animals, including snakes. Death from a hymenoptera sting is usually the result of anaphylaxis, which we have already discussed in the previous chapter. Here, we shall simply consider the management of the sting itself.

The diagnosis of a bee sting is usually not very obscure (the patient most often will have made the diagnosis himself). There is almost always an immediate local reaction, consisting of *pain, redness, swelling,* and sometimes *itching* at the site of the sting. If the perpetrator was a honeybee, the barbed stinger and its venom sac may still be attached to the patient's skin.

TREATMENT of a hymenoptera sting is aimed primarily at pain relief and trying to minimize the possibility of infection:

- Determine whether the stinger is still attached to the skin. If so, use a scalpel blade to SCRAPE THE STINGER AND ITS SAC FROM THE WOUND. Do *not* try to pluck the stinger out with a forceps or other instrument, for squeezing the stinger will only pump more venom into the wound.
- Once the stinger is out, CLEAN THE WOUND THOROUGHLY with soap and water or an antiseptic solution like povidone-iodine.
- Apply COLD PACKS to the sting for pain relief.

If the patient has no history of allergy to bee stings and shows no signs of a systemic reaction, it is not necessary to transport him to the hospital. He should, however, be advised of the warning signs of anaphylaxis and the urgency of getting to the hospital if any of those signs occur. He should also be instructed to have the wound checked by a doctor if it is not markedly improved within 24 hours. Bee stings, especially those on the extremities, often become infected and require antibiotic treatment. Infection is particularly likely after the stings of *fire ants*, which roam the southeastern United States throughout the late spring and early summer. Fire ant stings typically produce little pustules at the sting site about 6 hours after the sting. When the pustules get broken, as they invariably do when the patient starts to scratch, the affected area is very vulnerable to secondary infection.

Tick Bites

Ordinarily, tick bites are not a medical emergency, but they *are* of concern because ticks can transmit a variety of serious illnesses, including Lyme disease, Rocky Mountain spotted fever, and tularemia. In rare instances, furthermore, a tick bite on the back of the head, neck, or spine may produce a potentially life-threatening paralysis, which cannot be reversed unless the tick is removed. So it is something to keep in mind when there is a case of unexplained weakness or paralysis after a person (especially a child) has been out in the woods.

The principal treatment of a tick bite is simply to REMOVE THE TICK, but that must be done carefully. Ticks attach themselves quite tenaciously to their victims by their mouth parts (Fig. 27-1), and if you try to pull the tick away from the skin, the mouth parts may remain embedded there. To remove the tick, use a curved forceps (or *gloved* fingers) to grasp the tick by the head as close to the skin as possible and pull straight upward. Use even pressure as you pull; avoid twisting or jerking the tick. Do not squeeze or crush the tick's body, and do not handle the tick with bare hands, for doing so can result in disease transmission even without a tick bite. Dispose of the tick in a container of alcohol. Once the tick has been removed, wash the bitten area thoroughly with soap and water. In cases of tick paralysis, transport the patient to the hospital with supportive treatment, as needed, en route.

Spider Bites

Two types of spider are of medical concern in the United States: the black widow and the brown recluse.

It is only the female BLACK WIDOW SPIDER that poses a danger to humans. Her name derives from her rather disagreeable practice of devouring her mate, at least when she is able to catch him. She is glossy black, with a body about 10 by 15 mm (0.4 by 0.6 inch), a leg span of 4 cm (1.6 inches), and a characteristic orange or red "hourglass" on her abdomen (Fig. 27-2). She is found throughout the United States, but especially in the southeast, and makes her home in sheds, basements, woodpiles, and similar areas; because she also likes to hang about in outhouses, there is a tendency for bites to occur in some rather unusual, not to mention highly sensitive, areas of the human anatomy.

In the United States, most of the 500 to 1,000 black widow spider bites each year occur from April to October. A definite history of a spider bite is not often obtained. Instead, the patient reports having

FIGURE 27-1. TICK.

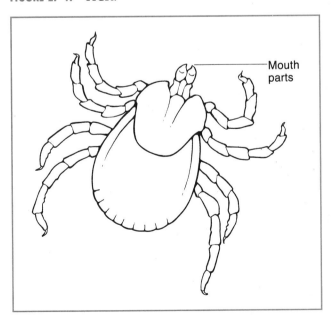

FIGURE 27-2. BLACK WIDOW SPIDER.

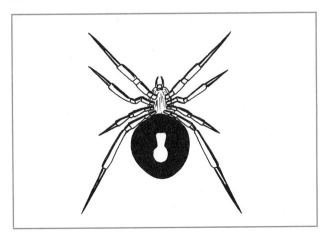

felt a *sudden, sharp prick* followed by a cramping or *numbing pain* that begins over the area of the bite and gradually spreads. Extreme *restlessness* is a hallmark of the reaction to a black widow spider bite. Excruciating pain and muscular rigidity may follow, with the abdomen becoming boardlike. The patient may, in addition, develop severe *respiratory distress, hypersalivation, nausea, vomiting, headache, sweating,* and *pins-and-needles sensations* (paresthesias) in the extremities. Sometimes the eyelids become puffy. A careful search on physical examination often reveals slight swelling in the area of the bite and tiny, red fang marks. Because the bite itself is not very obvious, however, many victims of black widow spider bite are initially thought to have an acute abdomen. Notably, though, the abdomen is *not* tender to palpation, despite the fact that it may be as rigid as a concrete slab from muscle spasms.

Black widow spider bites carry a mortality of 4 to 5 percent. TREATMENT OF BLACK WIDOW SPIDER BITES is mostly supportive:

- If the patient is in respiratory distress, administer OXYGEN.
- Place a COLD PACK over the bite wound, if you find it, to slow absorption of the spider's toxin.
- Start an IV LIFELINE with D5/W.
- The administration of 10% CALCIUM GLUCONATE often provides dramatic, though temporary, relief of muscle spasm. Give 10 ml of the 10% solution *slowly* IV.
- TRANSPORT to the hospital.

The BROWN RECLUSE SPIDER (Fig. 27-3) is about 15 mm (about ½ inch) long and 7 mm (¼ inch) wide. As its name implies, it is usually brown or tan, and it has a violin-shaped median band of darker shade that extends backward from its eyes—a feature responsible for its sometimes being called the "fiddleback" spider. Brown recluse spiders are found most commonly in the southern and midwestern United States, often in abandoned buildings.

The bite of a brown recluse spider may not result in immediate symptoms, and sometimes several hours may elapse before the local reaction is noticed. That reaction consists of a painful, reddened area with overlying blister formation and a surrounding area of ischemia. Over several days, the area turns dark and becomes deeply ulcerated—and it is usually at that point that the patient seeks care. Generalized reactions may accompany the local reaction and can be quite severe. Systemic reactions may include weakness, nausea, vomiting, rash, and a feeling of anxiety.

Prehospital TREATMENT of brown recluse spider bites consists simply in providing the general supportive measures given to any ill patient.

Scorpion Bites

Scorpions (Fig. 27-4) live in warm climates, principally in the southwestern states. The vast majority of scorpions in the United States are relatively harmless, although their bite can be very painful. The one exception is a species called *Centruroides sculpturatus,* or the bark scorpion, which is found principally in Arizona and across the border in Mexico, but also occasionally in New Mexico and southern California. Centruroides likes to live in the bark or rotted trunk of trees but will sometimes stray indoors. If touched or stepped on, the scorpion releases its venom from the stinger at the end of its whiplike tail. The sting

FIGURE 27-4.   SCORPION.

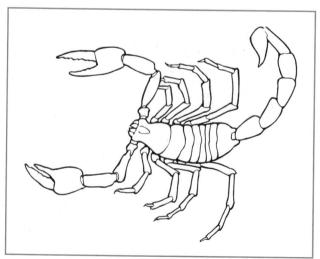

FIGURE 27-3.   BROWN RECLUSE SPIDER.

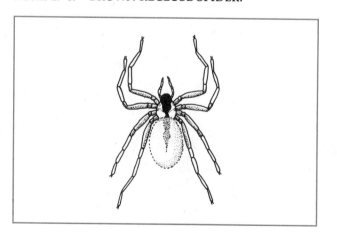

causes immediate pain at the site of the wound, followed by numbness or tingling. The pain is usually exacerbated by any pressure on the wound, and the whole area around the wound becomes hypersensitive to touch and to changes in temperature.

More worrisome, however, are the *systemic* effects of the Centruroides bite. Patients with severe envenomations may go on to develop very dramatic neuromuscular symptoms and signs. There may, for example, be uncontrolled roving movements of the eyes, difficulty in swallowing, drooling, muscle twitching, and—in the most severe cases—tetanic muscle spasms that literally bend the patient over backward.

The definitive TREATMENT for the bite of a bark scorpion is to administer a specific antivenin that counteracts the effects of the scorpion's venom. In the prehospital phase, all that can be done is to apply a cold pack to the sting, protect the airway, and treat seizures, if they occur, as in any other patient.

Snakebites

Ever since Eve had her memorable encounter with the serpent in the Garden of Eden, snakes have had a bad reputation. The vast majority of snakes are not poisonous, however, and in the United States, the poisonous varieties are limited to pit vipers (found everywhere except the extreme northeast of the country) and coral snakes (found chiefly in the mid-southern, southwestern, and western states). Only Alaska, Hawaii, and Maine are entirely free of venomous snakes.

Pit Vipers

The PIT VIPER class includes rattlesnakes (Fig. 27-5A), copperheads (Fig. 27-5B), and cottonmouth mocassins—the rattlesnake being by far the most common. Perhaps the most impressive rattlesnake is the diamondback, which reaches a length of 2.5 meters (8 feet) and a weight of 14 kg (30 lb)—clearly a creature best left in peace. The head of a pit viper is triangular, resembling an arrowhead. Just beneath the eyes on each side of the nostril is an indentation, or *pit.* The pit is a heat-sensing organ that helps the snake locate its prey. Also characteristic of snakes in the pit viper class are *vertical pupils* (most other snakes have round pupils). Long, erectile fangs are used to puncture the skin, leaving a distinctive mark (Fig. 27-6).

Pit vipers are not naturally aggressive, although some are more irritable than others, but they will strike in self-defense. When a pit viper does bite, it strikes with lightning speed. Its fangs snap forward and inject a variable amount of venom—anywhere

FIGURE 27-5. COMMON POISONOUS SNAKES. (A) Rattlesnake. (B) Copperhead. (C) Coral snake. Note the characteristic triangular head of the two viper species (A) and (B).

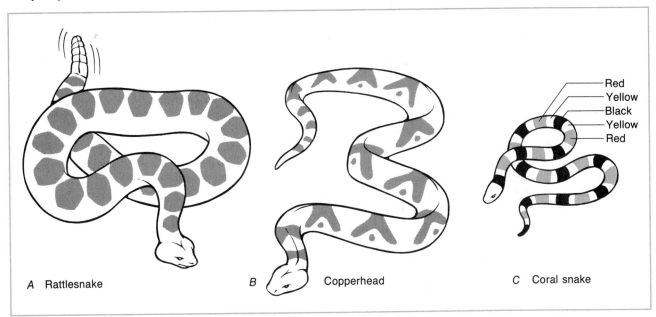

A Rattlesnake *B* Copperhead *C* Coral snake

Red
Yellow
Black
Yellow
Red

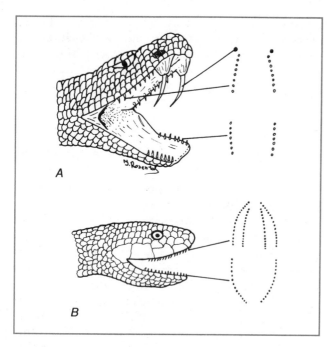

FIGURE 27-6.   CHARACTERISTICS OF PIT VIPERS AND NONPOISONOUS SNAKES.   (A) Pit vipers have vertical pupils, a pit between the eye and the nostril, a single row of teeth, and two erectile fangs. (B) Nonpoisonous snakes have round pupils and often a double row of upper teeth; they do not leave fang marks.

from no venom at all to a lethal dose—through the victim's skin. That brings up an important point:

> **NOT EVERY SNAKEBITE CONTAINS VENOM.**

If you want to be sure whether the bite was envenomed, look for fang marks: no fang marks, no venom, no matter how much it hurts. Furthermore, about 20 percent of patients bitten by pit vipers escape envenomation *despite* visible fang marks. When envenomation does occur, SYMPTOMS AND SIGNS begin almost instantaneously, starting with *burning pain* or *numbness* at the site of the bite. *Swelling* usually begins shortly thereafter and may spread within the next several hours to involve the whole extremity (the majority of snakebites are on the extremities, usually the lower extremities). *Ecchymoses* also occur early after pit viper envenomation, which together with swelling make the skin taut, shiny, and black and blue. A few hours later *hemorrhagic blisters* form in the area of the bite.

Meanwhile, as the venom is absorbed into the body, systemic symptoms start to occur. Many patients complain of *tingling* sensations in the scalp, face, or extremities, and there may be *twitching* of the muscles. *Signs of shock* may come on quite quickly, along with symptoms of the autonomic response to shock—*nausea, vomiting, sweating, weakness, lightheadedness.*

Coral Snakes

Coral snakes (Fig. 27-5C) belong to the Elapid family, which also includes the African cobras and mambas and all the Australian poisonous snakes. Coral snakes are small and brightly colored, with bands of yellow, red, yellow, and black (*in that order*). Their fangs are fixed, and unlike the pit vipers, they do not make a lightning-fast strike; instead, they hang on and chew! The venom of the coral snake is also quite different from that of a pit viper, for it produces a minimum of local tissue destruction and thus a minimum of pain or swelling at the site of the bite. SYMPTOMS, in fact, usually do not come on until about 3 hours after the bite, but symptoms then progress rapidly. Mood tends to be affected first, often starting with *euphoria* and then changing rapidly to *anxiety*. *Drowsiness* may be marked. Difficulty in swallowing leads to *pooling of saliva,* and nausea and vomiting are not uncommon. Paralysis may affect various muscle groups, including muscles of the eyelids, muscles of swallowing, and respiratory muscles. *Seizures* and *coma* may follow, and *death,* if it occurs, is usually within 24 hours of the bite.

Treatment of Envenomed Snakebites

The past 5 to 10 years have seen significant changes in the recommendations regarding prehospital treatment of envenomed snakebites. In general, the trend has been to do less and less in the field. It was previously recommended, for example, to apply ice or other cooling measures to snakebite, in an attempt to retard absorption of the venom. That technique, however, was found simply to increase local tissue destruction. Similarly, techniques such as incision and suction or the use of constricting bands have not been found to be of benefit in snakebite and may, in fact, lead to further complications. Notably, nearly all of the materials contained in commercially available snakebite kits are intended for procedures that can no longer be endorsed, such as incision and suction.

What *can* be recommended on the basis of our present knowledge of snakebites is the following:

• GET THE PATIENT AWAY FROM THE SNAKE. There is no code of ethics among snakes that says they may bite only once.

- CALM AND REASSURE THE PATIENT. More than one victim of snakebite has died of fright, not of the bite itself.
- REMOVE CONSTRICTING ITEMS, such as rings or bracelets, from a bitten extremity, so that they will not hamper distal circulation in the event of swelling.
- Keep the victim RECUMBENT and AT REST to minimize his metabolic needs and the spread of the venom.
- SPLINT THE BITTEN EXTREMITY in a dependent position, below the level of the heart.
- DO NOT ALLOW THE VICTIM TO WALK ON A BITTEN LEG, for exercise promotes blood flow and thereby enhances absorption of the venom.
- DO NOT PERMIT THE VICTIM TO DRINK ALCOHOL, for it may aggravate CNS depression. Indeed, GIVE NOTHING BY MOUTH, since the patient is very apt to vomit.
- DO NOT DELAY TRANSPORT. Definitive treatment requires administration of specific antivenin, and it should be given as early as possible.
- En route to the hospital:
  1. Administer OXYGEN.
  2. Start an IV LIFELINE with normal saline or lactated Ringer's in an uninvolved extremity. If there are signs of shock, run in fluids rapidly.
  3. GET A DESCRIPTION OF THE SNAKE, if you did not have a good look at it yourself. Some authorities recommend that the rescuer kill the snake and bring it along to the emergency room. That is left to the discretion of the paramedic, providing it will not take too much time. In the view of this author, chasing a poisonous snake has little to recommend it; one snakebite victim is enough.
  4. NOTIFY THE HOSPITAL of the type of snake thought to have caused the bite and your estimated time of arrival, so that they may meanwhile take steps to secure the specific antivenin required.

Marine Animal Envenomation

Paramedics working in coastal areas are apt to encounter patients who have suffered injury from various marine animals. Those marine creatures most likely to cause injuries in U.S. coastal waters are the stinging animals—coelenterates, echinoderms, and stinging vertebrates.

Coelenterates

The coelenterate group includes the JELLYFISH, PORTUGUESE MAN-OF-WAR, ANEMONES, and STINGING CORAL. All coelenterates are characterized by tentacles equipped with **nematocysts,** or stinging cells. Stings from coelenterates most commonly occur on the legs. The very young, the very old, and the very small tend to be most severely affected. There is usually intense, sometimes excruciating pain, which may be so severe as to disable a swimmer and cause him to drown. The pain generally radiates up from the site of the sting into the groin and abdomen. The stung area may turn brown or purple and develop blisters. Meanwhile systemic symptoms may occur, including faintness, weakness, chills, fever, and even shock and death.

TREATMENT of a victim of coelenterate stinging has three objectives: (1) to stabilize the patient's overall condition; (2) to relieve pain; and (3) to counteract the effects of the venom.

- Manage systemic reactions according to the usual priorities of ABC. If the patient is hypotensive, start an IV with lactated Ringer's, and give fluids.
- *RINSE* THE INJURED PART IN SEAWATER. Do *not* use fresh water. Do *not* scrub the injured area.
- Inspect the wound and try to REMOVE ANY TENTACLES adhering to it (wear gloves!).
- POUR VINEGAR OVER THE WOUND to fix the nematocysts onto the skin and prevent further stinging. If you don't have vinegar, use 40 to 70% alcohol. For sea nettles, use a slurry made from baking powder and water instead of vinegar or alcohol.
- After several vinegar rinses, apply a DRY POWDER to the area, which will make the nematocysts stick together. MEAT TENDERIZER is ideal because it also neutralizes the acid venom.
- Then use a knife or spatula to SCRAPE THE NEMATOCYSTS OFF THE SKIN. The best way to remove nematocysts, in fact, is to *shave* them off, using a razor and shaving cream. Once the nematocysts have been removed, RINSE THE INJURED PART AGAIN WITH SEAWATER.
- Usually inactivation and removal of the nematocysts will by itself provide considerable relief of pain. If, however, the patient is still in severe pain after nematocyst removal, first try a slow intravenous infusion of 10 ml of 10% CALCIUM GLUCONATE.

Any patient who has had a *systemic* reaction to a coelenterate sting—such as hypotension, wheezing, or vomiting—should be transported to the hospital for observation. Be alert for anaphylactic reactions in patients who have suffered similar stings in the past.

Echinoderms

Echinoderms are spiny sea creatures—such as sea urchins, starfish, and sea cucumbers. They produce their harmful effects by puncturing the victim's skin with a toxic material. Usually injury occurs when someone accidently steps on one of these creatures or injudiciously handles them. The resulting puncture may be extremely painful. With multiple punctures, there may be systemic symptoms, like nausea and vomiting, as well. Because of the usual mechanism of injury, most of these wounds occur on the feet.

In managing a puncture wound from an echinoderm, first check to see whether any of the creature's little spines have broken off in the wound. If so, try to REMOVE THE SPINE from the wound. The next step is to try to inactivate the venom, which will also provide pain relief. Echinoderm venoms are destroyed by high temperature. Therefore heat up a bucket of water to a temperature as hot as the patient can tolerate—usually around 113°F (45°C), and have the patient IMMERSE BOTH FEET (the injured *and* the uninjured foot) IN HOT WATER for 30 to 90 minutes. The uninjured foot serves as a safety device to warn if the water is too hot, for the injured foot may be numbed by pain and insensitive to temperature extremes.

Stinging Vertebrates

Stinging vertebrates include stingrays, scorpion fish, and catfish. STINGRAYS account for about 2,000 injuries in U.S. waters of both coasts each year. Because they burrow in the sand, they are easily stepped on, and the most common site of injury is therefore the lower extremities. SCORPION FISH injuries are most often seen off the Florida Keys, in the Gulf of Mexico, along the southern Californian coast and that of Hawaii. The most common victims of envenomation are divers. More than a thousand species of CATFISH inhabit both fresh and salt waters, and stings are most likely on the hands and arms of fishermen handling the fish. The stings of all of these vertebrates produce immediate, severe pain and are apt as well to cause a variety of systemic reactions including headache, nausea, vomiting, and hypotension. The treatment is the same as that for echinoderm injury—immersion of the stung extremity in very hot water and general supportive care.

Note that the treatment of various marine animal envenomations requires products not usually considered standard ambulance equipment, such as vinegar, meat tenderizer, and shaving cream. Paramedics working in coastal areas should therefore make up a special "seashore kit" containing the equipment and supplies relevant to the particular marine problems they are likely to encounter.

Mammalian Bites

Just about any creature with teeth can inflict a bite; but among the most common perpetrators of the nearly 2 million bites inflicted on Americans each year are domestic animals (mostly dogs) and undomestic people. We shall concentrate here on dog bites and human bites, those being the most prevalent. For information on the bites of other animals, see the list of Further Reading at the end of this chapter.

Dog Bites

Dogs inflict about a million bites on people (most commonly their owners) in the United States annually. Most of those bites are not serious, but the ever-present danger of rabies demands that the paramedic take a careful history of the injury. Be sure to find out at least the following:

- What were the CIRCUMSTANCES OF THE BITE? Was the bite provoked or unprovoked? Was the dog behaving strangely?
- Who is the OWNER OF THE DOG? Take down his address and telephone number. Health authorities may have to contact the dog's owner to obtain verification that the animal has been immunized against rabies.
- WHERE IS THE DOG NOW? The animal may have to be quarantined.

In examining the patient, look carefully to see if the bite penetrated the skin. Infection with rabies virus can occur only if the saliva of a rabid animal enters a person's body through a break in the skin surface.

TREATMENT of a dog-bite injury is aimed at preventing infection and neutralizing any rabies virus that might be present on the skin surface:

- WASH the wound thoroughly with LOTS OF SOAP AND WATER.
- RINSE the wound and surrounding skin with STRONG ALCOHOL (at least 40% strength).
- REMOVE CONSTRICTING JEWELRY from a bitten extremity.
- SPLINT a bitten extremity.
- TRANSPORT the patient to the hospital.
- NOTIFY public health authorities of the incident.

Human Bites

Human bites are much more dangerous than dog bites, because the human mouth contains a far more noxious collection of bacteria than a dog's mouth. Many human bites are not, strictly speaking bites; rather, they occur when the fist of one individual makes sudden, violent contact with the teeth of another individual. However they occur, though, human bites are potentially very serious, for infection often follows. For that reason, the most important step in treating a human bite wound is to CLEAN THE WOUND AS THOROUGHLY AS POSSIBLE WITH LOTS OF SOAP AND WATER. A quick, delicate dab with a povidone-iodine will *not* do. A good soap-and-water scrub is the mainstay of all wound care, and nowhere is it more important than in the treatment of a human bite.

Even if the wound looks trivial, TRANSPORT THE PATIENT TO THE HOSPITAL. He may need tetanus prophylaxis or antibiotic coverage, and he will certainly need arrangements for careful follow-up.

DRUG ABUSE

Drug abuse may be broadly defined as the self-administration of a drug or drugs in a manner that is not in accord with approved medical or social practice. Note that the definition is partially a cultural one, and there is considerable variation from culture to culture and from time to time as to what is regarded as drug abuse. Thus in our society, it is considered acceptable to administer narcotics under medical supervision for the relief of pain, but self-administration of the same drugs for the purpose of inducing euphoria is regarded as an abuse. In some Oriental societies, on the other hand, smoking of opium was, at least until recently, considered socially acceptable and was practiced among the wealthier classes. It is also notable that society's definition of abuse often has little relation to the potential harm from the abused substance. Thus in our culture, there are no restrictions on the chronic and compulsive use of tobacco, which is known to be a major contributor to death from cardiovascular and respiratory disease; yet the use of marijuana, whose damaging effects are not as clearly established, is in some regions punishable by fines and imprisonment.

Nonetheless, despite the inconsistencies and cultural variations, it is possible to identify certain patterns of drug use that are indeed harmful, patterns that can be classified under the general heading of *compulsive drug abuse*, or drug dependency. We need at this point to define some terms:

drug abuse   Any use of drugs that causes physical, psychologic, economic, legal, or social harm to the user or to others affected by the drug user's behavior.

physical dependence   A physiologic state of adaptation to a drug, usually characterized by *tolerance* to the drug's effects and a withdrawal syndrome if the drug is stopped.

psychologic dependence   The emotional state of craving a drug to maintain an individual's feeling of well-being.

tolerance   Physiologic adaptation to the effects of a drug such that larger and larger doses of the drug are required to achieve the same effect.

withdrawal syndrome   A predictable set of signs and symptoms, usually involving altered central nervous system activity, that occurs after the abrupt discontinuation of a drug or after rapidly decreasing the usual dosage of a drug.

drug addiction   A chronic disorder characterized by the compulsive use of a substance that results in physical, psychologic, or social harm to the user—and continued use despite that harm. Drug addiction almost always involves all of the other attributes mentioned—dependence, tolerance, and susceptibility to withdrawal.

Drug abuse is not limited to the younger generation nor to any particular stratum of society. It occurs in all age groups and at all social levels. The majority of the American population is vastly overmedicated in one way or another, owing partially to the widespread belief that there is a pharmacologic remedy for every problem. Even among people who would never consider themselves "junkies," therefore, the list of commonly abused substances is a long one, ranging from caffeine and tobacco (nicotine) to over-the-counter sleep medications.

Abused substances can be classified into four major categories:

- NARCOTICS, such as opium, heroin, morphine, hydromorphone (Dilaudid), meperidine (Demerol), codeine, and propoxyphene (Darvon)
- OTHER CNS DEPRESSANTS, such as alcohol, barbiturates, tranquilizers, and antihistamines
- CNS STIMULANTS, such as amphetamines and cocaine
- HALLUCINOGENS, such as LSD and mescaline

The specific syndromes resulting from abuse or overdose of agents in those groups will be described in the sections that follow.

The Implications of Drug Abuse for EMS

The wide prevalence of drug abuse among the population inevitably has an impact on EMS providers, especially those providing care in the prehospital sphere, who are literally on the front lines of the so-called war on drugs. Drug abuse has made it more complicated, medically and legally, and often more dangerous to provide the kind of humane and high-quality care that we all aspire to. The contingencies of the drug epidemic prompt certain general guidelines for the paramedic's work in the field:

- ALWAYS ASK EVERY PATIENT ABOUT THE USE OF MEDICATIONS, whether prescribed or self-administered. It is often useful, when in a patient's home, to check out the bathroom medicine cabinet and note what drugs are stored there. Be alert to the possibility that drugs may be contributing to the patient's difficulties when his medicine cabinet resembles the warehouse of a pharmaceutical company.
- ASK EVERY PATIENT ABOUT RECREATIONAL DRUG USE, not about addiction. Hardly anyone will admit to being an addict, but a user may be willing to concede, "Sure, I take a snort of coke now and then—doesn't everyone?"
- When dealing with teenagers whose problems you suspect may be related to drug use, maintain an interested, nonjudgmental attitude. Explain that you need to know about their use of drugs in order to give them the correct treatment and that it is not your job to report them to the authorities.
- CONSIDER THE POSSIBILITY OF A DRUG-RELATED PROBLEM in any patient presenting with unexplained behavioral changes, stupor, coma, or seizures.
- USE DISCRETION WITH THE DRUGS CARRIED IN THE EMERGENCY VEHICLE. Ideally, they should be in a cabinet or case that can be locked, especially if the ambulance service routinely carries morphine or other narcotics. It is wise, furthermore, not to refer to narcotic medications by name during radio communication with the physician, since doing so only serves to inform the interested bystander that there is a supply of the drug on board. For that reason, morphine is often referred to as a "Tubex"—a description of the type of syringe in which it is usually dispensed. Thus, the physician may order "half a Tubex," that is 5.0 to 7.5 mg of morphine, depending on the concentration of the drug routinely stocked.

- Make sure that your EMS service has ESTABLISHED, WRITTEN PROTOCOLS dealing with matters such as (1) transporting a patient you think to be under the influence of drugs against his will; (2) use of restraints in violent or potentially violent patients; and (3) cases that must be reported to the police.
- YOUR SAFETY COMES FIRST! If you get called for an "unconscious patient" and find yourself pulling up in front of a "crack house" in an unsavory part of town and you have a bad feeling about the place, call for police backup before you go in. It is not noble or brave to plunge into a situation that your instinct tells you might be dangerous; it is just plain stupid.

DRUG OVERDOSE AND DRUG TOXICITY

Before venturing out into the streets to save the legions of overdosed patients, the paramedic should acquire the vocabulary that will be necessary to communicate with the drug user and his friends. Table 27-5 presents some of the street names for commonly abused drugs, and Table 27-6 provides a small glossary of drug terminology. Those lists are not intended to be comprehensive but merely to serve as a guide. Street slang changes with time and place, and it is wise for the paramedic to make a glossary of terms current in his or her own community. A trip down to the local methadone clinic will usually turn up a few people who can provide very accurate and useful information about what substances are being used in your community and the local drug terminology.

General Principles

Overdose refers to the toxic effects that occur when a person takes a dose of a drug larger than he can tolerate. Overdose can occur by accident, by miscalculation (e.g., when a purer batch of heroin hits the streets), or by intention, in a suicide attempt. It can occur from a single drug or several drugs in combination. Regardless of the drug or drugs involved, there are certain general principles that apply to caring for any patient who has overdosed or experienced a toxic drug reaction.

Taking the History

Taking the history from a patient who has overdosed, to begin with, is similar to taking a history in a case of poisoning, for you need to find out the following:

TABLE 27-5.   STREET NAMES OF COMMONLY ABUSED DRUGS

TYPE OF DRUG	EXAMPLES	STREET NAMES
UPPERS		
Amphetamines	Benzedrine	A's, Bennies, Benzies, cartwheels, hearts, peaches, roses, speed
	Dexedrine	Dexies, footballs, oranges
	Methedrine	Bonita, bambita
	MDMA	Ecstasy, XTC, Adam, MDM
	MDEA	Eve
	Methamphetamine hydrochloride	Ice
Cocaine		Bernice, big C, blow, burese, C, Carrie, Cecil, Charlie, cholly, coke, corine, dama blanca, dynamite, flake, gin, girl, gold dust, green gold, happy dust, happy trails, heaven dust, jet, joy powder, lady, nose candy, paradise, snort, snow, stardust, star-spangled powder, sugar, toot, white dust, white girl, zoom
	Modified cocaine	Crack (freebase cocaine), liquid lady (cocaine + alcohol), rock (freebase cocaine), speedball (cocaine + heroin)
Antiasthmatics	Aminophylline	
	Isoproterenol	
	Adrenalin	
Caffeine	Coffee, cola	
DOWNERS		
Alcohol	Wine, beer, whiskey	Rose (wine), sneaky Pete (wine)
Narcotics	Heroin	China white, horse, Harry, smack, stuff, big H, blanco
	Morphine	Hard stuff, Miss Emma, big M, unkie
	Codeine	Fours
	Hydromorphone (Dilaudid)	Dillies
	Methadone	Amidone, dollies
	Opium	Auntie, black stuff, Greece
Barbiturates	Pentobarbital (Nembutal)	Yellow jackets, yellows, nimbies, nebbies
	Amobarbital (Amytal)	Blue devils, blue birds, blue heaven, blue bullets, jackup
	Seconal	Red birds, red devils, pinks, bala, M&Ms
Chloral hydrate		Mickey Finn, Mickey, Peter, chlorals, hog
Tranquilizers	Thorazine	
	Valium	
	Librium	Roche-tens
Marijuana and its products	Marijuana	Grass, pot, Acapulco gold, ace, Aunt Mary, bo-bo, broccoli, duby, gage, Mary Jane, tea, reefer
	Hashish	Black Russian, blue cheese, gram, hash, heesh, THC
HALLUCINOGENS		
Lysergic acid diethylamide (LSD)		Acid, blue cheers, California sunshine, crackers, cubes, ghost, heavenly blue
Phencyclidine (PCP)		Elephant, PeaCee Pill
Mescaline		Cactus buttons
Peyote		Bad acid, bad seed, big chief, button, half-moon

- WHAT was taken? If the patient took pills, bring the bottle and all its remaining contents with the patient to the emergency room. The label on the bottle may aid in identification, and the number of pills remaining may give a clue to how many were ingested.

- WHEN was it taken? Here again, as in poisoning, the timing of an ingestion will influence the decision about whether to induce vomiting.
- HOW MUCH was taken?
- Were there ANY OTHER DRUGS (INCLUDING ALCOHOL) TAKEN BY ANY ROUTE? Over-

TABLE 27-6. TERMS RELATING TO DRUG USE

TERM	REFERS TO
Amped	Hyperstimulated on cocaine
Bagging	Inhaling volatile substances from a bag
Blank	Low-grade narcotics
Bodypacker	Person who smuggles cocaine by ingesting latex containers (e.g., condoms) filled with the drug
Burned	Received phony narcotics
Coasting	Under the influence of drugs
Cold turkey	Sudden cessation of drug intake
Cut	Adulterated
Dynamite	High-grade heroin
Hit	2–200 mg of cocaine
Huffing	Inhaling through a cloth soaked in a volatile substance (such as glue)
Joy pop	Inject narcotics regularly
Layout	Outfit employed by opium user
Lemonade	Poor heroin
Mainlining	Injecting drugs IV
Mule	Same as a bodypacker
On the nod	Drowsy from narcotics
Panic	Shortage of narcotics on the streets
Quill	Matchbook cover for sniffing cocaine
Reader	Prescription order
Reader with tail	Forged prescription order
Run	Prolonged drug binge
Rush	Feeling of euphoric pleasure
Shooting gallery	Place where addicts inject themselves
Shooting up	Injecting narcotics IV
Snorting	Inhaling drugs in powdered form
Speedballing	Injecting drug combinations (especially cocaine plus alcohol)
Spoon	1 gm of cocaine
Stepped on	Diluted
Wired	Hyperstimulated on cocaine

doses are rarely "pure," but usually involve a combination of several drugs.

- WHAT HAS BEEN DONE to try to correct the situation? Has the patient vomited? Have any other "first aid" measures been applied?

Street resuscitation procedures are frequently as dangerous as the overdose itself, if not more so, and the rescuer needs to know exactly what the patient has been given. The most common form of street resuscitation is "stimulation"—cold showers, vigorous slapping, and the like. Check therefore for broken teeth, blood in the mouth, or other signs of injury. If the patient has taken an overdose of barbiturates, his helpful friends may have tried to reverse it by "shooting him up" with "speed" (methedrine). There is also a mythology prevalent on the streets that salt or milk given IV will reverse an overdose; those "remedies" will not reverse an overdose but may produce pulmonary edema. All such street remedies will, in any case, complicate the picture, and you must learn as much as possible about what has been done.

Physical Assessment

In carrying out the physical assessment of a patient known or suspected to be under the influence of drugs, probably the most important thing to evaluate is the patient's *state of consciousness*. When the patient presents with a depressed state of consciousness, use a neurologic checklist to record serial observations at frequent intervals. If the patient is unconscious, consider *all* possible causes of coma (AEIOU-TIPS), even in a known drug user. The *vital signs* are also of enormous importance in patients who have overdosed. Severe bradycardia and slow, deep respirations may be the tip-off to a narcotics overdose, while soaring blood pressure suggests that the patient has taken a toxic dose of amphetamines or cocaine. In the head-to-toe survey, check for evidence of *head injury*—a cause of altered consciousness that you will miss if you assume that the patient is "just another addict." Examine the *pupils* for the extreme miosis ("pinpoint pupils") characteristic of narcotics overdose. Check for unusual *odors on the breath*. Listen to the *chest* for equality of breath sounds (intravenous drug users may try the subclavian vein after they've destroyed all the arm veins, and a certain proportion of subclavian sticks end up producing pneumothorax). Examine the *extremities* for needle tracks. Have a quick look, as well, at the patient's *surroundings*, for drug paraphernalia like syringes or crack pipes.

General Principles of Management

In dealing with a victim of overdose, it is not always possible to know precisely what drug or drugs he took. If the patient is conscious, he may not give a reliable history. If he is unconscious, he won't give any history at all. But it *is* possible to give good general supportive care even when you don't know what the patient took.

- Maintain the AIRWAY. If the patient is unconscious, hold off endotracheal intubation until you've made a trial of naloxone (Narcan); should the naloxone be effective in rousing the patient, he will simply yank out the endotracheal tube that you went to so much trouble to insert. In coma unresponsive to naloxone and D50, however, intubate as soon as possible.
- Administer OXYGEN.
- If the drug was taken by mouth and the patient is still fully conscious, administer ACTIVATED CHARCOAL, at least 5 tablespoons mixed in tap water to make a slurry.
- Consult medical command regarding WHETHER TO INDUCE VOMITING. In any case, do *not* induce vomiting in

1. Any patient who is NOT FULLY ALERT.
2. Any patient who DOES NOT HAVE A GAG REFLEX.
3. Any patient having SEIZURES.
4. Any patient who is PREGNANT.

- If the drug was taken by mouth and the patient is *not* fully conscious, pass a NASOGASTRIC TUBE to lavage the stomach *after* the airway has been protected by a cuffed endotracheal tube.
- Where possible, start an IV LIFELINE with D5/W (in the intravenous drug user, you probably won't be able to find a vein).
- MONITOR cardiac rhythm.
- Observe full AIDS PRECAUTIONS when caring for any patient known or suspected to be an intravenous drug user (see Chap. 28).

It is beyond the scope of this book to deal with every possible overdose with every available drug. Rather, we shall look briefly at representative overdoses with each of the four general classes of drugs: narcotics, barbiturates, stimulant drugs, and hallucinogens. Basic principles of management are the same in all overdoses—the ABCs—but details differ. In specific overdose situations, consult your regional Poison Control Center.

Narcotic Overdose

The narcotic drugs include heroin, morphine, hydromorphone (Dilaudid), methadone, meperidine (Demerol), codeine, oxycodone (Percodan), propoxyphene (Darvon), and the newer "designer opiates" such as "China white." Taken in excess, they cause marked RESPIRATORY DEPRESSION, initially manifested by slow, deep breathing, but leading rapidly to apnea. Narcotic overdose also causes *hypotension, stupor,* and *coma*. The *pupils* characteristically become pinpoint, but that sign may be masked in a patient who has overdosed with a combination of drugs.

Maintain a high index of suspicion about any young patient found in unexplained coma, especially if there are needle tracks on the arms or elsewhere. Cigarette burns on the chest are also very suggestive when present; they occur when the addict "nods out" while smoking.

Heroin sold on the streets is usually "cut" (adulterated) with agents such as quinine, lactose, sucrose, baking soda, and talc, in a ratio of anywhere from 20 : 1 (adulterant : heroin) to 200 : 1. For that reason, heroin overdose tends to occur in small epidemics when an unusually "clean" (unadulterated) supply of the drug reaches the street and addicts miscalculate their dosage. Thus, when you encounter one patient with a heroin overdose, it is quite likely that you will encounter others before the day is over. Make sure the drug box is well stocked with naloxone.

Treatment of Narcotic Overdose

Treatment of the patient with narcotic overdose follows the principles of treatment for any comatose patient.

- Maintain the AIRWAY manually. Defer intubation until after you can assess the effects of naloxone (see below).
- Administer OXYGEN. Assist ventilations if the respiratory rate is less than about 12 per minute.
- LOOK FOR A VEIN IN WHICH TO START AN IV. If you can't find a vein on either arm because all the veins are sclerosed, you have good evidence that the patient is an intravenous drug user, and it is therefore worth going straight to a trial of naloxone. When there is no vein in which you can start an IV, give NALOXONE (NARCAN) 0.8 to 1.2 mg into the venous plexus on the underside of the tongue. Then keep the patient under observation for about 5 minutes. If he has not wakened by then, intubate him and proceed to the hospital.
- If you *are* able to start an IV, proceed as for any comatose patient and first give THIAMINE, 100 mg *slowly* IV, and 50% DEXTROSE, 50 mg IV. If the patient does not waken in response to the D50:
- Give NALOXONE. The safest way to give naloxone in the field is by slow titration. Draw up the contents of 3 or 4 ampules (1.2–1.6 mg) into a 10-ml syringe and fill the rest of the syringe with D5/W from the IV bag. Inject the diluted naloxone *slowly*, and stop the injection when the patient's respirations become normal. It is usually *not* desirable to waken the patient completely in the field because such patients often come out of their coma in a combative mood (and angry that the paramedic has just spoiled their $50 "fix"). So *titrate* the naloxone to the patient's respirations.
- If there is no response to naloxone, the patient may have taken a mixed overdose or his coma may be from another source altogether (e.g., head injury). Provide definitive airway care by intubating the trachea, and proceed to the hospital.

There are significant legal and ethical questions regarding whether to transport patients to the hospital after they have been resuscitated from a narcotics overdose. What very often happens is that the paramedics bring the overdosed patient to the emergency department (ED), having skillfully maintained the patient just below the threshhold of full consciousness. The people in the ED then give another dose of Narcan. The patient wakes up, becomes abusive, and storms out of the ED "against medical advice." After a few repetitions of that scene, the ED staff tend to greet paramedics bringing in a heroin overdose with something less than warmth and enthusiasm ("What did you have to bring him *here* for?"). So the paramedics become understandably reluctant to transport patients who have overdosed on narcotics but are inclined instead simply to give the patient a dose of Narcan and leave him at the scene.

The danger in that policy is that naloxone is a relatively short-acting drug, and its effect may wear off before the effect of the heroin does. The overdosed patient, therefore, is liable to slip back into coma and could die of an obstructed airway before you get to him the second time. What is needed is an *established policy*, worked out among all the health care providers concerned in a given community, for the prehospital management of narcotics overdose.

Barbiturate Overdose

Barbiturates are still among the most abused sedative/depressant drugs in the United States, even though there are now many other sedative/tranquilizer drugs available. They are used in more drug-related suicide attempts than any other single agent, and they are also widely abused on the streets.

The typical chronic "doper" is lethargic, disheveled, and frequently nodding off to sleep. He may be taking enormous doses of barbiturates to maintain his habit, and any decrease of his daily dose, because of some interruption in his source of supply, can lead to a dangerous withdrawal state.

Diagnosis of *acute* barbiturate poisoning may be difficult. The suicide-prone patient may have large supplies of a variety of drugs on hand, and it may not be readily apparent which drug or drugs the comatose patient ingested. In addition, suicide attempts frequently follow ingestion of large quantities of alcohol, and the odor of alcohol on the patient's breath may further confuse the picture. The rescuer will often have to rely on circumstantial evidence to make a presumptive diagnosis of barbiturate overdose—such as empty medication bottles near the patient or the characteristic color of tablets found in the mouth and gastric contents.

SIGNS AND SYMPTOMS of acute barbiturate poisoning are related chiefly to the central nervous system and cardiovascular system. Moderate overdose resembles alcohol intoxication, with general incoordination, slurred speech, emotional lability, and impaired thinking. In severe barbiturate toxicity, the patient is *deeply comatose.* The *pupils* may be constricted in the early stages, but later they will become *fixed and dilated.* (That is very important to remember during resuscitation efforts, for fixed and dilated pupils obviously do not have the same significance in the patient with a barbiturate ingestion as in the garden-variety cardiac arrest.) *Respirations* are affected early, becoming *very shallow,* so there is hypoventilation and consequent respiratory acidosis. Cheyne-Stokes respirations may be present. Aspiration is common, and if the patient survives his overdose, he is likely to develop pneumonia. Vasodilatation and depressed cardiac output result in *hypotension* and sometimes *shock* of a mixed neurogenic/cardiogenic variety. *Hypothermia* (abnormally low body temperature) is common. The muscles become flaccid, and deep tendon reflexes are markedly decreased. In a small percentage of cases, large blisters appear on the patient's legs—an important clue when present.

Treatment of Barbiturate Overdose

Treatment of a patient suspected of having taken an overdose of barbiturates follows the usual priorities of ABC.

- Maintain the AIRWAY. If the gag reflex is absent, intubate the trachea at the earliest opportunity.
- Administer OXYGEN. Assist ventilations to improve tidal volume.
- Start an IV LIFELINE with lactated Ringer's, and run in fluids at a rate sufficient to maintain the systolic blood pressure above 80 to 90 mm Hg.
- Consult medical command regarding administration of SODIUM BICARBONATE, 1 mEq per kilogram. Bicarbonate promotes more rapid urinary excretion of some barbiturates, such as phenobarbital, so it will be important to know precisely which barbiturate the patient ingested.
- MONITOR cardiac rhythm.
- After the airway has been secured with a cuffed endotracheal tube, insert a NASOGASTRIC TUBE. Withdraw and store in a closed container whatever is in the stomach. Then instill a slurry of ACTIVATED CHARCOAL, at least 5 tablespoons mixed with water. Gastric lavage is best carried out, if necessary, in the emergency room.
- If the patient is still alert, give activated charcoal by mouth. Do *not* give any stimulants, such as coffee.

Toxic Effects of Stimulant Drugs

The most commonly abused stimulant drugs are those in the amphetamine family and cocaine.

Amphetamine Toxicity

Amphetamine (Benzedrine), dextroamphetamine (Dexedrine), methamphetamine (Methedrine), and more recently the "designer drugs" methylenedioxyamphetamine (MDA, or "ecstasy"), methylenedioxyethamphetamine ("Eve"), and D-methamphetamine ("ice") are very commonly abused drugs. They can be taken orally or, in some formulations such as "ice," can be smoked for a very rapid onset of action. The chronic "speed freak" is easily recognized by his wild-eyed appearance, like someone who has just put his finger into a light socket. The patient has no appetite and may go for days scarcely eating. He shows *excitement, tachycardia, hypertension, sweating, dilated pupils,* and *tremors.* The body temperature may rise to dangerous levels (**hyperpyrexia**), and *seizures* are apt to occur. The patient may also demonstrate outright psychosis, with **paranoia** (an unwarranted sense that people have hostile intentions toward him) and hallucinations. Violent behavior is not uncommon, so be sure your crew is well-prepared, with plenty of assistance on hand, before you tackle a "hyperamped" amphetamine abuser.

In most instances, "speed" will burn itself out, and the user will "crash"; that is, he will go into a prolonged sleep followed by a period of extreme hunger and depression. When you are called to treat a toxic reaction to amphetamines in the field, priority goes to safety (yours and the patient's) and sustaining vital functions.

- Determine whether the patient is violent, and summon police assistance if needed.
- Do *not* induce vomiting, because the potential for seizures is very high. If the amphetamines were taken by mouth, administer ACTIVATED CHARCOAL, 5 tablespoons mixed into a slurry with water—if you can persuade the patient to drink the stuff!
- *If* the patient is fully alert, and *if* the vital signs are all normal, it is desirable to provide the patient with a place to "crash." The hospital is usually *not* a very good place for that. A quiet room in the house of a responsible friend, where concerned people will be available to reassure the patient, may be preferable if it can be arranged. Consult medical command, however, before any decision not to transport a patient to the hospital.

- If, on the other hand, there are abnormalities in the vital signs (elevated blood pressure, elevated temperature, irregularities in the pulse), or if the patient is entirely out of control, hospitalization will be necessary. Use police assistance, if needed, to facilitate transport.
- MONITOR cardiac rhythm.
- Treat seizures, if they occur, with diazepam, as described in a previous chapter.

Cocaine and Crack

Nowadays, by far the most commonly abused stimulant drug is cocaine, 30 to 60 tons of which are imported into the United States every year. An estimated 25 million Americans have tried cocaine at least once; 5,000 try it for the first time each day; and 4 million Americans use it regularly. What that means is that there is scarcely an ambulance service in America that will not have to deal with patients who are cocaine users.

Until recently, cocaine was most commonly sold as a fine, white, crystalline powder, which was taken either intranasally by inhalation ("snorting") or by injection into the skin, muscle, or a vein. Within the past few years, however, a much cheaper but more powerful form of cocaine, called **crack,** has become available that can be taken via the intrapulmonary route (smoked, or "freebased"). When cocaine powder is "snorted," the user feels a "high" within 1 or 2 minutes, which peaks around 15 to 60 minutes after use. When crack is smoked, by contrast, the user experiences a much more intense "high" in 8 to 10 *seconds.* It is probably because of the speed and intensity of the "high" it produces that crack is so addictive.

When the effects of a dose of cocaine, in whatever form, wear off, the user (like the user of amphetamines) experiences a "crash," a period of depression, irritability, sleeplessness, and exhaustion. To try to avoid the crash, the user will often seek more cocaine until he no longer has funds to buy more of the drug. At that point, he may try to escape the unpleasant effects of crashing by taking some kind of sedative drug (e.g., alcohol, heroin, Valium). Thus the chronic cocaine user is likely to be dependent on more than one drug—cocaine plus a combination of sedatives—and he may present to emergency services overdosed from "uppers" *or* "downers."

If the user has overdosed on cocaine, he may show any of the signs and symptoms described for stimulant drugs in general. Cocaine, furthermore, has been increasingly reported to cause a variety of very serious, sometimes fatal complications, including acute myocardial infarction, lethal cardiac dysrhythmias, seizures, stroke, apnea, hyperthermia, and a variety of psychiatric symptoms. What all that means in practice is that the paramedic must maintain a high index of suspicion regardless of the patient's chief complaint. Nowadays, a young person complaining of chest pain, for example, cannot be immediately written off as "probable hyperventilation syndrome"; he may indeed be suffering a myocardial infarction if he's been freebasing crack during the past hour. Make it a habit, therefore, to check out the patient's surroundings for drug paraphernalia, no matter what the chief complaint, and report any evidence of drug use to the doctor at the receiving hospital.

Toxic Effects of Hallucinogens

A hallucinogen is a substance that causes the user some distortion of sense perception—seeing, hearing, or feeling things that are not objectively present. A wide variety of substances have been in vogue at one time or another for their hallucinogenic properties, including lysergic acid diethylamide (LSD), phencyclidine (PCP), mescaline, psilocybin mushrooms, and the seeds of the jimson weed plant. LSD and PCP are fairly representative of the range of symptoms that hallucinogens may produce.

LSD Toxicity

The clinical picture of LSD intoxication includes excitement, panic, hallucinations (usually visual), unusual bodily sensations, and often psychotic reactions. Most authorities advocate trying to "talk the patient down" in such circumstances and to avoid needles and sedative drugs as much as possible. Needles can be frightening. And, in any case, EMS personnel need not foster the already too prevalent attitude that the solution to one drug problem is to give another drug. It is important to get the patient to a quiet place, away from crowds and noise. The emergency department atmosphere is far from ideal in that respect, and it is preferable to arrange for the patient to be looked after by a responsible friend, if he has any responsible friends. Consult medical command for advice.

Accidental ingestion of LSD by children or infants poses no physical danger to the victim, but the child may experience the same frightening sensations as an adult ingesting the drug. The treatment is simply for someone to fondle and play with the child for several hours. In most instances, the child will respond readily to close attention and physical contact.

PCP Toxicity

One particularly nasty drug that is sometimes taken for its hallucinogenic effects is phencyclidine (PCP). The patient intoxicated with PCP is apt to be violent, combative, and generally out of control. A blank stare is characteristic and only reinforces the zombie-like impression the patient creates. Pain perception may be depressed to the degree that the patient can carry out mutilating self-injury without apparent discomfort (PCP "zombies" have been known to gouge out their own eyes, for example). The patient may have feelings of superhuman strength, and indeed, it often requires much more than the usual amount of physical force to subdue a patient intoxicated with PCP. Severe PCP intoxication leads to cardiorespiratory collapse and even death.

The patient with PCP must be prevented from harming himself and others en route to the hospital. While medications and IV therapy will probably be required, invasive measures are nearly impossible to carry out in such patients outside the hospital. If the patient is at all manageable, it is desirable to persuade him to imbibe a slurry of activated charcoal, at least 5 tablespoons mixed in tap water. But if he is violent or out of control, emphasis should be on quiet, swift transport, with the patient fully restrained.

The clinical presentations of the major drug overdoses are summarized in Table 27-7.

ALCOHOL AND ALCOHOLISM

Despite all the attention given to other drugs, alcohol remains the most widely abused drug in the United States, and alcoholism ranks third—surpassed only by heart disease and cancer—as a cause of death in America. One hundred million Americans consume alcohol, of whom 12 million are alcoholics. Alcohol is directly involved in about 30,000 deaths and a half a million injuries from automobile accidents annually. One-third of pedestrians killed in traffic accidents are under the influence of alcohol. Furthermore, because of its harmful effects on a variety of organs, including the liver, stomach, pancreas, and central nervous system, alcoholism decreases the lifespan by 10 to 20 years.

Profile of the Alcoholic

The National Institute on Alcohol Abuse and Alcoholism defines an **alcoholic** as a person "whose drinking interferes with his health, his job, his relations with his family, or his community relationships—and yet he continues to drink." Note that in essence that is the same definition we gave previously for drug addiction, and indeed alcoholism is simply addiction to the drug alcohol. Like any addiction, it also involves physical and psychologic dependency, tolerance, and the emergence of withdrawal symptoms when the drug is stopped.

The alcoholic syndrome usually consists of *two phases*. The first is PROBLEM DRINKING, during which alcohol is used more and more often to relieve tensions or other emotional difficulties. The second phase is the state of TRUE ADDICTION, in which abstinence from alcohol causes major withdrawal symptoms. The form in which alcohol is consumed is irrelevant to the diagnosis. The heavy beer drinker may be as much an alcoholic as the patient who prefers the drug in the form of whiskey. A 12-ounce (360 ml) can of beer, a 1.5-ounce (45 ml) shot of 86-proof whiskey, and a 4-ounce (120 ml) glass of wine all contain about the same amount of alcohol; so the person who gets through a six-pack of beer while sitting in front of the television every night is taking the same dosage of alcohol as the drinker who downs six highballs in an evening.

TABLE 27-7. COMMON PRESENTATIONS OF DRUG OVERDOSE OR TOXICITY

DRUG TYPE	SIGNS OF OVERDOSE OR TOXICITY
Amphetamines and cocaine	Restlessness, agitation, jitters Incessant talking Insomnia, anorexia Dilated pupils Tachycardia, tachypnea, hypertension Extreme depression on withdrawal
Narcotics	Constricted "pinpoint" pupils Marked respiratory depression Needle tracks (heroin user) Sometimes bradycardia and hypotension Drowsiness, stupor, or coma
Barbiturates	Respiratory depression Dilated pupils Hypotension
Hallucinogens	Hallucinations Panic reactions, agitation Chills, shivering Tachycardia, elevated blood pressure PCP: Blank stare, muscular rigidity, sometimes extremely violent, self-destructive behavior

Alcoholism occurs in all social strata, and only a small minority of alcoholics fit the usual "skid row" stereotype. The majority of alcoholics are working men (only one in four alcoholics is a woman), and most do not consider themselves to be alcoholics at all but insist that they are only "social drinkers." However, the alcoholic differs in many significant respects from the true social drinker. First of all, the alcoholic usually begins drinking early in the day. He is more prone to drink alone or secretly, and he may periodically go on prolonged binges characterized by loss of memory ("blackout periods"). Abstinence from alcohol is likely to produce withdrawal symptoms, such as tremulousness, anxiety, or outright delirium tremens (DTs). As the alcoholic becomes more and more dependent on drinking, his performance at work and his relationships with friends and family deteriorate. Absences from work, emotional disturbances, and automobile accidents become more frequent.

Alcoholism may not only create medical problems in itself (see next section), it may also complicate any other medical problem that the patient develops. Therefore it is very important to try to establish whether a given patient has an alcohol problem. Because of the patient's denial of his problem, and often the family's reluctance to talk about it as well, it may be difficult to obtain an accurate history of alcohol dependence. There are, though, certain clues that should alert you to the possibililty that a patient has an alcohol problem:

Clues to Alcoholism

- An unexplained history of repeated gastrointestinal problems, especially gastrointestinal bleeding
- "Green tongue syndrome," caused by the use of chlorophyll-containing compounds to disguise the odor of alcohol on the breath
- Cigarette burns on clothing, from falling asleep with a lit cigarette
- Chronically flushed face and palms
- Tremulousness
- Alcoholic odor on the breath under inappropriate circumstances (e.g., at work, early in the morning)

A word of caution. While it is undeniably important to detect evidence of chronic alcoholism or acute intoxication in assessing a patient, it is equally important not to ascribe all of a patient's symptoms to alcohol until other causes have been ruled out.

THE PATIENT FOUND STUPOROUS WITH ALCOHOL ON HIS BREATH MUST NOT BE ASSUMED TO BE SIMPLY DRUNK.

His stupor may have resulted from anything that causes stupor in the sober individual, including head trauma, hypoglycemia, infection, and so forth. Furthermore, his stupor is no less a threat to life—indeed, it may be more so—than in the sober patient. Thus, whatever your suspicions about the patient's alcoholic intake, he deserves the same careful assessment and management as any other patient. In fact, the patient whose breath smells of alcohol merits even *more* careful assessment than a patient who appears sober, for it is very easy to miss significant illnesses and injuries in the alcoholic patient.

Medical Consequences of Alcohol

Because of the toxic effects of alcohol on a wide variety of tissues, the alcoholic is considerably more prone than his sober counterpart to a number of serious illnesses and injuries. Let us consider just a few of the organ systems that may be affected.

Chronic damage to the *central nervous system*, to begin with, leads to deterioration in higher mental functions, such as memory and logical thinking. Damage to the cerebellum results in problems of balance, which in turn contribute to the FREQUENT FALLS that produce a high percentage of injuries in the alcoholic. Especially common among those injuries are SUBDURAL HEMATOMAS. In many alcoholics, with or without injury, psychiatric symptoms, particularly of the paranoid type, often become prevalent. Meanwhile, damage to the *peripheral nerves* leads to a marked *decrease in sensation* in the extremities, which makes the alcoholic more prone to BURNS and similar injuries that an intact pain sense would ordinarily prevent. SEIZURES are a common manifestation of alcohol withdrawal. Finally, as noted in a previous chapter, administration of glucose-containing solutions to alcoholics may precipitate WERNICKE'S ENCEPHALOPATHY (ataxia, cranial nerve palsy, dementia), a result of the chronic thiamine deficiency common in alcoholics.

The toxic effects of alcohol on the *liver* produce a whole variety of complications because the liver is responsible for a whole variety of functions. It is in the liver, for example, that the body's major clotting factors are produced, so the patient whose liver has been poisoned by alcohol is likely to be deficient in clotting factors and therefore to BLEED EASILY. The liver also plays a key role in regulating blood sugar, by maintaining the body's sugar reserves in the form of glycogen. A liver impaired by alcohol cannot store and release glycogen normally, so alcoholics tend to develop HYPOGLYCEMIA, often severe enough to produce coma. Meanwhile, structural damage to the liver creates resistance to blood flow through it, which in turn increases the pressure in the portal circulation. Portal hypertension is felt most immediately in the blood vessels of the esophagus, which balloon out (**esophageal varices**) and become vulnerable to rupture. When varices do rupture, the result is usually massive GASTROINTESTINAL BLEEDING, exacerbated by the patient's clotting deficiencies.

If the patient doesn't bleed from his varices, he will almost certainly bleed from hemorrhagic gastritis, the result of alcohol's irritant effects on the gastric mucosa. Another vulnerable organ of the gastrointestinal system is the *pancreas*, and bouts of ACUTE PANCREATITIS are common among alcohol abusers.

Alcohol has a direct, suppressive effect on the *immune system*, reducing the numbers and activity of white blood cells and thereby rendering the alcoholic exceptionally SUSCEPTIBLE TO INFECTION. Among the most common infections is PNEUMONIA, precipitated by aspiration during an alcoholic stupor, when the gag reflex has been suppressed.

Toxic effects of alcohol on the *heart* lead to ALCOHOLIC CARDIOMYOPATHY, with dysrhythmias and a tendency to heart failure.

The medical problems to which alcoholics are particularly susceptible are summarized in Table 27-8. The lesson in that table is that

> **THE PATIENT WITH ALCOHOL ON HIS BREATH MAY BE ILL OR INJURED FROM OTHER CAUSES. DON'T LET THE SMELL OF ALCOHOL IMPAIR YOUR JUDGMENT AS WELL AS THE PATIENT'S.**

Be exceptionally thorough in assessing a patient who appears drunk. His life may depend on it.

TABLE 27-8. MEDICAL PROBLEMS TO WHICH ALCOHOLICS ARE PARTICULARLY SUSCEPTIBLE

CONDITION	CONTRIBUTING FACTORS
Subdural hematoma	Frequent falls; impaired clotting mechanisms
Gastrointestinal bleeding	Irritant effect of alcohol on the stomach lining (leading to gastritis); impaired clotting mechanisms; cirrhosis of the liver, leading to engorgement of esophageal veins (esophageal varices)
Pancreatitis	Indirect effect of alcohol on the pancreas
Hypoglycemia	Damage to the liver, which normally mobilizes sugar into the blood
Pneumonia	Aspiration of vomitus occurring during intoxication and coma; suppression of immune system by alcohol
Burns	Relative insensitivity to pain occurring during intoxication; falling asleep with a lit cigarette while intoxicated
Hypothermia	Insensitivity to extremes of temperatures while intoxicated; falling asleep outside in the cold
Seizures	Effect of withdrawal from alcohol
Dysrhythmias	Toxic effects of alcohol on the heart
Cancer	Mechanism not known (perhaps related to suppression of the immune system), but alcoholics are 10 times more likely than the general population to develop cancer

Alcoholic Emergencies

Any of the conditions previously mentioned may contribute to an emergency in an alcoholic. In addition, however, there are several emergencies related directly to the acute consumption of or abstinence from alcohol, including acute alcohol intoxication, withdrawal seizures, and delirium tremens.

Acute Alcohol Intoxication

Severe alcohol intoxication is a form of poisoning, and it therefore carries all the lethal potential of any other poisoning with a CNS-depressant drug. Death from alcohol intoxication has been reported with blood alcohol levels of 400 mg per deciliter, which can be attained by the relatively rapid consumption of half a pint of whiskey.

The most immediate danger to an acutely intoxicated person is DEATH FROM RESPIRATORY DEPRESSION. Furthermore, because the gag reflex is suppressed and the patient cannot therefore protect his airway, there is always a significant risk of ASPIRATION of vomitus and consequent pneumonia. Bear in mind as well that acute intoxication may be, and often is, complicated by a variety of coexisting conditions—the ingestion of other substances (especially barbiturates or tranquilizers), hypoglycemia, hypothermia, subdural hematoma—so evaluation of the apparently drunk patient must be painstakingly thorough.

In *assessing* the intoxicated patient, then, first make careful note of his *state of consciousness*, and use a neurologic checklist to record sequential observations. In measuring the *vital signs*, be alert for indications of increased intracranial pressure (bradycardia and hypertension) or internal bleeding (tachycardia and hypotension). The *head-to-toe survey* should be a careful search for signs of injury, especially head injury. Remember, the responses to pain are dulled by alcohol ingestion, so the patient may not react normally to injury (or may not be in any shape to report his symptoms reliably).

Treatment of the acutely intoxicated patient is aimed at protecting him from injury and safeguarding his vital functions. If he is conscious and agitated, he must be prevented from injuring himself and others. If that can be done without using physical restraints, all the better; many patients will, in fact, respond positively to a kind but firm approach. But if the patient is out of control and endangering those around him, do not hesitate to use restraints (see Chap. 38 for a discussion of dealing with the violent patient).

If the intoxicated patient is unconscious, he should be treated as any other unconscious patient:

- Establish an AIRWAY. If the gag reflex is still present, position the patient on his left side, and keep suction close at hand in the event of vomiting. If the gag reflex is absent, intubate the trachea.
- Administer OXYGEN, preferably by nasal cannula.
- If respirations are abnormally slow or shallow, ASSIST VENTILATIONS with a bag-valve-mask and oxygen.
- Start an IV LIFELINE with D5/W in a large vein.
- Administer THIAMINE, 100 mg slowly IV.
- Administer 50% DEXTROSE, 50 ml slowly IV.
- If there is any question of a mixed overdose, give a trial of NALOXONE, 0.8 to 1.2 mg IV.
- MONITOR cardiac rhythm.
- TRANSPORT to the hospital.

Take note of the last step. EVERY INTOXICATED PATIENT MUST BE TRANSPORTED TO THE HOSPITAL, no matter how unpopular that makes you in the emergency department. It is sheer negligence to leave a patient with impaired mental status at the scene on the assumption that he is "just drunk," even if the patient is one of your "regulars." *This* time around, he might just be in hypoglycemic shock or have a subdural hematoma.

Withdrawal Seizures

When a person who has been drinking heavily over an extended period suddenly stops drinking, for any reason, he may suffer a variety of withdrawal phenomena. One of the more common manifestations of withdrawal from alcohol is a seizure, sometimes referred to as alcoholic epilepsy, or "rum fits." Alcoholic withdrawal seizures usually occur, if they are going to occur at all, between about 12 and 48 hours after the patient took his last drink. The seizures are typically grand mal. Approximately 40 percent of patients with rum fits will have only one seizure; the rest have up to about four seizures over a 6-hour period. In a small number of cases—about 5 percent—there are more than four seizures and even status epilepticus.

Alcoholic withdrawal seizures should be treated like seizures from any other source (see Chap. 24):

- Protect the patient from injury.
- Maintain a patent AIRWAY. Suction secretions from the mouth.

- Administer OXYGEN in high concentration.
- Check the patient carefully for injuries after the tonic-clonic phase of the seizure abates.
- MONITOR cardiac rhythm.
- Start an IV LIFELINE with D5/W.
- Give 100 mg of THIAMINE slowly IV, followed by 50 ml of 50% DEXTROSE slowly IV.
- For *status epilepticus*, give DIAZEPAM in 2.5-mg increments, checking the blood pressure after each dose, up to a total of 10 mg.
- TRANSPORT to the hospital.

Delirium Tremens

One of the most serious syndromes resulting from alcohol withdrawal is **delirium tremens (DTs).** Not every alcoholic who stops drinking will experience DTs, but in those in whom DTs do occur—around 5 to 10 percent of alcoholics in withdrawal—the symptoms usually start somewhere between 48 and 72 hours after the last drink. In occasional patients, however, the onset of DTs may be delayed as long as 7 to 10 days from the time the patient stopped drinking.

Delirium tremens is a serious and potentially fatal syndrome, with a mortality as high as 15 percent, generally from exhaustion and dehydration. It is characterized by *confusion, tremors, restlessness,* and *hallucinations* that are usually very frightening (e.g., snakes, spiders, rats). *Fever, sweating,* and a greatly increased metabolic rate lead to marked *dehydration,* sometimes to the point of hypovolemic *shock.*

Treatment of a patient in DTs is aimed at protecting him from injury and supporting his cardiovascular system:

- PROTECT THE PATIENT FROM INJURY. Terrifying hallucinations may make him agitated and combative, and it is very important to try to calm and reassure him.
- If at all possible, AVOID THE USE OF PHYSICAL RESTRAINTS, which are likely to worsen the patient's agitation, especially if he feels himself to be in immediate danger from rats and snakes.
- Administer OXYGEN by nasal cannula.
- After carefully explaining to the patient what you are about to do, start an IV LIFELINE with lactated Ringer's, and run in fluids rapidly.
- Maintain a FLOW SHEET of neurologic and vital signs.
- KEEP TALKING to the patient throughout transport, to help orient and reassure him.
- TRANSPORT the patient to the hospital.

GLOSSARY

alcoholic A person whose drinking interferes with his health, his job, his relations with his family, or his community relationships but who nonetheless continues to drink.

antidote Substance used to counteract the effects of a drug or combat the effects of a poison.

antivenin Antiserum against an animal or insect venom.

carboxyhemoglobin Hemoglobin chemically combined with carbon monoxide rather than oxygen.

cholinesterase Enzyme that inactivates acetylcholine released at the nerve cell junction.

delirium tremens (DTs) Potential complication of alcohol withdrawal, characterized by agitation, frightening hallucinations, and sometimes cardiovascular collapse.

esophageal varices Widened, tortuous blood vessels in the esophagus that develop as a result of portal hypertension.

ethanol Ethyl alcohol; the type of alcohol consumed in alcoholic beverages.

Hymenoptera A family of insects that includes bees, wasps, yellow jackets, hornets, and ants.

lavage The washing out of a hollow organ, such as the stomach.

methanol Methyl alcohol; wood alcohol.

miosis Pupillary constriction.

nematocyst Stinging cell of a coelenterate, such as the jellyfish.

paranoia Mental disorder characterized by abnormal suspicions and other delusions (often of persecution or grandeur).

synapse The junction between two nerve cells.

tolerance Progressive diminution of susceptibility to a drug after repeated doses.

toxic Pertaining to a poison; harmful.

venom A poisonous substance derived from a snake, spider, bee, wasp, or other such creature.

APPENDIX: HOW TO PASS A NASOGASTRIC TUBE

Nasogastric intubation is indicated for decompression of a severely distended stomach and also for evacuation of stomach contents by lavage (rinsing), as in cases of poisoning or overdose. A nasogastric tube should be inserted *only* in a patient who is able to protect his or her airway, that is, a patient who is alert and has an intact gag reflex.

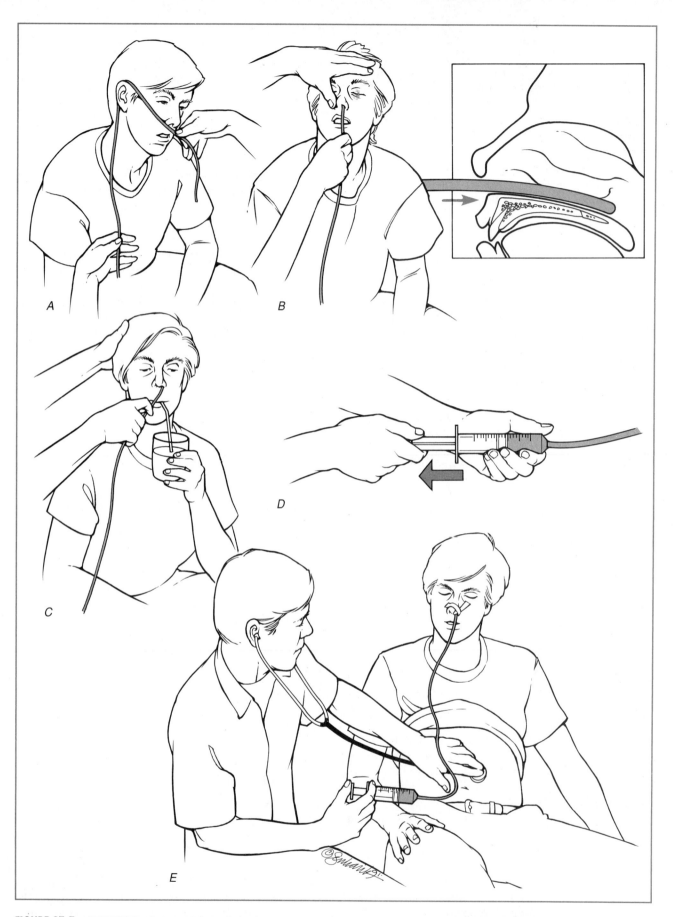

FIGURE 27-7.   INSERTING A NASOGASTRIC TUBE.   (A) Measure the tube alongside the patient. (B) Pass the tube along the floor of the nostril, holding it almost horizontal (*inset*). (C) Have the patient swallow sips of water as you advance the tube. (D) Aspirate the tube for return of gastric contents. (E) Confirm the location of the tube by injecting a small amount of air and listening for bubbling noise over the epigastrium.

IF NASOGASTRIC INTUBATION IS INDICATED FOR THE COMATOSE PATIENT, IT SHOULD ALWAYS BE PRECEDED BY INTUBATION OF THE TRACHEA WITH A CUFFED ENDOTRACHEAL TUBE, TO PROTECT THE AIRWAY FROM ASPIRATION.

For the conscious patient, nasogastric intubation is an unpleasant experience. Paramedics who are to be taught this skill should have an opportunity to practice on one another—to gain an appreciation of what the patient may feel during such a procedure. It is almost a certainty that the patient will look on the prospect of having a tube passed down his nose into his stomach with some misgivings, especially if—as may be the case with overdose victims—he has been through it before; therefore, it will be necessary to approach him with confidence and empathy, assuring him that the procedure is necessary. If you gain the patient's trust, half the battle is won, for cooperation is extremely important.

You will need an assistant to hold ancillary equipment, such as a container of water or emesis basin, and also in many instances to restrain the patient (especially if the patient is confused or is a child).

The steps in nasogastric intubation are as follows:

- ASSEMBLE THE EQUIPMENT:
  1. Levine tube (No. 16 French for adults, No. 12 French for children).
  2. Water-soluble lubricant.
  3. Adhesive tape, 1 inch wide.
  4. Small clamp.
  5. Irrigating syringe, 50 ml.
  6. Cup of water with straw.
  7. Emesis basin.
- EXPLAIN carefully to the patient exactly what is to be done and what will be expected of him. Obtain consent for the procedure. Then sit the patient up, leaning forward.
- WASH YOUR HANDS. Gloves are advisable for your own protection.
- MEASURE the nasogastric tube alongside the patient's face and chest (Fig. 27-7A) to get an idea of the length that will be required to reach the stomach. Note which marking on the tube corresponds to the right length.
- LUBRICATE the tip and the first few inches of the NASOGASTRIC TUBE generously, and ask your assistant to place the straw between the patient's lips. Tell the patient not to drink until instructed to do so, at which point he should drink as fast as he can, without stopping.

- PASS THE TUBE *gently* along the floor of the nasal passage; hold the tube almost horizontal to the ground to do this (Fig. 27-7B). A common mistake is to orient the tip upward, which causes it to get hung up in the turbinates and induce pain and bleeding.
- When the tube begins to enter the oropharynx—you will be able to feel this as a lessening of resistance to passage of the tube—tell the patient to drink and keep drinking (Fig. 27-7C). Advance the tip of the tube into the stomach as he swallows.
- The tube should go down about 20 inches, but the most reliable indication that the tube has reached the right place is a rapid return of gastric contents when the tube is aspirated with a syringe (Fig. 27-7D). Another method for checking tube position is to push about 20 ml of air into the tube with a syringe and auscultate over the epigastrium for the sound of bubbling (Fig. 27-7E).

Possible Problems in Nasogastric Intubation

Problems can arise in attempting nasogastric intubation. One problem is that the tube may inadvertently pass into the trachea. That should be readily obvious if it occurs, for the patient will begin to cough and choke. If in doubt, place the distal end of the tube under water; if the proximal end is in the trachea, there will be a steady bubbling as the patient exhales. If that is the case, withdraw the tube into the posterior oropharynx, and advance it again. Having the patient flex his neck slightly sometimes helps avoid the problem.

Another possible problem is that the tube may become hung up in the posterior pharynx. Suspect that has happened when the patient gags and retches excessively. It is very easy to check: Simply look in the patient's mouth. If there are half a dozen coils of nasogastric tube in his throat, pull back gently until the tip of the tube is visible in the posterior pharynx. Then try again to advance the tube.

FURTHER READING

INGESTED AND ABSORBED POISONS
Arena J. *Poisoning.* Springfield, Ill.: Thomas, 1979.
Arena J. Plants that poison. *Emerg Med* 21(11):20, 1989.
Bayer MJ. Reversing the effects of pesticide poisoning. *Emerg Med* 24(3): 61, 1992.
Becker C. Acute methanol poisoning. *West J Med* 135:122, 1981.
Caroline NL. Poison patrol. *Emerg Med Serv* 11(2):80, 1982.

Chodak GW, Passaro E. Acid ingestions. *JAMA* 239:225, 1978.

Corey EC. The treatment of poisonings. *Emergency* 26(2):20, 1994.

Daniels P, LePard A. Organophosphates: The pervasive poison. *JEMS* 16(11):76, 1991.

de Bleeker J et al. The intermediate syndrome in organophosphate poisoning: Presentation of a case and review of the literature. *Clin Toxicol* 30:321, 1992.

de Silva J, Wijewickrema R, Senananyake N. Does pralidoxime affect outcome of management in acute organophosphorous poisoning? *Lancet* 339:1136, 1992.

Dice WH et al. Pulmonary toxicity following gastrointestinal ingestion of kerosene. *Ann Emerg Med* 11:138, 1982.

Done AK. Petroleum industry specials. *Emerg Med* 15(1):237, 1983.

Ekins BR et al. Standardized treatment of severe methanol poisoning with ethanol and hemodialysis. *West J Med* 142:337, 1985.

Farrar HC, Wells TG, Kearns GL. Use of continuous infusion of pralidoxime for treatment of organophosphate poisoning in children. *J Pediatr* 116:658, 1990.

Goldfrank L, Weisman R, Flomenbaum N. Teaching the recognition of odors. *Ann Emerg Med* 11:684, 1982.

Gordon AM, Richards DW. Strychnine intoxication. *JACEP* 8:520, 1979.

Gumaste VV et al. Ingestion of corrosive substances by adults. *Am J Gastroenterol* 87:1, 1992.

Holliman CJ. Something's fishy: Prehospital management of toxic seafood ingestions. *Emerg Med Serv* 23(1):32, 1994.

Kirk MA, Bowers L. Cluing in on the acutely poisoned patient. *JEMS* 16(5):64, 1991.

Knopp R. Caustic ingestions. *JACEP* 8:329, 1979.

Kuhns DW, Dire DJ. Button battery ingestions. *Ann Emerg Med* 18:293, 1989.

Kulig K. Initial management of ingestions of toxic substances. *N Engl J Med* 326:1677, 1992.

Kunkel DB. Burning issues: Acids and alkalis. Part I: Ingestion. *Emerg Med* 16(17):167, 1984.

Kunkel DB. Burning issues: Acids and alkalis. Part II: Skin and eye exposures. *Emerg Med* 16(19):165, 1984.

Kunkel DB. Strychnine is still with us. *Emerg Med* 17(21):81, 1985.

Lampe KF, McCann MA. *AMA Handbook of Poisonous and Injurious Plants.* Chicago: American Medical Association, 1985.

Meadow R. Non-accidental salt poisoning. *Arch Dis Child* 68:448, 1993.

Midtling JE et al. Clinical management of field worker organophosphate poisoning. *West J Med* 142:514, 1985.

Moore WR. Caustic ingestions: Pathophysiology, diagnosis, and treatment. *Clin Pediatr* 25:192, 1986.

Moulin D et al. Upper airway lesions in children after accidental ingestion of caustic substances. *J Pediatr* 106:408, 1985.

Nelson R, Walson P, Kelley M. Caustic ingestion. *Ann Emerg Med* 12:559, 1983.

Penner GE. Acid ingestion: Toxicology and treatment. *Ann Emerg Med* 9:374, 1980.

Peterson CD. Oral ethanol doses in patients with methanol poisoning. *Am J Hosp Pharm* 38:1024, 1981.

Schiffman MA. Managing the toxic ingestion. *Emerg Med Serv* 21(4):28, 1992.

Schoolmeester WL et al. Arsenic poisoning. *South Med J* 73:198, 1980.

Smilkstein MJ. A rational approach to the unknown ingestion. *Emerg Med* 25(2):73, 1993.

Vance MV, Selden BS, Clark RF. Optimal patient position for transport and initial management of toxic ingestions. *Ann Emerg Med* 21:243, 1992.

Vasil EF. Pesticide poisoning. *Emerg Med Serv* 18(6):58, 1989.

Verrilli MR et al. Fatal ethylene glycol intoxication: Report of a case and review of the literature. *Cleve Clin J Med* 54:289, 1987.

Vesconi S et al. Therapy of cytotoxic mushroom intoxication. *Crit Care Med* 13:402, 1985.

Walton WW. An evaluation of the poison prevention packaging act. *Pediatrics* 69:363, 1982.

Zautcke JL, Schwartz JA, Mueller EJ. Chinese restaurant syndrome: A review. *Ann Emerg Med* 15:1210, 1986.

See also the excellent series by Dr. Donald Kunkel, "The Toxic Emergency," which appears in *Emergency Medicine.*

GASTRIC EMPTYING AND SYRUP OF IPECAC

Auerback PS et al. Efficacy of gastric emptying: Gastric lavage versus emesis induced with ipecac. *Ann Emerg Med* 15:692, 1986.

Bond GR et al. Influence of time until emesis on the efficacy of decontamination using acetaminophen as a marker in a pediatric population. *Ann Emerg Med* 22:1403, 1993.

Eason J et al. Efficacy and safety of gastrointestinal decontamination in the treatment of oral poisoning. *Pediatr Clin North Am* 26:827, 1979.

Flomenbaum NE, Hoffman R. GI evacuation: Is it still worthwhile? *Emerg Med* 22(2):80, 1990.

Freedman GE, Pasternak S, Krenzelok EP. A clinical trial using syrup of ipecac and activated charcoal concurrently. *Ann Emerg Med* 16:164, 1987.

Grande GA et al. The effect of fluid volume on syrup of ipecac emesis time. *Clin Toxicol* 25:473, 1987.

Ipecac syrup and activated charcoal for treatment of poisoning in children. *Med Lett* 21:70, 1979.

King WD. Syrup of ipecac: A drug review. *Clin Toxicol* 17:353, 1980.

Krenzelok EP et al. Preserving the emetic effect of syrup of ipecac with concurrent activated charcoal administration: A preliminary study. *Clin Toxicol* 24:159, 1986.

Krenzelok EP et al. Effectiveness of 15-ml vs 30-ml doses of syrup of ipecac in children. *Clin Pharm* 6:715, 1987.

Kulig K et al. Management of acutely poisoned patients without gastric emptying. *Ann Emerg Med* 14:562, 1985.

Levy DB. Syrup of ipecac review. *Emergency* 21(12):20, 1989.

Lipscomb JW et al. Response in children to 15-ml or 30-ml doses of ipecac syrup. *Clin Pharm* 5:234, 1986.

McDougal CB, Maclean MA. Modifications in the technique of gastric lavage. *Ann Emerg Med* 10:514, 1981.

Mofenson HC. Benefits/risks of syrup of ipecac. *Pediatrics* 77:551, 1986.

Pollack CV et al. Gastric emptying in the acutely inebriated patient. *J Emerg Med* 10:1, 1992.

Riegel JM et al. Use of cathartics in toxic ingestions. *Ann Emerg Med* 10:254, 1981.

Rosenberg H. The difficult NG intubation: Tips and techniques. *Emerg Med* 9(3):235, 1977.

Rumack BH. Ipecac use in the home. *Pediatrics* 75:1148, 1985.

Saetta JP et al. Gastric emptying procedures in the self-poisoned patient: Are we forcing gastric content beyond the pylorus? *J R Soc Med* 84:5, 1991.

Tandberg D, Diven BG, McLeod JW. Ipecac-induced emesis versus gastric lavage: A controlled study in normal adults. *Am J Emerg Med* 4:205, 1986.

Tenenbein M, Cohen S, Sitar DS. Efficacy of ipecac-induced emesis, orogastric lavage, and activated charcoal for acute drug overdose. *Ann Emerg Med* 16:838, 1987.

Wettach GE, Wettach RA. Effective utilization of nasogastric tubes in prehospital care. *EMT J* 4(3):50, 1980.

Wrenn K et al. Potential misuse of ipecac. *Ann Emerg Med* 222:1408, 1993.

Young WF, Bivins HG. Evaluation of gastric emptying using radionuclides: Gastric lavage versus ipecac-induced emesis. *Ann Emerg Med* 22:1423, 1993.

ACTIVATED CHARCOAL

Albertson T et al. Superiority of activated charcoal alone compared with ipecac and activated charcoal in the treatment of acute toxic ingestions. *Ann Emerg Med* 18:101, 1989.

Farley TA. Severe hypernatremic dehydration after use of an activated charcoal–sorbitol suspension. *J Pediatr* 109:719, 1986.

Greensher J et al. Ascendency of the black bottle (activated charcoal). *Pediatrics* 80:949, 1987.

Hoffman R. Choices in gastric decontamination. *Emerg Med* 24(10): 212, 1992.

Katona BG et al. The new black magic: Activated charcoal and new therapeutic uses. *J Emerg Med* 5:99, 1987.

Kornberg AE, Dolgin J. Pediatric ingestions: Charcoal alone versus ipecac and charcoal. *Ann Emerg Med* 20:648, 1991.

Krenzelok EP et al. Effectiveness of commercially available aqueous activated charcoal products. *Ann Emerg Med* 16:1340, 1987.

Levy DB. Activated charcoal update. *Emergency* 20(6):16, 1988.

McNamara RM et al. Efficacy of charcoal cathartic versus ipecac in reducing serum acetaminophen in a simulated overdose. *Ann Emerg Med* 18:934, 1989.

Park GD et al. Expanded role of charcoal therapy in the poisoned and overdosed patient. *Arch Intern Med* 146:969, 1986.

Tenenbein M. Multiple doses of activated charcoal: Time for reappraisal? *Ann Emerg Med* 20:529, 1991.

CARBON MONOXIDE AND OTHER INHALED POISONS

Baker MD et al. Carboxyhemoglobin levels in children with nonspecific flu-like symptoms. *J Pediatr* 113:501, 1988.

Ball RA. Carbon monoxide poisoning. *Emergency* 24(1):23, 1992.

Barret L et al. Carbon monoxide poisoning: A diagnosis frequently overlooked. *J Toxicol* 23:309, 1985.

Bascom R, Kennedy T. Toxic gas inhalation. *Emerg Med Serv* 13(7): 17, 1984.

Bass M. Sudden sniffing death. *JAMA* 212:2075, 1970.

Baud FJ et al. Elevated blood cyanide concentrations in victims of smoke inhalation. *N Engl J Med* 325:1761, 1991.

Beckerman B, Brody G. Smoke inhalation. *Emerg Med* 25(15):48, 1992.

Boutros AR, Hoyt JL. Management of carbon monoxide poisoning in the absence of a hyperbaric oxygen chamber. *Crit Care Med* 4:114, 1976.

Burney RE, Wu S, Nemiroff MJ. Mass carbon monoxide poisoning: Clinical effects and results of treatment in 184 victims. *Ann Emerg Med* 11:394, 1982.

Caplan YH et al. Accidental poisonings involving carbon monoxide, heating systems, and confined spaces. *J Forensic Sci* 31:117, 1986.

Caravati EM et al. Fetal toxicity associated with maternal carbon monoxide poisoning. *Ann Emerg Med* 17:714, 1988.

Centers for Disease Control. Chlorine gas toxicity from mixture of bleach with other cleaning products—California. *MMWR* 40:619, 1991.

Cobb N, Etzel RA. Unintentional carbon monoxide–related deaths in the United States, 1979 through 1988. *JAMA* 266:659, 1991.

Dan BB. The twilight zone: Death on a Sunday morning (editorial). *JAMA* 261:1188, 1989.

Done AK. Carbon monoxide: The silent summons. *Emerg Med* 5(2):268, 1973.

Done AK. It's a gas. *Emerg Med* 8(5):305, 1976.

Done AK. Sniffing, bagging and huffing. *Emerg Med* 9(7):187, 1977.

Edminster SC, Bayer MJ. Recreational gasoline sniffing. *J Emerg Med* 3:365, 1985.

Finck PA. Exposure to carbon monoxide: Review of the literature and 567 autopsies. *Milit Med* 131:1513, 1966.

Fine KC, Bassin RH, Steward MM. Emergency care for tear gas victims. *JACEP* 6:144, 1977.

Fortenberry JD. Gasoline sniffing. *Am J Med* 79:740, 1985.

Ginsberg MD. Carbon monoxide intoxication: Clinical features, neuropathology and mechanisms of injury. *J Toxicol* 23:281, 1985.

Greer WER, Giovacchini RP. Sniffing up trouble: Inhalation of volatile substances. *JAMA* 254:1721, 1985.

Hall AH. Cyanide poisoning: Dealing with an unexpected menace. *Emerg Med* 18(15):191, 1986.

Hampson NB, Norkool DM. Carbon monoxide poisoning in children riding in the back of pickup trucks. *JAMA* 267:538, 1992.

Hampson NB et al. Carbon monoxide poisoning from indoor burning of charcoal briquets. *JAMA* 271:52, 1994.

Heckerling PS. Occult carbon monoxide poisoning: A cause of winter headache. *Am J Emerg Med* 5:201, 1987.

Heckerling PS et al. Predictors of occult carbon monoxide poisoning in patients with headache and dizziness. *Ann Intern Med* 107:174, 1987.

Hedges JR, Morrissey WL. Acute chlorine gas exposure. *JACEP* 8:59, 1979.

Jackson DL. Accidental carbon monoxide poisoning. *JAMA* 243:772, 1980.

Jones J, Krohmer J. Injury through inhalation: Cyanide poisoning in fire victims. *JEMS* 15(4):36, 1990.

Kales SN. Carbon monoxide intoxication. *Am Fam Physician* 48:1100, 1993.

Kindwell EP. Hyperbaric treatment of carbon monoxide poisoning (editorial). *Ann Emerg Med* 14:1233, 1985.

King GS, Smialek JE, Troutman WG. Sudden death in adolescents resulting from the inhalation of typewriter correction fluid. *JAMA* 253:1604, 1985.

Kirk MA, Gerace R, Kulig KW. Cyanide and methemoglobin kinetics in smoke inhalation victims treated with the cyanide antidote kit. *Ann Emerg Med* 22:1413, 1993.

Kirkpatrick JN. Occult carbon monoxide poisoning. *West J Med* 146:52, 1987.

Kulig K. Cyanide antidotes and fire toxicology (editorial). *N Engl J Med* 325:1801, 1991.

Kunkel DB. Inhalant abuse update. *Emerg Med* 16(13):68, 1984.

Kunkel DB. Cyanide: Looking for the source. *Emerg Med* 19(9):115, 1987.

Levy DB. A breath of dead air. *Emergency* 20(11):18, 1988.

Levy DB, Peppers MP. Poisoning with cyanide. *Emergency* 22(9):18, 1990.

Manoguerra AS. Carbon monoxide poisoning. *Emergency* 12(1):29, 1980.

Marthieu D et al. Acute carbon monoxide poisoning: Risk of late sequelae and treatment by hyperbaric oxygen. *J Toxicol* 23:35, 1985.

Mrvos R et al. Home exposures to chlorine/chloramine gas: Review of 216 cases. *South Med J* 86:654, 1993.

Myers RAM, Linberg SE, Cowley RA. Carbon monoxide poisoning: The injury and its treatment. *JACEP* 8:479, 1979.

Myers RAM, Snyder SK, Emhoff TA. Subacute sequelae of carbon monoxide poisoning. *Ann Emerg Med* 14:1163, 1985.

Myers RAM, Snyder S, Majerus TC. Cutaneous blisters and carbon monoxide poisoning. *Ann Emerg Med* 14:603, 1985.

Norkool DM, Kirkpatrick JN. Treatment of acute carbon monoxide poisoning with hyperbaric oxygen: A review of 115 cases. *Ann Emerg Med* 14:1168, 1985.

Olson KR. Carbon monoxide poisoning: Mechanisms, presentation, and controversies in management. *J Emerg Med* 1:233, 1984.

Symington IS et al. Cyanide exposure in fires. *Lancet* 2:91, 1978.

Voigts A et al. Acidosis and other metabolic abnormalities associated with paint sniffing. *South Med J* 76:443, 1983.

Watanabe K et al. The role of carbon monoxide poisoning in the production of inhalation burns. *Ann Plast Surg* 14:284, 1985.

Wharton M et al. Fatal carbon monoxide poisoning at a motel. *JAMA* 261:1177, 1989.

Zarem HA, Rattenborg CC, Harmel MH. Carbon monoxide toxicity in human fire victims. *Arch Surg* 107:851, 1973.

DRUG ABUSE AND DRUG OVERDOSE: GENERAL

Aronson JK. The treatment of self-poisoning. *Emerg Med Serv* 18(5):51, 1989.

Berg MJ et al. Acceleration of the body clearance of phenobarbital by oral activated charcoal. *N Engl J Med* 307:642, 1982.

Callaham M. Tricyclic antidepressant overdose. *JACEP* 8:413, 1979.

Comstock EG et al. Assessment of the efficacy of activated charcoal following gastric lavage in acute drug emergencies. *J Toxicol* 19:149, 1982.

Done AK. Signs, symptoms, and sources. *Emerg Med* 14 (1):42, 1982.

Done AK. An update on antidepressants. *Emerg Med* 15 (3):225, 1983.

Fauman B et al. Psychosis induced by phencyclidine. *JACEP* 4:233, 1975.

Hooper RG, Conner CS, Rumack BH. Acute poisoning from over-the-counter sleep preparation. *JACEP* 8:98, 1979.

Koren G. Medications which can kill a toddler with one tablet or teaspoonful. *Clin Toxicol* 31:407, 1993.

Kriegman W, Peppers MP. Flumazenil for benzodiazepine overdose. *Emergency* 26(1):21, 1994.

Lafin SM et al. Dealing with drug abuse. *Emergency* 22 (7):42, 1990.

Leisner K. The EMS addict: Chemically dependent providers. *Emerg Med Serv* 17(8):12, 1988.

Levy G. Gastrointestinal clearance of drugs with activated charcoal. *N Engl J Med* 307:676, 1982.

MacDonald DI. Drug abuse in adolescents: When to intervene, how to help. *Postgrad Med* 78:109, 1985.

Madsen L et al. Acute propoxyphene self-poisoning in 222 consecutive patients. *Acta Anaesthesiol Scand* 28:661, 1984.

McCarron MM et al. Acute phencyclidine intoxication: Clinical patterns, complications, and treatment. *Ann Emerg Med* 10:290, 1981.

Mofenson HC, Greensher J, Gavin WJ. Acetaminophen overdose: Growing medical nemesis. *Emerg Med Serv* 7(2):64, 1978.

Olson KR. Taking care of the cardiotoxic emergency. *Emerg Med* 25(8):69, 1993.

Pond SM et al. Randomized study of the treatment of phenobarbital overdose with repeated doses of activated charcoal. *JAMA* 251:3104, 1984.

Rangno RE et al. Effect of ethanol ingestion on outcome of drug overdose. *Crit Care Med* 10:180, 1982.

Rappolt RT, Gay GR, Farris RD. Emergency management of acute phencyclidine intoxication. *JACEP* 8:68, 1979.

Shalansky SJ et al. Effect of flumazenil on benzodiazepine-induced respiratory depression. *Clin Pharm* 12:483, 1993.

Shih RD, Meggs WJ, Lewin NA. PCP. *Emerg Med Serv* 22(11):32, 1993.

Thornton WE. Sleep aids and sedatives. *JACEP* 6:408, 1977.

True RJ. Treatment of theophylline toxicity with oral activated charcoal. *Crit Care Med* 12:113, 1984.

Turner BM. Drug use: Myths, reality, and problems for EMS. *Emerg Med Serv* 12(3):49, 1983.

Wright N. An assessment of the unreliability of the history given by self-poisoned patients. *Clin Toxicol* 16:381, 1980.

NARCOTIC OVERDOSE AND NARCOTIC ANTAGONISTS

Bradberry JC et al. Continuous infusion of naloxone in the treatment of narcotic overdose. *Drug Intell Clin Pharm* 15:945, 1981.

Cahill JJ. Treatment of opioid overdose. *Emergency* 25 (12):20, 1993.

Cuss FM et al. Cardiac arrest after reversal of effects of opiates with naloxone. *Br Med J* 288:363, 1984.

Freitas PM. Narcotic withdrawal in the emergency department. *Am J Emerg Med* 3:456, 1985.

Handal KA, Schauben JL, Salamone FR. Naloxone. *Ann Emerg Med* 12:438, 1983.

Hoffman JR, Schriger DL, Luo JS. The empiric use of naloxone in patients with altered mental status: A reappraisal. *Ann Emerg Med* 20:246, 1991.

Kaplan JL, Marx JA. Effectiveness and safety of intravenous nalmefene for emergency department patients with suspected narcotic overdose: A pilot study. *Ann Emerg Med* 22:187, 1993.

Kunkel DB. Narcotic antagonist update. *Emerg Med* 19(5): 97, 1987.

Levy DB. Naloxone: Negating narcotics. *Emergency* 22(7): 16, 1990.

Martin M et al. China white epidemic: An eastern United States emergency department experience. *Ann Emerg Med* 20:158, 1991.

Moore RA et al. Naloxone: Underdosage after narcotic poisoning. *Am J Dis Child* 134:156, 1980.

Perry SW. Irrational attitudes toward addicts and narcotics. *Bull NY Acad Med* 61:706, 1985.

Yealy DM et al. The safety of prehospital naloxone administration by paramedics. *Ann Emerg Med* 19:902, 1990.

AMPHETAMINES, COCAINE, AND OTHER STIMULANTS

Brody G. Cardiovascular effects of cocaine. *Emerg Med* 21 (21):26, 1989.

Brody SL et al. Cocaine-related medical problems: Consecutive series of 233 patients. *Am J Med* 88:325, 1990.

Cregler LL et al. Medical complications of cocaine abuse. *N Engl J Med* 315:1495, 1986.

Dowling GP, McDonough ET, Bost RO. "Eve" and "Ecstasy": A report of five deaths associated with the use of MDEA and MDMA. *JAMA* 257:1615, 1987.

Fontanarosa PB, DiBartolomeo A. Cracking the case of the cocaine user. *JEMS* 14(5):42, 1989.

Gay GR. Clinical management of acute and chronic cocaine poisoning. *Ann Emerg Med* 11:562, 1982.

Gitter MJ et al. Cocaine and chest pain: Clinical features and outcome of patients hospitalized to rule out myocardial infarction. *Ann Intern Med* 115:277, 1991.

Goldfrank LR, Hoffman RS. The cardiovascular effects of cocaine. *Ann Emerg Med* 20:165, 1991.

Kunkel DB. Cocaine then and now. Part I: Its history, medical botany, and use. *Emerg Med* 18(11):125, 1986.

Kunkel DB. The divine plant of the Incas. *Emerg Med* 24(11):77, 1992.

Levine SR et al. Cerebrovascular complications of the use of the "crack" form of alkaloidal cocaine. *N Engl J Med* 323:699, 1990.

Lowenstein DH et al. Acute neurologic and psychiatric complications associated with cocaine abuse. *Am J Med* 85:841, 1987.

Marks EA, Arsura EL. Cocaine-induced rhabdomyolysis. *Emerg Med* 22(14):79, 1990.

Minor RL et al. Cocaine-induced myocardial infarction in patients with normal coronary arteries. *Ann Intern Med* 115:797, 1991.

Mittleman RE, Wetli CV. Death caused by recreational cocaine use: An update. *JAMA* 252:1889, 1984.

Pentel P. Toxicity of over-the-counter stimulants. *JAMA* 252:1898, 1984.

Rich JA, Singer DE. Cocaine-related symptoms in patients presenting to an urban emergency department. *Ann Emerg Med* 20:616, 1991.

Roehrich H, Gold MS. Emergency presentations of crack abuse. *Emerg Med Serv* 17(8):41, 1988.

Rothenberg R. Cocaine. *Emerg Med Serv* 13(2):29, 1984.

SNAKEBITES

Anker R et al. Retarding the uptake of "mock venom" in humans: Comparison of three first aid techniques. *Med J Aust* 6(5):212, 1982.

Boyden TW. Snake venom poisoning: Diagnosis and treatment. *Ariz Med* 37:639, 1980.

Burgess JL et al. Effects of constriction bands on rattlesnake venom absorption: A pharmacokinetic study. *Ann Emerg Med* 21:1086, 1992.

Curry SC et al. Death from a rattlesnake bite. *Am J Emerg Med* 3:227, 1985.

Glass TG. Cooling for first aid in snakebite (letter). *N Engl J Med* 305:1095, 1981.

Harvey WR. Black mamba envenomation. *S Afr Med J* 67:960, 1985.

Kunkel DB. Treating snakebites sensibly. *Emerg Med* 20 (12):51, 1988.

Kunkel DB et al. Reptile envenomations. *J Toxicol Toxicol* 21:503, 1984.

Mentor SA. Beware: Nonpoisonous snakes. *J Clin Toxicol* 15:259, 1979.

Pearn J et al. Efficacy of a constrictive bandage with limb immobilization in the management of human envenomation. *Med J Aust* 6(6):293, 1981.

Peppers MP, Bramhall P. Therapy for snakebites. *Emergency* 25(8):20, 1993.

Podgorny G. Snakebite in the United States. *Ann Emerg Med* 12:651, 1983.

Pruchnicki S. The serpent and the responder: Treating snakebites. *JEMS* 18(4):34, 1993.

Russell FE. *Snake Venom Poisoning.* Philadelphia: Lippincott, 1980.

Russell FE. Rattlesnake bite. *JAMA* 245:1579, 1981.

Russell FE. When a snake strikes. *Emerg Med* 22(12):21, 1990.

Steuven H et al. Cobra envenomation: An uncommon emergency. *Ann Emerg Med* 12:636, 1983.

Stewart ME et al. First-aid treatment of poisonous snakebite: Are currently recommended procedures justified? *Ann Emerg Med* 10:331, 1980.

Sutherland SK et al. New first aid measures for envenomation. *Med J Aust* 1:378, 1980.

Watt CW. Snakebite: Don't cool it. *Emerg Med Serv* 8(3):10, 1979.

Wingert WA, Chan L. Rattlesnake bites in southern California and rationale for recommended treatment. *West J Med* 148:37, 1988.

Winneberger TR et al. Snakebite treatment in the 80's. *NC Med J* 46:572, 1985.

OTHER BITES AND STINGS

Arnold R. Brown recluse spider bites: Five cases with a review of the literature. *JACEP* 5:262, 1976.

Auerbach PS. Marine envenomations. *N Engl J Med* 325:486, 1991.

Batista da Costa M, Bonito RF, Nishioka SA. An outbreak of vampire bat bite in a Brazilian village. *Trop Med Parasitol* 44:219, 1993.

Bengston K et al. Sudden death in a child following jellyfish envenomation by *Chiropsalmus quadrumanus. JAMA* 266:1404, 1991.

Beware the imported fire ant. *Emerg Med* 22(11):36, 1990.

Bond GR. Antivenin administration for *Centuroides* scorpion sting: Risks and benefits. *Ann Emerg Med* 21:788, 1992.

Burnett JW, Calton GJ. Jellyfish envenomation syndromes updated. *Ann Emerg Med* 16:1000, 1987.

Burnett JW et al. Environment vs. man: Gila monster bites. *Cutis* 35:323, 1985.

Candiotti KA, Lamas AM. Adverse neurologic reactions to the sting of the imported fire ant. *Int Arch Allergy Immunol* 102:417, 1993.

Clark RF et al. Clinical presentation and treatment of black widow spider envenomation: A review of 163 cases. *Ann Emerg Med* 21:782, 1992.

Curry SC et al. Envenomation by the scorpion *Centuroides sculpturatus. J Toxicol Clin Toxicol* 21:417, 1984.

DeShazo RD, Butcher BT, Banks WA. Reactions to the stings of the imported fire ant. *N Engl J Med* 323:462, 1990.

Erickson EH, Estes JB. The buzz on subduing bees and wasps. *JEMS* 18(3):119, 1993.

Erikson T et al. The emergency management of moray eel bites. *Ann Emerg Med* 21:212, 1992.

Feinberg SM. Allergic reactions to insect stings. *Hosp Med* 10:8, 1974.

Frazier CA. Emergency treatment of insect stings and bites. *Emerg Med Serv* 6(4):8, 1977.

Ginsburg CM. Fire ant envenomation in children. *Pediatrics* 73:689, 1984.

Green VA et al. Bites and stings of Hymenoptera, caterpillar and beetle. *J Toxicol Clin Toxicol* 21:491, 1984.

Groshong TD. Scorpion envenomation in Saudi Arabia. *Ann Emerg Med* 22:1431, 1993.

Gross ML, Millikan LE. The bite of the brown recluse spider. *Emerg Med* 23(12):45, 1991.

Jonas M, Cunha B. The ticks of summer. *Emerg Med* 14 (12):146, 1982.

Key GF. A comparison of calcium gluconate and methocarbamol (Robaxin) in the treatment of latrodectism (black widow spider envenomation). *Am J Trop Med Hyg* 30:273, 1981.

Kizer KW. Marine envenomations. *J Toxicol Clin Toxicol* 21: 527, 1984.

Kizer KW. Scorpaenidae envenomation: A five-year poison center experience. *JAMA* 253:807, 1985.

Kobernick M. Black widow spider bite. *Am Fam Physician* 29:241, 1984.

Kunkel DB. The myth of the brown recluse spider. *Emerg Med* 17(5):124, 1985.

Kunkel DB. The sting of the arthropod. *Emerg Med* 20 (12):41, 1988.

Manoguerra AS. Poisonous marine animals. *Emergency* 25(3):20, 1993.

McSwain NE. Brown recluse spider envenomation. *Emerg Med* 21(14):39, 1989.

Needham GR. Evaluation of five popular methods for tick removal. *Pediatrics* 75:997, 1985.

Powers RD. Taking care of bite wounds. *Emerg Med* 22(13):131, 1990.

Rauber A. Black widow spider bites. *J Toxicol Clin Toxicol* 21:473, 1984.

Raynor AC et al. Alligator bites and related infections. *J Fla Med Assoc* 70:107, 1983.

Rees R et al. The diagnosis and treatment of brown recluse spider bites. *Ann Emerg Med* 16:945, 1987.

Rossen CL et al. Management of marine stings and scrapes. *West J Med* 150:97, 1989.

Russell FE. Arachnid envenomations. *Emerg Med Serv* 20 (5):16, 1991.

Schultz K. Hazardous marine life. *Emerg Med Serv* 14(3):62, 1985.

Stein M et al. Portuguese man-o'-war (*Physalia physalis*) envenomation. *Ann Emerg Med* 18:312, 1989.

Streiffer RH. Bite of the venomous lizard, the gila monster (case report). *Postgrad Med* 79:297, 1986.

Sutherland SK. Lethal jellyfish. *Med J Aust* 143:536, 1985.

Thygerson A. Tick bites. *Emergency* 13(6):26, 1981.

Tu AT. Biotoxicology of sea snake venoms. *Ann Emerg Med* 16:1023, 1987.

Wasserman G. Wound care of spider and snake envenomations. *Ann Emerg Med* 17:1331, 1988.

MAMMALIAN BITES

Aghababian V et al. Mammalian bite wounds. *Ann Emerg Med* 9:79, 1980.

Anderson LJ et al. Human rabies in the United States, 1960 to 1970: Epidemiology, diagnosis and prevention. *Ann Intern Med* 100:728, 1984.

Baker MD, Moore SE. Human bites in children: A six-year experience. *Am J Dis Child* 141:1285, 1987.

Burdge D, Scheifele D, Speert D. Serious *Pasteurella multocida* infections from lion and tiger bites. *JAMA* 253: 3296, 1985.

Callaham M. Dog bite wounds. *JAMA* 244:2327, 1980.

Callaham ML. When an animal bites. *Emerg Med* 20(11):119, 1988.

Centers for Disease Control. Compendium of animal rabies vaccines 1985. *MMWR* 33:51–52, 1984.

Dire DJ. Cat bite wounds: Risk factors for infection. *Ann Emerg Med* 20:973, 1991.

Dreyfuss UY et al. Human bites of the hand: A study of one hundred six patients. *J Hand Surg* 10:884, 1985.

Early MJ et al. Human bites: A review. *Br J Plast Surg* 37:458, 1984.

Fishbein DB, Robinson LE. Rabies. *N Engl J Med* 329:1632, 1993.

Kizer KW. Epidemiologic and clinical aspects of animal bite injuries. *JACEP* 8:134, 1979.

Klein M. Nondomestic mammalian bites. *Am Fam Physician* 32:137, 1985.

Libby J, Meislin H. Human rabies. *Ann Emerg Med* 12:217, 1983.

Lindsey D et al. Natural course of the human bite wound: Incidence of infection and complications in 434 bites and 803 lacerations in the same group of patients. *J Trauma* 27:45, 1987.

Malinowski RW et al. The management of human bite injuries of the hand. *J Trauma* 19:655, 1979.

Ordog GJ et al. Rat bites: Fifty cases. *Ann Emerg Med* 14:131, 1985.

Peeples E, Boswick JA, Scott FA. Wounds of the hand contaminated by human or animal saliva. *J Trauma* 20:383, 1980.

Powers RD. Taking care of bite wounds. *Emerg Med* 22 (13):131, 1990.

Remington P, Shope T, Andrews J. A recommended approach to the evaluation of human rabies exposure in an acute-care hospital. *JAMA* 254:67, 1985.

Sacks JJ, Sattin RW, Bonzo SE. Dog bite-related fatalities from 1979 through 1988. *JAMA* 262:1489, 1989.

Tahzib A. Camel injuries. *Trop Doct* 14:187, 1984.

Taylor GA. Management of human bite injuries of the hand. *Can Med Assoc J* 133:191, 1985.

The who and how of rabies prophylaxis. *Emerg Med* 16 (14):159, 1984.

Zook EG et al. Successful treatment protocol for canine fang injuries. *J Trauma* 20:243, 1980.

ALCOHOL AND ALCOHOLISM

Adams SL, Mathews JJ, Flaherty JJ. Alcoholic ketoacidosis. *Ann Emerg Med* 16:90, 1987.

Alcouloumre E. The intoxicated patient. *Emerg Med Serv* 19(4):65, 1990.

Best J, Lawrence KE. Alcoholism in EMS: A management challenge. *Emerg Med Serv* 17(8):17, 1988.

Blume SB. Women and alcohol. *JAMA* 256:1467, 1986.

Brown CG. The alcohol withdrawal syndrome. *Ann Emerg Med* 11:276, 1982.

Caroline NL. *Emergency Medical Treatment: A Text for EMT-As and EMT-Intermediates* (3rd ed.). Boston: Little, Brown, 1991. Chap. 25.

Clark DE, McCarthy E, Robinson E. Trauma as a symptom of alcoholism (editorial). *Ann Emerg Med* 14:274, 1984.

Council on Scientific Affairs. Alcohol and the driver. *JAMA* 255:522, 1986.

Criteria Committee, National Council on Alcoholism. Criteria for the diagnosis of alcoholism. *Ann Intern Med* 77:249, 1972.

Ewing JA. Detecting alcoholism: The CAGE questionnaire. 252:1905, 1984.

Friedman IM. Alcohol and unnatural death in San Francisco youths. *Pediatrics* 76:191, 1985.

Goldfrank LR. A vitamin for an emergency. *Emerg Med* 14(16):113, 1982.

Johnson MW. Alcohol-related emergencies. *Emerg Med Serv* 12(3):51, 1983.

Knott DH, Fink RD, Morgan JC. Beware the patient with alcohol on his breath. *Emerg Med Serv* 6(3):40, 1977.

Kunkel DB. What do tests for ethanol intoxication mean? *Emerg Med* 17(7):103, 1985.

Lerner WD et al. The alcohol withdrawal syndrome. *N Engl J Med* 313:951, 1985.

Lundberg GD. Ethyl alcohol: Ancient plague and modern poison (editorial). *JAMA* 252:1911, 1984.

Madden JF. Calming the storms of alcohol withdrawal. *Emerg Med* 22(7):23, 1990.

Maull KI. Alcohol abuse: Its implications in trauma care. *South Med J* 75:794, 1982.

Maull KI, Kinning LS, Hickman JK. Culpability and accountability of hospitalized injured alcohol-impaired drivers. *JAMA* 252:1880, 1984.

McKinney HE Jr. Ethanol emergencies. *Emergency* 23(5):22, 1991.

Niven RG. Alcoholism: A problem in perspective (editorial). *JAMA* 252:1912, 1984.

O'Carroll BM. Alcohol and substance abuse emergencies: Handle with care. *Rescue* 3(5):21, 1990.

Regan TJ. Alcohol and the cardiovascular system. *JAMA* 264:377, 1990.

Scarano SJ. Emergency response: Alcohol-intoxicated patient. *Emerg Med Serv* 8(5):78, 1979.

Sellers EM, Kalant H. Alcohol intoxication and withdrawal. *N Engl J Med* 294:757, 1976.

Siscovick DS et al. Moderate alcohol consumption and primary cardiac arrest. *Am J Epidemiol* 123:499, 1986.

Smile DH. Acute alcohol withdrawal complicated by supraventricular tachycardia: Treatment with intravenous propranolol. *Ann Emerg Med* 13:53, 1984.

Stewart CE. Booze blues. *Emerg Med Serv* 21(4):39, 1992.

Taigman M. Just another drunk . . . *Emerg Med Serv* 17(8):8, 1988.

Taigman M. The battle scars of booze: Treating the chronic alcoholic. *JEMS* 14(10):45, 1989.

Thompson CJ et al. Alcoholic ketoacidosis: An underdiagnosed condition? *Br Med J* 292:463, 1986.

Thrasher MR, Thrasher CL. Prehospital treatment of acute adolescent alcoholism. *Emerg Med Serv* 14(1):32, 1985.

Treatment of alcohol withdrawal. *Med Lett Drugs Ther* 28:75, 1986.

Walker PF et al. The potentiating effects of alcohol on driver injury. *JAMA* 256:1461, 1986.

Young GP et al. Intravenous phenobarbital for alcohol withdrawal and convulsions. *Ann Emerg Med* 16:847, 1987.

28
Communicable Diseases

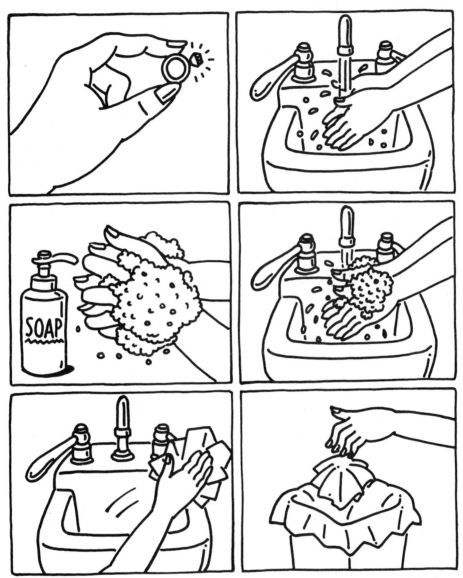

Adapted from Georgetown University Child Development Center. *Health in Day Care: A Manual for Day Care Providers*. Washington: 1986.

OBJECTIVES

Just ask for volunteers to undertake the next inter-hospital transport of a patient with meningitis or AIDS, and see how many hands *don't* go up. EMTs and paramedics who think nothing of plunging into the city's meanest streets to care for the victims of urban violence tend to suffer an acute attack of cold feet when it comes to dealing with patients who have communicable diseases. Such fears are mostly due to ignorance. A paramedic who understands how communicable diseases are transmitted and who knows how to take sensible precautions will not panic at the prospect of caring for a patient with AIDS or any other illness. In this chapter, we shall examine the ways in which communicable diseases are passed from one person to another. We shall look in particular at some of the communicable diseases that paramedics are most likely to encounter in the course of their work, as well as at those that cause the greatest anxiety among EMS personnel and the public at large. Finally, we shall review the measures that a paramedic can take to protect himself and others from contracting communicable diseases. By the end of this chapter, therefore, the student should be able to

1. List four ways in which communicable diseases may be passed from one person to another, and give an example of each
2. Define
   - Carrier
   - Communicable period
   - Incubation period
   - Fomite
   - Reservoir
3. List the usual mode(s) of transmission of
   - Rubella
   - Mumps
   - Meningitis
   - Tuberculosis
   - Syphilis
   - Type B hepatitis
   - AIDS

   and in each case state what measures the paramedic can take to minimize the risk of contracting the illness from a patient
4. Given a description of several patients with different clinical findings, identify a patient likely to be suffering from
   - One of the common contagious diseases of childhood
   - Meningitis
   - Tuberculosis
   - Hepatitis

   and describe the measures required to clean or disinfect the ambulance after each case
5. List the ways in which AIDS can be transmitted
6. List at least four universal precautions that should be taken during all procedures that involve contact with the blood or body fluids of *any* patient
7. Describe the procedure for
   - Routine cleaning of the ambulance after every call
   - Disinfection of the ambulance after transporting a patient with AIDS or hepatitis
8. List the immunizations that every paramedic should have had before starting employment

TRANSMISSION OF COMMUNICABLE DISEASES

"The only problem with being a doctor," observed a medical colleague, "is that you have to deal with sick people." That "problem," which is of course the very raison d'être of medicine, is shared by all health care workers, including paramedics. By the very nature of their work, health professionals come in contact with sick people; and a certain proportion of those sick people have contagious illnesses, that is, illnesses that can be transmitted from one person to another. It is inevitable therefore that paramedics, like other health personnel, will be exposed now and then to contagious diseases—so it is important to know what can be done to minimize the risk of contracting a contagious disease from a patient. To understand the principles of prevention, though, we need first to understand how contagious diseases are spread in the first place.

Contagious, or communicable, diseases are caused by microorganisms—usually bacteria or viruses, but sometimes also fungi. They spread from person to person by several mechanisms:

- DIRECT CONTACT with the infected person, that is, by touching. Direct contact may be as casual as a handshake or as intimate as sexual intercourse. Most cases of the common cold, for example, are now thought to be transmitted through casual direct contact. Venereal diseases, such as syphilis and gonorrhea, are transmitted principally by sexual contact and for that reason are now usually referred to as *sexually transmitted diseases,* or STDs for short.
- CONTACT WITH CONTAMINATED MATERIALS, such as a handkerchief containing the excretions of an infected person. Objects that har-

bor microorganisms and can transmit them to others are called **fomites.** Thus, for example, the towels used by a patient in the contagious period of chickenpox may serve as fomites.

- INHALATION OF INFECTED DROPLETS, such as those aerosolized into the surroundings when a person with measles coughs or sneezes.
- The BITE OF AN INFECTED ANIMAL, HUMAN, OR INSECT. The rabies virus, for example, is transmitted by the bite of an infected animal; malaria is transmitted by the bite of an infected mosquito.
- PUNCTURE BY A CONTAMINATED NEEDLE or other sharp instrument. This mode of transmission is responsible for a significant number of cases of AIDS and viral hepatitis. Puncture may happen by accident, when a health worker is careless with a needle that has been used on an infected patient; or it may happen when addicts, some of whom are infected with, say, AIDS, share needles to inject themselves with illicit drugs.
- TRANSFUSION OF CONTAMINATED BLOOD PRODUCTS. Screening tests for AIDS and viral hepatitis have vastly reduced the risks of contracting those illnesses from contaminated blood products in most developed countries, but the blood supply in much of the less developed world is still seriously compromised.

Knowing how a communicable disease is spread enables us to know what precautions we can take to avoid catching that disease and also what precautions are unnecessary. When a disease is contracted only by inhaling aerosolized droplets, for instance, wearing a surgical mask can be fully protective, while there is no need to incinerate all the linens and disposable equipment with which the patient had contact.

It is important to distinguish between exposure and infection. Simply being exposed to an infectious agent does not by any means guarantee that a person will become ill from that agent. Many other factors—including the infectivity of the agent, the intensity (dosage) of the exposure, the immune status of the exposed person—all play a role in determining whether a person exposed to a communicable disease comes down with the illness. Measles, for example, is extremely "catchy," and a majority of nonimmune individuals exposed to a person in the contagious stage of measles will break out in spots about 10 days later. Tuberculosis (TB), on the other hand, is much harder to contract; usually only those in intimate daily contact with the patient over a long period,

such as members of his immediate household, are at serious risk of catching TB from an infected person. However, a person whose immune system is compromised, perhaps by some other illness, will be more susceptible to contracting TB even after a much less intense and prolonged exposure.

Once a susceptible person has been exposed to a harmful microorganism, it still takes a certain amount of time for the microorganism to multiply within the person's body and produce symptoms. That time period—between exposure to the germ and the first symptoms of illness from it—is called the **incubation period.** In mumps, for example, it usually takes anywhere from 12 to 26 days from the time a susceptible person is exposed to the mumps virus until the patient begins to feel feverish and unwell. The incubation period for the influenza virus is much shorter—usually between 24 and 72 hours from the time of exposure to the time symptoms begin.

Most communicable diseases are *contagious* only during a portion of the illness. A person may, for instance, be sick with chickenpox for a couple of weeks, but he is capable of transmitting chickenpox to another individual only for about 1 week: from 1 day before the vesicles appear on the skin to about 6 days after. The portion of an illness during which a person can transmit the illness to someone else is called the **communicable period.**

Just as we made a distinction between exposure and infection, we also need to distinguish between contamination and infection. Any person or object that has harmful microorganisms on it or in it is **contaminated.** That applies to water, food, dressing materials, linens, other equipment, and even the ambulance. A person is not **infected,** however, unless the microorganisms involved produce an illness or other abnormal state. Some people walk around all the time harboring a whole collection of potentially harmful microorganisms but are not sick from those microorganisms. Such individuals are called **carriers;** that is, they *carry* an infectious agent—such as the bacteria that cause typhoid—and although they are not themselves ill, they can transmit the illness in question to others.

Another concept important in understanding disease transmission is that of a reservoir. In the context of communicable disease, a **reservoir** is a place where germs live and multiply. In institutional settings, for example, air-conditioning systems have been identified as reservoirs for the bacterial agent that causes Legionnaire's disease. In *ambulances*, the oxygen humidifier is commonly implicated as a reservoir for infection. The existence of things like fomites, carriers, and reservoirs means that health care personnel have a responsibility not only to protect *themselves* from contracting communicable diseases but also to ensure that they and their equipment do not become means for transmitting illness to others.

In the sections that follow, we shall look at some of the communicable diseases that are particularly common or that elicit particular anxiety among paramedics. The risks of handling patients with communicable diseases are real, but they should not be exaggerated, and certainly they should not be a source of fear and stress. Fear comes from ignorance, and there is no reason for a paramedic to be ignorant about health issues.

COMMON COMMUNICABLE DISEASES OF CHILDHOOD

The most striking thing about the "common" communicable diseases of childhood is that they are no longer so common, at least not in developed countries. Thirty years ago, it was the rare child who reached his teens without having had measles, chickenpox, and usually mumps as well. Now widespread immunization has drastically reduced the incidence of many of the communicable diseases of childhood. Nonetheless, there are still sporadic cases and even occasional epidemic outbreaks of those diseases, some of which may cause particular problems if contracted in adulthood.

Measles

Measles—also variously known as rubeola, hard measles, or red measles—is a highly communicable viral disease characterized by fever, conjunctivitis, cough, and a blotchy red rash. Measles is one of the most easily transmitted of the communicable diseases. TRANSMISSION is by aerosolized *droplets* or direct contact with the nasal or pharyngeal secretions of an infected person. Less commonly, measles is spread by contact with articles recently soiled by the patient's nasal or throat sections. The INCUBATION PERIOD is about 10 days from exposure to the onset of fever and about 14 days from exposure until the rash appears, and the COMMUNICABLE PERIOD starts at the time of the first symptoms (about 4 days before the rash) and then declines rapidly by about 2 days after the rash appears.

While wearing a mask may protect against droplet transmission, the only certain protection against measles is immunity. Any person who has had a documented case of measles or who received live measles vaccine after 1968 can be assumed to be immune to measles. Anyone else is susceptible, and

among health care workers, all susceptible individuals should be immunized.

No special disinfection measures are required for the ambulance after carrying a patient known to have measles. (Routine disinfection for the ambulance is described in a later section.) Simply washing and airing out the vehicle and laundering any soiled linens are sufficient.

> **WASH YOUR HANDS AFTER EVERY CALL.**

Rubella

Rubella, also known as German measles, is characterized by a low-grade fever, headache, runny nose, and usually a diffuse rash that may look a bit like the rash of measles. When it occurs in children, rubella is ordinarily a mild, uncomplicated illness. When it occurs in women during the first 3 to 4 months of pregnancy, however, rubella may cause severe abnormalities in the developing fetus, including deafness, cataracts, mental retardation, and heart defects.

Rubella occurs most commonly during the winter and spring and is highly communicable to susceptible individuals. It is TRANSMITTED by direct contact with the nasopharyngeal secretions of an infected person—either by droplet spread or by touching the patient or articles freshly contaminated with the patient's secretions. The INCUBATION PERIOD is 2 to 3 weeks, and the COMMUNICABLE PERIOD starts about a week before the rash appears and continues until 4 days after the rash becomes evident.

As in the case of measles, the only certain protection against rubella is immunity. All women working as paramedics should be immunized against rubella before starting their employment. No special measures are needed to disinfect the ambulance after carrying a patient known to have rubella.

> **WASH YOUR HANDS AFTER EVERY CALL.**

Mumps

If rubella is a matter of particular concern for female paramedics, mumps should worry any male paramedic who did not have the illness or receive immunization against it as a child. Mumps is a viral disease that occurs most commonly in winter and spring. In children, mumps is characterized by fever along with swelling and tenderness of one of the salivary glands, usually the parotid. When it occurs in males past the age of puberty, however, mumps causes a very painful inflammation of the testicles (**orchitis**) in up to 25 percent of cases, which may result in sterility.

TRANSMISSION of mumps is by droplet spread or direct contact with the saliva of an infected person. The INCUBATION PERIOD is 12 to 26 days, and the illness remains COMMUNICABLE for as long as 9 days after the salivary glands swell up.

All male paramedics should be immunized against mumps before starting employment if they did not have the illness as a child or undergo immunization in the past. Routine cleaning and airing of the ambulance are indicated after carrying a patient with mumps, and any articles soiled with the patient's nasopharyngeal secretions should be disinfected.

> **WASH YOUR HANDS AFTER EVERY CALL.**

Chickenpox

Chickenpox, or varicella, is a highly contagious viral disease that produces a slight fever, mild systemic symptoms, and a vesicular rash that gradually crusts over, leaving a series of scabs. The rash comes in crops, moving from one part of the body to another. The same virus—herpesvirus 3, or varicella virus— that produces chickenpox in children causes **herpes zoster** ("shingles") in adults. In herpes zoster, a crop of vesicles appears from time to time in the distribution of a single or associated group of spinal nerves (a dermatome). Zoster can be extremely painful and, when it occurs on the chest, can be mistaken for an acute myocardial infarction if the patient is seen before the characteristic vesicles pop up.

TRANSMISSION of varicella virus is by direct contact or droplet spread of respiratory secretions from patients with chickenpox. Contact with the vesicular fluid of patients with either chickenpox or zoster, and probably contact with articles recently contaminated by that fluid, can also transmit the virus. Contrary to popular belief, however, the dried scabs from varicella lesions are not infective. The INCUBATION PERIOD for chickenpox is 2 to 3 weeks, and the COMMUNICABLE PERIOD starts a few days be-

fore the appearance of the rash and lasts up to about 6 days after the first vesicles become apparent.

Having chickenpox as a child usually provides lifelong immunity against another infection. In a certain proportion of cases, however, the virus apparently remains latent (quiet) within the body only to reemerge years later, often after some stress, in the form of herpes zoster. When transporting a patient known to have chickenpox or shingles, paramedics should preferably wear mask and gown, which should be removed and disposed of (or laundered, if not disposable) immediately after the case. Gloves should also be worn and discarded after the case, and the paramedic should shower and change clothes on returning to base. Any articles soiled by the patient's nasopharyngeal secretions or fluid from the cutaneous vesicles should be thoroughly disinfected, and the ambulance should be cleaned and aired as usual.

> **WASH YOUR HANDS AFTER EVERY CALL.**

OTHER COMMON OR SERIOUS COMMUNICABLE DISEASES

Meningitis

Meningitis is an inflammation of the meninges, the membranes that cover the brain and spinal cord. With the exception of AIDS, few other illnesses provoke so much panic among ambulance personnel, although there is seldom any need for more than routine precautions in handling patients suspected to have meningitis.

Meningitis may be caused by a wide variety of different bacteria, viruses, and other microorganisms, and the contagiousness of the illness depends to a considerable extent on the type of microorganism involved. The type of meningitis most often involved in epidemic outbreaks is that caused by the meningococcus bacteria (*Neisseria meningitidis*) and hence called **meningococcal meningitis.** Sporadic cases of meningococcal meningitis occur most frequently during winter and spring, but epidemic outbreaks can occur any time, especially when there are young people living together under crowded conditions, as in military barracks. TRANSMISSION is by droplet spread or direct contact with the nasopharyngeal secretions of infected persons, most often from carriers rather than from people who are actually sick with the disease. Fomite transmission scarcely ever occurs, since the meningococcus is not a very hardy bacterium, and it is easily killed by chilling or drying. The INCUBATION PERIOD for meningococcal meningitis is between 2 and 10 days. The COMMUNICABLE PERIOD is variable; it lasts as long as meningococcal bacteria are present in the patient's nasal and oral secretions. Usually the microorganism disappears from the patient's upper respiratory tract within 24 hours of starting antibiotic treatment.

The classic SIGNS AND SYMPTOMS of meningitis include *fever, headache,* and *stiff neck*. There are almost always *changes in the state of consciousness,* ranging from apathy to delirium. *Vomiting* is common. In meningococcal meningitis, the onset of symptoms may be very sudden, and in addition, there is apt to be a characteristic *rash*, which may be blotchy red or bluish. Other types of meningitis tend to come on more slowly, preceded by a few days of sore throat, runny nose, and other upper respiratory symptoms.

SYMPTOMS AND SIGNS OF MENINGOCOCCAL MENINGITIS

- FEVER
- SEVERE HEADACHE
- STIFF NECK
- Some CHANGE IN THE STATE OF CONSCIOUSNESS
- VOMITING
- Sometimes a blotchy red or bluish RASH

If you are transporting a patient known or suspected to have meningitis, you can minimize your risk of catching the illness (which is not very great to begin with) by taking a few simple precautions:

- Since transmission occurs primarily through droplet spread, WEAR A SURGICAL MASK to protect yourself from inhaling infected droplets.
- When you have finished the call, place in a plastic bag all disposable materials that have come in contact with the patient's nasopharyngeal discharge and dispose of the bag as directed by hospital personnel. Then DISINFECT ARTICLES THAT HAVE COME IN CONTACT WITH THE PATIENT'S SECRETIONS (e.g., bag-valve-mask).
- AIR OUT THE VEHICLE, and send any used linens and bedding to the laundry.
- WASH YOUR HANDS THOROUGHLY (which you should do anyway after every call!).
- STAY IN TOUCH WITH THE HOSPITAL to

which you transported the patient, for follow-up on the patient's diagnosis. If it turns out that the patient has meningococcal meningitis, check with your medical director. Under certain circumstances people who have been exposed to meningicoccal meningitis are given sulfonamide drugs as a preventive measure.

WASH YOUR HANDS AFTER EVERY CALL.

Tuberculosis

Tuberculosis, or TB, was once widespread in the United States, taking an enormous toll, especially among people in the prime of life, and TB remains an important cause of disability and death in much of the world. In the United States and other industrialized countries, the incidence of tuberculosis started to drop dramatically during the 1940s. By the 1950s and 1960s, many specialized tuberculosis hospitals were closing down, and TB seemed on the way out. The past few years, however, have seen the opposite trend—a disturbing *rise* in the incidence of tuberculosis. In 1992, nearly 27,000 new cases of TB were reported in the United States, a 20 percent increase from 1985 (the year with the lowest number of TB cases). Part, but certainly not all, of the increase has been associated with AIDS. Other factors thought to contribute to the rising incidence of TB are substance abuse, poverty, limited access to health care, substandard housing, and homelessness.

Tuberculosis is *not* a highly contagious disease. It is *not* spread on hands, dishes, utensils, or other fomites, so the practice of incinerating the patient's linens or isolating his eating utensils is completely unnecessary. TRANSMISSION of the bacteria that cause tuberculosis usually occurs by droplet spread from a person with active disease. In general, that type of spread occurs among people who have continued and intimate exposure to the infected individual, chiefly those living in the same household. For the paramedic, such intense exposure is likely to occur only in cases when mouth-to-mouth ventilation is given to a patient with active tuberculosis.

The INCUBATION PERIOD for tuberculosis is 4 to 8 weeks. The disease becomes communicable, however, only when an active lesion develops in the lungs; from that point on, the COMMUNICABLE PERIOD lasts as long as infective tubercle bacilli are being discharged in the sputum, that is, until about 24 to 48 hours after antibiotic treatment has been started.

The SIGNS AND SYMPTOMS of a person's initial infection with TB are usually minimal. In fact, most patients don't have any symptoms at all when first infected, and the disease ordinarily lies dormant for many years before the signs that are commonly associated with TB—night sweats, headache, cough, and weight loss—occur. Early infection with TB can, however, be detected with a special skin test, called a **tuberculin test,** and also by chest x-ray. Every health worker, including paramedics, should have a tuberculin test at the beginning of his or her employment and annually thereafter, and should be x-rayed if the tuberculin test becomes positive ("converts") at any time.

Since the incubation period for TB is 4 to 8 weeks, the paramedic who suspects he or she has been exposed to TB should wait about 2 months from the time of the exposure before having a repeat tuberculin test. If the test has become positive at that time, the individual will usually be given a year's course of antibiotic therapy.

No special measures are required after transporting a patient suspected of having active TB. The vehicle should be thoroughly aired and cleaned, as usual. Linens should be laundered, and disposable equipment that was in contact with the patient should be safely disposed of.

> ## WASH YOUR HANDS AFTER EVERY CALL.

Sexually Transmitted Diseases

As the term implies, sexually transmitted diseases (STDs) are those that are usually acquired by sexual contact. While the term *STD* ordinarily conjures up diagnoses such as gonorrhea or syphilis, in fact the range of diseases that are transmitted sexually is very wide and includes such conditions as herpes, hepatitis, and AIDS. We shall consider hepatitis and AIDS separately. In this section, we shall review briefly the features of gonorrhea, syphilis, and herpes infections.

Gonorrhea

Gonorrhea is an infection caused by the gonococcal bacteria, *Neisseria gonorrhoeae.* It is TRANSMITTED sexually, by contact with the purulent exudates from mucous membranes of infected persons. The INCUBATION PERIOD is usually 2 to 7 days but may be

longer, and it can remain COMMUNICABLE for months if not treated. The SYMPTOMS AND SIGNS of gonorrhea differ between males and females. In *males,* there is usually a purulent discharge from the urethra and often pain on urination (dysuria) starting a few days after the exposure. In females, an initial inflammation of the urethra may be so mild that it passes unnoticed, and the illness may percolate quietly until it presents as **pelvic inflammatory disease,** with signs and symptoms of an acute abdomen. Depending on the sexual practices of the patient, gonorrheal infection may also involve the anus and throat.

The risk of acquiring any of the STDs, including gonorrhea, through anything but sexual contact is very small. Routine measures, including careful disposal or disinfection of materials soiled by discharge and thorough handwashing are all that is required for paramedic safety.

> ## WASH YOUR HANDS AFTER EVERY CALL.

Syphilis

Syphilis is an acute and chronic disease caused by the spiral-shaped bacteria *Treponema pallidum.* It is TRANSMITTED by direct contact with the infectious exudates of the disease lesions; it can be transmitted across the placenta from an infected mother to her fetus; and, rarely, it can be transmitted by contact with contaminated articles. Health workers have occasionally developed primary syphilis lesions after touching infectious cutaneous lesions of patients. The INCUBATION PERIOD for syphilis is 10 days to 10 weeks, and syphilis may remain COMMUNICABLE for as long as 3 or 4 years if untreated. Within about 48 hours of adequate treatment with penicillin, however, communicability ceases.

The initial infection with syphilis (primary syphilis) produces an ulcerative lesion, called a **chancre,** of the skin or mucous membrane, often with a painless, enlarged lymph node in the area draining the site of the lesion (e.g., the groin). Some weeks later, there may be a transient fever and rash. The signs and symptoms of syphilis are so variable, however, that the disease has traditionally been called "the great imitator."

Routine precautions are sufficient when transporting a patient suspected to have syphilis. Gloves and universal precautions for the disposal of needles, blood, and body fluids are all that is required.

WASH YOUR HANDS AFTER EVERY CALL.

Genital Herpes

Genital herpes is a chronic, recurrent illness produced by herpes simplex virus (HSV) type 2 and is characterized by vesicular lesions. In women, the vesicles occur initially on the cervix; during recurrent infections, vesicles may appear as well around the vulva, legs, and buttocks. In men, lesions are most common on the penis, as well as around the anus and mouth among homosexuals. TRANSMISSION is usually by sexual contact, but infants may become infected if delivered through the birth canal of a woman with active disease. The INCUBATION PERIOD is 2 to 12 days, and genital lesions remain COMMUNICABLE for 4 to 7 days. In about 50 percent of women with genital herpes, the disease is reactivated, often repeatedly over many years.

No special precautions are necessary in transporting a patient known or suspected to have genital herpes.

WASH YOUR HANDS AFTER EVERY CALL.

Viral Hepatitis

As the name implies, viral hepatitis is an inflammation of the liver produced by a virus. In fact, there are several distinct forms of viral hepatitis, produced by different viruses and varying somewhat from one another in their means of transmission and clinical manifestations. We shall consider here two types of viral hepatitis, known as type A and type B respectively, that account for the vast majority of hepatitis cases in the United States.

Type A, or **infectious hepatitis,** accounts for about 30 percent of hepatitis cases in the United States. It is TRANSMITTED by the fecal-oral route, that is, by ingestion of food or water that has been contaminated by infected feces. Epidemic outbreaks are most often traced to contaminated drinking water, milk, sliced meats, and undercooked shellfish. The INCUBATION PERIOD for hepatitis A is usually about 4 weeks, although it can range from 15 to 50 days after ingestion of the virus. The COMMUNICABLE PERIOD probably starts toward the end of the incubation period and continues for a few days after the patient becomes jaundiced. Ordinarily, illness from type A hepatitis starts rather abruptly and lasts for only a week or two, although it may take a long time before the patient feels "100 percent."

Type B, or **serum hepatitis,** accounts for about 50 percent of hepatitis cases in the United States. TRANSMISSION is almost always through sexual contact or through puncture of the skin with contaminated needles. (Occasionally other objects, such as shared razors, tattoo needles, or acupuncture needles have been implicated in transmission.) Type B hepatitis is therefore particularly common in intravenous drug users who share the same needles to "shoot up." Health care workers, especially those involved in surgery, dentistry, and emergency medicine, are also at particularly high risk of contracting hepatitis through accidental needlestick injuries and other exposures to the blood and body fluids of patients. The prevalence of antigenic markers of hepatitis B virus (HBV) among emergency physicians, for example, is five times higher than among the general population. Among EMTs and paramedics, 15 to 22 percent have been found to have been infected with HBV.

The INCUBATION PERIOD for type B hepatitis varies widely—usually somewhere from 45 to 180 days. The COMMUNICABLE PERIOD starts weeks before the first symptoms appear and may persist for years in chronic carriers. Type B hepatitis usually comes on gradually, with anorexia (loss of appetite), nausea, vomiting, vague abdominal discomfort, and sometimes aching in the joints. The very smell of food may provoke nausea, and smokers often notice a sudden distaste for cigarettes. After a week or two of such symptoms, the urine begins to turn dark, and then a day or two later, the patient develops **jaundice,** a yellowing of the skin, and scleral **icterus,** a yellowing of the eyes. (Not every patient with jaundice has hepatitis. But probably every patient with jaundice should be treated *as if* he had hepatitis, in terms of precautions with blood and body fluids.) There is usually a low-grade fever, and the patient feels very tired—"like a limp rag."

**SYMPTOMS AND SIGNS
OF HEPATITIS**

- ANOREXIA
- NAUSEA at the smell of food; sometimes VOMITING
- Sudden DISTASTE FOR CIGARETTES among smokers

- Generalized FATIGUE and MALAISE
- Low-grade FEVER
- DARK URINE
- JAUNDICE

Type B hepatitis usually lasts several weeks, although complete recovery may take 3 to 4 months. A significant proportion of patients, however, develop a chronic infection that may last a lifetime and that also predisposes to other serious illnesses, such as cancer of the liver. All told, hepatitis B is not a nice disease to contract.

Fortunately, there is a very safe and effective vaccine against hepatitis B, and every paramedic should be immunized against the virus before starting employment. Even those who are immunized, however, cannot afford to get sloppy in their care of hepatitis patients, for the vaccine protects only against hepatitis *B*; it offers no protection against hepatitis A or any of several other forms of viral hepatitis classified as non-A, non-B hepatitis.

The PRECAUTIONS necessary in transporting a patient suspected of having hepatitis follow logically from what we know of its means of spread:

- Most important of all, HANDLE WITH EXTREME CARE ALL NEEDLES AND IV EQUIPMENT USED FOR A PATIENT WITH JAUNDICE. Indeed, if you get into the habit of *always* exercising extreme care with needles and IV equipment, you won't need to start doing everything differently when you suddenly encounter a patient with yellow eyes. Those precautions include the following:
  1. Wear GLOVES to start an IV or whenever there is potential exposure to blood or other body fluids.
  2. *Never* recap, remove, bend, or break needles after use or manipulate them in any other way by hand.
  3. Dispose of syringes, needles, scalpel blades, and other sharp items in a puncture-resistant container kept within easy reach.
- WASH YOUR HANDS thoroughly after the call.
- DISINFECT all equipment contaminated with the patient's blood or saliva. Air out the ambulance. Send soiled linen to the laundry.
- STAY IN TOUCH WITH THE HOSPITAL to which the patient was transported for follow-up on the diagnosis. If the patient is found to have type A hepatitis, consult your medical director about getting a shot of immune globulin.

> **WASH YOUR HANDS AFTER EVERY CALL.**

Acquired Immunodeficiency Syndrome (AIDS)

No disease elicits so much panic among the general public and also among ambulance personnel as the acquired immunodeficiency syndrome, or AIDS. Perhaps that is because AIDS is still a relatively new disease and we do not know yet how to control it. Or perhaps because its victims are usually young people—people with whom paramedics can readily identify—and because they usually die. All of those factors combine to make AIDS one of the most feared conditions since the Black Death. Regrettably, that fear has prompted more than one instance of highly unprofessional and totally unacceptable behavior, such as refusal to provide ambulance services to AIDS patients.

Fear, as we noted earlier, comes mostly from ignorance, and ignorance about AIDS is unjustifiable for medical personnel. It is true that we do not yet know how to cure AIDS. But we have nonetheless learned a great deal about the illness in a very short time.

The Epidemiology of AIDS

During the past decade or so, AIDS has rapidly become a global health problem. Worldwide, it is estimated that between 5 and 10 million people are already infected with the virus that causes AIDS; in the United States, the number of people infected with the virus is 1.0 to 1.5 million. As of December 1991, 206,392 AIDS cases—that is, patients with clinical AIDS disease—had been reported in the United States, more than two-thirds of whom had died. By the end of 1992, there was an estimated cumulative total of 380,000 AIDS cases in the United States, among whom there were about 263,000 deaths. Furthermore, in 1993, when nearly 34,000 Americans died of AIDS, AIDS became the number one cause of death among American men aged 25 to 44 years. It is clear, therefore, that all health care providers will, at least during the next decade, be dealing with more and more patients who are either carrying the AIDS virus or actually ill with the disease.

As noted, AIDS is caused by a virus, now known as the **human immunodeficiency virus,** or **HIV.** The AIDS virus does its damage by attacking a person's immune system and thereby impairing the ability to fight off infections and other illnesses that depend on intact immune defenses (e.g., some cancers). The patient with AIDS, therefore, becomes extremely vulnerable to a whole variety of bacterial, viral, and fungal infections that would not afflict a person with a normal immune system.

TRANSMISSION of HIV can occur in three ways: sexually; parenterally, through contaminated blood or blood products; and across the placenta.

- In the United States, approximately 60 percent of patients with AIDS acquired the illness through SEXUAL CONTACT. The vast majority of patients who acquired the disease sexually, furthermore, have been *homosexual males* (56% of all AIDS cases).
- PARENTERAL TRANSMISSION accounts for most of the remaining cases. The largest group infected by this mode of transmission are *intravenous drug users* (about 25 percent of all AIDS cases), who contract the disease by sharing needles. Before 1985, a significant number of *patients requiring transfusion*—especially hemophiliacs—became infected by receiving blood or blood products contaminated with HIV. Since screening of all blood donors for HIV was implemented in 1985, transmission of HIV by transfusion is no longer a major source of infection, although there is still a very small but identifiable risk of HIV infection even after receipt of screened blood. Accidental exposure to blood products, as may occur as a result of needlestick injury, is another theoretical source of HIV infection, although to date it has not proved to be a significant source (see below).
- Finally, HIV can be transmitted from an infected mother to her fetus or newborn baby. Although HIV is present in the breast milk of infected mothers, most transmission probably occurs while the baby is still in the uterus. It is now estimated that between 1,500 and 2,000 new infections occur each year in newborns in the United States as a result of perinatal transmission.

It should be emphasized that after nearly 15 years of intensive investigation, there is still no evidence whatsoever of AIDS transmission by casual or even household contact. Even among individuals routinely sharing eating utensils, toothbrushes (!), and razors with HIV-infected patients, there has been no evidence of an increased rate of HIV infection. All of the evidence then, points to the conclusion that

AIDS IS NOT A HIGHLY COMMUNICABLE DISEASE.

The only means of transmission, as noted, are through sexual contact, contaminated blood products, or from infected mother to fetus.

In considering the INCUBATION PERIOD of AIDS, it is important to distinguish between patients who are infected with HIV but still asymptomatic (carriers) and those who have developed clinical signs of the disease. As noted earlier, it is estimated that there are currently as many as 1.5 million Americans who have been infected with HIV; of that number, a little over 250,000 have developed clinical manifestations of AIDS. So there are, in a sense, *two* incubation periods to consider. The first—from the time of exposure to the time a person's blood tests positive for AIDS (becomes **seropositive,** or HIV-positive)—may be anywhere from a few weeks to a few months. So a person who has had a possible exposure to AIDS—say, after an accidental needlestick injury—should be tested for HIV within 2 to 3 weeks after the exposure and then again at 6 weeks, 3 months, 6 months, and a year after.

The second incubation period is the time between documented infection (i.e., becoming HIV-positive) and the development of the disease AIDS. In patients who have contracted AIDS from contaminated blood transfusion, the mean incubation period after infection has been approximately 8 *years* for adults and 2 years for children. Among male homosexuals presumed to have become HIV-positive as a consequence of sexual activity, the mean incubation period is approximately 7 years. From those and other data, it has therefore been calculated that about half of seropositive patients will develop AIDS within 9 years and very nearly all seropositive patients will develop AIDS within 15 years. Once AIDS has developed, the life expectancy is not, as noted earlier, very cheerful, although there *are* patients who have survived AIDS, and new treatment approaches are constantly being tried.

The COMMUNICABLE PERIOD of AIDS is not known but is presumed to continue throughout the time that a patient is seropositive, *even before the patient develops clinically apparent AIDS.* That point is very important. Recall that for every patient with AIDS, there are nine asymptomatic HIV carriers, and as far as we know, those carriers are just as capable of transmitting the virus as patients with full-blown AIDS. What all of that means is that in the majority of cases, emergency personnel will not know when they are dealing with a patient capable of transmitting AIDS. Indeed, in quite a number of cases, the patients themselves may not know. Surveys of patients presenting to emergency departments have, in fact, shown that around 6 percent of seriously ill or injured patients turn out to be HIV-positive; and when you're working in a ditch by the side of the road, trying to resuscitate an unconscious, bleeding accident victim, there's *no way* you can know whether he is or is not HIV-positive. Clearly, there is only one safe course of action under such circumstances:

ASSUME THAT EVERY PATIENT YOU TREAT IS HIV-POSITIVE, EVEN YOUR GRANDMOTHER.

Precautions Necessary in Dealing with HIV-Positive Patients

For the reasons just mentioned, the precautions required in caring for HIV-positive patients are, in fact, precautions that should be taken in caring for *every* patient. For that reason, the safety measures involved are known as **universal precautions.** We shall detail in the next section *all* of the recommended universal precautions, but it should be mentioned that the precautions that are by far the most important are those dealing with the handling of sharp objects. As of this writing, there have been fewer than 50 documented cases worldwide of health workers becoming HIV-positive as a consequence of an occupational exposure to AIDS (only one of those health workers, incidentally, has been in EMS). Among those cases, the majority were a result of needlestick injury, and one resulted from being cut with a contaminated sharp object. Notably, very few of the needlestick injuries occurred during actual management of the patient. Usually they were the result of trying to recap a needle after use or of unsafe disposal of a needle after use.

In addition to employing universal precautions, there are some additional precautions applicable to situations in which the patient is *known* to have AIDS or is in a category at high risk for AIDS (e.g., a known intravenous drug user):

- Restrict pregnant EMTs from contact with known AIDS patients. While pregnancy does not increase susceptibility to AIDS, the potential consequences of HIV infection in a pregnant woman are grave—for if mother is infected, the chances are as high as 50 percent that her fetus will be infected. Furthermore, AIDS patients, because of their deficient immunity, often harbor other microorganisms, such as cytomegalovirus, that are potentially damaging to a developing fetus.

- It is a good idea for the known AIDS patient to WEAR A MASK while in your care and while waiting to be seen in the emergency room—for *his* protection, not yours! Recall that the patient suffering from AIDS has a severely compromised immune system and is therefore unusually vulnerable to every microorganism to which he might be exposed. Recall too that you spend all your time dealing with sick people, so you are very likely to be carrying around all kinds of microorganisms. Those microorganisms do not cause *you* any problems because you have a robust immune system, but they could cause devastating problems to the patient with AIDS. So PROTECT THE AIDS PATIENT FROM ACQUIRING AN INFECTION FROM YOU OR YOUR CREW.

- After the transport, air the vehicle and clean the interior thoroughly with disinfectant solution such as a 1:10 dilution of sodium hypochlorite (household bleach). Incinerate any disposable items, such as oxygen masks, that were in contact with the patient. Double-bag used linens, tag them with a "biohazard" label, and make sure the linens are laundered in hot water.

One other thing we forgot to mention:

WASH YOUR HANDS AFTER EVERY CALL.

STANDARD PRECAUTIONS AGAINST DISEASE TRANSMISSION

The immunization of all paramedics against communicable diseases they might encounter, the implementation of universal precautions, and a little common sense should reduce the risks of contracting a communicable disease from a patient to very near zero. Furthermore, simple routine measures for cleaning the ambulance and its equipment should also reduce the chances of the ambulance becoming a source of infection to the patients you care for.

Personal Precautions

There are basically two complementary strategies by which a paramedic can protect himself or herself from contracting a communicable disease. The first is, broadly speaking, to be healthy, that is, to pay attention to things like sufficient sleep, a good diet, a program of stress reduction, and a complete, up-to-date set of immunizations. The second is to observe universal precautions in dealing with the patients you care for in the field.

Immunizations

Before starting employment, every paramedic should have completed an immunization schedule. In general, the immunizations recommended for paramedics are the same as those recommended for the general public, with the addition of immunization against hepatitis B. But owing to the likelihood of exposure, it is particularly important that emergency care personnel make sure their immunizations are complete and up-to-date.

IMMUNIZATIONS FOR PARAMEDICS

- DPT (diphtheria-pertussis-tetanus) in childhood; tetanus booster every 10 years
- MEASLES
- MUMPS
- RUBELLA (German measles; mandatory for female paramedics)
- POLIO
- HEPATITIS B

In addition, paramedics should have a preemployment chest x-ray and tuberculin test followed up by an annual general checkup and a tuberculin test.

Universal Precautions

Universal precautions are, as mentioned, precautions that should be carried out in caring for *every* patient, no matter what the patient's chief complaint, age, sex, social or economic background.

UNIVERSAL PRECAUTIONS

- WEAR GLOVES whenever a case involves potential exposure to blood or other body fluids. Use heavy-duty rubber gloves for extricating accident victims or cleaning up contaminated areas. Wear surgical latex gloves for performing venipunctures, for touching mucous membranes or nonintact skin, or whenever there is a possibility of exposure to blood or body fluids. CHANGE GLOVES after contact with each patient. DISCARD USED GLOVES immediately after use in an appropriate receptable (e.g., a plastic bag with a "biohazard" label). WASH YOUR HANDS immediately after you remove your gloves.
- Use additional BARRIER PROTECTION (*mask, protective eyewear, face shield, gown*) during any procedure that is likely to generate splashes of blood or other body fluids.
- WASH YOUR HANDS or any other skin surfaces immediately and thoroughly if they become contaminated with blood or other body fluids. In the field, carry antiseptic wipes for that purpose. In the emergency room and at your base, use lots of soap and hot water to wash your hands.
- Handle all NEEDLES, INTRAVENOUS EQUIPMENT, and SHARP INSTRUMENTS with extreme care:
  1. *Never* recap, remove, bend, or break needles after use or manipulate them in any other way by hand.
  2. Dispose of syringes, needles, scalpel blades, and other sharp items in a puncture-resistant container kept within easy reach.
- Although saliva has *not* been implicated in HIV transmission, it is preferable for health workers to use a pocket mask (with one-way valve) or bag-valve-mask for artificial ventilation. Such devices, therefore, should always be immediately accessible—which you can ensure by always carrying a pocket mask where it was intended to be carried—in your pocket.

Ambulance Hygiene

Most of the emphasis in this chapter up to now has been on how the paramedic can protect himself or herself from contracting a communicable disease in the course of work. But the paramedic also has a responsibility to protect his or her patients from **nosocomial infection** (infection acquired from a health care setting—in this instance, an ambulance). One way, of course, to protect patients from contracting a contagious disease is not to have contact with patients when you are suffering from such a disease. Reporting for work when you have a cold or the flu is *not* a sign of dedication! It reflects total lack of regard for the welfare of the people you are supposed to treat (not to mention the rest of your crew). WHEN YOU'RE SICK, STAY AT HOME. Eat chicken soup, get better, and *then* go back to work.

The other way of protecting patients from nosocomial infections is to keep the ambulance interior and its equipment scrupulously clean. Specifically:

- After *every* call:
  1. Strip used LINENS from the stretcher immediately after use, and place them in a plastic bag or designated receptacle in the emergency room.
  2. In an appropriate receptacle, dispose of all DISPOSABLE EQUIPMENT used for care of the patient.
  3. DISINFECT all nondisposable equipment used in the care of the patient. For example, disas-

TABLE 28-1.   PROFILES OF COMMON COMMUNICABLE DISEASES

DISEASE	TRANSMISSION	INCUBATION PERIOD	COMMUNICABLE PERIOD	NECESSARY PRECAUTIONS	
				FOR PERSONNEL	FOR VEHICLE
AIDS	Sexual contact Contaminated needles or blood products Across the placenta	Months to years	Not known	Mask, gloves, gown, wash hands Extreme care with needles, IVs	Air; scrub, launder linen
Chickenpox (zoster)	Oral/nasal secretions Direct and droplet contact; fomites	2–3 weeks	1 day before rash to 6 days after	Shower, change clothes	Air; scrub; boil linen
German measles (rubella)	Oral/nasal secretions Direct, indirect, or droplet contact	14–21 days	7 days before rash to 4 days after	Mask if not immune PEI advised for all female paramedics	Air; scrub; launder linen
Gonorrhea	Sexual contact	3–4 days	Until treated	Routine	Air; launder linen
Hepatitis	Contaminated needles or blood products Oral/fecal secretions Contaminated food/water	15–180 days	Variable	PEI for hepatitis B Extreme care with needles, IVs Mask, gloves, gown	Air; scrub; launder linen
Measles	Droplet spread	10 days	4 days before rash to 5 days after	Mask if not immune PEI advised	Air; scrub; launder linen
Meningitis	Droplet spread	2–10 days	Variable	Mask Antibiotic prophylaxis for some types	Air; scrub; disinfect linen
Mumps	Saliva, droplet spread	12–26 days	9 days after swelling	Mask if not immune PEI for all male paramedics	Air; scrub; launder linen
Syphilis	Sexual contact Infected saliva, semen, vaginal discharge	10 days to 10 weeks	Variable	If scratched or bitten, consult MD	Air; launder linen
Tuberculosis	Droplet spread	4–8 weeks	Until treated	Mask Annual tuberculin test	Air; scrub; launder linen

PEI = preemployment immunization

semble the *bag-valve-mask* unit and place the components in a liquid sterilization solution as recommended by the manufacturer.

4. CLEAN THE STRETCHER with an EPA-registered germicidal/viricidal solution.
5. If there was any spillage or other contamination in the ambulance, clean it up with the same germicidal/viricidal solution.
6. AIR OUT THE AMBULANCE with all doors and windows open for 5 minutes. To save time, this can be carried out while the vehicle sits in the ambulance bay at the hospital and you are in the emergency room transferring the patient (assuming there is someone responsible outside to safeguard the ambulance contents from theft).

> **DON'T DRIVE A FOUR-WHEELED FOMITE. CLEAN AND AIR THE AMBULANCE AFTER EVERY CALL.**

- At least *once a day*:
1. EMPTY the ambulance of the stretcher and equipment boxes.
2. DISINFECT THE OXYGEN HUMIDIFIER, and refill it with sterile water.
3. SCRUB all interior surfaces with soap and water.
4. Scrub again with an EPA-registered GERMICIDAL/VIRICIDAL SOLUTION. Then air out the ambulance to let everything dry.

Finally, a reminder:

> **WASH YOUR HANDS AFTER EVERY CALL.**

The precautions needed in caring for patients with specific communicable diseases are summarized in Table 28-1.

GLOSSARY

carrier Person who harbors an infectious agent and, although not himself ill, can transmit the infection to another person.

chancre (Pronounced "shanker.") Ulcerated lesion characteristic of primary syphilis.

communicable disease Disease that can be transmitted from one person to another.

communicable period Period during which an infected person is capable of transmitting his illness to someone else.

contagious Describing a disease that is readily transmissible from one person to another.

contamination Presence of harmful microorganisms on or in a person, animal, or object.

dysuria Pain on urination.

fomite An inanimate object contaminated with microorganisms that serves as a means of transmitting an illness.

HIV Abbreviation for human immunodeficiency virus, the agent that causes AIDS.

HSV Abbreviation for herpes simplex virus, the agent that causes genital herpes.

icterus *Jaundice*; the yellow appearance of the skin and other tissues caused by an accumulation of bile pigments.

incubation period Period from infection until the appearance of the first symptoms of a disease.

jaundice The presence of excessive bile pigments in the bloodstream, which give the skin, mucous membranes, and eyes a distinct yellow color; jaundice is often associated with liver disease.

nosocomial infection Infection acquired from a health-care setting.

orchitis Inflammation of the testicles.

reservoir Place where germs live and multiply.

seropositive Having a positive blood test for an infectious agent, such as HIV or hepatitis B virus.

tuberculin test Skin test to determine if a person has ever been infected with tuberculosis.

vesicle Tiny fluid-filled sac; a small blister.

FURTHER READING

INFECTION CONTROL: GENERAL PRINCIPLES

Caroline NL. Chicken soup rebound and relapse of pneumonia: Report of a case. *Chest* 67:215, 1975.

Centers for Disease Control. General recommendations on immunization. *MMWR* 38:205, 1989.

Dettman G. Practicing infection control. *Emergency* 21(1):54, 1989.

Feiner B. Infectious diseases: Actual vs. perceived exposures. *Emerg Med Serv* 17(10):27, 1988.

Gardner P, Schafner W. Immunization of adults. *N Engl J Med* 328:1252, 1993.

LaForce FM. Immunizations, immunoprophylaxis, and chemoprophylaxis to prevent selected infections. *JAMA* 257:2464, 1987.

Olson RJ. Examination gloves as barriers to hand contamination in clinical practice. *JAMA* 270:350, 1993.

Read E et al. Occupational infectious disease exposure in EMS personnel. *J Emerg Med* 11:9, 1993.

Stern A, Dickinson E. Go wash your hands! *JEMS* 19(1):35, 1994.

Turner J. Handwashing behavior versus handwashing guidelines in the ICU. *Heart Lung* 22:275, 1993.

West KH. Infection control. *Emerg Med Serv* 12(1):53, 1983.

West KH. *Infectious Disease Handbook for Emergency Care Personnel.* Philadelphia: Lippincott, 1987.

CHILDHOOD DISEASES

Centers for Disease Control. Mumps—United States, 1983–1984. *MMWR* 33(38), 1984.

Centers for Disease Control. Measles prevention. *JAMA* 258:890, 1987.

Davis RM et al. Transmission of measles in medical settings: 1980–1984. *JAMA* 255:1295, 1986.

Greaves WK et al. Prevention of rubella transmission in medical facilities. *JAMA* 248:861, 1982.

Howard J et al. Rubella immunization policies for health care personnel. *J Fam Pract* 17:805, 1983.

Owens B. Rubella on the rise. *Emerg Med Serv* 21(11):62, 1992.

Schlech WF III et al. Bacterial meningitis in the United States, 1978 through 1981. *JAMA* 253:1749, 1985.

Strassburg MA et al. Rubella in hospital employees. *Infect Control* 5:123, 1984.

TUBERCULOSIS

Barnes PF et al. Tuberculosis in patients with human immunodeficiency virus infection. *N Engl J Med* 234:1644, 1991.

Centers for Disease Control. Tuberculosis morbidity—United States, 1992. *MMWR* 42:696, 1993.

Gaston B. Return of an old scourge. *JEMS* 19(1):70, 1994.

HEPATITIS

Bader T. A protocol for needle-stick injuries. *Emerg Med* 18(2):36, 1986.

Canadian National Advisory Committee on Immunization. Revised guidelines for booster vaccination against hepatitis B. *Can Med Assoc J* 14:1029, 1992.

Centers for Disease Control. Recommendations of the immunization practices advisory committee update on hepatitis B prevention. *MMWR* 36(23), 1987.

Clawson JJ et al. Prevalence of antibody to hepatitis B virus surface antigen in emergency medical personnel in Salt Lake City, Utah. *Ann Emerg Med* 15:183, 1986.

Francis DP et al. The safety of the hepatitis B vaccine: Inactivation of the AIDS virus during routine vaccine manufacture. *JAMA* 256:869, 1986.

Hollinger FB. Factors influencing the immune response to hepatitis B vaccine, booster dose guidelines, and vaccine protocol recommendations. *Am J Med* 87(Suppl 3A):3A, 1989.

Iserson KV, Criss EA. Hepatitis B prevalence in emergency physicians. *Ann Emerg Med* 14:119, 1985.

Kelen DG et al. Hepatitis B and hepatitis C in emergency department patients. *N Engl J Med* 326:1399, 1992.

Klontz KC, Gunn RA, Caldwell JS. Needlestick injuries and hepatitis B immunization in Florida paramedics: A statewide survey. *Ann Emerg Med* 20:1310, 1991.

Kunches LM. Hepatitis B exposure in emergency medical personnel: Prevalence of serologic markers and need for immunization. *Am J Med* 75:269, 1983.

Levine EA et al. Hepatitis prevalence in trauma patients. *Am Surg* 57:385, 1991.

Maddrey WC. Viral hepatitis today. *Emerg Med* 21(16):124, 1989.

Maniscalco PM. Hepatitis B. *Emerg Med Serv* 19(3):37, 1990.

Menegazzi J. A meta-analysis of hepatitis B serologic marker prevalence in EMS personnel. *Prehosp Disaster Med* 6:299, 1991.

Pepe PE et al. Viral hepatitis risk in urban emergency medical services personnel. *Ann Emerg Med* 15:454, 1986.

Peppers MP, Brown DR. Viral vaccines. *Emergency* 29(3):23, 1992.

Schiff ER. Viral hepatitis today. *Emerg Med* 24(15):115, 1992.

Schwartz JS. Hepatitis B vaccine. *Ann Intern Med* 100:149, 1984.

Snyder M. Management of health care workers remotely vaccinated for hepatitis B who sustain significant blood and body fluid exposures. *Infect Control Hosp Epidemiol* 9:462, 1988.

Tang E. Hepatitis C: A review. *West J Med* 155:164, 1991.

Valenzuela TD. Occupational exposure to hepatitis B in paramedics. *Arch Intern Med* 145:1976, 1985.

West KB. Non-A, non-B and delta hepatitis: Hepatitis C and D. *Emerg Med Serv* 19(3):37, 1990.

AIDS

American College of Emergency Physicians. AIDS: Statement of principles and interim recommendations for emergency department personnel and prehospital care providers. *Ann Emerg Med* 17:1249, 1988.

Baker J. What is the occupational risk to emergency care providers from the human immunodeficiency virus? *Ann Emerg Med* 17:700, 1988.

Becknell JM. The face of AIDS. *JEMS* 18(9):66, 1993.

Burrow GN. Caring for AIDS patients: The physician's risk and responsibility. *Can Med Assoc J* 129:1911, 1983.

Centers for Disease Control. Recommendations for prevention of HIV transmission in health-care settings. *JAMA* 258:1293, 1987.

Centers for Disease Control. Update: Human immunodeficiency virus infections in health-care workers exposed to blood of infected patients. *MMWR* 36:285, 1987.

Centers for Disease Control. Mortality attributable to HIV infection/AIDS—United States, 1981–1990. *MMWR* 40:41, 1991.

Centers for Disease Control. HIV seroprevalence among adults treated for cardiac arrest before reaching a medical facility. *MMWR* 41:381, 1992.

Centers for Disease Control. The second 100,000 cases of acquired immunodeficiency syndrome—United States. *MMWR* 41:28, 1992.

Chamberland ME et al. Health care workers with AIDS: National surveillance update. *JAMA* 266:3459, 1991.

Cueva KG. The AIDS factor. *Emergency* 21(1):48, 1989.

Curran JW et al. Acquired immunodeficiency syndrome (AIDS) associated with transfusions. *N Engl J Med* 310:69, 1984.

Flaherty M. Exposed? Now they have to tell you. *JEMS* 18(9):71, 1993.

Friedland G. AIDS and compassion. *JAMA* 259:2898, 1988.

Gerbert B et al. Why fear persists: Health care professionals and AIDS. *JAMA* 260:3481, 1988.

Go GW, Baraff LJ, Schriger DL. Management guidelines for health care workers exposed to blood and body fluids. *Ann Emerg Med* 20:1341, 1991.

Hahn RA et al. Prevalence of HIV infection among intravenous drug users in the United States. *JAMA* 261:2677, 1989.

Hammond JS et al. HIV, trauma, and infection control: Universal precautions are universally ignored. *J Trauma* 30:555, 1990.

Henderson DK et al. Prophylactic zidovudine after occupational exposure to the human immunodeficiency virus: An interim analysis. *J Infect Dis* 160:321, 1989.

Henry GL. Legal rounds: Treating AIDS patients. *Emerg Med* 24(3):118, 1992.

Hollander H. Neurologic and febrile syndromes in HIV. *Emerg Med* 25(4):27, 1993.

Kelen GD. Human immunodeficiency virus and the emergency department: Risks and risk protection for health care providers. *Ann Emerg Med* 19:242, 1990.

Landesman SH et al. The AIDS epidemic. *N Engl J Med* 31:521, 1985.

Lemp GF et al. Survival trends for patients with AIDS. *JAMA* 263:402, 1990.

Littlechild P et al. Contamination of skin and clothing of accident and emergency personnel. *Br Med J* 305:156, 1992.

Marcus R et al. Risk of human immunodeficiency virus infection among emergency department workers. *Am J Med* 94:363, 1993.

Nordberg M. AIDS/Infection control: Critical issues for EMS. *Emerg Med Serv* 17(10):35, 1988.

Ornato JP. Providing CPR and emergency care during the AIDS epidemic. *Emerg Med Serv* 18(4):45, 1989.

Quinn T. The epidemiology of the human immunodeficiency virus. *Ann Emerg Med* 19:225, 1990.

Redfield R et al. Frequent transmission of HTLV-III among spouses of patients with AIDS-related complex and AIDS. *JAMA* 253:1571, 1985.

Robinson EN. Arguments against the chemoprophylactic use of zidovudine following occupational exposure to the human immunodeficiency virus. *Clin Infect Dis* 16:357, 1993.

Rosen MJ. Acute pulmonary manifestations of AIDS. *Emerg Med* 22(1):67, 1990.

Sande MA. Transmission of AIDS: The case against casual contagion. *N Engl J Med* 314:380, 1986.

Soderstrom CA et al. HIV infection rates in a trauma center treating predominantly rural blunt trauma victims. *J Trauma* 29:1526, 1989.

Tokars JI et al. Surveillance of HIV infection and zidovudine use among health care workers after occupational exposure to HIV-infected blood. *Ann Intern Med* 118:913, 1993.

West K. Assessing the risks. *Emergency* 29(3):30, 1992.

29
Emergencies in the Elderly

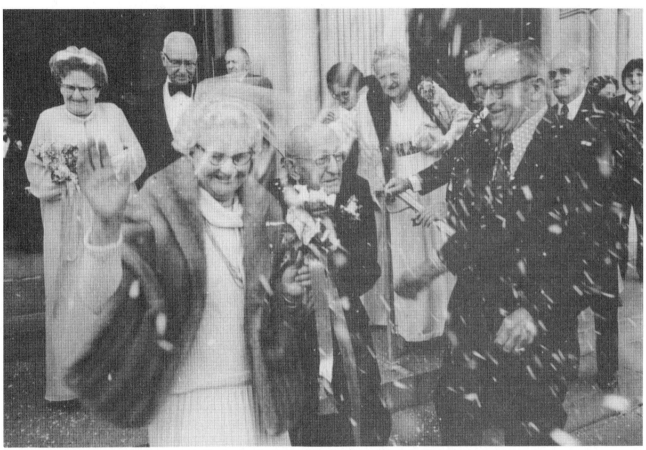

From J. Grimes, E. Burns. *Health Assessment in Nursing Practice* (3rd ed.). Boston: Jones & Bartlett, 1992. P. 521.

OBJECTIVES

Sometimes they call on some of us for help just to be able to talk to another person. We are their only link to the larger world. Our society runs too fast for them. All they have are memories of the past. In order for anyone to truly live, we must have a hope, a dream—something to make life worthwhile. For the elderly, if all their dreams fail, they will perish.

  Frank J. McMahan, Chief Paramedic Instructor, San Francisco Department of Public Health

Approximately 30 million Americans are over the age of 65. They make up 12 percent of the U.S. population today and account for approximately 30 percent of all ambulance calls. By the year 2000—not very far away—one out of every five Americans will be over 65. Furthermore, the elderly population is itself growing older; the most rapidly growing segment of the U.S. population is the group 85 years old and older, whose numbers are expected to reach over 5 million by the end of the century. Thus the old and the very old will constitute an ever increasing proportion of the patients presenting to the health care system and particularly to the emergency care sector of that system.

Older people have problems that are quantitatively and qualitatively different from the problems of younger people. They respond differently to illness and injury; they are more likely to develop toxic reactions to drugs; they do not tolerate fluid loads well; and in general many physiologic capacities are diminished. One cannot, therefore, simply transfer without any modification the principles of caring for the younger population to the care of the elderly. The special problems of the old require special approaches.

In this chapter, we shall first consider the changes that occur in normal anatomy and physiology as a person ages. We will then look at how those changes affect the way we take a history from an elderly patient and the things we need to be alert for in performing a physical examination in the elderly. We shall see how a variety of injuries and illnesses express themselves in the aged, and how the use of pharmacologic agents must be modified in treating older patients. By the end of this chapter, then, the student should be able to

1. List five attributes of the elderly that make their care more challenging than the care of younger patients
2. Identify true and untrue statements about the aging process, given a list of statements
3. List at least two psychosocial stresses that go along with growing old
4. List at least two alterations produced by the aging process in
   - The cardiovascular system
   - The respiratory system
   - The renal system
   - The digestive system
   - The musculoskeletal system
   - The nervous system
   - Homeostatic mechanisms
5. Distinguish between normal effects of aging and symptoms of disease given a list of clinical findings
6. List four common responses to illness among the elderly
7. List four obstacles to obtaining an accurate history from an elderly person, and indicate what steps can be taken to overcome each of those obstacles
8. List 10 questions you would ask in conducting a review of systems in an elderly patient
9. Indicate what information should be obtained regarding the elderly patient's past (or other) medical history
10. List five points of emphasis in conducting the physical assessment of an elderly patient
11. List three injuries to which the elderly are more vulnerable than younger patients, and explain why they are more vulnerable in each instance
12. Describe the steps in managing an injured elderly patient, given a description of the patient's clinical findings
13. List two atypical symptoms of
    - Acute myocardial infarction
    - Congestive heart failure
    apt to be found in an elderly patient suffering from one of those conditions
14. List five conditions that may present as acute confusion in the elderly
15. Describe how to evaluate the suicide risk in a depressed elderly patient
16. List four drugs used in prehospital emergency care that are likely to produce adverse reactions in the elderly

INTRODUCTION

The geriatric patient poses a unique set of problems (or challenges, depending on one's outlook) for health care professionals. To begin with, as we shall discuss in more detail later, the aging process is inevitably accompanied by CHANGES IN PHYSIOLOGIC FUNCTION, such as decline in the function of the liver and kidneys. The decrease in the functional capacity of various organ systems is perfectly normal, but it can nonetheless affect the way in which the patient responds to illness. It can also affect the way *health professionals* respond to the patient's illness; for a health worker who is unaware of the changes that are a normal part of aging may mistake those changes for signs of illness and be tempted to give treatment where no treatment is necessary. At the other end of the spectrum, there is a widespread tendency to attribute genuine disease symptoms to "just getting old" and therefore to neglect their treatment. Thus it is necessary at the outset to dispel some widely held misconceptions about aging. Here are the facts of the matter:

- Getting old is not something that happens only to "them," that is, people over 65. Human growth and development peaks in the late twenties and earlier thirties, at which point the aging process sets in. Aging is a *linear* process; that is, the rate at which we lose functions does not increase with age. A 35-year-old is aging just as fast as an 85-year-old, but in the latter we are simply seeing the cumulative results of a longer process.
- While illness is common among the elderly, it is *not* an inevitable part of the aging process. When an elderly patient complains of symptoms, therefore, those symptoms cannot be ascribed simply to "getting old."

> **GETTING OLD IS NOT A DISEASE, AND IT DOES NOT BY ITSELF PRODUCE SYMPTOMS OF DISEASE.**

- Along the same lines, there is a widespread misconception that elderly people tend to be hypochondriacs, with dozens of imaginary or minor complaints. The fact is that hypochondria is far less common among the elderly than among younger patients. Indeed, for reasons we shall discuss, most older patients tend *not* to complain even when they have very legitimate symptoms.

> **WHEN AN ELDERLY PERSON CALLS FOR AN AMBULANCE, THERE IS USUALLY A VERY GOOD REASON, EVEN IF IT IS NOT THE REASON THE PATIENT TELLS YOU.**

- Finally, a great many people, including health professionals, are under the impression that

mental decline is an invariable part of the aging process, and that sooner or later anyone who lives long enough will become demented. The data do not bear out that gloomy view. In fact, dementia occurs in no more than 10 percent of the elderly and is *not* part of the normal aging process.

> **SERIOUS MENTAL DECLINE IS NOT A NORMAL CONSEQUENCE OF AGING. WHEN DEMENTIA OCCURS, IT IS A SIGN OF DISEASE.**

Knowing what is and what is not part of the aging process constitutes, then, the first challenge in dealing with the elderly. A second challenge derives from the fact that the typical SIGNS AND SYMPTOMS OF DISEASE MAY, as a consequence of the aging process, BE MARKEDLY ALTERED in the elderly. Myocardial infarction may present without chest pain; fever may be minimal in pneumonia; diabetes gone out of control is more likely to present as hyperosmolar coma than as ketoacidosis. And a whole variety of acute illnesses—from congestive heart failure to an acute abdomen—present simply as an acute confusional state (delirium).

Yet another challenge in caring for the elderly involves the fact that the older the patient, the more likely he is to have multiple problems—medical, psychological, and social. One study of people over 65 living in the community found nearly 3.5 important disabilities per person; among elderly admitted to the hospital, the average is around 6 pathologic conditions per person. The conditions most likely to be present include arthritis, hypertensive disease, heart conditions, diabetes, depression, chronic renal failure, and venous insufficiency in the legs.

The COEXISTENCE OF A NUMBER OF PATHOLOGIC CONDITIONS has several consequences for the patient (and for those trying to figure out what is happening to the patient). To begin with, the symptoms of one disease or disability may alter or hide the symptoms of another. The patient with severe pain in his legs from arthritis, for example, may not pay much attention to the new, additional pain caused by thrombophlebitis in one leg. Secondly, when several organ systems are in borderline condition, a perturbation in function in only one of those systems may have repercussions throughout the body, leading to failure of one organ after the other. Needless to say, the presence of multiple underlying illnesses also makes it much more difficult for the health professional to sort out what problem is causing what symptom. Furthermore, the coexistence of several pathologic conditions may make it much more difficult to treat the patient's current, acute problem. The medication the patient needs for his cardiac problem may be contraindicated because of his renal or hepatic problem, or, at the least, may require major modifications in dosage.

That brings us to yet another challenge in caring for the elderly—the fact that the elderly are particularly PRONE TO ADVERSE REACTIONS FROM a variety of DRUGS at doses that would be perfectly safe in younger people. There seem to be several reasons for the increased incidence of adverse drug reactions among the elderly, including (1) changes in drug metabolism because of diminished hepatic function; (2) changes in drug elimination because of diminished renal function; (3) changes in body composition and the distribution of drugs through different body compartments; and (4) changes in the responsiveness to drugs of the central nervous system.

Finally, one of the greatest challenges in dealing with the elderly is to appreciate the degree to which PSYCHOSOCIAL FACTORS INFLUENCE PHYSICAL DISEASE. While mind and body operate as an inseparable whole throughout life, there are stresses uniquely associated with growing old that can markedly increase a person's susceptibility to illness. Age 65, first of all, often signals *retirement*, which means much more than not going off to work every morning. For many people, retirement is a symbol of being no longer useful or productive in society. Retirement, then, often means an enormous loss of self-esteem. It also means a loss of income and of the social network that had been provided by the workplace.

Age also brings *bereavement*—the loss of friends and loved ones—and bereavement is not good for health. Studies have shown, for example, that the likelihood of death increases sharply during the year following the death of one's spouse. As friends and family fall away, there is also a tendency among the elderly to increasing *loneliness and isolation*—again, factors that have been shown to have negative effects on health.

To summarize, then, there are several attributes of the elderly that make their care particularly challenging:

ATTRIBUTES OF ELDERLY PATIENTS

- Many physiologic functions are diminished.
- Typical signs and symptoms of disease may be absent.
- Physical illness often presents as a mental disorder (particularly as confusion).
- Multiple problems coexist in the same patient.
- Adverse reactions to drugs occur very commonly.
- Psychosocial factors have a dramatically increased impact on health.

THE ANATOMY AND PHYSIOLOGY OF GROWING OLD

Aging is a biologic process that begins when growth and development cease, usually around the age of 30. All tissues in the body undergo aging, but not all of them age at the same rate. Furthermore, as nearly everyone's personal observations will attest, there is enormous variation in the aging process from one person to another. Most of us can report having seen 60-year-olds who look terribly frail and elderly and 80-year-olds who run marathons. The general trends produced by aging, however, at whatever age the changes occur, can be summarized as follows.

Changes in the Cardiovascular System

A variety of changes occur in the cardiovascular system as one grows older, the net effect of them being to decrease the efficiency of the system. To begin with, the heart **hypertrophies** (enlarges) with age, probably in response to the chronically increased afterload imposed by stiffened blood vessels. Bigger is not better, however, and in fact CARDIAC OUTPUT DECLINES, mostly as a result of a decreasing stroke volume. ARTERIOSCLEROSIS is widespread among the elderly, and the stiffening of vessel walls contributes to systolic HYPERTENSION in a large number of older patients, which of course places an extra burden on the heart. At the same time, the ELECTRIC CONDUCTION SYSTEM OF THE HEART DEGENERATES. There is, for example, a profound decrease in the number of pacemaker cells in the sinoatrial (SA) node. In many cases, the changes in the conduction system lead to BRADYCARDIAS of one sort or another, which also then contribute to the decline in cardiac output.

Notably, at least part of the change in cardiovascular performance that occurs with age is probably not a direct consequence of aging at all, but rather reflects the deconditioning effect of a sedentary lifestyle. Whether because of other disabilities, such as arthritis, or for psychologic reasons, many people tend to limit their physical activity drastically as they grow older. The bodybuilder's slogan, "Use it or lose it," applies just as much to the cardiac muscle as to the biceps.

Changes in the Respiratory System

The respiratory capacity also undergoes significant reductions with age, largely due to decreases in the elasticity of the lungs and in the size and strength of the respiratory muscles. In addition, calcification of costochrondral cartilage tends to make the chest wall stiffer. As a result of all those changes, the VITAL CAPACITY, that is, the amount of air that can be exhaled following a maximal inhalation, DECREASES, while the **residual volume** (the amount of air left in the lungs at the end of a maximal exhalation) increases. What that means, in essence, is that while the total amount of air in the lungs does not change with age, the proportion of that air usefully employed in gas exchange progressively decreases. AIR FLOW, which depends largely on airway size and resistance, also DETERIORATES somewhat with age. Meanwhile, changes in the distribution of blood flow within the lungs result in a DECLINING ARTERIAL PO_2. At age 30, the PO_2 of a healthy person breathing ambient air is usually around 90 mm Hg; at age 80, the arterial PO_2 under the same conditions is 75 mm Hg. Furthermore, the RESPIRATORY DRIVE IS DULLED as a person gets older; either because of a decreased sensitivity to changes in arterial blood gases or because of a decreased central nervous system response to such changes, the reaction to hypoxemia or hypercarbia is slowed in the elderly.

Finally, there are IMPAIRMENTS IN THE LUNG'S DEFENSE MECHANISMS that occur as a natural consequence of the aging process. Both cough and gag reflexes decrease with age, thereby increasing the risks of aspiration. Furthermore, the ciliary mechanisms that normally help remove bronchial secretions are markedly slowed.

Changes in the Renal System

Age brings changes in the kidneys as well. In a young adult, the kidneys weigh 250 to 270 gm; in a healthy 70-year-old, they weigh 180 to 200 gm. The decline in weight represents a LOSS OF FUNCTIONING NEPHRON UNITS. What that translates into is a smaller effective filtering surface. At the same time, RENAL BLOOD FLOW DECREASES by as much as 50 percent.

Recall that the kidneys are responsible for maintaining fluid and electrolyte balance in the body and also play an important role in long-term acid-base balance. While the kidneys of an elderly person may be perfectly capable of dealing with day-to-day demands, they may not be capable of meeting unusual challenges, such as those imposed by illness. For that reason, acute illness in elderly patients is often accompanied by DERANGEMENTS IN FLUID AND ELECTROLYTE BALANCE. Aging kidneys, for example, respond sluggishly to *sodium deficiency*. An elderly patient can therefore lose a great deal of salt before the kidneys kick in to halt urinary salt excretion. The problem is exacerbated by the markedly DECREASED THIRST MECHANISM in the elderly. The net result is very often a rapid development of severe DEHYDRATION.

At the other end of the spectrum, elderly patients are also at considerable risk of OVERHYDRATION if exposed to large salt loads from any source (IV salt solutions, heavily salted foods). Because of its lower glomerular filtration rate, the aging kidney is less able than its younger counterpart to excrete a big load of salt. So the bagful of potato chips consumed while watching television, or the liter of lactated Ringer's administered by a paramedic, can lead very quickly to an acute volume overload.

The same factors that reduce the patient's ability to handle sodium also affect his ability to handle potassium, with the result that elderly patients are prone to HYPERKALEMIA, which can reach very serious and even lethal levels if the patient becomes acidotic or if his potassium load is increased from any other source. (How can you recognize hyperkalemia on an electrocardiogram?)

Changes in the Digestive System

The process of digestion begins in the mouth, which is also where changes in the digestive system can first be noted. A decrease in the number of taste buds with age along with changes in olfactory receptors lead to REDUCTION IN TASTE AND SMELL, which may in turn seriously interfere with the enjoyment of food. Consequent DECREASE IN APPETITE can lead over a period of time to various degrees of MALNUTRITION. Other changes in the mouth include reduction in the volume of saliva, with a resulting dryness of the mouth. DENTAL LOSS is *not* a normal result of the aging process but rather the result of disease of the teeth and gums; nonetheless, dental loss is widespread among the elderly population and also contributes to nutritional and digestive problems.

Like oral secretions, GASTRIC SECRETIONS are also REDUCED as a person ages—although there is still enough acid present to produce ulcer disease in predisposed individuals. There are also changes in gastric motility, which may lead to SLOWER GASTRIC EMPTYING—a factor of some importance when assessing the risk of aspiration.

Function of the small and large bowel changes little as a consequence of aging, although the incidence of certain disease conditions involving the bowel—such as diverticulosis—increases as a person grows older.

In the liver, there are CHANGES IN HEPATIC ENZYME SYSTEMS with age, some systems declining in activity, others increasing in activity. Notably, the enzyme systems most concerned with the detoxification of drugs are among those whose activities *decline* as a person grows older.

Changes in the Musculoskeletal System

Aging brings a widespread DECREASE IN BONE MASS, especially among women after menopause. Bones become more brittle and tend to break more easily. Narrowing of the intervertebral discs and compression fractures of the vertebrae together contribute to a DECREASE IN HEIGHT as a person ages, along with CHANGES IN POSTURE. Joints lose their flexibility and may be further immobilized by arthritic changes. MUSCLE MASS DECREASES throughout the body, with accompanying decreases in muscle strength. For EMS providers, the changes in the elderly patient's musculoskeletal system most often translate into fractures incurred as the result of falls.

Changes in the Nervous System

Anatomists and physiologists examining the brains of elderly humans tell us that brain weight declines as much as 17 percent by age 80, and cerebral oxygen consumption starts gradually decreasing from about the age of 30. The functional significance of such findings is not at all clear, however, for as noted earlier, dementia is *not* an inevitable part of normal aging. The human brain clearly has an enormous reserve capacity, and a 17-percent loss of brain weight certainly never interfered with the mental capabilities of Arthur Rubinstein or Pablo Picasso.

Undeniably, though, there is a progressive reduction in the performance of most of the sense organs with increasing age. We have already mentioned the reduction in the sense of taste and smell that occurs with aging. DECREASES IN VISUAL ACUITY are also common, even without disease processes such as cataracts. Night vision becomes impaired, as does the ability to adjust to rapid changes in lighting conditions.

HEARING DIMINISHES, particularly in the high frequencies, along with the ability to discriminate between a particular sound and background noise. The net effect is that it becomes harder for the older person to make out what other people are saying, especially in a noisy environment.

SENSE OF BODILY POSITION (**proprioception**) also BECOMES IMPAIRED with age. It is proprioception that enables us to maintain postural stability, through a variety of receptors in the joints as well as information provided by the eyes. As the proprioceptive mechanisms fail, a person becomes less and less steady on his feet, and the tendency to fall is markedly increased.

Homeostatic and Other Changes

We learned in an earlier chapter that all living organisms have mechanisms for maintaining **homeostasis**, that is, the constancy of the internal environment. Many of those homeostatic mechanisms work on a servo principle, like the thermostat in a house, whereby a change in the internal environment feeds back to the control system to induce a corrective response. Thus, for example, when the body temperature starts to rise, temperature sensors are activated, and they in turn activate compensatory responses: Cutaneous blood vessels dilate, and excess heat is shed from the body to the environment. Similarly, when the concentration of the sugar in the blood rises, the pancreas is stimulated to secrete insulin, which leads to the uptake of sugar by cells and the reduction of blood sugar levels back toward normal. Scores of such servo mechanisms operate to regulate scores of bodily responses. In the elderly, many of those servo mechanisms start to break down.

We have already mentioned how the THIRST MECHANISM, which ordinarily protects us from dehydration, BECOMES DEPRESSED in the elderly. TEMPERATURE REGULATING MECHANISMS also tend to BECOME DISORDERED. Poor temperature control renders elderly patients much more susceptible than the young to environmental stresses such as heat exhaustion or accidental hypothermia after relatively minor exposures. It is probably some defect in temperature regulation that also accounts for the ABSENCE OF A FEBRILE RESPONSE TO ILLNESS in many elderly people. Infections that would ordinarily produce high fever, such as pneumococcal pneumonia, may produce only a very low-grade fever in the elderly—or sometimes no fever at all.

The servo mechanism that enables CONTROL OF BLOOD GLUCOSE also BECOMES IMPAIRED with increasing age, and elevated levels of blood sugar occur quite commonly. Ordinarily moderate hyperglycemia does not do any harm, except when discovered by an overzealous doctor who decides that patient should receive treatment for "diabetes." The treatment, which is likely to produce periods of *hypo*glycemia, will almost certainly do harm.

Across the board, then, aging is accompanied by a PROGRESSIVE LOSS OF HOMEOSTATIC CAPACITY, that is, of the capacity to adjust to perturbations in the system. For that reason,

> **A SPECIFIC ILLNESS OR INJURY IN THE ELDERLY IS MORE LIKELY TO RESULT IN GENERALIZED DETERIORATION.**

In a young person, for example, a hip fracture will mean a certain circumscribed period of immobility, almost certainly followed by rehabilitation and recovery. For an elderly person, a fractured hip and the hospitalization it involves carry 10 times the risk of serious complication.

ASSESSMENT OF THE GERIATRIC PATIENT

The elderly patient is considerably less likely than his younger counterpart to present with a clearly defined symptom complex. More often, the history is vague—a little weakness, a little undefined pain or discomfort, a little fatigue. A variety of handicaps superimposed on old age—failing memory, diminished sight and hearing, sometimes depression—also make it more difficult to determine the precise nature of the patient's current problem. In this section, we shall look at some of the things we need to take into account when obtaining the history of an elderly patient and performing the physical assessment.

Taking the History

Taking the history from an elderly patient often presents a special set of problems. To begin with, COMMUNICATION PROBLEMS are common in the aged. Deficits in vision and hearing may make it difficult for the patient to catch what you are saying, and depression may cause him not to *care* what you are saying even if he *can* hear you. Dementia or the toxic effects of the patient's acute illness may, furthermore, make the patient confused and unable to provide reliable information. Nonetheless, it is important to start out with the assumption that you are dealing with a neurologically intact person. The majority of elderly people are *not* deaf or demented, and you will lose a lot of points with a lot of patients by making the assumption that they are.

> **ALWAYS ASSUME THAT AN ELDERLY PATIENT'S MENTAL STATUS IS NORMAL UNTIL YOU HAVE EVIDENCE TO THE CONTRARY.**

Because there *is* a significant incidence of hearing loss among the elderly, you should make every attempt to interview the patient in an environment where it will be easiest for him to hear you. In the field, that is sometimes difficult to arrange. But to the degree possible, try to INTERVIEW THE ELDERLY PATIENT IN A QUIET PLACE where there is a minimum of background noise. Sit directly opposite the patient, facing him, so that he can see you clearly and thereby read your lips or pick up other visual cues as you speak. The LIGHTING SHOULD also BE ADEQUATE to allow the patient to see you clearly, but should not be excessively bright. SPEAK SLOWLY AND CLEARLY. If the patient seems to be having difficulty hearing, move a little closer and try again. If you have to increase the volume of your voice, do so without increasing the pitch, for it is precisely the high tones that the elderly have difficulty hearing. In any event, DON'T SHOUT. Shouting merely distorts sound; it will not help the hearing-impaired patient make out what you are saying, and it certainly will not help establish a good relationship between you.

ASK ONE QUESTION AT A TIME, and keep the questions simple. Explain why you are asking all these questions and why the answers are important; otherwise the patient is apt to feel that things you are asking about are none of your business.

MAKE PHYSICAL CONTACT EARLY in your encounter with the patient. Take his hand, put a hand on his shoulder, put a finger on his pulse—any such gesture communicates warmth and provides reassurance.

The Chief Complaint

Obtaining the patient's chief complaint would seem to be a straightforward enough procedure, but in the elderly patient it may not be straightforward at all. A variety of studies conducted in several countries have all revealed a strong TENDENCY OF OLD PEOPLE *NOT* TO REPORT SIGNIFICANT SYMPTOMS. There are probably several reasons for that phenomenon. First of all, elderly people often share the widespread misconception, mentioned earlier, that illness and assorted aches and pains are simply part of the aging process. So an old person may not mention a significant symptom from the mistaken belief that it is "normal for someone my age."

Another reason that the old tend not to report their symptoms is that they are well aware of society's stereotype of the elderly—an inaccurate stereotype, as we have seen—that portrays the old person as a complaining hypochondriac. Many old people will therefore avoid mentioning even legitimate symptoms rather than risk being identified as old and hypochondriacal.

Depression is yet another reason that may prevent an old person from mentioning important symptoms. Depression is common in the elderly and brings with it a loss of concern for one's own health and well-being.

Elderly people, finally, are often fearful (and not without good reason) that mentioning a symptom will lead to a diagnosis or treatment that will jeopardize their independence. "If I mention those pains in my stomach," the old person may reason, "they'll put me in the hospital, and I may never come out of that place again."

If elderly patients tend to underreport serious symptoms, very often the symptoms they *do* report are vague and apparently trivial. Furthermore, the elderly patient is very likely to have SEVERAL CHIEF COMPLAINTS, and each of them may have a different source. Among the most common presenting complaints among the elderly are fatigue, weakness, dizziness, loss of appetite, difficulty sleeping, headache, and constipation. Once again, therefore, it is important to emphasize:

> **WHEN AN ELDERLY PATIENT CALLS FOR AN AMBULANCE, THERE IS USUALLY A VERY GOOD REASON, EVEN IF IT IS NOT THE REASON THE PATIENT GIVES YOU.**

When a patient's chief complaint seems trivial, it is necessary to go through a standard list of SCREENING QUESTIONS to be certain you are not missing some important piece of information. In medicine,

we call those screening questions the **review of systems** because the questions are designed to evaluate the functions of the body's major organ systems. In the field, there is not sufficient time to conduct a complete review of systems. But a few well-chosen questions can provide a lot of information about the function of the patient's more important systems:

ABBREVIATED REVIEW OF SYSTEMS

- CARDIOVASCULAR
  1. Have you had any pain or discomfort in your chest?
  2. Have you noticed any palpitations?
- RESPIRATORY
  1. Do you ever get short of breath?
  2. Have you had a cough lately?
- NEUROLOGIC
  1. Have you had any dizzy spells? Have you fainted?
  2. Have you had any trouble speaking?
  3. Have you had headaches recently?
  4. Have you noticed any unusual weakness or funny sensations in your arms or legs?
- GASTROINTESTINAL
  1. Have there been any changes in your appetite lately? Have you gained or lost any weight?
  2. Have there been any changes in your bowel movements?
- GENITOURINARY
  1. Do you have any pain or difficulty in urinating?
  2. Have you noticed any change in the color of your urine?

If any of your screening questions yields a positive answer, it should of course be followed up with further questions. If, for example, the patient states that he *has* been coughing lately, you will need to find out whether he is bringing up sputum and, if so, what the sputum looks like (e.g., Is there blood in the sputum?).

Once you have elicited what you believe to be the patient's chief complaint, go through the usual process of assembling the history of the present illness. Again, that will be more complicated than usual. Because it is very likely that the patient's current problem is superimposed on a background of other, more chronic problems, it may be hard to sort out which symptoms relate to the current chief complaint and which are part of the patient's more chronic difficulties. You might try asking questions such as, "How is this problem different now from what it was like last week?" or "What happened *today* to make you decide to get help?"

More than in the case of the younger patient, taking a history from the elderly patient requires PATIENCE. You must be prepared to listen, often for quite some length of time. But your listening will be rewarded—not only by helping you to find the patient's problem, but also by providing part of the solution to his problem. Listening is a demonstration of caring, and your caring can mean a great deal to a lonely old person.

Other Medical History

Just as it is not practical to go through a comprehensive review of systems in the field, similarly it is not usually feasible to obtain anything approaching a complete past medical history. Nonetheless, it is important to inquire about RECENT HOSPITALIZATIONS (For what? At what hospital? Who is the patient's doctor?) and ALLERGIES. Most important of all, however, is to obtain the most detailed history possible of the patient's MEDICATIONS. As we shall discuss in more detail later, medications account for a very significant percentage of medical problems in the elderly. Inquire about *all* medications, not just prescription drugs, for many people do not think to mention common over-the-counter preparations, such as aspirin or antacid tablets, when asked what medications they take regularly. Obtain the patient's permission to bring his medications with you to the hospital, and then collect them all—prescription and nonprescription drugs—in a bag and take them along. If the patient is not in condition to tell you where he keeps his medicines, check out the bathroom medicine cabinet, the bedside table, the kitchen table and counters, and the refrigerator.

BRING ALL THE PATIENT'S MEDICATIONS— PRESCRIPTION AND NONPRESCRIPTION—WITH HIM TO THE HOSPITAL.

Physical Assessment

The physical examination of an elderly patient may also be fraught with unique difficulties. Poor cooperation and easy fatigability may require that you re-

duce manipulations of the patient to a minimum. Often you will have to peel many layers of clothing off the elderly patient to examine him adequately, and there is always a certain temptation, on viewing all that clothing, to skip the whole thing. That temptation must be overcome! The ill or injured geriatric patient deserves as thorough an evaluation as his younger counterpart.

EXPLAIN everything you plan to do, especially if the patient seems confused. The object is to reduce his anxiety, not increase it—and if you simply whip out a lot of strange equipment and start, for example, gluing electrodes onto the patient's chest, the patient may well become frightened and wonder what is going to happen to him.

Begin, as usual, by observing the patient's GENERAL APPEARANCE. Under that heading, make note, first of all, of his *dress* and *grooming.* Sometimes, especially among women, inattention to appearance may be one of the first signs of depression or a serious medical condition. Evaluate the *level of consciousness* as you would for any other patient. In the critically ill or injured, use the AVPU scale. But when you have more time, try to make a more detailed assessment of the patient's cognitive function. Is he fully alert? Is he oriented to place and time? Does his affect seem appropriate to the situation? Are there any obvious disorders in his thinking, such as delusions (false beliefs)? As for every other patient, make a note of the patient's *position* and *degree of distress.* Check the color, moisture, and temperature of the *skin,* but bear in mind that the loss of elasticity in the skin of the elderly may produce apparent signs of dehydration (e.g., tenting) when hydration is in fact normal. To assess the STATE OF HYDRATION in the elderly, one must rely on other signs altogether:

SIGNS OF DEHYDRATION IN THE ELDERLY

- Dry tongue
- Longitudinal furrows in the tongue
- Dry mucous membranes
- Weak upper body musculature
- Confusion
- Difficulty in speech
- Sunken eyes

Measure the patient's VITAL SIGNS, preferably when he is recumbent and again when he is sitting upright and yet again when standing. Nearly all elderly people have some degree of postural change in blood pressure, but marked postural changes may indicate internal bleeding or overmedication with any of a variety of drugs. Bear in mind also as you measure the vital signs that what is normal blood pressure for a young person may represent significant *hypo*tension in the elderly, and consider the possibility of hypovolemia in any elderly patient whose systolic blood pressure is less than 120 mm Hg. Pay attention to the *respiratory rate.* Tachypnea over about 25 breaths per minute can be a very sensitive indicator of acute illness in the elderly, especially pulmonary infection, when there are few if any other signs.

Conduct the HEAD-TO-TOE SURVEY as you would for any other patient. When examining the *mouth,* make a note of any upper or lower dentures. In the chest examination, keep in mind that the elderly may have pulmonary crackles without apparent pathology—so don't lunge for the nitroglycerin and furosemide at the first crackle you hear in the chest. Similarly, edema in the legs may be the result of chronic venous insufficiency and not right-sided heart failure.

If you are examining the patient in his home, TAKE A GOOD LOOK AT THE PATIENT'S SURROUNDINGS as well as at the patient himself. Try to assess the patient's ability to care for himself. Is everything neat and well maintained? Or is the place a complete mess, with dishes piled in the sink and rubbish accumulating everywhere? Is there evidence of alcohol consumption (empty bottles lying around)? Are there signs of violence, such as broken glassware, that might provide clues to "elder abuse"? Are the patient's quarters adequately heated or cooled? Is he living alone? Does he have any pets? (If so, you should make arrangements for someone, like a neighbor, to assume their care until the patient returns.) Record all of those observations on the patient's trip sheet, to enable social service personnel at the hospital to make appropriate arrangements for the patient's follow-up care.

SPECIAL CONSIDERATIONS IN CARING FOR THE ELDERLY

The special problems confronting the elderly lead to special considerations in their emergency care. While the basic principles of care—especially the ABCs of the primary survey—are the same for all patients, there are inevitably differences of approach when the patient is very old.

Trauma in the Elderly

Trauma is the fifth leading cause of death among the elderly; and while people over 65 currently constitute only about 12 percent of the American population, they account for 25 percent of trauma deaths in the United States. A variety of factors place an elderly person at higher *risk* of trauma than a younger person—slower reflexes, visual and hearing deficits, equilibrium disorders, and an overall reduction in agility. Furthermore, for any given trauma, the elderly person is more likely to sustain serious injury, for stiffened blood vessels and fragile tissues tear more readily, and brittle, demineralized bone is more liable to fracture.

The Epidemiology of Geriatric Trauma

The vast majority of geriatric trauma occurs either in falls or as a result of motor vehicle accidents.

Approximately 9,500 elderly Americans die each year as a result of FALLS. In fact, falling is very common among the elderly—approximately 40 percent of individuals over the age of 65 will fall at least once per year, and the risk of falling markedly increases with age after 65. Most falls do *not* produce serious injury, but the likelihood of a significant fracture or death after a fall also increases sharply with age, particularly among women.

The *causes* of falls among the elderly are about evenly divided between extrinsic (accidental) causes, such as tripping on a loose rug or slipping on ice, and intrinsic causes, such as a dizzy spell or a syncopal attack. Osteoporosis in old bones means that the bones have lost their density; so when twisted, the bone of an elderly person can snap like a dried twig. A sudden, awkward turn, therefore, can fracture a bone, and for that reason, one must always consider the possibility that a patient's fall was the *result* of a fracture and not necessarily the cause. Some of the more common causes of falls in the elderly are summarized in Table 29-1. To distinguish among them, you need to take a careful history. While the patient will very often attribute the fall to an accidental cause ("I must have tripped over the rug."), meticulous questioning often reveals a period of dizziness or palpitations just before the fall, suggesting a different cause altogether.

MOTOR VEHICLE ACCIDENTS are the second leading cause, after falls, of accidental death among the elderly. Among the more than 13 million licensed drivers in the United States over the age of 65, the risk of being fatally injured in a road traffic accident is five times higher than among younger drivers. Im-

TABLE 29-1.   CAUSES OF FALLS IN THE ELDERLY

CAUSE	CLUES TO SUGGEST THIS CAUSE
Extrinsic (accidental)	Obvious environmental hazard at the scene, such as poor lighting, scatter rugs, uneven sidewalk, ice or other slippery surface.
Intrinsic	
Drop attacks	Sudden fall; patient found on the ground somewhat confused, often temporarily paralyzed and unable to get up; no premonitory symptoms.
Postural hypotension	Fall occurred on getting up from a recumbent or sitting position. (Check what medications the patient is taking, and ask about sources of occult blood loss, e.g., black stools. Measure blood pressure recumbent and sitting.)
Dizziness or syncope	Marked bradycardia or tachyarrhythmias.
Stroke	Other characteristic signs of stroke, such as hemiparesis or hemiplegia, aphasia.
Fracture	Patient felt something snap before falling.

paired vision, errors in judgment, and underlying medical conditions are all thought to contribute to that higher risk. Impairments in vision and hearing, along with diminished agility, probably contribute as well to the 2,000 pedestrian fatalities among the elderly in the United States each year.

Types of Trauma Commonly Seen in the Elderly

Changes associated with normal aging and with diseases of aging make the elderly particularly vulnerable to certain specific injuries. HEAD TRAUMA, for example, is an important problem in the elderly. Increased fragility of cerebral blood vessels along with an enlargement of the subarachnoid space and a decrease in the supportive tissue of the meninges all contribute to make the elderly person much more vulnerable than a younger person to intracranial bleeding, particularly **subdural hematoma.** In many instances, the hematoma develops slowly, over days or weeks; and by the time the patient has become symptomatic, he or his caretakers no longer remember the trauma incident, which may have been quite trivial anyway. A history of trauma may also be difficult to obtain when the patient's family or caretakers have feelings of guilt over their own negligence (or worse) in the incident. The most important early symptom of a subdural hematoma is *headache*, which may be worse at night. Sometimes the headache is on the same side of the head as the blood clot. With increasing intracranial pressure, the state of consciousness becomes depressed, and the patient is more and more drowsy.

The elderly are also much more vulnerable than the young to CERVICAL SPINAL CORD INJURY and cord compression, even after apparently minor trauma. Degenerative changes in the cervical spine, called **cervical spondylosis,** cause arthritic "spurs" and narrowing of the vertebral canal; the result is gradual compression of the nerve roots exiting from the cervical spine as well as pressure on the spinal cord itself. Any injury to the cervical spine, therefore, is much more likely to injure the already compromised spinal cord. Indeed, even when there is no fracture of the cervical vertebrae, a sudden movement of the neck may result in spinal cord injury.

Injuries to the chest in the elderly are much more likely to produce RIB FRACTURE and even flail chest, owing to the brittleness of the ribs and the overall stiffening of the chest wall as the costochondral cartilages become calcified. Abdominal trauma often produces LIVER INJURY, perhaps because the liver is less protected by abdominal musculature.

Falls, of course, are notorious for causing HIP FRACTURE in the elderly, although in some cases hip fracture may occur without any trauma at all, but simply because of vigorous contracture of the hip musculature. As noted, the most important risk factor for hip fracture is **osteoporosis,** a state in which the bone mass is so reduced that the skeleton becomes unable to perform its supportive function. Those most commonly affected by osteoporosis are postmenopausal white women, although men may be affected later in life. Among white women between the ages of 80 and 90, the incidence of hip fracture is nearly 10 percent.

Assessment and Management of Trauma in the Elderly

The initial management of the injured elderly patient follows the basic ABCDE of trauma care, with special attention to the following:

A   In securing the AIRWAY, be sure to check for *dentures*. If dentures are intact and in place, leave them where they are, but if they are broken or rattling around loose in the mouth, remove them and place them in a safe container. Otherwise, broken dentures may jeopardize the airway.

B   In assessing the injured patient's BREATHING, be sure to check for rib fracture. When assisted ventilation is required, use a bag-valve-mask gently; do not use a demand valve, which may blow out blebs in the lungs. Administer oxygen as early as possible, since even a "normal" PO_2 in an elderly person is very close to borderline.

C   In evaluating the patient's circulation, remember that what is a normal blood pressure in a younger person may be hypotension in an elderly person.

CONSIDER THE POSSIBILITY OF HYPOVOLEMIA IN ANY ELDERLY PERSON WHOSE SYSTOLIC BLOOD PRESSURE IS LESS THAN 120 MM HG.

D   The initial assessment of DISABILITY (neurologic status) should, as usual, include an evaluation of the pupils and the level of consciousness, according to the AVPU scale.

E   Once again, be sure to EXPOSE the entire injured area, even if that means having to peel away many layers of clothing.

Once the primary survey is complete, try to obtain as good a HISTORY as you can, both from the patient and from anyone who may have witnessed the accident. If the patient fell, from what height did he fall? Did he have any symptoms beforehand, such as dizziness? If he was struck by a car, how fast was the car moving? If he was the driver of a car involved in an accident, did he feel dizzy or black out before the crash? Did he have chest pain? Did witnesses notice the car moving erratically before it crashed? As usual, be sure to get a complete list of the *medications* the patient takes regularly. Inquire in particular about beta blockers, antihypertensives, and medications for diabetes, all of which may affect the patient's response to resuscitation measures and to anesthesia, if surgery is required.

Conduct the PHYSICAL EXAMINATION of the secondary survey as usual, being particularly alert for signs of the injuries mentioned earlier—injuries to the head, cervical spine, ribs, abdomen, and long bones.

The further steps of treatment will depend somewhat on the patient's specific injuries. There are, however, a few general principles to keep in mind:

- Start an IV with lactated Ringer's, but use EXTREME CAUTION IN ADMINISTERING INTRAVENOUS FLUIDS. Remember that it is very easy to overload an elderly person with salt and push him over into congestive heart failure. So keep the IV rate low—no more than about 100 ml per hour—until you reach the hospital. There, a line can be inserted to measure central venous pressure and to guide intravenous therapy more precisely.
- MONITOR cardiac rhythm throughout your care of the patient, and be alert for dangerous dysrhythmias.
- IMMOBILIZE THE CERVICAL SPINE before transporting the patient. When immobilizing an elderly person on a backboard, recall that loss of muscle mass means a relative lack of natural "padding," so the backboard may cause considerable pressure wherever bones are close to the surface of the body. Therefore PAD THE BACKBOARD GENEROUSLY with pillows or blankets. Probably the best splint for immobilizing an elderly patient is a whole-body vacuum splint.
- The frail elderly may not do very well with a traction splint for a femoral fracture. It is preferable simply to place the patient on a well-padded backboard and buttress him well with pillows strapped firmly in place.

Elder Abuse

One category of geriatric trauma that deserves special mention is "elder abuse," a syndrome involving the neglect or physical injury of elderly people by their care providers, which may be nursing home personnel or their own spouse or children. It is estimated that 10 percent of Americans over the age of 65 are victims of elder abuse. The average victim of elder abuse is 80 years old and has multiple chronic conditions, such as congestive heart failure, cancer, or incontinence. Those conditions render him unable to function on his own, so he is dependent on others for at least part of his care. The clue to elder abuse is *unexplained trauma* or injuries that do not fit the stated cause.

All 50 states have elder abuse statutes, and in very nearly all states the reporting of suspected elder abuse is mandatory under the law. However, the way elder abuse is defined varies considerably from state to state, so it is advisable to become familiar with the legislation that applies to your own area. Whatever the legislation, however, if you have any reason to suspect elder abuse in a given case of geriatric injury—if, for example, you found evidence of gross neglect of the patient in the place where he was living—report your findings and suspicions *in private* to the physician at the receiving hospital.

Medical Emergencies in the Elderly

Earlier in this chapter, we mentioned several factors that tend to modify the picture of illness in old age. To illustrate some of the problems involved in uncovering the underlying problem in an ill old person, let us consider two conditions that occur commonly in old age: myocardial infarction and congestive heart failure.

Acute Myocardial Infarction

Acute myocardial infarction (AMI) is very common in the elderly and occurs with about equal frequency in men and women in that age group. Only a minority of those patients, however, present with the classic picture of severe chest pain. More frequent is the slow development of *dyspnea* indicative of left heart failure. Frequently also, the elderly patient with an acute myocardial infarction will present simply with extreme *weakness, syncope, loss of bowel or bladder control,* associated *stroke,* or *confusion.* Indeed, a significant percentage of elderly patients with AMI will not experience any symptoms at all, and their infarction is detected only months or years later on routine electrocardiogram as a so-called silent MI. Some differences in the clinical presentation of myocardial infarction according to age are summarized in Table 29-2. What that table makes clear is that it is necessary to maintain a high index of suspicion for AMI when caring for any elderly patient who presents with vague symptoms of weakness, dizziness, or shortness of breath.

TABLE 29-2. PRESENTING SYMPTOMS OF MYOCARDIAL INFARCTION WITH INCREASING AGE

SYMPTOM	PERCENTAGE OF PATIENTS PRESENTING WITH THE SYMPTOM*		
	AGE UNDER 70	AGE 75–79	AGE 85 AND OVER
Chest pain	76	68	38
Dyspnea	38	41	43
Syncope	9	15	18
Stroke	2	5	7
Confusion	3	8	19
Weakness	7	8	10
Dizziness	6	4	5
Palpitations	4	2	1
Vomiting	18	18	16
Sweating	36	27	14
Silent	2	2	3

*Data adapted from Bayer AJ et al. Changing presentation of myocardial infarction with increasing old age. *J Am Geriatr Soc* 34:263, 1986.

MONITOR EVERY ELDERLY PATIENT, REGARDLESS OF CHIEF COMPLAINT.

Congestive Heart Failure

Congestive heart failure (CHF) is very common among the elderly, and again its presentation may be quite atypical. Heart failure is particularly likely to present in the form of an acute confusional state. (Why? Hint: What happens to the arterial PO_2 in heart failure? What is the effect of that change on cerebral oxygenation?) Often there is a history of multiple episodes of nocturnal confusion ("sundowning"). Another feature of heart failure in the elderly that is rarely encountered in younger patients is the occasional development of blisters on the legs. Those blisters, which are translucent, multiple, and sometimes quite large, develop when the elderly patient with orthopnea sleeps in his chair at night, thereby maintaining increased hydrostatic pressure in his already edematous legs. Classic signs of heart failure, on the other hand, may not have the same significance in an elderly person as in the young. Crackles, as noted earlier, are often heard in the lung bases of the elderly without any pulmonary pathology. So too, edema in the legs may be mechanical in origin, relating to inactivity and sitting with the feet dependent, and cannot always be assumed to be a sign of right heart failure.

Delirium in the Elderly

Delirium, or an acute confusional state, is one of the most common presenting signs in the elderly—occurring in up to one-quarter of all elderly patients admitted to the hospital with acute illness *of any cause.* Delirium may be associated with acute myocardial infarction, congestive heart failure, pneumonia, diabetes, dehydration, stroke, electrolyte imbalance, and—perhaps most importantly—the toxic effects of medications. Whatever the source of the delirium, it is a safe generalization that

> **DELIRIUM IN THE ELDERLY IS ALWAYS A SIGN OF PHYSICAL ILLNESS OR DRUG INTOXICATION AND IS ALWAYS AN EMERGENCY.**

Many elderly people suffer chronically from confusion and diminished mental function; that is to say, they suffer from **dementia**. Confusion in a patient with long-standing dementia may not have the same diagnostic significance as delirium, which by definition is an *acute* confusional state. It is important, therefore, when you find that an elderly patient is confused, to try to determine whether the patient is suffering from delirium or dementia (or, in some cases, both).

Delirium comes on relatively abruptly, often at night. It is of short duration, and the symptoms fluc-tuate in their severity over the course of a day, usually getting worse during the nighttime hours. All mental functions are disordered—thinking, memory, judgment, perception. Hallucinations, often vivid and frightening, are common. The patient is usually disoriented to time, and he may mistake unfamiliar people for people whom he knows. His level of consciousness may be depressed or hyperalert, and the sleep-wake cycle is often turned upside down—with the patient wide awake and agitated during the night and sleeping during the day. Some of the features that distinguish delirium from dementia are summarized in Table 29-3.

Depression and Suicide in the Elderly

Depression is common among the elderly, and one-quarter of all suicides occur among individuals over 65. Elderly men, especially those who are unmarried, divorced, or widowed, are at the highest risk. We shall discuss the evaluation of a depressed patient in more detail in Chapter 38. For our purposes here, suffice it to mention that any elderly person who appears depressed should be asked specifically about suicidal thoughts. It is best to start with a general sort of question, such as, "Have you ever felt that you just can't go on any more?" or "Have you ever felt that you'd be better off dead?" If the answer to a question of that sort is affirmative, try to determine if the patient has made any concrete plans for *how* he would do himself in. A patient who expresses suicidal thoughts and has formulated a concrete plan for killing himself is at very high risk for doing so. The patient's statements should be noted on the trip sheet and reported to the doctor at the receiving hospital.

TABLE 29-3.   DISTINGUISHING DELIRIUM FROM DEMENTIA

CHARACTERISTIC	DELIRIUM	DEMENTIA
Onset	Sudden, over hours or days	Gradual, over months or years
Daily course	Gets worse at night	Stable throughout 24 hr
Level of consciousness	Usually reduced	Normal
Hallucinations	Frequent, often vivid and frightening	Rare
Orientation	Disoriented as to time and sometimes as to place	May be impaired
Level of activity	Abnormally reduced or increased; agitation is common	Usually normal

Pharmacology for the Elderly

The elderly consume more than 25 percent of all prescribed and over-the-counter drugs sold in the United States. More than 80 percent of all elderly patients take at least one prescription drug, and more than one-third take three or more drugs every day. In surveys of nursing homes, patients have been found to be taking an average of anywhere from 5 to 12 different medications daily. Small wonder, then, that adverse drug reactions occur commonly in the elderly and account for as many as 30 percent of all hospital admissions among the aged. Indeed, a visitor arriving from another planet could easily get the impression that humans have a policy of routinely and systematically poisoning their elders.

A variety of factors contribute to the high incidence of adverse drug reactions among the old. The first, as already mentioned, is that elderly people are apt to be taking a variety of drugs, which their doctors may or may not know about. Patients may be taking medications prescribed by more than one physician, each dispensing prescriptions in blissful ignorance of the other. Patients may also be taking over-the-counter medications or medications prescribed for someone else in the family ("If it's good for Cousin Sadie, it must be good for me.").

A second factor contributing to drug toxicity in the elderly is the alteration in absorption, distribution, metabolism, and excretion of drugs that occurs as part of the aging process. Drugs such as digoxin that depend on the liver and kidney for their metabolism and excretion are particularly likely to accumulate to toxic levels in older patients. The fact is that we still know very little about the optimal dosage for the elderly of most drugs, since nearly all clinical trials carried out to establish the safe dosages of drugs are performed in young populations. For the most part, though, dosages for the elderly need to be *reduced* as compared to those for younger patients.

> **THE BEST DOSAGE OF A DRUG FOR AN ELDERLY PATIENT IS THE LOWEST DOSAGE THAT WILL ACHIEVE A THERAPEUTIC EFFECT.**

Just about any drug can produce toxic effects in an old person, but certain drugs are implicated more often than others—listed in Table 29-4 as the "Dirty Dozen." Of particular concern among those dirty

TABLE 29-4. THE DIRTY DOZEN: DRUGS MOST COMMONLY CAUSING TOXIC REACTIONS IN THE ELDERLY

1. Digitalis (most common cause of toxicity in the elderly)
2. Diuretics
3. Analgesics, including narcotics and aspirin
4. Sedative and hypnotic drugs
5. Phenothiazines
6. Tricyclic antidepressants
7. Anticoagulants
8. Theophylline
9. Propranolol
10. Quinidine
11. Lidocaine
12. Steroids

dozen for providers of prehospital emergency care are *lidocaine, diuretics, narcotic analgesics,* and *theophylline,* all of which should be given in reduced dosage when administered to elderly patients (if administered to them at all).

Summary

Approximately 3.3 million ambulance calls in the United States each year involve elderly patients, and the numbers will only increase as the proportion of the population over the age of 65 continues to grow. The elderly present a variety of challenges to EMS providers, not the least of which is learning to recognize when a serious emergency exists. For a variety of reasons—including dulled sensitivity to pain, blunted febrile response to infection, difficulty or reluctance in communicating distress—the signs and symptoms of potentially life-threatening problems may be obscured in the very old. Without a high index of suspicion, the paramedic is liable to be unaware of how very sick an elderly patient really is. For that reason, an elderly patient in any of the following categories should be considered seriously or critically ill until proved otherwise and should be given expeditious treatment and transport:

> **ELDERLY PATIENTS SHOULD BE CONSIDERED SERIOUSLY ILL IF THEY PRESENT WITH:**
>
> - Acute confusion, or any other sudden change in mental status
> - The acute onset or worsening of
>   1. Chest pain or discomfort

2. Dyspnea
3. Weakness or dizziness
- Syncope
- Fall
- Any significant trauma
- Nausea and vomiting

A word about transport and the use of sirens. Sirens are placed aboard emergency vehicles to assist in making a rapid response *to* the emergency scene. There is scarcely ever a justification for using sirens when proceeding *from* the emergency scene to the hospital with a patient in the vehicle. As noted in a previous chapter, the use of sirens under those circumstances gives the patient two clear messages: (1) There is something terribly wrong; and (2) those caring for him in the ambulance do not feel competent to handle the problem. Clearly those are *not* messages likely to improve the state of mind of a seriously ill person, nor will the howling and yapping of a siren enhance the mental clarity of a confused elderly person. Therefore, refrain from the use of sirens when you have *any* patient in the ambulance, but especially an elderly patient, unless a siren is absolutely necessary to get you expeditiously through traffic in a dire emergency. In that situation, *explain* to the patient that you are turning on the siren to enable a prompt transport and not because his condition is viewed as critical.

GLOSSARY

delirium An acute confusional state characterized by global impairment of thinking, perception, judgment, and memory.

dementia Chronic deterioration of mental functions.

geriatric Pertaining to the very old.

homeostasis Tendency to constancy or stability in the body's internal milieu.

hypertrophy Enlargement of an organ caused by an increase in size of its constituent cells (rather than an increase in the number of cells).

osteoporosis Pathologic reduction in bone mass to the degree that the skeleton can no longer perform its supportive function.

proprioception The ability to perceive the position and movement of one's body or its limbs.

residual volume Volume of air remaining in the lungs after a maximal exhalation.

review of systems Systematic survey of the patient's symptoms according to the major organ systems.

spondylosis Abnormal immobility and consolidation of a vertebral joint.

vital capacity The volume of air that can be forcefully exhaled from the lungs following a full inhalation.

FURTHER READING

Aronow WS. Prevalence of presenting symptoms of recognized acute myocardial infarction and of unrecognized healed myocardial infarction in elderly patients. *Am J Cardiol* 60:1182, 1987.

Bailey RB et al. Chronic salicylate intoxication: A common cause of morbidity in the elderly. *J Am Geriatr Soc* 37:556, 1989.

Bayer AJ et al. Changing presentation of myocardial infarction with increasing old age. *J Am Geriatr Soc* 34:263, 1986.

Birnbaumer DM. Abdominal emergencies in later life. *Emerg Med* 25(5):75, 1993.

Birrer R. Don't miss myocardial infarction in the elderly. *Emerg Med* 23(17):67, 1991.

Bonnin MG, Pepe PE, Clark PS Jr. Survival in the elderly after out-of-hospital cardiac arrest. *Crit Care Med* 21:1645, 1993.

Bosker G, Sequeira M. The 60-second geriatric assessment. *Emerg Med Serv* 17(7);17, 1988.

Bosker G et al. *Geriatric Emergency Medicine.* St. Louis: Mosby, 1990.

Brewer RA, Jones JS. Reporting elder abuse: Limitations of statutes. *Ann Emerg Med* 18:1217, 1989.

Bugliosi TF, Meloy TD, Vukov LR. Acute abdominal pain in the elderly. *Ann Emerg Med* 19:1383, 1990.

Clark-Daniels CL, Daniels RS, Baumhover LA. Abuse and neglect of the elderly: Are emergency department personnel aware of mandatory reporting laws? *Ann Emerg Med* 19:970, 1990.

Copeland AR. Fatal accidental falls among the elderly: The Metro Dade County experience, 1981–1983. *Med Sci Law* 25:172, 1985.

Counselman F. Two sides of acute abdomen in the elderly. *Emerg Med* 21(3):23, 1989.

Cunha BA. Infections in the elderly: Atypical clues to the puzzle. *Emerg Med* 22(1):56, 1990.

Denman SJ et al. Short-term outcomes of elderly patients discharged from an emergency department. *J Am Geriatr Soc* 37:937, 1989.

Dick T. Of "grunts" and "groids." *Emerg Med Serv* 20(7):13, 1991.

Eckstein D. Common symptoms and complaints of the elderly. *J Am Geriatr Soc* 21:440, 1973.

Eliastam M. Elderly patients in the emergency department. *Ann Emerg Med* 18:1222, 1989.

Garvin JM. Caring for the geriatric patient. *Emerg Med Serv* 9(2):75, 1980.

Gerson LW, Schelble DT, Wilson JE. Using paramedics to identify at-risk elderly. *Ann Emerg Med* 21:688, 1992.

Gerson LW, Skvarch L. Emergency medical service utilization by the elderly. *Ann Emerg Med* 11:610, 1982.

Godar T. Geriatric respiratory emergencies. *Emergency* 24(9):30, 1992.

Gross CR et al. Clinical indicators of dehydration severity in elderly patients. *J Emerg Med* 10:267, 1992.

Hamm B. If you could feel what I feel: Learning to care for the elderly. *JEMS* 18(10):57, 1993.

Hayflick L. The cell biology of human aging. *N Engl J Med* 295:1302, 1976.

Jones J et al. A geriatrics curriculum for emergency medicine training programs. *Ann Emerg Med* 15:1275, 1986.

Judd RL. Caring for the elderly. *Emergency* 21(6):38, 1989.

Kapoor W et al. Syncope in the elderly. *Am J Med* 80:419, 1986.

Keep the elderly cool. *Emerg Med* 17(13):155, 1985.

Kincaid DT, Botti RE. Myocardial infarction in the elderly. *Chest* 64:170, 1973.

Knudson MM. Trauma care in the elderly. *Emerg Med Serv* 19(4):52, 1990.

Lamy PP, Vestal RE. Drug prescribing for the elderly. *Hosp Pract* 11(1):111, 1976.

Lau WY et al. Acute appendicitis in the elderly. *Surg Gynecol Obstet* 16:157, 1985.

Lipowski ZJ. Delirium in the elderly patient. *N Engl J Med* 320:578, 1989.

McFadden JP et al. Raised respiratory rate in elderly patients: A valuable physical sign. *Br Med J* 284:626, 1982.

McMahan FJ et al. What special problems do geriatric patients present? *Emerg Med Serv* 14(2):19, 1985.

Mildenberger C et al. Abuse and neglect of elderly persons by family members: A special communication. *Phys Ther* 66:537, 1986.

Muller RT et al. Painless myocardial infarction in the elderly. *Am Heart J* 119:202, 1990.

O'Keefe ST, Noel J, Lavan JN. Cardiopulmonary resuscitation preferences in the elderly. *Eur J Med* 2:33, 1993.

Rockwood K. Acute confusion in elderly medical patients. *J Am Geriatr Soc* 37:150, 1989.

Rowe JW, Besdine RW. *Geriatric Medicine.* Boston: Little, Brown, 1988.

Schanzer HR. The emergencies of old age. *Emerg Med* 17(21):59, 1985.

Taylor BW. Altered factors in the assessment of the geriatric patient. *Emerg Med Serv* 14(2):26, 1985.

Wilder RJ. Trauma in the elderly. *Emerg Med Serv* 9(2):61, 1980.

Wilson LB, Simson SP, Baxter CR (eds.). *Handbook of Geriatric Emergency Care.* Baltimore: University Park Press, 1984.

Wroblewski M et al. Symptoms of myocardial infarction in old age: Clinical case retrospective and prospective studies. *Age Ageing* 15:99, 1986.

30
Pediatric Emergencies

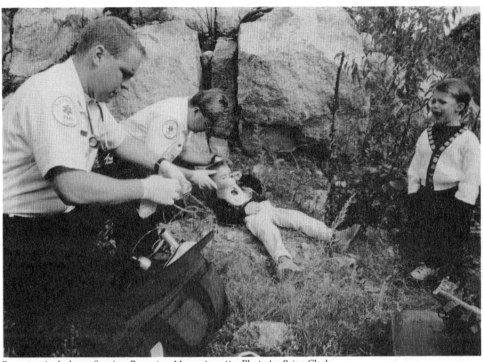

Brewster Ambulance Service, Brewster, Massachusetts. Photo by Brian Clark.

OBJECTIVES

Children are not simply miniature adults. They are different anatomically and physiologically from adults. And they are different from adults in the responses they elicit from paramedics. The same paramedic who can sail through the most grisly accident extrication without turning a hair may go completely to pieces when he has to deal with a kid who's been hit by a car. The fact is that critically ill and injured children are scary. Part of the reason they are scary is that relatively little time is spent on pediatrics in most paramedic training courses, so paramedics may feel inadequately prepared to deal with pediatric emergencies when they occur. Another reason is that, happily, we don't see as many very sick or severely injured children in prehospital care as we do adults. So most paramedics have less experience in dealing with children and tend to feel correspondingly less confident when it comes to handling a pediatric emergency. Furthermore, the pressures at the scene are invariably much greater when the patient is a child; parents, bystanders, law enforcement officials, and EMS personnel themselves all become much more upset when the critically ill or injured patient is a child than when he is an adult.

In this chapter, we shall address some of the special considerations that apply to caring for an ill or injured child. We shall first review the overall approach to the pediatric patient and see how that approach must take into account the child's age and also the mental state of his or her parents. We shall then look at a variety of emergencies that are unique to children or the treatment of which requires special modifications in children. Finally, we shall go over the steps of basic and advanced life support as they apply to children and learn some special techniques of airway control and intravenous access. By the end of this chapter, then, the student should be able to

1. Describe the anticipated responses to EMS personnel in an ill or injured child, given the child's age, and explain the approach that should be taken to a child of that age
2. Describe a strategy for dealing with aggressive or otherwise difficult parents that will be in the best interests of all concerned
3. Identify normal and abnormal vital signs, given several sets of vital signs from infants and children of different ages
4. Identify normal and abnormal physical signs, given a description of several infants and young children with different physical findings
5. Given a description of several children with different symptoms and signs, identify
   - A child who has choked on a foreign body
   - A child with epiglottitis
   - A child with croup
   - A child with a severe asthmatic attack
   - A child with bronchiolitis
   and describe the correct prehospital management of each
6. List the questions that should be asked in taking the history of an asthmatic attack and the points of emphasis in the physical assessment of the asthmatic patient
7. In a child having an acute asthmatic attack, explain the possible significance of
   - Drowsiness
   - Pulsus paradoxus
   - Skin tenting
   - Hyperresonance of the chest
   - A silent chest
8. List at least four characteristics of epiglottitis, and explain why epiglottitis is considered a life-threatening condition
9. Describe the management of a case of sudden infant death syndrome, given a description of the circumstances of the case
10. List five causes of seizures in children
11. List the questions that should be asked in taking the history of a child who has had a seizure and the points of emphasis in the physical assessment of that child
12. List the steps in the prehospital management of
    - A febrile seizure
    - Status epilepticus in a child
13. List at least 10 possible clues to child abuse, and describe
    - What to look for in examining a child who may be a victim of abuse
    - How to manage a case of suspected child abuse
    - How to document a case of suspected child abuse
14. Describe the injuries most likely to be present given a description of how a child was injured (i.e., given the mechanisms of injury)
15. State the differences in assessing and managing injured infants and children, as opposed to adults, with respect to
    - Use of airway adjuncts
    - Detection of pneumothorax
    - Signs of hypovolemic shock
    - Most frequent causes of hypovolemic shock
16. List at least 10 "load-and-go" situations in injured children
17. List the points of emphasis in performing the secondary survey of an injured child
18. Given a clinical description of several injured children with different injuries, identify a child who has suffered

- A serious head injury
- A serious chest injury
- A serious abdominal injury
- A critical burn

and describe the correct prehospital management of each

19. List five indications for immediate endotracheal intubation in a young child or infant who has suffered flame burns

20. Identify a child who has ingested an overdose of salicylates, given a description of several children with different clinical findings, and describe the correct prehospital management

21. Describe the prehospital treatment of children who put beans in their ears or commit similar offenses

22. For an infant and a young child undergoing cardiopulmonary resuscitation, state
    - The correct rate of artificial ventilation
    - The site for checking a pulse
    - The correct compression point
    - The correct rate of chest compressions
    - The defibrillation dosage
    - The dosage of epinephrine, atropine, and lidocaine

23. List the steps in intubating the trachea of a child, and describe the respects in which pediatric intubation differs from adult intubation

24. Identify correct and incorrect statements regarding intravenous and intraosseous infusions in children

25. List the therapeutic actions, indications, contraindications, possible side effects, and correct pediatric dosage of
    - Albuterol/salbutamol
    - Terbutaline
    - Epinephrine 1 : 1,000
    - Aminophylline
    - Diazepam

    after studying the relevant information about those medications in the Drug Handbook at the end of this textbook

APPROACH TO THE PEDIATRIC PATIENT

The sick or injured child presents unique challenges in evaluation and management, for the child's perception of his problem, of his world, and of the paramedic may be radically different from the perceptions of an adult. Depending on the child's age, he may or may not be able to report what is bothering him. Fear or pain may transform him into a howling banshee whose behavior evokes anxiety and confusion among all concerned. Furthermore, parents and bystanders

may be completely out of control, driven by guilt and anxiety to irrational and even aggressive acts. In the midst of all that, the paramedic is asked to be an island of calm and authority, carrying out his job systematically, carefully, confidently. It's a tall order.

The Ill or Injured Child: Special Considerations

In general, the ill or injured child is frightened. He is frightened by the disability itself and the discomfort it causes him; by the presence of strangers who may, for all he knows, have evil intentions toward him; and by the possibility of separation from his parents. A large percentage of the pediatric problems seen in the field, furthermore, result from accidents, which claim the lives of 12,000 children annually and render another 50,000 permanently disabled. Forty percent of those injuries occur in automobile accidents, in which other occupants are usually injured as well. Thus, the child may also be frightened by injuries to his parents or by noise, confusion, and an atmosphere of panic or distress. It is important to be aware of all those fears. For while you may see yourself as the knight in shining armor come to rescue those in distress, to the child you may appear to be a threatening stranger, who may hurt him or take him away from his mother and father.

Age-Related Responses to Illness, Injury, and You

The specific manner in which you approach the sick or injured child will depend to some extent on his age, for children of different ages react differently to illness and injury and also to strangers like yourself who appear on the scene in such circumstances.

We have no way of really knowing how the INFANT (the child younger than 1 year) perceives or remembers pain. However, we do know that infants are very distressed by separations from their mothers, so such separations should be kept to a minimum. The **neonate** (up to age 1 month) may be content to be held by a stranger and takes a rather undiscriminating interest in faces. But for the older infant, mother is mother, and substitutes will not be accepted cheerfully. The mother should therefore be allowed maximum contact with the infant at the scene and in transit, and wherever possible, she should hold and comfort the infant—both during your examination and en route to the hospital.

The 1 to 3 YEAR OLD is, as the designation **toddler** implies, a lot more mobile than the infant, having learned to crawl, walk, and then run; so typically this is the age when the child is "into everything"—

including household poisons. Language is starting to develop (the "terrible twos" are often characterized by an infatuation with the word "NO!"), and simple explanations can be understood. While somewhat more independent than the infant, the toddler nonetheless still wants to stay close to mother when there are strange people around and should also be permitted to take along a familiar blanket or teddy bear if the circumstances permit. Explain procedures to the toddler in very simple terms. Since children of this age have a limited time sense, there is no need to prepare them extensively for subsequent experiences in the emergency room; reciting to the toddler a list of all the things that might happen to him later will only increase his anxiety.

The 3 to 5 YEAR OLD (**preschooler**) lives in a world of many fears: fear of monsters, fear of aggression and retribution, and—for the first time—some awareness and fear of death. In addition, this is an age when fear of bodily mutilation is at its height. Even a minor cut sends the preschooler shrieking to his mother, and the sight of blood may precipitate utter panic. Furthermore, the child of this age tends to view illness and injury as punishment for his own aggressive feelings. And he is apt to interpret invasive procedures, such as starting an IV line, as outright acts of aggression by the forces of retribution. By this age, in addition, many children have learned to associate medical personnel with a variety of unpleasant experiences, such as getting shots, and they may not greet your arrival with very much enthusiasm. A lot of patience and tact are therefore required in dealing with preschoolers.

If the preschooler is injured, cover bleeding injuries rapidly, after assuring the child that none of his limbs or other vital structures have been lost or left at the scene (you may think that is obvious, but to the 3 year old it is of paramount concern). Reassure the child that it is all right to cry and that you would probably cry too if you hurt that much. (Using the old line about "big boys don't cry" is neither relevant nor fair to the child; at 3, one is not a big boy and should not be held to the dubious standards expected of big boys.) Explain everything you are doing, step by step.

Tell the preschooler a bit about what he can expect at the hospital, but do not overwhelm him; the amount of information you give should be guided by his expressed concerns (e.g., "Will I get a shot?")

Grade-school children (AGES 6 to 12) are not immune from the anxieties regarding pain, death, strangers, and separation from parents that preoccupy their younger brothers and sisters. They are also newly concerned with modesty and do not like to have their sexual parts exposed. However, the increased ability of grade-schoolers to communicate with adults helps them in dealing with such feelings. Furthermore, their natural curiosity can be mobilized effectively in helping them cope with illness or injury. The grade-school child likes to be treated with respect and ranks honesty high on his list of positive attributes in adults.

Attempt to make the grade-school child a partner in the examination and treatment process. Explain each procedure in detail. Some children may be especially interested in learning all about the equipment in the vehicle and may be usefully distracted by demonstrations of monitors or other gear.

As for younger children, clean and cover visible injuries as quickly as possible. Cover as well any other body parts whose exposure might offend the child's modesty. For school-age children, information tends to be reassuring rather than frightening, so you should prepare the child for what he will encounter in the emergency room. Where relevant, explain likely procedures such as x-rays or stitches. Again, the child's questions should help guide you toward topics of concern.

The **adolescent** (13 to 19 YEARS OLD) lives in a period of precarious self-esteem and is forever worrying over real and imagined bodily defects (pimples, stature, the shape of his or her nose, whether his or her sexual development compares favorably with that of friends, and so forth). Such fears are only compounded by an illness or injury. Paramount in the adolescent's thoughts may be a concern about how his current disability will affect him. Will a facial laceration leave a disfiguring scar? Will a fracture prevent competition in sports forever? Furthermore, the adolescent is in the difficult position of needing the support rendered a sick child yet at the same time wanting to be certain he or she receives the respect due an adult. Give the teenager the support and reassurance you would give a child; but be factual, and address the patient's questions as you would address those of an adult.

General Guidelines for Dealing with Children

Certain principles apply in dealing with children of any age who are sick or injured:

- STAY CALM.
- Kneel down or sit so that you DO NOT TOWER OVER THE CHILD.
- IDENTIFY YOURSELF, in simple terms. ("Hi, I'm Karen. What's *your* name?")
- SMILE a lot.
- Be PATIENT and GENTLE.

- DO NOT SEPARATE A CHILD FROM HIS PARENTS, even if they have been injured together with him in a multicasualty incident. In such circumstances, the child's normal anxieties about separation will only be heightened by worries that something terrible has happened to one or both parents. It is better that the child be allowed to remain with the injured parent, lest he become convinced that the parent is dead.

- When a child has been injured in a setting where neither parent is present (e.g., a child struck by a car some distance from home), ASSURE HIM THAT HIS PARENTS WILL BE NOTIFIED.

- Once you have ruled out life-threatening conditions, try to CONDUCT THE ASSESSMENT AT A RELAXED PACE. Rapid-fire questions and unexplained probings from a stranger can be very frightening to a child.

- Let the child hold onto HIS FAVORITE TOY, but KEEP YOUR FAVORITE TOYS DISCREETLY OUT OF SIGHT. If you come charging at a child with a stethoscope, sphygmomanometer, scissors, clamps, tubes, and all the other odds and ends that are so dear to your heart, he will inevitably wonder, "What on earth is this person going to do to me with all those things?" Save the instruments for last, and produce them one by one, as you need them.

- EXPLAIN EACH PROCEDURE, a step at a time. ("Now I'm going to put this funny balloon around your arm to measure your blood pressure. There. Now I'm going to inflate it by squeezing on this bulb, and it's going to feel tight for a few seconds. OK. Now I'm going to let all the air out, and it will feel loose again.")

- DON'T LIE! Do not tell a child that something won't hurt if it will hurt.

- Always keep a supply of LOLLIPOPS in the jump kit, to award to brave children (which, by definition, means all children who are not NPO because of their illness or injuries). The lollipops also come in handy for woozy diabetics and for acutely hypoglycemic paramedics who didn't manage to get a meal during a busy shift.

Dealing with the Parents of an Ill or Injured Child

The majority of children you will treat will come equipped with at least one parent. What that means, practically speaking, is that in many pediatric calls, you will be dealing with more than one patient, even if only the child is ill or injured. Serious illness or injury to a child is one of the most stressful situations a parent can face. As we learned in Chapter 4, people react to stress in different ways. One of the most common reactions to the stress of a sudden calamity to one's child is ANGER—anger at the driver of the car who struck the child, anger at the babysitter who wasn't paying enough attention, anger at the other parent, anger at anyone or anything that happens to be handy, which inevitably sometimes means anger at the unsuspecting and undeserving paramedics. Sooner or later it will happen to *you:* You will pull up at the scene of an accident where a child was struck by a car, and before you can even introduce yourself, you'll find yourself at the receiving end of a stream of verbal (and sometimes very nonverbal) abuse from a wildly distraught parent. And since it will happen sooner or later, it's a good idea to start thinking now about how you will deal with that situation. (We shall suggest some strategies shortly.)

Yet another common parental response is to indulge in an orgy of GUILT. "I knew I shouldn't have let him ride his bike to school," or "I kept thinking I ought to call the doctor about his fever, but then I'd say, 'Oh, you're just being silly, it's just a cold,' and now look how sick he is—if anything happens to him it will be all my fault."

Less commonly, the parent responds to the stress by withdrawing into a NUMBED DAZE, an extreme form of denial. While in such a condition, the parent may not be able to answer any of your questions or to provide any useful assistance.

Guidelines for Dealing with Parents Under Stress

Each paramedic will have to develop his or her own strategies for handling aggressive behavior, but there are some general guidelines that should govern your response:

- STAY CALM.
- THE PATIENT COMES FIRST. No matter what is going on around you, what names you are being called, what names you would like to apply in response, the most important person at the scene is the ill or injured child. Everything you say and do must be in the best interests of the child. As a general rule, antagonizing the child's parents, no matter how they are behaving, is not in the child's best interests, for you need their confidence—and, indeed, their consent—to treat the child.
- The best way to obtain the confidence of the parents is to behave in a calm, professional manner.
- If the parents are completely out of control and the child needs immediate attention for a life-

threatening condition, try to get other family members, bystanders, or law enforcement officers at the scene to RESTRAIN AND CALM THE PARENTS.

- As soon as the parents *are* calmed down, ENLIST THEIR HELP to hold, soothe, or talk to the child. ("Sir, I know this whole thing is terribly upsetting, but we're going to need your help in giving Timmy the care he needs.") The more active a role the parent can take in caring for the child, the better.

- When parents appear dazed and are unable to assist, don't put pressure on them to do so. Just EXPLAIN WHAT YOU ARE DOING, and offer HONEST REASSURANCE AND SUPPORT.

- Let the parents know that you DON'T BLAME THEM FOR WHAT HAPPENED. (If you *do* blame them, keep your thoughts to yourself!)

- Before you transport, ASK ABOUT OTHER CHILDREN at home. Sometimes a parent is so distraught about an injured child that he or she forgets the other small children left by themselves at home. Make sure arrangements are made to look after other children.

- TRANSPORT AT LEAST ONE PARENT WITH THE CHILD to the hospital, preferably the parent who seems to be coping *less* well (and who might therefore endanger himself or herself in getting behind the wheel of the family car to drive to the hospital).

- *If the child is dead at the scene,* give the parents time with the body. If the body is in a public place, such as on the street, move it into the ambulance so that the parents can have some privacy. Put a hand on the child's body, to signal the parents that it's all right for them to touch the body, hug it, and so forth. Then give them some time alone. Do not try to calm them down, and do not give sedatives; they need to feel and express their grief.

For a paramedic, especially a paramedic working in a busy urban service, one call blends into the next, and after a while most of the calls become hazy in memory. For the family of a seriously ill or injured child, on the other hand, the details of the emergency, and in particular the details of what happened before the child reached the hospital, will never be forgotten—especially if there was an unhappy outcome. What you want the family to remember about that stressful time is something like this: "Those paramedics really went all out for us." So when you have to deal with difficult behavior in the parents of an ill or injured child, think about the memories you are creating.

Assessment of the Ill or Injured Child

Assessment of the ill or injured child, like that of the adult, begins with the ABCs of the primary survey, which we shall discuss in some detail in the last section of this chapter. Assuming, however, that the primary survey does not reveal any immediate threats to life, the paramedic may proceed at once to the secondary survey. Here too, we find some modifications necessary according to the age of the child.

Taking the History

The basic goals in pediatric history-taking are identical to those in taking a history from an adult, that is, gathering information and establishing a relationship with the patient. However, there are significant differences in the way you achieve those goals with pediatric patients. To begin with, you can rarely obtain the whole history from the patient himself. Most commonly mother, or sometimes father, provides a good deal of the information. Bear in mind that some of that information may be colored by the parent's desire to present herself or himself as a "good parent." Try to be supportive of that tendency, for parents tend to feel excessively guilty when a child is ill or injured. Certainly the paramedic's attitude should *not* be accusatory ("Why did you wait so long to call?"). If the parents express guilt feelings, allow them to talk about those feelings; and reassure them that it is common, though rarely warranted, for parents to feel guilty under such circumstances.

In taking the history, do not discount the child as an important source of information. Even the very young child can sometimes provide valuable data if you ask about a neutral object (e.g., "Where does your dolly hurt?"). As children grow older, they become quite accurate in their reports of discomfort and indeed may provide that information with much more frankness than would an adult. Certainly once the child has reached school age, he should play an important part in the history, and his comments should be treated with respect. Many skilled pediatricians will devote their initial attention to the child's story, stating, "First, I'd like to talk with Johnny, and then we'll see what mother has to say." That indicates to both child and parent that the child has the floor and that his opinions are regarded as worth considering. In dealing with adolescents, it is particularly important to respect the patient's developing independence. The adolescent needs to feel that he is being treated as an adult and, further, that the paramedic will respect the confidentiality of his remarks. Whatever is told to the parent should first be discussed with the adolescent patient, who will want to be certain that the paramedic is acting on his behalf and not in the interests of his parents.

Facilitating the Physical Examination

Again, the goals of the physical examination in children are the same as in adults, but the techniques vary according to the age of the child. As noted, when a child of any age presents with an acute, life-threatening problem, conduct the primary survey rapidly and with a minimum of preliminaries, and manage life-threatening conditions as needed. When there is more time for assessment, however, certain techniques may facilitate the process.

The INFANT UNDER 6 MONTHS OLD will probably not object to being placed on a bed and having all his clothes taken off, so long as you provide entertaining distractions such as jangling keys, cooing, or making other pleasant noises. In infants and indeed in children up to school age, it is preferable to conduct the secondary survey in *toe-to-head* order, since small children as a rule do not like strangers poking at their faces.

> **IN INFANTS AND SMALL CHILDREN, CONDUCT THE PHYSICAL EXAMINATION IN TOE-TO-HEAD ORDER.**

The 6 to 24 MONTH OLD also may not object to having all his clothes removed, but he will not like it one bit if he is taken away from his mother and put on a bed or stretcher. It is usually most conducive to peace and goodwill to examine this child while he sits on mother's lap. The cooing routine is still worth a try, and it is worth taking time—if the situation is not extremely urgent—for a little play to allow the child to get accustomed to you. Your penlight is likely to be a good distraction. Again, in the body survey, start at the toes and work up.

The 2 to 3 YEAR OLD is usually difficult, no matter how charming the examiner may be. He does not like to have his clothing removed. He does not want to be touched, especially by a stranger. He doesn't have the slightest desire to play with the paramedic. And there is often nothing that anyone, including mother, can do to convince him that you are really a splendid person. The 2 to 3 year old is frightened and in no mood to be conciliatory. Sometimes, the physical examination may be rendered less traumatic for

all concerned if it is carried out in parallel on the child's teddy bear ("First we'll listen to Teddy's chest. Mm hm. Now we'll listen to Bobby's chest."). Often, however, the teddy bear ploy is met simply with an intransigent stare. In that situation, decide which parts of the physical examination are absolutely essential and get through them as best you can. Set the ground rules (crying is allowed; kicking and biting are not), and do what you have to as quickly as possible.

By comparison, the 4 to 5 YEAR OLD is often a delight. He is usually cooperative, except when inordinately frightened, and may often be examined on a chair or bed. He likes to help out (e.g., by listening to his own heart with the stethoscope). There is generally little problem in performing the physical assessment in the standard head-to-toe sequence in this age group.

The GRADE-SCHOOL CHILD is also likely to be cooperative. He appreciates being treated with respect and also appreciates explanations of what you are doing (e.g., "This instrument is called a stethoscope, and it helps me listen to the sounds that your heart makes.").

The ADOLESCENT, as noted earlier, is likely to be unusually concerned about his bodily integrity, and it is often helpful to assure him, as each part of the examination is completed, that things are OK (assuming that they *are* OK). After auscultating the chest, for example, an offhand comment such as, "Your lungs certainly sound good," may relieve many unspoken anxieties.

Special Considerations in the Physical Assessment

In this section, we shall deal with the general physical assessment of the infant and child; later on in the chapter we'll consider points of special emphasis when examining a child who has been injured. In performing the physical assessment of an infant or child, we evaluate mostly the same parameters as in an adult, but the measures we use and the criteria for normal sometimes differ.

As always, the first thing we assess is the child's GENERAL APPEARANCE, and the first thing to note in that category is the LEVEL OF CONSCIOUSNESS. Is the child awake, alert, and interested in his surroundings? Or is he drowsy, dull, and lethargic? (If he is sleeping, *don't* wake him yet! Wait until after you've had a chance to listen to his chest and heart in peace and quiet.) Start a neurologic flow sheet for any child with an altered level of consciousness, and record frequent observations.

Note the child's POSITION AND MOVEMENT. Is he moving all his extremities spontaneously? Is there abnormal posturing? Is there seizure activity?

The DEGREE OF DISTRESS may be difficult to gauge, especially in an infant, although often mother can identify a cry that means something other than "I'm wet" or "I'm hungry." Don't be lulled into complacency by a very quiet child. A severely ill child may be very quiet, and an abused child often will not cry even when in severe pain.

Assess the SKIN of the trunk and the extremities with the back of your hand for TEMPERATURE. If the distal extremities feel cold and the trunk is warm, consider the possibility of dehydration or shock. If the skin feels unusually hot or cold, measure the temperature with a thermometer (axillary temperatures will do—but be sure to record the fact that it's an axillary temperature when you record the vital signs).

In victims of trauma, scan quickly for OBVIOUS WOUNDS OR DEFORMITIES that need to be dealt with before any further manipulations are carried out.

After observing the child's general appearance, proceed to measurement of the VITAL SIGNS. Since that will mean deploying some sinister equipment, like a stethoscope and blood pressure apparatus, be prepared to spend a little time letting the child handle the equipment and explaining what you propose to do with it.

It is important to remember that VITAL SIGNS ARE AGE-SPECIFIC. What is normal for an infant may indicate hypovolemic shock in a 6 year old! Normal vital signs for six different age groups are shown in Table 30-1. Since it's nearly impossible to remember the information in that table, and certainly impossible to do so in an emergency, the best thing to do is make a copy of Table 30-1 and tape it to the case containing your pediatric sphygmomanometer. That way, you will be sure that the information is handy when you need it, that is, when you are actually measuring a child's vital signs.

Which brings us to another important point about measuring vital signs in infants and children: You need special equipment. The blood pressure cuff for an adult is far too large for a child. For an infant, you need a cuff that is 6 to 8 cm (about 2.5–3.0 inches) wide, and for a child you need a cuff that is 9 to 10 cm (about 3.5–4.0 inches) wide.

As noted earlier, whether the HEAD-TO-TOE SURVEY becomes the toe-to-head survey will depend on the age of the child. But in whatever order it is conducted, you need to look for certain things in particular.

When examining the HEAD of an infant, make certain to check the anterior "soft spot" (**fontanelle**) on the top of the head. The fontanelle may bulge out normally when the infant cries, but otherwise it should be relatively flat *when the infant is recumbent*—level with the surface of the skull or very slightly concave. It is often possible to observe pulsations in a normal anterior fontanelle. In conditions such as meningitis, the fontanelle may be tense and bulging, even when the infant is quiet and at rest, and pulsations will no longer be visible. In dehydration, on the other hand, the fontanelle becomes sunken.

In the infant, check the NOSTRILS to make sure they are not obstructed by secretions. Infants are obligate nose breathers, sometimes as long as up to the age of 6 months, and plugging of the nostrils may therefore lead to respiratory arrest.

When there is a question of foreign body aspiration, check the child's MOUTH. When the child is feverish, stridorous, and drooling, however, leave the mouth alone—he may have epiglottitis, and manipulation around the oropharynx may lead to complete airway closure.

In a child with fever, observe whether the NECK is stiff or moves freely.

Observe the CHEST for respiratory excursions and signs of respiratory distress. The child is a "belly breather," relying primarily on movements of his diaphragm to expand the thoracic cavity. That tendency

TABLE 30-1. NORMAL VITAL SIGNS IN CHILDREN AT REST

AGE	AVERAGE BP	PULSE	RESPIRATIONS
1 day–1 mo	74/40	120–150	30–70
1 mo–1 yr	85/60	115–130	20–40
2–6 yr	90/60	80–115	20–30
6–10 yr	95/62	85–100	20–25
10–18 yr	105/65	70–80	15–20

tends to be exaggerated in severe illness or injury, as the immature intercostal muscles tire rapidly. Listen to at least six symmetric lung fields, front and back, for abnormal breath sounds. Wheezes are usually a sign of bronchospastic lung disease (asthma, bronchiolitis), but localized wheezes may point to a foreign body blocking a bronchus. Before you remove your stethoscope from the chest, listen to the heart sounds, for clarity, rate, and regularity.

Inspect the ABDOMEN for distention and bulges that suggest hernias. Palpate for rigidity.

Observe the EXTREMITIES for normal spontaneous movements.

Throughout the physical assessment of the child, observe the following general guidelines:

- Respect the child's modesty. Undress only the part you are examining, and cover that part up again when you finish examining it.
- Postpone the use of instruments as long as possible.
- Examine injured or painful areas last.
- Be an opportunist! If an infant or small child is sleeping, seize the chance to auscultate the lungs and heart in quiet conditions; you may not have another opportunity to do so once the child wakens and decides he doesn't like you.

AIRWAY AND RESPIRATORY EMERGENCIES

Foreign Body Obstruction of the Airway*

The same things that produce upper airway obstruction in the adult—the tongue, swelling in the airway, and foreign bodies—may obstruct the airway of a child. Children are particularly prone to aspirate small objects, such as peanuts, coins, or small toys, into the air passages, with resulting partial or complete airway obstruction. The vast majority of deaths from foreign body aspiration in the pediatric set occurs in children under the age of 5 years, mostly in infants.

The first step in managing upper airway obstruction in the child is to TRY QUICKLY TO DETERMINE THE CAUSE. If there is reason to suspect croup or epiglottitis (see below), the measures used to dislodge a foreign body will be ineffective and may even

---

*The recommendations presented here are based on those of the Emergency Cardiac Care Committee and Subcommittees, American Heart Association. Guidelines for cardiopulmonary resuscitation and emergency cardiac care. *JAMA* 268:2171, 1992.

be dangerous. So find out under what circumstances the emergency occurred. A child who has been ill with fever, sore throat, a barking cough, or stridor needs rapid transportation to the nearest medical facility. A child who was previously healthy and who choked while eating or while playing with small toys needs immediate measures to relieve foreign body obstruction.

A foreign body in the upper airway may cause partial or complete airway obstruction. When there is partial obstruction, the child may still be capable of good air exchange. If so, the child will be able to cough forcefully and will have good color, although there may be wheezing between the coughs.

> **IF THE CHILD HAS GOOD AIR EXCHANGE, ENCOURAGE SPONTANEOUS COUGHING EFFORTS. DO *NOT* INTERFERE WITH THE CHILD'S ATTEMPT TO EXPEL THE FOREIGN BODY BY COUGHING.**

Poor air exchange, on the other hand, is characterized by an ineffective cough, high-pitched noises on inhalation, increased respiratory distress, and cyanosis. If air exchange is poor, manage the partial obstruction as if it were a complete airway obstruction.

COMPLETE AIRWAY OBSTRUCTION means there is no air exchange at all. The treatment of complete obstruction in the child utilizes a combination of back blows and *chest* thrusts. Abdominal thrusts are *not* recommended in infants less than 1 year old because of potential injury to abdominal organs.

If the victim is an INFANT, straddle him over your arm with his head lower than his trunk and supported with your hand around his jaw and chest (Fig. 30-1). To stabilize the baby, you may sit and rest your forearm on your thigh. Use the heel of your other hand to deliver UP TO FIVE BACK BLOWS between the infant's shoulder blades. *Don't overdo it!* Babies are very little, and not much force is required. Immediately after delivering the back blows, place your free hand on the infant's back, with your fingers supporting his head and neck, so that he is sandwiched between your two hands. Then flip him over, and place him supine on your thigh with his head lower than his trunk (Fig. 30-2). While he is in that position, give UP TO FIVE CHEST THRUSTS (performed just as you would perform external chest compressions on an infant—see the last section of this chapter). Then lift the baby's tongue and open his mouth. *If you see a foreign body,* hook it out with your finger, but

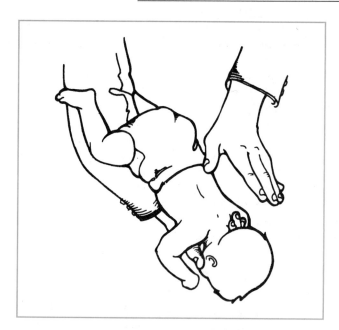

FIGURE 30-1. BACK BLOWS FOR THE CHOKING IN-FANT. Reproduced courtesy of the American Heart Association.

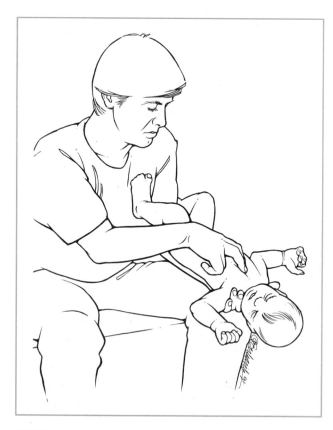

FIGURE 30-2. CHEST THRUSTS FOR THE CHOKING INFANT.

> **DO NOT PROBE BLINDLY FOR A FOREIGN BODY YOU CANNOT SEE.**

Especially in infants and children, blind poking about in the mouth and pharynx can easily push the foreign body farther back into the airway and worsen the obstruction.

The steps in managing foreign body obstruction of the airway in an infant are summarized in Figure 30-3 and in the performance checklists at the end of this chapter.

If the choking victim is a CHILD, the American Heart Association now recommends the use of abdominal thrusts only, without accompanying back blows. Perform the abdominal thrust as you would on an adult (Fig. 30-4), taking care that your hands are below the xiphoid process and the ribs. Give five thrusts in rapid sequence and attempt ventilation. As in infants, do not probe blindly into a child's mouth with your finger. Use a laryngoscope to visualize the larynx, and remove the foreign body with a Magill forceps under direct vision. If you have no equipment, grasp the child's tongue and lower jaw between your thumb and finger to *pull the tongue forward.* If you *see* the foreign body, pluck it out. The steps in treating a choking child are summarized in the performance checklists at the end of this chapter.

Acute Asthmatic Attacks and Status Asthmaticus

Asthma is a common problem among children, affecting between 5 and 10 percent of children under 10 years old. Nearly three-quarters of asthmatic children experience their first symptoms before the age of 5 years. About 50 percent of asthmatic children "outgrow" their asthma, while the remainder continue to experience attacks of varying severity into adulthood.

The Pathophysiology of an Asthmatic Attack

Recall that the acute asthmatic attack is characterized by reversible spasm and *constriction of the bronchi,* along with *inflammatory edema* and congestion *of their lining membranes* and *hypersecretion of mucus,* which comes to form tenacious plugs blocking the smaller airways. All those factors combine to interfere with the normal passage of air in and out of the lungs. *Exhalation* presents particular difficulty, and not all the air that is inhaled can be expelled; with each

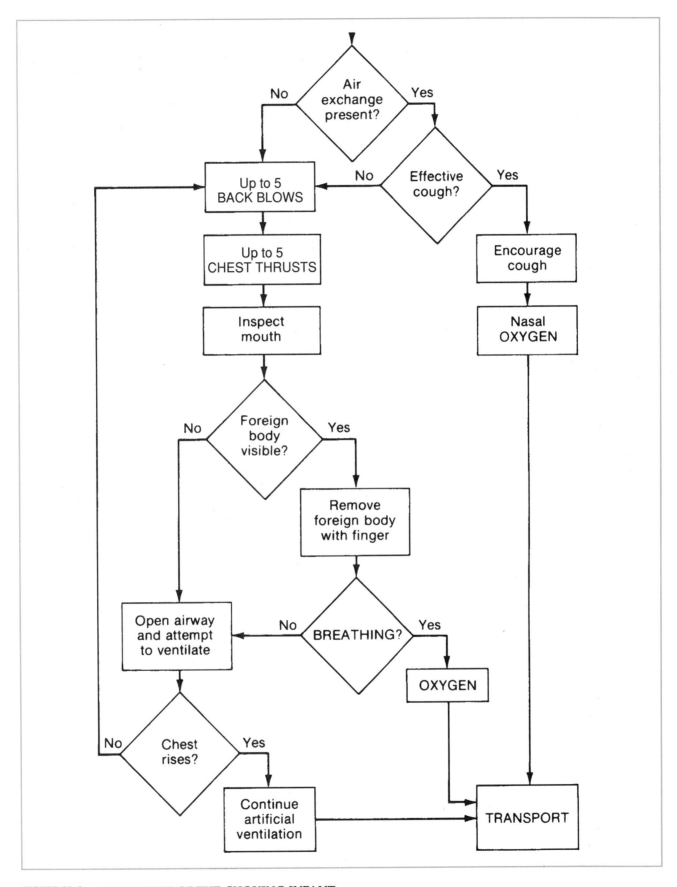

FIGURE 30-3. **TREATMENT OF THE CHOKING INFANT.**

processes are brought under control. As we shall see shortly, each of the measures we use in the treatment of an acute asthmatic attack is aimed at correcting one or more of the pathophysiologic conditions induced by the illness:

- BRONCHODILATORS are given to counteract bronchospasm and relax the bronchial musculature.
- OXYGEN is required to treat hypoxemia.
- In very severe cases, sodium BICARBONATE is given to treat acidosis, and STEROIDS are administered to diminish the edema and congestion of bronchial membranes.
- FLUIDS are sometimes administered to treat dehydration and loosen thick mucus collections.

Assessment of the Child Having an Acute Asthmatic Attack

Asthma is a chronic illness in children, and as a general rule, people with chronic illnesses do not call for an ambulance unless *something has changed*, changed for the worse. Thus when parents or school officials summon an ambulance for an asthmatic child, it is very often because the child is having an attack that is more severe than his usual attack or that has not been successfully controlled with the usual medications taken at home. Every call for an acute asthmatic attack should therefore be regarded as a serious medical emergency.

In evaluating the child having an acute asthmatic attack, a careful HISTORY should establish the following:

- What is the *chief complaint*? While wheezing is considered the hallmark of asthma, in fact many cases present with a persistent nonproductive cough or dyspnea on exertion.
- *How long* has the present attack been going on?
- *How much fluid* has the child been able to take during this time?
- Has the child (or anyone else in the family) had a *recent respiratory infection*? (As we shall see, recent respiratory infection, especially in a child under 2 years old, may point to bronchiolitis rather than asthma as the source of the child's wheezes.)
- What, if any, *medications* has the child been given for this attack? *When* were they given? *How much* was given? Ask about *all* medications, including syrups, tablets, and medications taken by inhalation. The types and dosages of medications already taken will influence the decision of what further medications can be safely administered.

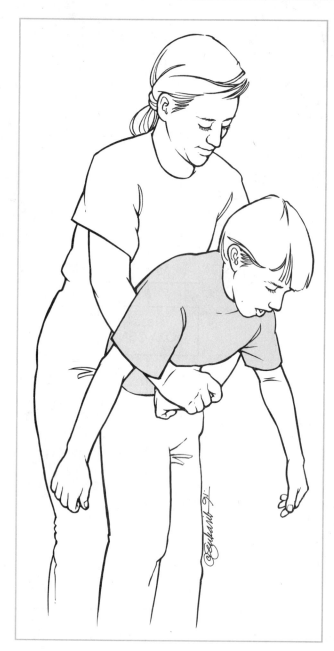

FIGURE 30-4.   **ABDOMINAL THRUSTS FOR A CHOKING CHILD.**

breath, some air remains trapped in the lungs. The chest, as a consequence, becomes hyperinflated and hyperresonant to percussion, and ventilation is progressively impaired. The child struggles more and more to breathe, with less and less to show for it. The net effect is increasing HYPOXEMIA, HYPERCARBIA, ACIDOSIS, and DEHYDRATION. Furthermore, as acidosis worsens, BRONCHOCONSTRICTION becomes even more severe, while dehydration causes the mucus plugs to become thicker and more tenacious. Thus a vicious cycle is set in motion, which cannot be reversed unless the underlying pathologic

- Does the child have any known *allergies* to drugs, foods, or inhalants?
- Has the child ever required *hospitalization* for an acute asthmatic attack? If so, how recently? How often? Where?

In the PHYSICAL EXAMINATION of the asthmatic child, pay particular attention to the following:

- GENERAL APPEARANCE: In what *position* is the child sitting or lying? In how much *distress* does he appear? The child with a mild asthmatic attack usually prefers to sit, but will lie down. He may be somewhat excited. The child with a severe attack will appear exhausted and may be unable to move from a preferred position, usually leaning forward with elbows braced.
- STATE OF CONSCIOUSNESS: Sleepiness, stupor, and coma are very grave signs in the asthmatic, usually indicating severe degrees of hypercarbia, hypoxemia, and acidosis. A depressed level of consciousness is therefore frequently the harbinger of cardiac arrest in the asthmatic child.

> ## THE SLEEPY ASTHMATIC IS AN ASTHMATIC IN TROUBLE!

- VITAL SIGNS: As the asthmatic attack worsens, the child's pulse grows faster and weaker, respirations become very shallow, and the blood pressure may fall. **Pulsus paradoxus** (the decrease or disappearance of the arterial pulse during inhalation) is a very reliable clue to the severity of an asthmatic attack. You can detect pulsus paradoxus in the field, without using a sphygmomanometer, simply by keeping a finger on the child's pulse through a few respiratory cycles. If pulsus paradoxus is present, you will notice that the pulse seems much weaker during exhalation.
- SKIN AND MUCOUS MEMBRANES: Look for evidence of *dehydration,* in tenting of the skin and dry mucous membranes. Check the lips and nail beds for *cyanosis.*
- LOOK AT THE CHEST to assess respiratory excursions, which will be increased in the mild asthmatic attack and may be entirely absent in the severe attack. *Hyperinflation* may give the chest a barrel shape and make it hyperresonant to percussion. LISTEN TO THE CHEST for crackles and *wheezes.* The chest is noisy in the mild to moderate asthmatic attack, with increased breath

sounds, loud expiratory wheezing, and sometimes crackles. Remember, though, that it takes two things to make a wheeze: narrowed airways *and* air flow through them. Thus, as the asthmatic attack progresses in severity, breath sounds become less and less audible, for less and less air is moving in and out of the chest. In the very severe attack, breath sounds cannot be heard at all. A silent chest means danger!

> ## A SILENT GRAVE AWAITS A SILENT CHEST.

Be sure to listen to the *entire* chest—at least six symmetric lung fields front and back. Wheezes localized to a small area suggest obstruction by a foreign body, not asthma. The wheezing in asthma is heard in all lung fields.

It is important to mention that *children under 2 years old* may not show the anxiety or positional preferences of older children during an asthmatic attack. The severely asthmatic infant may lie in an apparently comfortable supine position and sometimes, even if cyanotic, may smile and be easily distracted with toys and cooing. Children in this age group may also have extreme degrees of tachypnea (respiratory rates of 60–80/min) with abdominal breathing.

Treatment of the Acute Asthmatic Attack in Children

Specific protocols for the treatment of acute asthmatic attacks vary from place to place, and paramedics should be guided by local practice. All treatment regimens, however, are based on the principles mentioned earlier—attempting to improve oxygenation, correct dehydration, and reverse the processes that are inhibiting air flow within the lungs.

- Administer OXYGEN, initially by mask. If you are using a nebulization unit for giving bronchodilators, use oxygen (rather than compressed air) to deliver the aerosolized drug.
- Start an IV LIFELINE with normal saline. Use a butterfly needle in the hand veins of small children, and secure it well. Run the IV at the rate specified by the physician (usually in the range of 5–15 ml/kg/hr, depending on how dehydrated the child is). Use a microdrip administration set.
- For many years, epinephrine by subcutaneous injection was the preferred treatment for acute

asthmatic attacks. There is a growing trend, however, to initiate treatment with AEROSOLIZED BRONCHODILATORS, given either by metered-dose inhaler or by nebulizer. A number of agents are available for that purpose, including isoetharine (Bronkosol), albuterol/salbutamol (Ventolin), and terbutaline (Bricanyl). It should be pointed out that the use of those bronchodilators by aerosol, although increasingly widespread, is not yet FDA-approved for children under 12. Each ambulance service should, in any case, choose *one* of the **selective beta-2 bronchodilators**—that is, beta sympathomimetic agents that affect primarily the bronchial musculature and have minimal cardiac effects—and learn its pharmacology thoroughly. In the field, the most convenient and probably the most effective way to administer beta-2 bronchodilators, at least to children older than about 4, is by *metered-dose inhaler* (MDI) with a spacer (see Appendix I to Chap. 22). If you are using a *nebulizer*, follow the instructions on page 480 for setting up the equipment. The pediatric dosages of beta-2 agents given by nebulizer are summarized in Table 30-2. The flow rate of the nebulizer is adjusted to deliver the total dosage over a period of 5 to 15 minutes, usually about 6 liters per minute. The child should be encouraged to cough up secretions as he takes the treatment.

Ask the respiratory therapist at your base hospital to rig up a nebulizer that can be operated off your oxygen system and have him show you how to use it.

- If you do not have the means to give an agent such as albuterol by aerosol, administer TERBU-TALINE, 0.01 mg per kilogram subcutaneously. That dosage may be repeated once in 20 to 30 minutes. If the patient fails to respond to terbutaline, he should be considered to be in status asthmaticus and will need aggressive therapy with other agents.

- AMINOPHYLLINE is still sometimes given when there is little or no response to aerosolized bronchodilators or when the child is in severe distress from the outset. Find out first *what the child has taken at home,* for the loading dose of aminophylline will depend on whether the child has already taken a theophylline preparation (see Appendix II to Chap. 22):
  1. If the child is *not* taking a theophylline preparation at home, give a loading dose of **6 mg per kilogram** in 30 ml of IV fluid over 30 minutes. Use a Burotrol or similar device to regulate the infusion.
  2. If the child *is* taking a theophylline preparation at home, double-check with medical command whether you should go ahead with aminophylline in the field. If the answer is affirmative, give *no more than* 3 mg per kilogram in 30 ml of IV fluid over 30 minutes.

- For the child with a very severe asthmatic attack or status asthmaticus, you may also be asked to give:
  1. STEROIDS: Hydrocortisone (Solu-Cortef), 7 mg per kilogram IV over 5 minutes, *or* methylprednisolone (Solu-Medrol), 1 mg per kilogram over 5 minutes.
  2. SODIUM BICARBONATE: 1 mEq (1 ml) per kilogram IV over 5 minutes.

- DO NOT UNDER ANY CIRCUMSTANCES GIVE SEDATIVE MEDICATIONS to a child having an acute asthmatic attack. If the child is restless and hyperactive, it is because hypoxia is making him frantic. The solution to the problem is to improve

TABLE 30-2. PEDIATRIC DOSAGE OF DRUGS GIVEN BY NEBULIZER

DRUG	SUPPLIED AS	PEDIATRIC DOSAGE
Albuterol/salbutamol (Ventolin)	0.5% solution	0.15 mg/kg to a maximum dose of 5 mg, diluted in 3 ml of normal saline
Isoetharine (Bronkosol)	Usually 1 mg/ml	0.03 mg/kg to a maximum dose of 0.5 mg, diluted in 3 ml of normal saline
Metaproterenol (Alupent)	5% solution	Age < 10 yr: 0.1 ml in 3 ml of normal saline Age > 10 yr: 0.2–0.3 ml in 3 ml of normal saline
Racemic epinephrine (Vaponefrin)	2.25% solution	0.5 ml in 3 ml of normal saline
Terbutaline (Bricanyl, Brethine)	1 mg/ml	0.2–0.3 mg/kg in 3 ml of normal saline

the patient's oxygenation, not to depress his respiratory drive!

- MONITOR the cardiac rhythm of every child with an asthmatic attack. Hypoxemia, acidosis, and some of the drugs you are administering all increase the likelihood of cardiac dysrhythmias.
- TRANSPORT the child to the hospital in whatever position he finds most comfortable (which will usually be a sitting position).

Bronchiolitis

As the term implies, bronchiolitis is an inflammation of the bronchioles, most commonly caused by a virus. It occurs with greatest frequency in the winter and spring, among children under 2 years of age (males more often than females); the highest incidence is in infants between the ages of 2 and 6 months. Usually the child has had some contact with a family member suffering from an upper respiratory infection, and the history will reveal that the infant had a day or two of *low-grade fever, runny nose, sneezing,* and *poor appetite.* Over the course of a few days, signs of lower respiratory involvement—tachypnea, wheezes, sometimes cyanosis—then develop, although in severely ill infants those signs may develop more rapidly, over only a few hours.

On PHYSICAL EXAMINATION, the infant with bronchiolitis will typically be in mild to severe respiratory distress, as evidenced by *tachypnea* (respiratory rates as high as 60–80 /min), *nasal flaring, use of accessory muscles* of respiration, and *intercostal retractions.* As in asthma, progressive air trapping distends the chest and limits the tidal volume, so *respirations are shallow.* Auscultation of the chest usually reveals *wheezes,* but again, the volume of the wheezes depends on the amount of air flow: no air flow, no wheezes.

Bronchiolitis and infantile asthma are very similar in their clinical presentation, and in fact, there are some authorities who believe that bronchiolitis may be a forerunner of asthma in susceptible individuals. Some of the features that may help to differentiate bronchiolitis from asthma are the age of the infant (asthma is very rare in infants under 12 months old) and his recent medical and family history. If the infant had a recent low-grade fever and runny nose, or if someone else in the house was ill with an upper respiratory infection, bronchiolitis is a likely diagnosis. A history of recurring episodes of wheezes or coughing, on the other hand, or a positive family history for asthma or allergy favors the diagnosis of asthma—especially if the current attack came on without a preceding infection.

Because of the difficulty in distinguishing between bronchiolitis and asthma, many pediatricians will give the wheezing infant who is over 6 months old a trial of bronchodilators, to see whether those agents will relieve the bronchospasm. Bronchodilators tend to be effective in asthma and ineffective in bronchiolitis.

Treatment of Bronchiolitis

The prehospital treatment of bronchiolitis is aimed primarily at improving the infant's oxygenation. When the infant is nearing the end of his respiratory reserve, complete respiratory failure may occur very suddenly, so you must be prepared as well to take over the child's ventilations.

- Give humidified oxygen by mask. Assist ventilations *gently* with a pediatric bag-valve-mask as needed.
- Consult medical command or your protocol for bronchiolitis regarding whether to give an AEROSOLIZED BRONCHODILATOR. If so, administer the drug used by your service as described for the treatment of asthma.
- Keep a laryngoscope and endotracheal tube of the appropriate size ready in the event that the child stops breathing. If apnea occurs, oxygenate as well as you can by bag-valve-mask and then intubate.
- MONITOR the infant's cardiac rhythm. The occurrence of dysrhythmias should alert you to the probability that the child is not being adequately oxygenated and ventilated.

Croup

Croup (laryngotracheobronchitis) is a viral infection of the *upper* airways occurring in children between 6 months and 4 years of age; it occurs rarely in older children (and even more rarely in adults). The infection leads to airway obstruction by causing edema just beneath the glottis, with progressive narrowing of the airway. The child with moderate to severe croup is hoarse, with a high-pitched stridor and so-called seal bark. Often there is a peculiar whooping sound on inhalation. As the edema increases and the airway becomes more obstructed, the child uses accessory muscles of respiration, and the classic *signs of respiratory distress* are seen: nasal flaring, tracheal tugging, and retractions of intercostal and suprasternal muscles. Hypoxia may be evident as *restlessness* and agitation, a *rising pulse rate,* and eventually *cyanosis.*

Usually those signs and symptoms appear following a few days of symptoms of a cold or other infection. Typically, the child appears fairly well during the day, save for some hoarseness; but after he goes to bed, he develops a harsh, metallic cough—very slight at first, but progressing by around midnight to a barking noise alarming enough to wake the dead, not to mention the parents. The mild attack may subside by itself in a few hours, leaving the child and his parents exhausted, and it may recur on two or three successive nights. In the severe attack, signs of marked respiratory distress, as described above, are evident.

Treatment of the Child with Croup

Treatment of the child with croup is aimed at maintaining an airway and providing optimal oxygenation. Approximately 5 percent of children with croup require hospitalization in an intensive care unit because of severe airway obstruction, and up to half of children hospitalized for croup require a tracheostomy. So you need to keep in mind that the child's airway is in severe jeopardy and to move expeditiously to the hospital.

- Start administration of HUMIDIFIED OXYGEN immediately by mask while you set up your nebulizer.
- Use oxygen as the carrier gas to NEBULIZE RACEMIC EPINEPHRINE (Vaponefrin) into a face mask. Dilute 0.5 ml of racemic epinephrine in 2.5 ml of normal saline (0.25 ml of racemic epinephrine in the same volume of saline if the child is under 1 year of age). If you don't stock racemic epinephrine, you may use 5 ml of 1:1,000 L-epinephrine diluted in 5 ml of normal saline.
- AVOID PROCEDURES THAT WILL DISTRESS THE CHILD. Starting an IV is one such procedure; so unless there is a compelling reason to start the IV in the field (e.g., the child has severe cardiac dysrhythmias and may arrest at any moment), DEFER THE IV until the child reaches the emergency room.
- DO NOT ATTEMPT TO EXAMINE THE THROAT. If the child has epiglottitis and not croup, inserting a tongue blade into the mouth could be lethal.
- Let the child assume the POSITION IN WHICH HE IS MOST COMFORTABLE, which will usually be sitting up in mother's lap, and disturb him as little as possible.
- NOTIFY the receiving hospital of the nature of the case and your estimated time of arrival (ETA), so that the operating room can be alerted to the possibility of an emergency tracheostomy.
- TRANSPORT without delay.

Epiglottitis

Acute epiglottitis is a life-threatening bacterial infection of the epiglottis and sometimes the immediately surrounding tissues, leading to a swollen, "cherry red" epiglottis that may, from one moment to the next, totally obstruct the patient's airway. The clinical picture of epiglottitis differs from that of croup in several important respects:

- The child with epiglottitis is usually (but not invariably) somewhat *older* than the child with croup. Acute epiglottitis occurs most commonly between the ages of 2 and 6.
- The ONSET of epiglottitis tends to be quite ABRUPT, with the sudden occurrence of a severe sore throat. Indeed, the throat is so sore that the child *refuses to swallow anything*, even his own saliva, so DROOLING is characteristic.
- The child with epiglottitis usually has a HIGH FEVER, up to about 40.5°C (105°F) and looks very sick. He is apt as well to LOOK SCARED, but he will not show the agitation seen in croup because all of his effort is directed toward trying to obtain enough air.
- The child will usually be SITTING UPRIGHT and will resist any attempt to place him on his back. Often he is found in the "tripod position," leaning back on his hands with his elbows locked and with his chin thrust forward into the "sniffing position" and tongue protruding.
- The child's voice, if he speaks at all, is muffled, but the wheezing and coughing characteristic of croup are absent.

Epiglottitis is a dire medical emergency. Complete airway obstruction and respiratory arrest can occur with dramatic suddenness and may be precipitated by very minor irritation of the throat or even agitation. The goal of treatment, therefore, is to keep the child as calm and comfortable as possible until he reaches the hospital.

Prehospital Treatment of Epiglottitis

The potential benefit of any given intervention for epiglottitis must be weighed against the discomfort it causes the child. Don't try to force *anything* on him, for his becoming upset could be lethal.

- Administer humidified OXYGEN by mask if it does not disturb the child.
- Let the child assume the POSITION IN WHICH HE IS MOST COMFORTABLE, and disturb him as little as possible.

- Have a laryngoscope and an endotracheal tube of the appropriate size immediately at hand.
- NOTIFY the receiving hospital of your situation and ETA, so that a specialist team (which may include an anesthesiologist and an ear, nose, and throat specialist) can be standing by to receive the patient.
- TRANSPORT WITHOUT DELAY to the hospital.

NEVER, NEVER, NEVER PLACE ANY INSTRUMENT IN THE CHILD'S MOUTH. DO NOT ATTEMPT TO VISUALIZE THE EPIGLOTTIS WITH A LARYNGOSCOPE, TONGUE BLADE, OR ANY OTHER INSTRUMENT, SINCE INSTANT, LETHAL LARYNGOSPASM AND SWELLING MAY RESULT.

Children with acute epiglottitis are in grave danger from complete airway obstruction. More than half of such children end up requiring intubation or tracheostomy in the hospital, and their transport to a medical facility should not be delayed. It is extremely dangerous and difficult to try to intubate a child with epiglottitis in the field, so don't wait around until intubation becomes necessary!

If complete airway obstruction *does* occur before you reach the hospital, and you are unable to ventilate the child, you may be left with no choice but to attempt INTUBATION. First try as best you can to *preoxygenate* the child by forceful ventilation with a bag-valve-mask and 100% oxygen. High pressures may be required to push air past the swollen epiglottis. After at least 2 to 3 minutes of preoxygenation, gently *suction* the secretions from the child's mouth and insert the laryngoscope. If you are able to see the vocal cords, say a prayer of thanks and whip the endotracheal tube in through them. More probably, however, you will not be able to see the cords because of tissue swelling. In that case, have an assistant gently compress the child's chest to force air up through the trachea; as your assistant compresses, watch for air bubbles. The point where bubbles emerge from the swollen tissues is the site of the vocal cords, and you may try gently to slip the endotracheal tube through at that site.

If you are unable to intubate the trachea once complete obstruction has occurred, the child's only hope will be an immediate *cricothyrotomy*, the technique for which was described in Chapter 7.

SUDDEN INFANT DEATH SYNDROME

Sudden infant death syndrome (SIDS)—formerly known as "crib death" (or "cot death," to those of British persuasion)—is officially defined as the sudden death of any infant or young child that is unexpected by history and in which a thorough postmortem examination fails to demonstrate an adequate cause of death. Within that very formal-sounding definition lies the tragedy of SIDS; for what that definition tells us is that an apparently healthy infant is placed in his crib and, for no reason that anyone can determine, dies.

That indeed is precisely what happens to approximately 10,000 infants in the United States each year, making SIDS the leading cause of death in infants after the first few weeks of life. The cause of SIDS is not known, although studies have shown a higher incidence of SIDS in infants sleeping in the prone position. It cannot be predicted or completely prevented, and it usually occurs during sleep in an apparently normal, healthy infant. Victims range in age from 1 month to 1 year, with a peak incidence between the ages of 2 and 4 months.

In most cases of SIDS, the baby is not discovered until it has been dead for some time, and there will be little you can do to revive the infant. Nonetheless, it is worth starting CPR and continuing all the way to the hospital—even if the baby is cold and lifeless when you reach the scene—for it is enormously important for the family to feel that everything possible was done to save the child. In all probability, you will *not* save the child, but the family must see you trying to do so, for they are going to remember this day forever.

If the infant has obviously been dead for several hours and starting CPR would just be a meaningless charade in the circumstances, be prepared to spend some time helping the parents deal with their initial grief reaction. A whole range of feelings may burst forth in such a situation—disbelief, denial, anger, guilt, confusion, anxiety. Be prepared to deal with those feelings. Give the parents time as well to part from the baby. Find out if there is anyone you can contact who may be able to give continuing support, such as a relative, friend, or member of the clergy. And maintain a sympathetic, professional demeanor throughout.

Do *not* tell the parents what they should or should not have done prior to your arrival. Most parents confronted with the sudden, unexpected death of a child are already overwhelmed with unwarranted guilt. Your job is not to reinforce those guilt feelings, but rather to be as supportive as you can.

SEIZURES IN CHILDREN

Nearly all of the predisposing conditions that may lead to seizures in adults may also cause seizures in children, including *head trauma, meningitis, hypoxia, hypoglycemia,* and failure of a known epileptic to take his or her medications (see Chap. 24). Children, however, are also uniquely susceptible to **febrile seizures,** that is, seizures that come about in association with a sudden rise in body temperature.

Febrile seizures are common, occurring in about 3 to 4 out of every 100 children. The incidence is highest in children between 6 months and 3 years of age and is quite rare after the age of 6 years. Often there is a family history of similar seizures, in which case the parents are less likely to be terrified by the spectacle the first time it happens.

If a febrile seizure is going to occur at all, it usually occurs *early* in the illness, during a period when the child's temperature is rising rapidly, usually to above 39°C (about 102°F). Febrile seizures are most often generalized, grand mal seizures and last anywhere up to 20 minutes. Afterward, there is no lasting neurologic deficit.

Assessing the Child Who Has Had a Seizure

Except in the case of status epilepticus, the child's seizure will have usually stopped by the time you arrive on the scene, and you will not have a chance to witness it; it will therefore be important to take a HISTORY from those who did witness the seizure. The history should establish at least the following information:

- HAS THE CHILD EVER HAD SEIZURES BEFORE? How often? Have they always been associated with fever, or do they occur when the child is otherwise well?
- HOW MANY seizures has the child had today?
- Does the child have a history of HEAD TRAUMA, DIABETES, or recent FEVER, HEADACHE, or STIFF NECK?
- Is there any FAMILY HISTORY OF SEIZURES? Did any of the child's older brothers or sisters have seizures in association with fever when they were little?
- Is the child taking any MEDICATIONS? If he is a known epileptic for whom medications have already been prescribed, did he take his medications today?
- Could the child have INGESTED A TOXIC MATERIAL? Is there, for example, any evidence of

"breaking and entry" into a kitchen or bathroom cupboard?
- WHAT DID THE SEIZURE LOOK LIKE? Was it generalized or focal? Did it start in one part of the body and progress? Did the child's eyes deviate? In which direction?

It should be pointed out that if this was the child's first seizure, it may not be possible to obtain an accurate description of what happened, for the parents were probably too panic-stricken by the event to pay careful attention to such details as the direction in which the eyes deviated! But it is particularly important to find out about events preceding the seizure, such as complaints of headache or stiff neck. Not every seizure occurring in a febrile child is a febrile seizure. Serious illnesses such as meningitis or encephalitis must still be ruled out.

In performing the PHYSICAL EXAMINATION of the child who has had a seizure, pay particular attention to the following:

- Make a careful record of the STATE OF CONSCIOUSNESS, and start a flow sheet of neurologic and vital signs.
- Check the SKIN for evidence of *fever* or *dehydration.*
- Examine the HEAD for signs of *trauma,* sustained during the seizure itself or earlier. In an infant, be sure to check the fontanelle with the infant recumbent, and note whether it is bulging or sunken.
- Keep a record of PUPIL CHECKS on your neurologic flow sheet.
- Try gently to flex the child's NECK, and note whether there is any unusual stiffness.
- Complete the head-to-toe survey for SIGNS OF INJURY sustained during the seizure.

Prehospital Treatment of Seizures in Children

The SINGLE CONVULSION is usually self-limited and does not require any treatment other than protecting the child from injury and maintaining an airway. If you are present while the seizure is occurring, position the child left side down on a wide bed or on pillows, well away from any hard objects.

DO NOT TRY TO FORCE ANY OBJECT, INCLUDING AN OROPHARYNGEAL AIRWAY, INTO THE CHILD'S MOUTH DURING A SEIZURE.

If the child is feverish, sponging with *lukewarm* water may help bring down the temperature and reduce the likelihood of another seizure. Do *not*, however, sponge a feverish child with alcohol or cold water.

Take some time to calm the child's parents, for most parents are terrified by a child's first seizure. Reassure the parents that the majority of seizures in children are *not* a sign of serious disease and that, in any event, the child will be carefully evaluated in the emergency room to rule out any potentially dangerous source of the seizure.

A prolonged seizure or multiple seizures without a lucid interval between them (**status epilepticus**) represent a very serious medical emergency, and in that case you will have to take steps to try to stop the seizures:

- Place the child left side down on a wide bed or on cushions on the floor, away from furniture. Do *not* try to restrain him.
- Clear and maintain an AIRWAY. Do *not* attempt to jam a bite-block or any other object between a child's clenched teeth. Consider injuries that may have been sustained during the seizure, and take *cervical spine precautions* as needed.
- Administer OXYGEN. Assist ventilations with a pediatric bag-valve-mask if there are periods of hypoventilation or apnea. Remember: MOST DEATHS FROM SEIZURES ARE HYPOXIC DEATHS.
- Start an IV LIFELINE with D5/W by microdrip infusion. Secure the IV well against thrashing and pulling.
- Check a blood sample with Dextrostix. If the blood sugar is below 40 mg per deciliter, or if you are uncertain, give 25% DEXTROSE in a dosage of **1 ml per kilogram.** (To make up a solution of 25% dextrose, take a 50-ml prefilled syringe of 50% dextrose and expel half the contents, then draw 25 ml of sterile water into the syringe.)
- If the child is febrile, sponge him with tepid water to lower his temperature.
- If the seizures do not stop, the physician may order DIAZEPAM (Valium) in a dosage of **0.3 mg per kilogram,** up to a maximum of 10 mg (that usually works out to 1 mg per year of age). Give diazepam by *slow* intravenous infusion over 1 to 3 minutes with careful monitoring of vital signs. Apnea and cardiac arrest occasionally follow administration of diazepam, so watch the child closely, and have all the equipment necessary for resuscitation at hand. If you have been unable to start an IV, the DIAZEPAM MAY BE GIVEN RECTALLY. To do so, advance a 10F pediatric suction catheter or similar tube about 3 to 5 cm (1–2 inches) into the child's rectum. Draw up the appropriate dosage of diazepam in a syringe. For *rectal* administration, the dosage must be slightly higher—0.5 mg per kilogram—because absorption is not as complete. Inject the diazepam through the tube into the rectum. Then flush the tube by injecting 2 to 3 ml of normal saline through it, and remove the tube from the rectum.

Diazepam often produces respiratory depression, irrespective of the route by which it is given. Therefore, whenever you administer diazepam, *be prepared to intubate the trachea.* Have the intubation kit handy and all equipment checked and ready.

Because diazepam can produce marked respiratory depression, there is growing enthusiasm for the use of LORAZEPAM, a drug in the same family as diazepam, for the initial treatment of status epilepticus. Lorazepam is just as effective as diazepam in treating seizures, but it does not produce as much respiratory depression. It is given in a dose of 0.05 to 0.1 mg per kilogram IV. As of this writing, lorazepam has not been approved for use in children, but it is highly probable that this drug will soon find a place in prehospital care.

- Once you have administered diazepam, there is nothing to be gained by any further delay at the scene, even if the child is still seizing. Therefore, package the child in such a way as to minimize the possibility of injury (i.e., well padded with pillows), and TRANSPORT to the hospital.

CHILD ABUSE

Battered or abused children are children who are deliberately injured by adults. In the United States, there are an estimated 500,000 to 1,000,000 cases of child abuse annually, and they occur at every social and economic level. Child abuse may lead to serious mental and physical disabilities, and approximately 1 in 500 battered children die from their injuries each year.

Profile of Abuse

The Abusive Parent

The adult who abuses a child is usually a parent or other caretaker—often a person who was her- or himself abused as a child. The abusive parent tends to be poorly prepared for the task of bringing up a child and has unrealistic expectations of the child's behavior. Usually the parent has little social support, and he or she may be heavily involved with alcohol or drugs.

Sometimes specific events or stresses trigger the abuse. Marital difficulties, loss of a job, illness, a death in the family, overcrowding in the house—all of those factors have been linked to cases of child abuse.

If the abusive parent is at the scene with the child, he or she will often behave in an evasive manner, volunteering little information or giving contradictory information about what happened to the child. The parent may show outright hostility toward the child, toward the other parent, or toward the paramedic and rarely shows any guilt. Other parental indicators are lack of apparent concern for the child and haste to get away from the hospital before making certain the child is safe. A neglected or abused child is not cuddled by its parents, but rather carried "like a loaf of bread."

If you suspect child abuse, you may find yourself feeling hostile toward the child's parent. It is essential, however, to maintain a nonjudgmental attitude. The very act of calling for an ambulance may be an abusive parent's first cry for help, and the paramedic should be supportive of that impulse.

The Abused Child

The victim of abuse is likely to be a young child; approximately two-thirds of victims of physical abuse are under the age of 3. Often one child in the family is singled out for abuse—typically a child who is handicapped, slow in development, or for any other reason seen as special or different. Children who require a lot of extra attention, such as those with chronic illnesses, are at higher risk of abuse, as are those who had the misfortune to be born male when the parents wanted a girl, or vice versa.

Assessment of the Abused Child

Rarely if ever will a call come in to 911 neatly labelled "child abuse," nor are the abusers likely to volunteer the information that the child is a victim of abuse. Rather, child abuse is a diagnosis one begins to suspect on the basis of certain findings in the child's history and physical examination.

Clues to Abuse in the Child's History

Taking the history of the injury may provide the first clues that the "accident" was not an accident. If there was more than one witness to the event, try to find a discreet way to interview the different witnesses separately. Record precisely who said what, and quote statements verbatim, in quotation marks, on the trip sheet. The child himself, if old enough to speak, should also be questioned, preferably while your partner is interviewing the parent separately. A marked *discrepancy* between different versions of the event must be considered suspicious. Similarly, any discrepancy between the history and the physical findings is also a cause for concern. If the baby fell from his high chair, for example, he can be expected to have bruises *either* on the front of his body *or* on the back, depending how he fell, but *not on both* anterior and posterior surfaces. Be alert as well for a discrepancy between the account of the accident and the child's developmental capabilities. The child who is alleged to have pulled a pot of boiling water off the stove, for example, and who cannot yet stand unassisted doubtless sustained his burns in some other way than that stated. In general, any sort of *vague and contradictory history* should activate the flashing "alert" sign in the paramedic's brain.

Probably the most important historical clue in cases of child abuse is *delay in seeking treatment*. The vast majority of children who sustain accidental injuries will be presented for treatment immediately, while there is almost invariably a delay in seeking care for abused children.

The child's past medical history may also be revealing. *Repeated accidents* are suspect, especially if they began before the age of 1 year.

Physical Assessment of the Child Who May Have Been Abused

Irrespective of the child's chief complaint, once you have reason to suspect child abuse, you must conduct a painstaking examination of the child from head to toe. Do so in a professional, matter-of-fact way, and keep your suspicions to yourself. If asked why you are examining the child's head when his burn is on the leg, explain that the head-to-toe examination is standard operating procedure, part of the discipline of medical care that ensures you will not miss any important findings.

As usual, start with the child's GENERAL APPEARANCE. Even while you are still taking the history from the parents, observe the child's BEHAVIOR. The child who seems *apathetic* and doesn't cry despite his injuries, or the child who *does not turn to his parents for comfort* is likely to be a child who has been chronically abused. Observe as well the child's OVERALL HYGIENE AND CARE. Is he clean and well-dressed, or are there signs of neglect? Document the LEVEL OF CONSCIOUSNESS, and if it is depressed, start a neurologic flow sheet.

Check the SKIN from head to toe, for bruises and burns. Document the location and color of every BRUISE. Toddlers who are just learning to walk may have multiple bruises over the shins, forehead, or other bony prominences. Bruises on the sides of the face, behind the ears, on the buttocks, lower back, genitalia, and proximal extremities are more likely to have been inflicted intentionally. Similarly, bruises in different stages of healing or those that bear the imprint of the instrument used (e.g., a belt buckle) are highly suggestive of abuse. The age of the bruise can be gauged by its color (Table 30-3) and checked against the history. If a child is found to have a greenish bruise on the back, for instance, the injury that produced that bruise occurred around 5 to 7 days earlier, no matter what the parent or caretaker tells you.

BURN PATTERNS may also be revealing. Be suspicious when scald burns have a circumferential pattern and there are no splash marks. Burns in a stocking-and-glove distribution and burns of the buttocks are also much more likely to have been inflicted than accidental.

The head-to-toe survey should start with a very careful examination of the HEAD, for head injuries are the most common cause of death in abused children, particularly infants under 2 months of age. In infants, look for a *bulging fontanelle,* and in all children check for standard signs of head trauma and increased intracranial pressure. *Bald spots* may be a sign of hair having been yanked out. Swelling of the scalp can signal subgaleal hematoma from a skull fracture. Check for *bruises around the mouth* or lacerations of the oral mucosa, which may occur if a feeding bottle is jammed harshly into a baby's mouth.

Assume there has been injury to the cervical spine until proved otherwise, and avoid excessive motion to the NECK. Palpate for tenderness.

Palpate the CHEST for *tenderness and instability.* Rib fractures are extremely rare in accidental injuries in children but occur commonly in abuse.

Internal injuries to the ABDOMEN are the second most common cause of death secondary to child abuse. Inspect the abdomen for *distention,* and palpate for tenderness or rigidity. Signs of shock without an obvious cause suggest the presence of intra-abdominal bleeding.

Palpate the EXTREMITIES for swelling or deformity along the length of the bones. Accidental fractures are uncommon in children under 1 year of age.

Perhaps the most important contribution the paramedic can make to the assessment of the patient is a careful ASSESSMENT OF THE SCENE. The medical staff in the hospital will be able to repeat the examination of the child and perhaps the interview with at least one parent, but they will *not* have access to information about the child's environment. So take a careful look around. What is the condition of the child's home? Is it neat, clean, and well-maintained? Or does it reflect lives that are in disarray? Is there evidence of parental drug or alcohol abuse? All of those observations should be documented on the trip sheet.

TABLE 30-3. GAUGING THE AGE OF A SOFT TISSUE INJURY

TIME SINCE INJURY	COLOR OF THE BRUISE
0–2 hours	No discoloration (may be swollen and tender)
1–5 days	Reddish blue
5–7 days	Greenish
7–10 days	Yellow
10–14	Brown

SUMMARY: CLUES TO THE IDENTIFICATION OF A BATTERED CHILD

CLUES IN THE HISTORY
- Significant DELAY in seeking medical care
- Major DISCREPANCIES in the history:
  1. Discrepancy between different people's versions of the story
  2. Discrepancy between the history and the observed injuries
  3. Discrepancy between the history and the child's developmental capabilities
- History of multiple emergency room visits for various injuries
- A story that is VAGUE AND CONTRADICTORY

CLUES IN THE PHYSICAL EXAMINATION
- Child who seems apathetic and DOES NOT CRY despite his injuries
- Child who DOES NOT TURN TO HIS PARENTS FOR COMFORT
- Child who is POORLY NOURISHED and POORLY CARED FOR
- The presence of MULTIPLE BRUISES and abrasions, especially around the trunk and buttocks
- The presence of OLD BRUISES IN ADDITION TO FRESH ONES
- The presence of SUSPICIOUS BURNS:
  1. Cigarette burns
  2. Scalds without splash marks or involving the buttocks, hands, or feet but sparing skin folds

- Injuries about the MOUTH
- RIB FRACTURES
- FRACTURES in an infant under 1 year of age

Prehospital Management of the Physically Abused Child

Treatment of the abused child may ultimately require placing the child in a protected environment, away from the abuser. But that treatment will not be possible if abuse is not detected or, even if detected, not well documented. Thus the treatment of the battered child begins with the recognition that a child's injury may have been the result of abuse. From the moment you begin to suspect child abuse, you must carefully document everything, especially what the parents or caregivers told you (preferably in their own words) and what you observed at the scene.

Give whatever treatment at the scene is appropriate for the specific injuries you have detected (e.g., dress wounds, splint fractures), and TRANSPORT *every* child you suspect of having been abused, no matter how minor the current injury. When you arrive at the hospital, *privately* convey your suspicions and findings to the physician. It will be of particular value to him or her to learn what you have observed in the home. Remember, child abuse is a chronic problem. The battered child you bring into the emergency room this week may be DOA next week if the problem is not detected and dealt with. Furthermore, *you* may be held liable for that death if you did not speak up, for all 50 states have reporting requirements for child abuse, and in some states it is a criminal offense for any health care provider *not* to report suspected abuse. So if you have *any* suspicions, share them with the emergency department physician. In some regions, you may have to file a report with state or local agencies as well.

It is *not* the paramedic's responsibility, however, to confront the parents with a charge of child abuse, nor is it appropriate to do so. Be tactful and discreet in dealing with the parents of a child you think may be the victim of abuse, and save your comments for the professional staff in the emergency room.

Sexual Abuse of Children

A special case of child abuse is the sexually molested child. Reliable statistics on the extent of the problem are nearly impossible to come by. It has been estimated that anywhere from 1 to 25 percent of children have been sexually abused by the age of 18—usually by a close acquaintance or member of the family.

When sexual abuse is part of a chronic, ongoing pattern, you are not likely to hear about it. The child may be too numbed or afraid to speak of it. Often the mother is a very passive person and, if aware of the problem, is also afraid to say anything about it. So the problem goes undetected until the child presents for a related medical problem, such as vaginal discharge.

An ambulance is much more likely to be summoned for a more acute instance of sexual abuse, that is, the rape of a child by a stranger. A call of that sort requires utmost tact and composure. The child may be terrified and upset; but even more difficult to deal with may be the parents, who are apt to translate their feelings of guilt, helplessness, and distress into a demand for action—and to vent their anger on the paramedic. It is important to try to understand those feelings and to maintain a calm, understanding attitude. Explain to the child and his or her parents that you realize this has been a very frightening experience but that it is important that they be calm and give you as complete a report as possible. Telling the story will enable the child and parents to vent some of their feelings about what has happened, especially if the rescuer conveys to them a sense of interest and concern.

From the point of view of prehospital management, the most important thing to determine in the history is *what hurts*. The details of the attack can be elicited later in the emergency room. Limit the physical examination to a check for major injury requiring stabilization (e.g., bleeding, fractures). The child will in all probability have to undergo at least one complete physical examination in the emergency room, and that will be distressing enough. So simply do a rapid evaluation to make certain there are no injuries requiring immediate treatment in the field, and move on to the hospital. Inform the physician in the emergency department of your observations at the scene and of the history you obtained. Make a careful written record of the case, bearing in mind that your report is a legal document that may be used in court.

TRAUMA IN CHILDREN

Trauma is the leading cause of death among children over 1 year of age in the United States. Each year in the U.S., accidents claim the lives of 25,000 children. Another 100,000 children annually are permanently crippled from injuries, and 2 million children per year are incapacitated by injuries for periods of 2 weeks or longer. About 70 percent of accidents in preschool children occur in or around the home. The most common causes of traumatic deaths in children are *motor vehicle accidents* (55%), *falls* (27%), and *fires.* Nearly all of those are preventable causes. And what that means is that by the time you respond to an emergency involving an injured child, the EMS system has already failed. The accident should never have happened. If it did happen, health professionals have fallen down on the job—the job of educating the public; campaigning for more stringent safety regulations (e.g., mandatory seat beats and bike helmets for children); pressing for stricter enforcement of existing laws (e.g., penalties for drunk driving).

General Considerations in the Injured Child

Children are not simply miniature adults. Children are built differently and suffer different kinds of trauma. Take the *skin,* for example. A child has more skin (i.e., more surface area) in relation to body weight than an adult. Therefore a child loses more body heat across normal skin and more fluid across damaged skin after a burn. At the same time, the child's muscle and fat mass is smaller than that of an adult; that is to say, a child has less padding, so he is more vulnerable to blunt trauma. Furthermore, his diaphragm is lower and his abdominal organs relatively larger; thus he is much more likely than the adult to suffer injuries to the liver, spleen, and duodenum.

Children also *respond* differently to trauma. A child's blood vessels are capable of extreme vasoconstriction, for example, so hypotension may not occur until a child has lost a major proportion of his total blood volume.

Because children are different, many medical facilities have introduced specialized training in the care of injured children—courses in pediatric advanced life support (PALS), pediatric trauma life support (PTLS), and so forth. Paramedics are encouraged to take such courses to refine their skills in treating injured children.

Mechanisms of Injury

As in evaluating an adult victim of trauma, the evaluation of an injured child must first of all take into account the mechanism of injury (see Chap. 14). Indeed, when the patient is a child, the story of the accident can often establish with a high degree of certainty what injuries are present. An infant FALLING FROM A HEIGHT, for example, will almost invariably sustain head injuries, since babies fall head-first. BICYCLE HANDLEBAR TRAUMA typically produces compression injuries to retroperitoneal structures, like the pancreas and duodenum. The child STRUCK BY A CAR while crossing the street generally sustains three separate injuries (Fig. 30-5): a fractured left femur where the car's bumper hit the child's leg (a fractured *right* femur if the child is crossing a British street, where they drive on the wrong side); a bruised or ruptured spleen, where the car's fender came in contact with the left lower ribs; and an injury to the *right* side of the head produced when the child was thrown by the impact and landed on his head. Those three injuries occur together so often they even have a name: **Waddell's triad.**

On a statistical basis, when you get a call for a severely injured child you can assume that the child has sustained BLUNT TRAUMA, for more than 90 percent of mortality in children is the result of blunt

FIGURE 30-5. WADDELL'S TRIAD OF INJURIES. (1) Fractured left femur. (2) Ruptured spleen. (3) Injury to right side of head.

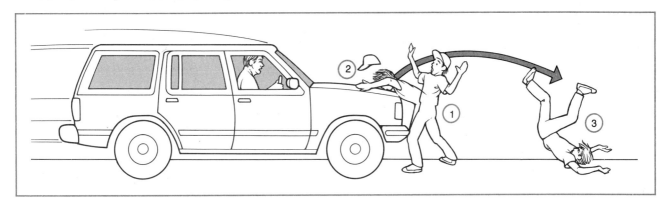

trauma. The head is going to be involved in a majority of cases, with the abdomen a close second. That's important to remember, because abdominal trauma often isn't obvious—so if you're not looking for it, you are likely to miss it.

The basic principles of advanced trauma life support for the pediatric patient are similar to those for the adult patient, but many details of assessment and management differ. It is therefore worthwhile to review the ATLS sequence for the injured child. As in the case of an injured adult, we need to proceed first through an expanded primary survey and then decide whether to "load and go" or to continue the secondary survey at the scene.

The Extended Primary Survey

Airway Management and Cervical Spine Stabilization

The airway of an infant is anatomically different from that of an adult. The infant's tongue is larger relative to his oral cavity; his larynx is higher; and, of considerable importance when intubating the infant, his trachea is very short—about 5 cm (2 inches) in a newborn and 7 cm (3 inches) in an 18 month old. Another point of importance is that neonates and infants sometimes even up to the age of 6 months are obligate nose breathers, so clearing a blocked nose with a bulb syringe may be lifesaving.

In a spontaneously breathing injured child, the airway should be opened by the *jaw thrust* maneuver (Fig. 30-6) while the head and neck are held steady in neutral, "sniffing" position. If the child is unconscious, an OROPHARYNGEAL AIRWAY can be very helpful in keeping the airway open. Nasopharyngeal airways are *not* useful in infants and children, because their internal diameters are inevitably very narrow and easily obstructed by secretions. Select the appropriate *size* oropharyngeal airway by measuring it alongside the child's face; it should extend from the corner of his mouth to his ear. Before inserting the airway, check the mouth for foreign bodies, such as dislodged teeth, and remove them; also suction out any secretions. Use a tongue blade to depress the tongue as you insert the airway. Inserting the airway upside down and then rotating it into place, as is customarily done in adults, is *not* recommended, for in children that technique may injure soft tissues or dislodge loose teeth and shove them down the pharynx.

In most cases, an oropharyngeal airway will be sufficient to maintain a patent airway in the injured child. It is preferable to avoid endotracheal intubation of the injured child in the field unless it is absolutely necessary, because the procedure may be quite difficult. If you *must* intubate at the scene, because you are unable to maintain an airway otherwise, use the orotracheal route and follow the procedure described later in this chapter.

Cricothyrotomy should *not* be performed on infants and small children. If no other means can be found to overcome an obstructed airway, percutaneous translaryngeal ventilation may be attempted (see Chap. 8).

Before leaving the airway, make sure to find some means for temporarily STABILIZING THE CERVICAL SPINE. Sandbags will do until you have completed the rest of the primary survey. Cervical collars are *not* effective when used alone in infants and children, so don't waste time trying to apply one.

Breathing

Look, listen, and feel to determine whether the child is breathing. If breathing is absent, provide artificial ventilation as described later in this chapter (section on cardiopulmonary resuscitation). Do *not* use a demand valve. If the child *is* breathing, note the RATE AND DEPTH OF RESPIRATIONS. Observe the face for NASAL FLARING, the neck for TRACHEAL DEVIATION, and the chest for INTERCOSTAL RETRACTIONS or OPEN WOUNDS. Listen without a stethoscope for GRUNTING (a sign of respiratory distress) and with a stethoscope for UNEQUAL BREATH SOUNDS, which may be much harder to detect in the infant or small child. Administer OXYGEN at the earliest opportunity. If there are signs of ventilatory failure (Table 30-4), assist ventilations with a bag-valve-mask.

Circulation

A small child has a small blood volume—about 80 to 90 ml per kilogram of body weight. That means that

FIGURE 30-6. **JAW THRUST** for opening the airway of an infant with suspected injury to the cervical spine. The head is supported in neutral position.

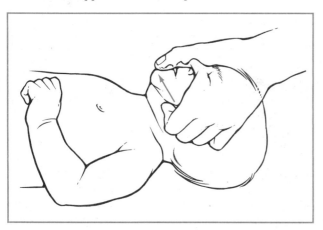

TABLE 30-4. SIGNS OF IMPENDING VENTILATORY FAILURE IN INFANTS AND SMALL CHILDREN

ASSESS	SIGN OF IMPENDING VENTILATORY FAILURE
Respiratory rate	Tachypnea
Respiratory effort	Labored breathing
	Gasping
	Grunting respirations
	Nasal flaring
	Suprasternal/intercostal retractions
	Seesawing of chest and abdomen
Auscultation	Little air movement
	Wheezes, stridor
Skin color	Dusky, gray, mottled, or cyanotic
Mental status	Restless, combative (early hypoxia)
	Lethargic, comatose (late hypoxia)

a 10-kg (22-lb) baby has less than a liter of blood, so he does not need to lose large quantities of fluid or blood to go into shock. A burn over 15 percent of his body or internal hemorrhage of a few hundred milliliters—either of those will do the job. And to complicate matters, signs of shock may be very subtle in children. Remember, the child will preserve his blood pressure nearly to the bitter end; most children will not develop hypotension until they have lost one-quarter of their total blood volume. So you need to be alert for earlier clues that shock is developing.

CLUES TO SHOCK IN CHILDREN

- Mechanism of injury: Blunt ABDOMINAL TRAUMA
- APATHY and listlessness
- COLD, PALE, MOTTLED SKIN (extremities cool first)
- PROLONGED CAPILLARY REFILL
- COLLAPSED VEINS (neck veins and peripheral veins)
- In abdominal trauma or suspected abdominal trauma, INCREASING ABDOMINAL GIRTH, as assessed with a tape measure
- TACHYCARDIA and TACHYPNEA (with respect to normal pulse and respiratory rates for the child's age—review Table 30-1)
- SCANTY URINE OUTPUT

External BLEEDING must of course be controlled as rapidly as possible. Use firm direct pressure on any bleeding wound, and apply a pressure dressing as you would for an adult.

Disability

A quick assessment of the child's neurologic status can at this point be made using the same AVPU scale as for adults:

A   Child is **alert.**
V   The child is not alert but can be wakened by **voice.**
P   The child cannot be wakened by voice but can be roused by a **painful** stimulus.
U   The child is **unconscious** and cannot be wakened.

Expose

The final step of the extended primary survey is to undress the injured child completely in order to permit a thorough assessment. All told, you should be able to carry out all five steps of the extended primary survey, from A to E, in under 2 minutes.

Transport Decision and Critical Interventions

As for the injured adult, we must at this point pause and decide whether the child is critically injured and must therefore be transported immediately ("load and go") or whether there is time to perform the secondary survey at the scene. Children may be classified in the load-and-go category either because of the *mechanism* of their injury or the injury itself:

LOAD-AND-GO SITUATIONS IN PEDIATRIC TRAUMA

- Ominous MECHANISMS OF INJURY:
  1. **Fall** from a height **over 20 feet** (about 6 meters)
  2. Involved in an **accident with fatalities**
  3. **Ejected** from an automobile in a vehicular accident
  4. **Struck by a car** (as a pedestrian or cyclist)
- When a child's AIRWAY is in jeopardy and you are **unable to secure the airway** (e.g., blunt laryngeal trauma)
- Children whose BREATHING is inadequate, including those with:
  1. **Respiratory arrest**
  2. **Open pneumothorax**
  3. **Tension pneumothorax**
- Children with CIRCULATORY insufficiency (i.e., SHOCK), including those with:
  1. Full **cardiopulmonary arrest**
  2. **Shock**
  3. **Uncontrollable bleeding**
- Children with severe neurologic DISABILITY:
  1. **Unconscious**
  2. **Deteriorating level of consciousness**
  3. Signs of **rising intracranial pressure**

Any child who falls into one of the categories listed must be immediately logrolled onto a pediatric backboard, properly secured, and transported, delaying only for critical interventions (airway control, control of external hemorrhage, sealing of open neck and chest wounds, and decompression of tension pneumothorax). Starting an IV is *not* considered a critical intervention; that is, it is not a procedure that should delay transport. If the child is in shock or in danger of shock, establish the IV while en route to the hospital and give a bolus of **20 ml per kilogram of normal saline**.

The Secondary Survey

If the primary survey does *not* reveal a load-and-go situation, proceed expeditiously to the secondary survey, which follows the same general sequence and method as for an adult.

Taking the History in Pediatric Trauma

When dealing with a seriously injured child, the history is usually obtained in snatches, while carrying out various interventions and en route to the hospital. As for the adult, the most convenient format for the trauma history in an infant or child is the AMPLE history:

A	ALLERGIES
M	MEDICATIONS that the child takes regularly or has taken today
P	PAST MEDICAL HISTORY
	• Previous hospitalizations
	• Operations/anesthetic complications
	• Serious underlying illnesses (e.g., asthma, diabetes)
L	LAST MEAL
E	EVENTS leading up to the incident (mechanisms of injury)

Physical Assessment

In performing the more detailed physical examination of the secondary survey, start by REASSESSING THE LEVEL OF CONSCIOUSNESS, and record your findings on the **neurologic flow sheet** already established for the child.

Measure and record the VITAL SIGNS. Surveys have shown that paramedics often skip that step in children, especially in injured children (precisely the children whose vital signs are most important to follow!), often because of unfamiliarity with pediatric vital signs. If you make it a habit to measure the vital signs of *every* pediatric patient you are called to treat, you will be less inclined to neglect the vital signs when you are under pressure.

MEASURE THE VITAL SIGNS IN EVERY CHILD YOU TREAT.

Proceed through the HEAD-TO-TOE SURVEY:

- Examine the HEAD for signs of injury as you would for an adult, but in the infant make sure you check the anterior FONTANELLE. A bulging fontanelle suggests increased intracranial pressure. Look for *ecchymosis*, blood or clear *fluid draining* from the nose or ears, and deformity suggestive of skull fracture. Palpate the infant's head for a soft, boggy mass beneath the scalp, a **cephalhematoma.** That is a collection of blood beneath the skull's outer lining, and it is usually a sign that the underlying bone of the skull has been fractured.

- Check the PUPILS for size, equality, and reaction to light. Remember, the presence of a fixed, dilated pupil or of Cushing's triad (bradycardia, hypertension, and irregular or slow respirations) suggests increased intracranial pressure.
- Take a more careful look at the CHEST now. Look for the **point of maximal impulse** (PMI) of the heart, that is, the spot where you can see the heart's pulsation on the chest wall, and mark that spot with an "X" using a ball-point pen or grease pencil. If the child develops a pneumothorax, the position of the heart will shift (*away* from the side of tension pneumothorax), so the PMI will move from the spot you have marked. If the child should subsequently develop respiratory distress, a shift in the position of the PMI can help you decide whether to whip in a catheter to decompress the chest. Once you have located and marked the PMI, inspect the chest for bruises.
- Inspect the ABDOMEN for bruises or distention. The development of abdominal distention may be the only clue to life-threatening internal hemorrhage, and it may not be obvious. To establish a baseline, MEASURE THE ABDOMINAL GIRTH with a tape measure at the level of the umbilicus, and record your finding along with the time of the measurement. Repeat the measurement of abdominal girth each time you obtain a set of vital signs. Look for contusions on the anterior abdominal wall in children who were involved in vehicular trauma and were wearing lap seat belts. Any child found to have a seat-belt contusion on the abdomen should be assumed to have suffered a seat-belt fracture of the lumbar spine and should not be manipulated further before being secured to a backboard.
- If there is no evidence of seat-belt injury, carefully logroll the child to examine the BACK for ecchymoses or swelling, and palpate for tenderness.
- Examine the EXTREMITIES for deformity, contusions, abrasions, swelling, or crepitus on palpation, and check for equality of peripheral pulses. The brachial and dorsalis pedis pulses are the easiest to check in an infant or small child. Upper extremity fractures are most likely after falls, while pedestrian injury classically produces a femoral shaft fracture.

As you proceed through the secondary survey, keep in mind that the "big three" in seriously injured children are—in order of frequency—head trauma (occurring in at least 40% of seriously injured children), abdominal trauma (30%), and chest trauma (15%).

Head Injuries in Children

The child's head is much larger in proportion to his body than that of an adult, and for that reason it is more often injured. Babies and small children suffer head injuries mostly from falls, automobile accidents, and parental battering. In school-age children, bicycles and skateboards start to enter the picture, but motor vehicle accidents still play the leading role.

From the standpoint of sustaining a blow to the head, there are advantages and disadvantages to being very little. On the minus side, the cranial bones of infants and young children are thinner, and the blood vessels within the skull are more fragile. Therefore any blow to the head is likely to send the brain banging back and forth against the inner surfaces of the skull, tearing blood vessels in the process. Furthermore, the infant or child is much more likely to respond to brain injury with a marked increase in cerebral blood flow (cerebral **hyperemia**), leading to rapid cerebral edema. On the plus side, however, at least in infants, the skull is not yet a rigid, closed box as it is in an adult; the sutures of the skull and the fontanelles allow a little bit of expansion in response to increased intracranial pressure. The neurologic deterioration from increased intracranial pressure can be more readily reversed in a child, and as a consequence the mortality from closed head injuries is considerably lower in children than in adults.

There is one other important respect in which head-injured infants differ from head-injured grown-ups. In adults and in older children, the rule is that if a head-injured patient has signs of hypovolemic shock, look for another source of bleeding elsewhere. The young infant is the exception to that rule. An infant under about 3 months of age *can* lose enough blood into the skull or scalp to produce shock.

As for adults, you must assume that

> **ANY CHILD WITH A HEAD INJURY OR FOUND UNCONSCIOUS AFTER GENERAL INJURY HAS A CERVICAL SPINE INJURY UNTIL PROVED OTHERWISE.**

Indeed, because of the flexibility of the child's spinal column and spinal ligaments, spinal *cord* injury may occur without any fracture of the vertebrae.

Treatment of the Head-Injured Child

A head-injured child whose level of consciousness is depressed is in the category of "load-and-go" patients, so the steps of management after spinal immobilization will have to be accomplished en route to hospital.

- Ensure an adequate AIRWAY.
- Administer OXYGEN. Children have a higher metabolic rate than adults and thus a higher oxygen need. With head injury, the cerebral metabolic rate increases further, so oxygen demand is correspondingly elevated.
- HYPERVENTILATE the comatose child at a rate of 25 to 30 per minute.
- IMMOBILIZE THE SPINE. Standard backboards and cervical collars, even when scaled down to pediatric size, are *not* effective in stabilizing the cervical spine in pediatric patients. Indeed, a standard backboard may aggravate a cervical injury in a young child because it forces the child's neck into flexion. Therefore it is recommended to use a special pediatric backboard that has a recess for the occiput. If you do not have such a backboard, place folded blankets onto a standard backboard to elevate the child's back and shoulders. In a pinch, a baby involved in a vehicular accident can be immobilized in the infant car seat in which it was presumably riding, although a specially designed pediatric immobilization device, such as the pediatric KED, gives more secure immobilization. Apply a *rigid* cervical collar. Buttress the sides of the head with a blanket roll or polystyrene blocks. And *tape* the collar and the head supports to the backboard. Also pad generously the child's sides and the edges of the backboard, to prevent lateral motion if the board must be tilted to the side during vomiting.
- Start TRANSPORT.
- NOTIFY the receiving hospital of your patient's injuries, condition, and estimated time of arrival.
- If the child is not in shock, ELEVATE THE HEAD end of the backboard about 30 degrees, to help lower intracranial pressure.
- Another measure that will help lower the intracranial pressure is to assist ventilations so as to produce MILD HYPERVENTILATION—a rate of about 45 per minute for an infant, 30 per minute for a child.
- ANTICIPATE VOMITING, and have suction at hand.

Chest Injuries in Children

Trauma to the chest occurs in about 15 percent of seriously injured children. The child's chest wall is much more pliable than that of an adult, so it can absorb a lot more kinetic energy. As a consequence, rib fractures are rare in children. But by the same token, injuries to the organs of the thorax may be more severe because the pliable rib cage is more easily compressed deep into the thoracic cavity during blunt trauma. Thus children are more vulnerable than adults to *pulmonary contusion, pericardial tamponade,* and *rupture of the diaphragm.* Furthermore, all of those injuries, along with massive *hemothorax,* may occur without any evidence of a fractured rib or sternum. The lesson in all of that is:

> **BE ALERT FOR SIGNS OF SHOCK OR RESPIRATORY INSUFFICIENCY IN ANY CHILD WHO HAS SUSTAINED BLUNT CHEST TRAUMA.**

As noted earlier, the signs of pneumothorax or hemothorax may be subtle, for inequality of breath sounds is much more difficult to detect in a small chest, especially under the conditions usually present in the field. Furthermore signs such as neck vein distention are not as reliable in children as in adults. So you may not have much to go by except respiratory distress and early indications of hypovolemia. A shift in the point of maximal impulse, as described earlier, may be the first indication that a tension pneumothorax is developing.

Treatment of the Child with a Chest Injury

Severe respiratory distress constitutes a "load-and-go" criterion, so most children with serious chest trauma will require transport immediately after the primary survey and chest decompression, if indicated.

- Ensure an adequate AIRWAY.
- Administer OXYGEN in high concentration by mask or bag-valve-mask (*not* demand valve).
- SEAL open chest wounds, if present.
- DECOMPRESS tension pneumothorax, if present. For a small child, use a 14-gauge Angiocath, and place it in the **fourth intercostal space in the anterior axillary line** at the level of the nipple. Puncture the skin just *above* the fifth rib, and proceed as you would for an adult (see Chap. 17).
- IMMOBILIZE the child on a backboard.
- Start TRANSPORT.
- NOTIFY the receiving hospital of your patient's injuries, condition, and estimated time of arrival.

- MONITOR cardiac rhythm. Myocardial contusion may produce serious dysrhythmias.
- If there are signs of shock, start an IV LIFELINE with lactated Ringer's solution at a rate of about 20 ml/kg/hr.

Abdominal Injuries in Children

The abdomen is involved in approximately 30 percent of major pediatric injuries, and abdominal trauma (usually rupture of the liver) is the second leading cause, after head injury, of pediatric trauma death. The relatively large size of a child's abdominal organs makes them particularly vulnerable to blunt trauma. The *liver and spleen*, furthermore, extend below the rib cage in children, so they do not have as much bony protection as those organs do in adults. The liver and spleen, in addition, are fragile organs, with a rich blood supply.

In the retroperitoneum, the *kidneys* are more vulnerable to injury in the child because they are more mobile and less well supported than in the adult. The *duodenum and pancreas* are likely to be damaged in handlebar injuries.

As noted earlier, sometimes the only clue to major abdominal trauma may be the presence of unexplained shock. But usually there will be other symptoms and signs as well. Complaints of pain in the right upper quadrant or right shoulder after blunt abdominal trauma should suggest injury to the liver, while the child complaining of left upper quadrant pain or pain in the tip of the left shoulder may have sustained a ruptured spleen. On examination, bruises over the abdomen, increasing abdominal girth, and a change in the breathing pattern (from belly breathing, which becomes painful, to thoracic breathing) are all highly suspicious signs. A mass or bruise in the flank suggests renal injury.

Treatment of a Child with Abdominal Injuries

Probably the most important contribution that a paramedic can make to the treatment of serious abdominal injury in children is to *suspect* that the injury is present and move with appropriate expeditiousness.

- Ensure an open AIRWAY. Anticipate vomiting, and keep suction at hand.
- Administer OXYGEN.
- IMMOBILIZE the child on a backboard.
- If use of the military anti-shock trousers (MAST) has become controversial in adults, it is even more so in small children. To date, there are no studies that establish a certain benefit from using a pneumatic anti-shock garment in children. If it is the policy of your service to use the MAST for children, however, INFLATE THE LEG SECTIONS ONLY.
- Start TRANSPORT.
- NOTIFY the receiving hospital of your patient's injuries, condition, and estimated time of arrival.
- Start an IV with lactated Ringer's en route, and administer fluids at a rate of about 20 ml/kg/hr.
- Continue making serial MEASUREMENTS OF ABDOMINAL GIRTH and vital signs.

A word of caution. A child who has suffered serious injury to one organ system has probably suffered serious injury to other organ systems as well.

IN THE SERIOUSLY INJURED CHILD, ALL ORGAN SYSTEMS MUST BE ASSUMED TO BE INJURED UNTIL PROVED OTHERWISE.

What that means is that injured children need to be moved to the hospital with all safe speed, for deterioration in overall condition may occur very rapidly.

Burns in Children

Thirty thousand children require hospitalization in the United States each year for serious burns, and thermal injury is the second leading cause of accidental death in children. Perhaps "accidental" is not the most accurate term, for nearly one-third of all pediatric burns are the result of child abuse.

The mechanisms of burn injury depend to a large extent on the child's age. *Infants* are more likely to be objects of abuse and to present with scald burns of the buttocks and feet from immersion in hot water or flame burns from a household fire they could not escape. The greater mobility of *toddlers* enables them to run away from a fire, but it also enables them to pull pots of hot liquid down off the stove. Toddlers are also most likely to suffer electric burns, often burns of the mouth incurred by chewing through an electric cord. *Preschoolers* are most often burned playing with matches, so their burns are typically flame burns.

Whatever the mechanism, burns in infants and children pose special problems. To begin with, the surface area in children is much larger in proportion to the total body mass than in adults; thus potential fluid loss through extensive burns can be massive. Furthermore, burn injuries create an enormous metabolic stress on the child, placing nearly every organ system in jeopardy. And burns have the capacity to create scars—both visible and not so visible—that a child will carry with him for the rest of his life.

Treatment of Burns in Children

The principles of treating burns in children are the same as for adults, but there must be a greater sense of urgency. The child's airway, for example, is very small to begin with and thus may obstruct within minutes of serious thermal injury. The potential for major heat and fluid loss across damaged skin is also far greater in pediatric patients and must therefore be addressed more aggressively.

- PUT OUT THE FIRE! Remove smoldering clothes or any other hot garments.
- Establish an AIRWAY, and immediately begin administration of 100% OXYGEN.
- Check for the presence of conditions that warrant IMMEDIATE INTUBATION:

INDICATIONS FOR IMMEDIATE INTUBATION

- Signs of imminent airway obstruction
  1. STRIDOR
  2. WHEEZING
  3. Signs of RESPIRATORY DISTRESS (nasal flaring, intercostal retractions)
- Signs that there are probably burns to the airway
  1. FACIAL BURNS
  2. SINGED NASAL HAIRS or eyebrows
  3. CARBONACEOUS SPUTUM
  4. RED, edematous MOUTH
- Fire victim with a DECREASED LEVEL OF CONSCIOUSNESS

- REMOVE CONSTRICTING OBJECTS from the extremities.
- Make a quick estimate of the DEPTH AND EXTENT OF THE BURN. The usual Rule of Nines is modified in infants, such that the head and neck account for 18 percent of the body, each upper extremity is 9 percent, each lower extremity 14 percent, and each surface of the trunk 18 percent (see Fig. 15-7). Then, with each year of age, we subtract 1 percent from the head and neck and add 1 percent to the lower extremity. Since that gets rather complicated, it's usually easier in an emergency to use the Rule of Palms: A child's palm covers an area roughly equivalent to 1 percent of body surface area (BSA).

- Check rapidly for OTHER INJURIES.
- COVER THE BURNS, preferably with wet, sterile dressings such as Water Jel. If the burns cover more than 15 percent BSA, wrap the whole child in a dry, sterile sheet after applying the wet dressings, to minimize heat loss from the body.
- Make a TRANSPORT DECISION. Children with critical burns should be transported to a pediatric burn center. The criteria for what constitutes a critical burn are the same in children as in adults (review Chap. 15). In addition, any burn in a child under 2 years old is best regarded as critical.
- Start TRANSPORT.
- NOTIFY the receiving hospital of your patient's injuries, condition, and estimated time of arrival.
- Start an IV with lactated Ringer's en route. There are all sorts of complicated formulas for calculating the intravenous fluid rate in burned children. None of those formulas are necessary in the field. For prehospital fluid resuscitation in burns, just remember the following:
- Children < 5 years old: 150 ml per hour
- Children 5 years and older: 500 ml per hour
  Inscribe those figures on a card, and tape the card to your pediatric trauma kit, along with the card containing normal vital signs for children of different ages.

Injuries to the Extremities

The bones of a child are quite pliable, being incompletely calcified, and are held together with strong collateral ligaments. It therefore takes quite *powerful forces* to produce skeletal trauma in children. When those forces are applied, injury is very likely to occur in the *growth plates* at the bone ends. Injury to growth centers in bone can lead to lifelong deformity if not treated correctly. Fractures near the elbows or knees, furthermore, are often associated with injury to nearby blood vessels. For those reasons, when the patient is a child, even skeletal trauma that looks minor needs to be evaluated in the hospital.

The most important information you can furnish to the emergency room staff are your observations at the scene. What was the likely *mechanism of injury*? *When* precisely did the injury occur? In what *position* was the child found? In what position was the injured limb? Were *pulses* and sensation present distal to the injury when you first examined the child?

EXTREMITY TRAUMA IN CHILDREN: POINTS TO REMEMBER:

- In the multiply injured child, *priority goes to the ABCs* no matter how alarming the extremity trauma looks.
- A child may lose a unit of blood into the thigh from a fractured femur. In a 7-year-old child, that may be a quarter of his total blood volume!
- Whenever the mechanism of injury involves massive forces (e.g., child struck by a car), *splint the whole child* on a backboard.
- Even apparently minor skeletal trauma in children requires evaluation in the hospital.

Summary: Management of the Injured Child

Taking care of injured kids is tough. It is tough because kids are built differently, respond to injury differently, and elicit different and usually very uncomfortable responses from rescuers. Nonetheless, taking care of injured children is part of the job, and if you want to do the job well, you will make sure you are prepared for dealing with the injured child.

One way to be prepared is to have a special pediatric kit that contains all the equipment and supplies you will need for pint-sized patients. The contents of such a kit are listed in Table 30-5. Experience will help you decide what you need to stock in *your* "Kiddie Kit."

Another way to be prepared is to get some experience with children. Try to arrange to do some shifts in a pediatric emergency department. And take advantage of occasions when you are caring for children who are *not* in critical condition to practice your skills in pediatric assessment. You will need those skills for the children who *are* seriously injured.

Remember: A severely injured child is in grave danger. His airway is apt to be compromised. He is likely to be hypoxemic at precisely the time when his oxygen demands are increased. And he cannot afford to lose much blood, because he doesn't have very much to begin with. For all those reasons, meticulous attention to the ABCs and prompt transport to the hospital are imperative.

TABLE 30-5.   SUGGESTED CONTENTS OF PEDIATRIC KIT

Pediatric BLOOD PRESSURE CUFFS: infant and child sizes

Airway and breathing equipment:
  Pediatric OXYGEN MASKS (partial rebreathing)
  Pediatric BAG-VALVE-MASK unit, with three mask sizes (newborn, infant, child)
  OROPHARYNGEAL AIRWAYS: newborn, infant, and child sizes (sizes 0 to 5)
  Bulb SUCTION for neonates
  Pediatric SUCTION CATHETERS (4, 6.5, and 8 Fr)
  ENDOTRACHEAL TUBES in graded sizes from 2.5 to 8.0 mm
  LARYNGOSCOPE handle and five straight blades (sizes 0, 1, 1.5, 2, 3)
  Magill forceps

Pediatric defibrillator paddles (20 cm²)

Pediatric monitoring electrodes

Intravenous equipment:
  Butterfly needles, sizes 14 through 23 gauge
  Over-the-needle catheters, sizes 18 through 24 gauge
  Intraosseous needles
  Pedatrol or Buratrol administration sets
  Microdrip infusion sets
  Nitroglycerin ointment
  250-ml and 500-ml bags of D5/W, D5/0.5 normal saline, and lactated Ringer's
  Mini-armboards
  Tape
  Self-adhering roller gauze

Tourniquet

Orthopedic and wound equipment (may be in a separate kit):
  Child-size splints
    Board splints
    Air splints
    Vacuum splint
  Pediatric MAST, if used by your service
  Pediatric BACKBOARD, preferably with head well
  Infant and child-size rigid plastic CERVICAL COLLARS
  Wide selection of bandages and dressings, including brightly colored Bandaids

Pediatric drug box

Information cards (preferably plasticized):
  Normal vital signs in children
  IV fluid rates for children
  Average pediatric weights
  Pediatric drug dosages

Lollipops

**SUMMARY: MANAGEMENT OF
THE INJURED CHILD**

- Establish an AIRWAY. More than half of all traumatic deaths in children are the direct result of asphyxia. ANTICIPATE VOMITING, and have suction at hand.
- Administer OXYGEN.
- ASSIST VENTILATIONS as needed with a bag-valve-mask. Do *not* use a demand valve in infants and small children.
- CONTROL EXTERNAL BLEEDING.
- IMMOBILIZE all seriously injured children on a specially designed or modified backboard.
- Make a TRANSPORT DECISION as soon as you have completed the extended primary survey.
- NOTIFY the receiving hospital of critical cases.
- When an IV is needed, start it EN ROUTE to the hospital.
- Keep the child WARM.
- TRANSPORT ALL children you suspect to be victims of CHILD ABUSE, even if the injuries are trivial.

MISCELLANEOUS PEDIATRIC EMERGENCIES

Common Childhood Poisonings

The general principles of managing a poisoning incident as well as the characteristics of some common poisonings have been discussed in detail in Chapter 27 and will not be repeated here. In this discussion we shall simply consider two specific poisonings that are so common in the pediatric age group as to merit particular attention: poisoning from aspirin products and poisoning from acetaminophen (paracetamol).

Aspirin Poisoning

Americans consume between 10,000 and 20,000 *tons* of aspirin annually, and aspirin or similar products (salicylates) are involved in nearly 20,000 poisonings in the United States each year. It is small wonder, then, that salicylate intoxication is one of the most frequently encountered overdoses in children, accounting for 25 percent of all pediatric poisoning deaths. Salicylate poisoning usually occurs as a result of the child's getting hold of a bottle of child or adult aspirin, but it may also occur after ingestion of oil of wintergreen (methyl salicylate) syrup or any of a va-

riety of other salicylate-containing products (e.g., Alka-Seltzer, Sine-Off, Pepto-Bismol, Doan's Pills, Compound W). In a significant number of cases, furthermore, salicylate poisoning in children is not the result of accidental ingestion but rather of parental administration of the drug. Well-meaning parents may give a feverish child adult aspirin or even children's aspirin at too frequent intervals, leading to a cumulative overdose. Anything over about 150 mg per kilogram should be considered a potentially toxic dose. (Question: How many 325-mg aspirin tablets would a 20-kg 4 year old have to swallow in order to have ingested a toxic dose?)

An accurate HISTORY of the poisoning may be very hard to obtain, because the parent may not even be aware that a poisoning has occurred. Unless the child is actually caught in the act of downing a bottle of oil of wintergreen, for example, the parent is more likely to call for an ambulance because of the symptoms the child develops *after* the ingestion. Often, therefore, the clinical picture will be all you have to go by.

Salicylate is an *acid* and causes a profound *metabolic acidosis*. The child tries to compensate with HYPERPNEA (why?), so the initial presentation may look a lot like that of diabetic keotacidosis. But as time passes, the child tires and respirations become depressed. Other symptoms and signs of salicylate intoxication include a paradoxical FEVER and SWEATING; VOMITING; DEHYDRATION, sometimes so severe as to lead to circulatory collapse; SEIZURES; and in severe cases, COMA.

ANY CHILD WITH UNEXPLAINED HYPERPNEA SHOULD BE SUSPECTED TO HAVE SALICYLATE POISONING.

When a child is breathing very deeply (but not necessarily very rapidly) and you don't know why, especially if he is also feverish and confused, it's a good idea to make a foray through the medicine cabinets and other places where salicylates may have been placed. Inquire as well whether the child has been ill lately and, if so, what the parents have been giving him for his illness.

Treatment of Salicylate Overdose

The treatment of a child you suspect of salicylate toxicity follows the same principles we learned in Chapter 27 for the treatment of any other ingestion:

- Maintain an open AIRWAY. If the child is sleepy or comatose and the gag reflex is absent, INTUBATE the trachea.
- Administer OXYGEN.
- If the child is alert and has an intact gag reflex, give ACTIVATED CHARCOAL, at least 5 tablespoons mixed into a slurry of tap water.
- If the child is fully alert and you arrived within 15 to 20 minutes of the ingestion, induce vomiting with SYRUP OF IPECAC, 15 ml PO for a child over 1 year old.
- If the child is stuporous or comatose, insert a NASOGASTRIC TUBE *after* the trachea has been intubated, withdraw (and save) the gastric contents, and instill activated charcoal prepared as described.
- If the child's temperature is elevated above 40°C (104°F), sponge his body with *tepid* tap water to bring down his temperature.
- Start an IV LIFELINE with D5/W.
- Consult medical command regarding the administration of SODIUM BICARBONATE, 1 mEq per kilogram, to alkalinize the child's urine and thereby speed up urinary excretion of the drug.
- If the child is having seizures, check with medical command regarding the administration of
  1. DEXTROSE 25%, 1 ml per kilogram IV.
  2. DIAZEPAM, 0.3 mg per kilogram IV.
- BRING THE CONTAINER of whatever it was that the child ingested with the child to the hospital.
- TRANSPORT the child to the hospital.

Acetaminophen Poisoning

Acetaminophen (paracetamol) is found in literally hundreds of analgesics, cough preparations, and cold medications—both prescription drugs and those available over the counter. Widely touted as a "safe" alternative to aspirin, acetaminophen is marketed as a single drug, in preparations like Anacin, Datril, Excedrin, Panadol, and Tylenol, or in combination with a whole range of other drugs (e.g., combined with propoxyphene as Darvocet, or with phenylephrine and chlorpheniramine as Dristan).

Overdose with acetaminophen produces severe, potentially fatal liver damage. It does not require a lot of acetaminophen to do so. For children, the minimum dosage capable of producing liver toxicity is 140 mg per kilogram, which means that a 15-kg toddler need swallow only four or five of Dad's extra-strength Tylenol tablets (500 mg each) to do a job on his liver.

As in the case of aspirin poisoning, there may or may not be an obvious history of ingestion. If the child was not caught in the act, the chances of guessing the cause of his problem are very small, for the early *symptoms and signs* of acetaminophen ingestion are quite nonspecific—a little nausea, vomiting, and perhaps some sweating during the first 24 hours after the overdose. It is quite unlikely that medical care will be sought for those symptoms.

You are more likely to be summoned when the child *is* caught in the act of swallowing the medication or caught shortly afterward with the telltale empty bottle.

Treatment of Acetaminophen Poisoning

There are variations in the treatment protocol for acetaminophen from region to region depending on the philosophy of the local poison control center toward induction of vomiting and giving activated charcoal. Nearly everyone agrees that if the child presents within 4 hours of the overdose, his stomach should be emptied. And everyone agrees that activated charcoal effectively adsorbs acetaminophen. So why the disagreement?

Regarding the induction of vomiting, first of all there are differences of opinion whether that is the preferred way to decontaminate the stomach in this particular instance. Several authorities point out that both the acetaminophen overdose itself and the drug that will be given as an antidote—*N*-acetylcysteine (NAC, or Mucomyst)—are themselves emetic, so if you give syrup of ipecac in addition, you may cause intractable vomiting. The consensus seems to be that gastric lavage is preferable if the child will tolerate it.

As to activated charcoal, the problem there is that the charcoal adsorbs not only acetaminophen but also NAC, the antidote to acetaminophen. So theoretically, activated charcoal might interfere with the action of the antidote. In practice, that effect does not appear to be clinically significant, but most authorities nonetheless advise that if given, charcoal should be rinsed out of the stomach before administering NAC.

- Try to find out as precisely as possible WHAT the child took and HOW MUCH he took. No treatment at all is necessary if the child swallowed less than 100 mg per kilogram of acetaminophen. But if there is any doubt whatsoever, assume that a toxic amount was ingested.
- Follow local protocol regarding the induction of vomiting and the administration of activated charcoal.

- TRANSPORT the child to the hospital. His subsequent treatment will depend on the concentration of acetaminophen detected in his blood.

Foreign Bodies

Infants and small children take a keen interest in all the nooks and crannies of their anatomy and in the various objects that can be inserted into those nooks and crannies. Foreign bodies in the EAR CANAL are thus a common problem among the pediatric age group. For reasons known only to the children who engage in such practices, there is some irresistible compulsion to stuff the ears with small objects, such as beans, peanuts, and the like. In general, the treatment in the field for the "bean-in-the-ear syndrome" is to LEAVE THE EAR ALONE! Calm the child's mother, if possible, and transport the child to the hospital, where good illumination and appropriate equipment are available to facilitate removing the foreign body from the ear. The one possible exception to the rule is the situation in which you are some distance from the hospital and the object in the ear is **hygroscopic** (absorbs water), such as corn or peas, and will thus swell rapidly within the ear canal. In that case, the physician may request that you try to flush out the foreign body before transport.

If so instructed, fill a 50-ml syringe or bulb syringe with *alcohol* (if you are using a hypodermic syringe, remove the needle!). Position the child lying down on his side, with the affected ear over a basin. In the case of a small child, some muscular assistance will doubtless be required to keep him still; toddlers in particular definitely do not like to have strange people fiddling with their ears. Place the tip of the syringe near the top part of the entrance to the ear canal, and rapidly flush the alcohol in. Use gentle pressure only, as forceful flushing can drive the object deeper into the canal. If you cannot flush out the object readily, move on to the hospital. Even if the object is removed, the child should be transported, for examination with an otoscope will be necessary to make certain the canal is entirely clear and that no damage was done.

The very same children who delight in putting beans in their ears also find satisfaction in putting FOREIGN BODIES IN THE NOSE. The treatment in that instance is to LEAVE THE NOSE ALONE. Safe removal of a foreign body from the nose requires special equipment and good lighting. Take the child to the emergency room, and reassure the parent, who is likely to be altogether distraught, especially—as is very often the case—if the child is a repeat offender.

SPECIAL TECHNIQUES FOR THE PEDIATRIC PATIENT

Cardiopulmonary Resuscitation*

In adults, cardiac causes are usually the precipitating factor in cardiopulmonary arrest. In infants and children, cardiac arrest is much more likely to occur *secondary to hypoxemia and respiratory arrest*. Thus, children merit meticulous attention to the airway and breathing; if those are assured, there may be no need for further resuscitative measures.

Situations that may require resuscitation in children include suffocation due to foreign body obstruction of the airway, near drowning, trauma, poisoning, smoke inhalation, near-miss SIDS, and certain infections, like croup and epiglottitis. A cursory inspection of that list makes it clear that

> **THE MAJORITY OF EMERGENCIES REQUIRING CPR IN CHILDREN ARE PREVENTABLE**

and paramedics have an important role in educating the public (not to mention their own children) in basic safety measures. Toys for young children should be inspected for small parts that could find their way into a toddler's windpipe. Matches and cigarette lighters should be kept out of the reach of children, as should all medications and potential poisons. Children must be taught to eat sitting down, not while running or playing. In the car, children should always be in the back seat, in a suitable infant seat where appropriate and restrained with seat belts. Children riding bicycles should wear helmets. Children who live near a swimming pool or a body of water must be instructed in water safety rules. CPR is very dramatic and sometimes very rewarding, but it cannot save nearly the number of young lives that could be saved by adequate preventive measures.

Respiratory or cardiac arrest in infants and children rarely occurs "out of the blue." Usually it is the final common pathway of a *process* of deterioration in

---

*The recommendations presented here are based on those of the Emergency Cardiac Care Committee and Subcommittees, American Heart Association. Guidelines for cardiopulmonary resuscitation and emergency cardiac care. *JAMA* 268:2172, 1992.

a severely ill or injured child. Cardiopulmonary arrest usually need *not* occur in a child if the signs of deterioration are detected and treated promptly.

ANTICIPATE RESPIRATORY ARREST IN INFANTS OR CHILDREN WITH

- Tachypnea or very slow respirations
- Gasping or grunting respirations, or any other sign that the child is struggling to breathe
- Inadequate chest movements
- Decreased breath sounds
- Depressed level of consciousness
- Poor muscle tone
- Cyanosis

The *principles* of CPR are the same in infants and children as in adults. However, the *techniques* of CPR differ somewhat due to differences in size and anatomy between babies and grown-ups.

The *first* step of CPR is the same in all age groups: ESTABLISH UNRESPONSIVENESS. An unconscious infant or child, like an unconscious adult, will not waken when tapped or shaken. Even the child who *is* conscious, however, may need to have his airway opened and, on occasion, his ventilation assisted as well. The need for rescue breathing alone (as opposed to rescue breathing combined with chest compressions) is much more common in infants and children than in adults.

A: Airway

Once you have established that the infant or child is unconscious *or* that he is having difficulty breathing, OPEN THE AIRWAY. If the child is struggling to breathe but his color is pink, the airway is probably adequate. *Let the child assume a position of comfort,* and transport him immediately. If however the child is blue or is not making respiratory efforts at all, you must first open the airway. The technique now favored for doing so is the HEAD TILT–CHIN LIFT (Fig. 30-7). Hold the child's head in slight extension by firm pressure with one hand on his forehead. Use the tips of the fingers of your other hand to lift the *bony* part of the jaw, under the chin, forward. Be careful not to press on the soft tissues under the chin, and do not close the infant's mouth entirely. Be careful

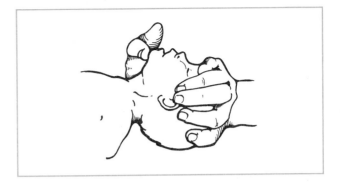

FIGURE 30-7. **HEAD TILT–CHIN LIFT** to open the infant's airway. Reproduced courtesy of the American Heart Association.

not to *hyper*extend the infant's head and neck, for hyperextension may itself produce airway obstruction.

As noted earlier, if there is any reason to suspect injury to the head or neck, use JAW THRUST with the head in neutral position to open the airway.

If manual procedures to open the infant's or child's airway are not sufficient, an artificial airway may be inserted. In the *unconscious* patient, use an OROPHARYNGEAL AIRWAY. Select the correct size by placing the airway alongside the child's face; the airway should be just long enough to reach from the corner of his mouth to his ear. Do *not* insert the airway upside down and rotate it into place as you would in an adult. Instead, use a tongue blade to depress the tongue as you insert the airway along the tongue's natural curvature.

In cardiac arrest, the best way to maintain a child's airway is by endotracheal intubation. Intubate as early as possible after you have started artificial ventilation with oxygen. (The technique of endotracheal intubation in children is described later.)

B: Breathing

As soon as the airway has been opened, immediately check whether the child is breathing, just as you would for an adult. That is, place your ear over the child's mouth and nose, look toward his abdomen, and then (1) LOOK for the rise and fall of the chest and abdomen; (2) LISTEN for the escape of air during exhalation; and (3) FEEL for air being exhaled against your cheek. If the child is not breathing *or* if breathing is not adequate (i.e., the child's lips are blue despite gasping efforts), you must provide artificial ventilation.

To apply rescue breathing to an infant or small child, you must cover the infant's nose *and* mouth with your mouth (Fig. 30-8); for a larger child, the

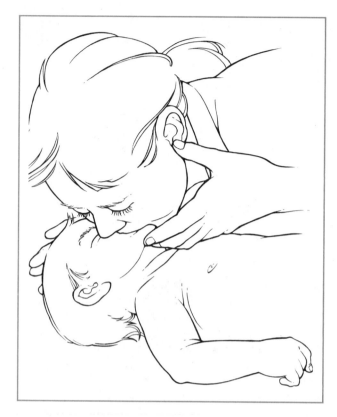

FIGURE 30-8.   MOUTH-TO-(NOSE-AND-) MOUTH VEN-TILATION OF THE INFANT. Cover the infant's nose and mouth with your mouth and give small puffs from your cheeks.

standard mouth-to-mouth technique is applicable. To start artificial ventilation, give TWO SLOW BREATHS (1.0–1.5 seconds/breath) with a pause in between them for you to take a breath and refresh the oxygen content of your exhaled air. Don't overdo the ventilations. Babies are smaller than adults, and their lungs are also smaller than those of grown-ups. Therefore

> **LIMIT VENTILATION VOLUME TO JUST THAT NECESSARY TO CAUSE THE CHEST TO RISE.**

That may take a bit of force, since the smaller airways of children provide greater resistance to air flow; but more force does not mean more volume. Keep your eye on the chest! As soon as you see the chest rise, stop blowing.

If air enters the chest freely with your first two breaths, check for a pulse as described below. If not,

reposition the baby's head and try again. If air still does not enter the child's lungs, suspect a foreign body obstruction and treat accordingly.

Administer OXYGEN at the earliest opportunity. Adjuncts such as a pediatric-size bag-valve-mask with oxygen may be used, but take care not to deliver too large a tidal volume; once again, use the rise and fall of the chest as your guide. The pocket mask turned upside down (so that it will fit with a good seal) enables finer control over tidal volume. If you do not use adjuncts, you can enrich the oxygen concentration you provide during mouth-to-mouth ventilation by placing a two-pronged nasal cannula or nasal catheter, run at low flow, in your own nose. DO NOT USE A DEMAND VALVE FOR AN INFANT OR SMALL CHILD.

When artificial ventilation is given too aggressively—with excessive force or excessive volume—the child's stomach may become distended and push the diaphragm upward, thereby reducing lung volume. You can minimize GASTRIC DISTENTION by maintaining an adequate airway and carefully limiting ventilation volumes to those just sufficient to cause the chest to rise. Do *not* attempt to relieve gastric distention when it occurs in an unintubated child because of the danger that the child's stomach contents will be aspirated into his lungs. If, however, the child's abdomen becomes so tense that effective ventilation is impossible, there will be little choice but to try to decompress the stomach. In that case, turn the child's whole body to the side, and then apply gentle pressure over the abdomen. Be prepared to sweep the child's mouth free of vomitus before turning him back supine and resuming artificial ventilation.

C: Circulation

Once you have opened the child's airway and have given two slow breaths, it is necessary to determine whether only breathing has stopped or whether the child's heart has stopped beating as well. That is, you must check for a PULSE. In a child, palpate for a carotid pulse, just as in an adult. In an infant, however, a short, thick neck may make the carotid pulse difficult to locate. For that reason, it is recommended that IN INFANTS, CHECK FOR THE BRACHIAL PULSE, which is located on the inside of the upper arm, midway between the elbow and shoulder (Fig. 30-9). To palpate for the brachial pulse, place your thumb on the outside of the baby's arm, between his elbow and shoulder, and lay the tips of your index and middle fingers along the volar (inside) surface of the arm, pressing *lightly* toward the bone.

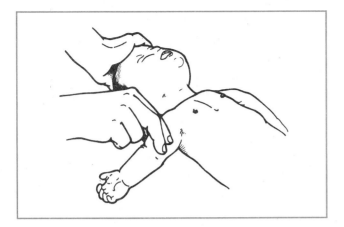

FIGURE 30-9. PALPATING FOR THE BRACHIAL PULSE in an infant. Reproduced courtesy of the American Heart Association.

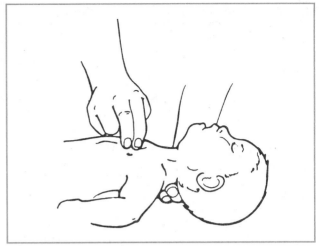

FIGURE 30-10. EXTERNAL CHEST COMPRESSIONS for the infant are performed with two fingers over the midline of the sternum, one fingerbreadth below the nipple line. Reproduced courtesy of the American Heart Association.

If you feel a pulse, cardiac activity is present, and the problem is only one of respiratory arrest; so continue rescue breathing—**20 times per minute** (once every 3 seconds). If the pulse is *absent*, then you must combine rescue breathing with external chest compressions to circulate the oxygenated blood.

The correct *compression point* for the INFANT is over the lower third of the sternum. You can locate that point by drawing an imaginary line between the infant's nipples (**intermammary line**); the compression point is one fingerbreadth below the center of that line. If you are on the infant's right side, place your right index finger on the midsternum just below the intermammary line. Then place your right middle and index fingers on the sternum beside your index finger; use those TWO FINGERS TO COMPRESS. (If that position is awkward, you may use the index and middle fingers for compression once you have identified the correct compression point as described.) The infant's chest is much more pliable than that of an adult, so two hands are not necessary to perform chest compressions. Two fingers are usually adequate.

To perform external chest compressions in the infant, then, place two fingers on the sternal compression point (Fig. 30-10) and compress one-third to one-half the depth of the chest, or about ½ to 1 inch (1.3–2.5 cm). The baby should be on a hard surface for compressions to be effective, and the head and neck should be supported. Because of the normally faster heart rate in infants, the compression rate should be a little faster than it is for adults: **at least 100 per minute**, with a **pause** of 1.0 to 1.5 seconds **after every fifth compression to interpose a breath**. While one hand is compressing the infant's chest, keep your other hand on his forehead to maintain head tilt. That will usually keep the airway open between ventilations and make it easier to switch back and forth between compressing and ventilating—which, even in the best of circumstances, is very tiring.

In the CHILD, the compression point is also over the lower third of the sternum. To apply compressions, use the HEEL OF ONE HAND, with the fingers kept well off the chest, and depress the sternum 1 to 1½ inches (2.5–3.8 cm). The compression rate in children is **100 per minute** with a **breath** interposed **after every fifth compression.** In both infants and children, reassess for a pulse after 20 cycles of compressions and ventilations (i.e., after about a minute) and every few minutes thereafter.

The differences between adult and infant CPR are summarized in Table 30-6, and the sequence of basic life support in the infant is shown in Figure 30-11.

THE ABCs IN CHILDREN: POINTS TO REMEMBER

- Cardiopulmonary arrest in children is usually due to hypoxemia, acidosis, or shock. Therefore,
- Most cardiac arrests in children are preventable.

TABLE 30-6. MODIFICATIONS IN CPR FOR INFANTS AND CHILDREN

TECHNIQUE	ADULT		CHILD	INFANT
	ONE-RESCUER CPR	TWO-RESCUER CPR		
A: Opening the AIRWAY	Maximum backward tilt of the head with neck lift or chin lift		Moderate backward tilt of the head with chin lift	Minimal backward tilt of the head with chin lift
B: Rescue BREATHING	Mouth-to-mouth or mouth-to-nose		According to size of child	Mouth-to-mouth-and-nose
	12–15/min		20/min	20/min
C: CIRCULATION				
Compression point	Lower third of sternum		Lower third of sternum	Lower third of sternum
Compress with	Two hands, one on top of the other		Heel of one hand	Two fingers
Compression depth	4–5 cm		2.5–3.5 cm	1.5–2.5 cm
Compression rate	80–100/min	80–100/min	100/min	> 100/min
Ratio of compressions to ventilations	15 : 2	5 : 1	5 : 1	5 : 1

- Most children in cardiac arrest are in asystole, not ventricular fibrillation.
- Bradycardia (heart rate < 80/min) in an infant or child is a grave sign and usually requires prompt treatment.

DEFIBRILLATION DOSAGES IN CHILDREN

Patient	Weight (kg)	Joules
Infant	12	25–50
Small child	13–25	100
Large child	>25	100–200

General rule: Start with **2 joules per kilogram.** If unsuccessful, double the energy dosage.

D: Definitive Therapy

As for adults, the sooner definitive therapy, particularly defibrillation, can be instituted, the better the chances for a successful outcome. Both defibrillation and drug therapy require significant dosage modifications for children. Pediatric defibrillation doses should be printed on a card that is taped to the defibrillator; drug dosages should be displayed prominently in the pediatric drug box.

- Administer OXYGEN as soon as it is available.
- While CPR is ongoing, one member of the team should start an IV LIFELINE (see section entitled Intravenous Techniques).
- MONITOR the cardiac rhythm, initially with quick-look pediatric paddles. If ventricular fibrillation is present, countershock, placing one paddle over the right chest at the junction of the clavicle and the sternum and the other over the apex of the heart. Pediatric paddles should be used for infants and children under 10 kg.

- The DRUGS used in advanced life support in children are principally the same as those used in adults, but the dosages are scaled downward according to the weight of the child. The pediatric dosages of first-line resuscitation drugs are
1. EPINEPHRINE 1 : 10,000, **0.1 ml per kilogram** (0.01 mg/kg) by IV push as the *initial dose* for asystole, fine ventricular fibrillation, and bradyarrhythmias. For *subsequent doses,* give 0.1 mg per kilogram (0.1 ml/kg of a *1 : 1,000* solution). When an IV has not been established, epinephrine may be given through the endotracheal tube (double or triple the dose) or by intraosseous infusion.
2. ATROPINE, **0.02 mg per kilogram** (up to a maximum single dose of 0.5 mg) by IV push as a second-line drug for bradycardias accompanied by poor perfusion or other signs of dis-

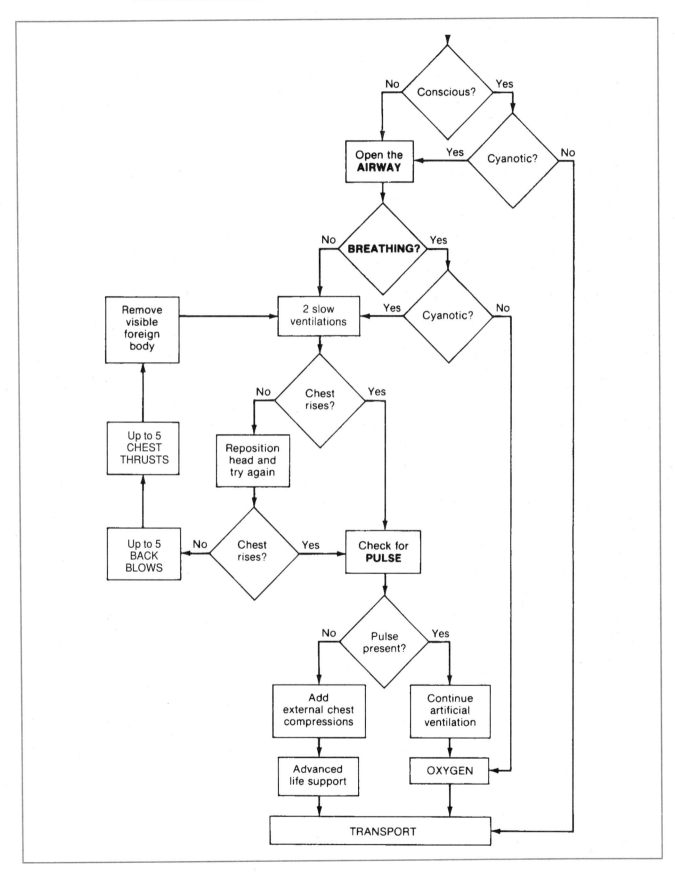

FIGURE 30-11. STEPS OF BASIC LIFE SUPPORT FOR THE INFANT.

tress and in some cases of asystole. (Epinephrine is now considered the first-line drug for those indications.) The dose may be repeated in 5 minutes, to a maximum *total dose* of 1.0 mg in a child and 2.0 mg in an adolescent.

3. LIDOCAINE, **1.0 mg per kilogram** by IV push for ventricular tachycardia, frequent premature ventricular contractions (PVCs), or recurrent episodes of ventricular fibrillation after countershock. The bolus may be followed by an *infusion* in which 120 mg of lidocaine is added to D5/W to make up a total volume of 100 ml. The infusion is run at 1.0 to 2.5 ml/kg/hr (thus delivering 20–50 μg/kg/min). When IV access cannot be obtained, bolus doses of lidocaine may be given by endotracheal tube.

Pediatric dosages of other drugs sometimes used in resuscitation can be found in the Appendix at the end of this chapter.

Endotracheal Intubation

The principles of endotracheal intubation in infants and small children are precisely the same as in adults. But there are differences in technique because of the differences in anatomy and size. To begin with, all of the structures in the pediatric airway are smaller than in the adult. While that point seems obvious, it has some important implications. Rough handling that produces trauma during adult intubation may create, say, 1 mm of edema within the wall of airway. If the diameter of the adult airway is about 8 mm, that edema will result in a 25-percent reduction in airway diameter; the same trauma to a child's tiny airway, however, producing the same millimeter of edema, may reduce the airway diameter by more than two-thirds. So having a small airway means having a very vulnerable airway.

Among the other anatomic differences encountered in pediatric intubation, the tongue of an infant is larger in relation to other structures of the airway, so there's less "working room" in the mouth. The glottis is higher (lying opposite the space between the third and fourth cervical vertebrae, rather than opposite the space between C4 and C5 as in adults), so slipping the end of a curved blade into the vallecula may simply fold the epiglottis down over the vocal cords and obscure the view. In addition, the vocal cords slant upward and backward behind a narrow, U-shaped epiglottis, so the endotracheal tube can become hung up as it passes into the larynx. Finally, the infant's trachea is very short, so mainstem bronchial intubation is a common complication. For all those reasons, the equipment and the approach must be somewhat modified in intubating infants and small children.

1. Gather the necessary **equipment:**
   • **Laryngoscope** and **blade:** The blade should be a *straight* blade; usually a Miller or Wis-Hipple blade is best. The size of the blade is determined by the size of the child, using the following rough guide:

SIZE OF LARYNGOSCOPE BLADE FOR CHILDREN

Age of Child	Blade Size
Premature newborn	0
Newborn to 8 months	1
8 months to 3 years	1.5
3 to 9 years	2
Over 9 years	3

In general, try to use the smallest blade that will do the job. **Check the light** on the blade; it should be bright white and steady.

   • **Endotracheal tube:** Endotracheal tubes for infants and small children do not have cuffs; the airway of the child is small, and if the endotracheal tube had a cuff, the internal diameter of the tube would have to be extremely narrow and thus would give a high resistance to air flow. **Choose the correct size tube** according to the size of the child, as detailed in Table 30-7. Since it is difficult to remember all those numbers, it is a good idea to make up a chart like that in Table 30-7 and tape it to the intubation kit. If you lose the chart, a rough guide to choosing the correct endotracheal tube is to use a tube of the same diameter as the fingernail of the baby's little finger ("pinkie"). A useful item to stash in the pediatric intubation kit is a *resuscitation tape*, a commercially available tape measure that identifies the appropriate tube size for a child based on the child's length. Since none of the methods for choosing the right size endotracheal tube is foolproof, though, have *three* endotracheal tubes ready: the tube you think is the right size, one that is 0.5 mm smaller, and another 0.5 mm larger.

TABLE 30-7. DIMENSIONS OF ENDOTRACHEAL TUBES

AGE	WEIGHT (LB)	INTERNAL DIAMETER (MM)	OPTIMAL LENGTH (CM)
Newborn	to 8	2.5	10
1–6 mos	8–12	3.5	11.5
6–12 mos	12–20	4.0	12
1 year	20	4.5	13
2 years	25	5.0	14
3–4 years	30–35	5.5	15
5–6 years	40–45	6.0	15
6–8 years	45–60	6.5	17
9–11 years	65–80	7.0	18–19
12–13 years	80–100	7.5	20
14–adult	100+	8.0	20–24
Adult female	100+	7.5–8.0	20–24
Adult male	100+	8.0–9.0	20–24

- **Suction catheters:** You will need one relatively large, preferably rigid catheter for suctioning secretions from the child's mouth and a sterile, flexible catheter of a size that will fit easily into your smallest endotracheal tube.
- **Tape** for securing the tube once it is in place.
- Water-soluble **lubricant** or sterile water for lubrication.

2. **Preoxygenate** the baby by bag-valve-mask with oxygen supplementation.

3. **Position** the baby on a firm surface with the neck flexed and the head in the "sniffing position." Very young babies, because of their large occiput, will lie normally in the sniffing position—indeed, sometimes in an exaggerated sniffing position that needs to be slightly modified by placing a small towel beneath the infant's back. Do *not*, however, *hyper*extend the baby's head, for that will make visualization of the cords more difficult.

4. **Open the baby's mouth** with your right index finger and thumb inserted in the right corner of the mouth.

5. **Grasp the laryngoscope** handle and blade as illustrated in Figure 30-12, and **insert the blade** into the baby's mouth.

6. As you **advance the blade,** you will first see the oropharynx and then the hypopharynx. Continue advancing the blade until you see the epiglottis. Slide the blade forward just a bit more so that it is beneath the epiglottis (*not* in the vallecula). Then **pick up the epiglottis** with the blade, and **lift gently upward** at a 45-degree angle to the floor, to elevate the tongue and jaw and bring the glottis into view. If you cannot see the cords, you can use the little finger of your left hand to **apply cricoid pressure** and push the larynx into view.

7. When you can see the vocal cords, watch them until they open spontaneously. Then take the endotracheal tube you selected, hold it so that its curve is in the horizontal plane (bevel sideways), and **insert the tube** from the right side of the baby's mouth. If the glottis is closed, wait for it to open; do not try to jam the tube through a closed glottis. Slip the tip of the tube about 5 to 10 mm below the vocal cords—stop when you see the double-ring marking on the tube pass the cords—and rotate the curve of the tube into the proper plane as you are advancing it. DO NOT TRY TO FORCE THE TUBE. The narrowest point in an infant's airway is at the cricoid ring (not at the cords, like an adult); if the tube will not pass the cricoid ring, the tube is too large. Remove it, reoxygenate the baby, and try again with a tube one size smaller.

8. Once the tube is in the trachea, you can **hold it firmly in place** by gripping it between your thumb and index finger against the baby's hard palate; that keeps your hand and the tube fixed in relation to the trachea, so movement of the patient will not cause the tube to be jerked out.

9. While holding the tube in place, **confirm the location of the endotracheal tube** by listening care-

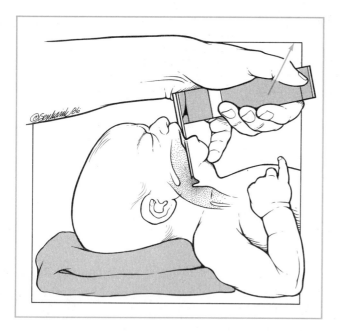

FIGURE 30-12.   INTUBATION OF THE INFANT. With the baby's head in the sniffing position, advance the straight laryngoscope blade slightly past the epiglottis. Use your little finger to apply cricoid pressure if necessary.

fully over both sides of the chest and over the stomach during ventilation through the tube.

10. Once you are satisfied that the tube is in the right position, **tape the tube securely in place,** and mark the point where it exits from the mouth so that slippage in or out can be detected. Because the infant's trachea is so short, even a small change in the baby's head position can result in bronchial intubation (with extension of the head) or complete extubation (with flexion of the head).

Infants and small children do not tolerate long periods of breath-holding. So

> **DO NOT SPEND MORE THAN 20 SECONDS ON ANY ONE INTUBATION ATTEMPT IN AN INFANT.**

If you are having difficulty, remove the laryngoscope, reoxygenate the baby for a couple of minutes, and then try again.

In children of early school age, there is one more very important consideration during endotracheal intubation: TEETH! The Tooth Fairy does not give rewards for teeth that are aspirated into a bronchus (although the courts often do!). So before you start to

intubate a school-age child, make a quick survey of his mouth, and note whether any teeth are already missing and whether there are any teeth that appear very loose. If so, you must take great care not to dislodge the loose teeth during intubation. Recheck the mouth after you've finished intubating the child, and make sure the tooth count is the same as that you recorded *before* intubation. If it isn't, start hunting for the missing tooth or teeth. Often a tooth dislodged during intubation can be found lying in the posterior pharynx. If it isn't there, notify the doctor on arrival at the hospital, for the child will have to be x-rayed to make certain the tooth has not found its way into the trachea or a bronchus.

Intravenous Techniques

Choice of the site and method of intravenous cannulation in a child depends on the age of the child as well as local practice. Four techniques will be described in this section; physicians in each community will have their own preferences among those techniques, and each service should establish its own protocols and opportunities for periodic refresher training in the locally preferred method.

Whatever technique is used to start the IV, intravenous fluid bags used for infusions in children should not exceed 250 ml in volume and should be equipped with a microdrip apparatus. Where possible, use a Pedatrol, Buratrol, or similar device for delivering small, measured quantities of fluid. Infusion rates should be according to local protocol or orders from medical command, but they usually will not exceed about 20 ml/kg/hr even in shock states.

Scalp Vein Cannulation

Scalp vein IVs are often well suited to the young infant, since the scalp veins are easily visualized and readily accessible. The steps in establishing a scalp vein IV are as follows:

1. Gather the necessary EQUIPMENT:
   - 21- or 23-gauge scalp vein **needle** (butterfly).
   - Adhesive **tape:** 1/2-inch width cut in lengths of 1 inch and 4 inches; 1-inch width cut in lengths of 3 inches.
   - 5-ml **syringe** filled with sterile saline.
   - Intravenous **fluid** and **infusion set** ready to be hooked up (IV bag containing no more than 250 ml of fluid, equipped with Pedatrol or Buratrol chamber and microdrip infusion set).
   - Wide **rubber band.**
   - **Skin prep** (alcohol or povidone-iodine swab).
   - Disposable **razor.**
   - Rubber **gloves.**

2. **Prepare the site** on the scalp with the alcohol swab, taking care not to let any alcohol run into the baby's eyes. Shave any hair overlying the vein you plan to puncture.

3. Place the **rubber band around the baby's forehead** to occlude venous return; however, it should not be so tight as to interfere with arterial supply to the scalp. Palpate the vein selected.

4. Attach the butterfly needle to the syringe, and **flush** with saline, leaving the syringe attached to the needle.

5. **Palpate the target vein** with a gloved finger of one hand, and grasp the plastic "wings" of the needle with the other. Hold the needle tangentially with the bevel up, and **pierce the skin** about 0.5 cm distal to the point of entry into the vein. Infants' veins, especially on the scalp, are very superficial, and a deep thrust will usually cause you to puncture right through the vein and produce a hematoma. With the needle under the skin, carefully **advance the needle into the lumen of the vein.** Blood should return through the tubing when the needle has entered the vein. If you think the needle is in the vein, but there is no blood return, draw back very slightly on the syringe. When good blood return is obtained, *slowly* inject about 1 ml of saline from the syringe to **clear the tubing,** and observe the puncture site for swelling. Should swelling occur, it means that the IV has infiltrated; in that event, the needle must be withdrawn and firm pressure applied over the site for several minutes thereafter.

6. Once there is good blood return and the tubing has been cleared, **tape the needle in place.** Do *not*

try to thread it farther into the vein, for you may perforate the other wall of the vein and produce a hematoma. Place the 1/2- by 1-inch strip of adhesive tape over the point of entry of the needle into the skin. Then loop the 1/2- by 3-inch strips of tape over the wings of the butterfly. Use the remaining tape to secure the rest of the tubing (Fig. 30-13). Detach the syringe, and **connect the infusion set.**

7. **Protect the infusion site** from accidental dislodgement of the needle by taping an inverted paper cup over the site, with a window cut in one side to permit passage of the IV tubing.

Hand Vein Cannulation

Hand veins are not always easy to find in small children, especially chubby little babies, but occasionally Fate is kind and the back of the little hand yields a plump, palpable vein for cannulation. The equipment used is the same as for scalp vein needle insertion, although a 22-gauge over-the-needle catheter (Medicut) may be used instead of the butterfly. In addition, an **armboard** and tape or **roller gauze** to secure the armboard in place are required.

1. First **restrain the arm** on an armboard in such a way that the target vein is readily accessible.

2. Place a small **tourniquet**—again, a rubber band will do—proximal to the puncture site.

3. If you have a little time, place a small dollop of nitroglycerin ointment on the dorsum of the child's hand and massage it in. Leave it for about 2 minutes, then wipe it off with an alcohol swab.

FIGURE 30-13.   SECURING A BUTTERFLY NEEDLE.

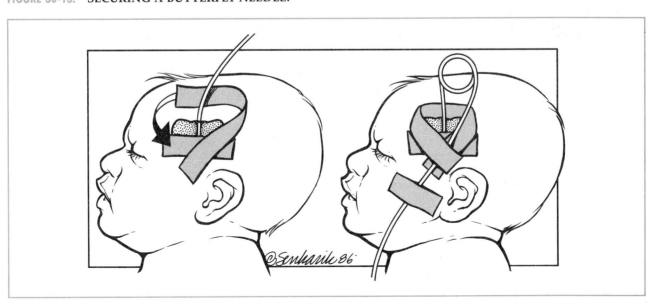

Nitroglycerin absorbed through the skin will dilate the veins just beneath and make them easier to cannulate.

4. **Prep** the puncture site with an alcohol or povidone-iodine swab.
5. Attach a saline-filled, 5-ml syringe to the butterfly needle, and **flush.**
6. **Pierce the skin** tangentially about 0.5 cm distal to the anticipated point of entry into the vein. Then advance the needle carefully into the vein until blood return is evident. *Slowly* inject 1 ml of saline to flush the line, and make certain the needle has not infiltrated.
7. **Tape** as described earlier (Fig. 30-14), and **connect the IV administration set.**

External Jugular Vein Cannulation

For cannulating the external jugular vein, the **over-the-needle catheter** is preferred; a 22-gauge Medicut, 3 to 4 cm in length, is well suited to this approach.

1. **Wrap the baby** securely in a sheet or blanket so that the arms and legs are restrained.
2. Place the baby on a table so that both its shoulders are touching the surface, and **rotate the head 90 degrees.** An assistant should hold the baby in position so that the head is extended 45 degrees over the end of the table (Fig. 30-15).
3. It will be very helpful if the infant is howling—and that is very likely to be the case—since his vigorous crying will distend the external jugular vein. **Palpate the vein** along its whole length so

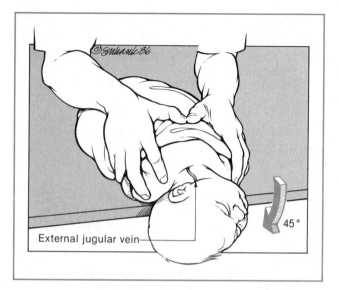

FIGURE 30-15. EXTERNAL JUGULAR VEIN CANNULATION IN THE INFANT.

that you will have a feeling for its direction. The IV catheter should be inserted so that flow will proceed in the normal caudad direction, that is, from the neck toward the feet.

4. **Prep** the puncture site with an alcohol or povidone-iodine swab.
5. With the gloved finger of one hand, **immobilize the vein** to keep it from rolling away from the needle.
6. Attach a saline-filled, 5-ml syringe to the needle, and **flush.** Keep the syringe attached. Then **pierce the skin** tangentially about 0.5 cm distal to the anticipated point of entry into the vein.
7. Gently **advance the needle** under the skin until free blood return is obtained.
8. Then, carefully **slide the catheter over the needle** into the vein.
9. **Remove the needle,** and swiftly **connect the IV tubing** to prevent entry of air into the catheter.
10. **Secure the catheter** firmly with tape, but do *not* use circumferential dressings around the neck!

Should you inadvertently puncture straight through the external jugular vein, swelling and discoloration will be immediately obvious. If that occurs, remove the needle and catheter as a unit, and apply pressure to the puncture site for 3 to 5 minutes with the child in a sitting position.

Intraosseous Infusions

The word *intraosseous* literally means "within the bone," and intraosseous infusion is a technique of administering fluids, blood, and medications into the

FIGURE 30-14. PERIPHERAL IV IN AN INFANT.

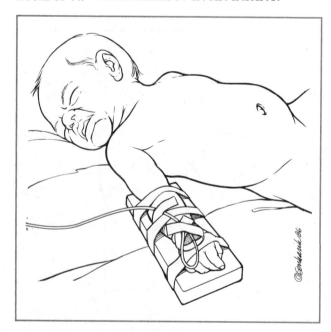

intramedullary space of a long bone, usually the tibia. It is a valuable method for emergency use in children when you are unable to start an IV and must have venous access to administer lifesaving fluids or resuscitation drugs. The method is simple, safe, and effective, with a very low rate of complications. It is indicated in cases of cardiac arrest in children under 6 years old in whom you cannot start an IV or intubate the trachea. Intraosseous infusions are *contra*indicated in fractured bones or when there is a cutaneous infection at the site where the needle would be inserted. (Different EMS services may have slightly different prerequisites and restrictions for employing intraosseous infusions.)

FIGURE 30-16. INTRAOSSEOUS CANNULATION. (A) The preferred site is usually in the proximal tibia, 2 cm below the tibial tuberosity. Use a to-and-fro boring motion to push through the bone. (B) An alternative site is the distal tibia, just above the medial malleolus.

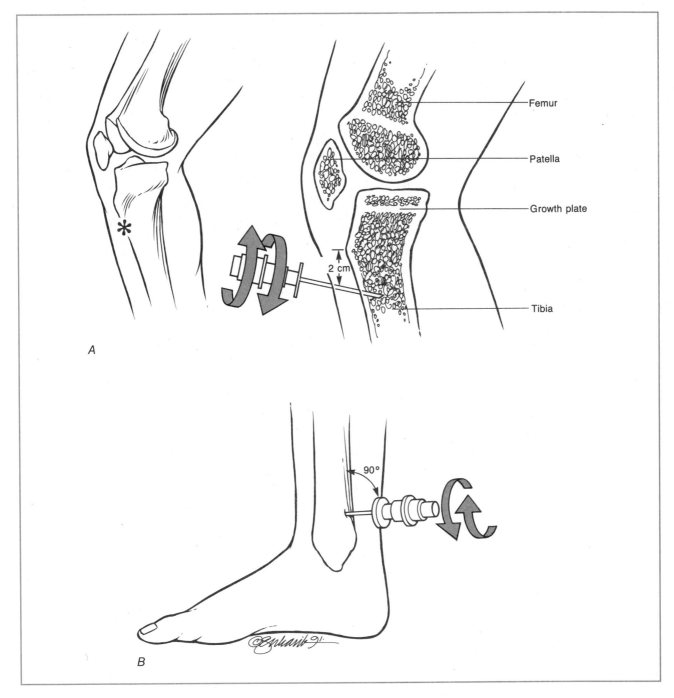

1. Gather the necessary **equipment:**
   a. Sterile 18-gauge 1½-inch **Jamshidi bone marrow needle.** Theoretically a spinal needle or standard metal IV needle can also be used, but the introduction of such needles is much more difficult. Spinal needles, because of their length, tend to bend. And standard IV needles, because they have no obturator, become plugged with bone spicules during placement. If your service plans to utilize the intraosseous infusion technique, it is worthwhile equipping yourselves to perform that technique optimally, which means using the right equipment.
   b. **Antiseptic swabs:** povidone-iodine and alcohol swabs.
   c. **IV fluid** and standard **administration set.**
   d. Sterile 5-ml **syringes,** one empty, one filled with sterile saline.
   e. Bulky **dressings** and self-adhering **roller gauze.**
   f. Sterile **gloves.**
2. **Prepare the site** selected, first with several povidone-iodine swabs, then with an alcohol swab. The most commonly used site for intraosseous infusions in children is the **proximal tibia,** on the flat part of the bone **one to two fingerbreadths (2 cm) below the tibial tuberosity** (Fig. 30-16A), to avoid injecting into the epiphyseal growth plate of the bone. Another site sometimes used is the distal tibia, just above the medial malleolus (Fig. 30-16B).
3. When using the proximal tibial site, place a **rolled towel under the knee** to help support it. Grasp the child's leg distal to the intended puncture site with one hand, and pick up the bone marrow needle with the other.
4. Hold the needle **at a 90-degree angle to the bone,** and **pierce the skin.**
5. When the needle reaches the bone, use a to-and-fro boring motion directed 60 degrees distally to **advance the needle into the marrow space.** You will be able to feel a very definite "give" when the needle pops through into the marrow.
6. **Confirm the location of the needle** in the bone marrow:
   a. Remove the stylet from the needle. Attach a syringe to the needle and see if you can aspirate blood and bone marrow.
   b. Attach the syringe containing sterile saline to the needle and try to flush. If the needle is seated in the marrow, it should flush easily, and there should not be any signs of infiltration.
   c. When the needle is in the bone marrow, it will be held rigidly in place and will not wobble.

7. If the needle is in the right place, **attach the administration set** and start the infusion at the rate ordered. It is usually possible to deliver fluids at rates up to about 200 ml per hour through an intraosseous infusion.
8. Loop the tubing of the administration set and tape it to the skin. Then **buttress the bone marrow needle** as you would an impaled object.

Several complications of intraosseous infusion are theoretically possible, but in fact the only complication that has been reported more than once or twice is **osteomyelitis** (infection of the bone) in about 0.6 percent of patients undergoing the procedure. Strict attention to aseptic technique should minimize the incidence of that complication. Infiltration rarely occurs, and it can be prevented altogether by confirming that the needle is within the marrow cavity, as described above, before infusing fluids through it.

> **OBSERVE UNIVERSAL PRECAUTIONS FOR ALL INTRAVENOUS PROCEDURES IN PEDIATRIC PATIENTS. SADLY, BABIES CAN ALSO BE CARRIERS OF HEPATITIS B AND AIDS.**

GLOSSARY

bronchiolitis   Condition seen primarily in children under 2 years old, characterized by dyspnea and wheezing.

cephalhematoma   Collection of blood beneath the periosteum of the skull, presenting as a boggy mass in the scalp.

croup   Common disease of childhood characterized by edema of the larynx and resulting upper airway obstruction.

epiglottitis   Common illness of childhood characterized by swelling of the epiglottis, high fever, severe pain on swallowing, and drooling.

febrile   Characterized by fever.

fontanelle   Opening between the bones of the skull in very young children.

hygroscopic   Tending to absorb water.

hyperemia   Increased blood flow to a region or tissue.

infant   A child less than a year of age.

intermammary line   Imaginary line between the nipples.

intraosseous   Within the bone.

TABLE 30-8.　DRUG DOSAGE GUIDELINES FOR INFANTS AND CHILDREN

DRUG	DOSAGE	ROUTE	ADMINISTRATION AND COMMENTS
Activated charcoal	<12 yrs: 15–30 gm >12 yrs: 1 gm/kg	PO PO	Mixed with water to form a slurry
Adenosine	0.1–0.2 mg/kg/dose	IV	Given as a rapid IV bolus in a *monitored* patient Do not exceed 12 mg in one dose
Albuterol/salbutamol (Ventolin)	0.01–0.03 ml/kg	Inhaled	Use 0.5% solution for inhalation in 3 ml of normal saline via nebulizer
Aminophylline	Loading dose: 6 mg/kg if none previously; 3 mg/kg with history of theophylline use	IV	Diluted in 30 ml IV fluid and infused over 30 minutes
Atropine sulfate			
For cardiac arrest	0.02 mg/kg/dose Minimum dose = 0.1 mg	IV	Give undiluted over 30 seconds; may be given through an endotracheal tube
For organophosphate poisoning	0.05 mg/kg/dose	IV	Half the dosage may be given IM
10% Calcium gluconate	0.2 ml/kg	IV	Slow push over 30 minutes; do not combine in same infusion with sodium bicarbonate
50% Dextrose (D50)	0.5 gm/kg	IV	Dilute 50% dextrose with equal parts of sterile distilled water to yield a 25% solution (0.25 gm/ml); infuse slowly through a good, free-flowing IV line
Diazepam (Valium)	0.3 mg/kg 0.5 mg/kg	IV Rectal	May cause hypotension and apnea when given IV The IV preparation can be given rectally via catheter
Diphenhydramine (Benadryl)	1 mg/kg	IV	Undiluted, by slow IV push over 5 minutes; use with caution in infants
Dopamine (Intropin)	2–20 μg/kg/min	IV	Indicated for treating post-resuscitation hypotension
Epinephrine			
For severe anaphylaxis	0.1 ml/kg of a 1 : 10,000 solution	IV	
For cardiac arrest	*First dose:* 0.1 ml/kg of a 1 : 10,000 solution (= 0.1 *mg*/kg) *Next doses:* 0.1 mg/kg	IV	May repeat q3–5 min as needed May be given through endotracheal tube
By infusion	0.1 μg/kg/min	IV	Infusions given in shock or bradycardia
For severe asthmatic attacks	0.01 ml/kg of a 1 : 1,000 solution (= 0.1 *mg*/kg)	SQ	Second-line drug for asthma Terbutaline now preferred for parenteral administation
Furosemide (Lasix)	1 mg/kg	IV	Slow push
Hydrocortisone (Solu-Cortef)	7 mg/kg	IV	Dilute to 1 mg/ml in D5/W and give over 30 minutes
Isoetharine (Bronkosol)	0.01 ml/kg	Inhaled	Diluted in 3 ml normal saline for use in nebulizer
Lidocaine (Xylocaine)	1 mg/kg	IV	Slow IV push as a loading dose; for an infusion, dilute 120 mg lidocaine in 100 ml D5/W and infuse at 1.0–2.5 ml/kg/min (20–50 μg/kg/min)

TABLE 30-8 (continued)

DRUG	DOSAGE	ROUTE	ADMINISTRATION AND COMMENTS
Mannitol	0.5 gm/kg	IV	The rate must be adjusted according to urine output
Methylprednisolone (Solu-Medrol)	1 mg/kg	IV	Slow IV push over 5 minutes
Morphine sulfate	0.1 mg/kg	IV	
Naloxone (Narcan)	0.01 mg/kg	IV	If ineffective, give 0.1 mg/kg/dose; if *that* is ineffective, increase to 0.2 mg/kg/dose
Sodium bicarbonate	1 mEq/kg	IV	Infuse slowly and ventilate briskly
Syrup of ipecac	6–9 months: 5 ml	PO	See contraindications in Chap. 27
	9–12 months: 10 ml	PO	Follow dose with 5 ml/kg water to maximum of 300 ml
	1–12 years: 15 ml	PO	
	>12 years: 30 ml	PO	
Terbutaline (Bricanyl)	0.03 ml/kg	Inhaled	Diluted in 3 ml normal saline for use in a nebulizer
	0.01 mg/kg	SQ	Given when an asthmatic is not moving enough air to inhale an adequate dose of a beta-2 drug

neonate   A newborn; an infant during the first few weeks of life.

osteomyelitis   Inflammation or infection of the bone.

PMI   Abbreviation for *point of maximal impulse,* the palpable beat of the apex of the heart against the chest wall during ventricular contraction.

pulsus paradoxus   Weakening or loss of a palpable pulse on inhalation, characteristic of a severe asthmatic attack in children (also seen in cardiac tamponade).

SIDS   Abbreviation for the sudden infant death syndrome.

status asthmaticus   Severe, prolonged asthmatic attack that cannot be broken with epinephrine.

status epilepticus   The occurrence of two or more seizures without a period of complete consciousness between them.

Waddell's triad   The syndrome of fractured left femur, ruptured spleen, and injury to the right side of the head in a child struck by a car while crossing the street.

APPENDIX: GUIDE TO PEDIATRIC DRUG DOSAGE

Nearly all pediatric drug doses are based on the child's weight in kilograms. It therefore does precious little good to know the correct dosage of a given drug if you don't know how much the child you are treating weighs. While there are many charts that provide *average* weights of children of different ages, best of all is to weigh the specific child to whom you are giving a drug. That can be accomplished fairly simply if you carry a bathroom scale, preferably one calibrated in kilograms, and just step on it first by yourself, then holding the child. The child's weight is the difference between the two.

Sometimes one of the parents can tell you the child's weight. In the United States, the parent will almost certainly report the weight in pounds, so make sure you convert the figure to kilograms (by dividing by 2.2).

If you do not carry a scale and the parents are not able to provide the information, you may use the chart below to obtain a rough estimate of the child's weight:

AGE-RELATED WEIGHTS IN CHILDREN

Age	Weight (kg)
Newborn	3–5
1 year	10
3 years	15

5 years	20
8 years	25
10 years	30
15 years	50

If you misplace your weight chart, you can use the following as a rough guide to estimating the weight of a child up to age 9:

$$\text{Weight (kg)} = [\text{Age (in years)} \times 2] + 9$$

Thus, for example, if the child is 3 years old:

$$\text{Weight (kg)} = [3 \times 2] + 9 = 6 + 9 = 15 \text{ kg}$$

The pediatric dosages for drugs commonly used in the prehospital care of children are summarized in Table 30-8. Make a copy of the dosage table, and tape it to the inside of your pediatric drug box. Even if you think you know the dosages by heart, always double-check against the dosage tables. Once you've injected a drug, you can't summon it back into your syringe—so GET IT RIGHT!

FURTHER READING

PEDIATRIC EMERGENCIES: GENERAL

American College of Emergency Physicians. Policy statement: Minimum pediatric prehospital guidelines. *ACEP News*, January 1992.

Baldwin GA (ed.). *Handbook of Pediatric Emergencies*. Boston: Little, Brown, 1989.

Berry FA Jr. The difficult child. *Emerg Med* 15(3):103, 1983.

Centers for Disease Control. Toy safety—United States, 1983. *MMWR* 33(50), 1984.

Costello L. When children die. *Emerg Med Serv* 19(4):16, 1990.

Finlay I et al. Your child is dead. *Br Med J* 302:1534, 1991.

Friedman H, Hill G. Feeling comfortable with pediatric transports. *JEMS* 17(12):44, 1992.

Gausche M, Henderson DP, Seidel JS. Vital signs as part of the prehospital assessment of the pediatric patient: A survey of paramedics. *Ann Emerg Med* 19:173, 1909.

Gratz RR. Children's responses to emergency department care. *Ann Emerg Med* 13:322, 1984.

Hagen-Moe D. Pediatric physical assessment. *Emergency* 24(10):32, 1992.

Hallock JA. Pediatric respiratory disease. *Emerg Med Serv* 8(1):13, 1979.

Henry GH, Cimino LE. Cardiac emergencies in pediatrics. *Emerg Med Serv* 9(10):53, 1980.

Holbrook PR. Prehospital care of critically ill children. *Crit Care Med* 8:537, 1980.

Jarvis DA. The unconscious child. *Emerg Med* 20(20):193, 1988.

Levine MI. On treating life-threatening emergencies. *Pediatr Ann* 15:11, 1986.

Lipton H. Parental care. *Emergency* 21(8):43, 1989.

Luten RC. For the sake of the child. *Emergency* 22(5):39, 1990.

Mackenzie A et al. Clinical signs of dehydration in children. *Lancet* 2:605, 1989.

Mellick LB, Dierking BH. One size doesn't fit all: Choosing pediatric equipment: Part II. *JEMS* 16(7):35, 1991.

Mellick LB, Guy JR. Approaching the infant and child in the prehospital arena. *JEMS* 17(3):126, 1992.

Oquist N. A child-proof assessment. *Emergency* 21(8):35, 1989.

Polakoff JM et al. The environment away from home as a source of potential poisoning. *Am J Dis Child* 138:1014, 1984.

Ramenofsky ML et al. EMS for pediatrics: Optimum treatment or unnecessary delay? *J Pediatr Surg* 18:498, 1983.

Reynolds SL, Jaffe DM. Quick triage of children with abdominal pain. *Emerg Med* 22(14):39, 1990.

Romig L. Parent-patience. *Emergency* 23(8):39, 1991.

Seidel JS. Emergency medical services and the pediatric patient: Are the needs being met? II. Training and equipping emergency medical services providers for pediatric emergencies. *Pediatrics* 78:808, 1986.

Seidel JS et al. Emergency medical services and the pediatric patient: Are the needs being met? *Pediatrics* 73:769, 1984.

Taylor M. The parent trap. *Emerg Med Serv* 22(3):37, 1993.

Tsai A, Kallsen G. Epidemiology of pediatric prehospital care. *Ann Emerg Med* 16:284, 1987.

CHOKING IN CHILDREN

Addy DP. The choking child: Back bangers against front pushers. *Br Med J* 286:536, 1983.

Badgwell JM, McLeod ME, Friedberg J. Continuing medical education article: Airway obstruction in infants and children. *Can Anaesth Soc J* 34:90, 1987.

Day RL. Differing opinions on the emergency treatment of choking. *Pediatrics* 71:976, 1983.

Day RL et al. Choking: The Heimlich abdominal thrust vs back blows: An approach to measurement of inertial and aerodynamic forces. *Pediatrics* 70:113, 1982.

Dierking BH. Pediatric notebook: Managing the obstructed airway. *JEMS* 15(7):89, 1990.

Emergency Cardiac Care Committee and Subcommittees, American Heart Association. Guidelines for cardiopulmonary resuscitation and emergency cardiac care. *JAMA* 268:2171, 1992.

Greensher J. Emergency treatment of the choking child. *J Pediatr* 70:110, 1982.

Harris CS et al. Childhood asphyxiation by food: A national analysis and overview. *JAMA* 251:2232, 1984.

Wiseman NE. The diagnosis of foreign body aspiration in childhood. *J Pediatr Surg* 19:531, 1984.

See also listings in the references to Chapter 7.

ASTHMA AND BRONCHIOLITIS

Bledsoe BE. Pediatric respiratory emergencies. *JEMS* 19(2):38, 1994.

Carden DL et al. Vital signs including pulsus paradoxus in the assessment of acute bronchial asthma. *Ann Emerg Med* 12:80, 1983.

Clark JR, Pringle RP. Pediatric respiratory drugs. *Emergency* 22(12):18, 1990.

Dawson K et al. The management of acute bronchiolitis. Thoracic Society of Australia and New Zealand. *J Paediatr Child Health* 29:335, 1993.

Fanta CH et al. Glucocorticoids in acute asthma: A critical controlled trial. *Am J Med* 74:845, 1983.

Groth ML, Hurewitz AN. Pharmacologic management of acute asthma. *Emerg Med* 21(7):23, 1989.

Harper TB et al. Techniques of administration of metered-dose aerosolized drugs in asthmatic children. *Am J Dis Child* 135:218, 1981.

Hurwitz ME et al. Clinical scoring does not accurately assess hypoxemia in pediatric asthma patients. *Ann Emerg Med* 13:1040, 1984.

Johnson AJ et al. Circumstances of death from asthma. *Br Med J* 288:1870, 1984.

Kampschulte S, Marcey J, Safar P. Simplified management of status asthmaticus in children. *Crit Care Med* 1:69, 1973.

Kattan M et al. Corticosteroids in status asthmaticus. *J Pediatr* 96:596, 1980.

Klassen TP et al. Randomized trial of salbutamol in acute bronchiolitis. *J Pediatr* 118:807, 1991.

Kravis LP et al. Unexpected death in childhood asthma. *Am J Dis Child* 139:558, 1985.

Lee H et al. Aerosol bag for administration of bronchodilators to young asthmatic children. *Pediatrics* 73:230, 1984.

Leffert F. The management of acute severe asthma. *J Pediatr* 96:1, 1980.

Mellis CM. Important changes in the emergency management of acute asthma in children. *Med J Aust* 148:215, 1988.

Nguyen MT et al. Causes of death from asthma in children. *Ann Allergy* 55:448, 1985.

Papo MC et al. A prospective, randomized study of continuous versus intermittent nebulized albuterol for severe status asthmaticus in children. *Crit Care Med* 21:1479, 1993.

Potter PC et al. Hydration in severe acute asthma. *Arch Dis Child* 66:216, 1991.

The proper use of aerosol bronchodilators (editorial). *Lancet* 1:23, 1981.

Ratto D et al. Are intravenous corticosteroids required in status asthmaticus? *JAMA* 260:527, 1988.

Reyes de la Rocha S, Brown MA. Asthma in children: Emergency management. *Ann Emerg Med* 16:79, 1987.

Schuh S et al. Nebulized albuterol in acute bronchiolitis. *J Pediatr* 117:633, 1990.

Silverman M. Bronchodilators for wheezy infants? *Arch Dis Child* 59:84, 1984.

Sly RM. Mortality from asthma in children 1979–1984. *Ann Allergy* 60:433, 1988.

Spiteri MA et al. Subcutaneous adrenaline versus terbutaline in the treatment of acute severe asthma. *Thorax* 43:19, 1988.

Springer C et al. Corticosteroids do not affect the clinical or physiologic status of infants with bronchiolitis. *Pediatr Pulmonol* 9:181, 1990.

Strunk RC et al. Physiologic and psychological characteristics associated with deaths due to asthma in childhood: A case-controlled study. *JAMA* 254:1193, 1985.

Victoria MS et al. Comparison between epinephrine and terbutaline injections in the acute management of asthma. *J Asthma* 26:287, 1989.

Wennergren G et al. Nebulized racemic adrenaline for wheezy bronchitis. *Acta Paediatr Scand* 80:375, 1991.

Wohl MEB, Chernick V. Bronchiolitis: State of the art. *Am Rev Respir Dis* 118:759, 1986.

EPIGLOTTITIS AND CROUP

Bass JW et al. Sudden death due to acute epiglottitis. *Pediatr Infect Dis* 4:447, 1985.

Chaisson RE et al. Clinical aspects of adult epiglottitis. *West J Med* 144:700, 1986.

Cohen E. Epiglottitis in adults. *Ann Emerg Med* 13:620, 1984.

Costigan DC, Newth DJL. Respiratory status of children with epiglottitis with and without an artificial airway. *Am J Dis Child* 137:139, 1983.

Denny FW et al. Croup: An 11-year study in a pediatric practice. *Pediatrics* 71:871, 1983.

Diaz JH, Lockhart CH. Early diagnosis and airway management of acute epiglottitis in children. *South Med J* 75:399, 1982.

Dierking BH. Respiratory distress! *Emergency* 21(1):27, 1989.

Husby S et al. Treatment of croup with nebulised steroid (budesonide): A double blind, placebo controlled study. *Arch Dis Child* 68:352, 1993.

Infectious Diseases and Immunization Committee, Canadian Paediatric Society. Steroid therapy for croup in children admitted to hospital. *Can Med Assoc J* 147:429, 1992.

Kelley PB, Simon JE. Racemic epinephrine use in croup and disposition. *Am J Emerg Med* 10:181, 1992.

Khilanani U et al. Acute epiglottitis in adults. *Am J Med Sci* 287:65, 1984.

Losek JD et al. Epiglottitis: Comparison of signs and symptoms in children less than 2 years old and older. *Ann Emerg Med* 19:55, 1990.

Lowenkron SE, Teitcher J, Fein AM. Acute epiglottitis: Adult vs pediatric. *Emerg Med* 25(14):54, 1992.

Mauro RD et al. Differentiation of epiglottitis from laryngotracheitis in the child with stridor. *Am J Dis Child* 142:679, 1988.

Mitchell DP et al. Secondary airway support in the management of croup. *J Otolaryngol* 9:419, 1980.

Newth CJL, Levison H, Bryan AC. The respiratory status of children with croup. *J Pediatr* 81:1068, 1972.

Schuh S, Huang A, Fallis JC. Atypical epiglottitis. *Ann Emerg Med* 17:168, 1988.

Sendi K, Crysdale WS. Acute epiglottitis: Decade of change—a 10-year experience with 242 children. *J Otolaryngol* 16:196, 1987.

Tintinalli J. Respiratory stridor in the young child. *JACEP* 5:195, 1976.

Waisman Y et al. Prospective randomized double-blind study comparing L-epinephrine and racemic epinephrine aerosols in the treatment of laryngo-tracheitis (croup). *Pediatrics* 89:302, 1992.

Zillger JJ et al. Assessment of intubation in croup and epiglottitis. *Ann Otol Rhinol Laryngol* 91:403, 1982.

SUDDEN INFANT DEATH SYNDROME

Beal S. Sudden infant death syndrome related to sleeping position and bedding. *Med J Aust* 155:507, 1991.

Brown KR. Sudden infant death syndrome: Part 1. Update for EMS providers. *Emerg Med Serv* 12(5):52, 1983.

Brown KR. Sudden infant death syndrome: Part 2. General theories of SIDS development. *Emerg Med Serv* 12(7):31, 1983.

Carpenter RG et al. Identification of some infants at immediate risk of dying unexpectedly and justifying intense study. *Lancet* 2:343, 1979.

Centers for Disease Control. Seasonality in sudden infant death syndrome. *MMWR* 39:891, 1990.

Centers for Disease Control. Sudden infant death syndrome—United States, 1980–1988. *MMWR* 41:515, 1992.

Chiodini BA, Thach BT. Impaired ventilation in infants sleeping facedown: Potential significance for sudden infant death syndrome. *J Pediatr* 123:686, 1993.

Gould JB et al. Management of the near-miss infant. *Pediatr Clin North Am* 26:857, 1979.

Guntheroth WG, Spiers PS. Sleeping prone and the risk of sudden infant death syndrome. *JAMA* 267:2359, 1992.

Hunt CE. Sudden infant death syndrome and sleeping position. *Pediatrics* 90:115, 1992.

James TN. Crib death. *Am Coll Cardiol* 5:1185, 1985.

Kleinberg F. Sudden infant death syndrome. *Mayo Clin Proc* 59:352, 1984.

Meadow R. Suffocation, recurrent apnea, and sudden infant death. *J Pediatr* 117:351, 1990.

Peterson DR. Evolution of the epidemiology of sudden infant death syndrome. *Epidemiol Rev* 2:97, 1980.

Poets CF, Southall DP. Prone sleeping position and sudden infant death (editorial). *N Engl J Med* 329:425, 1993.

Ponsonby AL et al. Factors potentiating the risk of sudden infant death syndrome associated with the prone position. *N Engl J Med* 329:377, 1993.

Shannon DC, Kelly DH. SIDS and near-SIDS. *N Engl J Med* 306:959 and 306:1022, 1982.

Southall DP, Samuels MP. Reducing risks in the sudden infant death syndrome (editorial). *Br Med J* 304:265, 1992.

Stanton AN. Overheating and cot death. *Lancet* 2:1199, 1984.

Strimer R, Adelson L, Oseasohn R. Epidemiologic features of 1,134 sudden unexpected infant deaths. *JAMA* 209:1493, 1969.

Weinstein SE. SIDS: The role of the EMT. *Emerg Prod News* 9(9):35, 1977.

SEIZURES IN CHILDREN

Albano A, Reisdorff EJ, Wiegenstein JG. Rectal diazepam in pediatric status epilepticus. *Am J Emerg Med* 70:168, 1989.

Berg AT et al. Predictors of recurrent febrile seizures: A metaanalytic review. *J Pediatr* 116:329, 1990.

Berg AT et al. A prospective study of recurrent febrile seizures. *N Engl J Med* 327:1122, 1992.

Camfield PR. Treatment of status epilepticus in children. *Can Med Assoc J* 128:671, 1983.

Chiulli DA et al. The influence of diazepam or lorazepam on the frequency of endotracheal intubation in childhood status epilepticus. *J Emerg Med* 9:13, 1991.

Crabb TJ. In the hot seat: Managing febrile seizures. *JEMS* 18(1):50, 1993.

Dieckmann RA. Rectal diazepam for prehospital pediatric status epilepticus. *Ann Emerg Med* 23:216, 1994.

Drawbaugh RE, Deibler CG, Eitel DR. Prehospital administration of rectal diazepam in pediatric status epilepticus. *Prehosp Disaster Med* 5(2):155, 1990.

Freeman JM. Febrile seizures: A consensus of their significance, evaluation, and treatment. *Pediatrics* 66:1009, 1980.

Fuchs S. Managing seizures in children. *Emergency* 22(12):47, 1990.

Gabor AJ. Lorazepam versus phenobarbital: Candidates for drug of choice for treatment of status epilepticus. *J Epilepsy* 3:3, 1990.

Glass BA. To sponge or not to sponge (letter). *Ann Emerg Med* 16:607, 1987.

Knudsen FU. Effective short-term diazepam prophylaxis in febrile convulsions. *J Pediatr* 106:487, 1985.

Knudsen FU. Rectal administration of diazepam in solution in the acute treatment of convulsions in infants and children. *Arch Dis Child* 54:855, 1979.

Lacey DJ et al. Lorazepam therapy of status epilepticus in children and adolescents. *J Pediatr* 108:771, 1986.

Littrell KA, Cantwell GP. Pediatric status epilepticus. *JEMS* 16(2):71, 1991.

Middleton DB. After a child's first seizure. *Emerg Med* 25(4):181, 1993.

Mitchell WG et al. Lorazepam is the treatment of choice for status epilepticus. *J Epilepsy* 3:7, 1990.

Newman J. Evaluation of sponging to reduce body temperature in febrile children. *Can Med Assoc J* 132:641, 1985.

Oppenheimer EY et al. Seizures in childhood: An approach to emergency management. *Pediatr Clin North Am* 26:837, 1979.

Orr RA et al. Diazepam and intubation in emergency treatment of seizures in children. *Ann Emerg Med* 20:1009, 1991.

Rosman NP et al. A controlled trial of diazepam administered during febrile illnesses to prevent recurrence of febrile seizures. *N Engl J Med* 329:79, 1993.

Rothner AD et al. Status epilepticus. *Pediatr Clin North Am* 27:593, 1980.

Sonander H et al. Effects of the rectal administration of diazepam. *Br J Anaesth* 5:578, 1985.

Tomlanovich MC, Rosen P, Mendelsohn J. Simple febrile convulsions. *JACEP* 5:347, 1976.

Vining EPG et al. Status epilepticus. *Pediatr Ann* 14:764, 1985.

Volpe JJ. Management of neonatal seizures. *Crit Care Med* 5:43, 1977.

CHILD ABUSE

AAP Committee on Hospital Care. Medical necessity for the hospitalization of the abused and neglected child. *Pediatrics* 79:300, 1987.

Akbarnia B et al. Manifestations of the battered-child syndrome. *J Bone Joint Surg [AM]* 56A:1159, 1974.

Anderson WA. The significance of femoral fractures in children. *Ann Emerg Med* 11:174, 1982.

Beals RK et al. Fractured femur in infancy: The role of child abuse. *J Pediatr Orthop* 3:583, 1983.

Bergman AB et al. Changing spectrum of serious child abuse. *Pediatrics* 77:113, 1986.

Buchanan MFG. The recognition of non-accidental injury in children. *Practitioner* 229:815, 1985.

Christoffel KK et al. Should child abuse and neglect be considered when a child dies unexpectedly? *Am J Dis Child* 139:876, 1985.

Council on Scientific Affairs. AMA diagnostic and treatment guidelines concerning child abuse and neglect. *JAMA* 254:796, 1985.

Henry GL. Legal rounds. Problem: Suspecting child abuse. *Emerg Med* 18(19):129, 1986.

Hobbs CJ. When are burns not accidental? *Arch Dis Child* 61:357, 1986.

Irons TG. Documenting sexual abuse of a child. *Emerg Med* 25(6):57, 1993.

Kaplan JM. Pseudoabuse: The misdiagnosis of child abuse. *J Forensic Sci* 31:1420, 1986.

King BR, Baker MB, Ludwig S. Reporting of child abuse by prehospital personnel. *Prehosp Disaster Med* 8(1):67, 1993.

King J et al. Analysis of 429 fractures in 189 battered children. *J Pediatr Orthop* 8:585, 1988.

Kirschner RH et al. The mistaken diagnosis of child abuse: A form of medical abuse? *Am J Dis Child* 139:873, 1985.

Kottmeier PK. Four clues to child abuse. *Emerg Med* 24(4):283, 1992.

Kunkel DB. The chemically abused child. *Emerg Med* 16(5):181, 1984.

Ledbetter DJ et al. Diagnostic and surgical implications of child abuse. *Arch Surg* 123:1101, 1988.

Leventhal JM et al. Fractures in young children: Distinguishing child abuse from unintentional injuries. *Am J Dis Child* 147:87, 1993.

Lipton H. Stepping into child abuse. *Emergency* 22(9):23, 1990.

Ludwig S, Warman M. Shaken baby syndrome: A review of 20 cases. *Ann Emerg Med* 13:104, 1984.

Merton DF et al. The abused child: A radiologic reappraisal. *Radiology* 146:377, 1983.

Millmire ME et al. Serious head injury in infants: Accident or abuse? *Pediatrics* 75:340, 1985.

Montrey JS et al. Nonaccidental burns in child abuse. *South Med J* 78:1324, 1985.

Pike KM. When a child cries. *Emergency* 25(9):39, 1993.

Purdue GF et al. Child abuse by burning: An index of suspicion. *J Trauma* 28:221, 1988.

Reynolds EA, Davidson L, Dierking BH. Delivering and documenting care in child abuse cases. *JEMS* 14(10):71, 1989.

Ricci R. Child sexual abuse: The emergency department response. *Ann Emerg Med* 15:711, 1986.

Robertson DM et al. Unusual injury? Recent injury in normal children and children with suspected non-accidental injury. *Br Med J* 285:1399, 1982.

Rosenberg N, Bottenfield G. Fractures in infants: A sign of child abuse. *Ann Emerg Med* 11:178, 1982.

Rosenberg N et al. Prediction of child abuse in an ambulatory setting. *Pediatrics* 70:879, 1982.

Shah CP, Holloway CP, Valkil DV. Sexual abuse of children. *Ann Emerg Med* 11:18, 1982.

Silverman FN. Child abuse: The conflict of underdetection and overreporting. *Pediatrics* 80:441, 1987.

Solomons G. Trauma and child abuse: The importance of the medical record. *Am J Dis Child* 134:503, 1980.

Thomas JL, Towberman DP. Responding to the child within: Child abuse and the EMS provider. *JEMS* 17(3):98, 1992.

Vey PK. Child abuse: Your standard of care. *Emerg Med Serv* 13(2):89, 1984.

TRAUMA IN CHILDREN

Agran PF, Winn DG, Castillo DN. Pediatric injuries in the back of pickup trucks. *JAMA* 264:712, 1990.

Apple JS et al. Cervical spine fractures and dislocations in children. *Pediatr Radiol* 17:45, 1987.

Baker MD et al. Household electrical injuries in children: Epidemiology and identification of avoidable hazards. *Am J Dis Child* 143:59, 1989.

Berger LR. Childhood injuries. *Public Health Rep* 100:572, 1985.

Bonadio WA, Hellmich T, Post-traumatic pulmonary contusion in children. *Ann Emerg Med* 18:1050, 1989.

Centers for Disease Control. Fatal injuries to children—United States, 1986. *MMWR* 39:442, 1990.

Clark JR. Managing burns in children. *JEMS* 15(4):90, 1990.

Clark JR. Babes & bullets. *Emergency* 24(10):43, 1992.

Davidson RI. Emergency care of pediatric head injuries. *Emerg Med Serv* 9(1):30, 1980.

Dierking BH. Burn injuries in children. *Emergency* 24(10):40, 1992.

Dyregrov A. Traumatized kids, traumatized rescuers? *Emerg Med Serv* 21(6):21, 1992.

Eichelberger MR et al. Pediatric trauma: An algorithm for diagnosis and therapy. *J Trauma* 23:91, 1983.

Frame SB, Hendrickson MF. Problem: Pediatric cervical-spine injuries. *Emerg Med* 19(19):47, 1987.

Fuchs S. Stocking your ambulance. *Emergency* 25(9):42, 1993.

Grant TA. Pediatric abdominal trauma. *Emergency* 24(10):36, 1992.

Gratz RR. Accidental injury in childhood: A literature review on pediatric trauma. *J Trauma* 19:551, 1979.

Graves TA et al. Fluid resuscitation of infants and children with massive thermal injuries. *J Trauma* 28:1656, 1988.

Hadley MN et al. Pediatric spinal trauma: Review of 122 cases of spinal cord and vertebral column injuries. *J Neurosurg* 68:18, 1988.

Haller JA. Trauma at an early age: A blow above the belt. *Emerg Med* 17(3):51, 1985.

Hazinski MF et al. Pediatric injury prevention. *Ann Emerg Med* 22:456, 1993.

Herzenberg JE et al. Emergency transport and positioning of young children who have an injury of the cervical spine: The standard backboard may be hazardous. *J Bone Joint Surg [Am]* 71-A:15, 1989.

Hoffman MA et al. The pediatric passenger: Trends in seatbelt use and injury patterns. *J Trauma* 27:974, 1987.

Hoy GA et al. Concurrent paediatric seat belt injuries of the abdomen and spine. *Pediatr Surg Int* 7:376, 1992.

Huerta C, Griffith R, Joyce SM. Cervical spine stabilization in pediatric patients: Evaluation of current techniques. *Ann Emerg Med* 16:1121, 1987.

Kaufmann CR et al. Evaluation of the pediatric trauma score. *JAMA* 263:69, 1990.

Lavery RF et al. The prehospital treatment of pediatric trauma. *Pediatr Emerg Care* 8:9, 1992.

Levine MI. On treating life-threatening emergencies. *Pediatr Ann* 15:11, 1986.

Lorentz WB. On pediatric fluid loss. *Emerg Med* 9(2):22, 1977.

Mathewson JW. Shock in infants and children. *J Fam Pract* 10:695, 1980.

McKoy C et al. Preventable traumatic deaths in children. *J Pediatr Surg* 18:505, 1983.

Merrell SW et al. Fluid resuscitation in thermally injured children. *Am J Surg* 152:664, 1986.

Myer CM. Damaged little heads and necks. *Emerg Med* 19(4):89, 1987.

Nakayama DK, Gardner MJ, Rowe MI. Emergency endotracheal intubation in pediatric trauma. *Ann Surg* 221:218, 1990.

Nypaver M, Treloar D. Neutral cervical spine positioning in children. *Ann Emerg Med* 23:208, 1994.

Ordog GJ. Gunshot wounds in children under 10 years of age: A new epidemic. *Am J Dis Child* 142:618, 1988.

Pyper JA et al. Orthopaedic injuries in children associated with the use of off-road vehicles. *J Bone Joint Surg [Am]* 70:275, 1988.

Ramenofsky ML. Trauma at an early age: To watch an injured child. *Emerg Med* 17(2):33, 1985.

Ramenofsky ML et al. Maximum survival in pediatric trauma: The ideal system. *J Trauma* 24:818, 1984.

Reynolds E, Dierking B, Ramenofsky ML. Head care for kids. *Emergency* 20(9):43, 1988.

Rivara FP et al. Injuries to children younger than 1 year of age. *Pediatrics* 81:93, 1988.

Romig L. Assessment of the traumatized child. *Emergency* 25(9):35, 1993.

Rosenthal BW, Bergman I. Intracranial injury after moderate head trauma in children. *J Pediatr* 115:346, 1989.

Ruge JR et al. Pediatric spinal injury: The very young. *J Neurosurg* 68:25, 1988.

Schutzman SA et al. Epidural hematomas in children. *Ann Emerg Med* 22:535, 1993.

Shoshany G et al. Safe immobilization of extremities for intravenous fluid administration in infants. *Surg Gynecol Obstet* 16:485, 1985.

Sparnon AL et al. Bicycle handlebar injuries in children. *J Pediatr Surg* 21:118, 1986.

Thompson BM et al. "PALS for Life!" A required trauma-oriented pediatric advanced life support course for pediatric and emergency medicine house officers. *Ann Emerg Med* 13:1044, 1984.

Thompson RS et al. A case-control study of the effectiveness of bicycle safety helmets. *N Engl J Med* 320:1361, 1989.

Throckmorton K, Throckmorton DW, Knight P. Number one killer. *Emergency* 20(5):20, 1988.

Valentine MW. Bicycle handlebar injuries in children. *Emerg Med* 20(21):37, 1988.

Weesner CL et al. Fatal childhood injury patterns in an urban setting. *Ann Emerg Med* 23:231, 1994.

Wheatley J et al. Traumatic deaths in children: The importance of prevention. *Med J Aust* 150:72, 1989.

Ziegler MM. Trauma at an early age: A blow below the belt. *Emerg Med* 17(3):65, 1985.

ASPIRIN AND ACETAMINOPHEN OVERDOSE

Chamberlain JM et al. Use of activated charcoal in a simulated poisoning with acetaminophen: A new loading dose for N-acetylcysteine? *Ann Emerg Med* 22:1398, 1993.

Chapman BJ et al. Adult salicylate poisoning: Deaths and outcome in patients with high plasma salicylate concentrations. *Q J Med* 72:699, 1989.

Done A. Acetaminophen: Beware the sleeper. *Emerg Med* 7(6):139, 1975.

Done A. Aspirin revisited. *Emerg Med* 9(9):151, 1977.

Gaudreault P et al. The relative severity of acute versus chronic salicylate poisoning in children: A clinical comparison. *Pediatrics* 70:566, 1982.

Henretig FM et al. Repeated acetaminophen overdosing: Causing hepatotoxicity in children. *Clin Pediatr* 28:525, 1989.

Hill JB. Salicylate intoxication. *N Engl J Med* 288:1110, 1973.

Hillman RJ et al. Treatment of salicylate poisoning with repeated oral charcoal. *Br Med J* 291:1472, 1985.

Kearney TE. Salicylate poisoning: Recognition and management. *Emerg Med Serv* 18(5):39, 1990.

Koch-Weser J. Acetaminophen. *N Engl J Med* 295:1297, 1976.

Kunkel DB. Updating acetaminophen toxicity. *Emerg Med* 17(13):111, 1985.

Litowitz T et al. Comparison of pediatric poisoning hazards: An analysis of 3.8 million exposure incidents. *Pediatrics* 89:999, 1992.

Mofenson HC, Greensher J, Gavin W. Acetaminophen overdose: Growing medical nemesis. *Emerg Med Serv* 7(2):64, 1978.

Peterson RG, Rumack BH. Toxicity of acetaminophen overdose. *JACEP* 7:202, 1978.

Prescott LF et al. Intravenous N-acetyl-cysteine: The treatment of choice for paracetamol poisoning. *Br Med J* 2:1097, 1979.

Prescott LF et al. Diuresis or urinary alkalinisation for salicylate poisoning? *Br Med J* 285:1383, 1982.

Rentzi FP et al. Concomitant use of activated charcoal and N-acetylcysteine. *Ann Emerg Med* 14:568, 1985.

Ruffalo RL et al. Cimetidine and acetylcysteine as antidotes for acetaminophen overdose. *South Med J* 75:954, 1982.

Rumack BH et al. Acetaminophen overdose: 662 cases with evaluation of oral acetylcysteine treatment. *Arch Intern Med* 141:380, 1981.

Temple AR. Pathophysiology of aspirin overdosage toxicity, with implications for management. *Pediatrics* 62(Suppl):873, 1978.

CARDIAC ARREST AND CPR IN CHILDREN

Atkins DL et al. Pediatric defibrillation: Importance of paddle size in determining transthoracic impedance. *Pediatrics* 82:914, 1988.

Benitz WE, Frankel LR, Stevenson DK. The pharmacology of neonatal resuscitation and cardiopulmonary intensive care: Part I. Immediate resuscitation. *West J Med* 144:704, 1986.

Berg RA. Emergency infusion of catecholamines into bone marrow. *Am J Dis Child* 138:810, 1984.

Brill JE. Cardiopulmonary resuscitation. *Pediatr Ann* 15:24, 1986.

Burchfield DJ et al. Medications in neonatal resuscitation. *Ann Emerg Med* 22:435, 1993.

Cavallaro D, Melker R. Comparison of two techniques for determining cardiac activity in infants. *Crit Care Med* 11:189, 1983.

David R. Closed chest cardiac massage in the newborn infant. *Pediatrics* 81:552, 1988.

Dierking BH. Pediatric notebook: Reviewing basic life support for children. *JEMS* 15(2):112, 1990.

Dishuk J. Cardiac care for kids. *Emergency* 21(8):29, 1989.

Eisenberg M, Bergner L, Hallstrom A. Epidemiology of cardiac arrest and resuscitation in children. *Ann Emerg Med* 12:672, 1983.

Finholt DA et al. The heart is under the lower third of the sternum: Implications for external cardiac massage. *Am J Dis Child* 140:646, 1986.

Freisen RM et al. Appraisal of pediatric cardiopulmonary resuscitation. *Can Med Assoc J* 126:1055, 1982.

Goetting MG, Paradis NA. High dose epinephrine in refractory pediatric cardiac arrest. *Crit Care Med* 17:1258, 1989.

Holbrook PR. On opening the airway. *Emerg Med* 14(1):137, 1982.

Holbrook PR. On restarting the heart. *Emerg Med* 14(1):126, 1982.

Holbrook PR et al. Cardiovascular resuscitation drugs for children. *Crit Care Med* 8:588, 1980.

Landwirth J et al. Ethical issues in pediatric and neonatal resuscitation. *Ann Emerg Med* 22:502, 1993.

Lewis JK et al. Outcome of pediatric resuscitation. *Ann Emerg Med* 12:297, 1983.

Lewis JM. Pediatric arrest card (letter). *Ann Emerg Med* 14:372, 1985.

Lubitz DS et al. A rapid method for estimating weight and resuscitation drug dosages from length in the pediatric age group. *Ann Emerg Med* 17:576, 1988.

Ludwig S, Kettrick RG, Parker M. Pediatric cardiopulmonary resuscitation: A review of 130 cases. *Clin Pediatr* 23:71, 1984.

McNamara RM et al. Pediatric resuscitation without an intravenous line. *Am J Emerg Med* 4:31, 1986.

Orlowski JP. Optimal position for external cardiac compression in infants and young children. *Ann Emerg Med* 15:667, 1986.

Phillips GWL et al. Relation of infant heart to sternum: Its significance in cardiopulmonary resuscitation. *Lancet* 1:1024, 1986.

Singer J. Cardiac arrests in children. *JACEP* 6:198, 1977.

Todres ID. Pediatric airway control and ventilation. *Ann Emerg Med* 22:440, 1993.

Torphy DE, Minter MG, Thompson BM. Cardiorespiratory arrest and resuscitation of children. *Am J Dis Child* 138:1099, 1984.

Williams DR. The heartsaver-baby: A CPR course for young parents. *Can Fam Physician* 31:1005, 1985.

Zaritsky A et al. Pediatric resuscitation pharmacology. *Ann Emerg Med* 22:445, 1993.

Zideman DA. Resuscitation of infants and children. *Br Med J* 292:1584, 1986.

ENDOTRACHEAL INTUBATION OF INFANTS AND CHILDREN

Aijan P et al. Endotracheal intubation of pediatric patients by paramedics. *Ann Emerg Med* 18:489, 1989.

Bloch EC et al. Tracheal intubation in children: A new method for assuring correct depth of tube placement. *Anesth Analg* 67:590, 1988.

Browning DH et al. Incidence of aspiration with endotracheal tubes in children. *J Pediatr* 102:582, 1983.

Clark JR. Pediatric intubation. *Emergency* 23(8):46, 1991.

Goitein KJ et al. Incidence of aspiration in endotracheally intubated infants and young children. *Crit Care Med* 12:19, 1984.

Hancock PH et al. Finger intubation of the trachea in newborns. *Pediatrics* 89:325, 1992.

King BR et al. Endotracheal tube selection in children: A comparison of four methods. *Ann Emerg Med* 22:530, 1993.

Losek JD et al. Prehospital pediatric endotracheal intubation. *Pediatr Emerg Care* 5:1, 1989.

Lutten RC et al. Length-based endotracheal tube and emergency equipment in pediatrics. *Ann Emerg Med* 21:900, 1992.

Pointer JE. Clinical characteristics of paramedics' performance of pediatric endotracheal intubation. *Am J Emerg Med* 7:364, 1989.

Wertz EM. Pediatric and infant intubation. *Emergency* 25(12):53, 1993.

Whitten CE. Intubating the child. *Emerg Med* 21(21):81, 1989.

INTRAVENOUS TECHNIQUES FOR INFANTS AND CHILDREN

Adelman S. An emergency intravenous route for the pediatric patient. *JACEP* 5:596, 1976.

Anderson TE et al. Intraosseous infusion: Success of a standardized regional training program for prehospital advanced life support providers. *Ann Emerg Med* 23:52, 1994.

Brickman K, Rega P, Guinness M. Intraosseous infusion: Rapid vascular access in critically ill children. *Emerg Med Serv* 18(7):56, 1989.

Brunette DD, Rischer R. Intravascular access in pediatric cardiac arrest. *Am J Emerg Med* 6:577, 1988.

Everidge JM. Achieving success in pediatric IV therapy. *JEMS* 14(7):94, 1989.

Friery JA. Pediatric intraosseous infusion. *Emergency* 24(10):47, 1992.

Fuchs S, LaCovey D, Paris P. A prehospital model of intraosseous infusion. *Ann Emerg Med* 20:371, 1991.

Garrison HG et al. A cost-effectiveness analysis of pediatric intraosseous infusion as a prehospital skill. *Prehosp Disaster Med* 7:221, 1992.

Glaeser PW, Losek JD. Emergency intraosseous infusions in children. *Am J Emerg Med* 4:34, 1986.

Glaser PW et al. Five-year experience in prehospital intraosseous infusions in children and adults. *Ann Emerg Med* 22:1119, 1993.

Hallen B et al. Does lidocaine-prilocaine cream permit pain-free insertion of IV catheters in children? *Anesthesiology* 57:340, 1982.

Hecker JF et al. Nitroglycerine ointment as an aid to venipuncture. *Lancet* 1(8320):332, 1983.

Iserson KV. Intraosseous infusions in adults. *J Emerg Med* :587, 1989.

Iserson KV, Criss E. Interosseous infusions: A usable technique. *Am J Emerg Med* 4:540, 1986.

Kanter RK et al. Pediatric emergency intravenous access: Evaluation of a protocol. *Am J Dis Child* 140:132, 1986.

Lillis KA, Jaffe DM. Prehospital intravenous access in children. *Ann Emerg Med* 21:1430, 1992.

Miner WF et al. Prehospital use of intraosseous infusion by paramedics. *Pediatr Emerg Care* 5:5, 1989.

Nott MR et al. Relief of injection pain in adults: EMLA cream for 5 minutes before venepuncture. *Anaesthesia* 45:772, 1990.

Orlowski JP et al. Comparison study of intraosseous, central intravenous, and peripheral intravenous infusions of emergency drugs. *Am J Dis Child* 144:112, 1990.

Parrish GA et al. Intraosseous infusions in the emergency department. *Am J Emerg Med* 4:59, 1986.

Roberge RJ. Facilitated intravenous access through local application of nitroglycerin ointment. *Ann Emerg Med* 16:546, 1987.

Rosetti VA et al. Intraosseous infusion: An alternative route of pediatric intravascular access. *Ann Emerg Med* 14:885, 1985.

Salassi-Scotter M, Fiser DH. Adoption of intraosseous infusion technique for prehospital pediatric emergency care. *Pediatr Emerg Care* 6:263, 1990.

Seigler RS, Tecklenburg FW, Shealy R. Prehospital intraosseous infusion by emergency medical services personnel: A prospective study. *Pediatrics* 84:173, 1989.

Simmons CM et al. Intraosseous extravasation complication reports. *Ann Emerg Med* 23:363, 1994.

Smith RJ et al. Intraosseous infusions by prehospital personnel in critically ill pediatric patients. *Ann Emerg Med* 17:491, 1988.

Vaksmann G et al. Nitroglycerine ointment as aid to venous cannulation in children. *J Pediatr* 111:89, 1987.

Vidal R et al. Compartment syndrome following intraosseous infusion. *Pediatrics* 91:1201, 1993.

PERFORMANCE CHECKLISTS

The following pages contain checklists for correct performance of some of the skills described in this chapter. The checklists can be used as a review and as a guide for practicing the respective skills.

Performance Test
Obstructed Airway: Conscious Infant

Student _____ Date _____

Instructor: Place an "X" in the Fail column beside any element that is done incorrectly, out of sequence, or omitted.

Step	Activity	Critical Performance	Fail
Assessment	Determine airway obstruction	Observes breathing difficulties	
Back blows	Deliver up to 5 back blows	Infant held prone straddling rescuer's forearm	
		Infant's head lower than trunk	
		Infant's head supported	
		Up to 5 back blows delivered between the shoulder blades with heel of one hand	
Chest thrusts	Deliver up to 5 chest thrusts	Infant sandwiched between rescuer's hands	
		Infant turned to recumbent position	
		Infant's head lower than trunk	
		Up to 5 chest thrusts over 3–5 seconds	
		Compression point: lower third of sternum	
Sequencing	Repeat sequence	Repeats back blows and chest thrusts until foreign body is expelled or infant becomes unconscious	
Infant with Obstructed Airway Becomes Unconscious			
Foreign body check	Tongue-jaw lift Removal of foreign body IF VISUALIZED	Performs tongue-jaw lift by placing thumb in infant's mouth over tongue	
		Lifts tongue and jaw forward with fingers wrapped around lower jaw	
		Removes foreign body IF VISUALIZED	
		Does NOT perform blind finger sweep	
Breathing attempt	Attempt ventilation	Opens airway with head tilt–chin lift	
		Seals mouth and nose properly	
		Attempts to ventilate	

Back blows	Deliver up to 5 back blows	Infant held prone straddling rescuer's forearm	
		Infant's head lower than trunk	
		Infant's head supported	
		Up to 5 back blows delivered between the shoulder blades with heel of one hand	
Chest thrusts	Deliver up to 5 chest thrusts	Infant sandwiched between rescuer's hands	
		Infant turned to recumbent position	
		Infant's head lower than trunk	
		Up to 5 chest thrusts over 3–5 seconds	
		Compression point: lower third of sternum	
Foreign body check	Tongue-jaw lift Removal of foreign body IF VISUALIZED	Performs tongue-jaw lift by placing thumb in infant's mouth over tongue	
		Lifts tongue and jaw forward with fingers wrapped around lower jaw	
		Removes foreign body IF VISUALIZED	
		Does NOT perform blind finger sweep	
Breathing attempt	Reattempt ventilation	Opens airway with head tilt–chin lift	
		Seals mouth and nose properly	
		Attempts to ventilate	
Sequencing	Repeat sequence	Repeats last four steps until successful*	

*After airway obstruction is removed, bheck for pulse and breathing. (1) *If pulse is absent:* Ventilate a second time, and start cycles of compressions and ventilations. (2) *If pulse is present:* Open airway, and check for spontaneous breathing. *If breathing is present,* monitor breathing and pulse closely; maintain open airway. *If breathing is absent,* perform rescue breathing 20 times/min, and monitor pulse.

Instructor _____

Based on the recommendations in Emergency Cardiac Care Committee and Subcommittees, American Heart Association. Guidelines for cardiopulmonary resuscitation and emergency cardiac care. *JAMA* 268:2172, 1992.

Performance Test
Obstructed Airway: Unconscious Infant

Student _____ Date _____

Instructor: Place an "X" in the Fail column beside any element that is done incorrectly, out of sequence, or omitted.

Step	Activity	Critical Performance	Fail
Assessment	Determine unresponsiveness	Taps or gently shakes shoulder	
	Position infant	Turns infant supine, supporting head	
		Places infant on firm, hard surface	
Airway	Open the airway	Head tilt–chin lift maneuver to sniffing or neutral position	
		Head not hyperextended	
Breathing	Determine breathlessness	Looks, listens, and feels for breathing (3–5 sec)	
		Ear over infant's mouth	
		Observes chest	
	Ventilation attempt (airway is obstructed)	Maintains infant's head position	
		Makes tight seal on mouth and nose of infant	
		Attempts to ventilate (1–1.5 sec/ventilation)	
	Second attempt (airway remains blocked)	Repositions infant's head	
		Seals mouth and nose properly	
		Reattempts to ventilate (1–1.5 sec/ventilation)	
Back Blows	Deliver up to 5 back blows	Infant held prone straddling rescuer's forearm	
		Infant's head lower than trunk	
		Infant's head supported	
		Up to 5 back blows delivered between the shoulder blades with heel of one hand	
Chest thrusts	Deliver up to 5 chest thrusts	Infant sandwiched between rescuer's hands	
		Infant turned to recumbent position	
		Infant's head lower than trunk	
		Up to 5 chest thrusts over 3–5 seconds	
		Compression point: lower third of sternum	
Foreign body check	Tongue-jaw lift Removal of foreign body IF VISUALIZED	Performs tongue-jaw lift by placing thumb in infant's mouth over tongue	
		Lifts tongue and jaw forward with fingers wrapped around lower jaw	
		Removes foreign body IF VISUALIZED	
		Does NOT perform blind finger sweep	

Breathing attempt	Reattempt ventilation	Opens airway with head tilt–chin lift	
		Seals mouth and nose properly	
		Attempts to ventilate	
Sequencing	Repeat sequence	Repeats last four steps until successful*	

*After airway obstruction is removed, check for pulse and breathing. (1) *If pulse is absent:* Ventilate a second time, and start cycles of compressions and ventilations. (2) *If pulse is present:* Open airway, and check for spontaneous breathing. *If breathing is present,* monitor breathing and pulse closely; maintain open airway. *If breathing is absent,* perform rescue breathing 20 times/min, and monitor pulse.

Instructor _____

Based on the recommendations in Emergency Cardiac Care Committee and Subcommittees, American Heart Association. Guidelines for cardiopulmonary resuscitation and emergency cardiac care. *JAMA* 268:2172, 1992.

Performance Test
Obstructed Airway: Conscious Child

Student _____ Date _____

Instructor: Place an "X" in the Fail column beside any element that is done incorrectly, out of sequence, or omitted.

Step	Activity	Critical Performance	Fail
Assessment	Determine airway obstruction	Asks, "Are you choking?"	
		Determines if child can cough or speak	
Abdominal thrusts	Perform abdominal thrust ONLY if child's cough is ineffective or there is increasing respiratory distress	Stands behind child	
		Wraps arms around child's waist	
		Makes a fist with one hand and places the thumb side against child's abdomen	
		Correct position: midline, slightly above umbilicus, well below tip of xiphoid	
		Grasps fist with other hand	
		Presses into the child's abdomen with quick upward thrusts	
		Each thrust distinct	
		Repeats thrust until either foreign body is expelled or child becomes unconscious	

Child with Obstructed Airway Becomes Unconscious

Step	Activity	Critical Performance	Fail
Additional assessment	Position the child	Turns child on back as a unit	
		Places faceup, arms by side	
Foreign body check	Tongue-jaw lift Removal of foreign body IF VISUALIZED	Performs tongue-jaw lift by placing thumb in infant's mouth over tongue	
		Lifts tongue and jaw forward with fingers wrapped around lower jaw	
		Removes foreign body IF VISUALIZED	
		Does NOT perform blind finger sweep	
Breathing attempt	Attempt ventilation (airway is obstructed)	Opens airway with head tilt–chin lift	
		Seals mouth and nose properly	
		Attempts to ventilate	
Heimlich maneuver	Abdominal thrusts	Kneels at child's feet	
		Places heel of one hand against child's abdomen	
		Correct position: midline, slightly above umbilicus and well below xiphoid	
		Second hand directly on top of first hand	
		Presses into abdomen with 5 quick upward thrusts	

Foreign body check	Tongue-jaw lift Removal of foreign body IF VISUALIZED	Performs tongue-jaw lift by placing thumb in infant's mouth over tongue	
		Lifts tongue and jaw forward with fingers wrapped around lower jaw	
		Removes foreign body IF VISUALIZED	
		Does NOT perform blind finger sweep	
Breathing attempt	Reattempt ventilation	Opens airway with head tilt–chin lift	
		Seals mouth and nose properly	
		Attempts to ventilate	
Sequencing	Repeat sequence	Repeats last four steps until successful*	

*After airway obstruction is removed, check for pulse and breathing. (1) *If pulse is absent:* Ventilate a second time, and start cycles of compressions and ventilations. (2) *If pulse is present:* Open airway, and check for spontaneous breathing. *If breathing is present,* monitor breathing and pulse closely; maintain open airway. *If breathing is absent,* perform rescue breathing 20 times/min, and monitor pulse.

Instructor ＿＿＿＿＿＿＿＿＿＿＿＿＿＿

Based on the recommendations in Emergency Cardiac Care Committee and Subcommittees, American Heart Association. Guidelines for cardiopulmonary resuscitation and emergency cardiac care. *JAMA* 268:2172, 1992.

Performance Test
Obstructed Airway: Unconscious Child

Student _____ Date _____

Instructor: Place an "X" in the Fail column beside any element that is done incorrectly, out of sequence, or omitted.

Step	Activity	Critical Performance	Fail
Assessment	Determine unresponsiveness	Taps or gently shakes shoulder	
Airway	Position the victim	Turns child supine as a unit, supporting head and neck (4–10 sec)	
	Open the airway	Head tilt–chin lift maneuver	
Breathing	Determine breathlessness	Ear over mouth; observes chest	
		Looks, listens, and feels for breathing (3–5 sec)	
	Attempt ventilation (airway is obstructed)	Maintains open airway	
		Seals mouth and nose properly	
		Attempts to ventilate (1–1.5 sec/breath)	
	Reattempt ventilation (airway still blocked)	Repositions child's head	
		Seals mouth and nose properly	
		Reattempts ventilation (1–1.5 sec/breath)	
		Total elapsed time so far: 15–35 seconds	
Heimlich maneuver	Abdominal thrusts	Kneels at child's feet	
		Places heel of one hand against child's abdomen	
		Correct position: Midline, slightly above umbilicus and well below xiphoid	
		Second hand directly on top of first hand	
		Presses into abdomen with 5 quick upward thrusts	
Foreign body check	Tongue-jaw lift Removal of foreign body IF VISUALIZED	Performs tongue-jaw lift by placing thumb in child's mouth over tongue	
		Lifts tongue and jaw forward with fingers wrapped around lower jaw	
		Removes foreign body IF VISUALIZED	
		Does NOT perform blind finger sweep	
Breathing attempt	Reattempt ventilation	Opens airway with head tilt–chin lift	
		Seals mouth and nose properly	
		Attempts to ventilate	
Sequencing	Repeat sequence	Repeats last four steps until successful*	

*After airway obstruction is removed, check for pulse and breathing. (1) *If pulse is absent:* Ventilate a second time, and start cycles of compressions and ventilations. (2) *If pulse is present:* Open airway, and check for spontaneous breathing. *If breathing is present,* monitor breathing and pulse closely; maintain open airway. *If breathing is absent,* perform rescue breathing 20 times/min, and monitor pulse.

Instructor _____

Based on the recommendations in Emergency Cardiac Care Committee and Subcommittees, American Heart Association. Guidelines for cardiopulmonary resuscitation and emergency cardiac care. *JAMA* 268:2172, 1992.

Performance Test
One-Rescuer CPR: Infant

Student _____ Date _____

Instructor: Place an "X" in the Fail column beside any element that is done incorrectly, out of sequence, or omitted.

Step	Activity	Critical Performance	Fail
Assessment	Determine unresponsiveness	Taps or gently shakes shoulder	
	Position infant	Turns infant supine, supporting head	
		Places infant on firm, hard surface	
Airway	Open the airway	Head tilt–chin lift maneuver to sniffing or neutral position	
		Head not hyperextended	
Breathing	Determine breathlessness	Looks, listens, and feels for breathing (3–5 sec)	
		Ear over infant's mouth	
		Observes chest	
	Two ventilations	Maintains infant's head position	
		Makes tight seal on mouth and nose of infant	
		Ventilates two times (1–1.5 sec/ventilation)	
		Observes chest rise	
		Allows deflation between breaths	
Circulation	Determine pulselessness	Palpates brachial pulse (5–10 sec)	
		Maintains head tilt with other hand	
	Begin compressions	Correct compression point (1 fingerbreadth below intermammary line)	
		Compression-relaxation ratio = 1:1	
		Compresses vertically ½ to 1 inch	
		Keeps fingers on sternum during upstroke	
		Completes chest relaxation on upstroke	
		Says mnemonic aloud	
		Compression rate: 100/min	
Compression-ventilation cycles	Do 20 cycles of 5 compressions and 1 ventilation	Proper compression-ventilation ratio = 5 compressions: 1 slow ventilation/cycle	
		Pauses for ventilation	
		Watches chest rise	
		1–1.5 seconds for each ventilation	
		10 cycles in 45 seconds or less	
Reassessment	Recheck pulse	Palpates brachial pulse (5 sec).* If absent:	

Continue CPR	Ventilate	Ventilates once	
		Observes chest rise	
		1–1.5 seconds for ventilation	
		Resumes chest compressions	

*If pulse is present, open airway and check for spontaneous breathing. (1) *If breathing is present,* monitor breathing and pulse closely; maintain open airway. (2) *If breathing is absent,* perform rescue breathing at 20 times/min, and monitor pulse.

Instructor _____

Based on the recommendations in Emergency Cardiac Care Committee and Subcommittees, American Heart Association. Guidelines for cardiopulmonary resuscitation and emergency cardiac care. *JAMA* 268:2172, 1992.

Performance Test
One-Rescuer CPR: Child (under about 8 years old)

Student _____ Date _____

Instructor: Place an "X" in the Fail column beside any element that is done incorrectly, out of sequence, or omitted.

Step	Activity	Critical Performance	Fail
Assessment	Determine unresponsiveness	Taps or gently shakes shoulder	
Airway	Position the victim	Turns child supine as a unit, supporting head and neck (4–10 sec)	
	Open the airway	Head tilt–chin lift maneuver	
Breathing	Determine breathlessness	Ear over mouth; observes chest	
		Looks, listens, and feels for breathing (3–5 sec)	
	Ventilate twice	Maintains open airway	
		Seals mouth and nose properly	
		Give two breaths (1–1.5 sec/breath)	
		Observes chest rise	
		Allows deflation between breaths	
Circulation	Determine pulselessness	Palpates carotid pulse on near side of child	
		Maintains head tilt	
	Begin chest compressions	Rescuer's knees by child's shoulders	
		Landmark check prior to hand placement	
		Uses heel of one hand for compression	
		Proper hand position throughout	
		Rescuer's shoulders over child's sternum	
		Compression-relaxation ratio = 1:1	
		Compresses 1 to 1½ inches	
		Keeps hand on sternum during upstroke	
		Completes chest relaxation on upstroke	
		Says mnemonic out loud	
		Compression rate = 100/min	
Compression-ventilation cycles	Do 20 cycles of 5 compressions and 1 ventilation	Proper compression-ventilation ratio = 5 compressions: 1 slow ventilation/cycle	
		Pauses for ventilation	
		Watches chest rise	
		1–1.5 seconds for each ventilation	
		10 cycles in 45 seconds or less	

Reassessment	Recheck pulse	Palpates carotid pulse (5 sec).* If absent:	
Continue CPR	Ventilate	Ventilates once	
		Observes chest rise	
		1–1.5 seconds for ventilation	
		Resumes chest compressions	

*If pulse is present, open airway and check for spontaneous breathing. (1) *If breathing is present*, monitor breathing and pulse closely; maintain open airway. (2) *If breathing is absent*, perform rescue breathing at 20 times/min, and monitor pulse.

Instructor ＿＿＿＿＿＿＿＿＿＿＿＿＿＿

Based on the recommendations in Emergency Cardiac Care Committee and Subcommittees, American Heart Association. Guidelines for cardiopulmonary resuscitation and emergency cardiac care. *JAMA* 268:2172, 1992.

Performance Test
Two-Rescuer CPR: Child

Student _____ Date _____

Instructor: Place an "X" in the Fail column beside any element that is done incorrectly, out of sequence, or omitted.

Step	Activity	Critical Performance	Fail
Assessment	One rescuer (ventilator): Determines unresponsiveness	Taps or gently shakes shoulder	
		Shouts, "Are you OK?"	
	Positions child	Turns child supine if necessary (4–10 sec)	
Airway	Opens the airway	Head tilt–chin lift	
Breathing	Determines breathlessness	Cheek over child's mouth; observes chest	
		Looks, listens, and feels for breathing (3–5 sec)	
		Says, "Not breathing."	
	Ventilator ventilates twice	Two slow ventilations each 1–1.5 seconds	
		Watches chest rise with each breath	
Circulation	Determines pulselessness	Palpates carotid pulse (5–10 sec)	
	States results	Says, "No pulse."	
	Second rescuer: Locates landmark	Finds correct point on lower third of sternum	
	Gets into position	Shoulders directly over sternum	
		Heel of hand correctly lined up	
		Fingers off chest	
Compression-ventilation cycles	Compressor begins chest compression	Compression-ventilation ratio = 5:1	
		Compression rate = 100/min	
		Says mnemonic out loud	
		Stops compressing for each ventilation	
	Ventilator ventilates after every 5th compression and checks effectiveness of CPR After 20 cycles:	Ventilator delivers each breath over 1–1.5 seconds	
		Periodically checks carotid pulse to assess compressions	
Reassessment	Pulse check	Compressor pauses 5–10 seconds	
		Ventilator rechecks pulse;* if pulse is absent, they resume CPR	

*If pulse is present, open airway and check for spontaneous breathing. (1) *If breathing is present,* monitor breathing and pulse closely; maintain open airway. (2) *If breathing is absent,* perform rescue breathing at 20 times/min, and monitor pulse.

Instructor _____

Based on the recommendations in Emergency Cardiac Care Committee and Subcommittees, American Heart Association. Guidelines for cardiopulmonary resuscitation and emergency cardiac care. *JAMA* 268:2172, 1992.

VI

ENVIRONMENTAL EMERGENCIES

31
Heat Exposure

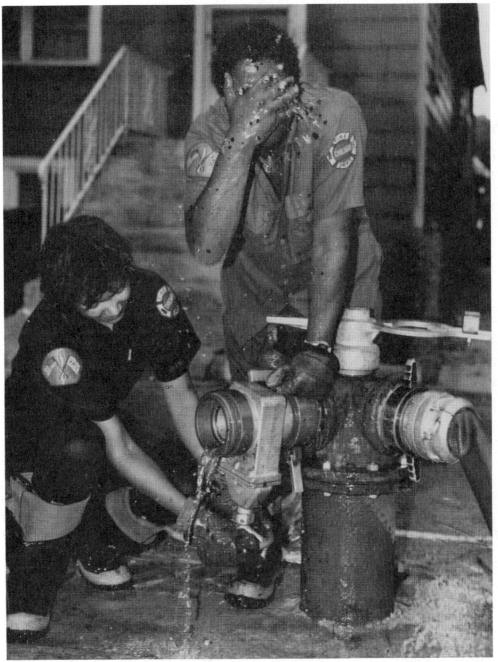

Chicago Fire Department, Chicago. Photo by Michael S. Kowal.

OBJECTIVES

Every year, the dog days of summer leave hundreds of casualties in their wake—people who succumb to one or another heat illness. The most vulnerable are the elderly, but the young are by no means immune to heat illness. Indeed, among teenagers, heat stroke is second only to spinal cord injury as a cause of death on the athletic field.

We shall begin this chapter by examining the techniques that the healthy body uses to shed excess heat. We shall then see what factors can interfere with the body's ability to shed heat and thereby increase a person's risk of suffering heat illness. We'll consider three forms of heat illness—heat cramps, heat exhaustion, and heat stroke—and review how each is manifested clinically and how each is treated in the field. Finally, we shall look at some of the ways that paramedics working in a hot environment can "keep their cool" and avoid becoming victims of heat illness themselves. By the end of this chapter, the student should be able to

1. List three sources of body heat
2. List four mechanisms by which the body can rid itself of excess heat, and describe the conditions necessary for each mechanism to be effective
3. Describe the normal physiologic response to entering a hot environment
4. List at least five factors that predispose a person to heat illness
5. Given a description of several patients with different symptoms and signs, identify a patient suffering from
   • Heat cramps
   • Heat exhaustion
   • Heat stroke
   and describe the correct treatment of each
6. List five measures a paramedic can take to help avoid heat illness when working under hot conditions

HOW THE BODY EXCRETES HEAT

The human body stubbornly defends a constant core temperature of 37°C (98.6°F) regardless of whether the body in question finds itself in the tropics or at the North Pole, for 37°C is the temperature at which all of the metabolic reactions of the body are programmed to proceed optimally. At lower body temperatures, many of the body's chemical reactions would proceed too slowly to be useful for anything that could be considered a process of life; and at higher temperatures, crucial proteins that govern the enzymatic reactions of the body would be damaged (denatured). So 37°C is just about perfect.

Sources of Body Heat

The core temperature of 37°C in fact represents a balance between the heat produced or absorbed by the body and the heat excreted to the outside. At rest, the body produces heat chiefly by the metabolism of nutrients and by other chemical reactions. The vast majority of *basal heat production* occurs in the liver and the skeletal muscles, and in the average adult the rate of heat production at rest is usually in the range of 75 kcal per hour.

Another way that the body generates heat is through *exercise*. A brisk walk can produce about 300 kcal of heat per hour; heavy physical work may generate two to three times that amount of heat.

Some of the heat generated by metabolism and muscular work is used to warm the body; the excess has to be excreted, ordinarily by taking advantage of the temperature gradient between the body and the outside environment. When, however, the environmental temperature is *higher* than the body temperature, there is a third potential source of body heat: *absorption of heat* from the outside. Standing in bright sunshine on a hot, breezeless day, for example, can add up to 150 kcal per hour to the internal heat load.

Excretion of Excess Heat

With the body churning out anywhere from 75 to 900 kcal of heat per hour, we would all be rapidly parboiled if we did not have some way of disposing of excess internal heat. Fortunately, we do have an efficient, although not infallible, system for shedding heat. Ensuring the balance between heat production and heat excretion is the job of a master thermostat located in a part of the brain called the anterior **hypothalamus**. Like the thermostat in a house, the one in the brain operates according to the principle of **negative feedback control:** A rise in core body temperature elicits responses to increase heat *loss;* a fall in core body temperature prompts heat *production* and *conservation*. Both responses depend on the body's ability to vary the blood flow from the core to the periphery. When the core temperature rises, peripheral blood vessels dilate; more blood (and thus more heat) reaches the skin, where the heat can be dissipated by three main mechanisms: convection, radiation, and conduction.

Convection refers to the loss of heat that takes place when moving air picks up heat and carries it away. Convection is the principle one instinctively uses in blowing on hot food to cool it down.

Radiation occurs when heat is simply emitted from the body into the surrounding atmosphere, without the help of moving air currents. A radiator used to heat a room is so named because it operates by this mechanism. Under ordinary circumstances, radiation and convection account for about 70 percent of heat excretion.

Conduction refers to the dissipation of heat into a solid object or a liquid rather than into air, as for instance when a person falls into cold water. As we shall see in the next chapter, heat loss by conduction may be extremely rapid.

All three mechanisms just described require a thermal gradient between the body and its surroundings; that is, the mechanisms work only so long as the skin surface temperature is higher than that of the outside environment (and also so long as metabolism does not produce an overwhelming heat load). When the outside temperature approaches or *exceeds* skin surface temperature, however, heat loss by radiation and convection diminishes and finally ceases altogether. Indeed, when the environmental temperature exceeds the skin temperature, heat is *absorbed* by the body. In those circumstances, the increase in blood flow to the skin becomes counterproductive, for it promotes an increase in the rate of heat absorption.

The only way that the body can dissipate heat when the ambient temperature approaches body temperature is by the **evaporation of sweat.** But that mechanism too has its limits. To begin with, the normal adult can sweat a maximum of about a liter per hour and cannot keep up that rate of sweating for more than a few hours at a time. Furthermore, for effective evaporation of sweat to occur, the ambient air has to be relatively unsaturated with water. As the relative humidity increases, the rate of evaporation decreases, until effective sweat evaporation ceases entirely when the relative humidity reaches about 75 percent.

Physiologic Responses to Heat

Now that we know something about how the body normally regulates its internal temperature, we can deduce some of the physiologic effects of exposure to high environmental temperature and humidity:

- Because of cutaneous vasodilatation, the effective volume of the vascular system is increased (when you increase the diameter of a tube, such as an artery, you increase its volume); the heart must therefore *increase its output* to compensate for vasodilatation. The heart does that by increasing its rate (tachycardia) and its stroke volume; but it pays a price in markedly increased cardiac work.

If vasodilatation is especially marked, there may be complete loss of vasomotor control, that is, the ability of the arteries to constrict in response to sympathetic stimulation. In that case, blood pools in the periphery, and the patient presents with the clinical picture of neurogenic shock.

- As the body pours more and more blood into the cutaneous circulation, less and less blood flows to internal organs. Thus *blood is shunted away from the brain,* and the blood that does reach the central nervous system may have an abnormally high temperature. The brain does not like to be deprived of blood; nor does it like to be parboiled. So it responds with headache, dizziness, impaired thinking, and emotional instability.
- As sweating increases, excessive amounts of sodium, chloride, and other electrolytes are lost through the skin, resulting in muscle cramps and *dehydration.*

When the thermoregulatory system is taxed beyond its limits or fails for any reason, the core body temperature soars, sometimes rising from normal to about 41°C (106°F) in less than 15 minutes. That is the situation in heat stroke, which represents a potentially lethal failure of the mechanisms by which the body rids itself of heat.

HEAT ILLNESS

Heat stress can produce a variety of different syndromes, depending on the type of heat (dry or humid), the intensity of the exposure, and the age and previous state of health of the victim.

Who Is at Risk

All of us will succumb to heat illness sooner or later if the exposure is sufficiently intense or prolonged. But certain factors increase a person's risk of suffering ill effects from any given heat stress. Some of those factors are summarized in Table 31-1. Note that, for a variety of reasons, the elderly are at particular risk. The elderly are more vulnerable to heat illness than the young because, first of all, they do not adjust as well to the heat: They perspire less; they acclimatize more slowly; they feel thirst less readily in response to dehydration. The elderly, in addition, are more likely to suffer from chronic conditions—such as diabetes, cardiovascular disease, or obesity—that interfere with normal heat excretion. And the elderly are more apt to be taking medications that disrupt the body's mechanisms for dissipating heat. The diuretics that so many older patients take for hypertension, for

TABLE 31-1.   FACTORS THAT PREDISPOSE TO HEAT ILLNESS

CATEGORY	EXAMPLES
Factors that increase internal heat production	Physical exertion Response to infection (fever) Hyperthyroidism Psychiatric condition with agitation
Factors that increase heat absorption	Living in confined, unventilated, hot quarters Working in hot conditions (bakeries, steel mills, construction sites) Locking children in parked automobiles in summer

Factors that interfere with heat dissipation	High ambient temperature
	High humidity
	Obesity (insulation effect)
	Impaired vasodilation mechanism
	    Diabetes
	    Alcoholism
	    Drugs: diuretics, tranquilizers, beta blockers
	Impaired ability to sweat
	    Cystic fibrosis
	    Skin diseases
	    Drugs: antihistamines, phenothiazines
	Heavy or tight clothing

Factors that impair the body's response to heat stress	Dehydration Hypokalemia Cardiovascular disease Previous stroke or other CNS lesion

example, may render an elderly person dangerously close to dehydration and also interfere with the peripheral vasodilatation necessary for heat transfer.

Among the young and healthy, those most vulnerable to heat stress are infants and young children exposed to a hot environment, such as children left unattended "for just a minute" in a parked automobile. Athletes and military recruits engaging in heavy exertion under hot conditions are also at increased risk.

Heat Cramps

Heat cramps are muscle pains, usually in the lower extremities, the abdomen, or both, that occur because of profuse sweating and consequent SALT DEPLETION. Heat cramps most often afflict people in *good physical condition* who are working or playing hard in conditions of high temperature or humidity. Usually a person exerting himself in a hot environment will become thirsty and increase his intake of fluids. But if the person is sweating heavily, he is losing both fluids *and* salt across his skin. A few drinks of water may replace the lost fluid but do not replace the lost salt. So as the person continues to sweat and to drink water, the concentration of salt within the body is progressively diluted, leading to the state of **hyponatremia** (deficiency of sodium in the blood) that seems to be a prerequisite for heat cramps.

Heat cramps usually come on suddenly during vigorous activity. They may be mild, with only slight abdominal cramping and tingling in the extremities. But more often they present with severe, incapacitating pain in the extremities and abdomen. The patient may become somewhat hypotensive and nauseated, but he remains alert. The pulse is generally rapid, the skin pale and moist, and the temperature normal. Untreated, heat cramps may progress to heat exhaustion.

Treatment of Heat Cramps

Treatment of heat cramps is aimed at eliminating the exposure and restoring lost salt and water to the body:

- Move the patient to a COOL ENVIRONMENT. Have him lie down if he feels faint.
- *If the patient is not nauseated,* give him one or two glasses of a salt-containing solution (e.g., lemonade with ½ teaspoon of salt added or a commercial preparation such as Gatorade). Instruct the patient to drink the solution slowly. Do *not*

give salt tablets, since they may precipitate or worsen nausea.

- If the patient is too nauseated to take liquids by mouth, start an IV with NORMAL SALINE, and infuse it rapidly. (Consult medical control for the IV rate.)
- Do *not* massage the cramping muscles. That rarely helps and may actually aggravate the pain.
- As the patient's salt balance is restored, his symptoms will abate and he may wish to resume his activity immediately, especially if he is a macho athlete keen to return to the playing field. He must be discouraged from doing so. A person who has suffered heat cramps should not return to strenuous activity for *at least 12 hours,* because further exertion may lead to heat exhaustion or heat stroke. The patient should also be instructed to drink salt-containing fluids like Gatorade rather than water during periods of exertion.

DO NOT PERMIT A PATIENT TO RETURN TO STRENUOUS ACTIVITY WITHIN 12 HOURS OF AN EPISODE OF HEAT CRAMPS.

Heat Exhaustion

Heat exhaustion occurs as a result of salt and water loss along with peripheral pooling of blood. Like heat cramps, heat exhaustion tends to occur in persons working in hot environments. In addition, however, heat exhaustion is common in dehydrated, elderly patients and in hypertensives. The elderly are more vulnerable because the thirst mechanism is dulled with age, so older patients may not increase their fluid intake sufficiently in the face of increased losses from sweating. Hypertensive patients, for their part, are often taking medications that deplete the body of fluids and electrolytes and that also interfere with reflex changes in the caliber of blood vessels.

Heat exhaustion may come on suddenly as SYNCOPE and collapse or may be heralded by symptoms such as HEADACHE, FATIGUE, DIZZINESS, NAUSEA, and sometimes abdominal CRAMPING. On examination, the patient is usually SWEATING PROFUSELY, and his skin is PALE and CLAMMY. He may be slightly disoriented. The TEMPERATURE may be low, normal, or elevated; the PULSE is RAPID and WEAK; the RESPIRATIONS are FAST and SHALLOW, and tachypnea may even be of such a degree to produce symptoms of hyperventilation

(carpopedal spasm, perioral numbness). The BLOOD PRESSURE may be DECREASED due to peripheral pooling of blood, and if not decreased at rest, it will almost certainly drop when the patient tries to sit up or stand up from a recumbent position (**orthostatic hypotension**).

Because it often presents with fatigue, headache, muscle cramps, and gastrointestinal symptoms, heat exhaustion is sometimes mistaken for "summer flu," and the patient may simply be sent off to bed with a couple of aspirin. Untreated, however, heat exhaustion may progress to heat stroke, with possibly fatal consequences.

Treatment of Heat Exhaustion

The treatment of heat exhaustion is aimed at removing the patient from exposure to heat and repairing the derangement in his fluid and electrolyte balance:

- Move the patient to a COOL ENVIRONMENT, take off his excess clothing, and place him supine with his legs elevated.
- If the patient's temperature is elevated (you won't know unless you measure it!), SPONGE him with tepid water and fan him gently to make him more comfortable. Don't overdo it though. In heat exhaustion, there is no necessity for heroic measures to lower body temperature rapidly, and chilling the patient will only compound the problem.
- Start an IV with LACTATED RINGER'S solution. If the patient is young and otherwise healthy, run the IV wide open. For an older patient, consult medical command for advice on the IV flow rate. Do *not* give fluids by mouth.
- MONITOR cardiac rhythm and vital signs.

Heat Stroke

Of all the heat illnesses, heat stroke is the least common but the most deadly. It is caused by a severe disturbance in the body's heat-regulating mechanism and is a *profound emergency,* with a mortality rate as high as 70 percent.

There are in fact two heat stroke syndromes, each affecting a distinct patient population. **Classic heat stroke** (passive heat stroke), which usually occurs during heat waves, is most likely to strike the very old, the very young, or the debilitated. Patients with chronic illnesses, such as diabetes or heart disease, are particularly susceptible, as are alcoholics and patients taking certain medications (diuretics, tranquilizers). In all of those patients, high environmental temperatures initially elicit the usual heat-shedding mechanisms, and the patient sweats profusely. But at a certain point, the patient becomes too dehydrated to sweat any more. The core body temperature then begins to soar, and the typical signs and symptoms of heat stroke appear. In classic heat stroke, then, the patient has two problems: a dangerously high temperature *and* dehydration. And, probably because of the typical patient's age and underlying medical problems, classic heat stroke carries a very high mortality—up to about 70 percent.

The second type of heat stroke, **exertional heat stroke,** is typically an illness of the young and fit—usually an athlete or a military recruit—exercising under hot *and* humid conditions. As noted earlier, when the ambient temperature approaches body temperature, radiation and convection are no longer effective means of shedding excess heat. When, in addition, the relative humidity rises above about 60 percent, evaporative cooling becomes ineffective as well. If a person continues exercising under such conditions, he will continue generating heat without any means of excreting that heat. So heat will build up within the body, once again causing the core temperature to rocket upward. In exertional heat stroke, however, unlike classic heat stroke, hyperpyrexia occurs *without* dehydration, for significant fluid loss through sweating has been prevented by the high humidity. Exertional heat stroke also has a somewhat better prognosis than classic heat stroke—the mortality rate rarely exceeds 20 percent—perhaps because the typical victim is young and otherwise healthy.

The Clinical Picture of Heat Stroke

Both types of heat stroke present with similar signs and symptoms, which may or may not be recognized as the consequence of heat exposure. The patient almost certainly won't be able to give you a coherent history, for he will be CONFUSED, DELIRIOUS, or even COMATOSE. Often the very earliest signs of heat stroke are changes in behavior—irritability, combativeness, signs that the patient is hallucinating—which may mislead bystanders and rescuers to conclude that the patient is "crazy" or "high on drugs." Elderly patients with heat stroke may present with signs resembling those of a cerebrovascular accident. If you don't *suspect* heat stroke in such patients, treatment may be fatally delayed.

SUSPECT HEAT STROKE, AND CHECK A TEMPERATURE, IN ANY PERSON BEHAVING STRANGELY IN A HOT ENVIRONMENT.

Other central nervous system disturbances—including tremors, seizures, fixed and dilated pupils, and decerebrate or decorticate posturing—may also be a prominent feature of heat stroke.

In assessing the patient's *vital signs,* the diagnostic vital sign is, of course, a markedly ELEVATED TEMPERATURE, usually to above 40.6°C (105°F). There is almost invariably a very RAPID PULSE, which may be strong and bounding in exertional heat stroke or weak and thready in classic heat stroke. RESPIRATIONS are usually RAPID. The BLOOD PRESSURE may be normal or even elevated in exertional heat stroke, but is apt to be depressed in classic heat stroke, where dehydration is a significant part of the picture. The SKIN tends to be FLUSHED and HOT. In about 50 percent of cases, the patient will still be sweating when first seen, so the classic picture of bone-dry skin that is burning hot to the touch is not universally present.

The diagnosis of heat stroke is easy to miss. It may develop rapidly in a patient whose heat exhaustion was mistaken for "the flu." Or it may present as coma of unknown cause. Unless you keep the possibility of heat stroke constantly in mind during the hot months of the year, and routinely take the temperature as part of the vital signs during those months, you may waste precious time searching for some other cause of the patient's symptoms. In heat stroke, you don't *have* time to spare.

Treatment of Heat Stroke

Treatment of heat stroke is aimed at supporting vital functions while bringing the patient's temperature down toward normal as rapidly as possible.

- Establish an AIRWAY and administer OXYGEN.
- Move the patient to a COOL ENVIRONMENT. Strip him to his underclothing, and place him in a semireclining position with the head elevated.
- COOL THE PATIENT AS RAPIDLY AS POSSIBLE. The most efficient way to do so without causing undesirable side effects, such as shivering, is by CONVECTION AND EVAPORATION, as follows:
  1. Apply ice packs to the patient's flanks while massaging his neck and torso to prevent a vasoconstrictive response to the ice.
  2. Spray the patient with tepid water while fanning him constantly to promote rapid evaporation. A portable fan should be carried in the ambulance during the summer months for this purpose.
- MONITOR THE RECTAL TEMPERATURE every 10 minutes. Cooling efforts should continue until

the rectal temperature has fallen *below* about 39°C (102°F).

- Start an IV LIFELINE. Use D5/W at a keep-open rate for exertional heat stroke; cautiously infuse normal saline or lactated Ringer's for classic heat stroke with signs of hypovolemia.
- MONITOR cardiac rhythm.
- Be prepared to treat seizures, as outlined in Chapter 24.

For those who may have taken a first aid or EMT course during the past decade, a word about some of the treatment measures that are no longer recommended. We used to suggest, for one thing, that if the patient was found at home, he should be immersed in a bathtub filled with ice water, to promote heat loss by conduction. There are, however, several major drawbacks to that method. First of all, it is unpleasant for the patient, who may not in any case be in a mood to cooperate. Furthermore, it is awkward for the rescuers to try to manage a patient in a bathtub, especially if the patient starts seizing or loses consciousness. Immersion in ice water, furthermore, is likely to cause shivering, which simply increases the patient's metabolic heat production. Finally, it is very difficult to transport a patient in a bathtub—so transport has to be delayed if cooling is carried out by conduction.

Another method of cooling by conduction—covering the patient with sheets soaked in ice water—has also gone out of favor. Covering the patient with wet sheets in fact *impedes* heat loss by evaporation.

> **USE CONVECTION AND EVAPORATION TO COOL THE PATIENT.**

The distinctions among various heat illnesses are summarized in Table 31-2.

PREVENTION OF HEAT ILLNESS

When the August heat wave has you racing from one victim of heat prostration to another, you need to take care that you don't become the next victim on the list. A little advance planning and common sense can help you "keep your cool" during the dog days of summer.

- Paramedics working in hot climates should have a summer uniform consisting of LIGHT-COLORED, LOOSE-FITTING CLOTHING that deflects the sun's rays and permits evaporation of sweat.
- STAY IN COOL PLACES as much as possible, and avoid sudden changes in temperature.
- PARK THE AMBULANCE IN THE SHADE.
- INCREASE YOUR DAILY INTAKE OF FLUIDS. Do not rely on thirst to gauge your need. Try to drink something every hour during very hot weather, aiming for an intake of about 3 to 4

TABLE 31-2. EMERGENCIES RESULTING FROM HEAT STRESS

PARAMETER	HEAT CRAMPS	HEAT EXHAUSTION	HEAT STROKE
Pathophysiology	Salt and water loss	Salt and water loss Peripheral blood pooling	Failure of heat-regulating mechanisms
Muscle cramping	Present	May be present	Absent
Mental status	Clear	May be disoriented	Delirium, stupor, or coma
Skin	Cool, moist	Pale, cool, moist	Flushed, hot, may be dry
Temperature	Normal	Low, normal, or elevated	Over 40.6°C (105°F)
Pulse	Rapid	Rapid, weak	Rapid; bounding or weak
Blood pressure	Normal or low	Normal or low	High in exertional heat stroke; normal or low in classic heat stroke
Treatment	Stop exertion Salt and water, orally if tolerated	Stop exertion IV lactated Ringer's Cool environment Monitor	ABCs Rapid cooling Oxygen IV (keep vein open for exertional heat stroke, fluid push for classic heat stroke) Monitor

quarts in 24 hours. Avoid beverages that contain a lot of sugar and (even when off duty) alcoholic drinks.

- Wear a COOL, DAMP TOWEL AROUND THE NECK.
- Install a portable fan on the dashboard of the ambulance to improve convection.
- Make it a practice to carry a PORTABLE COOLER, like those used for picnics, during very hot weather. Fill the cooler about half full with crushed ice, and stock it with Gatorade or other salt-containing drinks for both patients and ambulance crew. As the ice in the cooler melts, use some of the cold water to moisten the towel you are wearing around your neck.
- BE ALERT FOR EARLY SYMPTOMS OF HEAT ILLNESS, such as headache, nausea, cramps, and dizziness. If you experience any of those symptoms, get out of the hot environment immediately, and get medical attention. Or, to paraphrase the late Harry S. Truman:

> **IF YOU CAN'T STAND THE HEAT, GET OUT OF THE AMBULANCE.**

Don't try to be a hero or heroine by "toughing it out" until the end of the shift, for your crew won't appreciate it if you collapse in the middle of the next call.

GLOSSARY

conduction   Transfer of heat to a solid object or a liquid.

convection   Mechanism by which body heat is picked up and carried away by moving air currents.

hyponatremia   Deficiency of sodium in the blood.

hypothalamus   Portion of the brain that regulates a multitude of bodily functions, including core temperature.

orthostatic hypotension   Fall in blood pressure that occurs on going from a recumbent to a sitting or standing position.

radiation   Emission of heat from an object into surrounding, colder air.

FURTHER READING

Birrer RB. Heat stroke: Don't wait for the classic signs. *Emerg Med* 20(12):9, 1988.

Brill JC. Heat stroke. *Emerg Med Serv* 6(4):44, 1977.

Cantor RM. Heat illness. *Emerg Med* 23(11):93, 1991.

Caroline NL. *Emergency Medical Treatment: A Text for EMT-As and EMT-Intermediates* (3rd ed.). Boston: Little, Brown, 1991. Chap. 29.

Carter WA. Heat emergencies: A guide to assessment and management. *Emerg Med Serv* 9(4):29, 1980.

Centers for Disease Control. Heat-related deaths—United States, 1993. *JAMA* 270:810, 1993.

Clowes GHA, O'Donnell TF. Heat stroke. *N Engl J Med* 291:564, 1974.

Cummins P. Felled by the heat. *Emerg Med* 15(12):94, 1983.

Forester D. Fatal drug-induced heat stroke. *JACEP* 7:243, 1978.

Graham BS et al. Nonexertional heatstroke: Physiologic management and cooling in 14 patients. *Arch Intern Med* 146:87, 1986.

Hanson PG. Exertional heat stroke in novice runners. *JAMA* 242:154, 1979.

Hart GR et al. Epidemic classical heat stroke: Clinical characteristics and course of 28 patients. *Medicine* 61:189, 1982.

Jones TS. Morbidity and mortality associated with the July 1980 heat wave in St. Louis and Kansas City, Mo. *JAMA* 247:3327, 1982.

Kerstein MD. Heat illness in hot/humid environment. *Milit Med* 151:308, 1986.

Kilbourne EM et al. Risk factors for heatstroke. *JAMA* 247:3362, 1982.

Knochel JP. Environmental heat illness: An eclectic review. *Arch Intern Med* 133:841, 1974.

Knochel JP. Dog days and siriasis: How to kill a football player. *JAMA* 233:513, 1975.

Kunkel DB. The ills of heat. Part I: Environmental causes. *Emerg Med* 18(14):173, 1986.

Larkin JT. Treatment of heat-related illness. *JAMA* 245:570, 1981.

Parks FB, Calabro JJ. Hyperthermia: Performing when the heat is on. *JEMS* 15(8):24, 1990.

Porter AM. Heat illness and soldiers. *Milit Med* 158:606, 1993.

Sawka MN et al. Influence of hydration level and body fluids on exercise performance in the heat. *JAMA* 252:1165, 1984.

Slovis CM, Anderson GF, Casolaro A. Survival in a heat stroke victim with a core temperature in excess of 46.5°C. *Ann Emerg Med* 11:269, 1982.

Sprung CL. Heat stroke: Modern approach to an ancient disease. *Chest* 77:461, 1980.

Stine RJ. Heat illness. *JACEP* 8:154, 1979.

Surpure JS. Heat-related illness and the automobile. *Ann Emerg Med* 11:263, 1982.

Tintinalli JE. Heat stroke. *JACEP* 5:525, 1976.

Wettach JE, Smith DS, Stalling CE. EMS protocol for management of heat emergencies during a heat wave in an urban population. *EMT J* 5(5):328, 1981.

32
Cold Exposure

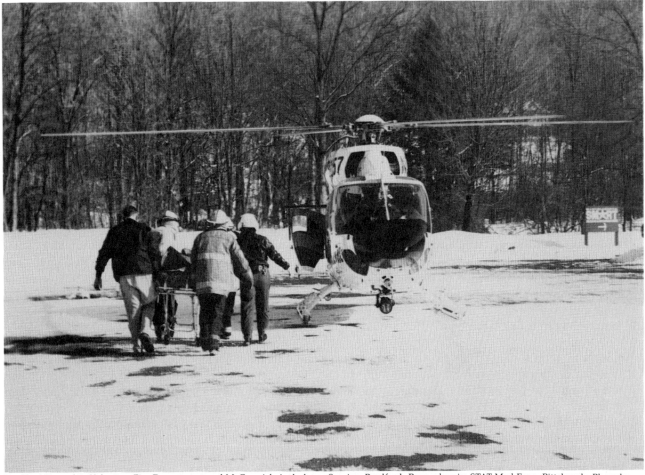

Bradford Township Volunteer Fire Department and McCormick Ambulance Service, Bradford, Pennsylvania; STAT Med Evac, Pittsburgh. Photo by Jay K. Bradish.

OBJECTIVES

Man was not designed for cold climates. Our forebears first appeared on earth in the equatorial regions; and although many of us have since strayed from the semitropical environment where mankind was born, we are not really well equipped to endure prolonged exposure to the cold. Approximately 700 Americans die each year from cold exposure. The vast majority of those deaths do not take place in exotic circumstances such as alpine blizzards. Most cold exposure deaths in fact occur in urban settings, often indoors, in poorly heated apartments. Thus cold exposure is of concern not only to paramedics on ski patrol but also to those patrolling the streets of the city.

In this chapter, we shall examine the ways that the body tries to defend itself from extremes of cold and the types of injuries that occur when the body's defenses against the cold are overwhelmed. By the end of this chapter, the student should be able to

1. Describe four ways in which heat is lost from the body, and describe how heat loss by each of those mechanisms can be retarded or prevented
2. List three mechanisms the body uses to defend itself against heat loss in a cold environment
3. List at least four risk factors for
   • Frostbite
   • Hypothermia
4. Given a description of several patients with different signs and symptoms, identify a patient with
   • Frost nip
   • Superficial frostbite
   • Deep frostbite
   and describe the correct prehospital management of each
5. Describe the changes that occur in the major systems of the body as the body temperature falls
6. Given a description of several patients with different signs and symptoms, identify a patient with
   • Moderate hypothermia
   • Severe hypothermia
   • Immersion hypothermia
   and describe the correct prehospital management of each
7. List five actions that can trigger ventricular fibrillation in a hypothermic patient
8. List at least five measures a paramedic can take to minimize his or her risk of suffering cold injury

KEEPING WARM IN A COLD WORLD

The human body likes to maintain an internal temperature very close to 37°C (98.6°F). In the previous chapter, we learned about some of the strategies the body uses to avoid overheating in a hot environment. We now need to look at some of the ways the body tries to defend its core temperature against cooling when exposed to cold temperatures.

How the Body Loses Heat

It is useful first to review how heat escapes from the body. When a person is placed in a cold environment, heat can be lost from the body in several ways, most of which we have already learned something about:

• RADIATION: Any object, including the human body, that is warmer than the surrounding environment can give off heat into the surrounding air as infrared radiation. Normally, the body dissipates about 65 percent of its heat by this mechanism. Heat loss from radiation can occur from any part of the body, but it is most prominent above the shoulders. Indeed, on a cold day, over half of the heat generated by the body can be lost through an uncovered head or neck—so when your mother wouldn't let you out the door on a winter day without a hat and scarf, she knew what she was talking about.
• CONDUCTION: Heat can also be lost by the direct transfer of heat from the body to a cold substance. Air is a poor conductor of heat. The ground is a good conductor. Water is even better, and a person who falls into a cold lake will lose heat 20 times faster than a dry individual exposed to air of the same temperature. You don't have to fall into a lake to get wet, however. Clothing soaked with rain, snow, or perspiration can be just as dangerous, for it will also rapidly conduct heat away from the body.
• CONVECTION: Still air is a poor conductor of heat. But air moving across the body surface can pick up heat and carry it away. The faster the air is moving, the faster it can remove heat from the body, so a windy, cold day is more likely to produce cold injury than a windless day of the same temperature. For that reason, we talk about the **windchill factor,** which measures the chilling effect of a given temperature at a given wind speed. For instance, the chilling effect of a 30°F temperature with a 35 mile per hour wind is −4°F; that is, the effect on an exposed person is

just as if the temperature were actually 4 below zero on a day without any wind. The windchill factor can be determined using a standard table (Table 32-1), which allows rescuers to estimate the degree of cold to which a person was exposed.

- EVAPORATION: Heat is required to convert water from a liquid to a gas; as moisture evaporates from the body surface, therefore, heat is lost from the body. Evaporative heat loss may occur, for example, when one's clothing becomes wet from sweating or from rain and then gradually dries. Wet clothes, then, are doubly hazardous in the cold: While they are still wet, they promote heat loss by conduction; as they dry, they cause further heat loss by evaporation.
- RESPIRATION: When cold air is inhaled into the lungs, its temperature is raised to body temperature. When that air is then exhaled, it carries the heat along with it out into the atmosphere.

Clearly the body has a variety of ways to lose heat, as befits an organism originally designed for a semitropical environment. How, then, does anyone living outside a semitropical environment ever manage to stay warm?

How the Body Defends Itself from Heat Loss

Fortunately, the human body does have some ways of keeping warm in a cold environment, so that a stroll on a winter day is not inevitably a fatal undertaking.

One way the body can maintain its internal temperature when exposed to the cold is to INCREASE HEAT PRODUCTION. The hypothalamus, which stays in close touch with both the body core and the skin, is programmed to reset the internal thermostat when the skin temperature falls considerably below the internal temperature. The rate of basal metabolism is increased, and more thermal energy is produced. In addition, increases in muscular activity can jack up heat production considerably. Shivering, for example, will increase the body's heat production about 500 percent, while strenuous exercise can bring about increases in heat production of anywhere from 1,000 to 2,000 percent.

Besides increasing the amount of heat it produces, the body can also DECREASE HEAT LOSS to the environment. To understand how that is accomplished, we need to think of the human body as consisting of two parts: a core and a shell (Fig. 32-1). The **core** comprises the vital internal organs, such as the brain, heart, lungs, and abdominal viscera, whose temperature must be maintained within very narrow limits to ensure normal function. The **shell** includes the skin, muscles, and the extremities, which can tolerate relatively wide temperature variations.

Because it is critical to maintain a stable core temperature, the body will do so at the expense of surface temperature. In conditions of cold, blood vessels supplying the surface of the body constrict, thereby reducing the amount of blood flow to the body's outer layer. Heat is thus hoarded deep within the

TABLE 32-1. WINDCHILL FACTOR

WIND SPEED (MPH)	DEGREES FAHRENHEIT													WIND DESCRIPTION
	35	30	25	20	15	10	5	0	−5	−10	−15	−20	−25	−30	
0–5	35	30	25	20	15	10	5	0	−5	−10	−15	−20	−25	−30	Calm; no breeze
5	33	27	21	16	12	7	1	−6	−11	−15	−20	−26	−31	−35	Leaves rustle
10	21	16	9	2	−2	−9	−15	−22	−27	−31	−38	−45	−52	−58	Leaves move
15	16	11	1	−6	−11	−18	−25	−33	−40	−45	−51	−60	−65	−70	Dust raised; paper blows
20	12	3	−4	−9	−17	−24	−32	−40	−46	−52	−60	−68	−76	−81	Small branches move
25	7	0	−7	−15	−22	−29	−37	−45	−52	−58	−67	−75	−83	−89	Small trees sway
30	5	−2	−11	−18	−26	−33	−41	−49	−56	−63	−70	−78	−87	−94	Large branches move
35	3	−4	−13	−20	−27	−35	−43	−52	−60	−67	−72	−83	−90	−98	Whole trees swaying
40	1	−4	−15	−22	−29	−36	−45	−54	−62	−69	−76	−87	−94	−101	Twigs torn from trees

VERY COLD   BITTER COLD   EXTREME COLD

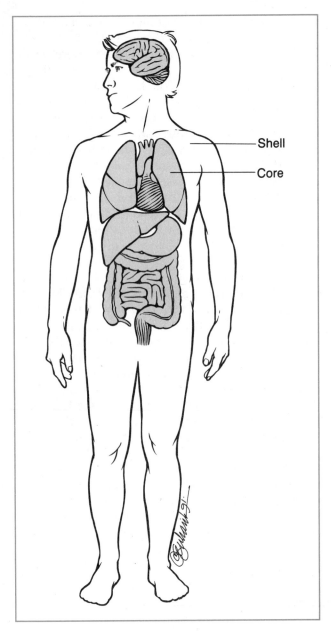

FIGURE 32-1.   THE BODY IN A COLD ENVIRONMENT shunts blood from the periphery to create an outer, insulating SHELL of skin, subcutaneous tissue, and skeletal muscle and an inner, warmed CORE of vital organs.

body and kept away from the skin, where it would otherwise be dissipated by convection, radiation, and so on. In addition, sweating is decreased or stops altogether in the cold. The net effect is that the skin and subcutaneous tissues function as a cool, dry shell that provides insulation for the vital core. The thicker the shell, the better the insulation, so fat people are relatively more protected from the cold than are skinny people.

The effects of exposure to cold on any given person will depend on the balance between the body's heat loss and heat production:

Heat Loss	Heat Production and Retention
RADIATION	INCREASED HEAT
CONVECTION	PRODUCTION
CONDUCTION	Increased basal metabolic rate
EVAPORATIVE	Shivering
COOLING	Muscular exertion
RESPIRATION	PERIPHERAL
	VASOCONSTRICTION

If heat loss occurs at a faster rate than heat production, injury from the cold will occur—either localized injury to an isolated part of the body or generalized cooling.

LOCAL COLD INJURY

Most injuries from the cold are localized to the extremities or exposed parts of the body, such as the face. Local freezing injuries fall under the general heading of **frostbite.** Like burns, frostbite can be superficial or deep, depending on the intensity of the cold and the duration of the exposure. The mildest form of cold injury, sometimes called **frost nip,** or first-degree frostbite, usually involves exposed or poorly insulated parts of the body, such as the tips of the ears, nose, upper cheek, and tips of the fingers or toes. Frost nip comes on slowly and generally is not painful, so the victim tends to be unaware of its occurrence unless he or she should glance into a mirror and notice an unusual pallor of the nose or ears. The problem is easily treated by placing a warm hand firmly over the chilled nose or ear or, when the fingers are frost-nipped, by placing the fingers into the armpit. The return of warmth to a frost-nipped area is usually signalled by some redness and tingling, but tissue damage rarely occurs.

Deeper degrees of frostbite involve actual freezing of tissues and can therefore occur only in ambient temperatures well below freezing. Cells are composed chiefly of water, and when cells are subjected to low enough temperatures, the water within them literally turns into ice crystals, which can damage or destroy the cells. Again, the most commonly affected areas of the body are the hands, feet, ears, and nose, all of which are distant from the warm body core and also prone to rapid heat loss because of large surface area.

There are several factors that *predispose* a person to develop frostbite:

HOW TO GET FROSTBITTEN

- Go out on a cold, windy day without earmuffs, mittens, a scarf, or a hat.
- Impede the circulation to your extremities:
  1. Wear tight gloves, tight shoes, and tight clothing.
  2. Lace your boots very tightly.
  3. Wear plastic boots that won't expand, preferably lined with felt, which *will* expand when wet.
  4. Smoke, so that your arteries will constrict.
- Go out in the cold when you are tired, dehydrated, or hungry.
- Hold onto cold metal objects.
- Spill organic solvents or gasoline on your clothing in subzero temperatures.
- Allow yourself to become thoroughly chilled; generalized hypothermia is the most effective way to sustain local cold injury.

Superficial Frostbite

Superficial, or second-degree, frostbite is by definition limited to the skin and subcutaneous tissues, like a second-degree burn. The *skin* typically appears WHITE AND WAXY. Because it is frozen, the skin is STIFF to palpation, but the *underlying tissues* remain soft. Sensation is generally absent, so the patient will usually report that the affected area feels NUMB. As *thawing* occurs, the injured area turns a MOTTLED BLUE, and the patient experiences a hot, stinging sensation. Leakage of plasma from damaged capillaries produces EDEMA in the frostbitten area, and BLISTERS develop within a few hours after thawing. Dull or throbbing pain may persist for days or even weeks after the injury, and the injured area usually becomes extremely sensitive to any subsequent exposure to cold.

The prehospital treatment of superficial frostbite differs significantly from that of deep frostbite, so it is very important to try to distinguish between the two. Usually it is difficult to determine the depth of the injury when you first see it, for even a shallow frostbite injury can appear like one that is frozen solid. If the tissues beneath the skin are soft when you press down on the skin surface, however, the

frostbite is probably superficial. If not, or if there is any doubt, treat the injury as deep frostbite (see next section).

Treatment of Superficial Frostbite

Once you have determined that the patient is suffering from superficial frostbite only, proceed as follows:

- GET THE PATIENT OUT OF THE COLD. Take him indoors or into a heated ambulance, so that the body can stop hoarding its warm blood in the core and can afford to send some of that warm blood out to the periphery, where it is urgently needed.
- REWARM THE INJURED PART WITH BODY HEAT. If an ear, nose, or foot is frostbitten, apply firm, steady pressure against the area with a warm hand. If a hand is frostbitten, have the patient insert the hand into his armpit and hold it there without moving. Do *not* try to rewarm a frostbitten part with radiant or dry heat.
- DO NOT RUB OR MASSAGE A FROSTBITTEN AREA, for massage will only cause further damage to injured tissues.
- COVER BLISTERS WITH A DRY, STERILE DRESSING, and protect the area from further injury. Do *not* put goo on frostbitten skin.
- TRANSPORT the patient to the hospital with the injured area elevated and protected from the cold.

Deep Frostbite

Deep frostbite usually involves the hands or the feet. It is a very serious injury, which can, if improperly handled, lead to the necessity to amputate part or all of a limb. A frozen extremity looks WHITE, yellow-white, or mottled blue-white, and it is HARD, COLD, and completely INSENSITIVE TO TOUCH. The major tissue damage occurs not from the freezing of the tissues but rather when the tissues thaw out, particularly if thawing occurs gradually. When tissues thaw slowly, there is often partial refreezing of melted water, and the new ice crystals produced tend to be much larger than those formed during the original freeze, so they cause even greater tissue damage. As thawing occurs, the injured area turns purple and becomes excruciatingly painful. Gangrene may set in within a few days, requiring amputation of the injured part.

Treatment of Deep Frostbite

The prehospital treatment of deep frostbite depends upon two factors: (1) whether the injured extremity has already been partially or completely thawed before you arrive and (2) how far the victim is from the hospital. Let us consider the possible scenarios one at a time.

- *If the extremity is still frozen* when you find the patient, it is preferable to leave it frozen until the patient reaches the hospital, for rapid rewarming is extremely difficult to carry out properly in the field. If, therefore, you are within about an hour's drive of a medical facility:
  1. LEAVE THE FROZEN EXTREMITY FROZEN. So long as the limb is not thawed, the patient may even walk on it if necessary.
  2. Once you get the patient into the ambulance, PAD THE INJURED EXTREMITY to protect the tissues from further trauma, and KEEP THE EXTREMITY AWAY FROM THE HEATER or any other sources of dry heat.
  3. DO NOT UNDER ANY CIRCUMSTANCES RUB SNOW OR ICE ONTO A FROSTBITTEN EXTREMITY.
  4. DO NOT MASSAGE THE EXTREMITY. The cells are full of ice crystals, and massaging the extremity will simply cause those ice crystals to lacerate delicate tissues.
  5. NOTIFY the receiving hospital of your estimated time of arrival (ETA), so that they can start preparing a rewarming bath for the patient.
  6. TRANSPORT without delay.
- *If the extremity is already partially thawed or if you are several hours from the hospital,*
  1. REWARM THE INJURED EXTREMITY before transport. To do so, you will need a water bath—a large, clean container in which the extremity can be immersed without touching the container's side or bottom. Water should be heated in a second container and then stirred into the water bath until the temperature of the bath is between 38 and 42°C (100–108°F). While you are heating the water, ADMINISTER MORPHINE SULFATE, 0.1 mg per kilogram IV. The patient will experience very severe pain as the limb thaws out, and you want to mitigate that pain as much as possible.

     When the water bath has reached the appropriate temperature, gently immerse the injured extremity. Keep a thermometer in the water, and when the water temperature falls below 38°C, temporarily remove the injured extremity from the bath while you add more

hot water to the container. Stir the water around and keep adding more hot water until the bath is again in the right temperature range; then reimmerse the injured extremity.

> **THE TEMPERATURE IN THE WATER BATH MUST BE KEPT AT A CONSTANT 38 TO 42°C.**

A temperature that is either lower or higher than that range will cause further damage to the limb.

   The rewarming procedure may require 30 to 60 minutes. It is complete when the frozen area is warm to the touch and is deep red or bluish in color (and remains red when you remove the limb from the water bath). While rewarming is in progress, the patient should be kept warm, preferably indoors, with insulated clothing and blankets. Do not permit the patient to smoke, for nicotine causes vasoconstriction and thus interferes with blood flow to the injured area.
  2. Once rewarming is complete, DRY THE EXTREMITY very gently with sterile dressings.
  3. APPLY STERILE DRESSINGS *lightly* over the thawed parts, taking care not to rupture any blisters. Use soft, sterile gauze or cotton to separate frostbitten fingers or toes. Do *not* put goo on frostbitten skin.
  4. TRANSPORT the patient supine, and ELEVATE THE INJURED EXTREMITY on soft pillows, well covered to protect it from the cold.

A word of caution:

> **DO NOT ATTEMPT REWARMING IN THE FIELD IF THERE IS ANY POSSIBILITY OF REFREEZING.**

The potential damage from refreezing is far greater than the potential damage from the limb remaining frozen. So if circumstances will not permit you to keep the extremity thawed out, leave it frozen.

To summarize, then, the principles of treatment in frostbite, remember the frostbite "don'ts":

THE FROSTBITE DON'TS

- DON'T rub snow on a frostbitten part.
- DON'T massage or rub a frostbitten area.
- DON'T rewarm with dry or radiant heat.
- DON'T rupture blisters.
- DON'T apply ointments.
- DON'T apply tight bandages.
- DON'T allow a thawed extremity to refreeze.
- DON'T handle a frostbitten extremity roughly.
- DON'T allow the victim to smoke.

GENERAL COOLING

Generalized cooling of the body, or **hypothermia,** is caused by prolonged or intense exposure to low temperatures. The old term for the condition, "exposure," conjures up images of a lone traveller stranded in a howling blizzard. The reality is, however, that most cases of hypothermia do not occur in howling blizzards, and in fact, temperatures need not even be below freezing for hypothermic death to occur. Indeed, most incidents of hypothermia take place in an urban environment in temperatures of between 30 and 50°F (−1 to 10°C). That fact has important implications for EMS personnel. For while it may not take a genius to suspect hypothermia in a hiker found unconscious in the snow, the diagnosis of hypothermia may be considerably less obvious to warmly dressed paramedics called to a slightly chilly apartment for an elderly woman with slurred speech.

People at Risk

Those at greatest risk of suffering hypothermia include the elderly, the very young, alcoholics, people with chronic illnesses, and those who engage in outdoor activities in winter (hikers, campers, hunters).

Most vulnerable to hypothermia are the ELDERLY, especially (but not exclusively) the impoverished elderly exposed to continuous cold in poorly heated homes. The capacity of an elderly person to *generate* heat is less than that of a younger person because of reduced muscle mass and a diminished shivering response. Atrophy of subcutaneous fat also reduces their insulation against heat *loss.* Medications commonly prescribed to the elderly may interfere with their ability to shunt blood away from the skin by vasoconstriction. Finally, the malnutrition and chronic illnesses that so often accompany the aging process may further contribute to an elderly person's vulnerability.

At the other end of the age spectrum, INFANTS AND VERY YOUNG CHILDREN are also at increased risk of hypothermia. Infants have a proportionally larger body surface area with respect to their mass than adults and thus a proportionally larger area exposed to cooling. They also have a less developed mechanism for temperature regulation and a less effective shivering response. So an infant will cool much faster than an adult at any given temperature. Furthermore, even at relatively warm ambient temperatures, infants and small children rapidly become hypothermic in response to shock.

Probably the highest incidence of hypothermia in any given community occurs among CHRONIC ALCOHOLICS. Intoxication dulls a person's sensitivity to cold, so the alcoholic may fall asleep in exposed areas. Alcohol interferes with internal heat *production* by inhibiting shivering. The poor nutritional status of most alcoholics further impairs metabolic heat generation. In addition, alcohol produces peripheral vasodilatation, so it undermines the body's attempts to create an insulating shell around a warm core. Finally, alcohol impairs judgment, which often leads to inappropriate behavior in cold conditions.

A variety of CHRONIC ILLNESSES can also render a person more vulnerable to hypothermia. Diabetes and hypothyroidism, for example, involve derangements in carbohydrate metabolism that impair the ability to adjust internal heat production in response to cold.

Finally, hypothermia can also occur in the young and fit—especially among CAMPERS, HIKERS, HUNTERS, and FISHERMEN—who are stranded outdoors in severe weather. In such individuals, poor judgment, poor survival skills, inadequate clothing and shelter, overexertion, and insufficient intake of water and carbohydrates all markedly increase the risk of suffering hypothermia. For that reason, hypothermia has earned the designation among outdoorsmen as "the killer of the unprepared."

The Pathophysiology of Cooling

Just as the body has mechanisms to protect itself from overheating, so too there are regulatory mechanisms to defend the core temperature against cooling. Even a slight drop in body temperature triggers the regulatory system to turn up the heat through (1) *shivering,* which generates heat through muscular activity, and (2) cutaneous *vasoconstriction,* which shunts blood away from the skin and the cold environment to which the skin is exposed. If the body temperature continues to drop, the *basal metabolic rate* is cranked up in a further effort to increase heat production.

The Descent into Hypothermia

There are limits to the body's ability to defend itself against the cold, and as the core temperature falls below about 95°F (35°C), the regulatory system falters. Ventilation slows as the respiratory control center becomes depressed. Progressive anoxia retards metabolism, and a vicious cycle is set in motion: As metabolic heat production decreases, the core temperature falls lower, respiration is further depressed, anoxia increases, and metabolism is thereby further impaired.

By the time the core temperature falls to around 83°F (28.3°C), the regulatory mechanisms are entirely overwhelmed, and the myocardium is in severe jeopardy. Atrial fibrillation is common at this point, and anoxic death is close by. Ventilation shortly ceases entirely; and lacking oxygen to fuel the metabolic heat generators, the body temperature begins dropping even faster. The lower limit of survival is said to be a core temperature of about 74°F (23.3°C), although most patients with accidental hypothermia succumb long before they reach that point. However, one survival has been reported of a patient whose core temperature plummeted to 50°F (10°C) and who, when found, had been in cardiac arrest for an hour. That case illustrates an important point: The hypothermic patient should not be written off even when, by ordinary standards, he seems entirely and irretrievably dead.

When the core temperature falls below 86°F (30°C), heart sounds may not be audible even if the heart is still beating, for tissues conduct sound poorly at low temperatures. Similarly, it may be impossible to hear the Korotkoff sounds to measure a blood pressure. Pupillary reflexes, furthermore, are likely to be blocked. Thus a patient who in fact still has a heart beat may present like one in cardiac arrest, without a detectable pulse and with fixed and dilated pupils. Even when true cardiac arrest has occurred, the usual prognostic indicators do not apply. At 86°F (30°C), the brain can survive without perfusion for about 10 minutes; at 68°F (20°C), it may be able to manage for 25 to 30 minutes without perfusion. The lesson is that patients with accidental hypothermia merit extraordinary resuscitative efforts; they may not be as dead as they appear.

The sequence of events described can develop within a few minutes when a person falls into cold water, within an hour or two of exposure to very cold weather, or over several days in elderly or chronically ill people who have continuous exposure to moderately cold temperatures. However rapidly or slowly hypothermia comes on, though, the underlying problem is the same: a depression in core body temperature that endangers the body's vital functions.

Effects of Hypothermia on Specific Body Systems

The net effect of hypothermia is to slow things down, but different body systems slow down in different ways.

The overall slowdown of function is perhaps most dramatically apparent in the CENTRAL NERVOUS SYSTEM, where just about everything slows down—thinking, feeling, speaking. The hypothermic patient is typically apathetic and often shows an impaired ability to reason. His speech is slow and may be slurred; his coordination is impaired; his gait is ataxic. All told, the picture can closely resemble that of stroke, head injury, or alcohol intoxication, which is probably the reason that so many cases of hypothermia are initially (and sometimes tragically) misdiagnosed.

In the CARDIOVASCULAR SYSTEM, hypothermia induces several changes, none of them salutary. To begin with, as peripheral vasoconstriction shunts blood to the body core, the body's volume receptors interpret the increased core blood flow as an increase in volume. So they telegraph the kidneys, "Dump some fluid; we're getting waterlogged here." Obediently, the kidneys start producing more urine (**cold diuresis**). At the same time, cooling of the tissues induces a flow of water from the intravascular to the extravascular spaces. The net effect is to increase the viscosity of the blood, thereby impairing circulation, and to produce a state of dehydration. Meanwhile, the heart is also suffering from the drop in body temperature. Cold slows the heart rate and disrupts the electric conduction system, producing a variety of cardiac dysrhythmias. Of most concern is *ventricular fibrillation* (VF), to which a hypothermic heart is extremely susceptible. It takes very little to cause a cold heart to fibrillate (Table 32-2); and once the heart does fibrillate, defibrillation is almost impossible until the heart has been rewarmed to near normal temperatures.

In the RESPIRATORY SYSTEM, as noted earlier, the respiratory rate slows, leading to a decrease in minute volume. Tracheobronchial secretions increase, but at the same time the cough and gag reflexes become sluggish; so secretions collect within the airway, producing loud, gurgling noises that usually send paramedics lunging for a suction catheter. In the hypothermic patient, however, the benefits of suctioning must be weighed against the potential

TABLE 32-2. TRIGGERS OF VENTRICULAR FIBRILLATION IN HYPOTHERMIA

- Physical exertion (by the victim who is still conscious)
- Insertion of an oropharyngeal airway
- Endotracheal intubation
- Respiratory alkalosis, from overzealous artificial ventilation
- Metabolic alkalosis, from sodium bicarbonate administration
- Insertion of a large-bore needle into a central vein
- Precordial thump
- Unwarranted cardiopulmonary resuscitation
- Sympathomimetic drugs, such as epinephrine or isoproterenol
- Rapid external warming
- Rough handling during lifting or transport

Source: Adapted from Wilkerson JA (ed). *Hypothermia, Frostbite, and Other Cold Injuries.* Seattle: Mountaineers, 1986.

danger of inducing ventricular fibrillation by stimulating the back of the throat.

The MUSCULAR SYSTEM also slows down in response to cold. Although the initial muscular reaction to cold is shivering, that reaction is a mixed blessing. It does generate heat. But it also makes skilled movements, such as lighting a fire, more difficult. Shivering, in any case, ceases when the body temperature falls below around 91°F (32.7°C). Thereafter, cold muscles become progressively weaker and stiffer, further impairing the exposed person's ability to take steps to save himself.

Finally, cold affects the body's METABOLISM. Shivering quickly depletes the body of glucose, leading to *hypoglycemia*. Meanwhile, insulin levels fall, making further glucose metabolism impossible, so the body switches to the metabolism of fat. In much the same way as it occurs in diabetics who have not taken enough insulin, the metabolism of fat in hypothermic patients results in the production of ketoacids, and the patient's breath therefore develops a fruity odor that can be mistaken for the odor of alcohol. The liver's metabolism of drugs is also affected by the cold, and medications administered to a hypothermic patient are metabolized much more slowly than normal, so the effects of medications last much longer.

Hypothermia, then, affects every system of the body and threatens the whole organism. Treatment depends on making an estimation of how cold the patient is. Most standard rectal thermometers do not register below around 92°F (33.3°C), so the prehospital determination of the patient's degree of hypothermia must usually be made on the basis of his signs and symptoms. For purposes of management,

it is useful to categorize victims of hypothermia according to whether they have suffered mild to moderate hypothermia or severe hypothermia.

Mild to Moderate Hypothermia

The patient with mild to moderate hypothermia (rectal temperature 94–84°F, or 34–29°C) is still CONSCIOUS, although he or she may be lethargic and apathetic. SHIVERING is often prominent. The *skin* is likely to be PALE AND COLD, and there may be an ACETONE ODOR on the patient's breath. That is the most common presentation when an elderly person is found in a poorly heated home, and the patient's confusion and lethargy are very likely to be mistaken for signs of a stroke.

Treatment of the Patient with Moderate Hypothermia

The treatment of moderate hypothermia is aimed at preventing further heat loss and rewarming the patient as rapidly as possible. To accomplish that, one must first

- MOVE THE PATIENT TO A PROTECTED AREA. If you cannot get the patient indoors, at least get him *out of the wind,* into a tent or other sheltered area. When triaging a group of exposure victims, PRIORITY GOES TO THE SKINNY, for they have the least natural insulation against the cold. Entrapped victims must be protected from further exposure until they can be moved; use any available materials to shield them from the wind and insulate them from cold surfaces.
- As soon as the victim is in a sheltered area, REPLACE ALL WET CLOTHING WITH DRY GARMENTS. Remember, moisture conducts heat away from the body much more efficiently than dry cloth; so long as the victim stays in his wet clothes, therefore, rapid heat loss will continue.
- Once the patient is in dry clothing, wrap him with any available INSULATING MATERIALS, and then cover the insulating materials with blankets. Do not place his arms and legs in direct contact with his body but rather outside the first layer of insulating material. Be sure to cover the patient's head and neck, but leave his face unobstructed.
- KEEP THE PATIENT RECUMBENT, with insulating material between him and the surface on which he is lying (e.g., several layers of folded blankets between the patient and the backboard).
- If you are at any distance from the hospital, PROVIDE EXTERNAL HEAT to prevent a further

drop in the patient's temperature. When the emergency occurs in the patient's home, the best rewarming method is to immerse the patient up to his neck in a tub of water at about 105°F (40.5°C), for conduction is the most efficient method of heat transfer. When the victim is in the wilderness, or anywhere else outdoors (e.g., trapped in a wrecked vehicle), immersion in a bathtub will not be feasible. In that case, apply hot water bottles or chemical hot packs, wrapped in towels, behind the victim's neck, in the armpits, and over the groin to promote core rewarming. Do *not* place hot water bottles or chemical heating pads over the extremities, and do *not* apply them directly to the skin.

- GIVE WARM FLUIDS CONTAINING LOTS OF SUGAR by mouth, along with other carbohydrate calorie sources, such as candy bars. The warm fluids probably do not, in fact, contribute very much to raising the patient's core temperature; but warm drinks make the patient *feel* warmer and therefore more at ease. Avoid hot drinks that contain caffeine, however, such as regular coffee, tea, or cocoa. Caffeine has diuretic actions, and most hypothermic patients are already dehydrated.
- DO NOT GIVE ALCOHOLIC BEVERAGES, no matter what you have seen in the movies about St. Bernard dogs carrying casks of brandy to snowbound victims. Alcohol impairs shivering, dilates peripheral vessels, and decreases the victim's level of consciousness.
- In patients rescued from exposure outdoors, CHECK CAREFULLY FOR OTHER INJURIES besides hypothermia, especially frostbite. Bear in mind that fractures are apt to go unnoticed in a hypothermic patient because cold renders the patient relatively insensitive to pain. So examine all the extremities, and check peripheral pulses and neurologic status. Splint suspected fractures before moving the patient.
- TRANSPORT the patient well insulated, from head to toe, ideally in a down sleeping bag or similar device.

Paramedics working in regions where winter wilderness rescue operations are routine should carry specialized gear for the prehospital management of moderate hypothermia. The *hydraulic sarong,* for example, is a thin, double-layered blanket with a network of plastic tubing running between the two layers. The blanket is wrapped around the hypothermia victim, and water heated over a camp stove is pumped through the tubing, thereby heating the blanket and warming the patient around whom it is wrapped. Other devices have been developed to facilitate the administration of *heated, humidified oxygen* in order to counteract respiratory heat loss from the body.

Severe Hypothermia

The patient with severe hypothermia (rectal temperature below 84°F, or about 29°C) is STUPOROUS OR UNCONSCIOUS. His skin is ice cold, his muscles are rigid (there is *no* shivering), and his heart sounds may be entirely inaudible (recall that cold tissues are poor conductors of sound). It may be impossible to obtain a blood pressure measurement; respirations are likely to be exceedingly slow, often only about 2 to 3 per minute; and the pupils are often entirely unreactive to light.

Rewarming is critical to save the life of such a patient, but the kind of core rewarming required is nearly impossible to carry out in the field. The only kind of rewarming that might be feasible in the field—slow external rewarming—will not help and can, in fact, make the situation even worse by precipitating a condition called **rewarming shock.** Rewarming shock occurs when the body shell is warmed before the core. As the shell rewarms, blood vessels near the body surface start to dilate, and blood from the core floods into them. The heart, however, is still too cold to rev up sufficiently to deal with the suddenly increased circulation, and it gets even colder as the blood that flooded out of the cool periphery returns to the right atrium. The result is a sharp drop in blood pressure and often ventricular fibrillation as well. The message in all that is:

DO NOT SPEND TIME IN THE FIELD TRYING TO REWARM A SEVERELY HYPOTHERMIC PATIENT.

Move the patient as expeditiously as possible to a medical facility, with stabilizing measures en route.

Treatment of Severe Hypothermia

Throughout your management of the severely hypothermic patient, keep in mind that he or she is very vulnerable to cardiac arrest from ventricular fibrillation and, mentally at least, place a large red sign over the patient reading, FRAGILE: HANDLE WITH CARE! The slightest jolt may trigger fibrillation.

- Maintain the AIRWAY by manual methods (head tilt–chin lift). DO NOT USE AIRWAY ADJUNCTS, such as an oropharyngeal airway, for they may stimulate the back of the throat and precipitate ventricular fibrillation. If endotracheal intubation is required to provide effective ventilation, preoxygenate the patient for at least 3 minutes with 100% oxygen via bag-valve-mask. Have everything set up and ready to go for a smooth, rapid intubation.
- If the victim is not BREATHING, you will have to provide artificial ventilation, but KEEP THE VENTILATORY RATE SLOW—no more than about 5 to 10 breaths per minute—for hyperventilation may also trigger cardiac arrest.
- Administer warmed, humidified OXYGEN if you have the means to do so, either by mask or, if you are assisting ventilations, by bag-valve-mask.
- MONITOR the patient's cardiac rhythm, and start external chest compressions if you see asystole or ventricular fibrillation on the 'scope. In severely hypothermic patients, you cannot rely on the pulse, because a pulse may not be palpable in cold tissues even when the heart is beating. So use the monitor to decide when to start CPR.
- *If ventricular fibrillation occurs*, GIVE BASIC LIFE SUPPORT ONLY. You may try a sequence of three defibrillatory shocks (200 joules → 300 joules → 360 joules); but if ventricular fibrillation persists after three shocks, do not make any further attempts to defibrillate, for repeated shocks will just damage the hypothermic myocardium. Don't bother either giving intravenous medications, because in all probability they are not going to work so long as the patient is hypothermic. Just continue CPR all the way to the the hospital. Once you have started CPR on a hypothermic patient, DON'T GIVE UP! Even if the patient appears entirely dead, there is every chance of a successful resuscitation; for the same low temperatures that put the heart into fibrillation protect the brain against the effects of hypoxia. The outcome of CPR cannot be properly assessed until after the patient has been fully rewarmed, thus the adage:

THE HYPOTHERMIC PATIENT ISN'T DEAD UNTIL HE IS WARM AND DEAD.

- If the victim's clothing is wet, CUT AWAY WET CLOTHING; don't try to pull it off. Undressing the patient in the usual fashion will cause too much motion.
- If you are able to do so, START A PERIPHERAL IV with NORMAL SALINE. Do not use lactated Ringer's because the cold liver may not be able to metabolize lactate. While you are getting set up, let the IV bag sit on the dashboard over the vehicle's heater or on any other warm object. Then tape a chemical hot pack around the IV bag, and coil the administration set tubing around another hot pack to warm the fluid reaching the patient. Run in about 300 ml with the IV wide open, and finish up the liter over the next 20 to 30 minutes.
- NOTIFY the receiving hospital of your patient's status and ETA, so that they can begin preparing rewarming equipment.
- TRANSPORT the patient in a slightly HEAD-DOWN POSITION, that is, with the foot of the stretcher tilted upward about 10 degrees so that the victim's head is lower than his feet. Whoever is doing the driving should avoid sudden stops and starts and watch out for bumps on the road. A bump in the road may literally "bump off" the patient!

The treatment of moderate and severe hypothermia is summarized in Table 32-3.

Immersion Hypothermia

One specific type of hypothermia deserves separate mention, and that is hypothermia caused by immersion in water. Immersion hypothermia is not exclusively a problem of cold climates or winter weather; for even in quite warm climates, water temperatures in oceans, lakes, or swift-running rivers can fall below 70°F (21°C), and that's all that is necessary to cause significant body cooling.

The problems in immersion hypothermia are basically the same as those in any other form of hypothermia, but they develop much faster. Only 15 to 20 minutes' immersion in water less than 50°F (10°C) can be sufficient to cause ventricular fibrillation and death. Furthermore, a person's instinctive behavior in water can actually hasten his own demise. Someone who attempts to swim, for example, will accelerate his body's cooling rate by at least 35 percent; and conventional "drown-proofing" techniques, which put the victim's head in the water, increase the rate of heat loss by about 80 percent. That is because every movement the victim makes requires him to perfuse his cold peripheral muscles with

TABLE 32-3.   MANAGEMENT OF MODERATE AND SEVERE HYPOTHERMIA

	MODERATE HYPOTHERMIA	SEVERE HYPOTHERMIA
Rectal temperature	94 to 84°F (34.4–28.9°C).	Below 84°F (28.9°C).
Signs	CONSCIOUS, but usually apathetic, lethargic. Often shivering; skin pale and cold to touch. May have acetone odor to breath. Suspect hypothermia in any elderly or chronically ill patient found in an environment less than 50°F (10°C).	UNCONSCIOUS OR STUPOROUS. Skin ice cold. Heart sounds inaudible; BP unobtainable. Pupils unreactive. Very slow respirations.
Field treatment	Get the patient out of the cold. Replace wet clothing with dry clothing. Cover with insulating materials and blankets. Heating pads (wrapped in towels) may be applied to armpits, groin, abdomen. If far from the hospital and facilities permit, immerse the patient in a tub of water at 105°F (40.5°C). Give sugar and sweet, warm fluids by mouth; DO NOT GIVE ALCOHOL. Wrap the patient from head to toe for transport. Transport the patient in a recumbent position.	VERY GENTLE HANDLING. Cut away wet clothing and replace with dry clothing. Maintain the AIRWAY, but DO NOT USE ADJUNCTS. Administer OXYGEN. Assist ventilations if respiratory rate is less than 5/min, but DO NOT HYPERVENTILATE; keep rate of artificial respiration around 8–10/min. MONITOR cardiac rhythm. START CPR FOR ASYSTOLE OR VENTRICULAR FIBRILLATION. Do not waste time trying to start an IV. For VENTRICULAR FIBRILLATION, try one series of DEFIBRILLATING SHOCKS (200 → 300 → 360 joules). Once you have started CPR, DO NOT GIVE UP. Transport the patient supine, in 10 degrees of head-down tilt.

warm core blood; the blood is thus cooled in the periphery and then returns, cold, to the core to lower the temperature there.

For all those reasons:

> **THE VICTIM MUST BE REMOVED FROM THE WATER WITH A MINIMUM OF PHYSICAL EXERTION ON HIS PART.**

If at all possible, do not allow the victim to swim or to climb out of the water himself. Throw him a rope and haul him ashore, or pull him into a boat.

After the victim has been removed from the water, his core temperature will continue to fall as cold blood from his extremities is pumped back into the core—a phenomenon termed **afterdrop.** After-

drop seems to be partly the result of purely physical, as opposed to physiologic, phenomena, since even an inanimate object like a watermelon will demonstrate afterdrop when fished out of cold water and subjected to external rewarming. Nonetheless, afterdrop will be increased by any maneuver that increases circulation to the extremities, such as moving about or rubbing one's arms and legs. Afterdrop is also increased if wet clothing is allowed to remain on the patient, permitting further heat loss by conduction and evaporation.

To minimize afterdrop, KEEP THE PATIENT AS STILL AS POSSIBLE. Do not permit him to sit, stand, or move in any way. Do not massage the victim's extremities. As soon as possible, remove his wet clothing, but do so with a minimum of patient movement; cut away the clothing if you have to, and replace it with dry garments. Protect the victim from the wind to lessen convective heat loss.

All of the additional measures discussed earlier for general hypothermia apply to immersion hypo-

TABLE 32-4. PREVENTION OF COLD INJURY

MECHANISM OF BODY COOLING	MEANS OF PREVENTING HEAT LOSS BY THAT MECHANISM
Convection	Wear insulating clothes, such as wool, down, Dacron, or foam linings.
	Take shelter from the wind; wear windproof garments.
	Keep ears and nose covered.
	Wear ointment over nose, cheeks, and lips.
Conduction	Don't sit in the snow.
	Don't touch cold metal with bare skin.
	Replace wet clothing with dry clothing.
Radiation*	Keep head and neck covered.
	Don't drink alcoholic beverages when out in the cold.
Evaporation	Change out of wet clothes immediately.
Inadequate heat production	Eat frequent snacks high in sugar and starch.
	Keep moving.
Interference with circulation	Avoid tight clothing, especially tight shoes and gloves.
	No cigarettes.

*Strictly speaking, radiant heat loss cannot be prevented; a hat and scarf actually prevent heat loss by convection.

thermia as well: gentle handling, rewarming for moderate degrees of hypothermia, and rapid evacuation to the hospital.

PREVENTING INJURIES DUE TO THE COLD

The majority of cold exposure injuries result from failure to take adequate safeguards against the elements. The "killer of the unprepared" should never be a threat to paramedics, who, like Boy Scouts and Girl Scouts, make it a practice to be prepared. The paramedic must know how to protect both himself or herself and the patient against heat loss in a cold environment. All it takes, really, is an understanding of the mechanisms by which heat is lost from the body and a little common sense (Table 32-4).

GLOSSARY

afterdrop Continued fall in core temperature after a victim of hypothermia has been removed from a cold environment, due at least in part to the return of cold blood from the body surface to the body core.

cold diuresis Secretion of large amounts of urine in response to cold exposure and the consequent shunting of blood volume to the body core.

core In reference to the human body, the part of the body comprising the heart, lungs, brain, and abdominal viscera.

frostbite Localized damage to tissues resulting from prolonged exposure to extreme cold.

frost nip First-degree frostbite, characterized by numbness and pallor without significant tissue damage.

hypothermia Condition in which the core body temperature is significantly below normal.

rewarming shock Shock caused by sudden expansion of the circulation that follows dilation of peripheral vessels as the body surface is warmed.

shell In reference to the human body, the skin, subcutaneous tissues, skeletal muscles, and extremities.

windchill factor Factor that takes into account both the temperature and wind velocity in calculating the effect of a given ambient temperature on living organisms.

FURTHER READING

Antretter H, Dapunt OE, Mueller LC. Survival after prolonged hypothermia (letter). *N Engl J Med* 330:219, 1994.

Arnold JW, Eichenberger CH. The hydraulic sarong: Emergency treatment device for accidental hypothermia. *JACEP* 4:438, 1975.

Auerbach PS. Some people are dead when they're cold and dead (editorial). *JAMA* 264:1856, 1990.

Avery WM. Hypothermia: The silent killer. *Emerg Med Serv* 8(1):26, 1979.

Bangs CC. Immersion hypothermia. *Emergency* 12(1):43, 1980.

Bangs CC. Caught in the cold. *Emerg Med* 15(21):29, 1982.

Besdine RW. Accidental hypothermia: The body's energy crisis. *Geriatrics* 34:51, 1979.

Brody GM, Elberger ST. Hypothermia and the heart. *Emerg Med* 23(2):81, 1991.

Daanen HAM et al. Comparison of four noninvasive rewarming methods for mild hypothermia. *Aviat Space Environ Med* 63:1070, 1992.

Danzl DF et al. Multicenter hypothermia study. *Ann Emerg Med* 16:1042, 1987.

DaVee TS et al. Extreme hypothermia and ventricular fibrillation. *Ann Emerg Med* 9:100, 1980.

Donner HJ. Out in the cold. *Emerg Med* 17(21):21, 1985.

Fergusson NV. Urban hypothermia. *Anaesthesia* 40:651, 1985.

Fishbeck KH, Simon RP. Neurological manifestations of accidental hypothermia. *Ann Neurol* 10:384, 1981.

Fitzgerald FT. Hypoglycemia and accidental hypothermia in an alcoholic population. *West J Med* 133:105, 1980.

Forgey WW. *Death by Exposure: Hypothermia.* Merrillville, Ind.: ICS Books, 1985.

Harnett RM, Pruitt JR, Sias FR. A review of the literature concerning resuscitation from hypothermia: Part I. The problem and general approaches. *Aviat Space Environ Med* 24:106, 1982.

Heggers JP et al. Experimental and clinical observations on frostbite. *Ann Emerg Med* 16:1056, 1987.

Holm PCA, Vaggaard L. Frostbite. *Plast Reconstr Surg* 54:544, 1974.

Lathrap TG. *Hypothermia: Killer of the Unprepared.* Portland, Ore.: Mazamas, 1975.

Leavitt M, Podgorny G. Prehospital CPR and the pulseless hypothermic patient. *Ann Emerg Med* 13:492, 1984.

Ledingham I, Mone J. Treatment of accidental hypothermia: A prospective study. *Br Med J* 280:1102, 1980.

McCauley RL et al. Frostbite injuries: A rational approach based on the pathophysiology. *J Trauma* 213:143, 1983.

McClean D, Emslie-Smith D. *Accidental Hypothermia.* Philadelphia: Lippincott, 1977.

Miller JW, Danzl D, Thomas DM. Urban accidental hypothermia: 135 cases. *Ann Emerg Med* 9:456, 1980.

Mills WJ. Out in the cold. *Emerg Med* 8(1):134, 1976.

Moss JF et al. A model for the treatment of accidental severe hypothermia. *J Trauma* 26:68, 1986.

O'Keefe KM. Accidental hypothermia: A review of 62 cases. *JACEP* 6:491, 1977.

Osborne L et al. Survival after prolonged cardiac arrest and accidental hypothermia. *Br Med J* 289:881, 1984.

Romet TT, Hoskin RW. Temperature and metabolic responses to inhalation and bath rewarming protocols. *Aviat Space Environ Med* 59:630, 1988.

Rossman L. Handling disasters in cold environments. *JEMS* 17(11):38, 1992.

Sherman FT et al. Hypothermia detection in emergency departments: How low does your thermometer go? *NY State J Med* 82:374, 1982.

Shields CP, Sizsmith DM. Treatment of moderate-to-severe hypothermia in an urban setting. *Ann Emerg Med* 19:1093, 1990.

Siebke H et al. Survival after 40 minutes submersion without cerebral sequelae. *Lancet* 1:1275, 1975.

Snadden D. The field management of hypothermic casualties arising from Scottish mountain accidents. *Scott Med J* 38(4):99, 1993.

Southwick FS, Dalglish PH. Recovery after prolonged asystolic cardiac arrest in profound hypothermia. *JAMA* 243:1250, 1980.

Steinemann S, Shackford S, Davis J. Implications of admission hypothermia in trauma patients. *J Trauma* 30:200, 1990.

Steinman AM. Immersion hypothermia. *Emerg Med Serv* 6(4):22, 1977.

Sterba J. Efficacy and safety of prehospital rewarming techniques to treat accidental hypothermia. *Ann Emerg Med* 20:896, 1991.

Stine RJ. Accidental hypothermia. *JACEP* 6:413, 1977.

Tacker WA et al. Transchest defibrillation under conditions of hypothermia. *Crit Care Med* 9:390, 1981.

Terr AL. Environmental illness. *Arch Intern Med* 146:145, 1986.

Volker C, Bunce G. Hypothermia: The cold weather killer. *Emergency* 10(2):46, 1978.

Webb JQ. Cold to the core: Treating the hypothermic patient. *JEMS* 14(12):30, 1989.

Weinberg AD. Hypothermia. *Ann Emerg Med* 22:370, 1993.

Weyman AE, Greenbaum DM, Grace WJ. Accidental hypothermia in an alcoholic population. *Am J Med* 56:13, 1974.

White JD. Hypothermia: The Bellevue experience. *Ann Emerg Med* 11:417, 1982.

White JD et al. Rewarming in accidental hypothermia: Radio wave versus inhalation therapy. *Ann Emerg Med* 16:50, 1987.

Wilkerson JA (ed.). *Hypothermia, Frostbite, and Other Cold Injuries.* Seattle: Mountaineers, 1986.

Zachary L et al. Accidental hypothermia treated with rapid rewarming by immersion. *Ann Plast Surg* 9:238, 1982.

Zell SC, Kurtz KJ. Severe exposure hypothermia: A resuscitation protocol. *Ann Emerg Med* 14:339, 1985.

33
Radiation Exposure

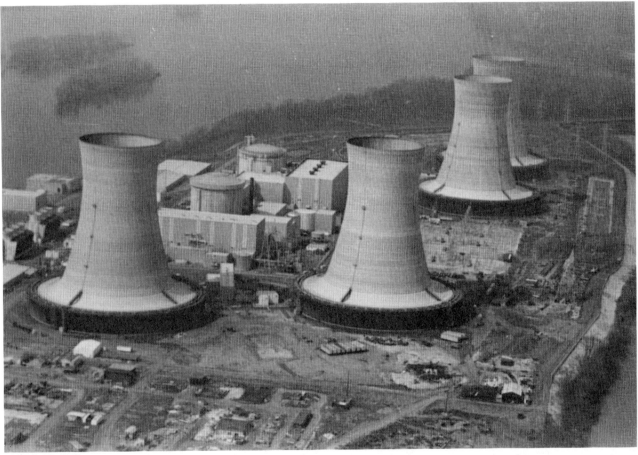

AP/Wide World Photos.

OBJECTIVES

EMS personnel gave scarcely any thought to radiation exposure until 1979, when the accident at Three Mile Island brought the potential dangers of a radiation accident suddenly into public consciousness. The 1986 accident at Chernobyl raised an even more dramatic specter of a radiation disaster. The upshot has been that, with the possible exception of AIDS, few subjects now elicit as much panic among the public and also among rescue personnel as radiation exposure. If an employee in a local radioisotope laboratory has chest pain and calls for an ambulance, the rescue crew is more likely than not to enter the premises as if they were walking on eggs. Such attitudes are mostly a reflection of inadequate information regarding the nature of ionizing radiation and the potential dangers of different types of radioactive materials.

Significant radiation accidents, in fact, are exceedingly rare. Perhaps for that reason, radiation accidents, when they do occur, tend to elicit panic all out of proportion to the dangers involved. The dangers are real, and they need to be understood. But panic is not warranted when one has a clear understanding of the risks and a definite plan of action. In this chapter, we shall learn a bit about the different types of ionizing radiation—where ionizing radiation comes from, what it can do to the body, and how a rescuer can minimize his or her exposure to ionizing radiation when responding to a "dirty" radiation accident. By the end of this chapter, the student should be able to

1. Identify the three principal forms of ionizing radiation, and indicate the means by which a person can be shielded from each
2. List three ways by which a person can protect himself or herself from excessive exposure to a radioactive source
3. Calculate the total dose of radiation received, given the emission rate from a radioactive source and the duration of exposure
4. Indicate how alpha and beta particles can gain access to the body, and list the means by which one can protect oneself from those particles
5. Identify an object or person who is radioactive, given a description of the circumstances of radiation exposure
6. Identify correct and incorrect procedures in dealing with a "dirty" radiation accident and its victims, given a list of various procedures
7. Indicate what signs and symptoms of radiation illness should be sought in persons exposed to a radioactive source

WHAT IS RADIATION?

For many people, the word *radiation* conjures up images of lethal rays that leave a trail of scorched earth and melting corpses in their wake. In fact, **radiation** is simply the transmission of energy in the form of waves or particles. We have already discussed, in the previous chapter, the radiation of thermal energy (heat) from the body. Both visible light and sound are also forms of radiation. The kind of radiation we are concerned about here, however, is **ionizing radiation,** that is, radiation capable of disrupting the atoms in the body into their component charged particles (ions). When ionizing radiation is absorbed by living tissues, it bumps ions loose from atoms, the smallest building blocks of all matter. The liberated ions in turn bump into other atoms, and the process continues—like the scattering of billiard balls—until the energy of the particles is dissipated. In the process, cell structures may be left in disarray.

There are three forms of ionizing radiation of importance to EMS providers (Fig. 33-1). Radiation can, first of all, be given off in the form of **alpha particles,** large, sluggish, positively charged particles that consist of two protons and two neutrons, equivalent to the nucleus of a helium atom. Alpha particles have a very short range and minimal penetrating ability—they can be stopped even by a sheet of paper—so they are unlikely to cause damage to the body *unless* they are inhaled or ingested.

Beta particles, corresponding to the electron of an atom, carry a negative charge. They are faster and slightly more penetrating than alpha particles, but they can be stopped by heavy clothing and, again, are unlikely to cause damage unless taken into the body through the nose, the mouth, or an open wound.

Gamma rays, as the name implies, are not particles but rather waves. Gamma rays are emitted from the nucleus of an atom and are, for practical purposes, the same as x-rays. Gamma rays can penetrate the whole thickness of the body without difficulty and can be stopped only by heavy lead shielding, thick concrete, and similar materials.

A substance that emits ionizing radiation is called **radioactive.** Radioactive emissions—whether alpha, beta, or gamma—cannot be seen, heard, or felt. They can be detected only with special instruments, such as a Geiger counter or an ionization chamber. Those

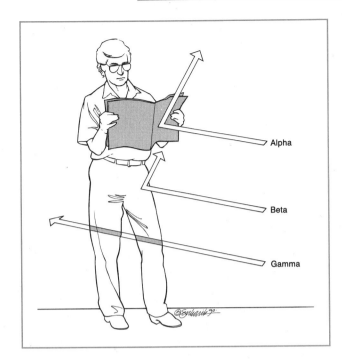

FIGURE 33-1. **THREE FORMS OF IONIZING RADIATION.** Alpha particles can be stopped by paper; beta particles can be stopped by clothing; but gamma waves can penetrate through the entire thickness of the body.

instruments measure the amount of ionizing radiation emitted by a radioactive source in **roentgens** (named for the man who discovered x-rays), or R. The energy actually *deposited* by ionizing radiation, or the radiation *dose,* is usually given in another unit of measurement called the *radiation absorbed dose,* or **rad.** (To make a rough conversion from rads to radiation measurements in roentgens, multiply the number of rads by 1.5.) Very small doses of radiation, like those in natural background sources, are usually given in *millirads* (thousandths of a rad), or *mrads* for short. You may also find another unit of measurement, the **rem** (roentgen equivalent man) referred to in some articles. That measurement takes into account the differing biologic effectiveness of different types of radiation and the fact, for example, that a given dose in rads of alpha particles may produce much more damage than the same rads of gamma rays. For x-rays, gamma rays, and beta particles, rads and rems are equivalent.

A person who has been exposed to ionizing radiation does *not* become radioactive—that is, he does not give off radiation—unless he has been contaminated by dust containing alpha or beta particles. Exposure to gamma radiation does not make a person radioactive, just as you do not become radioactive after you've had a chest x-ray. We shall return to that point later when we discuss the difference between a "clean" and a "dirty" radiation accident. For the moment, suffice it to bear in mind that

> **NO ONE GLOWS IN THE DARK AFTER A CHEST X-RAY.**

Thus in a radiation accident, a person who has been exposed to even a very high dose of ionizing radiation poses no hazard to rescue personnel, and the radiation victim may be handled just as any other patient.

HOW RADIATION AFFECTS THE BODY

Ionizing radiation attacks very minute targets—the atoms in its path. If the atoms disrupted by ionizing radiation happen to be part of a human cell, then the structure or function of that cell may be disrupted as well, just as the function of a watch is altered if you damage one of its springs or cogs. We cannot see the changes that occur in the body's atoms or molecules after a dose of radiation, but what we *can* observe (if the radiation exposure was significant) are the effects of those molecular changes on bodily function. The effects may be acute, occurring within hours or days, or they may be long-term, taking years or even generations to appear. In general, the larger the dose of radiation, the more acute the effects. For example, a person exposed to a dose of about 300 to 600 roentgens (R) over a short period has a 50-percent chance of dying within the next month; a person exposed to about 1,000R will probably die within a couple of weeks; and exposure to 2,000R can cause death within hours.

To put those doses into some kind of perspective, we need to consider the kinds of radiation exposure that a person encounters in the course of everyday life, for all of us are constantly exposed to minute amounts of radiation from cosmic rays and naturally occurring radioactive materials. Table 33-1 summarizes typical annual rates of exposure to radiation sources in the United States, which for most individuals is well below 100 mrad per year, or perhaps 10R over a lifetime.

TABLE 33-1.   RADIATION EXPOSURE FROM DIFFERENT SOURCES

SOURCE	DOSE (mrad)
ANNUAL EXPOSURES	
Cosmic rays	26/year
Terrestial background radiation	24/year
Stone/concrete/masonry buildings	7/year
Internal radiation (food, water, air)	24/year
Fallout from nuclear tests	4/year
Color television viewing	1/year
Approximate total =	86/year
OTHER EXPOSURES	
Chest x-ray	5/film
Upper GI series	100/series
Air travel	1/2,500 miles
Minimum dosage at which biologic effects are detectable	100,000 mrad

TABLE 33-2.   COLOR CODE FOR RADIOACTIVE MATERIALS

LEVEL	SURFACE RADIATION	RADIATION AT 3 FEET
White I	Less than 0.5 mR/hr	
Yellow II	0.5–50 mR/hr	Less than 1 mR/hr
Yellow III	50–200 mR/hr	1–10 mR/hr

Factors Influencing Radiation Dosage

The amount of radiation damage a person suffers depends on the dose of radiation he or she receives, and that in turn depends on several factors. To begin with, there is the STRENGTH OF THE RADIATION which is the number of roentgens per hour that the source is emitting. That emission rate can be measured with a Geiger counter and should, whenever possible, be determined before entering a radiation field. Every ambulance service should have quick access to radiation monitoring equipment (which is available from all Civil Defense authorities), and paramedics should receive instruction in the use of a simple Geiger counter. If you do not have a Geiger counter immediately available when you reach the scene of a *transport* acccident involving radioactive materials, the color coding of the radiation hazard sign will give you some indication of the strength of the emitter (Table 33-2).

A second factor determining the potential severity of radiation exposure is the DURATION OF EXPOSURE. By knowing how long a person was exposed to a radioactive source and how much radiation it was emitting, one can estimate the total dose of exposure with a simple equation:

$$\text{TOTAL DOSE} = \text{dose rate (R/hr)} \times \text{exposure time}$$

That equation tells us what is already intuitively obvious—that the longer the exposure to a radioactive substance, the bigger the dose of radiation the exposed person receives. The practical implications, furthermore, are clear: The exposure time of any one rescuer should be kept as short as possible. Say, for example, you are working near a radioactive source emitting 100R per hour (dose rate), and rescue is going to take 6 minutes, or 0.1 hour. If a single rescuer goes into the exposure zone for the whole 6 minutes, he or she will receive a radiation dose as follows:

$$
\begin{aligned}
\text{TOTAL DOSE} &= \text{dose rate} \times \text{exposure time} \\
&= 100\text{R/hr} \times 0.1 \text{ hour} \\
&= 10\text{R}
\end{aligned}
$$

But suppose there are six rescuers on the team, and they divide up the work so that each of them enters the radiation zone for only 1 minute (0.017 hr). Then each of them will receive a dose of radiation as follows:

$$
\begin{aligned}
\text{TOTAL DOSE} &= \text{dose rate} \times \text{exposure time} \\
&= 100\text{R/hr} \times 0.017 \text{ hour} \\
&= 1.7\text{R}
\end{aligned}
$$

That level of exposure is not very different from what one might receive in the course of a medical diagnostic procedure like a bone scan. The message, then, is clear:

> **KEEP EACH RESCUER'S EXPOSURE TIME TO A MINIMUM.**

Divide up the work among as many people as possible, and work as fast as you can to get yourself and the victim out of the exposure area. That will be possible only if there has been extensive practice beforehand in working in shifts, relay-race fashion.

A third factor influencing the amount of radiation damage a person sustains is the DISTANCE FROM THE RADIATION SOURCE. The exposure falls off as the inverse square of the distance, that is:

$$\text{EXPOSURE} = \frac{1}{(\text{distance})^2}$$

What that means is that if, for example, you double your distance from the radiation source, you get one-quarter the exposure, whereas if you halve the distance to the radiation source, you get four times the exposure.

Let's look at an example. Suppose we have a radioactive source whose emissions are measured as 1,000R per hour at 1 foot from the source, where the victim is lying. If we move the victim 20 feet from the source, his exposure will be reduced to 2.5R per hour ($1,000/20^2$). The practical significance of this relationship is very simple:

> **THE FARTHER AWAY YOU CAN GET FROM A RADIOACTIVE SOURCE THE BETTER, BUT MOVING EVEN A SMALL DISTANCE AWAY REDUCES EXPOSURE A GREAT DEAL.**

For practical purposes, we usually try therefore to establish a working zone at least *20 feet* from the radioactive source.

SHIELDING FROM THE RADIATION SOURCE is a fourth factor that influences a person's exposure and thus potential injury from radiation. Ordinary clothing provides adequate shielding from alpha and beta radiation. Shielding from gamma radiation, however, requires thick (1–2 inch) lead plate, and for that reason, it is more practical in the field to try to shield the *source* than to shield the rescuers. Any heavy accumulation of concrete, brick, or earth offers some protection, and rescuers can shelter behind a thick concrete wall or embankment while making preparations to enter the exposure area.

A fifth factor that determines how much radiation damage a person will suffer is the AREA OF THE BODY THAT RECEIVES RADIATION. Radiation exposure to the whole body is much more likely to produce systemic illness than an exposure limited to one small area of the body.

Finally, radiation damage is influenced by the TYPE OF RADIATION received—alpha, beta, or gamma. As noted earlier, a given dose in rads of alpha particles, for example, may produce many times more damage than the same dose in rads of beta particles or x-rays.

Protective Measures

Among the factors just described, three turn out to have practical implications for protecting ourselves and our patients from *direct* radiation exposure, namely, TIME, DISTANCE, and SHIELDING:

- Keep your exposure TIME to a minimum.
- Put the maximum DISTANCE between yourself and the radioactive source.
- SHIELD the source or shield yourself.

In addition, it is important to bear in mind that radiation can be transmitted *indirectly,* on particles of contaminated dust or smoke or in contaminated liquids. Inhaling or swallowing such contaminated materials is extremely dangerous, for it brings the radioactive material into direct contact with internal tissues, where ionizing radiation can wreak extensive cellular damage. Thus precautions are required to prevent accidental inhalation or ingestion of contaminated dust:

- Wear a FILTRATION MASK.
- NO SMOKING, EATING, OR DRINKING at the scene of a radiation accident.

RESPONDING TO A RADIATION ACCIDENT

The type of response required for a radiation accident, and the precautions necessary, will depend on the nature of the accident.

Types of Radiation Accidents

Radiation accidents can be categorized as "clean" accidents or "dirty" accidents. CLEAN ACCIDENTS are most likely to occur at nuclear power plants or industrial facilities where radioactive substances are routinely used. They occur when a radioactive source somehow becomes unshielded and personnel in the vicinity are thereby exposed to radiation. By definition, a clean accident is one in which there is no contamination or in which decontamination has already been carried out by radiation safety personnel before you arrive. In such cases, there is no hazard to the ambulance crew, and the exposure victims may be handled and transported as any other patients. Reactor sites and industrial users of radioactive materials generally have staff who are expert in dealing with ionizing radiation, and they will be able to provide you with a lot of logistic guidance at the scene. So when responding to a call at a facility that routinely uses radioactive materials, follow the instructions of the plant's radiation safety team.

A much more difficult problem in terms of rescue and patient care is that posed by a DIRTY ACCIDENT. The typical dirty accident is a transportation accident; and with the increasing delivery of radioactive substances by air, rail, and truck, transport accidents are likely to occur more and more frequently. The Interstate Commerce Commission has strict regulations regarding the packaging of radioactive materials, and radioactive shipments must carry the universal radiation symbol, a purple propellor on a white or yellow background (Fig. 33-2). Despite packaging precautions, however, a violent collision, especially if it results in fire or explosion, may permit release of radioactive materials, with contamination of the surrounding area.

It is in responding to a "dirty" radiation accident that special precautions are required. In the next section, we shall go step-by-step through the ambulance response to a "dirty" accident.

Managing a "Dirty" Radiation Accident

A typical "dirty" radiation accident is, as noted, a transport accident in which a vehicle carrying radioactive waste materials is involved in a violent collision, resulting in release into the air or spillage of radioactive substances. The response to the accident begins WHEN THE CALL COMES IN TO THE DISPATCHER. One of the jobs of the dispatcher is to try to determine what, if any, hazards are present at an accident scene; and with luck, the caller will report that the truck was carrying a radiation symbol. If the dispatcher is able to obtain such information ahead of time, he or she should (1) radio the responding ambulance to take necessary precautions at the scene and (2) telephone the appropriate local authorities, so that radiation safety experts can be sent to join you at the scene as soon as possible.

Arrival at the Scene

If the dispatcher has not been able to obtain any information about what the truck was carrying, your first job upon arrival at the scene will be to get a good look at the truck, *from a safe distance*, to check whether it bears the telltale purple and yellow radiation symbol. Every ambulance should carry a pair of binoculars as part of its hazmat (hazardous materials) gear to facilitate identification of dangerous cargoes from an area of safety. Should you see the radiation symbol, radio back to base immediately so that the dispatcher can notify the appropriate authorities.

PARK THE AMBULANCE UPWIND FROM THE ACCIDENT SCENE and upstream from any liquid spills or leaks from the disabled vehicle. If possible, park behind some kind of SHIELDING (a heavy concrete wall, an embankment, even a big semitrailer) and remain in that shielded location while you organize yourselves for the rescue process.

Quickly DON PROTECTIVE CLOTHING—surgical hood, mask, shoe covers, and gown or coveralls—which should ideally be kept in a special Radiation Emergency Kit (Table 33-3) in the vehicle. The kit should also contain a **dosimeter film badge,** a device for measuring your radiation exposure, which you should clip on *beneath* the protective outer clothing and wear for the duration of the call.

FIGURE 33-2.   UNIVERSAL RADIATION SYMBOL.

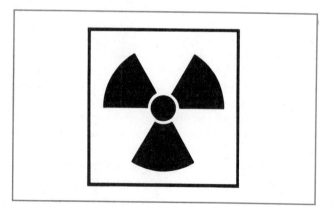

TABLE 33-3.   SUGGESTED RADIATION KIT FOR AMBULANCES

Geiger-Mueller (G-M) instrument
Dosimeter badge for each paramedic and EMT
5–10 heavy-duty plastic garbage bags
Packet of "radioactive" stickers to label
    contaminated articles
Several pairs of surgical gloves in various sizes
Several sets of surgical hoods, gowns, and shoe
    covers
Filtration masks
Masking tape
Special record-keeping forms for radiation accidents
Disaster tags

If you don't have protective clothing aboard the ambulance, you will have to adapt the clothes you are wearing to minimize contamination by alpha and beta particles carried in dust or smoke. If you have anything that will serve as a second layer of clothing, put it on, and don some kind of filtering mask. Button your shirt all the way up, and turn the collar up. Tape shirt cuffs and pant legs closed, and tape over buttonholes and other openings in your clothing through which dust might otherwise enter. Make sure to keep your head well covered, so that none of your hair is exposed, and protect your eyes with goggles.

Female paramedics who are or might be pregnant should stay on the sidelines, out of the radiation area. This is not male chauvinism; it is practical genetics. A developing fetus is much more sensitive to the effects of radiation than an adult, and even small exposures may result in birth defects.

BEFORE YOU ENTER THE "HOT" ZONE, REMEMBER: YOUR BEST ALLIES ARE TIME, DISTANCE, AND SHIELDING.

Extrication

Once you have suited up, first priority is to GET THE VICTIM(S) OUT OF THE EXPOSURE AREA AS RAPIDLY AS POSSIBLE, even at the risk of aggravating other injuries. If the victim is lying on top of a "hot" gamma emitter, for instance, there simply isn't time to apply a traction splint or undertake other stabilizing measures. For the patient's sake and your own, he or she must first be moved at least 20 feet away from the center of the "hot zone" (Fig. 33-3). Approach the wreckage from *upwind*, and try to stay clear of visible dust or smoke, which may be contaminated with alpha or beta particles. Disentangle the victim as fast as you can. If that will take more than a minute or two, WORK IN SHIFTS. As soon as the patient has been disentangled, move him rapidly to the most distant upwind edge of the contamination zone (zone B in Fig. 33-3).

Medical Care and Decontamination at the Scene

Once you are out of the "hot zone," the usual priorities of ABC apply. Don't worry at this point about decontamination. No one ever died from accidental surface contamination. Lots of people die from obstructed airways, respiratory arrest, bleeding, and

the like. So stop and give whatever medical care is urgently needed.

DECONTAMINATION CAN WAIT. AN OBSTRUCTED AIRWAY CANNOT.

Only when the airway is ensured, breathing is adequate, and external bleeding is under control should you turn your attention to the decontamination process.

To begin DECONTAMINATION, remove as much of the patient's clothing as possible. Doing so is usually sufficient to eliminate 70 to 80 percent of the patient's surface contamination. Place the contaminated clothing in a heavy-duty plastic garbage bag; seal the bag, and label it with a "radioactive" sticker. Then strip off your own protective clothing, and stash it in another plastic bag, which should be similarly sealed and labelled. All plastic bags containing contaminated or potentially contaminated items should be left in the contaminated work zone (zone B), to be checked and removed later by a radiation decontamination team.

If you have a Geiger counter, check the patient's whole body for radioactivity and make a record, on a body diagram, of how many counts were registered at each point you checked.

Usually it is *not* worthwhile to spend time trying to decontaminate the victim's skin in the field. Uptake of radioactive materials by intact skin is relatively slow, so cleaning the skin can ordinarily wait until the patient reaches the hospital. Furthermore, unskilled decontamination technique may simply aggravate the situation by flushing radioactive materials into open wounds, where radioactive uptake *is* rapid.

COMPLETE THE SECONDARY SURVEY. The most important thing to ask the conscious patient is whether he has experienced any NAUSEA OR VOMITING, for the gastrointestinal system is the most sensitive indicator of the intensity of radiation exposure. Low levels of radiation will frequently produce some nausea. If vomiting begins within a few hours, it is usually a sign of significant irradiation. Vomiting that begins within a few minutes may signify that the patient sustained a lethal radiation exposure.

Once the patient has been stabilized medically and his contaminated clothing has been removed, MOVE THE PATIENT FROM THE CONTAMINATION CONTROL AREA (zone B). Place him on a clean blanket spread out on top of a backboard in zone C, and fold the blanket over him, so that any

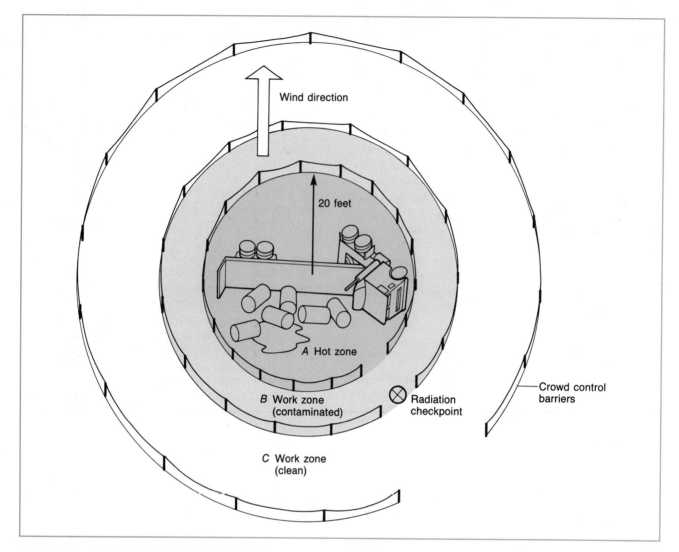

FIGURE 33-3.   HAZARD CONTROL ZONES AT A RADIATION ACCIDENT.
The patient must be quickly moved out of the "hot" zone (A) to a distance at
least 20 feet away and upwind. Only essential personnel should enter the
contaminated work zone (B). All contaminated items should be left in this
zone. Ambulances, extra supplies, and nonessential personnel should remain
in the clean work zone (C). Passage from zone B to zone C should be monitored by a radiation safety officer with a Geiger counter at a radiation check-
point (X).

residual contamination will be sealed inside. Then lift
the patient onto the wheeled stretcher for removal to
the ambulance.

Transport and Arrival at the Hospital

When you are ready for transport, NOTIFY THE RE-
CEIVING HOSPITAL of (1) the nature of the case, (2)
the number and condition of the victims, and (3) your
estimated time of arrival. The hospital will need lead
time to activate their own radiation accident protocol,
which involves setting up a separate area for reception and decontamination of victims.

When you reach the hospital, DO NOT WHEEL
THE PATIENT(s) IN THROUGH THE USUAL EMER-
GENCY ROOM ENTRANCE. Wait outside until you
receive instructions as to precisely where to unload
the victim(s). In general, the patient should be transferred from your stretcher to a hospital gurney *outside*
the hospital and then brought to a designated decontamination area.

BEFORE YOU MAY LEAVE THE HOSPITAL, you
and your vehicle will have to undergo thorough decontamination, so call out of service until you've been
officially released by the local radiation safety officer.
Follow the officer's instructions for showering and

for washing down the vehicle and its equipment. And don't leave the scene until you and your rig have been checked out for residual contamination.

Each state has a radiologic health department that can be contacted for assistance in radiation emergencies, and the dispatcher should know how to get in touch with state authorities in the event of a radiation accident. In addition, the Radiation Emergency Assistance Center/Training Site (REAC/TS) in Oak Ridge, Tennessee, maintains a hot line to provide telephone advice or even to dispatch a team of experts to the site of a radiation accident. REAC/TS can be reached 24 hours a day by calling (615) 481-1000 (Beeper 241).

GLOSSARY

alpha particle Positively charged subatomic particle corresponding to the nucleus of a helium atom with high ionizing ability but low penetration.

beta particle Negatively charged subatomic particle corresponding to the electron of an atom, with slightly greater penetrating ability than an alpha particle.

gamma ray Radioactive emission from the nucleus of an atom, with very high penetrating ability.

ion An electrically charged atom or molecule.

ionizing radiation Transmission of energy in the form of waves or particles that has the ability to disrupt atoms in its path into their component ions.

rad Abbreviation for *radiation absorbed dose*, a measure of radiation received at a given target.

radiation Transmission of energy in the form of waves or particles.

radioactive Having the property of emitting ionizing radiation.

rem Abbreviation for *roentgen equivalent man*, a measure of radiation dose that takes into account the potential destructiveness of the type of radiation emitted.

roentgen (R) Unit of measurement for radioactive emissions, named for the discoverer of x-rays.

FURTHER READING

Adelstein SJ. Uncertainty and relative risks of radiation exposure. *JAMA* 258:655, 1987.

Beane MJ et al. Radiation primer. *EMT J* 5(4):260, 1981.

Becker DV. Reactor accidents: Public health strategies and their medical implications. *JAMA* 258:649, 1987.

Deluca SA et al. Radiation exposure in diagnostic studies. *Am Fam Physician* 36:101, 1987.

English WE. Radioactive contamination. *Emergency* 14(1): 43, 1982.

Fabrikant JI. Health effects of the nuclear accident at Three Mile Island. *Health Phys* 40:151, 1981.

Gaffney J et al. Radiation: A rad response. *JEMS* 18(3)41, 1993.

Gale RP. Immediate medical consequences of nuclear accidents: Lessons from Chernobyl. *JAMA* 258:625, 1987.

Geiger HJ. The accident at Chernobyl and the medical response. *JAMA* 256:609, 1986.

Goldstein HA. Radiation accidents and injuries. *Emerg Med* 14(15):195, 1982.

Huebner KF. Decontamination procedures and risks to health care personnel. *Bull NY Acad Med* 59:1119, 1983.

In the shadow. *Emerg Med* 19(2):68, 1987.

Keller PD. A clinical syndrome following exposure to atomic bomb explosions. *JAMA* 131:504, 1946.

Ketchum LE. Lesson of Chernobyl: Health consequences of radiation released and hysteria unleashed. *J Nucl Med* 28:413, 1987.

Leaning-Link J. Emergency response to nuclear accident and attack. *Disaster Med* 1:386, 1983.

Leonard RB, Ricks RC. Emergency department radiation accident protocol. *Ann Emerg Med* 9:462, 1980.

Linnemann RE. Soviet medical response to the Chernobyl nuclear accident. *JAMA* 258:637, 1987.

Loken MK. Physicians' obligations in radiation issues. *JAMA* 258:673, 1987.

Lushbaugh CC, Huebner KF, Ricks RC. Medical aspects of nuclear radiation emergencies. *Emergency* 10(10):32, 1978.

MacLeod GK. Some public health lessons from Three Mile Island: A case study in chaos. *AMBIO* 10:18, 1981.

Macleod GK. The Three Mile Island (TMI) Accident. *Disaster Med* 1:399, 1983.

MacLeod GK, Hendee WR, Schwarz MR. Radiation accidents and the role of the physician: A post-Chernobyl perspective. *JAMA* 256:632, 1986.

Merz B. Physicians' reaction to Chernobyl explosion: Lessons in radiation—and cooperation. *JAMA* 256:559, 1986.

Merz B. REAC/TS handles "hot topics." *JAMA* 256:569, 1986.

Messerschmidt O. Combined radiation injuries and medical injuries. *Disaster Med* 1:398, 1983.

Mettler FA. Emergency management of radiation accidents. *JACEP* 7:302, 1978.

Mettler FA, Rocco FG, Junkins RL. The role of EMTs in radiation accidents. *Emerg Med Serv* 6(4):22, 1977.

Miller KL, Demuth WE. Handling radiation emergencies: No need for fear. *J Emerg Nurs* 9(1):41, 1983.

Milroy WC. Management of irradiated and contaminated casualty victims. *Emerg Clin North Am* 2:667, 1984.

Reid D. The Three Mile Island nuclear accident: Revisited. *Disaster Med* 1:402, 1983.

Richter LL et al. A systems approach to the management of radiation accidents. *Ann Emerg Med* 9:303, 1980.

Ricks RC. Radiation response. *Emergency* 21(2):28, 1989.

Trott KR. Nuclear power plant disasters: Health consequences and need for subsequent medical care. *Lancet* 2:32, 1981.

REAC/TS (the Radiation Emergency Assistance Center/Training Site) in Oak Ridge, Tennessee, has produced a 25-minute film, available on videotape, and an accompanying training manual, *Prehospital Management of Radiation Accidents*. For information, contact Office of Information Services, Oak Ridge Associated Universities, PO Box 117, Oak Ridge, TN 37831-0117.

34
Hazardous Materials

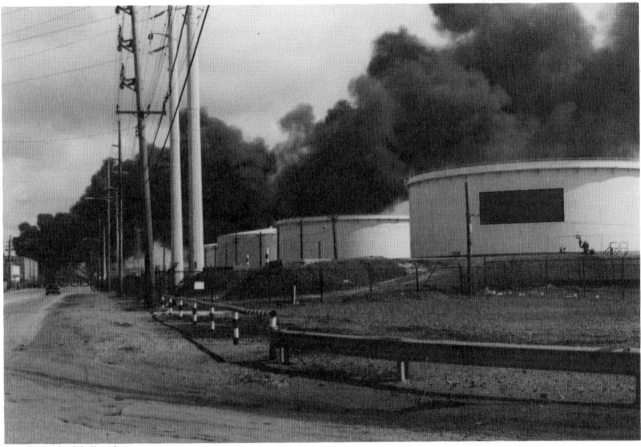

Photo by Michael S. Kowal.

OBJECTIVES

In the previous chapter, we looked at the response to one specific type of hazardous material ("hazmat") incident—that involving ionizing radiation. In fact, radiation accidents constitute only a small minority of hazmat incidents. One of the inevitable consequences of living in an industrialized world is the proliferation of hazardous materials all around us. The products of our civilization require the manufacture, transport, storage, use, and disposal of thousands of potentially toxic substances, which may be spilled or ignited at any stage between manufacture and disposal.

In this chapter, we shall take a broader overview of some of the special considerations involved in responding to any incident that may involve hazardous materials. We shall *not* attempt any sort of comprehensive coverage here of hazmat management; paramedics routinely involved in hazmat response should receive additional, specialized training as mandated by the Occupational Safety and Health Administration (OSHA). By the conclusion of this chapter, then, the student should be able to

1. Identify a potential hazmat incident, given a description of several incidents as reported to 911
2. List three potential sources of information regarding the identity of a hazardous cargo
3. List the steps in responding to a highway accident potentially involving hazardous materials given a description of the accident scene
4. Identify correct and incorrect decontamination procedures, given a description of several procedures

GENERAL CONSIDERATIONS

Some 35,000 dangerous commodities are produced in the United States, and there are nearly 200 *million* shipments per year in the U.S. of hazardous materials. Twenty-five percent of unintentional releases of those materials occur during transport; 75 percent occur during production, storage, or use. From 1971 to 1981, more than 108,000 hazmat events occurred on U.S. highways. What all those statistics mean is one simple rule: The first thing to remember when responding to a road accident or vehicular fire—especially if a truck or train is involved—is that a hazardous material may be part of the picture.

ALWAYS CONSIDER THE POSSIBILITY OF HAZARDOUS MATERIALS WHEN RESPONDING TO A ROAD OR RAIL ACCIDENT. EVERY CARGO SHOULD BE CONSIDERED DANGEROUS UNTIL PROVED OTHERWISE.

Dealing with hazardous materials requires special training and special equipment. The paramedic who plunges heedlessly forward to reach the casualties, without taking careful stock of the situation, is likely to become one of the casualties himself and therefore a burden to the rescue team.

DO NOT RUSH INTO A HAZMAT SCENE. STOP AND ASSESS THE SITUATION FIRST.

ESTABLISHING A HAZARD ZONE

As soon as you reach the scene of an accident that *might* involve hazardous materials, PARK THE VEHICLE UPWIND from any potential gas or liquid spill, preferably at least 50 to 100 yards away, and take action at once to establish a **hazard zone,** that is, an area from which unauthorized persons should be excluded. One quick method for estimating the extent of the hazard zone is to use the **Hazmat Rule of Thumb:** Hold your arm out straight in front of you, with your thumb pointing upward, and center your thumb over the hazardous area (the hazardous area will include, for example, an entire overturned vehicle and the whole area over which spilled materials are visible). If your thumb does not block out the entire hazardous area from your view, you are *too close!* Back up (in a direction upwind from the spill) until your thumb does obscure the whole area of potential hazard. That point is the border of the hazard zone. Do whatever you can to keep bystanders away from the hazard zone. And do not enter the hazard zone yourself until you have determined the identity of the hazardous material and your own capability to deal with it.

IDENTIFICATION OF THE HAZARDOUS MATERIAL

One of the most important contributions that the first ambulance on the scene can make to a hazmat response is to enable early identification of the hazardous substance involved. In the United States, trucks or trains carrying hazardous materials across state lines are required by law to follow federal regulations regarding markings on the vehicle and shipping documents.

The first thing to look for is a colored Department of Transportation **placard** (Fig. 34-1) on the side or back end of the vehicle (truck or railway car). The placard is a diamond-shaped sign, which is likely to be color-coded and which may contain some or all of the following:

- A pictorial representation of the hazard (e.g., a skull and crossbones to indicate poison, or a flame to indicate a flammable substance)
- A four-digit **identification number,** sometimes preceded by the letters *NA* (standing for "North American") or *UN* (standing for "United Nations"). Older placards may show the name of the chemical itself (e.g., "CHLORINE") rather than an identification number.
- A single number at the bottom, which refers to the United Nations classification system (Table 34-1).

TABLE 34-1.   UNITED NATIONS HAZARDOUS MATERIALS CLASSIFICATION CODES

NUMBER	MATERIAL
1	Explosives
2	Gases
3	Flammable and combustible liquids
4	Flammable solids
5	Oxidizers and organic peroxides
6	Poisons
7	Radioactive materials
8	Corrosives

We have already mentioned that paramedics arriving first at a potential hazmat incident should not cross into the hazard zone before the hazardous material has been identified. How, then, is a paramedic, who may be standing 100 yards from an overturned truck, supposed to be able to read the lettering on a placard at that distance? The answer is that your ambulance had better be equipped with BINOCULARS, or you will be out of luck. Do NOT risk personal exposure to a hazardous material in order to get close enough to read the placard on the side of a disabled truck or railway car.

Another source of information for identifying hazardous cargoes is the **bill of lading** carried in the cab of trucks or the **waybill** and **consist** carried by the conductor on trains. (The consist lists the order in which the cars are lined up in the train, and the waybill lists their contents.) Those shipping documents are usually not as helpful as the placard information, since it may not be possible at first to reach the truck cab or the engine car of a train. Furthermore, shipping documents may be lost or destroyed in the course of an accident. Nonetheless, it is useful to know what to look for in such a document if you should be fortunate enough to get access to it during a hazmat incident. The waybill or bill of lading will list the name of the shipper, the company to which the product is being shipped, the four-digit UN/NA identification number, and a description of all products being transported (e.g., "10 drums gasoline, flammable liquid, 4,500 lb").

Finally, the driver of the truck or the conductor of the train may, if conscious, be able to supply you with information regarding the cargo that was aboard.

From whatever source you obtain the information, RADIO YOUR DISPATCHER at once with the four-digit identification number of the cargo. Every

FIGURE 34-1.   USDOT PLACARD FOR HAZARDOUS MATERIALS. The placard shows a pictorial symbol of the substance carried (in this case, a poison), a four-digit UN/NA identification number (in this case, the number for chlorine), and the UN hazard class number (in this case, the number for a gas).

dispatch station should be equipped with the U.S. Department of Transportation's *Hazardous Material, The Emergency Response Handbook;* using that handbook, your dispatcher should be able to give you an initial identification of the substance involved in the incident and help you decide what to do until professional hazmat personnel reach the scene. Meanwhile, the dispatcher should contact CHEMTREC (the Chemical Transportation Emergency Center in Washington, D.C.), which maintains a 24-hour toll-free hotline to provide information on handling specific hazmat incidents. The telephone numbers of CHEMTREC are (800) 424-9300 from the continental United States, 483-7616 if dialling from the Washington, D.C., area, and (202) 483-7616 if calling from outside the continental United States (CHEMTREC will accept collect calls). The information that the dispatcher needs to furnish is as follows:

INFORMATION NEEDED BY THE CHEMTREC COMMUNICATOR

- Name of caller
- Call-back number
- Shipper*
- Manufacturer's name*
- Container type
- Rail car or truck number
- Carrier's name*
- Consignee*
- Product involved, if known, or 4-digit identification number
- Location of incident
- Condition at scene (including weather)
- Type of problem (e.g., spill, fire)

*Information from waybill or bill of lading.

RESCUE AND MEDICAL TREATMENT

As soon as paramedics have enough information and professional hazmat backup to enter the hazard zone, they should remove the injured from the zone to prevent further exposure—employing whatever protective equipment that the hazmat team instructs them to use (e.g., protective clothing, self-contained breathing apparatus). If you do not have the protective clothing and equipment required for the particular circumstances, do *not* enter the hazard zone. Different situations require different levels of protection,

and protective clothing is rated according to the level of protection it affords. Thus, for example, level I structural fire-fighting protective clothing will not suffice for hazmat environments that require full body protection from a hostile environment, such as a chlorine gas spill. For that situation, level III encapsulated protective clothing ("acid suit") is required.

IF YOU'RE NOT DRESSED FOR THE OCCASION, STAY ON THE SIDELINES.

Let someone who *is* properly dressed and equipped do the rescue, for otherwise you risk becoming one of the casualties.

As in the case of radiation incidents, once the casualty has been removed from the hazard zone, FIRST PRIORITY GOES TO URGENT MEDICAL PROBLEMS. The usual priorities of ABC apply. If either the casualty or the paramedic has come in contact with the hazardous material, then **decontamination** must also be carried out, preferably *before* transport.

DECONTAMINATION

Casualties or EMS personnel at a hazmat incident may become contaminated in a number of ways:

- Being splashed by materials during rescue operations
- Walking through puddles of hazardous liquids or across contaminated ground
- Coming in contact with gases, vapors, or particles of hazardous substances
- Touching contaminated persons or instruments

However contamination occurs, decontamination is required as soon as possible; otherwise exposure to the hazardous material will continue and the resulting injury will become progressively more severe. When highly toxic materials are involved, decontamination may have to be carried out simultaneous with medical stabilization of the patient.

Ideally, decontamination should be conducted by trained personnel using special equipment; but that may not always be possible, especially when a critically injured patient must be moved urgently to the hospital before the decontamination team has arrived and deployed its gear. In decontaminating casualties, the following general principles apply:

GENERAL PRINCIPLES OF DECONTAMINATION

- Remove all of the victim's clothing (including shoes, socks, underwear), and place it in a sealed container, such as a plastic bag.
- Flush the skin *gently* with water for at least 15 minutes. Start at the head and work downward. Make sure that hair and body folds are thoroughly rinsed as well. Pay special attention to fingernails, underarms, and groin. Then give a gentle wash with tincture of green soap, and rinse again.
- If there are open wounds on the skin, wash and rinse from the wound area outward, taking care not to flush contaminants into the wound. Once the wound area is clean, cover it with an occlusive dressing or plastic wrap.
- When flushing is complete, gently dry the patient with a clean towel. Cover him with a clean sheet for transport.
- No matter how thoroughly you think you have decontaminated the casualty, be sure to notify the receiving hospital in advance that the patient may still be partially contaminated—so that the hospital can implement its own hazmat protocols.

Whenever possible, it is preferable to have a separate team—paramedics who were not involved in the rescue and treatment of the casualty—transport the casualty to the hospital. In that way, the chances of bringing contaminants into the hospital are minimized, and the paramedics who did participate in rescue can, meanwhile, themselves undergo decontamination at the scene, without delaying the evacuation of the patient. All equipment, gear, and protective clothing used during the hazmat response must also undergo thorough decontamination before the rescue personnel leave the scene.

FURTHER READING

Barillo D. Hazmat response. *Emergency* 24(9):46, 1992.

Bronstein A, Currance P. *Emergency Care For Hazardous Materials Exposure.* St. Louis: Mosby, 1988.

Currance PL. Staging decon operations. *Rescue* 2(4):45, 1989.

Currance PL. Personal hazmat protection. *Rescue* 3(2):33, 1990.

International Fire Service Training Association. Personal protective equipment for hazardous incidents. *Emerg Med Serv* 18(10):44, 1989.

Isman WE. Emergency responders at a hazardous materials incident. *JEMS* 8(2):26, 1982.

Kurzeja W. HAZWOPER and you. *Emergency* 22(9):35, 1990.

Leonard RB. Chemicals in transit: Be prepared. *Emerg Med* 14(18):17, 1984.

Maniscalco PM. Hazardous-materials response. *Emerg Med Serv* 19(5):64, 1990.

McKenna R. Hazardous materials incidents and the EMT. *EMT J* 5(6):400, 1981.

Plante D, Walker J. EMS response at a hazardous material incident: Some basic guidelines. *J Emerg Med* 7:55, 1989.

Staten C. Hazardous materials: The EMS response. *Emerg Med Serv* 18(10):34, 1989.

Staten C. Could this happen to you? *Emerg Med Serv* 21(5):28, 1992.

Stutz DR, Janusz SJ. *Hazardous Material Injuries: A Handbook for Pre-Hospital Care* (2nd ed.). Beltsville, MD: Bradford Communications, 1988.

U.S. Department of Health and Human Services/U.S. Department of Labor. *IOSH/OSHA Pocket Guide to Chemical Hazards.* Washington, D.C.: NIOSH, 1986.

U.S. Department of Transportation. *1987 Emergency Response Guidebook, DOT-P-5800.4.* Washington, D.C.: USDOT, 1987.

Verdile VP, Full RA. EMS in the haz mat response. *Emergency* 22(9):42, 1990.

VII
OBSTETRICS/NEONATAL CARE/GYNECOLOGY

Obstetrics is the branch of medicine that deals with the pregnant woman throughout the stages of pregnancy, labor, and delivery. Gynecology deals with illnesses relating to the female reproductive tract. Neonatology concerns itself with problems of the newborn baby. In this section, we shall look at emergencies in all three categories: first, the usually happy "emergency" of childbirth, then some of the emergencies affecting the baby shortly after birth, and finally emergencies to which women are uniquely susceptible.

35
Obstetrics and Emergency Childbirth

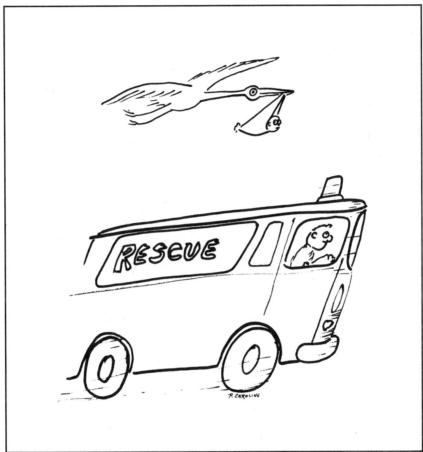

From N.L. Caroline. *Ambulance Calls: Review Problems for the Paramedic* (3rd ed.). Boston, 1991. Published by Little, Brown and Company.

OBJECTIVES

Long before there were paramedics, long before there were even doctors or nurses, women were having babies—for the most part quite successfully. The reason that women have managed to have babies without the help of medical professionals is that pregnancy and childbirth are not diseases; they are natural processes. And in the majority of cases, they proceed without serious complications. The paramedic called to assist in the birth of a baby, then, will most likely be participating in a happy event—a refreshing change from the paramedic's usual daily fare. But things *can* sometimes go wrong, and a happy event can turn into a tragic one if it is not managed correctly.

In this chapter, we shall first review the anatomy and physiology of the female reproductive system and learn where babies come from. We shall look at some of the complications that can occur during pregnancy. At the end of pregnancy comes delivery, so we shall consider the normal course of events during childbirth and then some of the things that can go wrong. By the end of this chapter, the student should be able to

1. Identify the major structures of the female reproductive system, given a diagram or a description of the structures
2. Explain where babies come from
3. List four functions of the placenta
4. Given a description of several pregnant women with different clinical histories, identify a woman with
   - Threatened abortion
   - Inevitable abortion
   - Incomplete abortion
   - Missed abortion
   - Septic abortion
   and describe the correct prehospital management of each
5. List three causes of third trimester bleeding, and describe the prehospital management of a woman who has vaginal bleeding during the later stages of pregnancy
6. Given a description of several pregnant women with different clinical findings, identify a woman with
   - Placenta previa
   - Supine hypotensive syndrome
   - Preeclampsia
   and describe the correct prehospital management of each
7. List five changes occurring in pregnancy that ren-

der a woman more vulnerable to serious injury, and outline the steps in treating a pregnant woman who has suffered trauma
8. List the measures that should be taken to assess and treat the fetus when a pregnant woman has been injured
9. Identify the stages of labor, given a description of the different stages, and state the approximate duration of each stage of labor in
   - A nullipara
   - A multipara
10. Determine whether there is time to transport a woman in labor to the hospital for delivery or whether delivery should be undertaken at the scene, given a description of the woman's symptoms and signs and an indication of the distance to the nearest hospital
11. Distinguish between true labor and false labor, given a description of the contractions experienced by a pregnant woman
12. Identify indications in the history or physical examination of a woman in labor that suggest her delivery may be complicated, given a description of several women in labor and their clinical findings
13. List the steps of
    - Preparing for delivery of a baby outside the hospital
    - Delivering the baby and the placenta
14. Describe what steps to take if
    - The amniotic sac is still intact around the baby's head as the head is delivered
    - The umbilical cord is wrapped around the baby's neck
15. Assign an Apgar score to a newborn, given a description of the newborn's appearance, vital signs, and activity at birth
16. Given a description of several women in labor with different physical findings, identify a woman in labor with
    - Buttocks breech
    - Footling breech
    - Prolapsed umbilical cord
    and describe the correct prehospital management of each
17. List the special measures that should be taken in dealing with
    a. Delivery of a small or premature baby
    b. Delivery of twins
18. List four risk factors for postpartum hemorrhage, and outline the steps in prehospital management of a woman who continues to bleed after delivery of the placenta
19. Identify a woman who is likely to have suffered a postpartum pulmonary embolism, given a description of several women with different clinical

findings, and outline the prehospital management

20. List the indications, contraindications, possible adverse side effects, and correct dosage of oxytocin, after studying the relevant section in the Drug Handbook at the end of this textbook

ANATOMY AND PHYSIOLOGY OF THE FEMALE REPRODUCTIVE SYSTEM

Structures of the Female Reproductive System

The female reproductive system (Fig. 35-1) comprises the ovaries, fallopian tubes, uterus, vagina, and external female genitalia.

Within the abdomen, lying in the right and left lower quadrants, are the **ovaries,** two walnut-size organs that produce female sex hormones. Each ovary also contains about 200,000 **follicles;** during each menstrual cycle, one of those follicles matures to release an egg, or **ovum.** Abutting each ovary is a **fallopian tube** whose job it is to collect each egg discharged from the ovary and conduct it to a pear-shaped, muscular organ in the center of the lower quadrant, the **uterus,** or womb. Note that the uterus lies posterior to the bladder, an anatomic relation that explains some of the urinary symptoms that commonly accompany the later stages of pregnancy. At

the distal end of the uterus is a narrow opening, called the **cervix,** by which the uterus is connected to the **vagina.** The vagina is a distensible tube that serves as a passageway between the uterus and the outside.

The EXTERNAL GENITALIA refer to the female structures visible from the outside of the body (Fig. 35-2). Two sets of "lips," the **labia majora** and **labia minora,** make up the **vulva,** which encloses and protects the vaginal opening together with the more anterior opening of the urethra. The area between the vaginal opening and the anus is referred to as the **perineum.**

The Menstrual Cycle

During early childhood, little girls are not a great deal different, physiologically, from little boys, but with the beginning of puberty, all that changes. Usually sometime between the ages of 12 and 14, girls experience **menarche,** that is, the onset of **menses** (menstrual flow). The menstrual cycle is, in fact, the result of a complex interaction of many different structures whose net effect is to prepare the uterus for possible pregnancy (and prepare it to try again if pregnancy does not occur). The story starts in the hypothalamus, the part of the brain concerned with regulating so many vital processes. Chemical messages released by the hypothalamus proceed to the anterior pituitary gland at the base of the brain, the so-called master gland of the body. The anterior pituitary gland produces two hormones important in the menstrual

FIGURE 35-1. **ORGANS OF THE FEMALE REPRODUCTIVE SYSTEM.** Note the bladder is anterior to the uterus.

FIGURE 35-2. **FEMALE EXTERNAL GENITALIA.**

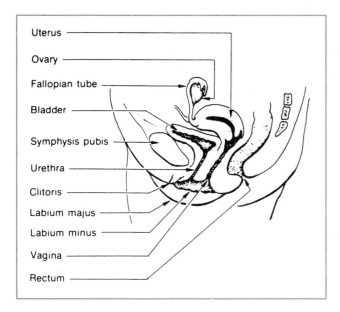

Uterus
Ovary
Fallopian tube
Bladder
Symphysis pubis
Urethra
Clitoris
Labium majus
Labium minus
Vagina
Rectum

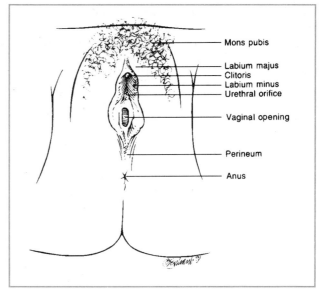

Mons pubis
Labium majus
Clitoris
Labium minus
Urethral orifice
Vaginal opening
Perineum
Anus

cycle: follicle-stimulating hormone (FSH) and luteinizing hormone (LH). It is not important for our purposes to remember their names. What *is* important is that those two pituitary hormones stimulate the ovaries to undergo certain changes. FSH, first of all, stimulates the ovarian follicle to develop into a mature egg, or ovum. That growing follicle in turn produces another hormone, **estrogen,** during the first 14 days of the 28-day cycle.

As the follicle starts developing and pumping out estrogen, the lining of the uterus, called the **endometrium,** is stimulated to increase its thickness in preparation for the reception and future growth of a fertilized egg. The phase of the menstrual cycle under estrogen control, when the endometrium is increasing in thickness, is called the **proliferative phase.** That phase lasts about 14 days from the beginning of menstruation, although the length varies among different women.

Around the fourteenth day of the cycle, the other pituitary hormone, LH, stimulates the growing ovarian follicle to rupture and release an egg, a process called **ovulation.** What is left of the follicle, after the egg has been released, becomes a special structure called the **corpus luteum,** which secretes another female hormone, **progesterone.** Under the influence of progesterone, the second phase of the menstrual cycle, the **secretory phase,** takes place. During the secretory phase, the glands of the endometrium increase in size and secrete the materials on which the fertilized egg will implant and grow. What happens next depends upon whether the ovum that was released at midcycle is fertilized or not.

If the ovum is *not* fertilized, it dies and degenerates 36 to 48 hours after being released. The corpus luteum also degenerates, about 10 days later, and the endometrium then breaks down and is shed as menstrual flow on about the twenty-eighth day of the cycle (i.e., about 14 days after ovulation).

If the ovum *is* fertilized, it will travel down the fallopian tube into the uterus and implant on the endometrium. Meanwhile, the corpus luteum will keep growing and producing hormones to sustain the pregnancy.

NORMAL PREGNANCY

When the ovarian follicle ruptures at midcycle and the ovum is released, it is ordinarily caught up by fingerlike fringes (fimbria) at the end of the fallopian tube and swept into the tube for its journey to the uterus. As in many other things in life, in the dating game between ovum and spermatozoa, timing is critical. The ovum, as mentioned, can stay alive for about 36 to 48 hours after ovulation. Sperm can stay alive for up to 72 hours in the vagina, cervical canal, and uterus. So if fertilization is to take place, sperm have to arrive on the scene very close to the time of ovulation. When it does take place, fertilization—the fusion of a spermatozoon with the ovum—usually occurs in the *fallopian tube.* The fertilized egg then remains in the tube, dividing and developing, for about 3 days before entering the uterus as a 30- to 40-cell mass, or blastocyst. (If the fallopian tube is scarred, from previous gonorrheal disease, for example, the fertilized egg may become stuck there and be unable to enter the uterus, as we shall see in Chap. 37.) The blastocyst nestles into the thickened endometrium of the uterus in a process called **implantation.**

During the first 3 weeks after fertilization, the developing structure is still called an ovum. From the third to the eighth week, it is referred to as an **embryo,** and thereafter until birth it is called a **fetus.**

The Specialized Structures of Pregnancy

At around the fourteenth day after ovulation, a special structure of pregnancy called the **placenta** begins to develop. The placenta, which becomes a quite substantial, fleshy organ, carries out a number of crucial functions during pregnancy:

- *Respiratory gas exchange*: The placenta serves the function of lungs for the developing fetus, enabling the fetus to exchange its carbon dioxide–laden blood for oxygen-rich blood.
- *Transport of nutrients* from the maternal to the fetal circulation.
- *Excretion of wastes*, some of which pass into the maternal circulation and others of which are excreted into the amniotic fluid.
- *Transfer of heat* from the mother to the fetus.
- *Hormone production*: A special hormone of pregnancy, chorionic gonadotrophin, is produced by the placenta to maintain the pregnancy and stimulate changes in the mother's breasts, vagina, and cervix that prepare her for delivery and motherhood.
- *Formation of a barrier* against harmful substances in the mother's circulation, such as chemicals or microorganisms. When a drug is excluded by the placenta from the fetal bloodstream, we say that the drug "does not cross the placenta." The placenta, however, is not able to exclude every harmful substance, so one has to be very careful about what drugs are administered to women during pregnancy.

Another specialized structure of pregnancy is the **umbilical cord,** which connects the placenta to the fetus via the fetal umbilicus (navel). The umbilical cord contains two arteries and one vein. The fetal circulation differs from that of the mother. The umbilical *vein* carries oxygenated blood from the placenta to the fetus, while the umbilical *arteries* carry arteriovenous blood to the placenta. Since the fetus obtains its oxygen via the placenta, the fetal circulation bypasses the lungs until birth. A duct connects the umbilical vein and the inferior vena cava; another duct connects the pulmonary artery and the aorta; and there is an opening between the right and left atria of the fetal heart. At birth, the lungs begin to function, and the various arteriovenous shunts close.

A third specialized structure of pregnancy is the **amniotic sac,** a membranous bag that encloses the fetus in a watery fluid (**amniotic fluid**). The amniotic fluid, whose volume reaches about a liter by the end of pregnancy, provides the fetus with a weightless environment in which to develop. In the latter stages of pregnancy, furthermore, the fetus swallows amniotic fluid and passes nitrogenous wastes out into the fluid, so amniotic fluid serves a role in fetal excretory function.

Fetal Development

Pregnancy, or **gestation,** normally takes 40 weeks, during which time the fetus is very busy growing and developing. If we were to peek inside the amniotic sac periodically during pregnancy, this is what we might find at different stages along the way:

- *At 3 weeks*: The embryo is the size of a grape and does not have any recognizable human features.
- *At 4 weeks*: The embryo is about the size of a robin's egg, has the shape of a kidney bean, and weighs about 1 gm. The beginnings of eyes are visible, and there is a primitive circulation.
- *At 8 weeks*: The embryo is about the size of a plum and weighs 4 gm. A good heart beat can be detected by ultrasound. Hands and feet are identifiable. There is about 10 ml of amniotic fluid.
- *At 12 weeks*: The fetus weighs about 60 gm (2 oz). Fingers and toes can be identified.
- *At 16 weeks*: The fetus weighs about 170 gm (5–6 oz). The sex can be distinguished.
- *At 20 weeks*: The fetus weighs about 400 gm (13 oz). The fetal heart sounds are audible with a stethoscope, and the mother can feel fetal movements (**quickening**).
- *At 28 weeks*: The fetus weighs 1 kg (2.2 lb) and has a good chance of surviving if born prematurely.

- *At 36 weeks*: The fetus still has little subcutaneous fat. It weighs about 2.5 kg (5.5 lb).
- *At 40 weeks* (**term**): The fetus is fully developed and well insulated with subcutaneous fat; the skin is not wrinkled.

It is customary to consider the progress of a pregnancy in terms of three 90-day periods, or **trimesters.** The first 90 days of pregnancy, or the FIRST TRIMESTER, see the most crucial stages of development, for it is during the first trimester that fetal cells undergo differentiation into specific tissues. Thus it is during the first trimester that the developing fetus is most vulnerable to damaging effects of certain drugs (e.g., thalidomide) or microorganisms (e.g., the rubella virus). In the SECOND TRIMESTER, the fetus develops bone structure. The mother's uterus begins to expand and becomes palpable above the pelvic rim. By the THIRD TRIMESTER, the last 90 days of pregnancy, the fetus is making its preparations to set forth into the world, and the uterus reaches its maximal expansion, eventually crowding up against the mother's diaphragm in the last weeks before delivery.

COMPLICATIONS OF PREGNANCY

Most pregnancies proceed uneventfully. But now and then complications occur, and it is when complications occur that paramedics are likely to be summoned.

Abortion

Abortion is defined as expulsion of the fetus, from any cause, before the twentieth week of gestation (in some versions of the definition, any loss of the pregnancy up to the the *twenty-eighth* week of gestation is considered an abortion). Most abortions in fact occur during the first trimester, before the placenta is fully mature.

Abortions can be broadly classified as either spontaneous or induced. A **spontaneous abortion** is one that occurs naturally and is often referred to by lay people as a *miscarriage.* Spontaneous abortion occurs in about 1 out of every 5 pregnancies. It may come about for any of a number of reasons, such as acute or chronic illness in the mother, abnormalities in the fetus, or abnormal attachment of the placenta. In many cases, the cause of a spontaneous abortion cannot be found.

In contrast to spontaneous abortion, an **induced abortion** is one that is brought about intentionally. When abortion is induced for justifiable medical reasons and carried out in an authorized medical setting, it is called a **therapeutic abortion.** When abortion is carried out illegally, which usually means under conditions that may pose a hazard to the mother's life, it is called **criminal abortion.**

Signs and Symptoms of Abortion

Detachment of the ovum or embryo from the uterine wall almost always results in bleeding. Indeed, abortion accounts for the vast majority of cases of bleeding in early pregnancy, and bleeding will doubtless be the reason that the woman called for an ambulance (i.e., the chief complaint). The bleeding may be very slight or profuse, and the woman may have noticed that she passed some tissue with the blood. Bleeding from an abortion, furthermore, is often accompanied by cramping abdominal pain.

In taking the *history,* then, try to find out more about the bleeding. WHEN did the bleeding start? HOW MUCH blood was lost (ask the woman how many sanitary napkins or tampons she used)? Ask also about abdominal pain and CRAMPING, using the usual PQRST-A formula to obtain details about the pain. On *physical examination*, the most important thing to look for is evidence of volume depletion from bleeding. Check, therefore, for ORTHOSTATIC CHANGES in vital signs; that is, check the pulse and blood pressure with the woman recumbent, and then check again about a minute after she sits up or stands up. A rise in pulse or fall in blood pressure in going from a recumbent to a sitting or standing position means that the woman has lost a significant volume of blood and must be treated for shock, as detailed in Chapter 9.

Stages of Abortion

The specific management of a spontaneous abortion will depend to some extent on the stage of the abortion at the time the patient presents for treatment.

A **threatened abortion** is characterized by vaginal bleeding during the first half of pregnancy—usually in the first trimester. There may be some abdominal discomfort, resembling menstrual cramps, but the woman ordinarily does *not* experience severe pain because there aren't any rhythmic uterine contractions. The cervix remains closed. Threatened abortion may progress to incomplete abortion, or it may subside, allowing the pregnancy to go to term. The treatment is usually bed rest for a week or for as long as the bleeding continues, but the woman should first be evaluated at the hospital. For the paramedic that means simply to transport and provide emotional support.

An **inevitable abortion** is a spontaneous abortion that cannot be prevented. Inevitable abortion is characterized by vaginal bleeding, sometimes quite massive; strong and painful uterine contractions; and dilatation of the cervix. When the patient's history is consistent with inevitable abortion, start an IV LIFELINE, and give normal saline or lactated Ringer's solution as rapidly as necessary to maintain blood pressure during transport.

An **incomplete abortion** occurs when part of the products of conception are expelled, but some remain in the uterus. Bleeding may be slight or profuse, but it is continuous, and the cervix remains dilated. Treatment is for shock, if present. In any event, start an IV LIFELINE with crystalloid. If products of conception are protruding from the vagina, consult medical command for instructions; gentle removal of protruding tissues may prevent or relieve signs of shock.

In a **missed abortion,** there is prolonged retention in the uterus of a fetus that died during the first 20 weeks of gestation. Generally the woman gives a history of threatened abortion that seemed to get better; the bleeding stopped, and everything seemed fine. But slowly the typical signs of pregnancy began to disappear: The breasts stopped developing; the uterus stopped enlarging. The mother may also report having had a brownish vaginal discharge. On examination, the uterus may be felt as a hard mass in the abdomen, and fetal heart sounds cannot be heard. The only management possible in the field for suspected missed abortion is TRANSPORT to the hospital, where the uterus will have to be evacuated surgically.

Septic abortion occurs when the uterus becomes infected following any type of abortion, but especially after an incomplete or an induced abortion. The patient will give a history of fever and bad-smelling vaginal discharge usually starting within a few hours after abortion. On physical examination, there is likely to be fever and abdominal tenderness. In severe cases, the woman may be in shock from septicemia. Prehospital management consists of starting an IV LIFELINE and administering crystalloids at a rate sufficient to maintain the blood pressure.

Third Trimester Bleeding

Vaginal bleeding is a bad sign at any stage of pregnancy, but it is particularly worrisome when it occurs during the third trimester, for the danger of exsanguinating hemorrhage is most acute as the woman approaches term. There are three main causes of significant **antepartum hemorrhage** (hemorrhage before delivery): abruptio placenta, placenta previa, and uterine rupture.

Abruptio Placenta

Abruptio placenta refers to a premature separation of a normally implanted placenta from the wall of the uterus during the last trimester of pregnancy. It occurs in about 1 out of every 400 pregnancies that go to term and is more likely in women who have been hypertensive during their pregnancy, who have had many pregnancies, or who have had abruptio placenta in a previous pregnancy. The patient will usually report *vaginal bleeding*, with loss of dark red blood, although in some cases the blood does not emerge through the cervix and the bleeding may remain concealed. With or without obvious bleeding, however, the woman will experience the sudden onset of severe *abdominal pain*, and she may report that she no longer feels the baby moving inside her. On physical examination, there may be signs of *shock*; indeed, shock is likely to be out of proportion to the apparent volume of blood loss. The abdomen will be *tender*, and the *uterus rigid* to palpation. Fetal heart sounds are often absent, since the fetus, partly or completely cut off from its blood supply, is likely to die.

Placenta Previa

In **placenta previa**, the placenta is implanted low in the uterus, so that it partially or completely covers the cervical canal. It is most likely in older women (over age 35) and in those who have had many previous pregnancies. Bleeding from placenta previa usually occurs late in the third trimester, as the cervix begins to dilate in preparation for delivery. The chief complaint of a woman with placenta previa is usually *painless vaginal bleeding*, with the loss of *bright red blood*. Since the blood supply to the fetus is not immediately jeopardized, fetal movements continue, and fetal heart sounds are still audible. On gentle palpation, the uterus is *soft* and nontender. (Do *not* try to palpate the abdomen deeply in any woman with third trimester bleeding; if she does have placenta previa, deep palpation may induce heavy bleeding.)

Uterine Rupture

Rupture of the uterus occurs, if it is going to occur at all, during labor. Those most at risk are women who have had many children and those with a scar on the uterus (e.g., from a previous cesarean section). In the typical scenario, you will be called for a "possible OB," and find a woman in active labor complaining of *weakness, dizziness, and thirst*. She may tell you that at first she had very strong and painful contractions, and then the contractions slackened off. On physical examination, there are *signs of shock*—sweating,

tachycardia, falling blood pressure. Significant vaginal bleeding may or may not be obvious.

Prehospital Management of Third Trimester Bleeding

In practice, it is not necessary in the field to make a precise diagnosis of the cause of third trimester bleeding. What *is* important is to recognize the gravity of the situation and move expeditiously:

> **ANY VAGINAL BLEEDING DURING THE THIRD TRIMESTER OF PREGNANCY MUST BE REGARDED AS A DIRE MEDICAL EMERGENCY UNTIL PROVED OTHERWISE.**

Regardless of the possible source of third trimester hemorrhage, the prehospital management is the same:

- Keep the woman RECUMBENT, lying on her left side.
- Administer OXYGEN.
- Begin TRANSPORT immediately, and NOTIFY the receiving hospital of the nature of the case.
- Start AT LEAST ONE LARGE-BORE IV en route to the hospital, and administer normal saline or lactated Ringer's solution as rapidly as needed to maintain blood pressure.
- DO NOT UNDER ANY CIRCUMSTANCES ATTEMPT TO EXAMINE THE PATIENT INTERNALLY.

Preeclampsia and Eclampsia

Preeclampsia

Preeclampsia is the first stage of a progressive condition called *toxemia of pregnancy*, which begins in susceptible women after the twentieth week of pregnancy. Toxemia most often affects women during their first pregnancy. Chronic hypertension and diabetes also seem to be predisposing factors. The term *toxemia* is not a very good one, because there are no toxins actually present in the blood, and in fact the cause of preeclampsia and eclampsia is not known. What toxemia does is produce derangements in the pregnant woman's circulation that particularly affect blood flow to her kidneys. The kidneys become very unhappy when their blood flow is disturbed. They start losing track of how much sodium they are supposed to excrete to maintain the body's salt balance, and they become rather overzealous as well about their role in regulating the blood pressure. As a result, what you see clinically in preeclampsia is EDEMA (from salt and water retention) and HYPERTENSION. The patient may also experience headaches, blurring of vision, and abdominal pain. But what makes preeclampsia so insidious is that very often there are NO SYMPTOMS AT ALL in the early stages. What that means is that you won't suspect preeclampsia if you don't specifically look for it. For that reason, it is imperative to

---

RECORD A BLOOD PRESSURE AND THE PRESENCE OR ABSENCE OF EDEMA IN EVERY PREGNANT WOMAN YOU EXAMINE—NO MATTER WHAT THE CHIEF COMPLAINT.

Blood pressure is normally somewhat low during the third trimester of pregnancy, and any blood pressure *over 130/80 mm Hg* should therefore be called to the attention of the doctor at the receiving hospital. If the patient's prepregnancy blood pressure is known, then any increase in the diastolic pressure of 15 mm Hg above that baseline should be considered suspect.

Preeclampsia is detrimental to the fetus as well as to the mother. The mother's peripheral vasoconstriction means impaired fetal perfusion. The result may be a slowing of fetal growth or even fetal death.

Eclampsia

Eclampsia refers to the full-blown toxemic syndrome of *headaches, visual disturbances, epigastric pain,* massive *edema* (especially of the face and hands), *proteinuria,* and *seizures.* It is the occurrence of seizures that most clearly marks the transition from preeclampsia to eclampsia. Preeclampsia may progress rapidly to eclampsia before, during, or after delivery. Eclampsia carries a mortality of 5 to 15 percent and is the second leading cause of maternal death.

The patient with eclampsia may present with a chief complaint of headache, blurring of vision, or abdominal pain. On physical examination, the patient usually appears pale and apprehensive with a puffy face and hands. Her blood pressure will be elevated, and if you check the deep tendon reflexes, you will find them hyperactive.

The goal of prehospital TREATMENT of toxemia

is to try to prevent the onset of seizures or, if seizures do occur, to control them rapidly.

- Keep the patient RECUMBENT on her left side in a QUIET, DARKENED ROOM until you are ready for transport.
- Administer OXYGEN.
- Start an IV LIFELINE with D5/W to keep a vein open.
- NOTIFY the receiving hospital of the patient's situation and your estimated time of arrival (ETA).
- Move the patient smoothly to the ambulance. TRANSPORT as gently as possible: NO SIRENS. NO FLASHING LIGHTS. Loud noises and flickering lights can precipitate seizures.
- Keep suction close at hand.
- Anticipate SEIZURES at any moment. If they do occur, safeguard the AIRWAY and notify the physician, who may order:
  1. DIAZEPAM (Valium), 5 to 10 mg slowly IV.
  2. MAGNESIUM SULFATE 10%, 2 to 4 gm SLOWLY IV. (The use of magnesium sulfate is now controversial in some quarters, so be guided by local protocol.)
  Have those medications at hand, ready to administer, as your protocol specifies. Bear in mind that magnesium sulfate may cause respiratory depression, so its antidote—calcium gluconate—should also be close at hand.
- Administration of MEDICATIONS TO LOWER THE BLOOD PRESSURE is best postponed until the woman reaches the hospital, for very careful titration is required to avoid causing a precipitous fall in blood pressure that could jeopardize placental circulation. When the woman is very far from the hospital, however, the physician may order HYDRALAZINE (Apresoline), 5 mg *slowly* IV.

Supine Hypotensive Syndrome

The pregnant woman near term has a large, heavy mass in her abdomen, and when she lies on her back, that mass—comprising the weight of the uterus, fetus, and placenta—compresses the inferior vena cava. Venous return to the heart is impaired, and as a consequence, cardiac output falls by as much as 30 to 40 percent. Those changes are especially pronounced if the mother's vascular volume is marginal to begin with, as, for example, in the setting of antepartum hemorrhage.

When you encounter a pregnant woman near term who is hypotensive or complaining of dizziness, the first thing to do, then, is to place her in a recumbent position, LYING ON HER SIDE. The lateral position will shift the weight of the gravid (pregnant) uterus off the vena cava. *Then* check her blood pressure. If hypotension persists, the problem is something more than supine hypotensive syndrome, and you must suspect internal bleeding and treat for impending shock.

Preexisting Illness

A variety of underlying, chronic medical conditions may affect a woman's pregnancy or be aggravated by the pregnancy, so it is important to ask the pregnant woman about underlying illnesses. Previously well-controlled *diabetes*, for example, may become unstable during pregnancy, requiring adjustments in insulin dosage that in turn may lead to episodes of hypoglycemia or hyperglycemia. Underlying *hypertension* is also likely to be aggravated during pregnancy and may be complicated by preeclampsia or eclampsia. Pregnancy places considerable demands on a woman's cardiovascular system, for she must increase her cardiac output by about 40 percent to supply the additional circulation required by the fetus. In a woman with preexisting *heart disease*, the increased cardiac output may place an excessive strain on her weakened heart, leading to heart failure.

Trauma During Pregnancy

Trauma affects 6 to 8 percent of pregnant women in America. The three major causes of injury to pregnant women are motor vehicle accidents, falls, and penetrating injuries such as gunshot wounds. Trauma to a pregnant woman is double trouble because there are *two* patients involved—the woman and her baby. Both patients are particularly vulnerable to trauma because of the unique features of pregnancy.

The Vulnerability of the Pregnant Woman to Trauma

Pregnancy involves major changes in a woman's anatomy and physiology, some of which put the woman at higher risk of injury and some of which may confuse the interpretation of trauma signs and symptoms.

The ANATOMIC CHANGES of pregnancy, many of which are obvious to all, have important implications for trauma. As the woman approaches term, her abdominal contents are compressed into the upper abdomen. The *diaphragm is elevated* by about 1.5 inches (4 cm), so there is a higher incidence of abdominal injuries in association with chest trauma. Meanwhile, because the peritoneum is maximally

stretched, significant abdominal trauma may occur without peritoneal signs.

As early as the second trimester, the *bladder is displaced* upward and forward so that it lies outside the pelvic cavity and is therefore at increased risk of injury, particularly deceleration injury from a lap seat belt. The uterus too becomes more vulnerable to injury as it increases in size; and deceleration forces, such as those produced by vehicular trauma, may bring about abruptio placenta or uterine rupture.

Along with the anatomic changes of pregnancy come important PHYSIOLOGIC CHANGES as well. To begin with, there are major alterations in cardiovascular function during pregnancy. The pregnant woman has to perfuse two circulations, her own and that of the fetus, so her *vascular volume increases* by nearly 50 percent over the first 6 months of pregnancy. To pump that increased vascular volume, the *cardiac ouput also increases*, by about 40 percent, both by increasing stroke volume and *increasing pulse rate*. The resting heart rate increases by 15 to 20 beats per minute over that in the nonpregnant state, so the resting pulse may be as high as 100 per minute by the end of the second trimester, making it much more difficult to interpret tachycardia. Furthermore, because of the vastly expanded blood volume, other signs of hypovolemia, such as a falling blood pressure, may not be evident until the woman has lost as much as 35 percent of her blood volume.

> **A PREGNANT WOMAN MAY LOSE A LOT OF BLOOD BEFORE SHE SHOWS SIGNS OF SHOCK. DON'T WAIT FOR SIGNS AND SYMPTOMS. SUSPECT SHOCK FROM THE MECHANISMS OF INJURY.**

Finally, there is a relative *redistribution of blood volume* during pregnancy, with a tenfold increase in blood flow to the pelvic region. If a pregnant woman sustains pelvic fracture, therefore, her chances of bleeding to death are significantly higher than those of a nonpregnant woman with the same injury.

On the respiratory side, the pregnant woman has a higher basal metabolism and therefore an increased need for oxygen. At the same time, she has more carbon dioxide to get rid of—hers and that produced by fetal metabolism. She responds by *increasing her tidal volume*, and thus her minute volume. And if she should for any reason need artificial ventilation, you will have to do the same *for* her; that is, ventilate her with supplementary oxygen at a higher minute volume than usual.

Yet another physiologic change during pregnancy is a *decrease in the rate of gastric emptying*, which, along with compression of the stomach by the uterus, increases the risk of aspiration.

The Vulnerability of the Fetus to Trauma

The muscular wall of the uterus cushions the fetus against the direct effects of blunt trauma. But fetal injury can occur as a result of rapid deceleration or secondary to impaired fetal circulation. The most common cause of fetal death in accidents is maternal death. But the fetus may also die when the mother survives, especially when abdominal trauma to the mother leads to abruptio placenta. Any injury that involves significant maternal bleeding, furthermore, will threaten the life of the fetus; for nature has designed things such that *maternal circulation will be maintained at the expense of the fetus*. If the mother is bleeding massively, therefore, her vascular system will shunt blood away from the fetal circulation in order to maintain her own blood pressure. By the time the mother is showing clinical signs of shock, fetal circulation will be so compromised that one can expect a 70- to 80-percent fetal mortality.

The best indication of the status of the fetus after trauma is the fetal heart rate. A **normal fetal heart rate** is between **120 to 160 per minute.** A rate slower than 120 per minute means fetal distress and therefore signals a dire emergency. (To measure the fetal heart rate, listen with the bell of the stethoscope over the abdomen. You may have to move your stethoscope around the abdomen a bit until you can hear the fetal heart tones. When you do hear fetal heart tones, palpate the mother's pulse at the same time as you count the fetal heart rate. If the fetal heart rate is identical to the maternal pulse, you are probably listening to an echo of the maternal heart beat and not the fetal heart, so change the position of your stethoscope and try again.) It takes a lot of practice to hear fetal heart tones and requires quiet surroundings as well. In most prehospital settings, the necessary quiet conditions are hard to come by.

Treatment of the Pregnant Trauma Victim

Although trauma in a pregnant woman involves *two* patients, we can treat only one of them directly: the mother. It is a safe generalization, however, that

Anything we can do to improve the mother's state of perfusion will inevitably improve fetal perfusion as well.

- Ensure an adequate AIRWAY. In the unconscious patient, that means early endotracheal intubation to isolate the airway, since regurgitation and aspiration are much more likely in a pregnant woman than in a nonpregnant patient.
- Administer OXYGEN. A pregnant woman's oxygen needs are 10 to 20 percent higher than normal.
- ASSIST VENTILATIONS AS NEEDED, and remember to provide a *higher minute volume* than usual. Because of the uterus pressing up against the diaphragm, it will be more difficult to ventilate a pregnant woman. Once the patient is intubated, therefore, you may want to use a demand valve periodically, to ensure an adequate tidal volume.
- CONTROL EXTERNAL BLEEDING promptly.
- NOTIFY the receiving hospital of the patient's status and your ETA.
- TRANSPORT the woman in the LATERAL RECUMBENT POSITION. If she is on a backboard, tilt the backboard 30 degrees to the left to take the weight of the woman's gravid (pregnant) uterus off the inferior vena cava and thereby improve venous return to her heart.
- Start AT LEAST ONE LARGE-BORE IV en route, and administer lactated Ringer's solution at a rate sufficient to maintain the blood pressure. In general, you will need to give larger volumes of fluid than you would in a nonpregnant woman.
- *If cardiac arrest occurs,* carry out CPR in the usual fashion, but wedge a pillow or inflatable splint underneath the woman's right hip, to displace her uterus off her inferior vena cava.

Potential damage to the other patient, the *fetus,* cannot be adequately assessed in the field. While a decreased fetal heart rate signals an emergency situation, a normal fetal heart rate does not guarantee that everything is all right. Even in cases where the mother sustained only minor injury, there may have been major trauma to the baby, especially in accidents involving significant deceleration forces (e.g., vehicular accidents). Thus

---

WHAT'S GOOD FOR THE MOTHER IS GOOD FOR THE FETUS.

***EVERY* PREGNANT WOMAN WHO HAS BEEN IN AN ACCIDENT MUST BE EVALUATED AT THE HOSPITAL, EVEN IF HER OWN INJURIES APPEAR TRIVIAL.**

At the other end of the spectrum is the pregnant woman who has been critically or hopelessly injured during her third trimester. Once again, one has to bear in mind that there are *two* lives involved. It may not be possible to save both lives, but sometimes the baby can be saved even when the mother cannot. Practically speaking, that means that you must go all out in the effort to resuscitate a pregnant woman, even when the situation seems hopeless. Good CPR—with endotracheal intubation, oxygen-supplemented artificial ventilation, and effective chest compressions—may keep the baby alive even after the mother is biologically dead and may thus permit the baby to be delivered alive by emergency cesarean section at the receiving hospital.

NORMAL CHILDBIRTH

Assisting in the birth of a baby is one of the few situations in which a paramedic has the opportunity to participate in a happy event rather than a tragic one. Usually Mother Nature will ensure that it *is* a happy event. But sometimes medical intervention is required to produce a happy outcome. Indeed, as Murphy's Law* would predict, the chances that complications will occur during delivery are significantly greater when delivery occurs in an unplanned fashion outside the hospital. So if there is going to be a problematic delivery, it won't happen to the obstetric specialist in the hospital; it will happen to the paramedic trying to deliver a baby in a movie theater. For that reason, providers of prehospital care need to be well schooled in how to assist at a normal delivery and what to do when complications arise.

Ordinarily, a woman will call for an ambulance at some point during her labor, so let us start by reviewing the stages of normal labor.

The Stages of Labor

Labor refers to the mechanism by which the **products of conception**—that is, the baby and the placenta—are expelled from the mother's uterus. It is called labor because it is hard work!

Some Definitions

In order to talk about the characteristics of labor and delivery in women with different obstetric histories, we need some special terminology. We need to be able to describe with precision how many times a woman has been pregnant before and how many times she has carried a fetus to a viable age. The term **gravida** refers to a uterus that contains a pregnancy, whatever the outcome (i.e., whether it resulted in an abortion, stillbirth, or live birth). **Parity** refers to delivery of a child after the twenty-eighth week of pregnancy, irrespective of whether it was born alive or dead. We classify a woman, then, according to the number of times her uterus has been occupied (gravidity) and the number of times she has carried a fetus more than 28 weeks (parity):

- A **primigravida** is a woman who is pregnant for the first time.
- A **primipara** ("primip" for short) is a woman who has had one delivery only.
- A **multigravida** is a woman who has had two or more pregnancies, irrespective of the outcome.
- A **multipara** ("multip" for short) is a woman who has had two or more deliveries. A woman who has had *lots* of deliveries (more than five) is referred to as a "grand multipara!"
- A **nullipara** is a woman who has never delivered.

Thus, for example, a woman who has had four pregnancies but carried only one of them to term—the three others ended in miscarriage—would be classified as gravida 4, para 1.

With those definitions in mind, let us consider the normal stages of labor.

Stages of Labor

Labor progresses through several, well-defined stages, whose duration depends in part on whether the mother is going through her first pregnancy or whether she is already a veteran at having babies. Labor starts with a PRODROMAL STAGE, which often goes unnoticed. In the prodromal stage, the woman begins to feel a relief of pressure in her upper abdomen and a simultaneous increase of pressure in her pelvis as the baby starts its descent toward the birth canal. A plug of mucus, sometimes mixed with blood, called the **bloody show,** is expelled from the dilating cervix and discharged from the vagina.

The FIRST STAGE OF LABOR begins with the onset of regular labor pains, crampy abdominal pains that may radiate into the small of the back and reflect the contractions of the uterus. Those early contractions come at about 5- to 15-minute intervals, and they serve to maneuver the baby into position, as well as to prepare the cervical opening through which the baby will have to make its exit. As the uterus contracts, its less muscular lower segment is pulled upward over the presenting part, resulting in

---

*Murphy's Law states that anything that *can* go wrong *will* go wrong.

effacement (thinning and shortening) of the cervix. Effacement is accompanied by progessive cervical **dilatation,** that is, stretching of the opening of the cervix until it is wide enough to accommodate passage of a baby. The first stage of labor lasts until the cervix is fully dilated, an average of about 12 hours in a nullipara and anywhere up to 8 hours in a multipara. It is usually toward the end of the first stage of labor that the amniotic sac ruptures, with a dramatic gush of fluid suddenly pouring out of the vagina.

The SECOND STAGE OF LABOR begins as the baby's head enters the birth canal. The mother's pains become more intense and more frequent, now occurring 2 to 3 minutes apart. Her pulse rate increases. Sweat appears on her face. She tends to bear down with each contraction, and because of the pressure of the baby's head against her rectum, she may feel as if she has to move her bowels. The cervix meanwhile becomes fully dilated and effaced, and the **presenting part** of the baby (the part that emerges from the mother first—normally the head) begins bulging out of the vaginal opening, a process called **crowning** (Fig. 35-3). When crowning occurs, delivery is imminent. The second stage of labor is concluded when the baby is fully delivered. Altogether, the second stage of labor takes about an hour in a nullipara and 20 to 30 minutes in a multipara.

The THIRD STAGE OF LABOR, also called the placental stage, is the period from the delivery of the baby until the placenta has been fully expelled and the uterus has contracted. Uterine contraction is necessary to squeeze shut all of the tiny blood vessels left exposed when the placenta separates from the uterine wall.

The stages of labor are summarized in Table 35-1.

Assessment of the Obstetric Patient

In assessing the pregnant woman who has called for an ambulance because of labor pains, the paramedic really needs to answer only two questions:

- Am *I* going to have to deliver this baby?!
- If so, what potential complications, if any, should I anticipate in this particular case?

Is There Time to Reach the Hospital?

To answer the first question, that is, to determine whether there will be adequate time to transport the woman to the hospital, find out the following:

- HAS THE WOMAN HAD A BABY BEFORE? As mentioned earlier, labor in a nullipara is usually

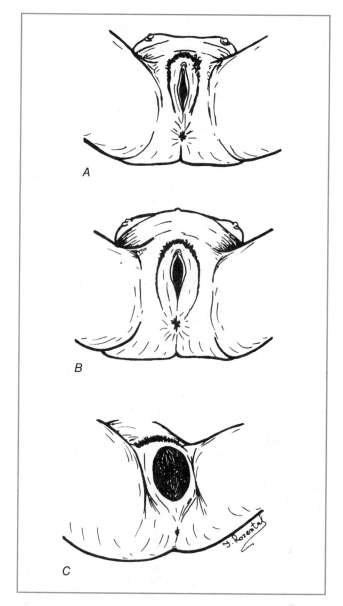

FIGURE 35-3. CROWNING. (A) Vaginal opening in a nonpregnant woman. (B) Early crowning. (C) Late crowning, just before delivery.

slower than in subsequent pregnancies, allowing more time for transport.
- WHAT ARE THE CONTRACTIONS LIKE? Some women experience **Braxton Hicks contractions** (sometimes called "false labor") toward the end of pregnancy, and it is important to distinguish those contractions from the real thing (Table 35-2). The pains of true labor are regularly spaced and increase in intensity over time.
- HOW FREQUENT ARE THE CONTRACTIONS? If contractions are more than 5 minutes apart, there is generally enough time to get the woman to a nearby hospital. Contractions less than 2

minutes apart signal impending delivery, especially in a multip.

- DOES THE MOTHER FEEL AN URGE TO MOVE HER BOWELS? That sensation occurring during labor is caused by the baby's head in the mother's vagina pressing against the rectum. It indicates that delivery is imminent. If the mother does report an urge to move her bowels, then:

> ## DO NOT ALLOW THE MOTHER TO GO TO THE TOILET.

The answers to those questions should give you a very good idea of whether there will be time to transport the woman to the hospital. To double-check, *inspect* (don't touch!) the mother for CROWNING (Fig. 35-3). Crowning indicates that the baby will be born within the next few minutes, whether you are ready or not!

Is this Likely to be a Complicated Delivery?

To answer the second question—what potential complications should be anticipated—you need to ask a few more questions and examine the woman further,

if the baby gives you time to do so. Even as you are setting up for delivery, try to find out:

- DID THE WOMAN RECEIVE PRENATAL CARE? The incidence of obstetric complications is higher in women who did not receive care during their pregnancy.
- WHEN WAS THE BABY DUE? Obstetric complications, such as breech delivery or prolapsed umbilical cord (see under Abnormal Deliveries), occur more frequently in a **premature birth** because the baby is smaller.
- HAS THE AMNIOTIC SAC ("bag of waters") RUPTURED, and if so, when? If rupture occurred many hours before, the likelihood of fetal infection is increased, and the hospital staff should be informed.
- HAS THE WOMAN HAD A PREVIOUS CESAREAN SECTION? Rupture of the uterus is more likely in a woman whose uterus has the scar of previous surgery.
- DID THE MOTHER HAVE ANY PROBLEMS WITH THIS PREGNANCY OR PREVIOUS PREGNANCIES?

If delivery is imminent, you will not have time to conduct an extensive physical examination, but try if possible to do the following:

- MEASURE THE VITAL SIGNS. If the blood pressure is elevated or the hands and face look puffy, test the *deep tendon reflexes* at the knees ("knee jerks") for hyperactivity. Any of those signs—elevated blood pressure, facial edema, or hyperactive reflexes—strongly suggest that the woman has preeclampsia, and you must be prepared to deal with seizures before, during, or after delivery.
- ESTIMATE THE GESTATIONAL AGE. Palpate the abdomen to estimate the height of the uterus.

TABLE 35-1. THE STAGES OF LABOR

STAGE OF LABOR	DURATION IN A NULLIPARA	DURATION IN A MULTIPARA
First stage	8–12 hours	6–8 hours
Second stage	1–2 hours	30 minutes
Third stage	5–60 minutes	5–60 minutes

TABLE 35-2. DISTINGUISHING FALSE VERSUS TRUE LABOR

PARAMETER	TRUE LABOR	FALSE LABOR
Contractions	Regularly spaced	Irregularly spaced
Interval between contractions	Gradually shortens	Remains long
Intensity of contractions	Gradually increases	Stays the same
Effects of analgesics	Do not abolish the pain	Often abolish the pain
Cervical changes	Progressive effacement and dilatation	No changes

If the top of the uterus (the **fundus**) is palpable just above the symphysis pubis, the gestational age is 12 to 16 weeks; if the fundus is palpable at the level of the mother's umbilicus, the gestational age is 22 weeks; if the fundus reaches all the way to the xiphoid, the fetus is at or near term.

- LISTEN FOR FETAL HEART TONES as described earlier. Remember, the normal fetal heart rate is 120–160 beats per minute.

> **A FETAL HEART RATE LOWER THAN 120 PER MINUTE MEANS FETAL DISTRESS.**

If the history and physical assessment indicate that there is ample time to reach the hospital, place the mother in the lateral recumbent position, remove any of her underclothing that might obstruct delivery in the event that the baby surprises you en route to the hospital, and then transport. In any event,

> **NEVER, NEVER, NEVER ATTEMPT TO DELAY OR RESTRAIN DELIVERY IN ANY FASHION.**

If you reach the conclusion that there is *not* enough time to get to the hospital, prepare to assist in delivery of the baby at the scene. In a crowded or public place, try to find an area of maximum privacy and cleanliness in which to work. In the patient's home, deploy nervous bystanders in such a way as to keep them occupied, preferably elsewhere. (Traditionally, for example, husbands have been dispatched to the kitchen to boil large volumes of water. There is no particular use for boiling water in carrying out a delivery, but the task keeps the husband busy in another room!) The mother may find it reassuring to have another woman (e.g., a friend, sister, mother, neighbor) or her husband present. But your own behavior, if calm and reassuring, will be the most effective sedative for patient and bystanders alike.

> **THE PARAMEDIC'S MOST IMPORTANT JOB AT A DELIVERY IS TO APPEAR CALM.**

Setting up for Delivery Outside the Hospital

When a paramedic has to assist in childbirth outside the hospital, it is because there isn't time to reach the hospital. And when there isn't time to reach the hospital, there generally isn't time for a lot of preparations. You may have only a minute or two to get the mother into position, open the OB kit, and catch the baby! So the sequence of actions in emergency childbirth needs to be well planned and well rehearsed before it is deployed in the field.

- POSITION THE MOTHER-TO-BE. If childbirth is to take place in the patient's home, the mother is usually delivered lying supine in her bed, preferably with a Reeves stretcher and sheet beneath her to facilitate moving her after delivery. It should be pointed out, however, that while placing the mother in the supine position makes things much easier for the paramedic assisting delivery, it makes things harder for the mother, for she has to push against gravity. Some women therefore prefer to sit at the edge of a chair or to squat for delivery—positions that enable the woman to take advantage of gravity. If that is the mother's preference, don't argue! Assign someone to stand behind her and support her back, and position yourself such that you will be able to "catch" the baby when it comes.

  In the ambulance, there generally isn't enough working space to permit the woman to sit or squat for delivery, and you will need to position the mother on her back on the stretcher, with a folded sheet under her buttocks. She should then bend her knees and spread her thighs apart (Fig. 35-4).

FIGURE 35-4. POSITION FOR DELIVERY. When the mother is to be delivered in bed or on a stretcher, position her supine with her knees and hips flexed and her buttocks slightly elevated on folded towels.

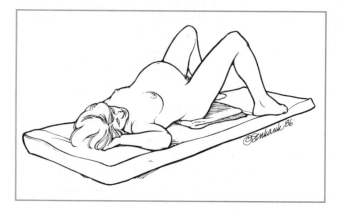

- OPEN THE STERILE OBSTETRIC KIT, touching only the outside. Every ambulance should carry such a kit that contains all of the equipment needed for a delivery (Table 35-3).
- WASH YOUR HANDS THOROUGHLY. Keep povidone-iodine scrub solution with the kit for this purpose.
- DON STERILE GLOVES.
- Don goggles and a disposable surgical mask and gown. Remember, deliveries are messy, so there is always a risk of contamination from infected blood or bodily fluids.
- DRAPE THE MOTHER with sterile towels. Place the first sterile towel beneath her buttocks, taking care not to touch her or the sheet beneath her as you do so. Lay a second sterile towel flat on the bed or stretcher between the mother's legs, just below the vaginal opening. A third sterile towel or drape should be laid across the mother's abdomen, and each thigh should be draped as well. When you finish, everything should be covered with sterile drapes except the vaginal opening.

> **IF THE BABY IS COMING FAST, IT IS MORE IMPORTANT TO CONTROL THE DELIVERY THAN TO PUT ON STERILE DRAPES.**

While you are getting set up as described, your partner should be tending to the emotional preparation of the woman and bystanders. Remember, most women don't *plan* to have their babies in a movie theater or a football stadium, so the mother and her ret-

inue may be understandably upset. Your partner's job is to calm them down and then to take up a position at the mother's head, with an emesis basin and portable suction at hand. If there is a spare moment, your partner should also START AN IV LIFELINE with D5/W to keep a vein open, especially if your local OB protocol calls for giving oxytocin after delivery.

The mother should be encouraged to rest between contractions and to resist bearing down until you are ready to assist with the delivery. If she finds it difficult not to bear down, instruct her to "pant like a dog" during each contraction. Panting makes it nearly impossible to push, since bearing down requires a closed glottis.

Assisting Delivery

With the mother prepared as described, take up a position just distal to her buttocks (on her right side if you are right-handed, on her left side if you are left-handed). Then proceed as follows:

- CONTROL THE DELIVERY. That is, when crowning occurs, place *gentle* pressure on the baby's head with the palm of your hand, to prevent the head from delivering too quickly and tearing the mother's vagina.
- As the baby's head begins to emerge from the vagina, it will start to turn. SUPPORT THE HEAD AS IT TURNS (Fig. 35-5). Do *not* attempt to pull the baby from the vagina! If the membranes cover the head after it emerges, tear the amniotic sac with your fingers or forceps to permit escape of amniotic fluid and enable the baby to breathe.

FIGURE 35-5. **SUPPORT INFANT'S HEAD** as it delivers.

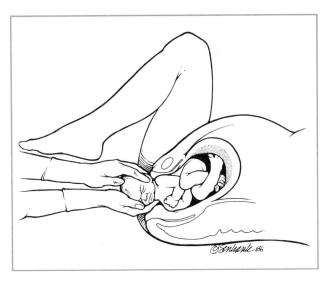

TABLE 35-3. STERILE OBSTETRIC KIT FOR AMBULANCES

QUANTITY	EQUIPMENT
1 pair	Surgical scissors
4	Cord clamps
4–6	12-inch lengths of umbilical tape
4–6	Towels
2–3 pair	Surgical gloves
1	Surgical gown
1–2	Surgical masks
12	4- by 4-inch gauze sponges
1	Bulb syringe
1	Baby blanket
2	Large plastic bags

- Slip your middle finger alongside the baby's head to his neck to CHECK THAT THE UMBILICAL CORD IS NOT WRAPPED AROUND THE BABY'S NECK. If it is, try to slip it gently over the shoulder and head (Fig. 35-6). Should that maneuver fail, and if the cord is wrapped tightly around the neck, place umbilical clamps 2 inches apart and cut the cord between the clamps.
- With the baby's head cradled and supported in your hand, CLEAR THE BABY'S AIRWAY with the bulb syringe. (For technique, see below.)
- Gently guide the baby's head downward to ALLOW DELIVERY OF THE UPPER SHOULDER (Fig. 35-7). Remember, *it is not necessary to pull!*

- Gently guide the head upward to ALLOW DELIVERY OF THE LOWER SHOULDER (Fig. 35-8).
- Once the shoulders are delivered, the baby's trunk and legs will follow rapidly. Be prepared to grasp and support the infant as it emerges, keeping in mind an important fact:

BABIES ARE SLIPPERY!

Therefore, lay the baby along your arm, and grasp it like a football, with one arm and shoulder between your fingers and the head held dependent to aid drainage (Fig. 35-9).
- Wipe any blood or mucus from the baby's nose and mouth with a sterile gauze. Then use the rubber bulb aspirator to SUCTION THE MOUTH AND NOSTRILS. Be sure to squeeze the bulb *before* inserting the tip, *then* place the tip in the baby's mouth or nostril and release the bulb slowly (Fig. 35-10). Withdraw the bulb, expel its contents into a waste container, and repeat suctioning as needed.
- DRY THE BABY with sterile towels (heat loss is much faster from a wet baby than a dry baby, remember?), and COVER THE BABY with a blanket.
- RECORD THE TIME OF BIRTH.

FIGURE 35-6. **LOOSEN CORD** from around neck.

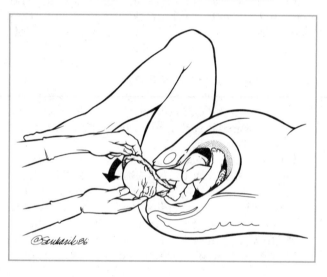

FIGURE 35-7. Gently guide head downward to **HELP UPPER SHOULDER DELIVER.**

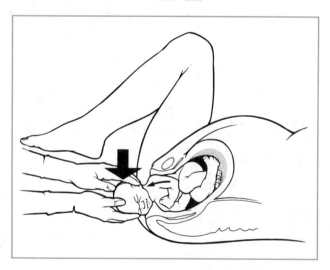

FIGURE 35-8. Guide head upward to **HELP LOWER SHOULDER DELIVER.**

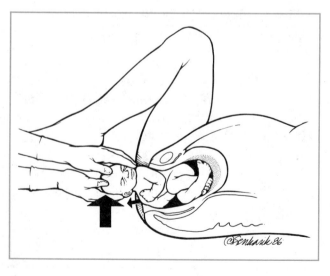

In a normal delivery, the baby will usually be breathing on its own, if not shrieking, by the time you finish suctioning the airway. Babies are usually born blue, but with a few good howls, the baby should turn a nice pink, although its extremities may remain dusky. It will be useful to those who take over the care of the baby if you are able to quantitate the baby's status right after birth. A standardized way of doing so is called the **Apgar** scoring system.

Apgar Scoring

The scoring system devised by Virginia Apgar is a useful means of evaluating the adequacy of a newborn's vital functions immediately after birth. Five parameters—heart rate, respiratory effort, muscle tone, reflex irritability, and color—are each given a score from 0 to 2. The majority of infants are vigorous and have a total score of 7 to 10; they cough or cry within seconds of delivery and require no further resuscitation. Infants with a score in the 4 to 6 range are moderately depressed; they may be pale or blue 1 minute after delivery, with poorly sustained respirations and flaccid muscle tone. Such infants will require some form of resuscitation.

The five signs to be evaluated in Apgar scoring are most easily remembered with the mnemonic "APGAR":

A   Appearance (color)
P   Pulse (heart rate)
G   Grimace (reflex irritability to a gentle slap)
A   Activity (muscle tone)
R   Respiratory effort

Sixty seconds and 5 minutes after the complete birth of the infant, evaluate those five signs according to the scoring system shown in Table 35-4. Give each sign a score of 0, 1, or 2. A total score of 10 indicates that the infant is in the best possible condition. A

FIGURE 35-10.   **SUCTIONING THE NEWBORN.** (A) *First* squeeze the bulb. (B) Then insert the tip of the aspirator into the baby's nostril or mouth. (C) *Then* slowly release the bulb.

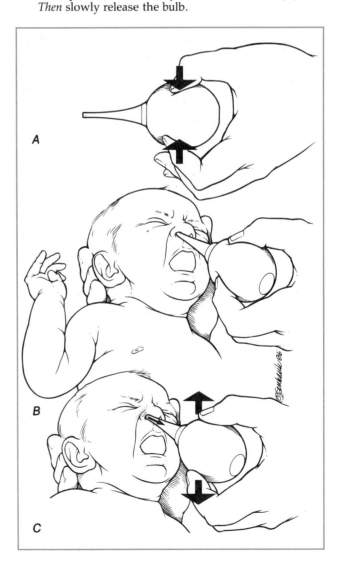

FIGURE 35-9. Babies are slippery! **HOLD THE BABY FIRMLY,** with its head dependent to facilitate drainage of secretions.

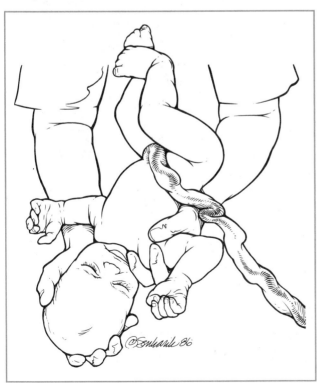

TABLE 35-4. APGAR SCORING SYSTEM

CLINICAL SIGN		POINTS GIVEN ACCORDING TO STATUS		
		0 POINTS	1 POINT	2 POINTS
A	Appearance	Blue, pale	Body pink, extremities blue	Completely pink
P	Pulse	Absent	Below 100	Over 100
G	Grimace	No response	Grimaces	Cries
A	Activity	Limp	Some flexion of extremities	Active motion
R	Respiratory effort	Absent	Slow, irregular	Good, strong cry

score of 4 to 6 indicates moderate depression and a need for resuscitative measures. (We shall deal with the resuscitation of a depressed infant in Chap. 36.)

Cutting the Umbilical Cord

Once the infant has been delivered and is breathing well, the umbilical cord can be clamped and cut, since it is no longer necessary for the infant's survival. There is no particular hurry about cutting the cord. In fact, it is preferable to wait a minute or two after the baby has delivered before cutting the cord, to enable the contracting uterus to squeeze the maximum volume of blood from the placenta into the baby. So take your time.

- HANDLE THE CORD GENTLY. It tears easily.
- Tie or CLAMP THE CORD about 8 inches from the infant's navel, with two ties (or clamps) placed 2 inches apart. Cut the cord between the two ties or clamps (Fig. 35-11).
- EXAMINE THE CUT ENDS OF THE CORD to be certain there is no bleeding. If the cut end attached to the infant is bleeding, tie or clamp the cord *proximal* to the previous clamp, and examine it again (do *not* remove the first clamp). There should not be any oozing from the infant's end of the cord.
- Once the cord is clamped and cut, WRAP THE BABY IN A BLANKET, and place it on the mother's abdomen to keep warm while you await the delivery of the placenta.

Delivery and Management of the Placenta

With the delivery of the baby, the second stage of labor is complete, and the third stage—delivery of the

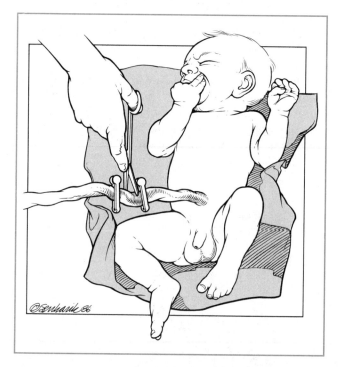

FIGURE 35-11. CUTTING THE UMBILICAL CORD. Place clamps about 2 inches apart along the cord after it has stopped pulsating, and cut between them.

placenta—begins. The placenta is usually delivered within about 20 minutes of the baby's arrival. Your job is to make stimulating conversation with the mother and bystanders as you wait patiently for the placenta to begin to separate spontaneously.

> **NEVER PULL ON THE UMBILICAL CORD TO TRY TO HASTEN DELIVERY OF THE PLACENTA.**

If you're in a hurry—perhaps because you have a depressed infant—or if the placenta does not deliver within about 15 minutes of the baby's delivery, then start transport before the placenta has delivered. But *don't* try to hasten the descent of the placenta.

There are several SIGNS that will tell you THAT THE PLACENTA IS SEPARATING FROM THE UTERINE WALL. The patient may report that she feels her contractions starting up again. The uterus rises in the abdomen and feels hard to palpation. The end of the umbilical cord protruding from the vagina lengthens, and there is usually a gush of blood from the vagina. When those signs occur:

- Instruct the patient to bear down to expel the placenta. As she does so,
- Hold the placenta with both hands and *gently* twist it so that the membranes will peel completely off the uterine wall.
- *Gently* MASSAGE THE ABDOMEN over the uterus to aid in its contraction (Fig. 35-12).
- PUT THE BABY TO THE MOTHER'S BREAST, which also stimulates the uterus to contract and thereby helps to control bleeding.
- If it is part of your local OB protocol to do so, this is the time to add 10 units of OXYTOCIN (Pitocin) to the mother's IV bag and drip it in *slowly*, no faster than about 30 gtt per minute. Before you start oxytocin, make absolutely sure the woman isn't harboring a second baby!

When the placenta is delivered, place it in a basin or plastic bag to be taken to the hospital, where it must be examined for completeness; retained pieces of placenta will cause persistent bleeding. Examine the perineum for lacerations, and apply pressure to any bleeding tears. Clean up and place a sanitary pad over the mother's vaginal opening, lower her legs, and prepare for transport.

ABNORMAL DELIVERIES

Most deliveries are normal. The baby arrives headfirst, followed shortly by the placenta; the mother and paramedics come through the ordeal like champs; and everyone lives happily ever after. Occasionally, however, there are complications, and the paramedic who wants to be able to deal with obstetric complications successfully must know when to anticipate them, how to recognize them when they do occur, and what action to take to ensure that everyone will still live happily ever after.

Breech and Other Abnormal Presentations

Most term babies enter the world headfirst (vertex presentation), according to the well-known principle of football: Follow your blockers. The baby's head serves as a fine blocker to open a path through the cervix for the narrower shoulders and hips. In a **breech presentation,** however, it is another part of the body that leads the way, usually the buttocks (the word *breech* means "buttocks"), but sometimes one of the feet. Breech presentations occur in about 4 percent of all deliveries and are more common with premature births.

The best place for a breech presentation to be delivered is in the hospital. But sometimes you won't realize that you are dealing with a breech until the mother is crowning and you notice that the presenting part does not have any hair but rather has a suspicious indentation down the middle. By the time you have made that astute observation, it's usually too late to get the woman to the hospital.

Buttocks Breech

If you have determined that the buttocks is the presenting part and that delivery is imminent, proceed as follows:

- POSITION THE MOTHER with her buttocks at the edge of the bed or stretcher and her legs flexed.
- Allow the buttocks and trunk of the baby to deliver spontaneously. DON'T PULL!
- Once the baby's legs are clear, SUPPORT THE BABY'S BODY on the palm of your hand and volar surface of your arm (Fig. 35-13).
- Now lower the baby slightly so that it very nearly

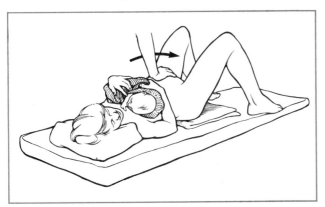

FIGURE 35-12. UTERINE MASSAGE. Gentle massage of the uterine fundus and putting the baby to the mother's breast both stimulate uterine contraction and help control postpartum bleeding.

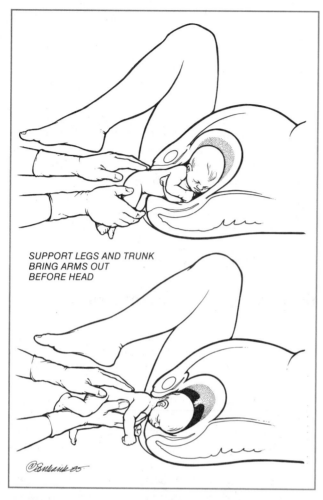

FIGURE 35-13. DELIVERING A BUTTOCKS BREECH. Support legs and trunk; bring arms out before head.

SUPPORT LEGS AND TRUNK
BRING ARMS OUT
BEFORE HEAD

hangs by its own weight downward; that will help the head pass through the pelvic outlet. You can tell when the head is in the vaginal canal because you'll be able to see the baby's hairline at the nape of his neck just below the mother's symphysis pubis.

- *When you can see the baby's hairline,* grasp him by his ankles and lift him upward in the direction of the mother's abdomen. The head should then deliver without difficulty.
- IF THE HEAD DOES NOT DELIVER WITHIN 3 MINUTES, YOU MUST TAKE ACTION TO PREVENT SUFFOCATION OF THE BABY. Suffocation may occur when the baby's umbilical cord is compressed by his head against the birth canal, which cuts off his supply of oxygenated blood from the placenta, and his face is pressed against the vaginal wall, which prevents him from breathing on his own. Place your gloved hand in the vagina, with your palm toward the baby's face. Form a V with your fingers on either

side of the baby's nose, and push the vaginal wall away from the baby's face until the head is delivered.
- DO NOT ATTEMPT TO PULL THE BABY OUT. DO NOT ALLOW EXPLOSIVE DELIVERY. If the head does not deliver within 3 minutes of establishing the airway, TRANSPORT rapidly to the hospital, with the mother's buttocks elevated on pillows. If at all possible, try to maintain the baby's airway throughout transport in the manner described. En route, alert the hospital so that they can have the appropriate personnel on hand when the mother arrives.

Other Abnormal Presentations

There are a variety of other abnormal ways in which the baby may present for delivery, most of them fortunately quite rare. In a **footling breech** (Fig. 35-14A), one or both feet will be dangling down through the vaginal opening. In a **transverse presentation,** or transverse lie (Fig. 35-14B), the fetus lies crosswise in the uterus and may wave at the paramedic with one hand protruding through the vagina. Even the baby who is coming headfirst may deflex his head and thus present with his *face* or *brow* instead of the top of his head (vertex). The only thing a paramedic really needs to know about all of those abnormal presentations is *not to attempt delivery in the field.* Nearly all of the abnormal presentations mentioned, except for a buttocks breech, will require delivery by cesarean section, so the prehospital management is simply to TRANSPORT.

> **ANY BABY WHO IS NOT COMING HEADFIRST OR FANNY-FIRST MUST BE DELIVERED IN THE HOSPITAL.**

Prolapsed Umbilical Cord

A prolapsed umbilical cord means that the cord emerges from the uterus ahead of the baby. As a result, with each uterine contraction the cord is compressed between the presenting part and the bony pelvis, shutting off the baby's supply of oxygenated blood from the placenta. Fetal asphyxia may ensue if circulation through the cord is not rapidly reestablished and maintained until delivery.

Cord prolapse occurs in about 1 out of every 300 deliveries. It is more likely in circumstances when the presenting part does not completely fill the pelvic

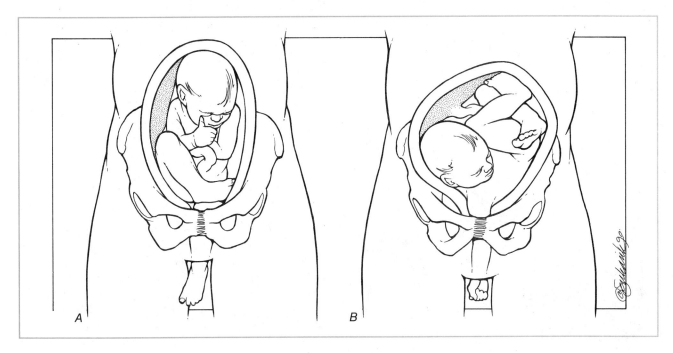

FIGURE 35-14. **ABNORMAL PRESENTATIONS.** (A) Footling breech. (B) Transverse lie.

brim, such as in abnormal presentations or with small babies (premature births, multiple births).

Treatment of cord prolapse is clearly urgent. If you see the cord protruding (Fig. 35-15A), take the following steps:

- POSITION THE MOTHER supine with her hips elevated as much as possible on pillows.
- Administer OXYGEN to the mother.
- Instruct the mother to pant with each contraction, which will prevent her from bearing down.
- If you are trained and authorized to do so, catheterize the mother's bladder; instill 500 ml of saline into the bladder through the catheter; then clamp the catheter shut. The full bladder helps keep the presenting part off the cord.
- With two fingers of a gloved hand, gently PUSH THE *BABY* (NOT THE CORD) BACK up into the vagina until the presenting part is no longer pressing on the cord (Fig. 13-15B).
- While you maintain pressure on the presenting part, have your partner COVER THE EXPOSED CORD WITH A STERILE DRESSING MOISTENED IN SALINE.
- Somehow, you're going to have to try to maintain that position, with a gloved hand pushing the presenting part away from the cord, throughout URGENT TRANSPORT to the hospital.

Premature and Small Infants

Any baby born before 37 weeks' gestation *or* weighing less than 2.5 kg (5.5 lb) needs special care. We shall discuss the care of neonates in more detail in the next chapter. For our purposes here, suffice it to state the following guidelines for dealing with small, red, wrinkled babies:

- KEEP THE BABY WARM. Babies lose heat by the same mechanisms that big people do—radiation, convection, conduction, and evaporation. But babies—and especially premature babies—have less natural insulation and a larger surface area in relation to mass, so they are much more vulnerable to rapid heat loss. To keep a "premie" warm, therefore:
1. DRY THE BABY THOROUGHLY as soon as possible after birth.
2. WRAP THE BABY IN ALUMINUM FOIL, from head to toe.
3. Cover the baby with a BLANKET.
4. Place the baby on the mother's chest, and cover them both with another blanket.
Keep the ambulance interior nice and warm. If it's comfortable for *you*, it's too cold for the premie!
- MAINTAIN THE BABY'S AIRWAY. Use a bulb

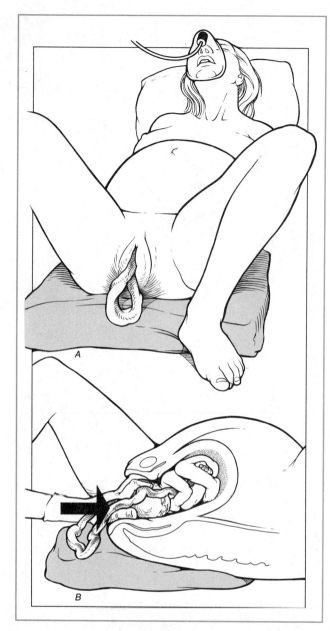

FIGURE 35-15. PROLAPSED UMBILICAL CORD.
(A) Cord prolapsed through the vaginal opening.
(B) Maintain firm pressure against the baby's head to keep it from compressing the cord. The mother's buttocks are elevated as much as possible on pillows.

syringe to keep the baby's nose and mouth clear of fluid.
- PREVENT BLEEDING from the umbilical cord; a very little baby cannot afford to lose even a very little bit of blood. If the cord is oozing, apply another clamp.
- Administer OXYGEN through a tent above the infant's head; do *not* blast oxygen directly into the baby's face. Use low flow—less than 4 liters per minute.
- PREVENT CONTAMINATION. Premature babies are highly susceptible to infection. Wear a surgical gown and mask, and keep bystanders—especially relatives who want to "give the new baby a big kiss"—at a distance.

Twins

About 1 in every 90 pregnancies produces multiple births (i.e., more than a single baby), so the chances of having to assist in the delivery of twins during your career as a paramedic are not all that remote. As a rule, the delivery of twins does not pose any special problems, except that you have to do a few things twice. There is, granted, a higher incidence of breech presentations in twin deliveries, but because the babies are usually smaller, delivery is easier than in a single breech birth.

If the mother has had prenatal care, she will doubtless know that she is carrying more than one baby (and will, one hopes, share that information with the paramedics). If she has not had prenatal care, suspect the possibility of a twin (or worse!) pregnancy if the abdomen remains very large after delivery of the (first) baby. Whenever you have reason to suspect there is more than one baby, proceed as follows:

- PREPARE FOR DELIVERY as described earlier.
- Twins are usually delivered single file, one after the other. When the first baby is born, clamp and cut the cord in the usual fashion. Inspect *both* ends of the cord for oozing, and apply a second clamp if necessary, to prevent hemorrhage from the twin.
- Contractions will usually start up again within about 5 to 10 minutes after the birth of the first baby, and baby number two can be expected to arrive within 30 to 45 minutes of its twin. That usually gives you time to transport before the birth of the second baby, if you are so inclined.
- Usually both babies are born before the first placenta is delivered (there may be only one placenta).
- Since twin babies tend to be smaller than single term babies, TREAT THEM AS YOU WOULD PREMATURE BABIES, with meticulous attention to keeping them warm, well-oxygenated, and protected from germs.

COMPLICATIONS OF LABOR AND DELIVERY

Postpartum Hemorrhage

The average blood loss during the third stage of labor is normally about 150 ml. When blood loss exceeds 500 ml during the first 24 hours after giving birth, it is considered postpartum hemorrhage (bleeding after birth). Anything that interferes with the contractions of the interlacing uterine muscle fibers after delivery of the placenta will promote postpartum bleeding:

RISK FACTORS FOR POSTPARTUM HEMORRHAGE

- PROLONGED LABOR, which leads to a "tired" uterus.
- RETAINED PRODUCTS OF CONCEPTION: The uterus cannot contract fully until it is empty.
- GRAND MULTIPARITY: After many pregnancies, the muscle tissue in the uterus is gradually replaced with fibrous tissue, which does not contract.
- TWIN PREGNANCY: The placental site is larger, and the overstretched uterine muscles don't contract as well.
- PLACENTA PREVIA: Muscles in the lower segment of the uterus, where the placenta is implanted, do not contract efficiently.
- A FULL BLADDER, which may prevent proper placental separation and uterine contraction.

The only measures feasible in the field to manage postpartum hemorrhage are those that encourage uterine contraction and help restore circulating volume. Some of those measures are part of our routine care of any woman after delivery:

- Continue UTERINE MASSAGE, as described earlier.
- PUT THE BABY TO THE MOTHER'S BREAST.
- If you have not already done so, add 10 units of OXYTOCIN to the IV bag (1,000 ml), and start infusing it at a rate of 20 to 30 gtt per minute.
- NOTIFY the receiving hospital of the mother's status and your ETA.
- TRANSPORT without delay.

- Start another LARGE-BORE IV en route, and infuse normal saline or lactated Ringer's wide open.
- DO NOT ATTEMPT TO EXAMINE THE VAGINA.
- DO NOT INSERT PACKS INTO THE VAGINA.
- Manage *external* bleeding from perineal tears with firm pressure. It may be necessary to open the labia and place packs at the bleeding site.

Pulmonary Embolism

Sudden dyspnea, tachycardia, or hypotension developing in the mother postpartum may signal pulmonary embolism, which is one of the most common causes of maternal death during childbirth. The embolism most frequently is in the form of a blood clot arising in the pelvic circulation, but leakage of **amniotic fluid** into the maternal circulation during delivery may also produce a clinical picture of pulmonary embolism. The patient may complain of sudden, sharp chest pain. Physical examination may reveal nothing unusual save for an increased pulse rate, tachypnea, and hypotension—signs that are apt to be mistaken for those of shock.

The prehospital management of suspected pulmonary embolism in the postpartum period is the same as that for pulmonary embolism under any other circumstances:

- Ensure an adequate AIRWAY.
- Administer OXYGEN in high concentration.
- MONITOR vital signs and cardiac rhythm.
- TRANSPORT without delay to the hospital.

Uterine Inversion

Inversion, or turning inside out, of the uterus is a rare complication of delivery, usually resulting from mismanagement of the third stage of labor. It may occur from excessive pressure on the uterus during fundal massage or from strong traction on the umbilical cord in an attempt to hasten delivery of the placenta. Shock commonly accompanies this condition. Should uterine inversion occur, take the following measures:

- Keep the patient RECUMBENT.
- Administer OXYGEN.
- Start TWO IV LIFELINES with normal saline or lactated Ringer's, and run them as rapidly as necessary to maintain blood pressure.
- If the placenta is still attached to the uterus, do NOT attempt to remove it.

• TRY *ONCE* TO REPLACE THE UTERUS MAN-UALLY, exerting pressure first on the area closest to the cervix. If that is not easily accomplished, pack all protruding tissues lightly with moist, sterile towels, and move rapidly to the hospital.

GLOSSARY

abortion The expulsion from the uterus of an embryo or fetus before the twenty-eighth week of gestation.

abruptio placenta Premature separation of a normally implanted placenta from the uterine wall, sometimes with massive hemorrhage, occurring during the third trimester of pregnancy.

amniotic fluid Fluid that surrounds the fetus in the uterus.

amniotic sac Thin, transparent sac that holds the fetus suspended in amniotic fluid; popularly called the bag of waters.

antepartum Before delivery.

bloody show Mucus and blood passed from the vagina when labor begins.

Braxton Hicks contractions Intermittent contractions of the uterus after the third month of pregnancy.

breech presentation Delivery in which the presenting part is the buttocks or foot.

cervix Lower portion, or neck, of the uterus.

corpus luteum Part of the ovarian follicle that remains and produces progesterone after release of the ovum.

crowning Stage of birth when the presenting part of the baby becomes visible at the vaginal opening.

eclampsia Toxic condition of pregnancy that includes all the symptoms of preeclampsia plus seizures.

effacement Thinning of the cervix as the lower segment of the uterus retracts during the first stage of labor.

embryo The developing egg from the third to eighth week after conception.

endometrium Lining cells of the uterus on which the fertilized ovum implants.

estrogen Female sex hormone that governs the proliferative phase of the menstrual cycle.

fallopian tube Tube extending from an ovary to the uterus.

fetus The unborn human after the second month of pregnancy.

follicle (graafian follicle) Immature ovum and the epithelial cells that surround it.

footling breech Delivery in which the presenting part is one or both of the baby's feet.

fundus (uterine) Part of the uterus above the entrance of the fallopian tubes.

gestation Pregnancy.

gravid Pregnant.

gravidity The number of times a woman has been pregnant, regardless of the outcome of the pregnancies.

implantation Process by which the fertilized egg attaches to the endometrium.

labia The folds of skin and mucous membrane that make up the vulva, comprising the labia majora and labia minora.

labor Mechanism by which the fetus is expelled from the uterus.

menarche The onset of menstrual periods.

menses The monthly flow of blood from a woman's genital tract.

multigravida Woman who has had two or more pregnancies.

multipara Woman who has had two or more deliveries ("multip" for short).

nullipara A woman who has never delivered.

ovary Female sex organ in which eggs and female hormones are produced.

ovulation Process by which an ovum is released from an ovarian follicle, usually occurring once a month in nonpregnant women of childbearing age.

ovum Egg (plural: ova).

parity The number of times a woman has carried a fetus at least to 28 weeks' gestation.

perineum The region between the vaginal opening and the anus.

placenta Special, vascular organ of pregnancy that supplies oxygen and nutrients to the fetus; popularly called the afterbirth.

placenta previa Situation in which the placenta is implanted low in the uterus, so that it partially or completely covers the cervical os.

postpartum After delivery.

preeclampsia Syndrome of hypertension, edema, and proteinuria sometimes seen in late pregnancy.

presenting part The part of the baby that comes out first during delivery.

primigravida Woman who is pregnant for the first time.

primipara Woman who has had only one previous delivery.

products of conception The fetus and placenta.

progesterone Female hormone produced by the corpus luteum that governs the secretory phase of the menstrual cycle.

quickening The first recognizable movements of the fetus in the uterus, usually occurring around the sixteenth to twentieth week of pregnancy.

term Forty weeks' gestation; the time when the fetus is fully mature and ready to be born.

toxemia of pregnancy Preeclampsia/eclampsia.

transverse lie Abnormal presentation in which the fetus lies crosswise in the uterus.

trimester Three-month period.

umbilical cord Muscular tube containing two arteries and one vein that connects the fetus to the placenta.

uterus Muscular organ in the female pelvis that houses the developing fetus; the womb.

vagina Genital canal in the female, extending from the uterus to the vulva; the birth canal.

vulva The external parts of the female genitalia.

FURTHER READING

ANTEPARTUM BLEEDING

Celebrezze EM. Third trimester predelivery hemorrhage. *Emergency* 13(10):48, 1981.

Gilling-Smith C et al. Management of early pregnancy bleeding in the accident and emergency department. *Arch Emerg Med* 5(3):133, 1988.

Nixon RG. Third trimester obstetric complications: Part I. Antepartum hemorrhage and fetal distress. *Emerg Med Serv* 10(3):53, 1981.

ECLAMPSIA AND PREECLAMPSIA

Ferris TF. Hypertensive and pregnant. *Emerg Med* 15(7):29, 1983.

Jayda A, Riggio S. Emergency department approach to managing seizures during pregnancy. *Ann Emerg Med* 20:80, 1991.

Kaplan PW et al. No, magnesium sulfate should not be used in treating eclamptic seizures. *Arch Neurol* 45:1361, 1988.

Miller K, Levy DB, Peppers MP. Toxemia of pregnancy. *Emergency* 22(4):10, 1990.

Nixon RG. Third trimester obstetric complications: Part II. Eclampsia and postpartum hemorrhage. *Emerg Med Serv* 10(4):52, 1981.

Ogle ME, Sanders AB. Preeclampsia. *Ann Emerg Med* 13:368, 1984.

Pritchard JA. Standardized treatment of 154 consecutive cases of eclampsia. *Am J Obstet Gynecol* 123:543, 1975.

Pritchard JA. The use of magnesium sulfate in preeclampsia-eclampsia. *J Reprod Med* 23:107, 1979.

Sibai BM et al. Eclampsia: Observations from 67 recent cases. *Obstet Gynecol* 58:609, 1981.

White JD. Treatment for hypertension with eclampsia. *Ann Emerg Med* 10:166, 1981.

TRAUMA DURING PREGNANCY

Agran PF et al. Fetal death in motor vehicle accidents. *Ann Emerg Med* 16:1355, 1987.

American College of Obstetrics and Gynecology. Trauma during pregnancy. ACOG Technical Bulletin #162. *Int J Gynecol Obstet* 40:165, 1993.

Bocka JJ. OB trauma: Prehospital care of the pregnant trauma patient. *JEMS* 13(10):51, 1988.

Bocka JJ et al. Trauma in pregnancy. *Ann Emerg Med* 17:829, 1988.

Brown K et al. The case of the pregnant MVA victim. *JEMS* 16(7):99, 1991.

Brown K et al. The case of the mortally wounded pregnant patient. *JEMS* 17(3):38, 1993.

Fatovich DM. Electric shock in pregnancy. *J Emerg Med* 11:175, 1993.

Haydel M, McSwain N. Trauma in pregnancy. *Emerg Med* 25(9):41, 1993.

Katz VL, Dotters DJ, Droegenmueller W. Perimortem cesarean delivery. *Obstet Gynecol* 63:571, 1986.

Muller RJ. Cesarean section in the street. *Emerg Med* 16(15):143, 1984.

Palmer CJ, Williams PP. Trauma primer: The obstetrical patient. *Emergency* 23(7):47, 1991.

Williams JK et al. Evaluation of blunt abdominal trauma in the third trimester of pregnancy: Maternal and fetal considerations. *Obstet Gynecol* 75:33, 1990.

OTHER COMPLICATIONS OF PREGNANCY

Biggs JSG et al. Medications and pregnancy. *Drugs* 21:69, 1981.

Field DR et al. Maternal brain death during pregnancy: Medical and ethical issues. *JAMA* 260:816, 1988.

Kaunitz AM et al. Causes of maternal mortality in the United States. *Obstet Gynecol* 65:605, 1985.

Lee RV et al. Cardiopulmonary resuscitation of pregnant women. *Am J Med* 81:311, 1986.

Murphy P. Problem pregnancies: Hemorrhagic complications in the third trimester. *JEMS* 17(9):44, 1992.

Selden BS, Burke TJ. Complete maternal and fetal recovery after prolonged cardiac arrest. *Ann Emerg Med* 17:346, 1988.

Smith JC et al. An assessment of the incidence of maternal mortality in the United States. *Am J Public Health* 74:780, 1984.

NORMAL CHILDBIRTH

Anderson B, Shapiro B. *Emergency Childbirth Handbook.* Albany, N.Y.: Delmar, 1979.

Brunette DD, Sterner SP. Prehospital and emergency department delivery: A review of eight years experience. *Ann Emerg Med* 18:1116, 1989.

Gage JE et al. Suctioning of upper airway meconium in newborn infants. *JAMA* 246:2590, 1981.

Higgins SD. Emergency delivery: Prehospital care, emergency department delivery, perimortem salvage. *Emerg Med Clin North Am* 5:529, 1987.

Kilgore JR. Management of an obstetric patient by the EMT. *EMT J* 4(2):50, 1980.

Roush GM. Abdominal examination of the pregnant uterus. *EMT J* 3(2):33, 1979.

Weir PE, Beischer NA. Birth before arrival in hospital. *Med J Aust* 2:31, 1980.

Williams C. Emergency childbirth. *Emerg Med Serv* 14(3):100, 1985.

Wojslawowicz JM. Emergency childbirth for emergency medical technicians. *EMT J* 1(4):66, 1977.

ABNORMAL AND COMPLICATED DELIVERIES

Boulton FE et al. Obstetric haemorrhage: Causes and management. *Clin Haematol* 14:683, 1985.

Corey EC. High-risk deliveries. *Emergency* 25(9):28, 1993.

Doan-Wiggins L. Oxytocin use in prehospital care. *Emerg Med Serv* 21(8):27, 1992.

Harris BA. Dealing with a difficult delivery. *Emerg Med* 16(11):22, 1984.

Katz Z et al. Management of labor with umbilical cord prolapse: A 5-year study. *Obstet Gynecol* 72:278, 1988.

Levy DB, Peppers MP, Miller K. A last resort for postpartum hemorrhage. *Emergency* 22(5):16, 1990.

Nixon RG. Third trimester obstetric complications: Part III. Problems during fetal delivery. *Emerg Med Serv* 10(5):80, 1981.

Sperry K. Amniotic fluid embolism: To understand an enigma. *JAMA* 255:2183, 1986.

Steiner PE, Lushbaugh CC. Maternal pulmonary embolism by amniotic fluid: As a cause of obstetric shock and unexpected deaths in obstetrics. *JAMA* 117:1245, 1941.

Sterner S, Campbell B, Davies S. Amniotic fluid embolism. *Ann Emerg Med* 13:343, 1984.

Turner R, Gusack M. Massive amniotic fluid embolism. *Ann Emerg Med* 13:359, 1984.

36
Neonatal Care and Transport

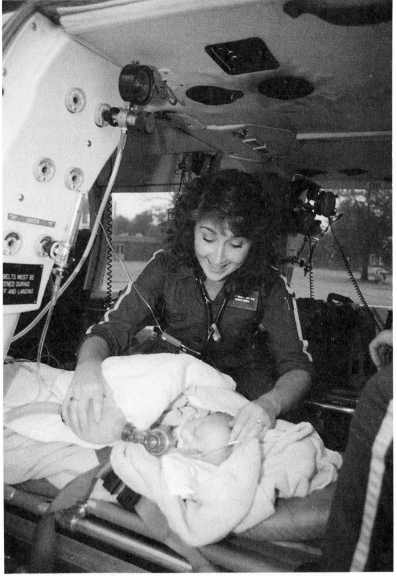

University of Chicago Aeromedical Network, University of Chicago Hospitals, Chicago. Photo by Michael S. Kowal.

OBJECTIVES

The human newborn, or **neonate,** is not equipped to survive on its own. While a newborn colt, for example, will soon scramble to its feet and take its first faltering steps, a newborn human will require many months of additional development before it is ready to undertake such a project, usually to wild cheering and applause. In the interim, the infant is totally dependent on others to keep it from harm. For the newborn baby, harm comes principally in the form of fluids obstructing the airway and cold or wet environmental conditions. One of the reasons that grown-ups were invented was to protect newborns from those threats.

In this chapter, we shall first look at the anatomic and physiologic changes that occur in a newborn as it makes the transition from the watery world of the womb to the world in which it must start breathing air. We'll review the care that should be given to every newborn infant during and immediately after delivery and consider the special needs of premature or very small babies. We shall then go over the steps involved in neonatal resuscitation, which differs in several important respects from resuscitation of older children and adults. Finally, we shall consider what is involved in undertaking the interhospital transport of a critically ill newborn. By the end of this chapter, the student should be able to

1. List two anatomic or functional changes that must occur in the fetal circulation immediately after birth
2. Indicate at what point in the delivery of a baby the baby's mouth and nostrils should be suctioned, and describe the technique for doing so
3. List two risk factors for meconium staining of the amniotic fluid, and describe the measures that should be taken when a baby is born covered with meconium
4. Identify correct and incorrect procedures for cutting the umbilical cord, given a list of different procedures
5. List four ways in which a newborn can lose body heat, and describe the measures to take in preventing excessive heat loss in a neonate
6. List two adverse effects of hypothermia on a newborn baby
7. Identify a premature infant, given a description of several newborn infants, and list the special measures required in its care after birth
8. List six factors in the mother's obstetric history or the circumstances of labor and delivery that suggest a baby will be at increased risk for conditions that require resuscitation
9. Identify an infant who requires resuscitative measures, given a description of several infants immediately after birth, and list in order the steps in resuscitating a newborn
10. List the indications for
    * Artificial ventilation of a newborn baby
    * Chest compressions in a newborn infant
    and describe the correct technique for each
11. List the drug(s) that may be required for neonatal resuscitation in the field, and for each list
    * The indications
    * The dosage
    * The route of administration
12. List the preparatory steps necessary before a critically ill newborn may be transferred from one medical facility to another

CARDIORESPIRATORY FUNCTION AT THE THRESHOLD OF BIRTH

A baby at the threshold of birth must prepare to enter a new world, a world that is altogether different from the one in which it has spent the previous 40 weeks. For its entire intrauterine life, the fetus has lived underwater, deriving its oxygen not through its lungs but ultimately from its *mother's* lungs, via the placental circulation. All that has to change, and change in a matter of seconds, during the second stage of labor, when the baby emerges from the watery deep of the womb and takes its first breath of air.

The Fetal Circulation

The fetal circulation is more complex than that of a baby after birth and must undergo some crucial changes immediately at birth in order to adapt to life outside the water. Recall that the fetus is attached to the placenta by the *umbilical cord* and that the cord contains one vein and two arteries. Those three vessels spiral around one another, rather like the cable to a telephone receiver, and thus enable the umbilical cord to be stretched without jeopardizing the fetal circulation.

The fetal circulation is perhaps best described by following the course of blood flow from the placenta to the fetus and back (Fig. 36-1). It is the umbilical *vein* that carries oxygenated blood from the placenta to the fetus. The umbilical vein enters the abdomen through a muscular ring, the **ductus venosus,** and empties (primarily via the hepatic circulation) into the inferior vena cava of the fetus. Upon entering the heart, most of the blood from the inferior vena cava is diverted through an opening (**foramen ovale**) into

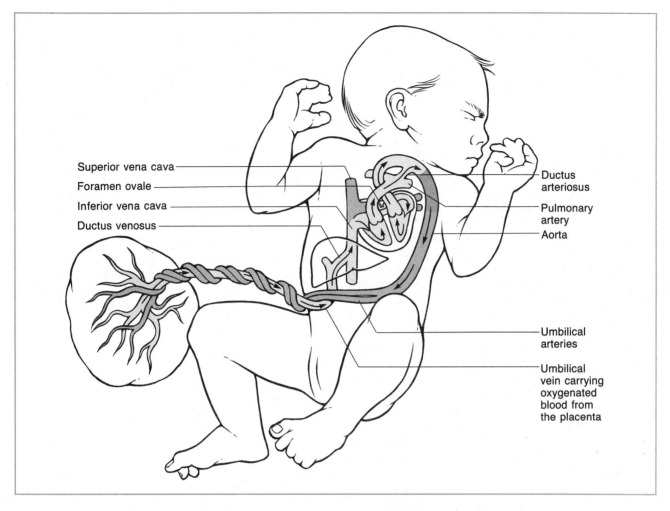

FIGURE 36-1. **THE FETAL CIRCULATION.** Oxygenated blood from the placenta reaches the fetus through the umbilical vein. Blood returns to the placenta via two umbilical arteries. Right-to-left shunts occur at the foramen ovale and the ductus arteriosus.

the *left atrium.* The small amount of inferior vena caval blood that does reach the *right atrium* mixes with blood coming from the superior vena cava; and with each atrial systole those two streams of blood—that from the right atrium and that from the left atrium—are directed into the respective ventricles. In contrast to the adult, then, whose right and left ventricles pump in series, in the fetus the ventricles essentially work in parallel.

Recall that in the adult, ventricular systole squeezes the blood that was in the right ventricle into the pulmonary arteries and thence into the lungs. In the fetus, however, the lungs are virtually nonfunctional; they are not taking in air because the fetus is in a watery environment. So there is no point sending the output of the right ventricle to the lungs, for there is no oxygen to be picked up there. Accordingly the

vascular resistance of the lungs is very high—that is, the pulmonary arteries are tightly constricted—which prevents most of the output of the right ventricle from entering. Instead, most of the blood leaving the right ventricle goes through a shunt, the **ductus arteriosus,** that connects the pulmonary artery directly with the aorta.

The aorta also receives blood pumped from the left ventricle, as in the adult. Oxygenated blood pumped into the aortic arch perfuses the head and upper extremities. Blood flowing in the descending aorta perfuses the kidney and travels to the two umbilical *arteries* and thence back to the placenta.

It is not necessary to remember all the details of fetal circulation. What is important is to realize that until a few moments after birth, the fetus has collapsed, nonfunctional lungs and a circulation designed to bypass the lungs almost entirely. With the baby's first breath, both its anatomy and physiology must undergo a radical change. Understanding how that change occurs helps us to understand what can go wrong in the moments immediately following birth.

Cardiorespiratory Changes That Occur at Birth

The newborn has two crucial tasks to accomplish as it emerges from the birth canal: (1) to get rid of the fluid filling his lungs so that they can expand and fill with air, and (2) to close off the two right-to-left shunts in the circulation—at the foramen ovale and at the ductus arteriosus—so that venous blood will no longer bypass the lungs.

The normal sequence of events is usually as follows: As the baby emerges from the womb, the umbilical cord, in response to its contact with the air, undergoes changes. The muscular walls of the umbilical vessels start to constrict (clinically, what we see is the gradual cessation of pulsations in the cord). Constriction of the umbilical vessels in turn triggers spasm of the ductus venosus, the muscular sphincter of the umbilical vein. Now, oxygenated blood from the placenta can no longer reach the baby, so asphyxia starts to develop in the newborn. The asphyxia activates the baby's respiratory center, which in turn stimulates the lungs to expand. The baby has, in fact, been practicing for this moment for quite a while, making respiratory movements for weeks while still in the uterus. But in utero, the fetus was "breathing" amniotic fluid. With baby's first respiratory effort in the outside world, by contrast, its lungs fill for the first time with air.

While everyone in the delivery room is cheering the baby's first cry, dramatic changes are now occurring within the baby's body. The presence of air in the lungs causes the pulmonary arteries to dilate, thereby abolishing the state of high vascular resistance that had kept pulmonary circulation to a minimum during fetal life. Now blood leaving the right ventricle can flow unimpeded to the lungs. Furthermore, the decrease in pulmonary vascular resistance alters the pressure gradients within the heart itself, enabling the two right-to-left shunts to close off. The foramen ovale is closed almost immediately after the baby's first breath; within several minutes, the ductus arteriosus begins to constrict as well and is usually fully closed within 24 to 48 hours after birth. (Rarely, the foramen ovale or ductus arteriosus fails to close after birth, and the baby must have surgery to repair the "hole in his heart.")

Normally, all of the changes described—the lungs filling with air, the right-to-left shunts closing off—occur spontaneously during the first seconds after birth. But a number of things may interfere with that spontaneous process. A newborn that suffered distress in the hours preceding birth, for example, may not have the energy to take the all-important first breath. Or, when he does so, he may aspirate fluid that accumulated in his mouth and upper airway. Hypothermia, hypoxia, or acidosis may, furthermore, interfere with the process by which intracardiac shunts close off and result in persistence of right-to-left shunting. (What effects will a persisting right-to-left shunt have on the baby's oxygenation? Think about the concept of shunt that we studied in Chap. 8.)

Much of what we do in the routine care of the newborn is aimed at ensuring that the baby makes a success of his first breath (and of those that follow).

ROUTINE CARE OF THE NEWBORN

In the previous chapter, we mentioned the steps in caring for the newborn. We shall now look at each of those steps in a bit more detail, to gain a better understanding of why and how they are performed.

The Newborn Airway

Suctioning

When the baby first pokes his head out into the world, before the trunk delivers, is the time to suction out the airway. At that point, the baby will not yet be breathing, for the chest and therefore the lungs are still squeezed down by the birth canal. So it is the ideal moment to try to remove fluid, mucus, or meconium (see following section) from the airway, *before* the baby takes its first deep breath and sucks all that material into its lungs.

Use a rubber bulb aspirator to suction the baby's mouth and nose as described in Chapter 35 (see Fig. 35-10). Suction the mouth first, then each nostril. Take care, though, not to push the tip of the aspirator too deeply into the baby's mouth; pressure against the back of the baby's throat is a very powerful vagal stimulus and may lead to severe bradycardia.

Suction the mouth and nostrils again after the baby is fully delivered. Do *not*, however, suction for more than 10 seconds at a time; as in the adult, suctioning removes oxygen as well as secretions.

DO NOT SUCTION DEEP INTO THE OROPHARYNX. DO NOT SUCTION FOR MORE THAN 10 SECONDS AT A TIME.

Positioning

Immediately after delivery, hold the baby head downward, to drain the fluid and blood from his mouth, nose, and oropharynx (Fig. 36-2). Gently wipe the mouth and nostrils clean with a gauze pad or sterile towel, then carry out suctioning as described.

When you set the baby down, place it with its head to the side and slightly lower than the rest of the body, to facilitate continued drainage of fluid.

Prevention of Meconium Aspiration

Meconium is fetal stool. It is composed of swallowed amniotic fluid, bile acids, cholesterol, and other sub-

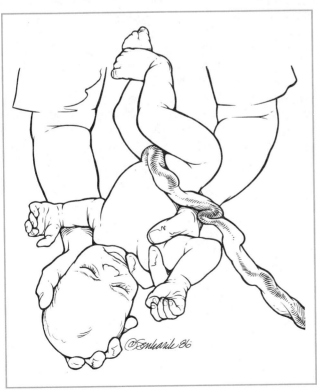

FIGURE 36-2. **POSITIONING.** Immediately after delivery, hold the baby with its head dependent to facilitate drainage of secretions.

stances, and usually it stays within the fetal intestinal tract until after birth. Should there be a problem during labor, however, causing some interference with the fetal blood supply, the meconium may become a source of problems. Anything that disrupts blood flow to the fetus will produce fetal hypoxia. Fetal hypoxia in turn causes spasm of the fetal colon, which leads to the passage of meconium into the amniotic fluid. At the same time, developing asphyxia stimulates the fetus to take deep gasps. As it does so, it is likely to pull meconium-containing amniotic fluid into the larger airways. Having meconium in the airway is no problem *before* birth, since the fetus isn't breathing anyway. It becomes a very serious problem immediately *after* birth however, for if the large airways are filled with fetal fecal material, the newborn baby will not be able to take its first breaths and inflate its lungs.

Meconium staining of amniotic fluid occurs in 8 to 10 percent of deliveries. Fortunately, it is often possible to anticipate which babies will be born in a meconium-stained fluid and to take some measures to prevent massive meconium aspiration.

First of all, we know that certain situations increase the risk of meconium spillage. *Postmature* infants, that is, infants born after the fortieth week of pregnancy, are particularly at risk. The complication also occurs commonly when the mother is a *heavy smoker.* Preterm problems that jeopardize the placental circulation, such as preeclampsia, also predispose to meconium staining.

Any time you detect signs of *fetal distress* during labor, which essentially means any time you auscultate a **fetal heart rate less than 120 per minute,** you need to take immediate steps to try to improve the fetal circulation.

**STEPS TO IMPROVE
FETAL CIRCULATION**

- Roll the mother onto her side, to take the weight of her uterus off the great vessels.
- Administer 100% OXYGEN by mask to the mother.

Whether or not you have advance warning of meconium staining, you must be prepared to take immediate action at the first indication that meconium is present in the amniotic fluid. That indication will usually occur when the amniotic sac ruptures late in the first stage of labor. Normally, amniotic fluid is clear, colorless, and odorless. The presence of meconium will give amniotic fluid a yellow-green hue. Heavy meconium staining gives the amniotic fluid the color and consistency of pea soup. When you see a greenish amniotic fluid, especially if it is heavily stained, you must take action. (If the "bag of waters" broke before your arrival, ask the mother to describe what the fluid looked like.)

- Assemble some additional EQUIPMENT, beside that for the delivery itself. (If you are already busy with the delivery, have your partner gather the equipment.)
  1. Pediatric INTUBATION KIT, including several 3.0- or 3.5-mm endotracheal tubes and a No. 1 Wis-Hipple laryngoscope blade (for cases of heavy meconium staining only).
  2. DELEE SUCTION trap.
  3. GAUZE pads.
  4. OXYGEN.
  5. Pediatric BAG-VALVE-MASK.

  All of that equipment should be laid out in an orderly fashion on a sterile drape that has been placed on a table close to the bed or stretcher on which delivery is taking place.
- *As soon as the baby's head delivers,* wipe the nostrils and mouth clean with gauze pads, and use the bulb aspirator to SUCTION the baby's mouth and nostrils. Then use the DeLee aspirator to suction the oropharynx *gently*.
- After the mouth and oropharynx have been well suctioned, DELIVER THE REST OF THE BABY, immediately clamp and cut the cord, and hand the baby off to your partner. (You will have to stay right where you are, to monitor delivery of the placenta.)
- When there has been heavy meconium staining (pea-soup variety), your partner should swiftly place the baby supine on the table previously prepared for that purpose and immediately INTUBATE THE TRACHEA, preferably before the baby has had a chance to take his first breath. If there are three in your crew, the third team member should apply monitoring electrodes to the baby's chest to help detect bradycardia.
- Once inserted past the vocal cords, the endotracheal tube will be used essentially as a suction catheter. A device called a meconium aspirator, which controls the amount of suction applied, is hooked up between the endotracheal tube and the suction tube. Then the endotracheal tube is slowly withdrawn from the trachea as suction is applied. If there is a lot of meconium in the trachea, a second intubation and suction with a

clean endotracheal tube may be necessary, *after* the infant has been reoxygenated with 100% oxygen. It is not worthwhile to try to insert a suction catheter *through* the endotracheal tube, for any suction catheter tiny enough to slip through a 3.0- to 3.5-mm tube will be too tiny to remove thick goop from the trachea.
- After one or two quick tracheal suctions, or as soon as the baby starts breathing, give supplemental oxygen for a few minutes, and carry out whatever resuscitative measures may be necessary (see later section of this chapter).

Cutting the Cord

Under ordinary circumstances, there need not be any rush to clamp and cut the baby's umbilical cord. The optimal time for clamping the cord is still somewhat controversial. Those who advocate waiting several minutes point to the fact that infants with late-clamped cords have higher iron stores throughout infancy than infants whose cords were clamped immediately and are thus less prone to anemia. The proponents of early clamping argue that babies whose cords were clamped more than 3 to 5 minutes after birth have a higher incidence of hyperbilirubinemia and less efficient lung function during the first days of life. Probably the best solution is a middle-of-the-road approach. It will, in any case, probably take about 45 to 60 seconds after the baby is fully delivered to suction the airway and get him or her dried off. The cord can then be clamped and cut, and the 1-minute Apgar score evaluated. Thereafter, inspect the cord periodically to make sure it isn't oozing.

Whether you are an "early clamper" or a "late clamper," do *not* try to "strip" or milk the cord to squeeze the last drops of blood out into the baby. Stripping the cord simply disrupts the red blood cells within it, so what gets infused into the baby is a lot of red blood cell breakdown products, such as bilirubin.

> **DON'T MILK THE UMBILICAL CORD.**

Keeping the Baby Warm

One of the most important steps in caring for the newborn, and one of the steps most easily forgotten in the confusion of a delivery in unexpected circumstances, is prevention of heat loss from the baby.

Why Hypothermia Is Harmful to the Newborn

As we learned in Chapter 32, when any human is placed in a cold environment, he will attempt to preserve his core body temperature by (1) increasing heat *production*, through shivering and jacking up the metabolic rate, and (2) decreasing heat *loss*, through peripheral vasoconstriction. The newborn responds in largely the same way, but in trying to maintain core temperature through those mechanisms, the newborn may get into a lot of physiologic trouble.

To *increase heat production*, the neonate has only one available strategy—an increased metabolic rate—for it is not yet capable of shivering. There is a price to pay for increasing the metabolic rate, however, and that is an increase in oxygen consumption. If the baby is already in a state of borderline oxygenation, the increased oxygen demand may jeopardize oxygenation of vital organs. Furthermore, a drop in tissue oxygenation forces a shift from aerobic to anaerobic metabolism. Anaerobic metabolism produces lactic acid. And lactic acid in the blood produces ACIDOSIS.

The increased metabolic rate also increases the demand for *fuel*, and in the newborn, especially the premature newborn, the principal fuel is glucose, which is stored in limited quantities in the baby's liver. The faster the metabolic rate, the faster that glucose will be consumed, leading to HYPOGLYCEMIA.

To *decrease heat loss*, the neonate uses the same mechanism that an adult uses—peripheral vasoconstriction. But the decrease in peripheral perfusion also has a cost: Metabolism in the periphery, deprived of oxygen, switches to the anaerobic mode, thereby worsening the acidosis.

In trying to protect itself from cold stress, therefore, the newborn may rapidly become *hypoxemic, hypoglycemic,* and *acidotic*—a recipe for serious and sometimes fatal complications. In the premature infant, for example, acidosis may be followed quickly by shock, and the combination further predisposes the infant to the respiratory distress syndrome. Even in the term infant, acidosis may cause an increase in pulmonary vascular resistance that reestablishes the right-to-left shunts of the fetal circulation, thereby worsening the baby's hypoxemia. Such complications should not happen, even in deliveries occurring outside the hospital, because there is no reason to allow a newborn to become chilled.

How a Newborn Loses Heat

Newborn babies lose heat by the same four mechanisms that grown-ups lose heat:

- RADIATION, the transfer of heat from the baby to the surrounding air.
- CONDUCTION, the transfer of heat from the baby to surrounding liquid or solid objects with which it is in physical contact.
- CONVECTION, the loss of heat caused by moving air currents.
- EVAPORATION, the loss of heat by transforming water from a liquid to a gas. Evaporative heat loss is a major problem so long as the infant is wet.

By understanding the mechanisms by which a newborn loses heat, we ought to be able to devise ways to prevent heat loss.

Radiant heat loss is prevented in the hospital delivery suite by placing the baby under a source of radiant heat, such as hot lights. In the field, that is unlikely to be possible, and radiant heat loss is difficult to prevent. In the ambulance, the heater should be turned on and the ambient temperature should be raised to about 33°C (about 91°F) for a term infant and to 35°C (95°F) for a premie.

Conductive heat loss can be prevented by making sure that the baby does not lie on a cold surface. In a chilly environment, conductive heat loss can be prevented by placing *well-insulated* hot water bottles (or, if you don't carry a hot water bottle, rubber gloves filled with hot water) alongside the infant. DO NOT USE CHEMICAL HOT PACKS.

Heat loss by convection is prevented by keeping the newborn out of drafts.

Finally, *evaporative heat loss* is prevented by drying the infant as rapidly as possible after birth, preferably with a towel that has been warmed beforehand, and then covering him with a dry blanket.

One excellent method for preventing the newborn from losing heat while you are waiting for the placenta to deliver is to place the baby on the mother's abdomen and cover them both with a blanket. Mother's body heat will warm the baby, and meanwhile mother and baby have their first opportunity to "get the feel of one another" (a process that has been going on as long as women have been having babies, but that has recently acquired a name: "bonding").

CARE OF THE PREMATURE NEWBORN

For purposes of prehospital care, a premature baby ("premie") can be considered any baby born before 38 weeks' gestation or weighing less than 2.5 kg (5.5 lb). Unless you carry a scale around in the ambulance, you will usually have to make an educated guess about the baby's weight. Practice making those estimates when you do your clinical rotation through the obstetric service; guess each baby's weight, and then check your guess against the measurement on the scale. After a while, you should be able to come within about half a pound of the correct weight. Other clues to prematurity come from the history provided by the mother: If the mother says that she wasn't "due" for another 2 months, the baby is doubtless premature.

Premies are fragile babies and need special care to survive. Because their surface area is large with respect to their mass and because they have so little subcutaneous fat as insulation, premies lose heat much faster than do full-term babies, so they can become hypothermic with alarming rapidity. Because their glucose stores are smaller, they become hypoglycemic faster. A limited blood volume makes them exquisitely sensitive to even small amounts of bleeding, and immature immune mechanisms render them more susceptible to infection. All of those facts govern the special care needs of the preterm infant.

- KEEP THE PREMIE WARM! Prevent heat loss by all the mechanisms described earlier, and provide an ambient temperature in the ambulance of 35°C (95°F).
- Give meticulous attention to the baby's AIRWAY. Check the airway frequently after delivery, and use the bulb aspirator to suction mucus from the nostrils and mouth as needed.
- Administer humidified OXYGEN. Use a baby blanket to make a tent above the baby's head, and pipe the oxygen—at about 2 to 3 liters per minute—into the tent. Aim the flow toward the top of the tent, not directly into the baby's face.
- EXAMINE THE UMBILICAL CORD CLOSELY, to make absolutely certain it isn't oozing. If there *is* oozing, add another clamp proximal to the first one, and check again.
- PROTECT THE BABY FROM CONTAMINATION. Wear a mask and surgical gown when handling the baby. Keep bystanders and family members, especially small children (who are always full of GERMS!), away from the baby.

NEONATAL RESUSCITATION

Approximately 6 percent of babies born in U.S. hospitals each year require life support immediately or shortly after birth. Probably the percentage is higher when one considers babies born *outside* the hospital. In one of the few studies carried out to assess complications of prehospital deliveries, 25 percent of infants delivered outside the hospital required resuscitation! (See Brunette DD under Further Reading.) The chances are therefore quite high that a paramedic working in a busy EMS system will sooner or later have to resuscitate a newborn.

High-Risk Babies

It is impossible to predict with absolute certainty which infants will require resuscitation immediately after birth. But it *is* possible to identify situations in which the infant is at increased *risk* of needing resuscitative measures. And by knowing ahead of time— before delivery is complete—that resuscitation may be required, you can at least take steps to prepare for carrying out a resuscitation, that is, assemble the necessary equipment, set up a resuscitation table in a warm place, and so forth. Then, if it is indeed necessary to resuscitate the infant during those hectic moments right after delivery, you can do so in an orderly, systematic way, without having to rummage frantically for the equipment you need. And if it turns out that you don't, after all, have to carry out a resuscitation, you can simply pack up your gear and be grateful you didn't have to use it.

Some of the risk factors that should alert you to the possibility of a depressed or asphyxiated newborn are summarized in Table 36-1. Note that some of those risk factors pertain to the mother's obstetric history, which you may not find out about unless you ask the right questions. Other risk factors do not become evident until delivery is in progress, and you may need to find a code by which you can communicate to your partner—without terrifying the

TABLE 36-1.   FACTORS ASSOCIATED WITH A HIGH RISK FOR NEONATAL RESUSCITATION

PROBLEMS IN THE MOTHER
- Age > 35 years
- Diabetes
- Alcohol or drug abuse
- Previous history of stillbirth or neonatal death

PROBLEMS DURING THE PREGNANCY
- Antepartum hemorrhage
- Preeclampsia
- Multiple (twin) pregnancy
- No antenatal care

PROBLEMS DURING DELIVERY
- Abnormal presentations (e.g., breech)
- Preterm or post-term delivery
- Prolonged labor
- Prolapsed umbilical cord
- Meconium-stained amniotic fluid
- Fetal distress from any cause (fetal heart rate < 120/min)

mother—that he or she should start setting up for a resuscitation.

Deciding When Resuscitation Is Necessary

In the previous chapter, we learned that any baby whose Apgar score is less than about 5 will need resuscitation. While that is certainly true, the problem is that the Apgar score is first evaluated at 1 minute after birth—and one should not delay resuscitation that long just to measure an Apgar score.

> **DO NOT WAIT UNTIL YOU HAVE MEASURED THE 1-MINUTE APGAR SCORE BEFORE YOU START RESUSCITATION.**

In practice, what determines the need for resuscitation and the specific measures required is the baby's *heart rate,* most easily measured by listening to the apical beat with a stethoscope. Before evaluating the heart rate, however, there are a few things we have to do first. Let us consider, then, the steps in dealing with the distressed newborn in sequence, for often the timely performance of the early steps of resuscitation eliminates the necessity for carrying out the later steps.

Positioning, Suctioning, and Stimulation

The initial steps in dealing with a potentially depressed neonate are part of the routine care of *every* newborn that we have already discussed. To review briefly, those steps are

- POSITIONING: After delivery, the baby should be placed in a position that will enhance drainage of secretions from the mouth, which usually means lying with a slight head-down tilt and the head turned to the side.
- SUCTIONING is carried out twice—initially right after delivery of the head, then a second time after the whole baby has delivered.
- STIMULATION: Usually the process of suctioning and drying off the baby by itself produces enough stimulation to induce the newborn to take its first breath. If those stimuli are not sufficient, a small puff of air delivered to the infant's lungs (mouth-to-mouth) usually does the trick. The American Heart Association recommends

rubbing the infant's back or gently flicking the soles of its feet. More vigorous measures, however, like the traditional spank delivered by the obstetrician, are never indicated and may be harmful.

> **A NEWBORN HAS NOT COMMITTED ANY OFFENSE, SO DOES NOT DESERVE A SPANKING.**

Ventilation of the Newborn

The measures outlined above—positioning, suctioning, and stimulation—ordinarily will not take more than about 15 to 20 seconds. If the infant has not begun breathing spontaneously and effectively by the time you have accomplished those measures, he or she is going to need some respiratory assistance.

If the baby is breathing spontaneously but is still cyanotic or bradycardic (pulse less than 100/min), the first thing to try is simply the administration of OXYGEN. Set up an oxygen mask at a flow rate of 4 to 6 liters per minute, and hold it near the infant's face. Often a minute or two of breathing an enriched oxygen mixture is all that is required to enable a depressed baby to "pink up."

If the newborn does not establish effective respiration with oxygen, assisted ventilation will be required. Specifically, the *indications for artificial ventilation* of a newborn are as follows:

> **INDICATIONS FOR ARTIFICIAL VENTILATION OF THE NEWBORN**
>
> - Apnea
> - Heart rate less than 100 per minute
> - Persisting central cyanosis despite breathing 100% oxygen

If any of those conditions is present, begin artificial ventilation immediately. Usually it is necessary to *start* with MOUTH-TO-MOUTH (and nose) ventilation, while someone else gets the pediatric bag-valve-mask assembled and connected to oxygen. While giving mouth-to-mouth ventilation, remember to give only SMALL PUFFS FROM YOUR CHEEKS and only that volume sufficient to cause the infant's chest to rise. The first few inflations may be quite difficult, but subsequent breaths should not require as much pressure.

If you do not have a pediatric bag-valve-mask and must therefore continue artificial ventilation by mouth-to-mouth methods, you will need to supplement your own exhaled air with oxygen. The easiest way to do so is to don a two-pronged nasal cannula running at about 6 liters per minute. Then, each breath you give the infant will be enriched with the oxygen that you are breathing.

Much more satisfactory oxygen concentrations can be delivered via BAG-VALVE-MASK. Use *only* a bag-valve-mask specially designed for infants. To ventilate an infant with a bag-valve-mask, hold the infant's head in very slight extension. Grasp the mask between the thumb and index finger of the left hand, and place it firmly over the infant's mouth and nose. Use the middle finger of your left hand to exert coun-

terpressure on the bony part of the infant's chin, as shown in Figure 36-3, while your fourth and fifth fingers can be used to perform slight jaw thrust.

Ventilate the newborn at a rate of **40 to 60 breaths per minute.** Gauge the effectiveness of ventilations as you would in an adult—by watching the chest to see if it rises and by auscultating for breath sounds during ventilations. If you are unable to provide effective ventilation via bag-valve-mask, you may have to intubate the baby. The *indications for endotracheal intubation* are as follows:

INDICATIONS FOR ENDOTRACHEAL INTUBATION OF THE NEWBORN

- Inability to ventilate effectively by bag-valve-mask

FIGURE 36-3.   BAG-VALVE-MASK VENTILATION OF THE NEWBORN. Hold the mask securely to the face with your thumb and index finger; apply countertraction under the bony part of the chin with your middle finger.

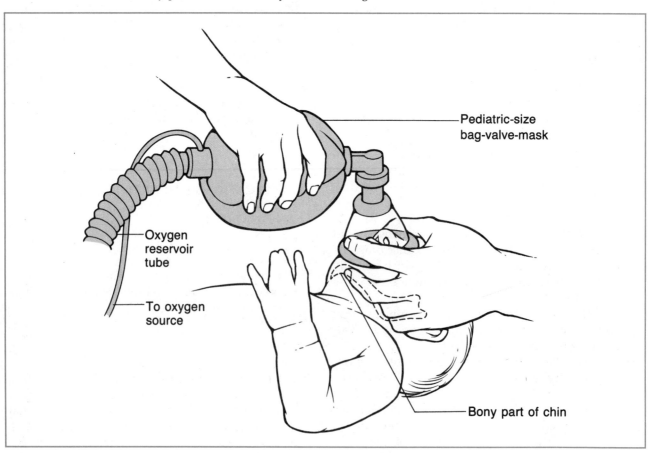

Pediatric-size bag-valve-mask

Oxygen reservoir tube

To oxygen source

Bony part of chin

- Necessity to perform tracheal suctioning, especially for thick meconium
- When prolonged ventilation will be necessary

The technique of intubating a baby was described in Chapter 30.

Once you have established good artificial ventilation, by whatever means, ventilate the baby for 30 seconds, and then REASSESS.

- *If the baby's heart rate is greater than 100 per minute and the baby is breathing spontaneously,* you may discontinue artificial ventilation and simply give supplemental oxygen.
- *If the heart rate is between 60 and 100 per minute,* continue artificial ventilation.
- *If the heart rate is less than 60 per minute,* continue artificial ventilation and start external chest compressions as well.

Chest Compressions in the Newborn

External chest compressions are required in only a very small percentage of neonatal resuscitations. Severe bradycardia and cardiac arrest come about only after a period of extreme tissue hypoxia and acidosis, which can ordinarily be prevented or corrected by prompt artificial ventilation and oxygenation. When, however, the heart rate does fall below 60 beats per minute, chest compressions must be performed.

There are two techniques for applying external chest compressions to the newborn. When there are two rescuers, one giving chest compressions, the other ventilating, the easiest compression technique employs the rescuer's two thumbs placed side by side on the sternum, as shown in Figure 36-4A. The thumbs are positioned on the sternum just below an imaginary line drawn between the two nipples, and the rescuer's fingers encircle the baby's torso. When a single rescuer is performing CPR, or when the infant is large, it is usually easier for the rescuer to compress the chest using two fingers of one hand (Fig.

FIGURE 36-4. **CHEST COMPRESSIONS IN THE NEWBORN.** (A) When there are two rescuers, use your thumbs side by side, placed just below an imaginary line drawn between the two nipples. (B) When working alone, or when the baby is large, use two fingers to depress the sternum.

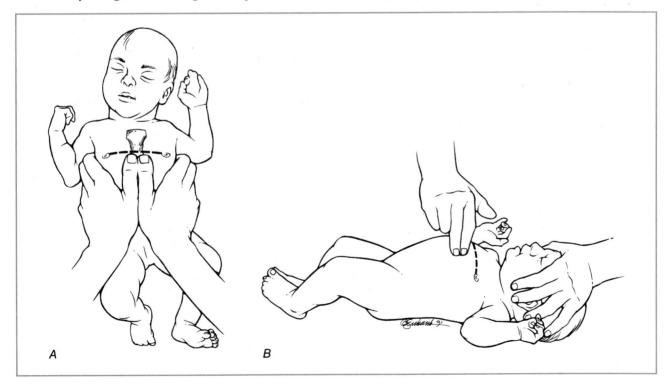

A   B

36-4B). In either case, the sternum should be compressed ½ to ¾ inch at a rate of **120 per minute,** with compression and relaxation times about equal. As always, external chest compressions must be accompanied by artificial ventilation (with 100% oxygen) at a rate of 40 to 60 breaths per minute. That means you will have to pause after every *third* chest compression to interpose a ventilation.

REASSESS the baby's pulse rate after the first minute of chest compressions and periodically thereafter. Chest compressions may be discontinued when the baby's spontaneous heart rate reaches 80 per minute or higher.

Medications in Neonatal Resuscitation

If it is rare that external chest compressions are required in the resuscitation of an infant, it is rarer still that drug therapy has to be employed. In the vast majority of cases, the establishment of adequate ventilation and oxygenation will do the job. What that means is:

> **BEFORE YOU LUNGE FOR A SYRINGE, RECHECK THE EFFECTIVENESS OF ARTIFICIAL VENTILATION.**

In the field, there is only one drug that might, on rare occasions, be needed in neonatal resuscitation, and that is EPINEPHRINE. It is indicated for

- Asystole
- Spontaneous heart rate less than 80 per minute *despite adequate ventilation with 100% oxygen and chest compressions*

Check with medical command before administering epinephrine to a newborn. When epinephrine *is* ordered, the dosage is **0.01 to 0.03 mg per kilogram** (0.1–0.3 ml of a 1 : 10,000 solution). In the field, the only feasible route of administration will be **via the endotracheal tube,** since trying to start an IV in the newborn will take too much time. When giving epinephrine via the endotracheal tube, dilute the dose in 1 to 2 ml of normal saline to ensure that it is effectively delivered down the tube. The dose may be repeated every 3 to 5 minutes.

A reminder: While all of these resuscitative measures are going on,

> **DON'T NEGLECT TO KEEP THE BABY WARM.**

In the panic and confusion that often surround neonatal resuscitation, the need to protect the baby from heat loss is very often forgotten, and the rescuers cannot understand why the baby's condition is deteriorating. It is nearly impossible to resuscitate a hypothermic baby! Hypothermia leads to acidosis, hypoglycemia, hypoxemia, and shock—all of which make successful resuscitation unlikely.

NEONATAL TRANSPORT

Transport of the high-risk or critically ill newborn requires many specialized skills and thorough training in a neonatal intensive care unit. It is beyond the scope of this textbook to provide all the information necessary for such an undertaking. Those paramedics who will be involved in the transport of high-risk neonates should receive additional, hospital-based training under the supervision of qualified pediatricians and neonatal intensive care nurses. This section is provided only to familiarize the paramedic with some of the unique problems involved in neonatal transport.

The development of new and sophisticated techniques for the care of newborn infants, especially premature infants, together with round-the-clock care by expert medical personnel, has significantly reduced the mortality among high-risk newborns in those hospitals where such facilities are available. However, the average community hospital cannot—and should not—provide the specially trained doctors and nurses or the expensive equipment needed for such care. Thus, it is sometimes necessary to transfer the critically ill infant to a regional center, where the infant may benefit from greater resources of skilled manpower and sophisticated equipment. The survival of such infants depends in large measure on their management during transport. That management will be optimal if it is conducted by a stable medical transport team skilled in techniques of neonatal intensive care. Highly successful neonatal transport teams consisting of nurses and paramedics are now functioning in several regions of the United States.

In the well-organized regional referral system, transport of a high-risk neonate proceeds through several steps:

- The REQUEST FOR TRANSPORT is initiated by the physician at the referring hospital. A physician in the regional control center decides which intensive care nursery can accommodate the patient and gives the referring physician advice on management of the baby until the transport team arrives.

- A MODE OF TRANSPORTATION IS CHOSEN. It may be ground transportation, helicopter, or fixed-wing aircraft, depending on the distance, availability of services, and weather conditions. The mode of transport is selected with a view to keeping transport time to a minimum while providing an optimal environment for care of the newborn en route.

- The TRANSPORT TEAM IS MOBILIZED, and EQUIPMENT IS ASSEMBLED. The ideal team probably consists of a pediatrician with special training in neonatal intensive care, a nurse with similar special training, and a paramedic who has spent a period of apprenticeship in a neonatal intensive care unit. The equipment is also highly specialized, requiring appropriately designed ventilation and oxygenation units and an incubator meeting stringent criteria.

- On arriving at the referring hospital, THE TRANSPORT TEAM STABILIZES THE INFANT BEFORE EMBARKING ON TRANSPORT. Conditions such as hypoxemia, acidosis, hypoglycemia, and hypovolemia must be treated before leaving the referring hospital. Since that may require a few hours, the transport team must be prepared to spend a good deal of time on their mission.

  While stabilizing the infant, the team COLLECTS INFORMATION and materials including
  1. A copy of the mother's and infant's charts.
  2. Any x-rays taken of the infant.
  3. The names of the infant, the parents, and the referring physician and a phone number where the parents may be reached.
  4. Specimens of maternal and umbilical cord blood.
  5. A consent form, indicating that the parents consent to the transfer.
  If the distance to the receiving hospital is not too great, it is often a good idea to encourage the infant's father to follow in his car. In that way, he can become acquainted with the staff who will be caring for the infant and can communicate his impressions back to the mother.

- Once the infant has been stabilized, TRANSPORT IS BEGUN. A detailed transport record is initiated, and the receiving hospital is notified of the estimated time of arrival.

GLOSSARY

ductus arteriosus Direct communication between the pulmonary artery and the aorta in the fetal circulation.

ductus venosus Muscular tube through which the umbilical vein enters the abdomen.

foramen ovale Opening between the right and left atria of the fetal heart.

meconium Fetal stool.

neonate A newborn.

FURTHER READING

Brunette DD, Sterner SP. Prehospital and emergency department delivery: A review of eight years experience. *Ann Emerg Med* 18:1116, 1989.

Carson BS et al. Combined obstetric and pediatric approach to prevent meconium aspiration. *Am J Obstet Gynecol* 126:712, 1976.

Cloherty JP, Stark AR (eds.). *Manual of Neonatal Care.* Boston: Little, Brown, 1980.

Dierking BH. Neonatal resuscitation. *Emergency* 21(8):19, 1989.

Dunlap TM. Grasping the principles of neonatal resuscitation. *JEMS* 19(1):46, 1994.

Emergency Cardiac Care Committee and Subcommittees, American Heart Association. Guidelines for cardiopulmonary resuscitation and emergency cardiac care. *JAMA* 268:2171, 1992.

Ferrara A, Harin A. *Emergency Transfer of the High-Risk Neonate.* St. Louis: Mosby, 1979.

Gregory GA. Resuscitation of the newborn. *Anesthesiology* 43:225, 1975.

Hackel A. A medical transport system for the neonate. *Anesthesiology* 43:258, 1975.

Hood JL et al. Effectiveness of the neonatal transport team. *Crit Care Med* 11:419, 1983.

Kanto WP, Calvert LJ. Thermoregulation of the newborn. *Am Fam Physician* 16:157, 1977.

Lindemann R. Resuscitation of the newborn: Endotracheal administration of epinephrine. *Acta Paediatr Scand* 73:210, 1984.

MacDonald MG, Miller MK (eds.). *Emergency Transport of the Perinatal Patient.* Boston: Little, Brown, 1989.

Milner AD et al. Efficacy of facemask resuscitation at birth. *Br Med J* 289:1563, 1984.

Montgomery WH et al. Neonatal advanced life support. *JAMA* 255:2969, 1986.

Nixon RG. Intubation of the newborn. *Emerg Med Serv* 6(2):21, 1977.

Palme C, Nystrom B, Tunell R. An evaluation of the efficiency of face masks in the resuscitation of newborn infants. *Lancet* 1:207, 1985.

Segal S (ed.). *Transport of High-Risk Newborn Infants.* Sherbrooke, Quebec: Canadian Pediatric Society, 1972.

The sick newborn. *Emerg Med* 15(17):26, 1983.

Simon J, Goldberg A. *Prehospital Pediatric Life Support.* Baltimore: Mosby, 1989.

Transporting a sick newborn. *Emerg Med* 16(17):95, 1984.

Wirth FH, Millhouse CA. Evaluation of a neonatal transport system. *Emerg Med Serv* 8(3):74, 1979.

37
Gynecologic Emergencies

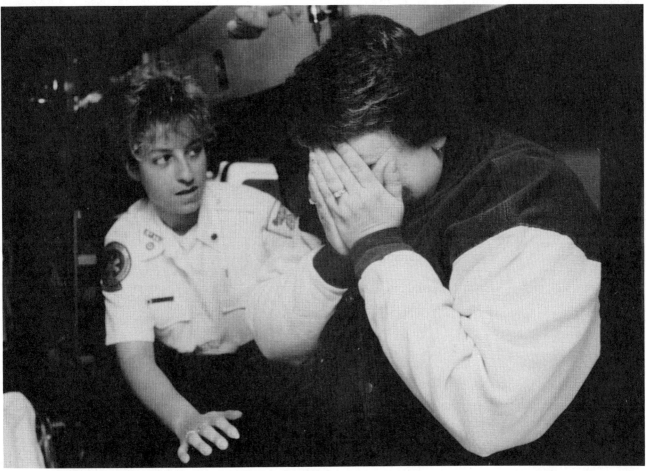

Brewster Ambulance Service, Brewster, Massachusetts. Photo by Brian Clark.

OBJECTIVES

Women are designed differently from men. The special design features of women enable them to bear children but also render them vulnerable to a variety of problems that do not beset men. In this chapter, we shall look at a few of those problems. We shall first consider the gynecologic causes of abdominal pain in women and look in detail at those causes that may constitute a threat to life. We shall look briefly at vaginal bleeding and how it should be managed in the field. And finally, we shall consider the principles of managing a woman who has been the victim of sexual assault. By the end of this chapter, the student should be able to

1. List ten questions that should be asked in taking the history of a woman whose chief complaint is abdominal pain
2. List the points of emphasis in performing the physical assessment of a woman whose chief complaint is abdominal pain
3. Given a description of several women with different clinical findings, identify a woman likely to be suffering from
   • Pelvic inflammatory disease
   • Ectopic pregnancy
   and describe the correct prehospital management of each
4. List two risk factors for ectopic pregnancy
5. List the "classic triad" of symptoms of ectopic pregnancy
6. Describe the prehospital management of a patient whose chief complaint is vaginal bleeding
7. Identify correct and incorrect procedures in the management of a woman who has been sexually assaulted, given a list of procedures

ABDOMINAL PAIN IN WOMEN

It is axiomatic in medicine that any woman between the ages of 8 and 80 who presents with lower abdominal pain has a gynecologic problem—a problem related to the female reproductive organs—until proved otherwise. The statement is, of course, an exaggeration. Women are subject to nearly all of the causes of acute abdomen that affect men—such as renal colic, ulcers, gastroenteritis, diverticulitis, pancreatitis, appendicitis, mesenteric ischemia, and dissecting aneurysm. Nonetheless, there is wisdom in the old medical axiom; for anyone who neglects to consider a gynecologic cause in a woman of childbearing age complaining of abdominal pain is going to miss

the diagnosis at least 50 percent of the time. Missing the diagnosis may be fatal for the patient.

Patient Assessment

A careful assessment of the woman complaining of abdominal pain will ensure appropriate prehospital management. It may not always be possible to make a specific diagnosis in the field; but a careful assessment will enable the paramedic at least to gauge how sick the woman is and to initiate lifesaving measures where necessary.

Taking the History

As we learned in Chapter 11, taking a patient's history involves, first of all, an elucidation of the chief complaint. When the chief complaint is abdominal pain, therefore, we need first to find out more about the pain itself. The most efficient way to do so is with the PQRST-A formula we have used to ask about other kinds of pain:

P What PROVOKES the pain? Did something in particular bring it on? Does anything make it better or worse? A patient with a ruptured ovarian cyst may report that the pain came on during exercise. A patient with pelvic inflammatory disease (PID) may (or may not!) volunteer that the pain is made worse by sexual intercourse.

Q What is the QUALITY of the pain? Dull? Sharp? Crampy? A patient having a spontaneous abortion usually has crampy pain. The pain of pelvic inflammatory disease is more likely to be dull and steady.

R In what REGION is the pain? Does it RADIATE? The pain of an ectopic pregnancy is usually localized at first to one side of the abdomen. Radiation to the shoulder indicates large amounts of blood in the abdomen. The pain of spontaneous abortion is in the midline. Pelvic inflammatory disease presents with diffuse aching in the lower abdomen.

S How SEVERE is the pain? Excruciating pain points to a *non*gynecologic cause, such as ureteral colic or aortic dissection.

T What is the TIMING of the pain? When did it start? What is the temporal relation between the pain and the last menstrual period? The pain of pelvic inflammatory disease often comes shortly after the last menstrual flow. What symptoms came first? In ectopic pregnancy, pain usually develops *before* bleeding. In spontaneous abortion, pain is more likely to *follow* bleeding.

A Are there ASSOCIATED SYMPTOMS? Ask specifically about bleeding (see below) and symptoms of significant blood loss, such as dizziness.

Once we have a feeling for the patient's pain, we can then proceed to obtain the rudiments of a GYNECOLOGIC HISTORY. Find out:

- When was the patient's LAST MENSTRUAL PERIOD (LMP)? That is probably the single most important question in the gynecologic history. Record the date that the last menstrual flow began. Ask whether the period was normal or unusual in any way (more or less bleeding than usual, more or less cramping then usual, duration of flow shorter or longer than usual). Very heavy menstrual flow is termed **menorrhagia.** Has there been any spotting or *bleeding between periods* (**metrorrhagia**)? Be sure to make note of a menstrual period that did not come on time. A missed period (**amenorrhea**) in a woman of childbearing age means pregnancy until proved otherwise.

> **THE MOST COMMON CAUSE OF AMENORRHEA IS PREGNANCY.**

- Does the woman think she might be PREGNANT? A negative response to that question is not always entirely reliable, but an affirmative response provides useful information. Ask specifically about *symptoms of pregnancy,* such as breast enlargement or tenderness, urinary frequency, and nausea or vomiting in the mornings.
- Does the woman use any form of CONTRACEPTION? Woman using the intrauterine contraceptive device (IUCD), often referred to as "the loop" or "the coil," are more prone to pelvic inflammatory disease and ectopic pregnancy. Women who do not use *any* form of contraception and are sexually active are, needless to say, at higher risk of becoming pregnant.
- Has there been any VAGINAL BLEEDING? If so, what color was it (bright red or dark)? When did it start? How much blood was lost? One way to try to quantitate the amount of blood loss is to ask how many sanitary pads were used. For each

soaked pad, estimate a blood loss of about 20 to 30 ml.
- Has she had any VAGINAL DISCHARGE? If so, how much? What color was it? Did it have a bad smell?
- What is the woman's OBSTETRIC HISTORY? How many times has she been pregnant (gravidity)? How many times has she delivered (parity)?
- Has she had GYNECOLOGIC PROBLEMS IN THE PAST, such as bleeding, infections, or miscarriages?
- Does she have any UNDERLYING ILLNESSES, such as diabetes, hypertension, or other cardiovascular disease?

Remember: Women who present with problems referable to the reproductive tract may be embarrassed or apprehensive. Tact, understanding, and a professional manner on the part of the paramedic are necessary in taking the gynecologic history.

The Physical Examination

In examining the woman whose chief complaint is abdominal pain, there is fundamentally just one question that needs to be answered in the prehospital setting: Is this woman suffering from a potentially life-threatening situation? As we shall learn shortly, there are only three gynecologic conditions that can pose an immediate threat to life, and all of them present with similar findings.

> **IN THE WOMAN WITH ABDOMINAL PAIN, THE MOST IMPORTANT THINGS TO LOOK FOR ARE SIGNS OF SHOCK.**

Therefore, the points of emphasis in the secondary survey are as follows:

- Note the woman's GENERAL APPEARANCE. Does she seem *restless* or *apprehensive*?
- Note the CONDITION OF THE SKIN AND MUCOUS MEMBRANES. Is the skin warm and dry? Cold and clammy? Is there pallor or cyanosis?
- Check the VITAL SIGNS in both the SITTING AND STANDING positions. If there are orthostatic changes, the woman must be presumed to be in shock.
- *Briefly* examine the ABDOMEN. All that you need determine in the field is whether the abdomen is *distended* and whether it is *rigid*.

Pelvic Inflammatory Disease

Pelvic inflammatory disease (PID) is the most common infection and one of the most common sources of abdominal pain among women of reproductive age. In the United States, there are about 1 million cases of PID every year, of which one-quarter are severe enough to require hospitalization.

PID results from infection of the female reproductive organs and occurs almost exclusively in sexually active women. Microorganisms introduced into the vagina migrate up through the cervix and uterine cavity to the fallopian tubes, where they infect the mucosa. Infection may then spread out through the open end of the fallopian tubes to involve the ovaries (tubo-ovarian abscess) or even the peritoneal cavity.

PID is most prevalent in *women under 30* years of age, with a peak incidence between the ages of 20 and 24. Risk factors for developing PID include frequent sexual activity with *multiple partners,* the use of an *IUCD* for contraception, and a *history of previous PID.* Although PID is rarely if ever life-threatening, it may have serious consequences. To begin with, PID may lead to the development of a tubo-ovarian abscess, which *can* be life-threatening. By producing scars in the fallopian tubes, furthermore, PID increases a woman's later risk of ectopic pregnancy (also life-threatening) or of infertility.

Clinical Findings in PID

The woman with PID nearly always presents with a chief complaint of *abdominal pain.* Very often, the pain comes on *during or immediately after menstruation.* The pain is described as *achy,* and involves both quadrants of the lower abdomen. When there is severe involvement of the cervix, the patient will experience a worsening of pain during sexual intercourse or even when trying to walk. Spread of infection into the abdominal cavity may produce peritoneal pain, sometimes localized to the right upper quadrant. Associated symptoms may include *vaginal discharge, fever and chills,* and pain or burning on urination (*dysuria*).

The physical findings in PID vary from no findings at all to findings consistent with severe toxicity from infection. As a general rule, women with PID who feel sick enough to call for an ambulance will be those with more severe infections. They are likely to be *febrile* and to *look ill.* The lower abdomen will be diffusely and sometimes exquisitely tender, and there may be signs of peritoneal irritation (e.g., the woman wincing each time the ambulance takes a bump).

Prehospital Treatment

The definitive treatment of PID requires administration of appropriate antibiotics over 10 to 14 days. In the field, all that can be done is to make the patient as comfortable as possible and transport her atraumatically to the hospital. Allow her to assume a PO-SITION OF COMFORT in the ambulance, and drive in a manner that will minimize swings and bounces of the stretcher.

Ectopic Pregnancy

There are only three potentially life-threatening gynecologic emergencies, and ectopic pregnancy is the most common among them. (The other two, ruptured ovarian cyst and ruptured tubo-ovarian abscess, present with symptoms similar to those of ectopic pregnancy, and it is of no value to try to distinguish them from ectopic pregnancy in the field.) Ectopic pregnancy has reached epidemic proportions in the United States and currently accounts for 1.4 percent of all pregnancies. Furthermore, ectopic pregnancy is the most common cause of maternal death in the first trimester.

The word **ectopic** means "occurring in an abnormal position." (Question: What are "ectopic beats" on the electrocardiogram?) An ectopic pregnancy occurs when a fertilized egg implants in an abnormal position, that is, somewhere other than inside the uterus. In 95 percent of cases, ectopic implantation occurs in a fallopian tube, where the egg is fertilized, in which case it is referred to as a tubal pregnancy. Tubal pregnancy is more likely when the tube is scarred from previous infection or tubal surgery. The fertilized egg may then get hung up at an obstruction in the tube and be unable to make the normal descent into the uterus.

When the fertilized egg implants in the fallopian tube, it draws nourishment from the maternal blood supply and begins to grow and to produce hormones just as a normally implanted egg would do. The hormones bring about the early physiologic changes of pregnancy—amenorrhea, stimulation of the uterine endometrium, enlargement and tenderness of the breasts. The tube, however, has very little capacity to stretch, so the growing embryo soon starts to run out of room. Eventually—usually sometime between the fifth and sixth week after the last menstrual period—pressure exerted by the embryo on the wall of the tube starts to cause crampy, unilateral, lower abdominal pain. If the embryo continues to grow within the tube, the tube is likely to rupture, producing massive intra-abdominal hemorrhage and shock.

Clinical Findings

The presenting complaint in nearly all women with ectopic pregnancy is *abdominal pain.* The pain is initially *localized* to one side of the lower abdomen, and early on it is intermittent and *crampy.* As the pregnancy develops, the tube will either rupture or abort the embryo out of its fimbriated end, either of which will produce severe pain, again localized to one side of the abdomen. By the time the patient is seen by paramedics, however, the pain is likely to be constant and felt diffusely throughout the abdomen, especially if there is significant **hemoperitoneum** (blood in the peritoneal cavity). *Shoulder pain* is a particularly ominous symptom, for it suggests the presence of massive hemoperitoneum.

Approximately 65 percent of women with ectopic pregnancy will have also *vaginal bleeding*. In contrast to the bleeding that occurs in spontaneous abortion,

> **IN ECTOPIC PREGNANCY, BLEEDING USUALLY OCCURS *AFTER* THE ONSET OF PAIN.**

It is important, therefore, to establish the temporal relationship between the patient's symptoms. Bleeding in ectopic pregnancy comes, at least in part, from shedding the uterine lining as the embryo is disrupted from its implantation site and ceases producing hormones. The volume of bleeding from the vagina may be slight ("spotting") or considerable and in no way indicates how much blood the woman may have lost *internally*.

In inquiring about the woman's LMP, a history of *amenorrhea* will be found in about 75 percent of patients with ectopic pregnancy. And those three symptoms—ABDOMINAL PAIN, VAGINAL BLEEDING, and AMENORRHEA—are considered the classic diagnostic triad for ectopic pregnancy. The history is also likely to reveal previous PID, previous ectopic pregnancy, or use of an IUCD for contraception.

On physical examination, look for SIGNS OF HYPOVOLEMIC SHOCK: restlessness and anxiety; cold, moist skin; pulse rate greater than 100 per minute; and systolic blood pressure less than 90 mm Hg.

Prehospital Management of Suspected Ectopic Pregnancy

Any woman presenting with a history of abdominal pain and vaginal bleeding must be treated for impending shock, whether or not she has signs of shock when you first examine her.

- Ensure an adequate AIRWAY, and administer OXYGEN.
- Keep the patient RECUMBENT, preferably lying on her left side.
- Start at least one LARGE-BORE IV with lactated Ringer's solution, and be prepared to run it wide open if signs of shock develop.

- Give NOTHING BY MOUTH.
- Anticipate vomiting. Have an emesis basin and suction close at hand.
- Keep the patient WARM.
- MONITOR cardiac rhythm.
- NOTIFY the receiving hospital of the patient's suspected diagnosis, her condition, and your estimated time of arrival.
- TRANSPORT.
- Recheck VITAL SIGNS frequently during transport.

VAGINAL BLEEDING

Abnormal bleeding from the vagina is the most frequent complaint for which women of all ages consult a gynecologist. The assessment and management of a patient whose chief complaint is vaginal bleeding will depend to some extent on whether there is a history of injury.

In evaluating the woman who has VAGINAL BLEEDING WITHOUT A HISTORY OF TRAUMA, it is a useful generalization that

> **ABNORMAL VAGINAL BLEEDING IS A COMPLICATION OF PREGNANCY UNTIL PROVED OTHERWISE.**

By remembering that generalization, you will not overlook the possibility of ectopic pregnancy or inevitable abortion.

For the purposes of prehospital care, the most important things to find out from a woman whose chief complaint is vaginal bleeding are the date of her last normal menstrual period and the volume of her bleeding. Here again, try to quantitate the blood loss by asking how many sanitary pads or tampons the woman has used. In the physical examination, look for *postural changes* in vital signs. As a general rule, a normal menstrual period will not prompt a woman to dial 911; so it's usually a safe assumption that a woman who has called for an ambulance because of vaginal bleeding is having A LOT of bleeding— enough to scare her. That's a good enough reason to TREAT EXPECTANTLY FOR SHOCK:

- Keep the patient RECUMBENT.
- Administer OXYGEN.
- START AN IV with a large-bore catheter and normal saline or lactated Ringer's solution.
- MONITOR cardiac rhythm.

- Follow the VITAL SIGNS closely, and open up the IV wide at the first indication of developing shock (e.g., restlessness, increasing pulse rate).

A somewhat different approach is required WHEN THERE HAS BEEN TRAUMA TO THE FEMALE GENITALIA. Lacerations to the external female genitalia sometimes occur from rape or other trauma and may bleed heavily. Usually the bleeding can be controlled simply by external pressure applied over the laceration. Bleeding from the *internal* genitalia, on the other hand, can be massive and very difficult to control. In general, it is both useless and dangerous to introduce packs blindly into the vagina in an attempt to control bleeding. A woman with exsanguinating hemorrhage per vagina must be treated as any other injured patient with exsanguinating hemorrhage, that is, as a *load-and-go* emergency:

- Ensure an adequate AIRWAY.
- Administer OXYGEN.
- Start TRANSPORT and NOTIFY the receiving hospital.
- En route, start AT LEAST ONE LARGE-BORE IV for rapid infusion of lactated Ringer's solution.
- MONITOR cardiac rhythm.
- Recheck VITAL SIGNS frequently.

SEXUAL ASSAULT

Rape has become one of the most common violent crimes in America, and it is estimated that one in every three to six women experiences a rape or attempted rape sometime during her life. For the paramedic called to treat a victim of sexual assault, rape or alleged rape presents a complex problem, one with serious medical, psychologic, and legal ramifications. Usually the paramedic will be the first representative of the community with whom the victim has contact. That initial contact can do a great deal of good or a great deal of harm. Tact, kindness, and sensitivity are essential. Wherever possible, the female rape victim should have the option of being managed by a female paramedic if she wishes, for the victim may have ambivalent feelings toward men in the wake of having been assaulted.

There are several important principles to observe in dealing with any victim of sexual assault. The first is that A PARAMEDIC IS NOT A POLICE OFFICER.* Your primary job is to provide urgent medical care,

---

*Even paramedics who *are* police officers have a primary responsibility, when working as paramedics, to the patient's *medical* needs.

not to cross-examine the patient, *not* to collect evidence, and certainly *not* to pass judgment one way or the other on the patient's story. In taking the *history*, concentrate on the medical aspects of the case: What is the patient's chief complaint? Does anything hurt? Was she struck anywhere? The details of the incident itself will be elicited in the emergency room or by law enforcement authorities, and you need not concern yourself with obtaining information that does not relate to the patient's immediate medical problem. Many rape victims report feeling "re-raped" when subjected to a lengthy interrogation, and conducting such an interrogation will not enhance your prospects for gaining the patient's trust and confidence.

> **FIND OUT IF THE WOMAN HAS BEEN INJURED. DO *NOT* ASK QUESTIONS ABOUT THE INCIDENT ITSELF.**

Limit the *physical examination* to a brief survey for life-threatening injuries. Do not examine the vaginal area unless there is obvious bleeding that must be controlled. It is important to try to preserve evidence, which means that the patient should be discouraged from changing clothes, showering, urinating, moving her bowels, gargling, or drinking any fluids before coming to the emergency room. Some rape victims, however, have a strong need to "clean up" before presenting themselves at the hospital, as a way of trying to wash away the feelings of humiliation that sexual assault engenders. If the patient cannot be persuaded by tactful explanations to defer her "clean up," respect her feelings. Indeed, if the patient refuses transport to the hospital, that is also her right. In the event that the patient does not want to be examined in the hospital, though, do not simply abandon her at the scene. Transport her instead to the home of a friend or relative, so that she will not have to be alone after such a frightening experience.

Throughout your contact with the rape victim, do your utmost to PROTECT THE PATIENT'S PRIVACY. If the victim is in a public place, move her into the ambulance as quickly as possible, to shield her from the stares of curious bystanders. Avoid using the word *rape* in your radio communications to the hospital; a preestablished code, such as "Case A," is preferable.

When you write up your report, keep in mind that THE TRIP SHEET IS A LEGAL DOCUMENT. In recording the history, state only what the patient said, in her own words; use quotation marks or some other means of indicating that you are reporting the patient's version of events. Do not volunteer your own opinion as to whether the patient was or was not raped. Record all of your observations on physical examination—the patient's emotional state, the condition of her clothing, obvious injuries, and so forth. Bear in mind that rape is a *legal* diagnosis, not a medical diagnosis. The medical team can establish only whether sexual intercourse occurred; a court must decide whether intercourse was inflicted forcibly on the victim, against her will.

Managing the Victim of Rape: Summary

One of the most important needs of anyone who has just suffered an assault is to feel that she is safe now, among people she can trust, people who will see to it that no further harm comes to her. That is the message you need to convey, through word and behavior, as you care for the victim of rape.

- Wherever possible, give the rape victim the option of being cared for by a female paramedic. (The patient may or may not wish to exercise that option.)
- Your primary responsibility is to TAKE CARE OF THE PATIENT'S URGENT MEDICAL PROBLEMS:
  1. Take a *medical* history, not a history of the assault.
  2. *Limit the physical examination* to a search for injuries requiring immediate stabilization.
- TRY TO PRESERVE EVIDENCE, but respect the patient's feelings.
  1. Handle the patient's clothing as little as possible.
  2. Place bloodstained articles in separate, *paper* (not plastic) bags (plastic containers favor bacterial growth).
  3. Do not disturb the crime scene.
  4. Discourage the patient from changing clothes, bathing, gargling, and so forth.
- PROTECT THE PATIENT'S PRIVACY. Respect her confidentiality.
- DO NOT ABANDON THE PATIENT AT THE SCENE.
- Remember that YOUR TRIP SHEET IS A LEGAL DOCUMENT. Stick to the facts. Do not record your opinions.

GLOSSARY

amenorrhea   Absence of menstruation.
ectopic   Occurring in an abnormal location.

ectopic pregnancy   A pregnancy in which the ovum implants somewhere other than the uterine endometrium.
hemoperitoneum   Blood in the peritoneal cavity.
IUCD   Abbreviation for intrauterine contraceptive device.
LMP   Abbreviation for last menstrual period.
menorrhagia   Very heavy menstrual flow.
metrorrhagia   Vaginal bleeding between menstrual periods.
PID   Abbreviation for pelvic inflammatory disease.
rape   Sexual intercourse that is inflicted forcibly on another person, against that person's will.

FURTHER READING

American College of Emergency Physicians. Management of the patient with the complaint of sexual assault. *Ann Emerg Med* 21:732, 1992.

American College of Obstetrics and Gynecology. Sexual assault. ACOG Bulletin #172. *Int J Gynecol Obstet* 42:67, 1993.

Bitterman RA. Pelvic inflammatory disease. *Emerg Med* 22(8):33, 1990.

Brenner PF et al. Ectopic pregnancy: A study of 300 consecutive surgically treated cases. *JAMA* 243:673, 1980.

Carson S, Buster J. Ectopic pregnancy. *N Engl J Med* 329:1174, 1993.

Centers for Disease Control. Ectopic pregnancy—United States, 1981–1983. *MMWR* 35(17), 1986.

Dickinson ET. Gynecologic emergencies. *JEMS* 15(3):20, 1990.

Dorfman SF et al. Ectopic pregnancy mortality, United States, 1979 to 1980: Clinical aspects. *Obstet Gynecol* 64:386, 1984.

Hicks DJ. The patient who's been raped. *Emerg Med* 20(20):106, 1988.

Hughes GJ. The early diagnosis of ectopic pregnancy. *Br J Surg* 66:789, 1979.

Little A. Dressing the emotional wounds: The sexual assault case. *Emergency* 24(5):44, 1992.

Mayer R, Boggio N. The adolescent rape victim. *Emerg Med* 24(3):98, 1992.

Niemi TA et al. Vaginal injuries in patients with pelvic fractures. *J Trauma* 25:547, 1985.

Powers DN. Ectopic pregnancy: A five-year experience. *South Med J* 73:1012, 1980.

Rainbow B et al. Female sexual assault: Medical and legal implications. *Ann Emerg Med* 21:727, 1992.

Rubin GL et al. Ectopic pregnancy in the United States: 1970 through 1978. *JAMA* 249:1725, 1983.

Santiago JM et al. Long-term psychological effects of rape in 35 rape victims. *Am J Psychiatry* 142:1338, 1985.

Snyder JR. Defusing the deadly ectopic. *Emerg Med* 14(20):92, 1983.

Steinkampf MP, Nichols JE. Ectopic pregnancy: The deadly gestation. *Emerg Med* 22(10):17, 1990.

Whitehead C. After the violation: Treating rape victims. *Emerg Med* 16(4):48, 1991.

Young WW et al. Sexual assault: Review of a national model protocol for forensic and medical evaluation. *Obstet Gynecol* 80:878, 1992.

VIII
BEHAVIORAL EMERGENCIES

38
Disturbances of Behavior

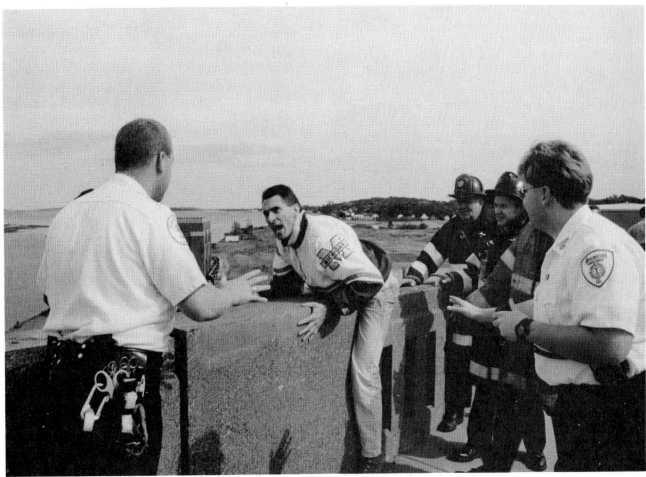

Brewster Ambulance Service, Brewster, Massachusetts. Photo by Brian Clark.

OBJECTIVES

This chapter is about problems that present as disturbances in behavior. Such problems are commonly classified as "mental problems," implying that they originate in some ephemeral place called the mind, as opposed to "real" medical problems, which originate in the solid, tangible structures of the body. In fact, however, the mind and the body are not separate entities; they are two inseparable parts of a whole human being. When a person becomes ill with any disease, his illness will inevitably affect his mood and behavior—often making him anxious and depressed. Similarly, changes in mental state influence the body's physical health. A depressed person, for example, may lose his appetite or become more susceptible to bodily disease. Thus, whenever we examine a patient—no matter what his or her complaint—it is important to view the patient as a whole person and try to understand both the physical and mental factors that contribute to the patient's distress.

In this chapter, we shall take a closer look at some of the conditions that manifest themselves as disturbances of behavior. We shall consider some of the causes of disturbed behavior and the methods of assessing a disturbed patient. We shall then look at some specific behavioral emergencies and their prehospital management. Finally, we shall consider some of the medicolegal aspects of dealing with disturbed patients. By the conclusion of this chapter, the student should be able to

1. List eight conditions other than psychiatric illness that can cause disturbed behavior, and indicate what signs and symptoms would suggest that a patient's disturbed behavior has an organic cause
2. Identify productive and less productive approaches to a disturbed patient, given a description of several approaches
3. List four principles of interviewing a disturbed patient
4. List the components of the mental status examination, and describe which components are characteristically impaired in
   - Psychosis
   - Depression
   - Mania
5. Given a description of several patients with different clinical findings, identify a patient likely to be suffering from
   - Psychosis
   - Depression
   - Mania
   - A panic attack
   - Disorganization or disorientation

     • An organic brain syndrome
   and describe the most appropriate prehospital management of each
6. List six symptoms and signs characteristic of
   - Psychosis
   - Depression
   - Mania
   - Panic disorder
7. List five factors that increase a person's risk of suicide
8. List five scenarios or classes of patients that carry an increased risk of violence
9. List five warning signals of impending violent behavior
10. Outline the steps that should be taken in managing a violent patient

WHAT IS A PSYCHIATRIC EMERGENCY?

Psychiatric, or behavioral, emergencies are those in which the patient's presenting problem is some disorder of mood, thought, or behavior that is dangerous or disturbing to himself or others. As we learned in Chapter 4, almost all disordered behavior represents the individual's effort to adapt to some stress, internal or external; and in most cases the disruptive behavior is a temporary action, abating when the person has managed to mobilize his or her psychologic defense mechanisms.

No matter what definition of a psychiatric emergency a textbook may furnish, however, the *operative* definition of a psychiatric emergency is, in fact, provided by the person who dials 911. Psychiatric emergencies are in the eyes of the beholder. No matter what the textbooks say, it is ultimately the person who calls for help who decides that an emergency exists. And often what makes a psychiatric emergency an "emergency" is panic on the part of the patient, his family, bystanders, or all of the above. That panic, in turn, frequently translates into a demand for action, and the paramedic responding to a psychiatric emergency may therefore be under intense pressure to "do something."

Paradoxically, it is precisely in this situation—when the patient is behaving strangely and bystanders are clamoring for action—that the paramedic usually feels least *able* to "do something." Most paramedics would vastly prefer to deal with a train wreck than with the tangle of confused and frayed feelings presented by a psychiatric emergency. There are probably at least two reasons for that fact. First, nearly every person prefers to operate in areas in which he or she feels competent, and paramedics come to feel competent in dealing with broken legs, cardiac dysrhythmias, narcotic overdoses, and the like. They feel much less confident of their ability to deal with emotional disturbances—especially when most paramedic training programs scarcely mention such matters. Second, paramedics are action-oriented people. They like to see tangible results of what they do—a hypoglycemic patient coming around after a bolus of glucose, a clinically dead patient restored to life by cardiopulmonary resuscitation (CPR). What comparable rewards can there be in escorting a confused, hallucinating patient to the hospital, let alone in dealing with a belligerent and violent patient who is screaming obscenities at the rescuer?

The fact is that useful prehospital intervention *is* possible and often critical in psychiatric emergencies. Paramedics *can* make a big difference in the life of a disturbed patient, and the skills required for doing so can be learned just as the skills for performing CPR can be learned. Indeed, it can be argued that the skills for dealing with disturbed behavior will be much more important to the paramedic's work than skills ordinarily receiving much more emphasis, such as endotracheal intubation. After all, how many calls require an intubation? Compare that figure with the number of calls in which the paramedic must deal with people who are angry, depressed, agitated, panicky, out of control. So it is worthwhile learning an organized and systematic approach to emergencies that involve disturbances in behavior.

CAUSES OF DISTURBED BEHAVIOR

Anyone who has seen a paranoid, belligerent diabetic transformed into a paragon of courtesy and charm by the mere addition of 25 gm of glucose to his bloodstream knows that not everyone who acts crazy *is* crazy. Similarly, no one would diagnose mental illness in a person who walked about stunned and mute after the unanticipated death of a husband or wife. Intuitively we all realize that there are a variety of things that can cause disturbances of behavior. We can consider those causes in three broad categories: (1) situational causes, (2) organic causes, and (3) intrapsychic (psychiatric) causes.

Situational Causes of Disturbed Behavior

Normal individuals may develop abnormal reactions to stressful events. In Chapter 4, we considered the responses of patients, their families, bystanders, and rescue personnel to the stresses of emergencies. We examined as well the ways in which people react to death and dying. In Chapter 21, we looked at some of the behaviors commonly seen in response to mass casualty situations. Nearly anyone can "go to pieces" if subjected to enough stress, but some people are more vulnerable than others.

When a person's basic needs are threatened, that person faces a crisis. The severity of the crisis will depend on the individual's ability to deal with his own feelings. There are two alternatives open to a person in crisis: (1) He may cope with it, finding ways to alter his situation or his perception of it so that it is no longer so stressful, or (2) he may attempt to decrease his discomfort by escaping from the stress. Escape may take many forms, including alcohol, drugs, suicide, and even psychiatric symptoms. Symptoms thus represent a compromise for the patient, a means of reducing the anxiety that his internal crisis created.

Organic Causes of Disturbed Behavior

Many patients presenting with psychiatric symptoms are in fact suffering from a physical illness or are under the influence of a substance that interferes with normal cerebral function. Such patients are generally classified under the heading "organic brain syndrome." We have already seen, in previous chapters, how diabetes, seizure disorders, severe infections, metabolic disorders, head injury, stroke, alcohol, and drugs may all cause derangements in behavior. Table 38-1 summarizes some of the conditions and substances that can produce psychiatric symptoms. Probably the most common offenders on the list are alcohol and drugs. Indeed, when dealing with disturbed patients, if you assume that their behavior is due to alcohol or another drug, you will be correct about 50 percent of the time.

Two other common forms of organic brain syndrome, beside intoxication with alcohol or drugs, are delirium and dementia. Recall from Chapter 29 that *delirium* is characterized by a global impairment of cognitive function that comes on quite rapidly and may fluctuate in severity over the course of a day. In delirium, furthermore, there is almost always a disturbance in the state of consciousness. *Dementia* is a more chronic process that produces severe deficits in memory, abstract thinking, and judgment.

All of the organic brain syndromes, then, can produce profound behavioral disturbances. The point to remember is:

ABNORMAL BEHAVIOR MAY BE DUE TO MANY CONDITIONS OTHER THAN MENTAL ILLNESS.

TABLE 38-1.   DISEASE STATES THAT MAY PRODUCE PSYCHOTIC SYMPTOMS

TOXIC AND DEFICIENCY STATES
- Drug-induced psychoses, especially from
  Digitalis
  Steroids
  Disulfiram
  Amphetamines
  LSD, PCP, and other psychedelics
- Alcoholic hallucinosis
- Wernicke's encephalopathy
- Korsakoff's psychosis
- Poisoning with bromide or other heavy metals
- Pellagra and other vitamin deficiencies
- Uremia
- Liver failure

INFECTIONS
- Syphilis
- Toxoplasmosis
- Viral encephalitis
- Brain abscess

NEUROLOGIC DISEASE
- Seizure disorders (especially temporal lobe seizures)
- Primary and metastatic tumors of the brain
- Presenile and senile dementias
- Postencephalitic states (e.g., after measles encephalitis)

CARDIOVASCULAR DISORDERS
- Low cardiac output (e.g., in heart failure)
- Hypertensive encephalopathy

ENDOCRINE DISORDERS
- Thyrotoxicosis
- Myxedema
- Adrenal hyperfunction (Cushing's syndrome)

METABOLIC DISORDERS
- Electrolyte imbalances (e.g., after severe diarrhea)
- Hypoglycemia
- Diabetic ketoacidosis

This list is not intended to be comprehensive. It is provided simply as a reminder that "psychiatric" symptoms may be the result of physical illness. Assess every "psychotic" patient carefully!

As we proceed through this chapter, we shall learn some clues to help distinguish between the organic brain syndromes and psychiatric causes of disturbed behavior.

Psychiatric Causes of Disturbed Behavior

Finally, patients may present with disturbances of behavior as a result of psychiatric problems, that is, problems that arise within the mind of the patient, by mechanisms that we do not yet understand. It is with those intrapsychic causes of disturbed behavior that we shall be concerned for the remainder of this chapter, for the situational and organic causes have been largely covered in other chapters throughout the book. For purposes of our discussion here, we shall divide the psychiatric syndromes into the following categories:

- Psychotic disorders: disorders characterized by an impaired view of reality
- Affective disorders: disorders of mood
- Anxiety disorders: disorders involving overwhelming fear
- Disorientation and disorganization
- Hostile and violent patients

Before we consider those categories in detail, however, we need to learn a little about the approach to a disturbed patient.

ASSESSMENT OF THE DISTURBED PATIENT

Assessment of the disturbed patient differs in at least two ways from the methods of patient assessment we have studied so far. In assessing the victim of trauma or acute illness, to begin with, you use a variety of diagnostic instruments to measure vital functions and detect abnormalities—a stethoscope to evaluate breath sounds, a sphygmomanometer to measure the blood pressure, and so forth. In assessing the disturbed patient, *you* are the diagnostic instrument. You must use your thinking processes to evalute someone else's thinking processes, your perceptions to test the validity of someone else's perceptions, your feelings to measure someone else's feelings. All of that takes a little practice, for most people are not accustomed to *using* their feelings for anything. In ordinary social encounters, for example, if someone makes you feel very angry, your reaction is apt to be, "That guy infuriates me. I'd like to knock his teeth in." In conducting the psychiatric examination, a more useful paradigm is, "That guy infuriates me, so it's quite likely he is paranoid, because paranoid patients often elicit anger in others."

A second way in which the assessment of a disturbed patient differs from that of a patient with a more straightforward medical problem is that the assessment is part of the treatment! As soon as you speak to the patient, your voice and manner will influence his condition, for better or worse. And the very process of listening to him describe his problem can itself mitigate the problem.

General Principles

In later sections, we shall consider the different approaches to patients who are behaving in particular ways—patients who are sad and withdrawn, patients who are angry and violent, and so on. There are, however, certain general guidelines for dealing with *any* patient with a psychiatric problem:

- BE PREPARED TO SPEND TIME WITH THE DISTURBED PATIENT. Don't be in a hurry, but rather convey to the patient that you have the time and concern to learn what is bothering him.
- BE AS CALM AND DIRECT AS POSSIBLE. Disturbed patients are often frightened of losing self-control. Your behavior should indicate to the patient that you have confidence in his ability to maintain control. Indeed, one of the main purposes of the interview is to help the patient reestablish some mastery of himself. If you show anxiety or panic, you will only fortify the patient's conviction that the situation is overwhelming.
- IDENTIFY YOURSELF CLEARLY. Tell the patient who you are and what you are trying to do for him. If the patient is confused or delusional, you may have to explain who you are at frequent intervals. Do so without arguing, in an emotionally neutral tone of voice. ("No, Mr. Jones, I'm not from the CIA. I'm a paramedic with the city ambulance service, and I'm here to see if I can help you.")
- ASSESS THE PATIENT WHEREVER THE EMERGENCY OCCURS. Don't rush off immediately to the hospital, since the hospital is likely to be a strange, intimidating place for the patient, and haste to get him there will also reinforce his belief that something is terribly wrong. Let the patient recover his bearings in familiar surroundings.
- EXCLUDE DISRUPTIVE PERSONS FROM THE INTERVIEW. In most cases, that means interviewing the patient alone, while relatives and bystanders are asked to wait in another room (your partner can interview *them*). Some patients, however, will become anxious if separated from an important other person—a parent or friend. If another person has a calming effect on the patient, ask that person to remain.
- SIT DOWN to interview the patient, preferably at a 45-degree angle from him so that you do not encroach on his "personal space."
- SET THE GROUND RULES. Let the patient know what you expect of him and what he may expect of you. ("It's OK to cry or even scream, but we aren't going to let you hurt yourself or anyone else.")
- LET THE PATIENT TELL HIS STORY IN HIS OWN WAY. Do not attempt to direct the conversation, but allow the patient to give vent to his feelings. Sometimes offering a cup of coffee or a soft drink will facilitate a more relaxed atmosphere. (We shall have more to say shortly on how to interview a disturbed patient.)
- MAINTAIN A NONJUDGMENTAL ATTITUDE. Accept the patient's right to have his own feelings about things, and don't blame or criticize him for feeling as he does.
- PROVIDE HONEST REASSURANCE. Give supportive information that is truthful. ("Many people experience periods of hopelessness like you are having, but today there are effective treatments for those feelings.") Avoid excessive reassurance, however—statements such as, "Everything is going to be all right." Such statements will only convince the patient that you don't understand how bad things are.
- After the patient has finished telling his story and you have concluded your assessment, TAKE A DEFINITE PLAN OF ACTION. That gives the patient the feeling that something is being done to help, which in turn relieves anxiety. Furthermore, persons in crisis need direction. Do not confront the patient with an array of decisions ("Do you want to go to the hospital, or would you rather stay at home and call your doctor tomorrow?"); rather, state what you think is the best course of action (e.g., "I think it's important for you to go to the hospital. There are doctors there who can help you."). Do not, however, preempt *all* initiative from the patient. To the extent that the patient seems capable of doing so, allow him to make choices and thereby to exercise some control over his situation. You might ask him, for example, whether he prefers to be carried on a stretcher or to walk to the ambulance on his own. It is a minor decision, granted; but it allows the patient a measure of self-respect.
- ENCOURAGE SOME MOTOR ACTIVITY. Moving about often helps ease anxiety. If you are taking the patient to the hospital, have him gather up the things he wishes to bring along with him. Let him do as much for himself as possible, which will again reinforce his feeling that you expect him to improve.
- STAY WITH THE PATIENT AT ALL TIMES. Once you have responded to the emergency, the patient's safety becomes your responsibility. If he politely excuses himself, locks himself in the bathroom, and swallows the contents of a bottle

of sleeping pills, you'll have a lot of explaining to do—at least to your own conscience.

- BRING ALL THE PATIENT'S MEDICATIONS WITH HIM TO THE HOSPITAL. If the patient is under treatment for psychiatric problems, knowing what medications he has been prescribed can help the doctors at the receiving hospital identify the condition for which the patient has been treated.
- NEVER ASSUME THAT IT IS IMPOSSIBLE TO TALK WITH ANY PATIENT UNTIL YOU HAVE TRIED. Even the patient who sits mutely and appears unaware of your presence must be assumed to hear and understand everything you say.

Interviewing Techniques

In evaluating the victim of trauma, one can generally obtain enough information to provide appropriate initial treatment just from the physical examination, even if the patient is unconscious and cannot give a history. In evaluating the patient with a behavioral emergency, by contrast, virtually all of the diagnostic information (and a lot of the therapeutic benefit) must come from talking with the patient. Skill in interviewing a disturbed person, therefore, is central to dealing with psychiatric emergencies. Here are some guidelines:

- After obtaining basic, identifying information about the patient (full name, age, address), BEGIN THE INTERVIEW WITH AN OPEN-ENDED QUESTION, such as, "It's clear you've been feeling bad. Tell me something about the kind of troubles you've been having." (The only circumstance in which you should begin with more direct questioning is when it is essential to obtain specific information in a hurry, e.g., "What kind of pills did you take? How many?")
- LET THE PATIENT TALK and tell his story in his own way, even if it takes a little more time. Letting him talk enables him to gain some control over himself and his situation. At the same time, it enables *you* to begin assessing the patient's speech, affect, and thought processes.
- LISTEN, and show that you are listening. Your facial expression, your posture, an occasional nod—all of those things can convey to the patient that you are paying close attention to what he is saying.
- DO NOT BE AFRAID OF SILENCES, even though they may sometimes seem intolerably long. Just maintain an attentive and relaxed attitude until the patient takes up his story again. It is especially important to be silent when the patient has stopped speaking because he is overwhelmed by emotion. Avoid the temptation to jump into the silence with a hasty "There, there," to forestall the patient's expressions of emotion, such as crying. The expression of feelings is often therapeutic in itself—that's why people speak of having "a good cry"—and it is likely that the patient will be better able to express himself after intense emotion has been released. Furthermore, your silence gives the patient a chance to get control of himself in his own way.
- ACKNOWLEDGE AND LABEL THE PATIENT'S FEELINGS. The disturbed patient may feel overwhelmed by intense and chaotic feelings. Identifying those feelings, and giving them a name (e.g., "You seem very angry"), helps the patient gain control over them.
- DON'T ARGUE. If the patient misperceives reality, it is your job to make note of his misperceptions, not to try to talk him out of them. When a misperception is very frightening or distressing to the patient, it may be worth trying once to provide a simple and accurate statement, in a neutral tone of voice ("Yes, that does look a lot like a snake, but actually it's just a shadow."). But don't get into a dispute on the nature of reality.
- FACILITATION means encouraging the patient to communicate by using gestures or noncommittal words, such as a nod of the head or a phrase like, "Go on," or "I see," or "What happened after that?" You can also use facilitation to return the patient to a topic on which you would like him to elaborate. For example, a patient may have made passing reference to suicidal thoughts and then moved on to another subject. When he finishes, you might say, "You say you have had thoughts of suicide?" This tells the patient that you've been paying attention to what he has been saying and would like to learn more.
- CONFRONTATION refers to pointing out to the patient something of interest in his conversation or behavior and thereby directs the patient's attention to something of which he may not have been aware. Confrontations describe how the patient appears to the interviewer, based on observations, *not* judgments. For example, the interviewer might remark, "You seem worried" or "You look very sad." Such comments often elicit a freer expression of feelings from the patient. Confrontations must, however, be carefully phrased, lest they sound nagging or condescending.

- Eventually, when the patient finishes giving his initial account of the problem, you will have to ask QUESTIONS. Keep the questions as NON-DIRECTIVE as possible. Avoid asking questions that can be answered with a yes or no ("Are you very angry?"). Avoid leading questions ("Do you think that your husband is a part of the problem?"). *How* and *what* questions are to be preferred ("What did you feel when that happened?").

It should be mentioned that some patients find it difficult to deal with the unstructured situation of nondirective questioning and may become very anxious during silences. That is particularly likely among adolescents, severely depressed patients, and patients who are confused or disorganized. When your open-ended questions are met with uncomprehending silence, try another approach and provide more structure to the interview.

Psychiatric Symptoms and Signs

When the function of a bodily organ is disturbed, the body mobilizes various defenses to correct the disturbance. The patient experiences those corrective measures as symptoms, and the doctor observes their effects as signs. Thus, for example, when streptococcal bacteria take up residence on a tonsil, the body responds by increasing blood flow to the tonsil and dispatching white blood cells there. A fierce battle ensues, and soon the battlefield is strewn with the corpses of dead streptococci and dead white blood cells. What the patient *feels*, however, is not a Homeric struggle between the forces of illness and health, but just a sore throat. And what the examining physician sees are red, swollen tonsils covered with pus. Physical symptoms and signs, then, although sometimes painful and distressing to the patient, reflect the body's attempts to maintain the best possible balance in the face of some physical stress.

Psychiatric symptoms and signs serve the same function for the mind: They show us the personality trying to maintain the optimal internal balance in the face of a stress.

Like the symptoms and signs of physical illness, psychiatric symptoms and signs can be grouped according to the "systems" they affect. In the case of psychiatric symptoms, however, we are talking about systems of psychologic rather than physiologic functioning. The psychologic functions involved are consciousness, motor activity, speech, thought, affect, memory, orientation, and perception.

Disorders of Consciousness

Consciousness refers to the degree to which a person is aware of and attentive to the world around him. We are already familiar with disorders of consciousness such as **delirium, stupor,** and **coma,** which usually indicate an organic basis for the patient's disorder. There are, however, other disorders of consciousness seen in psychiatric patients. **Inattention** means that it is difficult to gain the patient's attention; **distractibility** means that the patient's attention is easily diverted; **confusion** refers to an impaired understanding of one's surroundings.

Disorders of Motor Activity

Motor activity in a disturbed patient may be increased, decreased, or bizarre in some way. **Restlessness** refers to the situation in which the patient can't sit still; when restlessness occurs in association with extreme anxiety, we call it **agitation.** At the other end of the spectrum, one may find a very depressed or psychotic patient whose movements are exceptionally slow (**retarded**). In some cases, the patient appears to have little or no control over his motor activity. **Stereotyped activity** involves a repetition of movements that don't seem to serve any useful purpose, for instance a patient's repetitive touching of his elbow, nose, and forehead in succession. **Compulsions** are repetitive actions that are carried out to relieve the anxiety of obsessive thoughts, like Lady Macbeth washing her hands over and over again.

Disorders of Speech

Like motor activity, speech may be abnormally fast or abnormally slow. **Retardation of speech** is seen in severely depressed patients, while manic patients often show **accelerated speech** and **pressure of speech** (i.e., the words pour out like water escaping under pressure). The words the patient uses may themselves be strange or unusual. **Neologisms** are words that the patient invents. In **echolalia,** the patient echoes the words of the examiner. When the patient doesn't speak at all, we call it **mutism.**

Disorders of Thinking

Thinking is the highest of the mental functions, requiring integration of knowledge, perception, memory. Thinking may be disordered in its progression or in its content.

The *progression* of thought, like motor activity and speech, may be speeded up or slowed down. **Flight of ideas,** which occurs in some manic conditions, refers to accelerated thinking, in which the mind skips so rapidly from one idea to another that it is very difficult for the listener to grasp the connection between them. At the other end of the spectrum, in depression, **retardation of thought** is more characteristic, and the patient seems to take a very long time to get from one thought to the next. In **circumstantial thinking,** the patient includes many irrelevant details in his account of things. **Perseveration** refers to the repeating the same idea over and over again. (Go back and review Chap. 28; you will find an example of intentional perseveration there!)

The *content* of thought may also be abnormal in a patient with psychiatric problems. The patient may, for example, express **delusions,** that is, fixed beliefs that are not shared by others of his culture or background and that are not amenable to change by reasonable explanation. Among the more common types of delusions, for example, are *delusions of persecution,* in which a person believes that others are plotting against him. In *delusions of grandeur,* the person believes himself to be someone of great importance. Other delusions that suggest psychosis include *thought broadcasting* (the belief that others can hear one's thoughts) and *thought control* (the belief that outside forces are controlling one's thoughts).

Obsessions are thoughts that won't go away, despite attempts to forget them. Usually the person with an obsession knows that the idea is unreasonable, but he can't stop thinking about it. A person may, for example, have an obsessional belief that the gas stove hasn't been turned off, so he will return again and again to the kitchen to make sure. Each time he does so, his anxiety will be relieved for a short time, but then he'll have to go back and check yet again.

Phobias are obsessive, irrational fears of specific things or situations, such as fear of heights, fear of open places, fear of confined places, or fear of certain animals.

Disorders of Mood and Affect

Mood refers to a person's sustained and pervasive emotional state; **affect** is the outward expression of a person's mood. Thus a person's mood may be described as *depressed, euphoric,* or *anxious.* The affect is described as *appropriate* or *inappropriate.* A patient who puts on a waxy smile as he tells you of a parent's death would be considered to be showing inappropriate affect; that is, the emotion he seems to be expressing is out of synch with the situation. Affect is characterized as *labile* when it shifts rapidly, as in the patient who is laughing one moment and crying the next. It is termed *flat* when the patient doesn't seem to feel much of anything at all.

Disorders of Memory

The most profound disorder of memory is **amnesia,** the loss of memory. Memory is, in fact, a complex process consisting of four separate functions: *registration,* the ability to add new items to the cerebral data bank; *retention,* the ability to store those items in an accessible place in the mind; *recall,* the ability to retrieve a specific piece of stored information on demand; and *recognition,* the ability to identify information that one has encountered before. Amnesia may reflect the disruption of any one or several of those functions. In delirium, for example, a person may be unable to register events properly, so he will not later be able to recall what happened while he was delirious. When painful memories are *repressed,* on the other hand, it is not registration but recall that is impaired.

Sometimes patients with severe memory deficits from organic brain disease will invent experiences to "paper over" the gaps in memory. We call that **confabulation.**

Disorders of Orientation

Orientation refers to a person's sense of who he is (person), where he is (place), and at what point in time he finds himself (time). A person who is confused as to any of those particulars is said to be disoriented. Disorientation is most common in organic brain syndromes.

Disorders of Perception

Perception refers to the way a person processes the data supplied by the five senses. There are two disorders of perception: illusions and hallucinations. An **illusion** is a misinterpretation of sensory stimuli, for example, mistaking a piece of rope for a snake or a cat's meowing for a human voice. An **hallucination** is a perception that has no basis in reality and occurs without any external stimuli. Hallucinations may reflect any of the five senses—a person may hear, see, feel, taste, or smell something that isn't there. Auditory hallucinations, such as hearing voices, are the most common. Hallucinations involving other sense modalities—like the frightening visual hallucinations in delirium tremens—suggest an *organic* cause.

The types of psychiatric symptoms and signs are summarized in Table 38-2. The table, and the foregoing discussion, seem to involve a lot of new terminology. In fact, most of the new terms are simply technical names for phenomena that are familiar from everyday experience. Anyone who has a child (or has been a child) who wants a new bicycle will know, for example, what perseveration is all about. The tech-

TABLE 38-2.   CLASSIFICATION OF PSYCHIATRIC SYMPTOMS AND SIGNS

DISORDERS OF CONSCIOUSNESS
- Distractibility and inattention
- Confusion
- Delirium
- Stupor and coma
- Fugue state

DISORDERS OF MOTOR ACTIVITY
- Restlessness
- Stereotyped movements
- Compulsions

DISORDERS OF SPEECH

DISORDERS OF THINKING
- Disordered thought *progression*
  Flight of ideas
  Retardation of thought
  Perseveration
  Circumstantial thinking
  Fragmented thinking
  Thought block
- Disordered thought *content*
  Delusions
  Obsessions
  Phobias

DISORDERS OF MOOD AND AFFECT
- Anxiety
- Panic
- Euphoria
- Depression
- Inappropriate affect
- Flat affect
- Ambivalence

DISORDERS OF MEMORY
- Amnesia
- Confabulation

DISORDERS OF ORIENTATION

DISORDERS OF PERCEPTION
- Illusions
- Hallucinations

DISORDERS OF INTELLIGENCE
- Mental retardation

nical terms simply help us to communicate our impressions of the patient more precisely and succinctly.

The Mental Status Examination

Knowing the different "systems" of mental function enables us to conduct what is called a mental status examination (MSE). The MSE is a way of measuring the "mental vital signs" in a disturbed patient. For just as the temperature, pulse, respirations, and blood pressure reflect the functions of the body's most critical organ systems, so the parameters we assess in the MSE reflect the vital functions of an intact mind.

To conduct the mental status examination, we need to check each of the "systems" of mental function in an orderly way. Since paramedics like mnemonics, the mnemonic for the elements of the mental status examination is COASTMAP (if you can think of a better one, the author will be happy to hear about it!):

C   CONSCIOUSNESS: Note the patient's ability to *pay attention* to a discussion and *concentrate.* Is he easily distracted?

O   ORIENTATION: Ask what is the year, season, month, date, and day of the week. Ask the patient to state where he is at the moment—the country, state, town, and specific location. A lot of us have to take a furtive look at the calendar to remember the date and even sometimes the day of the week, but a person who doesn't know that it's summer or thinks it's 1942 has a more serious problem, often organic.

A   ACTIVITY: Is the patient restless and agitated, pacing up and down? Or is he sitting very still, scarcely moving at all? Is he making any strange or repetitive movements?

S   SPEECH: Note the rate, volume, articulation, and intonation of speech. Is there pressure of speech? Is the speech garbled or slurred (dysarthria)? Is the patient using any strange words? Slurring of speech suggests an organic problem. Accelerated or retarded speech suggests an affective disorder.

T   THOUGHT: Listen to the patient's story. What's on his mind? Is he making sense? Is there anything unusual about his reasoning? Is he expressing apparently false ideas (delusions), such as a belief that the CIA is after him?

M   MEMORY: You can form an impression of the patient's memory by listening to his reconstruction of events. A more precise assessment requires asking a few questions. Ask the patient if you may test his memory. If he assents, slowly say the names of three unrelated objects (e.g., apple, bicycle, sewing machine). After you have named all three, ask the patient to repeat them; that will test *registration*. A few minutes later, ask the patient if he can remember the three words you named before; that tests *retention* and *recall*.

A   AFFECT and mood: The patient's mood may be most apparent in his body language. The patient sitting with shoulders drooping and head bent, for example, conveys depression. Note whether the affect—the expression of inner feelings—seems appropriate to the situation.

P   PERCEPTION: Detecting disorders of perception may be difficult, since patients are often hesitant to answer direct questions about hallucinations. Sometimes it is helpful to ask the patient, "Do you ever hear things that other people can't hear?"

Note that you can conduct nearly all of the mental status examination just by watching and listening (and knowing what to watch and listen *for*!). Only the assessment of memory, orientation, and perhaps perception requires you to ask some direct questions. So practice being an observer. As you sit in the all-night diner drinking your coffee, eavesdrop on the waitress talking to the customer next to you and go systematically through the COASTMAP sequence to evaluate *her* mental status. Or try it out on a date! Get into the habit, that is, of *noticing* how other people talk, move, and express their feelings, and practice describing those things to yourself.

The Rest of the Examination

The patient's overall condition and the nature of his or her psychiatric problem will determine how much of the usual secondary survey you are able to perform. (The primary survey is, of course, performed in *every* patient.) A disturbed patient may prefer not to be touched, and that wish must be respected unless there is a compelling medical reason for doing otherwise (e.g., profuse bleeding from slashed wrists). At the very least, however, you should be able to make an assessment of the patient's GENERAL APPEARANCE. In the psychiatric patient, assessing the general appearance means taking note of the patient's *dress, cleanliness,* and *grooming,* all of which provide clues to the way the patient perceives himself.

If the patient permits you to examine him or her further, what you will be looking for in particular are SIGNS OF AN ORGANIC CAUSE of the patient's behavior, as well as anything that may provide more clues to the patient's personality:

- Measure the VITAL SIGNS for *fever* or indications of *increased intracranial pressure*. (What abnormalities in the vital signs would you expect if the intracranial pressure is elevated?)
- Examine the SKIN temperature and moisture, and take the opportunity to note any prominent tattoos. Tattoos proclaiming "Born to Kill" or similar sentiments suggest it may be unwise to proceed any further with the physical examination.
- Inspect the HEAD for evidence of trauma.
- Check the PUPILS for size, equality, and reaction to light. Pupillary abnormalities may indicate a toxic ingestion or an intracranial process as the source of the patient's behavior.
- Note any unusual ODORS ON THE PATIENT'S BREATH.
- In examining the EXTREMITIES, check for needle tracks, tremors, and unilateral weakness or loss of sensation.

Now that we have learned a bit about how to assess patients who present with psychiatric symptoms, we can consider a few specific psychiatric emergencies. In a psychiatric emergency, the patient may present with disorders of thinking, mood, behavior, or any combination of the three.

PSYCHOSES

A psychotic, by definition, is out of touch with reality. He is tuned in to his own internal reality of ideas and feelings, which he mistakes for the reality of the world outside himself. That internal reality may make him belligerent and angry toward others. Or he may become mute and withdrawn as he gives all his attention to the voices and feelings within.

The Mental Status Examination in Psychosis

The most characteristic feature of psychosis is a profound thought disorder, often accompanied by disorders of mood and perception:

C   CONSCIOUSNESS: The psychotic is awake and alert, but he may be easily distractible, especially if he is paying attention to hallucinations. If the level of consciousness is fluctuating, suspect an organic brain syndrome.

O ORIENTATION: Disturbances in orientation are more common in organic disorders than in psychoses, but the severely psychotic patient may be disoriented as to time and place.

A ACTIVITY: Most commonly accelerated, with agitation and hyperactivity, although it can be retarded. Bizarre, stereotyped movements are also common.

S SPEECH: May be pressured or sound strange because of unusual words that the patient has invented (neologisms).

T THOUGHT: Disturbed in progression and content, and likely to show any or several of the following disorders:
- *Flight of ideas*, the headlong plunge from one thought to another.
- *Loosening of associations*, in which the logical connection between one idea and the next becomes obscure, at least to the listener. In extreme cases, the patient's speech may as a consequence be entirely incomprehensible to the listener.
- *Delusions*, especially of persecution (e.g., people are plotting against him, his telephone is tapped, people are following him).
- *Thought broadcasting*, the belief that his thoughts are broadcast aloud and can be heard by others.
- *Thought insertion*, the belief that thoughts are being thrust into his mind by another person, and *thought withdrawal*, the belief that his thoughts are being removed.

M MEMORY: Memory can be relatively or entirely intact in psychosis, but it may be difficult to obtain the cooperation of the patient for formal memory testing.

A AFFECT AND MOOD: Mood is likely to be disturbed in psychosis. The disturbance may take the form of euphoria, sadness, or wide swings in mood; affect may reflect those inner states or be flat.

P PERCEPTION: Auditory hallucinations are common in psychosis. The patient hears voices coming from outside himself commenting on his behavior or instructing him what to do. Suspect that the patient is hearing such voices when he seems to be attending a conversation other than yours or when he is talking to himself.

WARNING! THE PATIENT WHO HEARS VOICES COMMANDING HIM TO HURT HIMSELF OR OTHERS MUST BE CONSIDERED DANGEROUS.

Management of the Patient with Psychotic Symptoms

Dealing with a psychotic patient is difficult. The usual methods of reasoning with a patient are unlikely to be effective, since the psychotic has his own rules of logic quite different from those that govern everyday thinking. Furthermore, the paramedic is likely to feel acutely uncomfortable in the presence of a psychotic—anxious, helpless, often angry as well. Remember, those uncomfortable feelings are one of your built-in diagnostic instruments. They are elicited by the fear, suspicion, and hostility that the patient is broadcasting through his body language. *Use your uncomfortable feelings to help make a tentative diagnosis of a psychotic problem.* Once you have made that tentative diagnosis, proceed as follows:

- ASSESS THE SITUATION FOR DANGER to yourself or others. (We shall discuss this matter in more detail later, in the section on dealing with the violent patient.)
- IDENTIFY YOURSELF CLEARLY, and explain your mission. ("I'm Gloria Goodheart. I'm a paramedic with the ambulance service, and this is my partner, Stan Steadfast. We've come to see if we can help. Can you tell us about your problem?")
- BE CALM, DIRECT, AND STRAIGHTFORWARD. Your calm and confidence will do a great deal toward calming the patient.
- MAINTAIN AN EMOTIONAL DISTANCE. Do not touch the patient. Do not be overfriendly or effusively reassuring. The attitude you want to convey is one of emotional neutrality.
- DON'T ARGUE. Don't challenge the patient regarding the reality of his beliefs or the validity of his perceptions. Don't go along with the patient's delusions simply to humor him, but don't make an issue of them either. Talk about real things.
- EXPLAIN YOUR EXPECTATIONS OF THE PATIENT. ("We're not going to let you hurt anyone with that baseball bat. . . .")
- EXPLAIN EACH STEP OF MANAGEMENT. ("Now we're going downstairs to the ambulance.")

- Wherever possible, INVOLVE PEOPLE WHOM THE PATIENT TRUSTS, such as family or friends, in managing the patient and gaining his cooperation.

AFFECTIVE DISORDERS

Affective disorders, or disorders of mood, are among the most prevalent psychiatric disorders. It has been estimated that 10 to 15 percent of the population will experience an affective disorder, such as a major depression or a manic-depressive illness, at some point in their lives. Affective disorders differ from the normal bouts of sadness or happiness that all of us experience. In affective disorders, the changes in mood are attended by other symptoms, and the net effect is to cause a major disturbance in the patient's ability to function.

Depression and Suicidal Behavior

The depressed patient is often readily identified by his sad expression, bouts of crying, and listless or apathetic behavior. He expresses feelings of worthlessness, guilt, and pessimism. He may want to be left alone, asserting that no one understands or cares and that his problems are hopeless anyway.

The diagnostic features of depression are most easily remembered by the mnemonic GAS PIPES—a mnemonic that also underscores the greatest danger in depression, namely, that the patient will "take the gas pipe" (i.e., commit suicide):

G   GUILT and self-reproach are characteristic features of depression. One way to try to get at the patient's guilt feelings is to ask a question like, "Are you down on yourself?" or "Do you ever feel as if you're worthless?"

A   APPETITE is disturbed in depression. Usually appetite is *decreased*, but a minority of depressed patients may report increases in appetite.

S   SLEEP DISTURBANCE usually takes the form of insomnia. The typical depressed patient will report that he or she wakens at 3:00 or 4:00 in the morning and cannot get back to sleep again.

P   The depressed patient has difficulty in PAYING ATTENTION, that is, the ability to concentrate is impaired, sometimes severely. Ask the patient, "When you are reading a book or a newspaper, can you get all the way through what you're reading, or does your mind start to wander after a couple of minutes?"

I   The depressed patient loses INTEREST in things that were formerly important to him. He can no longer summon enthusiasm for his work or hobbies. You might ask him, for example, "Are you a Celtics fan?" (Substitute the name of your local team.) If the answer is yes, ask, "How are they doing this season?" The depressed patient will tell you, "Well, I haven't really been following them lately."

P   PSYCHOMOTOR abnormalities in the depressed patient can take the form of either retardation or agitation. Usually we think of depressed patients doing everything in slow motion. But a significant percentage show agitated behavior, such as pacing, wringing their hands, or picking at themselves.

E   Depressed people have no ENERGY. They are tired all the time and don't feel like doing anything.

S   Finally, and most worrisome, depressed people tend to have pervasive and recurrent thoughts of SUICIDE.

Assessing the Risk of Suicide

Suicide is defined as any willful act designed to bring an end to one's own life. Suicide is the tenth leading cause of death in the United States; it is the third leading cause of death among the 15- to 25-year-old age group and the fourth leading cause of death among those between the ages of 25 and 45 years. Suicide predominates among *men*, especially those who are *single, widowed, or divorced*. The risk of suicide is also high among *depressed patients*, 15 percent of whom will succeed at some point in taking their own lives. *Alcoholism* is another important risk factor. Notably, at least 60 percent of successful suicides have a *history of a previous attempt*, and 75 percent have given some *clear warning* of their intent to kill themselves. The risk factors for suicide are summarized in Table 38-3.

Suicide attempts typically occur when a person feels that close emotional attachments are endangered or when a person has lost someone or something important in his or her life. The suicidal patient, in addition, often has feelings characteristic of depression: feelings of worthlessness, lack of self-esteem, and a sense of being unable to manage his or her life.

The assessment of *every* depressed patient must include an evaluation of the suicide risk.

TABLE 38-3.   RISK FACTORS FOR SUICIDE

Depression, or sudden improvement in depression

Expresses suicidal thoughts and concrete plans for carrying them out

Male sex, age > 55

Single, widowed, or divorced

Social isolation

Alcohol or drug abuse

Previous suicide attempt

Recent loss of spouse or significant relationship

Financial setback or job loss

Chronic, debilitating illness

Family history of suicide

Schizophrenia

EVALUATE THE SUICIDE RISK IN EVERY DEPRESSED PATIENT.

Many paramedics are reluctant to ask a patient directly about suicidal thoughts, because they are fearful they might "put ideas into the patient's head." The paramedic should realize, however, that suicide is not such an original idea that a depressed patient will not have thought of it himself. Most depressed patients, in fact, are relieved when the topic of suicide is brought up and they are thereby given "permission" to talk about their suicidal ideas. Often it is easier, for both the paramedic and the patient, to broach the subject in a stepwise fashion. You might start, for example, by asking, "Have you ever thought that life was not worth living?" From there, you may proceed by degrees with questions like these: "Did you ever feel that you would be better off dead? Have you ever thought of harming yourself? Do you feel that way now? Do you have a plan of how you would go about it? Do you have the things you need to carry out the plan? Has anyone in your family ever committed suicide? Have you ever tried to kill yourself before?" Patients who have made previous attempts, who have fashioned detailed, concrete plans for suicide, or who have a history of suicide among close relatives are all at particular risk and must be evaluated at the hospital.

Many patients make last-minute efforts to communicate their suicidal intentions. When a patient phones to threaten suicide, someone should stay on the line with him until the rescue squad has reached the scene. On arrival, quickly survey the area for any implements that the patient might use to injure himself, and discreetly remove those implements. Talk with the patient, and encourage him to discuss his feelings. Ask the same questions outlined above regarding the patient's suicidal ideas and plans.

EVERY SUICIDAL ACT, GESTURE, OR THREAT MUST BE TAKEN SERIOUSLY.

Management of the Patient at Risk of Suicide

Whenever you find a patient to be severely depressed or when you have any other reason to suspect that a patient is at risk of suicide, observe the following guidelines:

- DO NOT LEAVE THE PATIENT ALONE. Once you have responded to the call, the patient's well-being is your responsibility until he is transferred to the care of another medical professional.
- Bring to the hospital whatever implements of potential self-destruction you may have found at the scene (pill bottles, weapons).
- Acknowledge the patient's feelings. Do not argue with his wish to die, but provide honest reassurance. ("It's not unusual for a person to feel as you do after losing someone close to them. Sometimes it helps to talk about it.")
- If the patient refuses transport, try to involve persons close to him in eliciting his cooperation. If he still resists, it may be necessary to obtain police assistance. (We shall return to the matter of involuntary transport in the last section of this chapter.)

When a patient has *attempted* suicide, his medical treatment has priority. The patient who has taken an overdose of sedative or depressant drugs must be managed for possible respiratory depression or circulatory collapse; the patient who has slashed his or her wrists must be treated to control bleeding and restore circulating volume. Nonetheless, if the patient is conscious, try to establish communication and enable the patient to talk about his situation.

There is a tendency among EMS personnel to resent patients who attempt suicide. Doctors, nurses, and paramedics working in busy services are often inclined to feel that the person who attempts suicide does so with the express intent of creating more work for already overburdened medical personnel. Such beliefs on the part of EMS personnel belong in the category of delusions, for they are false beliefs. Furthermore, such beliefs often lead to inappropriate behavior, such as hostile remarks to the patient. A person who attempts suicide—whatever you may think of his or her reason for doing so—is a person in enormous distress. One of the most important skills that any health worker can acquire is the ability to see beyond another person's irritating behavior to the distress that lies beneath it. When called to treat a patient who has attempted suicide, therefore, it is worthwhile to say to the patient, in order to remind yourself, "You must have been very unhappy to do a thing like this."

Manic Behavior

In psychiatric terminology, patients with mania are said to suffer from *bipolar disorder* or *manic-depressive illness*, but *mania* remains a more descriptive term. The manic syndrome is one of the most striking psychiatric conditions. It will usually be a bystander or family member who calls for an ambulance, for the patient himself is unlikely to feel that he has any problem at all. To the contrary, the manic patient is more apt to tell you that he is "on top of the world—never felt better in my life." The mental status examination, however, tells a different story.

The Mental Status Examination in the Manic Patient

If we proceed systematically through the mental status examination of the manic patient, we are likely to find the following:

C   CONSCIOUSNESS: Awake and alert, but easily distracted. The patient may complain of an inability to concentrate.

O   ORIENTATION to both time and place is commonly disturbed in manic patients.

A   ACTIVITY: Markedly *hyper*active. Almost all manic patients report a significantly *decreased need for sleep*, and they may go for days without sleeping.

S   SPEECH is *pressured* and rapid, and the patient is very talkative.

T   The most prominent disorders of THOUGHT are *flight of ideas* and *delusions of grandeur*. The patient may report that his thoughts are racing, and the listener will note that the patient's monologue skips rapidly from one topic to another.

The patient's ideas are often grandiose, such as unrealistic plans to embark on large business ventures or to run for high public office. Or the patient may believe himself to have special powers or to be famous and wealthy.

M   MEMORY is usually intact in manics, although it may be distorted by underlying delusions.

A   The hallmark of mania is the apparently elated AFFECT. The patient seems to be on a "high," unusually and infectiously cheerful. His good cheer, however, may be quite brittle, and he may quickly become irritable, sarcastic, and hostile with very little provocation.

P   PERCEPTION may also be disturbed, and a person having an acute manic episode may show psychotic symptoms such as hallucinations.

Prehospital Management of the Manic Patient

Patients experiencing acute manic episodes have a high probability of getting themselves into trouble of one sort or another—going on wild spending sprees, making foolish business investments, driving recklessly, committing sexual indiscretions, picking fights. Generally it is when the patient has gotten into some sort of trouble, or when his behavior has become intolerably disruptive, that an ambulance is summoned. As noted, it is highly unlikely that the patient will view himself or herself as ill. It is therefore equally unlikely that the patient will agree that he or she needs treatment. In dealing with the manic patient, follow these guidelines:

- BE CALM, FIRM, AND PATIENT. Do not argue or get into a power struggle with the patient.
- MINIMIZE EXTERNAL STIMULATION. Talk to the patient in a quiet place, away from other people. (Meanwhile, have your partner obtain the history separately from relatives or bystanders.) When it comes time to transport, do not use sirens.
- If the patient refuses transport, consult medical command. Obtain police assistance to transport the patient if your medical director indicates that hospital evaluation is necessary.

ANXIETY DISORDERS

Anxiety disorders are those mental disorders in which the dominant mood is fear and apprehension.

All of us experience anxiety from time to time, and a certain amount of anxiety is useful and even necessary in helping us adapt constructively to stress. But patients with anxiety disorders experience persistent, incapacitating anxiety in the absence of external threat. There are several types of anxiety disorder, of which two are most likely to elicit a call for an ambulance or affect the delivery of prehospital care: panic disorder and phobia.

Panic Disorder

Panic disorder is characterized by sudden, usually unexpected, and overwhelming feelings of fear and dread, accompanied by a variety of other symptoms that come about from massive discharge of the autonomic nervous system. It is estimated that between 3 and 10 percent of the population have suffered from panic attacks. Women are at least twice as commonly affected as men, and the disorder tends to run in families. The attacks usually begin when the patient is in her twenties. Most patients can identify a stressful event that preceded their first attack, such as an illness or loss of a loved one. Thereafter, however, the attacks may come on "out of the blue," without any apparent precipitating stress. If allowed to continue, panic attacks may cause severe restrictions in the patient's life-style. The victim of panic attacks rapidly becomes afraid to go to work, to go shopping, or to leave the house at all, out of fear that an attack will occur away from home. We call that fear of going into public places **agoraphobia,** which literally means "fear of the marketplace."

The classic signs and symptoms of panic disorder are summarized in Table 38-4. Note that a large percentage of those signs and symptoms—like palpitations and sweating—are a consequence of autonomic nervous system discharge, while others (chest discomfort, paresthesias) may reflect hyperventilation. The symptoms usually peak in intensity within about 10 minutes and last about an hour altogether.

Anxiety is catchy. So usually by the time the paramedics arrive at the scene, the patient having a panic attack is surrounded by a horde of anxious and excited people, who themselves contribute to the problem. You will therefore need to take control of the situation quickly:

- IDENTIFY YOURSELF in a calm, confident manner.
- SEPARATE THE PATIENT FROM PANICKY BYSTANDERS, but if you can find a calm friend or member of the patient's family, it is often helpful to have such a person present.

TABLE 38-4. SIGNS AND SYMPTOMS OF A PANIC ATTACK

Shortness of breath or a sensation of being smothered

Dizziness or feeling faint

Palpitations or tachycardia

Trembling

Sweating

Choking

Nausea or abdominal distress

Paresthesias

Flushes or chills

Chest pain or discomfort

Fear of dying

Fear of going crazy

Feelings of unreality or of stepping apart from oneself

Source: Adapted from American Psychiatric Association, *Diagnostic and Statistical Manual of Mental Disorders, Third Edition, Revised.* Washington, D.C.: APA, 1987.

- BE TOLERANT OF THE PATIENT'S DISABILITY. The patient having an anxiety attack may not be able to cooperate or answer questions initially, because of intense fear and distress. Your manner must convey that everything is under control.
- GIVE THE PATIENT'S SYMPTOMS A NAME. Once you have checked the vital signs and the electrocardiogram (ECG) monitor, you should be in a position to reassure the patient that he or she is not having a heart attack or in immediate danger of dying. You might say something like this: "I know that the symptoms you are having are very distressing, but they are not symptoms of a life-threatening condition. Most patients with symptoms like yours have a condition called panic disorder, for which there are very effective treatments."
- Encourage the patient to do things for herself to the extent that she is able, in order to help her regain a sense of being in control.

Because of the many symptoms produced by anxiety, panic attacks may mimic a whole range of physical disorders. Conversely, symptoms of anxiety may be the presenting complaint in many medical conditions, such as cardiac dysrhythmias, withdrawal states, anaphylaxis, hyperthyroidism, and certain tumors. For that reason, any patient experiencing a panic attack, especially a first panic attack, should be fully evaluated in the hospital. For that reason as well, we no longer recommend that patients found hyperventilating be treated with "paper bag therapy." The patient whose anxiety is the result of an unsuspected pulmonary embolism or cardiac problem may suffer serious complications and even die from the hypoxemia induced by rebreathing into a paper bag. Hyperventilation is best managed by coaching the patient to slow his or her breathing.

Phobias

Phobic disorders involve an unreasonable fear of a specific situation or thing. We have already mentioned *agoraphobia,* the fear of places from which it might be difficult to escape. The patient with a *simple phobia* focuses all his anxieties onto one class of objects (e.g., mice, spiders, dogs) or situation (e.g., high places, flying). When confronted with the feared object or situation, the phobic person experiences intolerable anxiety and all the autonomic symptoms that anxiety brings. The patient usually recognizes that the fear is unreasonable but is unable to do anything about it.

It is unlikely that anyone will call for an ambulance because of a phobia. However, a patient's phobia may complicate your efforts to provide appropriate management of other problems. An elderly patient suffering an acute myocardial infarction, for example, needs to be transported to the hospital. But if that patient is terrified of leaving the house, simply carting him or her out the door without first dealing with the phobia may have fatal consequences.

In managing a phobic patient, then, REHEARSE EACH STEP OF TREATMENT IN DETAIL before you carry it out. "First we'll give you this oxygen to help you breathe. Then we're going to move you onto the stretcher, so that we can carry you downstairs. Then, once we have all our equipment together, we'll take you downstairs and out to the ambulance. You don't have to worry, because we'll be with you every step of the way. . . ." The description should then be repeated as the actions occur. "Now we're going to take you down the stairs. . . ."

DISORGANIZATION AND DISORIENTATION

Disorganization and disorientation are *not* diagnoses; they are ways in which various conditions, such as schizophrenia or organic brain syndromes, may present themselves. We are considering them separately, however, because those presentations account for a large number of ambulance calls. The paramedic does not need to make a specific diagnosis in such cases;

the paramedic *does* need to know how patients presenting with disorganization or disorientation should be managed in the field.

The DISORGANIZED PATIENT is characterized by uncontrolled and disconnected thought. He is usually incoherent or rambling in his speech, although he may be oriented to person and place. Often such patients are found wandering aimlessly down the center of the street, dressed peculiarly, uttering meaningless words and sentences. It will rarely be possible to conduct a thorough examination of such a patient, and the principal objective is to get the patient to the hospital in an atraumatic fashion.

The disorganized patient needs structure. The paramedic should explain in a simple way what is being done and specify exactly what the patient's role will be. Directions should be simple, consistent, and firm. It will be useless to try to take a detailed history; a name and address (if there *is* an address) may be all that can be obtained. Explain to the patient that he needs to be seen by a doctor and that you are going to take him to a hospital where he can be helped.

The DISORIENTED PATIENT does not know where he is or what day it is, and he may not even know his own name. Disorientation is most common among the elderly, who may lapse back into memories and behave as if they were still living in an earlier period of their lives. Disorientation is also characteristic of a variety of organic brain syndromes, including head injury, drug ingestion, and metabolic disorders.

In managing the disoriented patient, the key is to KEEP ORIENTING THE PATIENT to time, place, and the people around him. Tell the patient who you are, and explain what you are doing. You may have to identify yourself several times en route. Reassure the patient, and point out landmarks that will help him orient himself while en route to the hospital.

HOSTILE AND VIOLENT PATIENTS

Few situations are as difficult for the paramedic as dealing with a HOSTILE, ANGRY PATIENT. It takes a lot of maturity and a lot of experience to understand that anger can be a response to illness, and aggressive behavior may be the patient's way of dealing with feelings of helplessness. Sometimes the patient seems to be implying, "There's something very wrong with me, and you are not doing everything possible to help." The temptation is to respond with anger, but doing so rarely serves any useful purpose.

Most angry patients can be calmed by a trained person who conveys an impression of confidence that the patient will behave well. Sometimes it is useful to ask the patient directly about his anger, with a question such as, "Can you explain why you're so angry at me?" Giving the patient a chance to talk about his feelings often enables him to get mastery of those feelings.

The PATIENT WHO IS VIOLENT OR THREATENING VIOLENCE poses one of the most difficult management problems for EMS personnel. To begin with, most EMTs and paramedics see themselves as caregivers, not as "heavies," and often they find themselves unprepared—psychologically and tactically—to deal with hostile and even violent behavior. Furthermore, the encounter with a violent patient carries the constant risk that someone may get hurt—the patient himself, a bystander, the paramedics, or all of the aforementioned. The best way to try to ensure that no one does get hurt is to take preventive action—that is, to assess the potential for violence in *every* call and take steps to prevent violence from happening.

Assessing the potential for violence is not, unfortunately, merely an academic exercise. A 1993 survey of EMS agencies in 25 American cities reported high rates of violence against on-duty EMS personnel. In Chicago, for example, 92 percent of the fire department paramedics surveyed reported that they had been assaulted at least once while on duty (68% sustained blunt trauma, 33% were cut or stabbed, and 64% were shot at). The paramedic who does *not* look out for a possible violent encounter, therefore, may become a statistic like those just cited.

Identifying Situations with a Potential for Violence

Preventive action starts with being psychologically prepared for a possible violent encounter and keeping that possibility somewhere in the back of your mind in your response to *every* call. Do not rely too heavily on the information you get from your dispatcher—the "old woman with a possible stroke" may have a disgruntled son with an M-16 rifle! Being psychologically prepared for violence does *not* mean becoming paranoid or treating every patient with distrust. It *does* mean developing a "nose for danger," or what has been called "survival awareness."

How do you identify potentially dangerous calls? Which scenarios, and which kinds of patients, are most likely to be associated with violence?

RISK FACTORS FOR VIOLENCE

SCENARIOS
- Any place where alcohol is being consumed (e.g., tavern, party)
- Crowd incidents
- Incidents where violence has already occurred (e.g., shooting, stabbing, "domestic")

DIAGNOSTIC GROUPS
- Intoxicated with alcohol
- Intoxicated with drugs (especially PCP, LSD, amphetamines, cocaine)
- Withdrawal from alcohol or drugs
- Psychosis (especially manic and paranoid types)
- Delirium from any cause (e.g., hypoglycemia, sepsis)

The risk factors listed provide a general guideline to situations in which you need to be alert for possible violence. In any given specific case, however, the most important clues to the patient's potential for violence are found in his behavior and body language. Look for the following **warning signals:**

- POSTURE: The patient who sits tensely at the edge of his chair or grips at the armrest.
- SPEECH: Loud, critical, threatening, a lot of profanity.
- MOTOR ACTIVITY: Unable to sit still; paces back and forth or in circles; startles easily.
- OTHER BODY LANGUAGE: Clenched fists, avoidance of eye contact, turning away when spoken to.
- YOUR OWN FEELINGS: One of the most sensitive detectors of impending violence is your own "gut" response to the patient. If your instinct tells you that you are in danger, pay attention!

Those signals should alert you to the possibility of imminent violence and should therefore trigger an almost automatic set of "survival awareness" actions on your part.

Management of Violent Patients

Once you have, for any reason, concluded that there is a potential for violence in a situation, take the following steps:

- ASSESS THE WHOLE SITUATION. Are there factors in the surroundings that are contributing to the escalation of violence (e.g., friends who are egging the patient on)? Can those factors be removed? Is there evidence to suggest drug use, alcohol use, head injury, or diabetes? Is there anyone present who can give you some background information? (Did the patient's behavior come on gradually or suddenly? Does he have a history of violent behavior? Does he have any known medical problems, such as diabetes?)
- OBSERVE YOUR SURROUNDINGS. Make sure you have access to an *escape route.* Place yourself between the patient and the door, but do not move *behind* an agitated patient. And do not turn your back on the patient, even for a moment. Make note of furniture and other potential barriers. Scan the area quickly for anything that could be used as a weapon (e.g., heavy or sharp objects) if the level of violence escalates. If a violent patient is armed with a dangerous weapon, don't try to deal with the situation yourself; back off and notify law enforcement authorities. Try to ensure that others at the scene are not endangered while you await the arrival of the police. If the patient is not armed, you may attempt to deal with him.
- MAINTAIN A SAFE DISTANCE. Moving too close to a potentially violent patient is likely to increase his anxiety level. In general, maintain a safety zone of two arm lengths; but if the patient is backing away from you, that's a sign that you're too close. Let him find a comfortable distance. Do not position yourself directly face-to-face with the patient but rather slightly to the side.
- TRY VERBAL RESTRAINTS FIRST. Remember, often anger and aggressive behavior are a response to illness or to feelings of helplessness, and just talking to the angry person in a calm, sympathetic way may defuse some of his anger.
  1. Take a moment to CONCENTRATE YOUR OWN THOUGHTS, for you will need to convey an impression of calm and self-control to the patient. You can't fake it, because the agitated patient will see right through your act.
  2. IDENTIFY YOURSELVES as medical personnel who are there to try to help him. Keep your voice low—that forces the patient to stop what he is doing in order to focus on what you are saying to him.
  3. Acknowledge the patient's behavior, and restate your willingness to help (e.g., "You look very upset. How can we help you?").

4. ENCOURAGE THE PATIENT TO TALK about what is bothering him. *Listen* to what he says, and *show* him that you are listening by paraphrasing his words back to him ("I think I understand. Are you saying that . . . ?").
5. ASK THE PATIENT specifically if he feels he might lose control or if he is carrying any sort of weapon.
6. DEFINE YOUR EXPECTATIONS of the patient's behavior. Acknowledge his potential to do harm ("You could really hurt someone with that crowbar. . . ."), but assure him that he will not be permitted to lose control.
7. If "verbal de-escalation" isn't working, BACK OFF AND GET HELP. You can simply say to the patient, "Look, I've been trying to talk with you for the past 15 minutes and we're just going in circles. So I'm going to leave you alone for a few minutes and see if you can get hold of yourself. When I come back, we'll try again to talk, but if talking still doesn't work, I'm going to have some people with me to help prevent you from hurting anyone."
- WHEN VERBAL RESTRAINT FAILS, USE PHYSICAL RESTRAINT.
  1. Make sure you have SUFFICIENT PERSONNEL before you attempt to overpower the patient. You will need police assistance, since in most jurisdictions it is not legal for a paramedic (or anyone else) to restrain or transport a person against his will except at the express order of the police. You must, furthermore, have overwhelming force, which means a *minimum* of five trained, able-bodied people—one for each limb (a specific limb assigned in advance to each responder, so there won't be any confusion at the time action is initiated) and one for the head. Appoint one leader, who will direct the team and maintain verbal contact with the patient.
  2. Sometimes the SHOW OF FORCE may in itself be sufficient to calm the patient. The mere sight of five 250-pound police officers, for example, has been known to have a remarkably tranquilizing effect on even the most belligerent patient. Don't move in on the patient right away; give him a chance to make a graceful retreat to a nonviolent alternative behavior.
  3. If the show of force does not by itself calm the patient down—which may occur, for example, in a patient under the influence of drugs such as PCP—you will have to move quickly to restrain the patient. First, remove any equipment or jewelry from your own person that could be used as a weapon against you (e.g.,

name badge, scissors worn on the belt, key chain, earrings). Make sure you have adequate restraining devices—preferably padded leather or nylon restraints—immediately available. Then, at a signal from the leader, move in *fast* from the patient's sides. Grasp him at the elbows, knees, and head, and apply restraints to all four extremities. Probably the best position in which to secure him to the stretcher is supine, with his legs spread-eagled and both his arms secured to one side of the stretcher. That position will turn his head to the side, so that he won't aspirate if he should vomit.

4. Throughout the whole restraint procedure and transport, MAINTAIN VERBAL CONTACT with the patient, even if he does not appear to be paying attention to what you are saying. Once he is restrainted, DO NOT REMOVE THE RESTRAINTS. Don't negotiate. Don't make deals.

5. Once restraints have been applied, CHECK THE PERIPHERAL CIRCULATION every 5 minutes to make sure the restraints are not too tight. Check the radial pulses in the arms and the dorsalis pedis pulses in the feet.

6. DOCUMENT EVERYTHING in the patient's chart—the reasons for using restraints (be specific—give examples of the patient's behavior and the indications of his violent potential); the number of people used to subdue him; the restraining devices used; the status of the peripheral circulation after restraints were applied.

Dealing with the Aftereffects of Violence

As noted earlier, most paramedics do not enjoy dealing with violent patients. The type of person who chooses a career in EMS is usually oriented toward rescue and care, not toward martial arts and the use of force. So the call that involves a violent patient is likely to leave the ambulance team feeling tired, angry, guilty, and just plain upset. It should, therefore, be the policy of every ambulance service to provide for a debriefing after every call that involved violence—a time when those who took part in the incident can get together and talk it over and share their feelings about what happened. Paramedics who are not given such opportunities to debrief after tough calls are paramedics who will "burn out" very quickly.

LEGAL ASPECTS OF MANAGING DISTURBED PATIENTS

Patients who are seriously disturbed—whether or not the paramedic is able to put a precise label on the disturbance—should be seen by a physician and evaluated for possible hospitalization. In most regions, there are four different ways in which patients can be admitted for psychiatric observation and treatment. First, there is *voluntary admission,* in which the patient of his own accord signs himself into the hospital and is free to leave whenever he chooses. The second kind of admission is *voluntary commitment,* in which the patient again of his own free will agrees to be admitted to the hospital; but in this case he is not necessarily free to leave whenever he wants. Voluntary commitments usually expire in a period of 10 to 30 days, unless the patient agrees to extend his commitment.

For seriously disturbed patients who do not agree to enter the hospital of their own accord, there are usually mechanisms of *involuntary* detainment. One such procedure is *emergency detention,* in which a family member or the police bring the patient to the hospital, where he is examined by a psychiatrist. If the psychiatrist feels that the patient is a danger to himself or others, he may authorize hospitalization for a limited period, usually about 10 days. In some regions, the psychiatrist must obtain permission from the county mental health authorities to invoke an emergency detention and must show cause for the patient's admission. Finally, most regions also have a procedure known as *court commitment,* in which one or more psychiatrists must provide evidence in court that a patient is mentally ill and needs treatment. Some courts further require that the patient be considered dangerous to himself or others before they will commit the patient against his will.

There are serious questions involved in such decisions, for involuntary commitment represents a deprivation of civil liberties and must never, therefore, be undertaken lightly. It is not always easy, even for the experienced psychiatrist, to define what kind of behavior justifies removing a person from society, what constitutes "dangerous behavior," and so forth. Furthermore, laws pertaining to involuntary commitment vary from one region to another, and it is important to be familiar with the legal requirements in your community. As a general rule, a conscious adult must consent to be taken to the hospital. If the patient does not consent, he may be taken against his will only on the express request of the police. The same applies to the use of forcible restraint. Where such measures are deemed necessary, therefore, law enforcement officers should be summoned. In addition, every ambulance service should have clearly defined protocols, drawn up with legal advice, for dealing with patients who require involuntary commitment. Paramedics should follow those protocols to the letter and consult medical command whenever any doubt exists.

GLOSSARY

affect   The outward expression of a person's mood.

agitation   Extreme restlessness and anxiety.

agoraphobia   Literally, "fear of the marketplace"; fear of entering a place from which escape may be impeded.

compulsion   A repetitive action carried out to relieve the anxiety of obsessive thoughts.

confabulation   The invention of experiences to cover over gaps in memory, seen in patients with certain organic brain syndromes.

confrontation   Interviewing technique in which the interviewer points out to the patient something of interest in his conversation or behavior.

delirium   An acute confusional state characterized by global impairment of thinking, perception, judgment, and memory.

delusion   Fixed belief that is not shared by others of a person's culture or background and that cannot be changed by reasonable argument; a false belief.

dementia   Chronic deterioration of mental function.

echolalia   Meaningless echoing of the interviewer's words by the patient.

facilitation   Interviewing technique in which the interviewer encourages the patient to proceed by noncommital words and gestures.

flight of ideas   Accelerated thinking in which the mind skips very rapidly from one thought to the next.

hallucination   A sense perception not founded on objective reality.

illusion   A misinterpretation of sensory stimuli.

mania   Mental disorder characterized by hyperactivity, insomnia, and grandiose ideas.

mood   A person's sustained and pervasive emotional state.

mutism   The absence of speech.

neologism   An invented word that has meaning only to its inventor.

obsession   Persistent idea that a person cannot dismiss from his thoughts.

perseveration   Repeating the same idea over and over again.

phobia   An abnormal and persistent dread of a specific object or situation.

pressure of speech   Speech in which words seem to tumble out under immense emotional pressure.

psychosis   Mental disorder characterized by loss of contact with reality.

stereotyped activity   Repetitive movements that don't appear to serve any purpose.

APPENDIX: DRUGS COMMONLY PRESCRIBED TO PATIENTS WITH PSYCHIATRIC PROBLEMS

Patients with psychiatric problems may receive any of several types of so-called *psychotropic drugs*, that is, drugs that affect mood, thought, or behavior. The psychotropic drugs are among the most widely prescribed medications in the United States. They can be broadly divided into four classes, according to the problems they are designed to treat: (1) antipsychotic drugs, (2) tranquilizers, (3) antidepressant drugs, and (4) drugs to control mania.

ANTIPSYCHOTIC DRUGS

Antipsychotic drugs, also called *neuroleptics*, are given to control psychotic symptoms, from whatever cause. It is important for paramedics to be aware of one particular syndrome that may occur in patients (usually male) taking antipsychotic agents, and that is the **acute dystonic reaction.** Typically, the patient develops muscle spasms of the neck, face, and back within a few days of starting treatment with the drug. An acute dystonic reaction can be rapidly corrected by giving *diphenhydramine* (Benadryl), 25–50 mg IV, but the muscle spasms are apt to recur after the diphenhydramine wears off. Neuroleptics also have **atropine-like effects** (anticholinergic effects), so patients taking antipsychotic medications may suffer all the same side effects that atropine produces, such as dry mouth, blurred vision, urinary retention, and cardiac dysrhythmias.

ANTIPSYCHOTICS (NEUROLEPTICS)	
Generic Name	*Trade Name*
Acetophenazine	**Tindal**
Chlorpromazine	**Thorazine**

Chlorprothixene	**Taractan**
Droperidol	**Inapsine**
Fluphenazine	**Prolixin, Permitil**
Haloperidol	**Haldol**
Loxapine	**Loxitane, Daxolin**
Mesoridazine	**Serentil**
Molindone	**Moban**
Perphenazine	**Trilafon**
Pimozide	**Orap**
Thiothixene	**Navane**
Thioridazine	**Mellaril**
Trifluoperazine	**Stelazine**
Triflupromazine	**Vesprin**

Antihistamines	Diphenhydramine	**Benadryl**
	Hydroxyzine	**Atarax, Vistaril**
	Promethazine	**Phenergan**
Miscellaneous	Chloral hydrate	**Noctec***
	Ethchlorvynol	**Placidyl**

*Prescribed chiefly as a *hypnotic* (sleep medicine).

Tranquilizers (Anxiolytics)

Drugs that exert a tranquilizing or sedative effect, and thus calm anxiety, are the most commonly prescribed (and overprescribed) psychotropic agents. In 1982, for example, nearly 28 million prescriptions for diazepam (Valium) were filled in the United States. There are basically three types of drugs used for their tranquilizing effects: (1) benzodiazepines, (2) barbiturates and barbiturate-like drugs, and (3) antihistamines.

Antidepressant Drugs

Antidepressants, as the name implies, are prescribed to combat the symptoms of depressive illness. There are three categories of antidepressants: (1) *Tricyclic and related drugs*, like the neuroleptics, produce atropine-like side effects and may also cause orthostatic hypotension. (2) *Monoamine oxidase (MAO) inhibitors*, usually prescribed when tricyclics have not been effective, are notable for one particular potential side effect—**hypertensive crisis,** which may occur in patients taking MAO inhibitors if they receive certain other drugs (e.g., sympathomimetics, narcotics) or even if they eat certain foods (cheese, yogurt, sour cream, beer, wine, chopped liver). (3) *Other agents* include the very widely prescribed fluoxetine (Prozac).

TRANQUILIZERS (ANXIOLYTICS)

Class	Generic Name	Trade Name(s)
Benzodiazepine	Alprazolam	**Xanax**
	Chlordiazepoxide	**Librium**
	Clonazepam	**Klonopin**
	Clorazepate	**Tranxene**
	Diazepam	**Valium**
	Flurazepam	**Dalmane***
	Halazepam	**Paxipam**
	Lorazepam	**Ativan**
	Oxazepam	**Serax**
	Prazepam	**Centrax**
	Temazepam	**Restoril***
	Triazolam	**Halcion***
Barbiturates and related drugs	Amobarbital	**Amytal**
	Butabarbital	**Butisol**
	Pentobarbital	**Nembutal***
	Phenobarbital	**Luminal**
	Secobarbital	**Seconal**
	Glutethimide	**Doriden**
	Methyprylon	**Noludar**
	Meprobamate	**Equanil, Miltown**

ANTIDEPRESSANTS

Class	Generic Name	Trade Name(s)
Tricyclics and related drugs	Amitriptyline	**Amitril, Endep, Elavil**
	Amoxapine	**Asendin**
	Desipramine	**Norpramin, Pertofrane**
	Doxepin	**Adapin, Sinequan**
	Imipramine	**Imavate, Janimine, Pramine, Presamine, Tofranil**
	Maprotiline	**Ludiomil**
	Nortriptyline	**Aventyl, Pamelor**
	Protriptyline	**Vivactil**
	Trimipramine	**Surmontil**
MAO inhibitors	Isocarboxazid	**Marplan**
	Phenelzine	**Nardil**
	Tranylcypromine	**Parnate**

Others	Bupropion	**Wellbutrin**
	Fluoxetine	**Prozac**
	Trazodone	**Desyrel**

Drugs to Control Mania

Drug therapy of bipolar (manic-depressive) disorder is generally undertaken with lithium carbonate. Some patients taking lithium preparations develop symptoms of toxicity, including nausea and vomiting, dysarthria, tremors, and lethargy. Lithium toxicity may lead to brain damage if not treated, so patients showing signs of toxicity require medical attention.

DRUGS TO CONTROL MANIA

Generic Name	*Trade Name(s)*
Lithium carbonate	**Eskalith, Lithane, Lithobid, Lithonate, Lithotabs**
Lithium citrate	**Cibalith**
Carbamazepine	**Tegretol**

FURTHER READING

PSYCHIATRIC EMERGENCIES: GENERAL

Bassuk EL, Fox SS, Prendergast KJ. *Behavioral Emergencies: A Field Guide for EMTs and Paramedics.* Boston: Little, Brown, 1983.

Boggio N, Cohall AT. Evaluating the adolescent: The search for the hidden agenda. *Emerg Med* 22(2):18, 1990.

Cusack JR, Malaney KR. The diagnostic psychiatric interview. *Emerg Med* 21(14):27, 1989.

Dernocoeur K. How to beat hysteria. *Rescue* 3(1):32, 1990.

Dubin WR. Sudden unexpected death: Intervention with the survivors. *Ann Emerg Med* 15:54, 1986.

Edwards FJ. Psychiatric emergencies, Part 1. *Emerg Med Serv* 14(3):46, 1985.

Edwards FJ. Psychiatric emergencies, Part 2. *Emerg Med Serv* 14(4):45, 1985.

Enelow AJ, Swisher S. *Interviewing and Patient Care.* New York: Oxford, 1972.

Hyman SE, Tesar GE (eds). *Manual of Psychiatric Emergencies* (3rd ed). Boston: Little, Brown, 1994.

Judd RL. A matter of behavior. *Emergency* 22(6):33, 1990.

Koenig RR. Handling grief in the emergency department. *Emerg Med Serv* 4(4):18, 1975.

Levine RJ. Mass hysteria: Diagnosis and treatment in the emergency room. *Arch Intern Med* 144:1945, 1984.

Lipscomb WR. Acute paranoia: A medical emergency. *Emerg Med* 20(8):123, 1988.

Lund JW. Social work in EMS. *Emerg Med Serv* 9(2):41, 1980.

Milgram BA. Psychiatric emergencies. *Emerg Med* 5(2):174, 1973.

O'Rear J. Post-traumatic stress disorder: When the rescuer becomes the victim. *JEMS* 17(1):30, 1992.

Peterson L. The psychological impact of trauma: Recognition and treatment. *Am J Emerg Med* 1:102, 1983.

Pisarcik GK. Psychiatric emergencies and crisis intervention. *Nurs Clin North Am* 16:85, 1981.

Rabin PL, Hussain G. Crisis intervention in an emergency setting. *Ann Emerg Med* 12:300, 1983.

Rabin PL et al. Acute grief. *South Med J* 74:1468, 1981.

Rund DA. Alcohol use and psychiatric illness in emergency patients. *JAMA* 245:1240, 1981.

Scarano S. The mentally disordered patient: A legal model for field management. *JEMS* 6(3):37, 1981.

Selden BS. Adolescent epidemic hysteria presenting as a mass casualty, toxic exposure incident. *Ann Emerg Med* 18:892, 1989.

Shore D. White House cases: Psychiatric patients and the Secret Service. *Am J Psychiatry* 142:308, 1985.

Soreff S, Olsen P. Emotional emergency. *Emerg Med* 7(10):224, 1975.

Tkach T. Psychiatric emergencies. *Emerg Med Serv* 22(1):21, 1993.

Twerski AJ. Over the edge. *Emerg Med* 8(11):27, 1976.

Wood KA et al. The need for hospitalization as perceived by emergency room patients and clinicians. *Hosp Community Psychiatry* 35:830, 1984.

DEPRESSION AND SUICIDE

Brent DA, Perper JA, Allman CJ. Alcohol, firearms, and suicide among youth. *JAMA* 257:3369, 1987.

Brooksbank DJ. Suicide and parasuicide in childhood and early adolescence. *Br J Psychiatry* 146:459, 1985.

Cassem E. When symptoms seem groundless. *Emerg Med* 24(8):191, 1992.

Centers for Disease Control. Premature mortality due to suicide and homicide—United States, 1984. *MMWR* 36:(32,33), 1987.

Centers for Disease Control. Youth suicide—United States, 1970–1980. *MMWR* 36:(6,10,17), 1987.

Crumley FE. Adolescent suicide attempts. *JAMA* 241:2404, 1979.

Crumley FE. Substance abuse and adolescent suicidal behavior. *JAMA* 263:3051, 1990.

Deykin EY et al. Non-fatal suicidal and life-threatening behavior in 13- to 17-year-old adolescents seeking emergency medical care. *Am J Public Health* 75:90, 1985.

Ekker T. When hope is lost: Dealing with the suicidal patient. *JEMS* 16(11):65, 1991.

Garfinkel BD, Froese A, Hood J. Suicide attempts in children and adolescents. *Am J Psychiatry* 139:1257, 1982.

Goldacre M et al. Repetition of self-poisoning and subsequent death in adolescents who take overdoses. *Br J Psychiatry* 146:395, 1985.

Jenike MA. Depressed in the ER. *Emerg Med* 16(6):102, 1984.

Leisner K. Trauma: Accident or attempted suicide? *Emerg Med Serv* 18(5):30, 1989.

Minoletti A et al. Suicidal behavior in the emergency room: 2. Treatment and disposition. *Can Fam Physician* 31:1668, 1985.

Motto JA et al. Development of a clinical instrument to estimate suicide risk. *Am J Psychiatry* 142:680, 1985.

Murphy GE. Suicide and attempted suicide. *Hosp Pract* 12(11):73, 1977.

Pallis DJ et al. Estimating suicide risk among attempted suicides: I. The development of new clinical scales. *Br J Psychiatry* 141:37, 1982.

Patterson WM et al. Evaluation of suicidal patients: The SAD PERSONS scale. *Psychosomatics* 24:343, 1983.

Perez E et al. Suicidal behavior in the emergency room: 1. Assessment of risk. *Can Fam Physician* 31:1663, 1985.

Rotheram MJ. Evaluation of imminent danger for suicide among youth. *J Orthopsychiatry* 57:102, 1987.

Roy A. Risk factors for suicide in psychiatric patients. *Arch Gen Psychiatry* 39:1089, 1982.

Rund DA. Assessment of suicide risk. *Emerg Med Serv* 18(5):27, 1989.

Ruple JA. Honing skills for suicide intervention. *JEMS* 15(1):149, 1990.

Schmidt TA. Evaluating and transporting patients at risk for suicide. *Emerg Med Serv* 17(8):48, 1988.

Simmons K. Adolescent suicide: Second leading cause of death. *JAMA* 257:3329, 1987.

Soreff S, Cadigan R. Depression and suicide: A semester in hell. *Emerg Med Serv* 22(4):66, 1993.

Solomon J. The suicide scenario: Rewriting the final act. *Emerg Med* 21(4):75, 1989.

Solomon J. Decoding signals from the suicidal patient. *Emerg Med* 24(2):201, 1992.

ANXIETY AND PANIC STATES

Cameron OG. The differential diagnosis of anxiety: Psychiatric and medical disorders. *Psychiatr Clin North Am* 8:3, 1981.

Raj A et al. Medical evaluation of panic attacks. *J Clin Psychiatry* 48:309, 1987.

Recognizing panic disorder. *Emerg Med* 22(12):97, 1990.

Schweizer E. Calming panic disorder in primary care. *Emerg Med* 25(2):106, 1992.

Weissman MM et al. Suicidal ideation and suicide attempts in panic disorder and attacks. *N Engl J Med* 321:1209, 1989.

Yingling KW et al. Estimated prevalences of panic disorder and depression among consecutive patients seen in an emergency department with acute chest pain. *J Gen Intern Med* 8:231, 1993.

VIOLENCE AND VIOLENCE CONTAINMENT

Atkinson WK, Bassett AW. Dodging bullets: Gang violence and EMS. *JEMS* 18(7):55, 1993.

Dernocoeur K. Tips on defusing a violent situation. *JEMS* 18(7):78, 1993.

Dick T. Rules of restraint. *JEMS* 5(7):22, 1980.

Dick T. Gloves without fingers: Using stockinette as a restraint. *JEMS* 14(12):25, 1989.

Dubin WR. Evaluating and managing the violent patient. *Ann Emerg Med* 10:481, 1981.

Dubin WR et al. Rapid tranquilization of the violent patient. *Am J Emerg Med* 7:313, 1989.

Goldstein SN. Family feud. *Emerg Med Serv* 20(10):12, 1991.

Gorski T. Managing the violent patient. *Emerg Med Serv* 10(5):6, 1981.

Infantino JA. Controlling violent patients. *Emerg Med Serv* 13(5):23, 1984.

Leisner K. Managing the pre-violent patient. *Emerg Med Serv* 18(7):18, 1989.

Makadon HJ, Gerson S, Ryback R. Managing the care of the difficult patient in the emergency unit. *JAMA* 252:2585, 1984.

Nordberg N. Hate in the streets. *Emerg Med Serv* 18(8):24, 1989.

Rhoads J. Restraint restrictions. *Emerg Med Serv* 22(1):16, 1993.

Rund DA. Emergency management of the difficult patient. *Emerg Med Serv* 13(3):17, 1984.

Salzman C et al. Parenteral lorazepam versus parenteral haloperidol for the control of psychotic disruptive behavior. *J Clin Psychiatry* 52:177, 1991.

Schiavone FM, Salber PR. Hitting close to home: Domestic violence and the EMS responder. *JEMS* 19(2):112, 1994.

Shanaberger CJ. What price patient restraint? *JEMS* 18(6):69, 1993.

Smith M. Are you gaining by restraining? *JEMS* 17(9):36, 1992.

Taylor C. Domestic violence: The medical response. *Emerg Med Serv* 13(5):35, 1984.

Thomas H et al. Droperidol versus haloperidol for chemical restraint of agitated and combative patients. *Ann Emerg Med* 21:407, 1992.

Tintinalli JE. Violent patients and the prehospital provider. *Ann Emerg Med* 22:1276, 1993.

IX

RESPONDING TO THE CALL

39
Communications and Dispatching

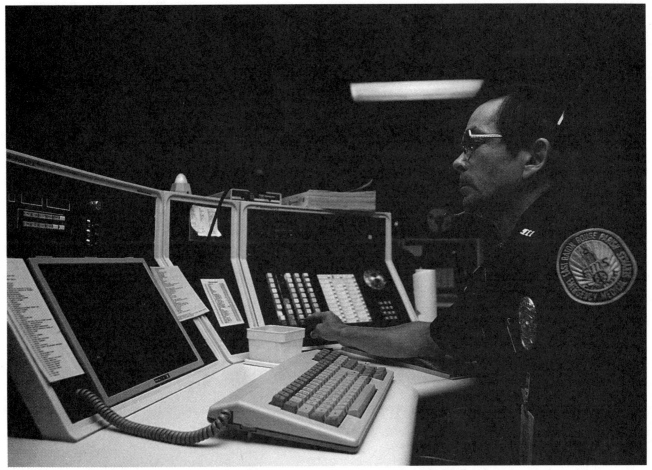

East Baton Rouge Parrish Emergency Medical Services, East Baton Rouge, Louisiana. Photo by Michael S. Kowal.

OBJECTIVES

Communication has to do with getting information from one person to another. In EMS, that information may be extremely urgent (e.g., "My husband just collapsed and isn't breathing."); so it needs to move rapidly and efficiently. Indeed, the very rapid transfer of information in various directions is one of the things that distinguishes *emergency* medical services from routine medical services. If a patient had to send a letter in order to request an ambulance, there wouldn't be much point to the system.

In this chapter, we shall examine what constitutes an EMS communications system: who needs to be able to talk with whom, what technical resources are available to make those conversations possible, and what we can do to make communications as efficient as possible. We shall also consider the crucial role that the dispatcher plays in facilitating all phases of EMS communications. By the end of this chapter, the student should be able to

1. List the links that are needed to form an effective EMS communications system (i.e., specify who needs to be able to talk to whom)
2. Identify the type of communications equipment (e.g., telephone, radio, pager) most suitable for
   - Dispatching
   - Ambulance-to-hospital communication
   - Ambulance-to-other-agency communication
3. List the most appropriate uses, in prehospital emergency care, for
   - Cellular telephones
   - VHF radio frequencies
   - UHF radio frequencies
   - Biotelemetry
4. List the components of an EMS communications system and describe the function of each
5. Identify correct and incorrect procedures for radio communications, given a description of several procedures
6. List three reasons for using radio codes
7. Spell out several words in the international phonetic alphabet
8. Report a patient's case history in the correct format
9. List four tasks the dispatcher performs
10. Specify the information that should be gathered by the dispatcher from a caller requesting an ambulance

WHO NEEDS TO COMMUNICATE WITH WHOM?

For the EMS system to work, a number of people have to be able to contact a number of other people.

Let's follow an emergency call from its inception to its conclusion in order to see who needs to reach whom:

- The first stage of the EMS response is NOTIFICATION; that is, someone has to notify the EMS agency that an emergency exists. Usually notification is carried out by **landline** (telephone), whereby THE PERSON REQUESTING HELP COMMUNICATES WITH THE DISPATCHER. Telephone notification is greatly facilitated by the existence of a universal emergency telephone number—911 in the United States—and the availability of public telephones, on highways and elsewhere, that do not require a coin to obtain a dial tone. Notification may, less frequently, come by radio, when the emergency is detected by a patrolling law enforcement vehicle.
- The next step is DISPATCH, wherein the DISPATCHER COMMUNICATES WITH THE UNIT THAT IS TO RESPOND, directing that unit to the scene of the emergency. Dispatch may be accomplished by telephone, radio pager, or two-way radio (usually the last).
- As the ambulance starts to roll, the dispatcher may have to speak with the ambulance team en route, to provide additional information about the call. For their part, the ambulance personnel may need to request other resources, such as police or fire officials. Those COMMUNICATIONS BETWEEN THE DISPATCHER AND RESCUE PERSONNEL are usually carried out by mobile and portable radios; recently cellular telephones have also been used for that purpose.
- Once the rescuers are at the scene, COMMUNICATIONS BETWEEN RESCUE PERSONNEL AND A PHYSICIAN (the latter usually hospital-based, but not invariably so) are necessary to enable orders for invasive procedures to be transmitted and to facilitate the care of the patient at the scene and in transit. Communications with the medical command physician are also necessary to transmit telemetered data like the patient's electrocardiogram when the protocol calls for doing so. Communications with the physician in charge, whether by voice or telemetry, require two-way radios, a telephone patch (telephone-to-radio connection), or cellular telephones.
- Finally, once the patient is packaged and ready to be moved, there must be a means of COMMUNICATION BETWEEN RESCUE PERSONNEL AND THE RECEIVING HOSPITAL, so that the hospital can be notified of what type of case to expect. Once again, most ambulance-to-hospital communications today are by radio, but cellular telephones also play an increasingly important role.

Those are the communications links essential to ensure an efficient response to the average emergency call. However, a full-scale EMS commmunications system ideally requires a few other components as well:

- It is highly desirable to have a means of linking all area hospitals into the communications network, so that, in the event of a disaster, multiple casualties may be appropriately distributed and hospitals may be informed of the number of victims they will be receiving. INTERHOSPITAL COMMUNICATIONS can be accomplished through landline networks or by radio, preferably both.
- There should also be a means by which various OTHER AGENCIES that may be involved in an emergency response (police, fire, public utilities, civil defense, poison control) CAN COMMUNICATE WITH ONE ANOTHER. Here again, cellular technology has made such communications much more accessible, but a backup radio network is still desirable in the event that telephone lines and frequencies become overloaded during a mass casualty.
- Finally, it is important—especially in mass disasters—to be aware of OTHER BROADCAST SYSTEMS that may be recruited to assist in communications within the community:
  1. The Amateur Radio Public Service Corps (ARPSC) may be available in your community. If so, it should be involved in planning for disaster communications. The Radio Amateur Civil Emergency Services (RACES) is another group that can be of assistance.
  2. Even in areas where there isn't any formally organized amateur radio service, it is useful for the EMS dispatcher to monitor channel 9 on the Citizen's Band (CB) frequency, the channel reserved for emergency communications (or other channels, such as channel 15 for marine emergencies, where applicable).
  3. BUSINESS RADIO SERVICE SYSTEMS, such as taxi dispatching and trucking services, can be used in a disaster to extend communications capabilities.
  4. Finally, managers of COMMERCIAL BROADCAST SERVICES (radio and television) should be assigned specific communications responsibilities in the event of a disaster.

COMPONENTS OF AN EMS COMMUNICATIONS SYSTEM

Most EMS communications systems today are still based primarily on the use of radios, so we need to learn a little bit about what radio signals are and what equipment is available for propagating and receiving radio signals.

Radio Communications and Telemetry

Radio refers to the transmission of signals by electromagnetic waves. Recall that energy can be emitted in the form of waves or particles. When energy is emitted in the form of waves, the nature of that energy can be characterized by the length of the waves it produces. Energy of relatively long wavelength produces audible sound; energy of shorter wavelength is in the infrared light spectrum. In between sound and infrared light are the wavelengths for radio transmission.

It is customary to refer to radio wavelengths by their reciprocals, called **frequencies.** The word refers to how frequently the wave recurs in a given period of time (a second). Clearly, the shorter the wavelength, the more times the wave will be repeated in a second, so the higher the frequency. Radio frequencies are designated by their *cycles per second*, or **hertz** (named for the man who first described the propagation of electromagnetic waves). The following abbreviations are commonly used:

DESIGNATIONS OF RADIO FREQUENCIES

hertz (Hz)	cycles per second
kilohertz (kHz)	1,000 cycles per second
megahertz (MHz)	1,000,000 cycles per second
gigahertz (GHz)	1,000,000,000 cycles per second

Radio waves are confined to that part of the electromagnetic frequency spectrum extending from 3 kHz to about 3,000 GHz. A normal voice channel requires a minimum of 3 kHz. **Frequency bands** are portions of the radio frequency spectrum assigned for specific uses. The most commonly used bands for medical communications are the **very high frequency (VHF) band** and the **ultrahigh frequency (UHF) band.**

The VHF BAND extends from roughly 30 to 175 MHz and has been arbitrarily divided into what is referred to as low band (30–50 MHz) and high band (150–175 MHz). The *low band* frequencies may have ranges up to 2,000 miles but are unpredictable, since changes in ionospheric conditions may cause "skip interference," with patchy losses in communication. The *high band* frequencies are almost wholly free of skip interference but the price you pay for less interference is a much shorter transmission range. The most commonly used of the VHF high band frequencies for emergency medical purposes are in the 150 to 160 MHz range.

The UHF BAND extends from 300 to 3,000 MHz, with most medical communications occurring around 450 to 470 MHz. At those frequencies, communications are entirely free of skip interference and have minimal noise (signal distortion). The UHF band has better penetration in dense metropolitan areas, and UHF reception is usually quite adequate inside buildings. The UHF band, however, has a shorter range than the VHF band, and energy at UHF is more readily absorbed by rain and environmental objects, such as trees and brush.

The Federal Communications Commission (FCC), which controls frequency allocation in the United States, has set aside medical VHF band assignments for general emergency radio communications and UHF band assignments for ambulance-to-hospital telemetry systems, especially where communications from physicians to rescue personnel are needed to furnish instructions for patient care. Those band assignments tend to be rather liberally interpreted in most EMS systems.

Radio equipment used for both VHF and UHF bands is **frequency modulated (FM),** which more easily eliminates noise and interference than amplitude-modulated (AM) stations.

Biotelemetry

Biotelemetry (usually called simply *telemetry*) is the technique of measuring vital life signs and transmitting them to a distant terminal, as, for example, when the pulse and respiratory rate of an astronaut are measured in space and transmitted to a receiving station on earth. When the term *telemetry* is used in emergency medical care, it usually refers to the transmission of an electrocardiogram (ECG) signal from the patient to a distant receiving station. The standard ECG is composed of low-frequency signals (100 Hz or less), which would be filtered out by a voice communications system. Thus, the ECG signal must be *encoded* if it is to be sent over the same radio channels used to transmit voice. The ECG signal is encoded by using a reference audio tone, for example at 1,000 Hz, which is made to vary with the voltage generated by the electric events in the heart. The varying 1,000-Hz tone is used to frequency modulate the transmitter. When the signal is received at the distant terminal, it is amplified and *decoded* to produce a voltage that is an exact replica of the original. That voltage is then converted to the graphic plot seen on the oscilloscope or printout.

ECG telemetry over UHF frequencies is confined to one lead of a 12-lead ECG, so it can be used only to interpret cardiac rhythms; it is not of value in trying to determine whether a patient has suffered acute injury to the heart, as in myocardial infarction. To make that determination, one must examine all 12 leads of the ECG.

Distortion of the ECG signal by extraneous spikes and waves is known as **noise** and may arise from a variety of sources:

SOURCES OF NOISE IN ECG TELEMETRY

- Loose ECG electrodes
- Muscle tremor
- Sources of 60-cycle alternating current (AC), such as transformers, power lines, and electric equipment
- Attentuation of transmitter power, caused by either weak batteries or transmission beyond the range of the transmitter.

ECG telemetry had a very important role in establishing the paramedic profession, for it made it possible for doctors based in the hospital to supervise paramedics caring for patients in the field. It was the technical feasibility of such supervision that convinced the medical community and the public to accept the idea of paramedics carrying out procedures such as defibrillation or the administration of cardiac drugs, and many states made it mandatory for all advanced life support units to have telemetry capabilities.

In the past several years, as paramedics have become more and more skilled in dysrhythmia recognition, the trend has been to make less and less use of ECG telemetry; most systems, rather, rely solely on the paramedic's assessment of the patient's cardiac rhythm and do not require confirmation of the assessment by a physician. Just as ECG telemetry seemed headed for the fate of the horse-drawn ambulance, however, two developments occurred to bring about a reassessment of prehospital ECG telemetry. First, research on the use of thrombolytic agents indicated that the earlier those agents were given in the course of an acute myocardial infarction, the better the chances of myocardial reperfusion. Second, cellular telephone technology made it possible to transmit a 12-lead ECG from a moving ambulance to a hospital and therefore to diagnose myocardial infarction before the patient reaches the hospital. At the least, such early diagnosis enables the hospital to gear up for administration of thrombolytic therapy immediately as the patient arrives; and in some EMS systems trials are now under way to assess the efficacy of starting thrombolytic therapy in the *pre*hospital phase (see Chap. 23). It is likely, therefore, that ECG telemetry in one form or another will remain a part of prehospital emergency care for some time to come.

Modes of Radio Operation

Assigned radio frequencies may be employed in any of a variety of systems. In a **simplex** system, portable units can transmit only in one mode (voice or telemetry) *or* receive (voice) at any given time. A simplex system requires only a single radio frequency. When a network uses two different frequencies at the same time, to permit simultaneous transmission and reception (like a telephone), it is referred to as **duplex**. Another alternative is to combine, or **multiplex**, two or more signals—such as the paramedic's voice and the patient's ECG—for simultaneous transmission on one frequency.

Suppose, for example, that an ambulance service wanted the possibility of voice communications as well as continuous telemetry. There are at least four ways they could design their communications system to meet those requirements:

- The ambulance could transmit on two frequencies of a UHF-frequency pair (**channel**) allocated for telemetry (DUPLEX). On one frequency, they would transmit the voice signal and on the other the telemetry signal. Such a system requires that the ambulance have two UHF transmitters (one for voice, one for telemetry) and one receiver (voice).
- The ambulance could MULTIPLEX (combine) both telemetry and voice on one frequency of the allocated UHF pair and receive voice communications on the other frequency of the pair. That requires only one UHF transmitter on the vehicle, but the base station must be fitted with demultiplexing equipment to separate out the two signals coming in on one frequency.
- The ambulance could transmit telemetry data on one frequency of the allocated telemetry pair and transmit voice data on a VHF frequency. That requires both a UHF and a VHF transmitter on the vehicle (hence TWO SIMPLEX SYSTEMS).
- As noted, there is now an increasing trend toward using CELLULAR TELEPHONES for ECG

telemetry. Cellular phones have full duplex capability, a multitude of available channels, a very high quality signal that is unlikely to degrade over distance, and a much lower capital and maintenance cost.

Building Blocks of a Communications System

While EMS communications systems vary considerably among one another, most systems serving moderate to large populations are constructed of the following components.

Base Stations

The base station is a collection of radio equipment consisting, at minimum, of a transmitter, receiver, and antenna. The base station serves as a dispatch and coordination area and ideally should be in contact with all other elements of the system. Base stations generally use relatively high power output (45–275 watts); the maximum allowable power is determined by the FCC and printed on the station's license.

The base station must be equipped with an antenna sited in suitable terrain, preferably on a hill or high building, close to the base. The antenna system plays a vital part in transmission and reception efficiency. A good antenna system can compensate for FCC limits on power output and man-made signal distortion in the area.

Mobile Transmitter/Receivers (Transceivers)

A mobile transmitter/receiver, or mobile transceiver, is a two-way radio mounted in a vehicle. Mobile transmitter/receivers come in a variety of power ranges, and the power output largely determines the distance over which the signal can be effectively transmitted. A transmitter in the 7.5-watt range, for example, will transmit for distances of 10 to 12 miles over slightly hilly terrain. Transmission distances are greater over water or flat terrain and reduced in mountainous areas or where there are many tall buildings. Mobile transmitters with higher outputs have proportionally greater transmission ranges. Today, the typical mobile transmitter operates at between 20 and 50 watts.

Portable Transmitter/Receivers

Portable, hand-held radios are useful when paramedics must work at a distance from their vehicle but need to stay in communication with the base or with one another. Portable units may also be used by physician consultants when not stationed at the hospital. Portable units usually have power outputs of up to 5 watts and thus have limited range by themselves, although the signal of a hand-held transmitter can be boosted by retransmission through the vehicle (see below).

Repeaters

A repeater is essentially a miniature base station used to extend the transmitting and receiving range of a telemetry or voice communications system. Repeaters may be stationary in one location (**fixed repeaters**) or carried in the emergency vehicles (**mobile repeaters**). What a repeater does is to pick up a weak signal and retransmit it at a higher power on another frequency, so it extends the range of low-power portables and allows more members of the system to hear one another.

Remote Consoles

A remote console, usually located in the emergency room of a hospital, is a terminal that receives transmissions of telemetry and voice from the field and transmits messages back, usually through the base station. Remote consoles are connected to the base station by dedicated telephone lines, microwave, or radio. They contain an amplifier and speaker for incoming voice reception, a decoder for translating the telemetry signal into an oscilloscope trace or printout, and a microphone for voice transmission.

Backup Communications Systems

In addition to radio communications, most systems employ landline (telephone) backup to link various fixed components of the system, such as hospitals, public safety services, and poison control. Telephones may also be "patched" into radio transmissions through the base station, enabling, for example, communication between paramedics using radios in the field and a physician using his or her telephone at home. Finally, as mentioned earlier, cellular telephones are becoming an increasingly important part of EMS communications, overcoming many of the problems of overcrowded EMS radio frequencies. Cellular phones are cheaper than radios and generally give a much clearer signal. Furthermore, they enable a paramedic in the field to communicate with anyone who has a telephone—the patient's family physician, an injured child's parent, an expert in another state who can advise on a particular hazmat situation. The possibilities are as varied as the listings in the telephone directory.

A sample communications system is shown in Figure 39-1.

COMMUNICATING BY RADIO

The effectiveness of an EMS communications network depends less on the technical hardware than on the people who use it. Communicating effectively by radio under emergency conditions requires skill and experience. Some paramedics "freeze" at the microphone, while others find themselves acting out their latent ambitions as disc jockeys. Neither behavior is appropriate or useful. Effective radio communications in EMS require a knowledge of the rules that govern those communications and an understanding of conventions for transmitting medical information by radio. All of that need not be very complicated if you bear in mind:

> **THE PURPOSE OF TALKING ON THE RADIO IS TO TRANSMIT PERTINENT INFORMATION.**

FCC Regulations

The Federal Communications Commission (FCC) is the agency of the United States government assigned to regulate all radio and television communications in the United States. Its functions are (1) licensing and frequency allocation, (2) establishing technical standards for radio equipment, and (3) establishing and enforcing rules and regulations for the operation of radio equipment. To carry out the last-mentioned task, the FCC monitors transmissions on various frequencies and conducts spot checks of base stations to ensure that they are properly licensed.

The FCC requires that communications over frequencies allocated for emergency medical use be confined to that use. According to the FCC, "Except for test transmissions, stations licensed to ambulance operators or rescue squads may be used only for the transmission of messages pertaining to the safety of life or property and urgent messages necessary for the rendition of an efficient ambulance or emergency rescue service." While that regulation may be somewhat liberally interpreted, the use of obscenity or the transmission of messages unrelated to provision of medical services is forbidden. When it is necessary to communicate a personal message to a paramedic in the field, it is best simply to notify her or him by radio to contact the base by phone. Similarly, the paramedic who wants the dispatcher to order a pizza with double cheese and mushrooms should use a tele-

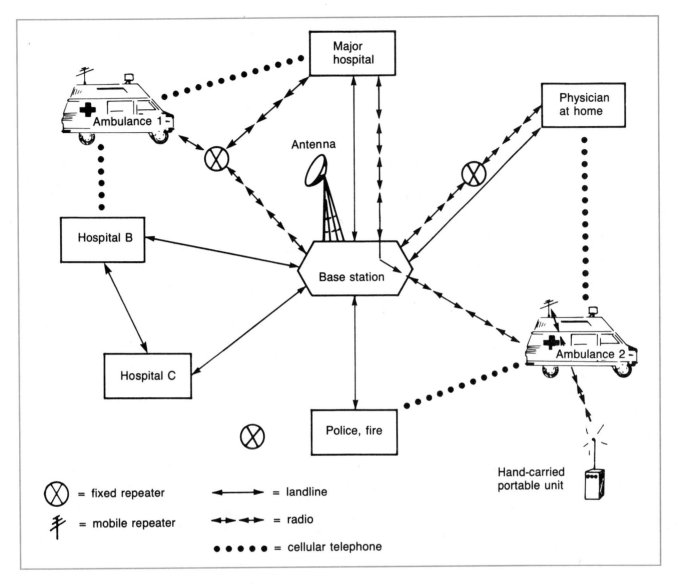

FIGURE 39-1. **SAMPLE COMMUNICATIONS SYSTEM.**

phone, not a two-way radio to communicate that message; it may be urgent, but it is *not* medical.

All EMS radio communications are regulated by the Special Emergency Radio Service provisions of the FCC Rules and Regulations, Part 90, and a copy of the Part 90 regulations should be available for reference at every base station.

Clarity of Transmission

The purpose of communications equipment is to permit communication. That sounds obvious, and yet it is often forgotten. Simply blurting something into a microphone is not communicating. For communication to occur, someone at the other end of the radio has to be able to hear and understand what you say.

Therefore the first principle of communicating by radio is CLARITY.

There are a number of guidelines that can help the radio user improve the clarity of a transmission:

- Before you begin to transmit, LISTEN TO MAKE SURE THAT THE CHANNEL IS CLEAR. If another radio transmission is in progress, *wait* until the parties have finished transmitting before you try to get on the air. Cutting in on someone else's transmission will only ensure that *neither* of you will be adequately heard.
- Once the channel is quiet, PRESS THE TRANSMIT KEY FOR AT LEAST 1 SECOND BEFORE SPEAKING, to ensure that the beginning of your message is not lost.

- Start your transmission with the identifying information: GIVE THE NUMBER OR NAME OF THE UNIT *BEING CALLED* FIRST, then your own identification (e.g., "Montefiore Hospital from Medic 3"). In that way, the unit being called is alerted immediately and will already be listening when you give your own identification, so they can reply at once, "Go ahead, Medic 3." If you do it the other way around ("Medic 3 calling Montefiore Hospital"), chances are that the recipients will prick up their ears only when you've mentioned *their* identification and therefore will already have missed *your* identification. So what inevitably happens then is, "This is Montefiore Hospital. What unit is calling?" That extra transmission is an unnecessary waste of everyone's time.
- KEEP YOUR MOUTH CLOSE TO THE MICROPHONE, BUT NOT TOO CLOSE—about 2 to 3 inches is usually ideal.
- SPEAK CLEARLY AND DISTINCTLY, pronouncing each word carefully.
- DON'T SHOUT! Shouting just distorts the signal. Speak in a normal pitch, for very high pitched or low-pitched sounds do not transmit well either.
- DON'T TALK WITH YOUR MOUTH FULL. It muffles transmission, and besides, you might choke.
- KEEP YOUR VOICE FREE OF EMOTION. You don't have to imitate a talking computer; a normal conversational tone is fine. Just keep your voice free of panic, anger, excitement, and other feelings that can distort both your transmission and your judgment.
- KEEP YOUR TRANSMISSIONS BRIEF. Air time is precious, and emergency medical frequencies are not the place for long philosophic dialogues.
- If you have a long message to transmit, BREAK UP THE MESSAGE INTO 30-SECOND SEGMENTS, checking at the end of each segment to determine whether it was received and understood.
- DON'T WASTE AIR TIME WITH SUPERFLUOUS PHRASES, such as "be advised." Also bear in mind that courtesy is taken for granted; there is no need to use air time for social graces such as "please," "thank you," and "how nice to hear your voice."
- When speaking a word or name that might be misunderstood, SPELL IT OUT, using the international phonetic alphabet (Table 39-1) or a similar system. Suppose, for example, you are asking the hospital to notify the patient's family doctor whose name might be mistaken for that of another doctor on the staff; you might say, "Notify Dr. Wilby. That's Dr. WHISKEY-INDIA-LIMA-BRAVO-YANKEE, Wilby."
- When presenting numbers that might be misunderstood, TRANSMIT THE NUMBER AS A WHOLE, THEN DIGIT BY DIGIT. For instance, if the respirations are 15, you would say, "The respirations are fifteen, that is, one-five."

Content of Transmissions

Radio transmissions for emergency medical services should be brief, to the point, and professional in tone. Here are some guidelines about what should and should not be included in EMS radio communications:

- The first thing to remember when you get "on the air" is that your words are, quite literally, in the air, floating around for anyone to hear. Remember:

TABLE 39-1.   INTERNATIONAL PHONETIC ALPHABET

A	ALPHA	J	JULIETTE	S	SIERRA
B	BRAVO	K	KILO	T	TANGO
C	CHARLIE	L	LIMA	U	UNIFORM
D	DELTA	M	MIKE	V	VICTOR
E	ECHO	N	NOVEMBER	W	WHISKEY
F	FOXTROT	O	OSCAR	X	X-RAY
G	GOLF	P	PAPA	Y	YANKEE
H	HOTEL	Q	QUEBEC	Z	ZEBRA (or ZULU)
I	INDIA	R	ROMEO		

> **ANYONE MAY BE LISTENING!**

The medical staff at the local emergency room, a patient signing in at the front desk of another emergency room, a 12-year-old ambulance buff playing with his scanner at home—any of them may be listening with rapt attention to your transmission. For that reason, it is essential to PROTECT THE PRIVACY OF THE PATIENT. Do not use the patient's name on the air, and do not transmit personal information about the patient. Certain types of cases, such as rape or psychiatric problems, are best identified on the air by an established code (see next section).

Don't assume, by the way, that your cellular telephone offers you protected conversations. There are now scanners on the market that can tune into the local cellular frequencies too. So don't say anything on the radio *or* the cellular phone that you don't want everyone in town to hear.

- BE IMPERSONAL. Use "we," not "I," to refer to yourself, and use proper names and titles ("Sergeant York," not "Billy") to refer to others where necessary.
- DON'T TRY TO BE A COMEDIAN. There is no place for wisecracks, sarcasm, or other non-professional conduct on emergency medical radio frequencies.
- DON'T USE PROFANE LANGUAGE ON THE AIR (or off the air, for that matter). The penalty specified by the FCC for doing so—quite aside from the reflection on your professional character—is a fine of $10,000 or 2 years in prison or both.
- USE PROFESSIONAL LANGUAGE, BUT DON'T SHOW OFF. Once again, remember that the object of the exercise is to communicate information, not to stun your listener into awe and admiration.
- AVOID USING WORDS THAT ARE DIFFICULT TO HEAR. The word "yes," for instance, is easily lost in transmission; use "affirmative" instead. Similarly, use "negative" instead of "no."
- USE STANDARD FORMATS FOR TRANSMISSION. The patient's history, for example, should always be presented in the same order (which we shall review shortly). When the listeners know what they are listening *for,* they are less likely to miss parts of the transmission.
- When you finish transmitting, OBTAIN CON-

FIRMATION THAT THE TRANSMISSION WAS RECEIVED.
- When you receive instructions by radio from the dispatcher or from medical command, ECHO THE ORDER BACK to make certain you have understood it correctly. Thus, for example, if the physician instructs you to administer 75 mg of lidocaine slowly IV, you would respond, "That is lidocaine 75 milligrams, repeat, seven-five milligrams, slowly IV. Is that confirmed?"
- QUERY ANY ORDERS YOU DID NOT HEAR CLEARLY.
- USE EMS FREQUENCIES ONLY FOR EMERGENCY MEDICAL COMMUNICATIONS. Order your pizza by telephone.

Codes

Some ambulance services make extensive use of radio codes; others rely exclusively on plain English. Usually some combination of the two is preferable. Codes are used for several reasons:

- To maintain security of communication
- To keep "air time" as brief as possible
- To diminish the likelihood of misunderstanding or noise
- To prevent the patient, his family, and bystanders from understanding what is being said

The last-mentioned reason is particularly important when the information you need to convey to the dispatcher or physician may be alarming to the patient. Suppose, for example, that you wish to indicate to the physician that your patient is probably having an acute myocardial infarction and is in very serious condition. It is preferable that the patient *not* be privy to that assessment, for it will only further his anxiety and thereby possibly worsen his condition.

For a code to be of any use, everyone using the radio must know the meaning of the code words. It doesn't do much good to radio the hospital that you have a "case 3, condition 2" if no one at the other end of the radio has the foggiest notion of what you are talking about. When codes are used, therefore, they should be simple as well as standardized within a given region, and a copy of the code should be posted at every radio terminal.

The so-called **ten-codes** are one commonly used system of codes (Table 39-2). Ten-codes vary somewhat among different public safety agencies, but all ten-codes utilize the number 10 plus another number to indicate a given message. Numbers are used because they are brief and easily understood.

TABLE 39-2.   COMMONLY USED TEN-CODES

CODE	MEANING
10-1	Signal weak.
10-2	Signal good.
10-3	Stop transmitting.
10-4	O.K.
10-6	Busy; please stand by unless urgent.
10-7	Out of service; unavailable for a call.
10-8	In service; available for a call.
10-9	Please repeat.
10-12	Stand by.
10-17	En route.
10-18	Urgent.
10-20	What is your location?
10-22	Disregard.
10-23	Arrived at the scene.
10-24	Completed the assignment.
10-33	Help me quick! Emergency!

The 10-33 code deserves particular mention. When a unit gets on the air with a 10-33 or any other indication of an emergency ("May Day" or just "Help!"), all other radio users should get off the air. Emergency communications always have priority.

WHEN YOU HEAR SOMEONE ON THE RADIO CALLING FOR HELP, GET OFF THE AIR!

When you use ten-codes, remember that one of their main purposes is to shorten air time. You defeat that purpose if you stick a ten-code into a long sentence. There is no need, for example, to say, "What is your 10-20?" It is enough simply to say, "10-20." Similarly, it's a waste of time to say "10-6 for a minute." Just say, "10-6."

Ten-codes from 10-40 onward may be designated for special local use. For instance, the various public safety services in your region may agree that 10-53 will mean a case of rape or 10-76 will designate a psychiatric case. Alternatively, one may design a separate code system for medical information. A sample medical code system, that designed by the pioneering Freedom House ambulance service in Pittsburgh more than 25 years ago, is illustrated in Figure 39-2.

Using the Freedom House code, one might notify the hospital of the possible acute myocardial infarction described earlier in this way: "Unit 3 is 10-98 to Montefiore Hospital with a case 7, condition 2," which means "Unit 3 is en route to Montefiore Hospital with a possible heart attack victim in serious condition." The information is thus conveyed tersely, with a minimum possibility of misinterpretation and without alarming the patient or his family.

Whenever codes are used, they should be kept simple and reserved for cases in which they are really needed. During mass casualties, when personnel unfamiliar with the codes may be manning radios and when everyone is apt to be anxious, it is usually best to abandon codes and stick to plain English.

Relaying Information to Medical Command

Radio communications between paramedics in the field and their medical director need to be terse and accurate. A standard format for communicating patient information over the radio will ensure that the significant data are related in a consistent manner and that nothing is omitted. The most effective format follows the order of the classic medical case presentation that we learned in Chapter 13. Medical professionals are accustomed to hearing information presented in that format and will sometimes fail to hear important details if the details are given in a different sequence.

FORMAT FOR REPORTING MEDICAL INFORMATION

- The patient's AGE and SEX
- The patient's CHIEF COMPLAINT
- A brief, pertinent HISTORY OF THE PRESENT ILLNESS
- Anything the physician needs to know about the patient's OTHER MEDICAL HISTORY, including major underlying medical conditions, medications, and important allergies
- The patient's STATE OF CONSCIOUSNESS and DEGREE OF DISTRESS
- The VITAL SIGNS
- The PERTINENT PHYSICAL FINDINGS in head-to-toe order
- ECG findings
- TREATMENT given so far

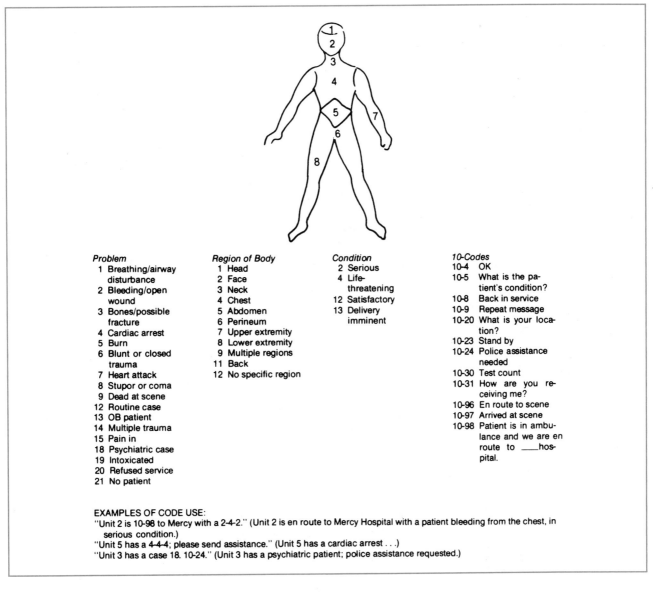

Problem
1 Breathing/airway disturbance
2 Bleeding/open wound
3 Bones/possible fracture
4 Cardiac arrest
5 Burn
6 Blunt or closed trauma
7 Heart attack
8 Stupor or coma
9 Dead at scene
12 Routine case
13 OB patient
14 Multiple trauma
15 Pain in
18 Psychiatric case
19 Intoxicated
20 Refused service
21 No patient

Region of Body
1 Head
2 Face
3 Neck
4 Chest
5 Abdomen
6 Perineum
7 Upper extremity
8 Lower extremity
9 Multiple regions
11 Back
12 No specific region

Condition
2 Serious
4 Life-threatening
12 Satisfactory
13 Delivery imminent

10-Codes
10-4 OK
10-5 What is the patient's condition?
10-8 Back in service
10-9 Repeat message
10-20 What is your location?
10-23 Stand by
10-24 Police assistance needed
10-30 Test count
10-31 How are you receiving me?
10-96 En route to scene
10-97 Arrived at scene
10-98 Patient is in ambulance and we are en route to ___ hospital.

EXAMPLES OF CODE USE:
"Unit 2 is 10-98 to Mercy with a 2-4-2." (Unit 2 is en route to Mercy Hospital with a patient bleeding from the chest, in serious condition.)
"Unit 5 has a 4-4-4; please send assistance." (Unit 5 has a cardiac arrest . . .)
"Unit 3 has a case 18. 10-24." (Unit 3 has a psychiatric patient; police assistance requested.)

FIGURE 39-2. **FREEDOM HOUSE AMBULANCE SERVICE RADIO CODE.**

For example, here is a transmission regarding a patient in congestive heart failure:

> We have a 53-year-old man complaining of severe shortness of breath, which wakened him from sleep and is worse when he is lying down. He has a history of high blood pressure and takes Diuril at home. He is alert but in a lot of respiratory distress, with a pulse of 130 and regular, respirations 36 per minute, and BP 190/120. His neck veins are not distended. He has crackles and wheezes in both lung fields. There is 2+ pitting edema of the ankles. We are sending you an ECG.

The above transmission can be relayed in less than 30 seconds, and any physician hearing that information will immediately recognize that this is a hypertensive patient in moderately severe left heart failure.

When paramedics call in without a standard reporting format, the physician will often have to waste a lot of time trying to glean the information he or she needs in order to know what is going on. Consider the following dialogue:

EMT: *We have a patient with a pulse of 130, a blood pressure 190/120, and respirations of 30. We're sending you a strip.*
Doc: *Fine, but what's his problem?*
EMT: *He's short of breath.*
Doc: *How long has this been going on?*

EMT: *Just a minute (pause). He says it woke him up from sleep about an hour ago.*
Doc: *Does he have any underlying medical problems?*
EMT: *He takes medicine for hypertension.*
Doc: *Is he in any distress?*
EMT: *Yeah, he's having a hard time breathing.*
Doc: *What do his lungs sound like?*
EMT: *He has crackles and wheezes all over.*

Clearly, that type of communication is much less efficient. It wastes time and gets everyone frustrated and annoyed. To avoid dialogues like the one just quoted, you should gather your information thoroughly at the scene, *organize* it clearly in your mind, and only then get on the air to the physician. Since even the best of us can get rattled under pressure, it's a good idea to write the reporting format on a card and affix the card to your hand-held transmitter or the dashboard of the ambulance, so you may refer to it while reporting in.

DISPATCHING

The verb, *to dispatch* means "to send out on a mission," but the EMS dispatcher does a lot more than just send ambulances out to emergencies. It is the job of the dispatcher, first of all, to obtain as much information as possible about the emergency, then to direct the appropriate vehicle to the scene and to provide the caller with whatever advice may be needed to manage the situation until help arrives. The dispatcher also monitors and coordinates communication with the field and maintains written records pertaining to the response to the call. Let us consider the dispatcher's tasks according to the phases of the call.

Receipt of the Call for Help

Whenever someone telephones for an ambulance, one has to assume that the caller needs help, even if the caller is too upset to be very clear about the nature of the problem. The dispatcher, therefore, has to be able to put himself or herself in the caller's place and understand the caller's distress. That means the dispatcher must

- ANSWER THE TELEPHONE PROMPTLY, within two or three rings, for each ring may seem like an eternity to a person who is panicky.
- IDENTIFY HIMSELF AND HIS AGENCY. The caller needs immediate confirmation of having reached the right number.

- SPEAK DIRECTLY INTO THE MOUTHPIECE, clearly and without mumbling.
- OBSERVE TELEPHONE COURTESY. The dispatcher must be calm and professional over the phone, informing the caller exactly what is being done and how soon assistance can be expected.
- TAKE CHARGE OF THE CONVERSATION. Once the dispatcher has identified the ambulance service, he or she must start asking the caller questions to which immediate answers are needed.

Information Gathering

The method used to gather information from a caller is most often a series of short questions asked by the dispatcher. When the call for an ambulance comes in, the dispatcher needs to elicit at least the following information:

- THE EXACT LOCATION OF THE PATIENT(S), including the street name and number. The dispatcher must obtain the proper geographic designation (e.g., whether the street is East Maple or West Maple) and the name of the community, since adjacent towns may have streets by the same name. If the call comes from a rural area, the dispatcher should try to establish landmarks, such as the nearest crossroad or business establishment, water tower, antenna, or other readily identifiable structure by which the rescue team can orient themselves.
- THE TELEPHONE NUMBER ("CALL-BACK NUMBER") OF THE CALLER, in case the call is disconnected or there is a need to phone the caller back for more information (e.g., if the rescue team cannot find the address and needs better directions). Asking for the caller's telephone number also helps discourage nuisance calls, since prank callers are generally reluctant to supply their phone numbers. Finally, the caller's telephone exchange may help to pinpoint his location if he is unfamiliar with the region, as in the case of a traveller calling from the road. In services equipped with an **enhanced 911 system,** a lot of the information mentioned—such as the phone number and location of the caller—is recorded automatically through sophisticated telephone technology, and the dispatcher need not take the time to ask.
- The NAME OF THE PATIENT, if known. That will help the rescue team identify the patient when they reach the scene.

- The caller's perception of the NATURE OF THE PATIENT'S PROBLEM.
- Specific information concerning the PATIENT'S CONDITION that will help evaluate the urgency of the situation and the need to provide the caller with first aid instructions by phone. The dispatcher should ask specifically:
  1. Is the patient conscious?
  2. If not, is he still breathing?
  3. Is the patient bleeding badly?
- If the emergency is a VEHICULAR ACCIDENT, further important information should be sought:
  1. The KINDS OF VEHICLES INVOLVED (i.e., cars, trucks, motorcycles, buses). If a truck is involved, is there any indication what CARGO it is carrying, since a truck carrying dynamite will require a different approach from one carrying bananas?
  2. The NUMBER OF PERSONS INJURED and the EXTENT OF INJURIES. Even if the caller can only guess, the dispatcher can at least get some idea of the magnitude of the problem.
  3. Apparent HAZARDS AT THE SCENE. Since the caller probably will not be schooled in evaluating hazards, the dispatcher should ask specifically about
     a. Traffic hazards
     b. Downed electric wires
     c. Fire
     d. Spilled materials
     e. Peculiar odors
     Information about such hazards enables the dispatcher to contact other agencies that may have to be involved, such as utility workers to take care of downed wires or an engine company to deal with spilled fuel.

A preprinted form, such as that shown in Figure 39-3, can help guide the dispatcher through the necessary questions, so that no questions are omitted, and also provides a lasting record of the call.

Dispatch

At the point when the dispatcher has obtained the address of the emergency and the telephone number of the caller, the dispatcher should ask the caller to wait on the line. The dispatcher must then decide, assuming the call is a medical emergency within his service's jurisdiction, which crew(s) and vehicle(s) will be dispatched. That decision will be governed by the nature and location of the call as well as the availability of various units at the time. The appropriate crew is then contacted and informed of the nature of the call and its exact location ("Medic 5, possible

heart attack at 573 East Main Street, that's five-seven-three East Main Street"). Once the ambulance is rolling, the dispatcher may return to the telephone to obtain the rest of the information previously outlined. Further questioning may elicit information about special conditions that might affect travel to the scene or the paramedics' actions at the scene. If so, that information should be relayed to the ambulance crew while they are en route, for two reasons:

- So that the rescuers may know if the response requires travel under emergency conditions, using emergency warning devices
- So that the rescuers may anticipate the situation and prepare while en route for tasks to be performed at the scene (e.g., suit up for a hazmat incident, assemble the equipment to deliver a baby)

Advice to the Caller

Having directed the rescue crew(s) to the scene and alerted them of any special conditions, the dispatcher should return to the telephone and tell the caller what is being done ("An ambulance is on the way and should be there in about 5 minutes."). If the patient is suspected to have a life-threatening emergency, the dispatcher should also provide instructions to the caller *in very simple terms* concerning emergency care techniques (e.g., airway maintenance, mouth-to-mouth ventilation, cardiac compressions, hemorrhage control). The caller is likely to be in an agitated state, so instructions must be clear and simple. Excellent protocols have been developed for giving such instructions by telephone, and all dispatchers should undergo training in those procedures.

Ongoing Communications with the Field

It is important for the dispatcher to monitor the communications of the ambulance and to be aware of what is occurring in the field, for the dispatcher must coordinate communications between the ambulance and medical command as well as contact any other agencies (e.g., fire, police) whose presence may be required at the scene. The dispatcher should also receive and record communications from the field regarding

- The time the ambulance DEPARTED for the scene
- The time the ambulance ARRIVED AT THE SCENE

Date _____   Log # _____

Times
Call received _____ A.M./P.M.
Car out _____
Arrived at scene _____
Left scene _____
Arrived at hospital _____
Back in service _____

Patient's name _____
Address _____
City/town _____

Patient status
Conscious? _____
Breathing? _____
Bleeding? _____
Other _____

If vehicular accident
Number and kinds of vehicles involved
_____cars   _____trucks   _____buses   _____other
Number of persons injured _____
Extent of injuries _____
Are persons trapped? _____
Hazards
_____traffic   _____wires down   _____fire   _____hazardous cargo
_____unstable vehicle   _____debris   _____submerged vehicle

Caller: Name _____   Phone no. _____

Vehicle dispatched _____
    Crew _____   Other units called _____
          _____   _____
          _____   _____

FIGURE 39-3.   **SAMPLE DISPATCH RECORD.**

- The time the ambulance LEFT THE SCENE
- The time the ambulance ARRIVED AT THE HOSPITAL
- The time the ambulance went BACK IN SERVICE

Paramedics involved in giving emergency care simply don't have time to keep looking at their watches and recording the moment that each of those events occurred. But the times cited, along with the time the call was received, must be recorded accurately at the base station. The easiest way to accomplish that is to have the paramedics radio in at each time indicated (e.g., "Leaving for hospital") and for the dispatcher to record the times. One of the most common complaints received by providers of emergency services is that response time—the time it took to get an ambulance to the patient—was too long. By recording the times mentioned, it is possible to determine the response time precisely and thereby support or refute the claim of slow ambulance service. Furthermore, a record of those times permits a whole gamut of medical and administrative evaluations: Supervising medical personnel can evaluate whether paramedics are spending too long at the scene; managers can assess how long it takes a unit to get back in service after a call.

The phases of the dispatcher's work are summarized in Table 39-3.

TABLE 39-3. PHASES OF DISPATCH

INFORMATION GATHERED	DISPATCHER ACTION
	Answers telephone promptly
	Identifies agency
Address of incident	
Call-back number	
Perceived problem	Dispatches (first) ambulance
Patient's name	
Patient's condition	Gives first-aid instruction by phone if required

For road accident:
    Number of vehicles
    Kinds of vehicles
    Number of victims
    Hazards at the scene
	Notifies responding ambulances of special situations

	Dispatches additional ambulances as needed
	Contacts other agencies as needed
	Monitors communications from the field

GLOSSARY

base station Assembly of radio equipment consisting of at least a transmitter, receiver, and antenna connection at a fixed location.

biotelemetry Transmission of physiologic data, such as an ECG, from the patient to a distant point of reception.

channel In EMS radio systems, a pair of radio frequencies (one for transmitting, the other for receiving).

duplex Radio system employing more than one frequency to permit simultaneous transmission and reception.

FCC Abbreviation for Federal Communications Commission.

FM Abbreviation for frequency modulation.

frequency The number of cycles per second of a radio signal, inversely related to the wavelength.

hertz (Hz) Unit of frequency equal to one cycle per second.

landline Communications system linked by wires, usually in reference to a conventional telephone system.

multiplex Method by which simultaneous transmission of voice and ECG signals can be achieved over a single radio frequency.

noise Interference in a radio signal.

patch Connection between a telephone line and a radio communications system, enabling a caller to get "on the air" by dialling into a special telephone.

repeater Miniature transmitter that picks up a radio signal and rebroadcasts it, thus extending the range of a radio communications system.

simplex Method of radio communication utilizing a single frequency that enables either transmission or reception of either voice or an ECG signal but is incapable of simultaneous transmission and reception.

ten-code Radio code system using the number 10 plus another number.

transceiver A radio transmitter and receiver housed in a single unit; a two-way radio.

UHF Ultrahigh frequency; the portion of the radio frequency spectrum between 300 and 3,000 mHz.

VHF Very high frequency; the portion of the radio frequency spectrum between 30 and 150 mHz.

wavelength The distance in a propagating wave from one point to the corresponding point on the next wave.

FURTHER READING

COMMUNICATIONS

Bush SG. Sending and receiving signals: The "art" of communicating. *Emergency* 10(3):34, 1978.

Butler N. Communications: Making a good thing better. *Emerg Med Serv* 10(5):101, 1981.

Cayton CG et al. The effect of telemetry on urban prehospital cardiac care. *Ann Emerg Med* 14:976, 1985.

Committee on Regional Emergency Medical Communications Systems. *Final Report.* Washington, D.C.: National Academy of Sciences, 1978.

Drury CD, Schiro SG. Evaluation of an EMS communications system. *JACEP* 6:133, 1977.

Felt J. A primer on radio communications: Or, how do I get from here to there? *JEMS* 5(6):22, 1980.

Garza MA. Cellular technology: Revolutionizing EMS communications. *JEMS* 15(5):46, 1990.

Gaull E. Scene communications pitfalls. *Emerg Med Serv* 21(8):23, 1992.

Grim P et al. Cellular telephone transmission of 12-lead electrocardiograms from ambulance to hospital. *Am J Cardiol* 60:715, 1987.

Henke S, Orcutt L. Portable radio communications for emergency medical services. *Emerg Med Serv* 12(4):32, 1983.

Hirschman JC, Nussenfeld SR, Nagel EL. Mobile physician command: A new dimension in civilian telemetry-rescue systems. *JAMA* 230:255, 1974.

Howell JE. Amateur radio: An alternative means of emergency communication. *Emerg Med Serv* 14(4):28, 1985.

Kulp R. Basic considerations in implementing a medical consultation radio system. *EMT J* 1(4):61, 1977.

Lambrew CT. The experience in telemetry of the electrocardiogram to a base hospital. *Heart Lung* 3:756, 1974.

Lewbel N, Felt HG. The care and feeding of communications equipment. *Emergency* 11(5):50, 1979.

McCorkle JE et al. *Basic Telecommunications for Emergency Medical Services.* Cambridge, Mass.: Ballinger, 1978.

National Highway Traffic Safety Administration. *Communications: Guidelines for Emergency Medical Services.* Washington, D.C.: U.S. Government Printing Office, 1972.

Pozen MW et al. Studies of ambulance patients with ischemic heart disease: The outcome of pre-hospital life

threatening arrhythmia in patients receiving electrocardiographic telemetry and therapeutic interventions. *Am J Public Health* 67:527, 1977.

Shapiro RA et al. Signal system for ambulance-to-hospital communication. *EMT J* 2(2):73, 1978.

Uhley HN. Electrocardiographic telemetry from ambulances: A practical approach to mobile coronary care units. *Am Heart J* 80:838, 1970.

U.S. Department of Transportation. *EMS Communications Design Manual.* DOT HS805749. Washington, D.C.: U.S. Government Printing Office, 1980.

Yandell DC. 911 update. *Emerg Med Serv* 18(7):36, 1989.

DISPATCH AND ADVICE BY TELEPHONE
Brodsky H. Delay in ambulance dispatch to road accidents. *Am J Public Health* 82:873, 1992.

Carter WB et al. Development and implementation of emergency CPR instruction via telephone. *Ann Emerg Med* 13:695, 1984.

Clawson J. Dispatch priority training. *JEMS* 6(2):32, 1981.

Cully L et al. An educated response. *Emergency* 25(7):29, 1993.

Curka P et al. Emergency medical services priority dispatch. *Ann Emerg Med* 22:1688, 1993.

Eisenberg MS et al. Emergency CPR instruction via telephone. *Am J Public Health* 75:47, 1985.

Eisenberg MS et al. Identification of cardiac arrest by emergency dispatchers. *Am J Emerg Med* 4:299, 1986.

Keene K. Emergency medical dispatch: The holistic approach. *Emerg Med Serv* 18(7):48, 1989.

Krumperman K. Humanistic dispatch. *Emerg Med Serv* 20(8):24, 1991.

Sampsel RE. Telephone-directed CPR: Does it work? *Emerg Med Serv* 18(4):49, 1989.

Slovis CM et al. A priority dispatch system for emergency medical services. *Ann Emerg Med* 14:1055, 1985.

Stratton SJ. Triage by emergency medical dispatchers. *Prehosp Disaster Med* 7:263, 1992.

40
Rescue and Extrication

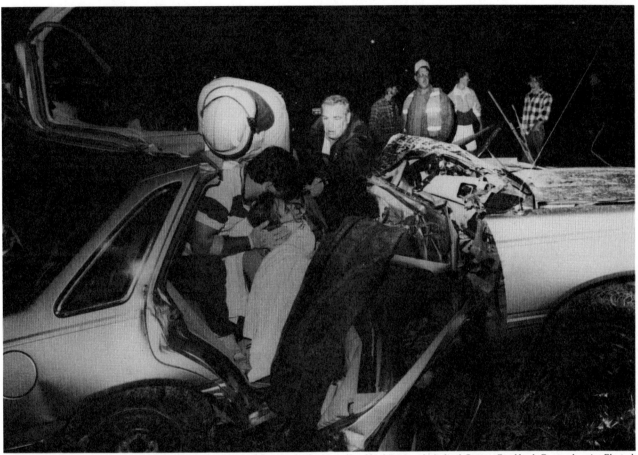

Bradford City Fire Department and Ambulance Service, and Paramedic Services, Bradford Regional Medical Center, Bradford, Pennsylvania. Photo by Jay K. Bradish.

OBJECTIVES

Rescue and extrication refer to the process by which an entrapped, injured person is approached, treated, and safely removed from the area of entrapment. There are a whole variety of situations in which an accident victim may require rescue. The most common scenario is the road accident in which one or more victims may be trapped within the twisted wreckage of a car. But rescue is also required for the person buried in the rubble of a collapsed building; for the construction worker crushed beneath earth and equipment at a building site; for the miner trapped in a damaged shaft; for the utility worker unconscious at the top of an electric power pole; for the skater who fell through the ice on the local pond. Each of those situations poses unique challenges for those who must reach the patient and provide emergency medical care.

Paramedics who plan to engage in rescue activities on a full-time basis will need additional training. Each rescue scenario—automobile extrication, extrication from fallen debris, high-angle rescue, wilderness rescue—requires its own complement of tools and its own particular skills, skills that can be acquired only in the course of specialized training. It is not useful to provide that specialized training as a routine part of a paramedic course, for each geographic area has its own special needs. There is little to be gained by teaching a Florida paramedic the fine points of winter mountain rescue or teaching a Nevada paramedic ocean scuba rescue. Paramedics should learn about the kinds of rescue that will be relevant to the particular regions where they work.

In this chapter, then, we shall concentrate mainly on the general principles of rescue and extrication. We shall use as our model the most commonly encountered extrication scenario—extrication from a wrecked motor vehicle—for that is a scenario that nearly every paramedic is likely to encounter sooner or later, no matter what his or her geographic location. By the end of this chapter, the student should be able to

1. Identify the primary function of a paramedic in a rescue situation, given a list of functions
2. List five measures a paramedic can take to ensure personal safety and the safety of others at an accident scene
3. Identify the most appropriate rescue tool for a particular purpose, given a list of tools
4. List the five stages of rescue and extrication
5. List six types of hazards that should be sought at every road accident scene

6. Identify hazardous conditions at an accident scene, given a description or picture of the scene, and indicate what measures should be taken to control each hazard
7. Choose the best method of gaining access to an entrapped patient, given a description of the patient's situation
8. List the treatment measures that should ordinarily be taken before an entrapped casualty is removed from a disabled vehicle
9. List the measures that should be taken after a seriously injured patient has been rescued and delivered safely to the emergency room

GENERAL PRINCIPLES OF EXTRICATION

No matter what the extrication problem—be it entrapment in a wrecked vehicle or entombment under a pile of rubble—there are certain general principles that always apply:

- THE PARAMEDIC'S PRIMARY RESPONSIBILITY IS TO PROVIDE EMERGENCY MEDICAL CARE. Everything else is secondary. If specialized rescue personnel are not on the scene when you arrive, you may have to use whatever means you have to gain access to the patient and even, rarely, to begin disentangling the patient from the wreckage. But the technical details of rescue should never distract the paramedic from his or her basic mission: administering *medical* care to the patient and ensuring that the patient's removal from the wreckage is carried out in a way that will not cause additional injury. When specialized rescue personnel *are* available, step aside and let them do their job. If you're working as a paramedic, *your* job is caring for the patient, not wielding the Hurst tool.

THE PARAMEDIC'S JOB AT THE SCENE OF AN ACCIDENT IS TO TAKE CARE OF THE PATIENT(S).

- A second fundamental principle of rescue and extrication is that if there is both an easy and a hard way to do something, TRY THE EASIER WAY FIRST. That may seem obvious, but it is extraordinary how many times one will find a rescue crew deploying all their heavy-duty power tools to pry and cut open a damaged car door when the opposite door is undamaged and unlocked and could be opened simply by pulling the handle.

- Extrication should be ORDERLY AND SYSTEMATIC. To be orderly and systematic, an extrication must be preplanned, even if only for a minute or two. The paramedic who comes barrelling out of the ambulance and immediately starts hacking away at a wrecked car is unlikely to do much good for the victim inside. Each extrication poses its own unique problems, and one must step back for a few moments to analyze those problems and determine the best way to solve them.
- As we shall learn shortly, there are five stages in any extrication, starting with a size-up of the scene and concluding with the packaging and removal of the patient. PATIENT CARE MUST ALWAYS PRECEDE REMOVAL OF THE PATIENT FROM THE WRECKAGE except when delay in removal would endanger the life of the patient or rescuers. When the victim of a motor vehicle accident is pinned behind the steering wheel screaming, "Get me out of here, get me out of here!" and bystanders and perhaps law enforcement officials are also urging haste, there is a strong temptation to remove the patient from the wreckage as fast as possible. Haste may impress the bystanders (at least those who are not knowledgeable in prehospital care), but haste is rarely in the best interests of the patient.
- Finally, ALWAYS KEEP YOUR OWN SAFETY AND THE SAFETY OF THE PATIENT UPPERMOST IN YOUR MIND. This last principle is so important that we need to spend a little more time considering it.

Safety First

Most rescue scenarios are dangerous. The untrained or inexperienced person may not notice the dangers. That is probably how the old saying "Fools rush in where angels fear to tread" originated. What the old saying doesn't mention is that fools are usually carried back *out* on stretchers—or in body bags. At every stage of the extrication, from arrival at the scene to removal of the patient, the paramedic needs to ask, "Am I safe? Is my patient safe?" If the answer to either question is no, you have to do something about it.

PERSONAL SAFETY of rescue personnel requires, at a minimum, protective headgear, protective coats and pants or coveralls, gloves, eye protection, protective boots or shoes, and in some cases breathing apparatus. The special circumstances of the rescue will dictate what other protective gear is needed, such as, specially insulated clothing for winter mountain rescue or fully encapsulated suits for some hazmat incidents.

The patient too must be protected from injury that might arise during the extrication process. PATIENT SAFETY may require a blanket or board to shield the patient from flying glass. Breathing apparatus may be needed if the patient is trapped in an environment of poisonous fumes. Protection against extremes of heat or cold, against fire, against spilled chemicals—any of those may be necessary under some circumstances.

Clearly, ensuring both personal safety and the safety of accident victims requires that the rescuer make an inventory of the HAZARDS AT THE SCENE. As we shall see shortly, hazard identification and control therefore constitute the first steps of the rescue response.

Tools of the Trade

Professional rescue crews have whole trucks full of specialized rescue equipment and usually need very little encouragement to show that equipment off. For the most part, paramedics who are not specializing in rescue need not become experts in the use of all of that equipment. There are, however, a number of simple rescue tools that every paramedic should know how (and, equally important, when) to use. The American College of Surgeons has compiled a list of items for use in rescue that they regard as essential equipment for *every* ambulance (Table 40-1), not just for specialized rescue teams. In general, the tools used in extrication fall into four broad categories: disassembly tools, spreading tools, cutting tools, and pulling tools.

- DISASSEMBLY TOOLS are those used to take things apart, such as screwdrivers, wrenches,

TABLE 40-1. ESSENTIAL RESCUE EQUIPMENT FOR AMBULANCES

QUANTITY	ITEM	TYPICAL USES
4	Triangular reflectors or battery-operated flares	To demarcate the danger zone and caution oncoming traffic
1	12-in. adjustable wrench	Disassembly
1	12-in. regular screwdriver	Disassembly
1	12-in. Phillips screwdriver	Disassembly; breaking tempered glass
1	Hacksaw with 12-in. carbide blades	Cutting through corner posts, steering wheel
1	10-in. pliers with vise grip	Breaking away covering of steering wheel
1	5-lb hammer with 15-in. handle	Making openings with cutting tools
1	Fire axe butt with 24-in. handle	Cutting roof section
1	51-in. crowbar with pinch point	Displacing and prying operations
1	Bolt cutter with 1¼-in. jaw opening and 36-in. handles	Breaking padlocks; cutting chains, fences
1	Portable power jack and spreader tool	Prying open doors, breaking seats loose
1	49-in. shovel with pointed blade	Removing debris
1	Double-action tin snip (at least 8 in.)	Cutting seat belts, removing metal trim
2	Manilla ropes, each 50 ft long and ¾ in. in diameter	Stabilizing a vehicle, raising or lowering a stretcher
1	Heavy-duty hand winch (come-along) with 15-ft rated chain and grab hook	Displacing steering columns, widening door openings, pulling front seat back
4	Shoring blocks	Supporting an unstable vehicle, preventing collapse of hood when come-along is in use
1 set/EMT	Hard hat, goggles, heavy gloves	Safety

Source: Adapted from the American College of Surgeons, Committee on Trauma, Essential equipment for ambulances. *Bull Am Coll Surg,* Sept., 1977.

and pliers. They are the tools you will probably be using most often.

- SPREADING TOOLS are usually hydraulic and may be either manual, like the Porto-power, or power-driven, like the Hurst or Lukas tool. Spreading tools are used to force open a door, break a car seat loose, and perform other operations that require prying one object away from another.
- CUTTING TOOLS include a variety of manually operated devices, such as bolt cutters, hacksaws, and giant can-openers, as well as power-driven tools, such as the air chisel. As the name of the category implies, cutting tools are used for operations that require cleaving through a hard object—for instance, severing a steering wheel rim, sawing through roof posts, or even opening up the roof of a car as one would a can of soup.
- PULLING TOOLS are exemplified by the hand winch, or "come-along," and employ a ratchet-driven drum to shorten a steel cable or chain. Pulling tools are used for displacing a steering column or pulling back a door or seat.

It cannot be overstressed that sophisticated extrication tools, such as the "Jaws of Life," should be used only by personnel who have been thoroughly trained in their proper operation. *Every tool has operational limits and hazards.* The paramedic must know what each of his or her tools can and cannot do and what potential dangers they create. And, once again, remember that you don't get extra points for doing things the hard way:

DON'T USE A SLEDGEHAMMER TO CRACK A WALNUT.

STAGES OF EXTRICATION

It is customary to divide extrication into five stages: (1) assessing the scene and controlling hazards, (2) gaining access to the patient, (3) providing urgent medical care to the patient, (4) disentangling the patient, and (5) packaging the patient and removing him from entrapment. In the real world, those five phases often overlap; assessing the situation and controlling hazards, for example, are ongoing activities that must continue throughout the whole rescue process. Nonetheless, for purposes of planning a rescue operation, it is useful to think of the operation in terms of those five separate phases.

Assessment and Stabilization of the Scene

Rescue and extrication begin even before you reach the accident scene. The process in fact begins as soon as you get the call from the dispatcher informing you of the incident. Ideally, the dispatcher will have supplied you with information regarding the number and types of vehicles involved in the accident, the number of persons estimated to be injured, the weather and road conditions, the traffic problems you may encounter, and the other emergency equipment or agencies that have already been dispatched. So even as you are en route to the scene, you should be able to begin planning your response. If, for example, you've been notified of a head-on collision on the interstate, you need to start assembling the equipment essential for a "load-and-go" trauma case (see Chap. 20) and strap it to the backboard along with a fire extinguisher and your rescue kit, so that you can carry the whole lot to the damaged vehicle on your first trip. If your information is that there is an overturned truck at the scene, get out your binoculars so that you'll be able to scan the truck from a safe distance for a hazardous material warning placard.

As soon as you do reach the accident scene, the phase of assessment, or size-up, begins. Recall from our discussion of the primary survey in Chapter 6 that the assessment of the scene seeks to answer four questions:

**ASSESSMENT OF THE SCENE:
QUESTIONS TO BE ANSWERED**

1. Is it safe for *me* to approach the victim?
2. Is there any hazard to the *patient*?
3. Am I going to need any help?
4. Do I need any special equipment to reach the patient?

Identification and Control of Hazards

The first two questions in the survey of the scene require you to determine whether there are hazards present and to do something about them if you find them.

Identification of Hazards at the Scene

In order to find hazards, you need to know what you are looking for! That is, you need a mental checklist of potential hazards. That checklist should include at least the following if the scenario is a vehicular accident:

- Are there TRAFFIC HAZARDS at the scene? Are the disabled vehicles out in the flow of traffic, where they might cause additional accidents?
- Are there DOWNED ELECTRICAL WIRES on or near the disabled vehicles?
- Is there a FIRE OR IMMINENT DANGER OF FIRE or explosion? If fire is going to occur, it usually occurs at impact or very soon thereafter; so by the time you reach the scene, the vehicle will already be engulfed in flames and the diagnosis of fire will not be difficult to make. Fires that occur some time *after* impact are usually the result of carelessness in the vicinity of SPILLED FUEL or flammable materials. Any vehicle that has been struck from the rear or is lying on its side or upside down should be assumed to have spilled gasoline and therefore constitutes a fire risk.
- Are any of the vehicles carrying HAZARDOUS MATERIALS? Note all details on a truck's warning placards, such as the UN/NA identification number. Also make note of any peculiar odors that might signal a hazardous spill.
- Is any VEHICLE IN AN UNSTABLE POSITION? In fact, the safest assumption is that *every* vehicle that has been involved in an accident is unstable, but asking yourself the question will remind you to take the appropriate action.
- Are there BYSTANDERS in vulnerable positions?

Control of Hazards

Once you have asked yourself the previous questions, you will be in a position to take steps to control the hazards at the scene. Here are a few guidelines for hazard control:

- ALL DOWNED WIRES ARE LIVE ELECTRICAL WIRES UNTIL PROVED OTHERWISE by qualified personnel (i.e., personnel from the power company). Paramedics should *not* attempt to deal with downed wires. If a downed wire is draped across a disabled vehicle, use the PA system of your ambulance to instruct the occupants to *stay inside the vehicle*. Move bystanders back at least 50 meters in all directions.

- Park your vehicle in a protective and warning position, with warning lights flashing. If necessary to protect the scene, use your vehicle to obstruct traffic. Consider using flares if you are sure there is no danger of fire or explosion.
- During every vehicle extrication, there should be at least one CHARGED FIRE HOSE manned until all patients have been removed from the vehicle to a safe place.
- STABILIZE *EVERY* DISABLED VEHICLE, even those standing upright on all four wheels. Use tire **chocks** for vehicles that are upright (if you don't have tire chocks, let the air out of the vehicle's tires).
- Do *not* try to disconnect the BATTERY of a disabled vehicle; you may spark an explosion. The best way to prevent an electric short-circuit is simply to TURN OFF THE IGNITION of the disabled car.
- KEEP BYSTANDERS AT A DISTANCE, ideally by roping off the zone around the accident. If you don't have the means to set up barriers, deputize a few of the bystanders to keep the others back until the police arrive in sufficient numbers to take over control of the scene.

Assessing the Need for Help

The next question you need to answer is whether you are going to need help in dealing with this emergency. Specifically, you need to decide:

- WILL ONE AMBULANCE BE ENOUGH to deal with the number of victims immediately apparent? If you have any doubts, call for help. Remember, you will need at least one ambulance and two rescuers for every seriously injured victim; the less seriously injured can be accommodated two to an ambulance. Clearly, to evaluate the need for help, you have to estimate the number of patients, which means that first you have to *locate* all the patients. If a car rolled over, one or more patients may have been thrown from the vehicle. So scan the path that the vehicle took as it left the road, and be alert for clues that there are missing victims (e.g., clothing or personal items in the vehicle that clearly don't belong to the victim you have found).
- Are any OTHER SERVICES needed here?
  1. POLICE, for crowd or traffic control.
  2. FIRE personnel, for virtually any accident that will require extrication.
  3. HAZMAT specialists.

  4. POWER COMPANY technicians, for downed wires.

Put in the call for help as soon as possible after your arrival on the scene, for it's going to take those additional resources time to get to you.

Deciding What Equipment You Need to Reach the Patient

Depending on the patient's location and situation, you may need special equipment to reach him. That includes protective equipment for yourself, such as breathing apparatus and protective clothing in a smoky environment. It also includes equipment for gaining access to a patient and for protecting the patient during access (e.g., a blanket to shield the patient from shattered glass if access must be obtained by breaking through a window). And that brings us to the next phase of rescue.

Gaining Access to the Patient

Having secured the scene, your next priority is to get to the patient as quickly as possible, so that you can begin any urgently needed treatment. To be rapid, access should be accomplished with the minimum of tools and procedures. The object of this step is simply to provide a space large enough for the paramedic to reach the patient and begin stabilizing treatment.

Access Through Doors

Like every other stage of extrication, gaining access requires that most uncommon of virtues, common sense.

> **THE EASIEST WAY TO ENTER AN AUTOMOBILE IS THROUGH A DOOR.**

Try first to open the door nearest the victim. If that door is jammed, try *all the other doors*. That may sound elementary, but rescuers engrossed in trying to open a car door with all their fancy equipment may neglect to check other doors that are unlocked and perfectly functional. The moral of the story is:

> **TRY BEFORE YOU PRY.**

If all the doors are locked and the victim inside is conscious, ask the victim to unlock the door. If the victim is unconscious in a locked car, the quickest solution is usually to break a window and unlock the door from the inside. Side and rear windows of automobiles are made of **tempered glass,** which can be broken if punctured with a sharp object. A spring-loaded center punch specially designed for breaking windows is a handy addition to the ambulance rescue kit; but if you don't have a center punch, any sharp-pointed tool, like a Phillips screwdriver, will do the job. Select a window away from the victim, and strike the glass in a lower corner, taking care not to displace it toward the victim. Once the glass is broken, pull it out of the frame (that's why you're wearing gloves!), and then reach inside the car and unlatch the door. If the door does not open after unlocking it, try releasing the inside and outside door handles simultaneously. Should those maneuvers fail, it will require more complicated, and therefore more time-consuming measures to get the door open; so leave the doors to the rescue crew and look for another means of gaining access to the patient.

Access Through a Window

When you can't get to the patient quickly through a door and the patient's condition seems to warrant urgent treatment, try to get in through a window. The fastest window access is achieved by breaking a rear or side window with a center punch. First, apply strips of masking or adhesive tape to the window to minimize the dispersion of broken glass over the interior of the vehicle. If the patient is conscious, warn him that you are about to break a window. Then fire the center punch in a lower corner of the window. Pull the broken glass out of the window frame. If shattered glass does fall within the vehicle, drop a heavy blanket or canvas tarp over it before you crawl in.

Access to an Overturned Vehicle

A vehicle found upside down or lying on its side presents special problems of access, for an improper approach may jeopardize the safety of both victim and rescuer. *The vehicle should be stabilized in the position in which it is found.* Attempts to right the vehicle may cause additional injuries to those inside. A vehicle that is fully upside down is relatively stable and so may be entered, cautiously, if necessary. When the vehicle is lying on its side, however, it is highly *unstable* and must be stabilized in place before entry. Most rescue squads carry **cribbing** materials for that purpose.

Providing Emergency Care

The whole point of gaining rapid access to the patient is to be able to start giving medical care as soon as possible. The paramedic who enters the vehicle should carry a blanket and a small jump kit with basic equipment such as airways, bag-valve-mask, dressings, and triangular bandages. Other equipment, such as an oxygen mask or suction, can be handed in to the paramedic as it is required.

Inside the wreckage, first make sure the ignition is turned off. If there is more than one victim, quickly identify which victim is most critically injured and start with her or him. The usual priorities apply: the ABCs, hemorrhage control, and cervical spine management.

If the victim is unconscious, open the AIRWAY by placing one hand beneath the victim's chin and the other behind his neck and then slowly raising the head into neutral position. Apply a cervical collar as soon as you can, and if at all possible, get someone into the back seat to hold the patient's head steady until the patient can be stabilized on a backboard.

Assessment of BREATHING means not only checking for apnea and respiratory distress, but also making sure there are no signs of tension pneumothorax or a sucking chest wound. If a tension pneumothorax *is* present, it may have to be decompressed before the patient is disentangled and removed from the vehicle. All seriously injured patients should receive OXYGEN at the earliest opportunity.

In assessing the CIRCULATION, bear in mind that cardiopulmonary resuscitation (CPR) is effective only when a patient is supine on a hard surface; CPR cannot be carried out on a patient who is sitting or lying on a car seat. Thus, if the pulse is absent, the patient must be removed as quickly as possible from the vehicle, even if hasty removal may aggravate other injuries. Injured is better than dead.

External BLEEDING should be controlled with direct pressure. Any patient in a vehicle that was sufficiently damaged to cause entrapment must be considered at high risk of shock, so at least one LARGE-BORE INTRAVENOUS INFUSION should be started at once. Don't wait for the patient to show signs of shock, because by then you won't find a vein!

Once the ABCs are under control, COVER OPEN WOUNDS and SPLINT FRACTURES. So long as the patient is still in the vehicle, it's preferable to stabilize fractures manually, for bulky splints are very difficult to apply in cramped quarters and may, in addition, impede removal of the patient from the wreckage. Body splinting is therefore preferable until after the patient is removed—securing a broken arm to the chest with a sling and swath or a broken leg to the uninjured leg.

Throughout the remainder of the disentanglement and removal procedures, the paramedic in the car with the victim will have three principal tasks:

- To maintain the victim's AIRWAY
- To KEEP THE VICTIM'S HEAD AND NECK STABLE
- To PROTECT THE VICTIM from further injury

Those tasks require the paramedic not only to monitor the patient closely but also to remain alert to what other rescuers are doing. If the rescue team is about to knock in a window, for instance, the paramedic must warn the patient and see to it that the patient is shielded from flying glass. The paramedic should also provide reassurance to the conscious patient and a running explanation of what is being done. And remember, throughout the entire rescue procedure, keep asking yourself, "Am I safe? Is the patient safe?"

Disentanglement

Disentanglement is the process of removing those parts of the wrecked vehicle that are keeping the victims pinned or entrapped. The basic principle of disentanglement is very simple:

> **REMOVE THE VEHICLE FROM THE PATIENT, NOT THE PATIENT FROM THE VEHICLE.**

While the principle may be simple, however, the execution is not. Disentanglement is the most highly technical of the phases of rescue and requires the highest degree of specialized training. In vehicular accidents, doors, steering wheels, windshields, dashboards, pedals, and seats all require specific approaches and specific skills. If you will be working in a service where you will need those skills—for example, in a community that does not have a separate rescue division—you should take special training in vehicle rescue.

Packaging and Removal

The final stage of rescue, packaging and removal, requires the most coordination among all those involved. PACKAGING the patient consists of

- Dressing open wounds
- Splinting fractures

- Making sure that IV lines, straps, and the patient's clothing are free from entanglement
- Securing the patient to a backboard

With those tasks accomplished, the paramedic inside the vehicle with the patient must verify that the EXIT PATH is secure. The route you used to gain access to the patient may not be the best route for removing the patient. You may have entered the vehicle through a side window, for example, while it is nearly always preferable to get the patient out through a door.

Once the patient is out of the disabled vehicle, the terrain will largely determine how he is moved to the ambulance. If the vehicle is right by the side of the road, the backboard may be placed directly onto the wheeled stretcher. When the accident sent the vehicle to a less accessible location, like the bottom of a ravine, a different approach will be required. While you remain with the patient throughout removal, another member of your crew should make a final check of the scene to be doubly sure that no victims have been overlooked. The final check also helps your crew retrieve equipment accidentally left behind.

Afterward

You've just finished a big-time trauma call—a five-car pileup on the interstate. You've spent nearly an hour in a muddy ditch by the side of the road in the pouring rain, and you and three other ambulance teams delivered five seriously injured patients to the hospital in stable condition. Now you feel tired and grubby and all you want to do is clean up and sink into an easy chair in front of the television with a nice cup of hot chocolate.

Not so fast.

The call isn't over yet. Before you retire to the easy chair, you have to go through all the equipment in the vehicle. Everything that got muddy or wet has to be cleaned and dried. The trauma kit, the medication kit, and any other kit you opened has to be restocked. You may fervently believe that it wouldn't be fair to get called to yet another big-time trauma case right after the one you just finished dealing with. But there is an important fact of existence that paramedics must learn to appreciate:

> **LIFE ISN'T FAIR.**

There are no guarantees that you won't get called in 10 minutes for the next accident on the interstate. Do you want to get there with an empty oxygen cylinder, a muddy bolt cutter, and a trauma kit that looks like a hurricane hit it? If not, CLEAN UP YOUR ACT before you pour that cup of hot chocolate and sink into your easy chair.

GLOSSARY

chock   A block of wood or similar object placed in front of or behind a wheel of a vehicle to prevent the vehicle from rolling.

cribbing   Timber used to provide a support or framework, usually wooden 2 × 4s or 4 × 4s.

tempered glass   Glass that breaks into small pieces when struck by a sharp-pointed object; safety glass.

FURTHER READING

Bailyn L. Subway and bus extrication. *Emergency* 10(4):62, 1978.

Bouvier KF. Industrial rescue: Not just routine. *Emergency* 22(5):35, 1990.

Briese GL. Elevator extrication. *EMT J* 3(3):45, 1979.

Carr T. Vehicle rescue in the '90s: New cars, new challenges. *Rescue* 36(6):38, 1990.

Carr T. Vehicle rescue in the '90s: New challenges in patient care. *Rescue* 4(2):47, 1991.

Dickenson E. Small spaces, big challenges: Treating the entrapped victim. *JEMS* 16(11):56, 1991.

Farrington JD. Extrication of victims: Surgical principles. *J Trauma* 8:493, 1968.

Grant H. *Vehicle Rescue* (2nd ed.). Bowie, Md.: Brady, 1990.

Hunt D. Ten common automobile-extrication errors. *Emerg Med Serv* 18(1):15, 1989.

Hunt DW. The ins and outs of automobile extrication. *Emerg Med Serv* 14(1):38 and 14(2):50, 1985.

Jarboe T. Surviving the tensions of trench rescue. *Rescue* 2(4):55, 1989.

Jarboe T. Building collapse rescue: Treating safety as a duty. *Rescue* 3(1):46, 1990.

Kruft SR. Rescue equipment and techniques: Lessons from wilderness search and rescue. *Emerg Med Serv* 14(6):40, 1985.

Linton SJ, Rust D. Ice rescue. *Emerg Med Serv* 12(1):26, 1983.

Moore R. *Vehicle Rescue and Extrication*. St. Louis: Mosby, 1990.

Moore R. Glass evolutions. *Emerg Med Serv* 21(6):60, 1992.

Schottke DE. A systematic approach to extrication. *EMT J* 3(3):76, 1979.

Stanford TM. Rescue from the dungeon. *Emergency* 21(4):24, 1989.

Tomlinson D. Taking time to do it right. *Rescue* 2(4):22, 1989.

U.S. Department of Transportation. *Emergency Medical Technician: Crash-Victim Extrication Training Course*. Publication No. 5003–00164. Washington, D.C.: U.S. Government Printing Office, 1976.

Vomacka R. Rapid extrication. *Emergency* 25(8):45, 1993.

DRUG HANDBOOK

Drugs Used in the Field

This first section of the Drug Handbook contains a detailed description of the majority of drugs used by paramedic services in the United States. Specifically, we shall consider the following drugs (listed alphabetically by generic name):

Activated charcoal USP
Adenosine (Adenocard)
Albuterol/salbutamol (Ventolin)
Aminophylline
Amyl nitrite (Vaporole)
Atropine sulfate
Bretylium tosylate (Bretylol)
Calcium preparations
50% Dextrose (D50)
Diazepam (Valium)
Diphenhydramine (Benadryl)
Dopamine (Intropin)
Epinephrine (Adrenalin)
Epinephrine, racemic (Vaponefrin)
Furosemide (Lasix)
Hydrocortisone and other corticosteroids
Isoetharine (Bronkosol)
Isoproterenol (Isuprel)
Labetalol (Normodyne, Trandate)
Lidocaine (Xylocaine)
Magnesium sulfate
Mannitol (Osmitrol)
Metaraminol (Aramine)
Morphine sulfate
Naloxone (Narcan)
Nifedipine (Adalat/Procardia)
Nitroglycerin
Nitrous oxide (N₂O) (Nitronox, Entonox)
Norepinephrine (Levophed)
Oxygen
Oxytocin (Pitocin, Syntocinon)
Propranolol (Inderal)
Sodium bicarbonate
Streptokinase (Streptase)
Succinylcholine (Anectine)

Syrup of ipecac
Terbutaline (Bricanyl)
Thiamine
Tissue plasminogen activator (rt-PA)
Verapamil (Isoptin, Calan)

For each of those drugs, information is provided regarding

- The **trade name(s)** of the drug
- The **therapeutic effects** of the drug
- The **indications** for giving the drug
- The **contraindications** to use of the drug
- The possible **side effects** of the drug
- The **form in which** the drug is **supplied**
- The usual **route of administration** of the drug and **correct dosage** (Note: **All dosages in this appendix are adult dosages unless otherwise specified. For pediatric dosages, see Appendix to Chapter 30.**)
- Any major **incompatibility** between the drug and other drugs
- The chapter(s) in this book in which to find **further discussion** of the use(s) of the drug
- **References** to the medical literature, for those interested in learning about the drug in greater depth.

Undoubtedly, not every drug used by every paramedic service is included in this Handbook. Where several alternative drugs share all or most of the same indications, we have—for purposes of reducing confusion—selected only one or two of those drugs for detailed consideration (usually the one with more documented benefit, wider application, or fewer potential hazards). Thus, for example, we have provided information on morphine as a strong analgesic, but not on meperidine (Demerol), because meperidine has no demonstrated advantages over morphine, and morphine has additional uses in emergency medicine (e.g., in the treatment of congestive heart failure). Similarly, lidocaine and procainamide have nearly the same indications (prevention and treatment of ventricular dysrhythmias); since lidocaine is regarded by the American Heart Association as the first-line drug for those indications, we have presented information on lidocaine only.

This Handbook is provided for reference, but the paramedic should *learn by heart* all of the information regarding those drugs that are in use by his or her ambulance service. That is not quite so overwhelming a task as it may first appear. For while the list of drugs covered in this Handbook is somewhat long, there are still several drugs on the list that serve much the same purpose. For example, dopamine, isoproterenol, metaraminol, and norepinephrine are all used in the field principally as vasoconstrictors, to raise the blood pressure. There is no need for an ambulance service to carry all four of those drugs. It is far better to stock just one of them and learn its pharmacology thoroughly.

Do not try to learn all the information in this Handbook at one time. The information will have much more meaning to you as you learn about the specific conditions for which the various drugs are used. It is recommended, therefore, that each time you finish studying a given condition—for example, asthma or congestive heart failure—you return to this Handbook and *then* learn by heart the properties of the drugs used to treat that condition.

A word of caution. Even though, by the time you finish your paramedic course, you should be able to recite in your sleep the dosages of the drugs your service uses,

---

DO NOT TRUST YOUR MEMORY IN AN EMERGENCY.

Whether you are giving medications according to voice orders or protocols, ALWAYS RECHECK THE CORRECT DOSAGE BEFORE YOU ADMINISTER A DRUG. The most convenient way to do so is to make up a file card listing all of the drugs used by your service and the correct dosage of each and to keep that file card taped to your drug box, so that the dosages will be right there in front of you when you need them.

ACTIVATED CHARCOAL USP

TRADE NAMES	Charcodote, SuperChar
THERAPEUTIC EFFECTS	Adsorbs many poisonous compounds to its surface, thereby reducing their absorption by the body. Particularly effective in binding aspirin, amphetamines, strychnine, Dilantin, theophylline, and phenobarbital.
INDICATIONS	To treat certain cases of POISONING and OVERDOSE.
CONTRAINDICATIONS	There are no absolute contraindications to activated charcoal, but there are a number of poisonings in which it is ineffective and may create more problems than it solves: • Of no value in poisoning due to *methanol, caustic acids and alkalis, iron tablets,* and *lithium.* • Do not use in *cyanide poisoning.* Activated charcoal should not be used if the container in which it was stored was not tightly sealed.
SIDE EFFECTS	No serious adverse side effects.
HOW SUPPLIED	Fine black powder in bottles of 25 gm and 50 gm.
ADMINISTRATION AND DOSAGE	Given by mouth or through a nasogastric tube. *Dosage*: A good rule of thumb for both children and adults is **1 gm/kg.** The charcoal is **mixed in tap water** to make a slurry.
INCOMPATIBILITY	None. Previous concerns that activated charcoal might interfere with the action of syrup of ipecac or *N*-acetylcysteine have not been substantiated by clinical experience.

Further Discussion

Chapter 27.

References

Albertson TE et al. Superiority of activated charcoal alone compared with ipecac and activated charcoal in the treatment of acute toxic ingestions. *Ann Emerg Med* 18:56, 1989.

Berg MJ et al. Acceleration of the body clearance of phenobarbital by oral activated charcoal. *N Engl J Med* 307:642, 1982.

Burton BT et al. Comparison of activated charcoal and gastric lavage in the prevention of aspirin absorption. *J Emerg Med* 1:411, 1984.

Comstock EG et al. Assessment of the efficacy of activated charcoal following gastric lavage in acute drug emergencies. *J Toxicol* 19:149, 1982.

Corby DG, Decker WG. Management of poisoning with activated charcoal. *Pediatrics* 54:234, 1974.

Freedman GE, Pasternak S, Krenzelok EP. A clinical trial using syrup of ipecac and activated charcoal concurrently. *Ann Emerg Med* 16:164, 1987.

Greensher J et al. Ascendancy of the black bottle (activated charcoal). *Pediatrics* 80:949, 1987.

Hayden JW, Comstock EG. Use of activated charcoal in acute poisoning. *Clin Toxicol* 8:515, 1975.

Hoffman R. Choices in gastric decontamination. *Emerg Med* 24(10):212, 1992.

Katona BG et al. The new black magic: Activated charcoal and new therapeutic uses. *J Emerg Med* 5:99, 1987.

Kornberg AE et al. Pediatric ingestions: Charcoal alone versus ipecac and charcoal. *Ann Emerg Med* 20:648, 1991.

Levy DB. Activated charcoal update. *Emergency* 20(6):16, 1988.

Levy G. Gastrointestinal clearance of drugs with activated charcoal. *N Engl J Med* 307:676, 1982.

Mofenson HC et al. Gastrointestinal dialysis with activated charcoal and cathartic in the treatment of adolescent intoxications. *Clin Pediatr* 24:678, 1985.

Park GD et al. Expanded role of charcoal therapy in the poisoned and overdosed patient. *Arch Intern Med* 146:969, 1986.

Pollack MM et al. Aspiration of activated charcoal and gastric contents. *Ann Emerg Med* 10:528, 1981.

Tennebein M. Multiple doses of activated charcoal: Time for reappraisal? *Ann Emerg Med* 20:529, 1991.

Tennenbein M, Cohen S, Sitar DS. Efficacy of ipecac-induced emesis, orogastric lavage, and activated charcoal for acute drug overdose. *Ann Emerg Med* 16:838, 1987.

True RJ, Berman JM, Mahutte CK. Treatment of theophylline toxicity with oral activated charcoal. *Crit Care Med* 12:113, 1984.

ADENOSINE

TRADE NAME	Adenocard
THERAPEUTIC EFFECTS	Adenosine is a chemical that occurs naturally throughout the body as part of DNA and other substances. When given as a drug, adenosine slows discharge of the sinoatrial node and, more importantly, *delays conduction through the atrioventricular node.* Because it is metabolized rapidly, adenosine has a very short half-life in the body (less than 10 seconds), so its effects are brief and it is less likely than other drugs to cause hypotension.
INDICATIONS	• First-line drug for narrow-complex PAROXYSMAL SUPRAVEN-TRICULAR TACHYCARDIA (PSVT). • May be used diagnostically (*after* lidocaine) in wide-complex tachycardia of uncertain type.
CONTRAINDICATIONS	• **Second- or third-degree heart block** • Sick sinus syndrome • Patients taking **incompatible drugs** (see below)
SIDE EFFECTS	Very common, but transient. The following side effects usually resolve spontaneously within 1 to 2 minutes: • *Flushing* • *Dyspnea* • *Chest pain or tightness* • *Headache* In addition, adenosine often causes brief cardiac *dysrhythmias* immediately after conversion of PSVT, especially: • *Sinus bradycardia* and even brief asystole • Premature ventricular contractions Finally, because adenosine has a very short half-life, *PSVT may recur.*
HOW SUPPLIED	In vials containing 6 mg in 2 ml. (The vials should not be refrigerated, as the solution may crystallize in cold temperatures.)
ADMINISTRATION AND DOSAGE	The patient should be recumbent, with the stretcher tilted slightly head up. Adenosine is given through the IV line at the *most proximal* injection port. • The initial dosage is 6 mg by rapid IV bolus over 1 to 3 seconds, followed immediately by 20 ml of saline to flush the drug into the circulation. • If there is no response within 1 to 2 minutes, a repeat dose of 12 mg by rapid IV bolus may be given. • A third dose, of 12 mg, may be given after 1 to 2 minutes if needed. • If PSVT is corrected by adenosine but then keeps recurring, try verapamil or propranolol.
INCOMPATIBILITY	Do *not* give adenosine to patients taking either *dipyridamole* (Persantine) or *carbamazepine* (Tegretol), both of which prolong and potentiate adenosine's effects. Adenosine is *less* effective in patients taking *theophylline* preparations (which many asthmatics use) or other xanthines, such as *coffee.*

Further Discussion

Chapter 23.

References

Belardinelli L et al. The cardiac effects of adenosine. *Progr Cardiovasc Dis* 32:73, 1989.

Cairns C, Niemann J. Intravenous adenosine in the emergency department management of paroxysmal supraventricular tachycardia. *Ann Emerg Med* 20:717, 1991.

Duffy SP et al. Adenosine: An old drug learns a new trick. *JEMS* 17(4):58, 1992.

Hood MA et al. Adenosine versus verapamil in the treatment of supraventricular tachycardia: A randomized double-crossover trial. *Am Heart J* 123:1453, 1992.

Levy DB. Adenosine: A new drug for PSVT. *Emergency* 22(11):18, 1990.

McCabe JL et al. Intravenous adenosine in the prehospital treatment of paroxysmal supraventricular tachycardia. *Ann Emerg Med* 21:358, 1992.

Melio FR et al. Successful conversion of unstable supraventricular tachycardia to sinus rhythm with adenosine. *Ann Emerg Med* 22:709, 1993.

Rankin AC et al. Verapamil or adenosine for the immediate treatment of supraventricular tachycardia. *Q J Med New Series* 74:203, 1990.

ALBUTEROL/SALBUTAMOL

TRADE NAMES	Proventil, Ventolin
THERAPEUTIC EFFECTS	Selective beta-2 sympathomimetic drug, that is, a beta agent that acts primarily on the *bronchial* musculature rather than the myocardium. Therefore, albuterol relaxes bronchial smooth muscle and thereby relieves bronchospasm.
INDICATIONS	Drug of first choice for the relief of bronchospasm associated with ACUTE ASTHMATIC ATTACKS or acute exacerbations of CHRONIC BRONCHITIS or emphysema.
CONTRAINDICATIONS	• **Tachyarrhythmias.** • Should be used with *caution* in patients with **hypertension, angina,** or **diabetes.**
SIDE EFFECTS	• Palpitations, tachycardia. • Tremor, nervousness. • Dizziness. • Nausea, heartburn.
HOW SUPPLIED	• Metered-dose inhaler • Bottles of 0.5% solution for use in nebulizer
ADMINISTRATION AND DOSAGE	• If using a *metered-dose inhaler,* attach a spacer. The patient should take **1 to 2 inhalations.** The dose may be repeated in 15 minutes. • By *nebulizer:* *Dosage for adults and children over 12:* **Dilute** 0.5 ml of 0.5% solution (**2.5 mg**) in **3 ml of sterile saline** and place that solution in the nebulizer. Regulate the flow rate of the nebulizer to deliver the 3 ml over 5 to 15 minutes. *Pediatric dosage:* **0.01 to 0.03 mg/kg in 3 ml of sterile saline** via nebulizer.
INCOMPATIBILITY	May be ineffective in a patient taking beta blockers (e.g., propranolol).

Further Discussion

Chapters 22 and 30.

References

Becker AB et al. Inhaled salbutamol (albuterol) vs injected epinephrine in the treatment of acute asthma in children. *J Pediatr* 102:465, 1983.

Bedell GN et al. Safety and efficacy of albuterol aerosol in the relief of bronchospasm. *Ann Allergy* 475:392, 1981.

Colacone A et al. Continuous nebulization of albuterol (salbutamol) in acute asthma. *Chest* 97:693, 1990.

Emmerman C et al. A randomized controlled comparison of isoetharine and albuterol in the treatment of acute asthma. *Ann Emerg Med* 20:1090, 1991.

Godfrey S. Worldwide experience with albuterol (salbutamol). *Ann Allergy* 475:423, 1981.

Kerem E et al. Efficacy of albuterol administered by nebulizer versus spacer device in children with acute asthma. *J Pediatr* 123:313, 1993.

Lee HS et al. Albuterol by aerosol and orally administered theophylline in asthmatic children. *J Pediatr* 101:632, 1982.

Olshaker J et al. The efficacy and safety of a continuous albuterol protocol for the treatment of adult asthma attacks. *Am J Emerg Med* 11(2):131, 1993.

Pearlman DS et al. A comparison of salmeterol with albuterol in the treatment of mild-to-moderate asthma. *N Engl J Med* 327:1420, 1992.

Yates T et al. A comparison of isoetharine and albuterol: Report of changes in pulmonary functions over 1 hour. *J Am Osteopath Assoc* 81:546, 1982.

AMINOPHYLLINE

THERAPEUTIC EFFECTS
Xanthine drug derived from theophylline with the following actions:
- Stimulation of the myocardium to increase heart rate and cardiac output.
- Bronchodilation and vasodilation (by smooth muscle relaxation).
- Strengthening of diaphragmatic contractions.
- Stimulation of respiratory drive.
- Increase in coronary blood flow.
- Mild diuretic.
- Central nervous system stimulation.

INDICATIONS
A second-line drug for the following indications:
- For bronchodilation in acute attacks of ASTHMA and in decompensated CHRONIC OBSTRUCTIVE PULMONARY DISEASE.
- To relieve bronchoconstriction in ANAPHYLAXIS.
- To relieve bronchoconstriction in selected cases of CONGESTIVE HEART FAILURE and PULMONARY EDEMA from other causes.

CONTRAINDICATIONS
Relative contraindications:
- Cardiac **dysrhythmias.**
- **Hypotension.**
- Massive **myocardial infarction.**

SIDE EFFECTS
- Myocardial irritability and *dysrhythmias*, especially in the presence of hypoxemia; palpitations.
- *Hypotension.*
- *Nausea* and *vomiting.*
- *Headache.*
- *Excitement, confusion, seizures.*

Because of the high risk of dangerous side effects, aminophylline is not a drug of first choice for any indication.

HOW SUPPLIED
Ampules of 250 mg or 500 mg

ADMINISTRATION AND DOSAGE
Given **intravenously** through a peripheral IV line. For patients who are not already taking theophylline, start with a **bolus of 5 mg/kg in 50 ml of D5/W over 20 minutes;** follow with an infusion:
- *For acute asthmatic attacks*: Add 250 mg to 1 liter of D5/W, to make a solution of 0.25 mg/ml. **Infuse** at a rate of **0.5 mg/kg/hr.**
- *For pulmonary edema*: Add 250 mg to 250 ml D5/W, to yield a solution of 1 mg/ml. **Infuse** at a rate of **0.5 mg/kg/hr.**

Further Discussion

Chapters 22, 23, 26, and 30.

References

Appel D et al. Comparative effect of epinephrine and aminophylline in the treatment of asthma. *Lung* 159:243, 1981.

Canavan JW et al. Intravenous administration of aminophylline in asthmatic children taking theophylline orally. *J Pediatr* 97:301, 1980.

Carter E et al. Efficacy of intravenously administered theophylline in children hospitalized with severe asthma. *J Pediatr* 122:470, 1993.

Coleridge J et al. Intravenous aminophylline confers no benefit in acute asthma treated with intravenous steroids and inhaled bronchodilators. *Aust NZ J Med* 23:348, 1993.

DiGiulio GA et al. Hospital treatment of asthma: Lack of benefit from theophylline given in addition to nebulized albuterol and intravenously administered corticosteroid. *J Pediatr* 122:464, 1993.

Kelly HW et al. Should we stop using theophylline for the

treatment of the hospitalized patient with status asthmaticus? *Ann Pharmacother* 23:995, 1989.

Lam A et al. Management of asthma and chronic airflow limitation: Are methylxanthines obsolete? *Chest* 98:44, 1990.

Littenberg B. Aminophylline treatment in severe, acute asthma. *JAMA* 259:1687, 1988.

Piafsky KM, Ogilvie RI. Dosage of theophylline in bronchial asthma. *N Engl J Med* 292:1218, 1975.

Rossing TH. Methylxanthines in 1989. *Ann Intern Med* 110:502, 1989.

Seidenfeld JJ et al. Intravenous aminophylline in the treatment of acute bronchospastic exacerbations of chronic obstructive pulmonary disease. *Ann Emerg Med* 13:248, 1984.

Self TH et al. Inhaled albuterol and oral prednisone therapy in hospitalized adult asthmatics: Does aminophylline add any benefit? *Chest* 98:1317, 1990.

Sessler CN. Theophylline toxicity: Clinical features of 116 consecutive cases. *Am J Med* 88:567, 1990.

Stewart MF et al. Risk of giving intravenous aminophylline to acutely ill patients receiving maintenance treatment with theophylline. *Br Med J* 288:450, 1984.

Taylor DR et al. Parenteral aminophylline in acute severe asthma. *NZ Med J* 102:402, 1989.

Viskin S et al. Aminophylline for bradysystolic cardiac arrest refractory to atropine and epinephrine. *Ann Intern Med* 118:279, 1993.

AMYL NITRITE

TRADE NAME	Vaporole
THERAPEUTIC EFFECTS	• Oxidizes hemoglobin to methemoglobin, a form that competes with cytochrome oxidase for the cyanide ion; therefore helps inactivate the cyanide ion. • Vasodilatation, including coronary artery dilation (in the same family of drugs as nitroglycerin). • As a smooth muscle relaxant, can relieve spasms of the biliary tract.
INDICATIONS	To treat CYANIDE POISONING.
CONTRAINDICATIONS	**None** when used to treat cyanide poisoning.
SIDE EFFECTS	• Marked *hypotension* due to sudden vasodilation, with syncope if the patient is not recumbent. • Reflex *tachycardia* secondary to the drop in blood pressure. • Cutaneous *flush* involving the head, neck, and clavicular regions. • Pounding *headache*. • Nausea and vomiting.
HOW SUPPLIED	Perles (small ampules) of 0.2 to 0.3 ml.
ADMINISTRATION AND DOSAGE	Start treatment *urgently* in suspected cyanide poisoning. KEEP PATIENT RECUMBENT. Break a perle into a gauze pad or handkerchief; hold it over the patient's face for **20 seconds,** then give **100% oxygen for 40 to 100 seconds.** Continue alternating amyl nitrite and 100% oxygen in that fashion all the way to the hospital.

CAUTION: Amyl nitrite is a frequently abused drug (street name: "Amy"). Keep it under lock and key.

Further Discussion

Chapters 22 and 27.

References

Baud FJ et al. Elevated blood cyanide concentrations in victims of smoke inhalation. *N Engl J Med* 325:1761, 1991.

Blanc P et al. Cyanide intoxication among silver-reclaiming workers. *JAMA* 253:367, 1985.

Hall AH. Cyanide poisoning: Dealing with an unexpected menace. *Emerg Med* 18(15):191, 1986.

Johnson RP, Mellors JW. Arteriolization of venous blood gases: A clue to the diagnosis of cyanide poisoning. *J Emerg Med* 6:401, 1988.

Jones J, Krohmer J. Injury through inhalation: Cyanide poisoning in fire victims. *JEMS* 15(4):36, 1990.

Kirk M et al. Cyanide and methemoglobin kinetics in smoke inhalation victims treated with the cyanide antidote kit. *Ann Emerg Med* 22:1413, 1993.

Kulig K. Cyanide antidotes and fire toxicology (editorial). *N Engl J Med* 325:1801, 1991.

Kunkel DB. Cyanide: Looking for the source. *Emerg Med* 19(9):115, 1987.

Levy DB, Peppers MP. Poisoning with cyanide. *Emergency* 22(9):18, 1990.

Silverman SH et al. Cyanide toxicity in burned patients. *J Trauma* 28:171, 1988.

ATROPINE SULFATE

THERAPEUTIC EFFECTS

By blocking parasympathetic (vagal) action on the heart, atropine
- Increases the rate of discharge by the sinus node.
- Enhances conduction through the atrioventricular (AV) junction.
- Accelerates the heart rate, thereby improving cardiac output.

In addition, by speeding up a slow heart to a normal rate, atropine reduces the chances of ectopic activity in the ventricles and thus of ventricular fibrillation. Atropine is most effective in reversing bradycardia due to increased parasympathetic tone, morphine, or organophosphates; it is less effective in treating bradycardias due to actual damage to the AV or sinoatrial (SA) node.

INDICATIONS

- SINUS BRADYCARDIA *when accompanied by premature ventricular contractions or hypotension.*
- TYPE I SECOND-DEGREE AV BLOCK (Wenckebach) when accompanied by bradycardia.
- Third-degree heart block when accompanied by symptomatic bradycardia in the context of *inferior*-wall acute myocardial infarction.
- In some cases of ASYSTOLE.
- As an antidote in ORGANOPHOSPHATE POISONING.

CONTRAINDICATIONS

None when used for life-threatening emergencies. Use with *caution* in patients with
- **Atrial flutter** or **atrial fibrillation** where there is a rapid ventricular response.
- **Type II second-degree AV block.**
- **Complete** (third-degree) **AV block** in the context of *anterior*-wall myocardial infarction.
- **Glaucoma.**
- **Chronic obstructive pulmonary disease.**

SIDE EFFECTS

The patient should be warned that he or she may experience some of the following side effects and that these side effects are part of the drug's usual and expected actions:
- *Blurred vision, headache, pupillary dilatation.*
- *Dry mouth, thirst.*
- *Flushing* of the skin.
- *Difficulty in urination* (especially in older men).

Paradoxical *bradycardia* may occur if a dose less than 0.5 mg is given or if even the correct dose is given too slowly.

HOW SUPPLIED

Prefilled syringes in a variety of volumes and concentrations; CHECK THE VOLUME AND CONCENTRATION on every preloaded syringe before giving the drug!
Ampules with 1 mg in 1 ml.
Multidose vials with a concentration of 1 mg/ml.

ADMINISTRATION AND DOSAGE

In the field, atropine is given **intravenously** for bradycardia; for organophosphate poisoning, a combination of **intravenous and intramuscular** administration is commonly used. In resuscitation from cardiac arrest, if an intravenous route cannot be established, atropine may be given through the **endotracheal** tube.
- For *bradycardia*: **0.5 to 1.0 mg IV,** repeated at 5-minute intervals until the desired heart rate is achieved; *the total dose should not, however, exceed 2.0 mg.*

- For *organophosphate poisoning*: **2 mg IM and 1 mg IV.** The IV dose may be repeated every 5 to 10 minutes as needed, until a decrease in secretions is observed.
- For *asystole*: **1 mg IV,** repeated in 5 minutes if asystole persists.

The patient suffering from POISONING by atropine or other anticholinergics is classically described as:

Hot as a hare,

Blind as a bat,

Dry as a bone,

Red as a beet,

Mad as a hen.

Further Discussion

Chapters 23 and 27.

References

Averill JH, Lamb LE. Less commonly recognized actions of atropine on cardiac rhythm. *Am J Med Sci* 237:304, 1959.

Bray BM et al. Tracheal versus intravenous atropine: A comparison of the effects on heart rate. *Anaesthesia* 42:1188, 1987.

Brown DC, Lewis AJ, Criley JM. Asystole and its treatment: The possible role of the parasympathetic nervous system in cardiac arrest. *JACEP* 8:448, 1979.

Coon GA et al. Use of atropine for brady-asystolic prehospital cardiac arrest. *Ann Emerg Med* 10:462, 1981.

Cooper MJ, Abinader EG. Atropine-induced ventricular fibrillation: Case report and review of the literature. *Am Heart J* 97:255, 1979.

Dauchot P, Gravenstein JS. Bradycardia after myocardial ischemia and its treatment with atropine. *Anesthesiology* 44:501, 1976.

Gonzalez ER. Pharmacologic controversies in CPR. *Ann Emerg Med* 22:317, 1993.

Greenberg MI et al. Endotracheal administration of atropine sulfate. *Ann Emerg Med* 11:546, 1982.

Howard RF et al. Endotracheal compared with intravenous administration of atropine. *Arch Dis Child* 65:449, 1990.

Kottmeier CA, Gravenstein JS. The parasympathomimetic action of atropine and atropine methylbromide. *Anesthesiology* 29:1125, 1968.

Massumi RA et al. Ventricular fibrillation and tachycardia after intravenous atropine for treatment of bradycardias. *N Engl J Med* 287:336, 1972.

Myerburg RJ et al. Outcome of resuscitation from bradyarrhythmic or asystolic prehospital cardiac arrest. *J Am Coll Cardiol* 4:1118, 1984.

Steuven HA et al. Atropine in asystole: Human studies. *Ann Emerg Med* 13:815, 1984.

BRETYLIUM TOSYLATE

TRADE NAMES	Bretylol, Bretylate
THERAPEUTIC ACTION	• Raises the threshold of heart muscle for ventricular fibrillation. • May reduce energy required for defibrillation. • Occasionally converts ventricular fibrillation to an effective rhythm without electric countershock.
INDICATIONS	• VENTRICULAR FIBRILLATION that has not been successfully converted with countershock and lidocaine or that recurs despite lidocaine treatment. • VENTRICULAR TACHYCARDIA that has been unresponsive to first-line therapy (i.e., lidocaine and/or countershock).
CONTRAINDICATIONS	None when used for life-threatening dysrhythmias.
SIDE EFFECTS	• *Hypotension* (by beta blocking action); patients should be kept supine after receiving bretylium to minimize this effect. • *Nausea* and *vomiting,* when the drug is given rapidly IV.
HOW SUPPLIED	10-ml ampules containing 500 mg (50 mg/ml).
ADMINISTRATION AND DOSAGE	Bretylium tosylate is given intravenously for life-threatening dysrhythmias. • For *refractory ventricular fibrillation*: Give **5 mg/kg** as a **bolus IV** followed by electric defibrillation. If ventricular fibrillation persists, the dose may be increased to 10 mg/kg and repeated at 15- to 30-minute intervals. Do not exceed a **maximum total dose of 30 mg/kg.** • For *refractory or recurrent ventricular tachycardia*: Dilute 500 mg of bretylium tosylate in 50 ml of D5/W (to yield a concentration of 10 mg/ml) and give **10 mg/kg** by **IV infusion over 8 to 10 minutes.** Once that loading dose has been given, bretylium may be administered as a continuous drip at 1 to 2 mg/min. *Note*: Bretylium may require 15 to 30 minutes before taking full effect.
INCOMPATIBILITY	• May interact with *antihypertensive* medications to cause hypotension. • May interact with *sympathomimetic* agents to potentiate their pressor effects.

Further Discussion

Chapter 23.

References

Bernstein JG, Koch-Weser, J. Effectiveness of bretylium tosylate against refractory ventricular arrhythmias. *Circulation* 45:1024, 1972.

Bryan CK et al. Bretylium tosylate: A review. *Am J Hosp Pharm* 36:1189, 1979.

Chow MSS. Antifibrillatory effects of lidocaine and bretylium immediately postcardiopulmonary resuscitation. *Am Heart J* 110:938, 1985.

Harrison EE, Amey BD. The use of bretylium in prehospital ventricular fibrillation. *Amer J Emerg Med* 1:1, 1983.

Haynes RE et al. Comparison of bretylium tosylate and lidocaine in management of out of hospital ventricular fibrillation: A randomized clinical trial. *Am J Cardiol* 48:353, 1981.

Holder AH et al. Experience with bretylium tosylate by a hospital cardiac arrest team. *Circulation* 55:541, 1977.

Koch-Weser J. Bretylium. *N Engl J Med* 300:473, 1979.

Koo CC, Allen JD, Pantridge JF. Lack of effect of bretylium tosylate on electrical ventricular defibrillation in a controlled study. *Cardiovasc Res* 18:762, 1984.

Murphy KM et al. Endotracheal bretylium tosylate in a canine model. *Ann Emerg Med* 13:87, 1984.

Nowack RM et al. Bretylium tosylate as initial treatment for cardiopulmonary arrest: Randomized comparison with placebo. *Ann Emerg Med* 10:404, 1981.

Olson DW et al. A randomized comparison study of bretylium tosylate and lidocaine in resuscitation of patients from out-of-hospital ventricular fibrillation in a paramedic system. *Ann Emerg Med* 13:807, 1984.

Sanna G, Raffaele A. Chemical ventricular defibrillation of the human heart with bretylium tosylate. *Am J Cardiol* 32:982, 1973.

Stang JM et al. Treatment of prehospital refractory ventricular fibrillation with bretylium tosylate. *Ann Emerg Med* 13:234, 1984.

Terry G et al. Bretylium tosylate in treatment of refractory ventricular arrhythmias complicating myocardial infarction. *Br Heart J* 32:21, 1970.

Torresani J. Bretylium tosylate in patients with acute myocardial infarction. *Am J Cardiol* 54:20A, 1984.

CALCIUM PREPARATIONS

THERAPEUTIC EFFECTS	• Reverses overdose with magnesium sulfate or calcium channel blockers (such as verapamil). • Relieves some types of muscle spasm. • Increases the strength of myocardial contractions.
INDICATIONS	• To oppose the actions of potassium in HYPERKALEMIA. • As an ANTIDOTE TO MAGNESIUM sulfate. • As an ANTIDOTE TO VERAPAMIL overdose. • To relieve muscle spasm and pain from the BITES of BLACK WIDOW SPIDER, SCORPION, and PORTUGUESE MAN-O-WAR.
CONTRAINDICATIONS	Should be used with extreme caution and in reduced dosage in patients taking **digitalis.**
SIDE EFFECTS	• When given to a patient who has been taking digitalis or when given too rapidly, calcium can cause *sudden death* from ventricular fibrillation. • Rapid IV administration may cause metallic or chalky taste, paresthesias, vasodilation, hypotension, and a feeling that a "wave of heat" is passing through the body.
HOW SUPPLIED	Calcium chloride: 10 ml of a 10% solution in prefilled syringes (13.6 mEq Ca^{++}). Calcium gluconate: 10 ml of a 10% solution in prefilled syringes (4.8 mEq Ca^{++}).
ADMINISTRATION AND DOSAGE	Calcium preparations are given as a **slow intravenous injection.** • For severe muscle pain after *black widow spider bite*: calcium gluconate, **10 ml of a 10% solution IV.** • For *magnesium sulfate overdose*: calcium gluconate, **10 ml of a 10% solution IV.** • For *verapamil toxicity*: Calcium gluconate, **10 ml of a 10% solution slowly IV.**
INCOMPATIBILITY	Should not be given in the same infusion with *sodium bicarbonate,* since calcium chloride will combine with sodium bicarbonate to form an insoluble precipitate (calcium carbonate, i.e., chalk).

Further Discussion

Chapters 25 and 27.

References

Dembo DH. Calcium in advanced life support. *Crit Care Med* 9:358, 1981.

Harrison EE et al. Use of calcium in electromechanical dissociation. *Ann Emerg Med* 13:844, 1984.

Hughes WG et al. Should calcium be used in cardiac arrest? *Am J Med* 81:285, 1986.

Kuhn M et al. Low-dose calcium pretreatment to prevent verapamil-induced hypotension. *Am Heart J* 124:231, 1994.

Morris DL et al. Calcium infusion for reversal of adverse effects of intravenous verapamil. *JAMA* 249:3212, 1983.

Redding JS, Haynes RR, Thomas JD. Drug therapy in resuscitation from electromechanical dissociation. *Crit Care Med* 11:681, 1983.

Steuven HS et al. The effectiveness of calcium chloride in refractory electromechanical dissociation. *Ann Emerg Med* 14:626, 1985.

Steuven HS et al. Lack of effectiveness of calcium chloride in refractory asystole. *Ann Emerg Med* 14:630, 1985.

Steuven HS et al. Use of calcium in prehospital cardiac arrest. *Ann Emerg Med* 12:136, 1983.

Woie L et al. Successful treatment of suicidal verapamil poisoning with calcium gluconate. *Eur Heart J* 12:239, 1981.

50% DEXTROSE (D50)

THERAPEUTIC EFFECTS	• Rapidly restores blood sugar level to normal in states of hypoglycemia. • Acts transiently as an osmotic diuretic.
INDICATIONS	• To treat suspected HYPOGLYCEMIA. • To treat COMA OF UNKNOWN CAUSE. • In STATUS EPILEPTICUS OF UNCERTAIN CAUSE.
CONTRAINDICATIONS	• Intracranial hemorrhage. • Known **stroke** (CVA).
SIDE EFFECTS	• May precipitate severe neurologic symptoms of *Wernicke's encephalopathy* in alcoholics. For that reason, administration of D50 should be preceded by *thiamine* (50 mg IV plus 50 mg IM), which will prevent the neurologic syndrome from emerging. • Will cause *tissue necrosis* if it infiltrates; should therefore be given only through a RAPIDLY FLOWING IV LINE IN A LARGE VEIN.
HOW SUPPLIED	Prefilled syringes and vials containing 50 ml of 50% dextrose (= 25 gm dextrose).
ADMINISTRATION AND DOSAGE	Given **intravenously through a free-flowing line,** preferably in a large vein. If possible, draw blood for serum glucose determinations before administering the dextrose. *Dosage*: 50 ml of 50% solution (**25 gm**) slowly IV.

Further Discussion

Chapters 24 and 27.

References

Andrade R et al. Hypoglycemic hemiplegic syndrome. *Ann Emerg Med* 13:529, 1984.

Baker FJ et al. Diabetic emergencies: Hypoglycemia and ketoacidosis. *JACEP* 5:119, 1976.

Browning RG et al. 50% dextrose: Antidote or toxin? *Ann Emerg Med* 19:683, 1990.

Cox DJ et al. Symptoms and blood glucose levels in diabetics (letter). *JAMA* 253:1558, 1985.

Helgason CM. Blood glucose and stroke. *Stroke* 23:1, 1988.

Hoffman J et al. The empiric use of hypertonic dextrose in patients with altered mental status: A reappraisal. *Ann Emerg Med* 21:20, 1992.

Iscovich AL. Sudden cardiac death due to hypoglycemia. *Am J Emerg Med* 1:28, 1983.

Jones JL et al. Determination of prehospital blood glucose: A prospective, controlled study. *J Emerg Med* 10:679, 1992.

Kunian L, Wasco J, Hulefeld L. Sweets for the alcoholic. *Emerg Med* 5(a):45, 1973.

Lanier WL et al. The effects of dextrose infusion and head position on neurologic outcome after complete cerebral ischemia in primates: Examination of a model. *Anesthesiology* 66:39, 1987.

Longstreth WT Jr, Inui TS. High blood glucose level on hospital admission and poor neurologic recovery after cardiac arrest. *Ann Neurol* 15:59, 1984.

Pulsinelli WA et al. Increased damage after ischemic stroke in patients with hyperglycemia with or without established diabetes mellitus. *Am J Med* 74:540, 1983.

Stapczynski JS, Haskell RJ. Duration of hypoglycemia and need for intravenous glucose following intentional overdoses of insulin. *Ann Emerg Med* 13:505, 1984.

Thurston JH. Blood glucose: How reliable an indicator of brain glucose? *Hosp Pract* 11:123, 1976.

DIAZEPAM

TRADE NAME	Valium
THERAPEUTIC EFFECTS	• Suppresses seizure activity in the motor cortex of the brain. • Generalized central nervous system depressant. • Muscle relaxant.
INDICATIONS	• To treat STATUS EPILEPTICUS. • To provide sedation prior to CARDIOVERSION. • In very selected cases, to relieve SEVERE ANXIETY.
CONTRAINDICATIONS	• Should not be given during **pregnancy** because of possible toxic effects on the fetus. • Should not be given to patients who have taken **alcohol** or other **sedative drugs.** • Should not be given to patients with **respiratory depression** from any source. • Should not be given to patients with **hypotension.**
SIDE EFFECTS	• Possible *hypotension.* • Depression in the *level of consciousness.* • In the elderly, the very ill, and patients with pulmonary disease, may cause *respiratory arrest* and/or *cardiac arrest.*
HOW SUPPLIED	Prefilled syringes and ampules of 2 ml and vials of 10 ml, in a concentration of either 5 mg/ml or 10 mg/ml.
ADMINISTRATION AND DOSAGE	• For *status epilepticus*: Given intravenously in slow, titrated doses. Before administering the drug, check and record the patient's vital signs. Then give **2.5 mg** (0.5 ml of a 5 mg/ml concentration) **slowly IV.** Wait a few minutes, and recheck the blood pressure (BP); if it has fallen, do *not* give any more of the drug. If the BP is stable, and the patient is still seizing, give another 2.5 mg slowly IV. Then recheck the BP. Continue until the seizures have stopped or the BP drops, but **do not exceed a total dose of 10 mg** in the field. (In children, may be given *rectally* for status epilepticus, in a dosage of 0.5 mg/kg.) • For *severe anxiety* that must, for some reason, be treated in the field: Given intramuscularly. *Dosage*: **2 to 5 mg IM.** • For *premedication prior to cardioversion*: **5 to 10 mg slowly IV.**
INCOMPATIBILITY	Should not be mixed with any other drugs because of possible precipitation.

Further Discussion

Chapters 16, 23, 24, and 30.

References

Canfield PR. Treatment of status epilepticus in children. *Can Med Assoc J* 128:671, 1983.

Drawbaugh RE, Deibler CG, Eitel DR. Prehospital administration of rectal diazepam in pediatric status epilepticus. *Prehosp Disaster Med* 5(2):155, 1990.

Knudsen RU. Rectal administration of diazepam in solution in the acute treatment of convulsions in infants and children. *Arch Dis Child* 54:855, 1979.

Nicol CF. Status epilepticus. *JAMA* 234:419, 1975.

Sonander H et al. Effects of the rectal administration of diazepam. *Br J Anaesth* 5:578, 1985.

DIPHENHYDRAMINE

TRADE NAME	Benadryl
THERAPEUTIC EFFECTS	• Blocks histamine effects. • Reverses some untoward effects of phenothiazine tranquilizers. • Inhibits motion sickness (antiemetic). • Mild sedative.
INDICATIONS	• As an adjunct to epinephrine in the treatment of ANAPHY-LACTIC SHOCK and SEVERE ALLERGIC REACTIONS. • To treat ACUTE DYSTONIC REACTIONS caused by phenothiazines like thorazine (Compazine).
CONTRAINDICATIONS	• **Asthma** or **chronic obstructive pulmonary disease.** • **Prostatic enlargement.** • Narrow-angle (acute) **glaucoma.** • Ulcer disease with symptoms of obstruction (vomiting). • **Pregnancy.** • **Nursing mothers.**
SIDE EFFECTS	Resemble those of atropine: • *Drowsiness, confusion.* • *Blurring of vision.* • *Difficulty in urination* (especially in older men). • *Dry mouth.* • *Wheezing;* thickened bronchial secretions. • *Headache.* • *Palpitations.*
HOW SUPPLIED	• Vials of 10 or 30 ml containing 10 mg/ml. • Vials of 10 ml containing 50 mg/ml. • Ampules of 1 ml containing 50 mg/ml • Prefilled syringes containing 50 mg in 1 ml. CHECK THE LABEL CAREFULLY!
ADMINISTRATION AND DOSAGE	For most purposes, diphenhydramine can be given by **deep intramuscular injection.** *Dosage:* **10 to 50 mg.**

Further Discussion

Chapters 26 and 38.

References

Greenblatt DJ, Shader RI. Anticholinergics. *N Engl J Med* 288:1215, 1973.

DOPAMINE

TRADE NAMES	Intropin, Revimine
THERAPEUTIC EFFECTS	Beta sympathomimetic drug—hence causes an increase in the force and rate of cardiac contractions as well as dilatation of mesenteric and renal arteries. The latter effect promotes urine flow, and for that reason, dopamine is sometimes preferred over norepinephrine (which constricts renal arteries) in shock. Dopamine causes less increase in oxygen consumption by the myocardium than does isoproterenol. At low doses (less than 10 µg/kg/min), the beta effects of dopamine predominate; at higher doses, dopamine has alpha effects as well and thus causes vasoconstriction.
INDICATIONS	• In resuscitation, to treat HYPOTENSION that comes with bradycardia or with the return of spontaneous circulation. • To increase cardiac output in CARDIOGENIC SHOCK while maintaining good renal perfusion.
CONTRAINDICATIONS	• Should not be used as a first-line therapy in hypotension caused by **hypovolemia** (e.g., hemorrhagic shock), where volume replacement should precede the use of vasopressors. • **Pheochromocytoma** (a tumor that produces epinephrine and/or related substances). • Should not be given in the presence of uncorrected **tachyarrhythmias** or **ventricular fibrillation.**
SIDE EFFECTS	• *Ectopic beats, tachycardia, palpitations.* • *Nausea, vomiting.* • *Angina.* • *Headache.* • Leakage around the vein (extravasation) may cause local *tissue necrosis.*
HOW SUPPLIED	• 5-ml ampules containing 200 mg (40 mg/ml). • 5-ml vials containing 400 mg (80 mg/ml). READ THE LABEL CAREFULLY!
ADMINISTRATION AND DOSAGE	Given by **titrated intravenous infusion** (microdrip infusion set). *Dosage*: Transfer the contents of one ampule (200 mg) of dopamine into a 250-ml bag of D5/W to yield a concentration of 800 µg/ml. START the infusion at a rate of **2 to 5 µg/kg/min** (e.g., 140–350 µg/min for a 70-kg man, or roughly 0.25 ml/min of the above dilution). TITRATE the infusion according to the state of consciousness, blood pressure, and urine flow. If a dosage higher than 20 µg/kg/min is needed, add a norepinephrine infusion instead of increasing the dopamine dosage any further. When blood pressure support is no longer required, dopamine should be tapered slowly, not discontinued abruptly.
INCOMPATIBILITY	Do not mix with *sodium bicarbonate*, since alkaline solutions may inactivate dopamine.

Further Discussion

Chapter 23.

References

Goldberg W. Dopamine: Clinical use of an endogenous catecholamine. *N Engl J Med* 291:707, 1974.

Goldbert LI, Hsieh YY, Resnekov L. Newer catecholamines for treatment of heart failure and shock: An update on dopamine and a first look at dobutamine. *Prog Cardiovasc Dis* 19:327, 1977.

Holzer J et al. Effectiveness of dopamine in patients with cardiogenic shock. *Am J Cardiol* 32:79, 1973.

MacCannell KI et al. Dopamine in the treatment of hypotension and shock. *N Engl J Med* 275:1389, 1966.

Otto CW et al. Comparison of dopamine, dobutamine and epinephrine in CPR. *Crit Care Med* 9:366, 1981.

EPINEPHRINE

TRADE NAME   Adrenalin

THERAPEUTIC EFFECTS

Beta-1 sympathetic effects:
- May restore electric activity in asystole.
- Increases myocardial contractility.
- Lowers the threshold for defibrillation.

Beta-2 sympathetic effects:
- Acts as a bronchodilator.

Alpha sympathetic effects:
- Produces vasoconstriction, which elevates perfusion pressure and may thus improve coronary blood flow during external chest compressions.
- Vasoconstriction also helps support the blood pressure in anaphylactic shock.

INDICATIONS

- In CARDIAC ARREST, to restore electric activity in asystole or to enhance defibrillation potential in ventricular fibrillation; also to elevate systemic vascular resistance and thereby improve perfusion pressure during cardiopulmonary resuscitation (CPR).
- To treat the life-threatening symptoms of ANAPHYLAXIS.
- To treat acute attacks of ASTHMA (second-line drug).

CONTRAINDICATIONS

- Must be used with caution in patients with **angina, hypertension,** or **hyperthyroidism.**
- **Tachyarrhythmias.**
- THERE ARE NO CONTRAINDICATIONS TO THE USE OF EPINEPHRINE IN CARDIAC ARREST OR ANAPHYLACTIC SHOCK.

SIDE EFFECTS

In the patient who is not in cardiac arrest, may cause
- *Palpitations* from tachycardia or ectopic beats.
- **Hypertension.**
- **Angina.**

HOW SUPPLIED

- Prefilled syringes containing 1 mg of epinephrine in 10 ml (1 : 10,000 solution).
- Ampules containing 1 mg epinephrine in 1 ml (1 : 1,000 solution).

ADMINISTRATION AND DOSAGE

- In *cardiac arrest*, epinephrine is given **intravenously.** If an IV route cannot be established quickly, the drug may be instilled in the tracheobronchial tree via **endotracheal tube.**

IV dosage: 1.0 mg (**10 ml of 1 : 10,000 solution**); repeat at 3- to 5-minute intervals throughout resuscitation. After each dose by peripheral V, *flush* the line with 20 ml of IV fluid to ensure delivery of the drug into the central circulation.

For *endotracheal instillation*, use 2 to 2½ times the intravenous dose (i.e., **2.0–2.5 mg**).
- For *mild anaphylactic reactions:* **0.3 to 0.5 ml of 1 : 1,000 solution SQ.** If the reaction is due to an injection or an insect sting, also inject 0.1 to 0.2 ml of the same solution at the injection site (but not on fingers, toes, ears, nose, or genitalia).
- For *severe anaphylactic reactions in a patient < 35 years old*: Give **0.1 ml/kg of 1 : 10,000 solution slowly IV.** If you have neither IV nor endotracheal access, give 0.5 ml of 1 : 1,000 solution into the vascular plexus at the base of the tongue.

- For *severe anaphylactic reactions in a patient > 35 years old*: Dilute **0.1 ml of 1 : 1,000 solution in 10 ml of saline,** and **infuse over 5 to 10 minutes.**
- For *asthmatic attacks*: **0.3 to 0.5 ml of a 1 : 1,000 solution SQ.**

INCOMPATIBILITY
- Do not mix with sodium bicarbonate, since alkaline solutions may inactivate epinephrine.
- May cause severe hypertension and reflex bradycardia if given to a patient taking *beta blockers,* such as propranolol.

Further Discussion

Chapters 7, 10, 22, 23, 26, and 30.

References

EPINEPHRINE IN CARDIAC ARREST

Amey BD et al. Paramedic use of intracardiac medications in prehospital sudden cardiac death. *JACEP* 7:130, 1978.

Brown CG et al. A comparison of standard-dose and high-dose epinephrine in cardiac arrest outside the hospital. *N Engl J Med* 327:1051, 1992.

Callaham M, Barton CW, Kayser S. Potential complications of high-dose epinephrine therapy in patients resuscitated from cardiac arrest. *JAMA* 265:1117, 1991.

Callaham M et al. A randomized clinical trial of high-dose epinephrine and norepinephrine vs. standard-dose epinephrine in prehospital cardiac arrest. *JAMA* 268:2667, 1992.

Chernow B et al. Epinephrine absorption after intratracheal administration. *Anesth Analg* 63:829, 1984.

Gonzalez ER et al. Dose-dependent vasopressor response to epinephrine during CPR in human beings. *Ann Emerg Med* 18:920, 1989.

Marwick TH et al. Adverse effect of early high-dose adrenaline on outcome of ventricular fibrillation. *Lancet* 2:66, 1988.

McCrirrick A et al. Haemodynamic effects of tracheal compared with intravenous adrenaline. *Lancet* 340:868, 1992.

Ornato JP. Use of adrenergic agonists during CPR in adults. *Ann Emerg Med* 22:411, 1993.

Otto CW, Yakaitis RW, Blitt CD. Mechanism of action of epinephrine in resuscitation from asphyxial arrest. *Crit Care Med* 9:321, 1981.

Paradis NA, Koscove EM. Epinephrine in cardiac arrest: A critical review. *Ann Emerg Med* 19:1288, 1990.

Pearson JW, Redding JS. Epinephrine in cardiac arrest. *Am Heart J* 66:210, 1963.

Peppers MP. High-dose epinephrine. *Emergency* 24(2):23, 1992.

Quinton DN, O'Bryre G, Aitenhead AR. Comparison of endotracheal and peripheral intravenous adrenaline in cardiac arrest. *Lancet* 1:828, 1987.

Roberts JR, Greenberg JI, Baskin SI. Endotracheal epinephrine in cardiorespiratory collapse. *JACEP* 8:515, 1979.

Rothenberg MA. Reviewing high-dose epinephrine in cardiac arrest. *JEMS* 15(4):43, 1990.

Schneider SM et al. Endotracheal versus intravenous epinephrine in the prehospital treatment of cardiac arrest. *Prehosp Disaster Med* 5(4):341, 1990.

Stiell IG et al. High-dose epinephrine in adult cardiac arrest. *N Engl J Med* 327:1045, 1992.

Yakaitis RW, Otto CW, Blitt CD. Relative importance of alpha and beta adrenergic receptors during resuscitation. *Crit Care Med* 7:293, 1979.

EPINEPHRINE FOR ANAPHYLAXIS AND ASTHMA

Appel D et al. Comparative effect of epinephrine and aminophylline in the treatment of asthma. *Lung* 159:243, 1981.

Barach EM et al. Epinephrine for the treatment of anaphylactic shock. *JAMA* 251:2118, 1984.

Ben-Zvi Z et al. An evaluation of repeated injections of epinephrine for the initial treatment of acute asthma. *Am Rev Respir Dis* 127:101, 1983.

Cydulka R et al. The use of epinephrine in the treatment of older adult asthmatics. *Ann Emerg Med* 17:322, 1988.

Elenbaas RM et al. Subcutaneous epinephrine vs. nebulized metaproterenol in acute asthma. *Drug Intell Clin Pharm* 19:567, 1985.

Gandy W. Severe epinephrine-propranolol interaction. *Ann Emerg Med* 18:98, 1989.

Gotz VP et al. Bronchodilatory effect of subcutaneous epinephrine in acute asthma. *Ann Emerg Med* 10:518, 1981.

Grandstetter RD et al. Optimal dosing of epinephrine in acute asthma. *Am J Hosp Pharm* 37:1326, 1980.

Karetzy MS. Acute asthma: The use of subcutaneous epinephrine in therapy. *Ann Allergy* 44:12, 1980.

Owney DR et al. Response to epinephrine in children receiving oral beta-agonists. *Am J Dis Child* 140:122, 1986.

Peppers MP. Updating epinephrine. *Emergency* 22(3):18, 1990.

Pliss LB et al. Aerosol vs. injected epinephrine in acute asthma. *Ann Emerg Med* 10:353, 1981.

RACEMIC EPINEPHRINE

TRADE NAME	Vaponefrin
THERAPEUTIC ACTIONS	Bronchodilator.
INDICATIONS	• Upper airway problems in children, especially CROUP.
	• To buy time to secure the airway in ANAPHYLAXIS with rapidly progressive laryngeal edema (as evidenced by stridor).
CONTRAINDICATIONS	• Severe **tachyarrhythmias.**
	• **Epiglottitis.**
SIDE EFFECTS	• *Tachycardia, dysrhythmias, palpitations.*
	• *Angina.*
	• *Headache, dizziness.*
	• Paradoxical *bronchospasm* if used excessively.
HOW SUPPLIED	30-ml bottle of 2.25% solution for nebulization.
ADMINISTRATION AND DOSAGE	Dilute **0.5 ml in 3 ml of normal saline** and **nebulize** over 10 to 15 minutes. DO NOT REPEAT DOSAGE. (The inhalation therapist at your base hospital can help you rig up a nebulizer for the ambulance.)
INCOMPATIBILITY	May induce hypertensive crisis in patients taking tricyclic or monoamine oxidase inhibitor *antidepressant drugs*

Further Discussion

Chapters 26 and 30.

References

Gardner HG et al. The evaluation of racemic epinephrine in the treatment of infectious croup. *Pediatrics* 52:52, 1973.

Kelley P, Simon J. Racemic epinephrine use in croup and disposition. *Am J Emerg Med* 10:181, 1992.

Waisman Y et al. Prospective randomized double-blind study comparing L-epinephrine and racemic epinephrine aerosols in the treatment of laryngotracheobronchitis (croup). *Pediatrics* 89:302, 1992.

Westley CR et al. Nebulized racemic epinephrine by IPPB for the treatment of croup. *Am J Dis Child* 132:484, 1978.

FUROSEMIDE

TRADE NAME	Lasix
THERAPEUTIC EFFECTS	• Potent diuretic, causing the excretion of large volumes of urine within 5 to 30 minutes of administration, thus useful in ridding the body of excess fluid in conditions of fluid overload (e.g., congestive heart failure). • Vasodilator, allowing temporary "internal phlebotomy" in conditions of fluid overload.
INDICATIONS	• For the treatment of fluid overload in CONGESTIVE HEART FAILURE. • For some cases of transfusion reaction.
CONTRAINDICATIONS	• **Pregnancy.** • **Hypovolemic states.** • **Hypokalemia** (suspect in patients on chronic diuretic therapy with prominent P waves and flattened T waves on the electrocardiogram).
SIDE EFFECTS	Acute side effects may include • *Nausea* and *vomiting.* • Potassium depletion, leading to *cardiac dysrhythmias.* • *Dehydration.* • Acute *urinary retention* in an uncatheterized male. • Adverse reactions more likely in the elderly, so avoid giving furosemide to elderly patients in the prehospital phase.
HOW SUPPLIED	• Prefilled syringes of 2 ml, 4 ml, and 10 ml containing 10 mg/ml. • Ampules of 2 ml, 4 ml, and 10 ml containing 10 mg/ml.
ADMINISTRATION AND DOSAGE	In the field, furosemide is given **intravenously.** If transport time will be more than 15 minutes, the patient should have a urinary catheter. *Dosage*: **20 to 40 mg slowly IV** (injected over 1–2 minutes).
INCOMPATIBILITY	Should not be given to patients taking *lithium* (furosemide may block the renal excretion of lithium and thereby cause lithium to accumulate in the body to toxic levels).

Further Discussion

Chapters 9, 16, and 23.

References

Bigg RW, Bapat N. Furosemide in acute pulmonary edema. *Lancet* 1:849, 1967.

Cotrell JE et al. Furosemide and head injury. *J Trauma* 21:805, 1981.

Davidov M, Kakviatos N, Finnerty F Jr. Intravenous administration of furosemide in heart failure. *JAMA* 220:824, 1967.

Dikshit K et al. Renal and extrarenal hemodynamic effects of furosemide in congestive heart failure after acute myocardial infarction. *N Engl J Med* 288:1087, 1973.

Francis GS et al. Acute vasoconstrictor response to intravenous furosemide in patients with chronic congestive heart failure. *Ann Intern Med* 103:1, 1985.

Genton R, Jaffe AS. Management of congestive heart failure in patients with acute myocardial infarction. *JAMA* 256:2556, 1986.

Hoffman JR, Reynolds S. Comparison of nitroglycerin, morphine and furosemide in treatment of presumed pre-hospital pulmonary edema. *Chest* 92:586, 1987.

Kirkendall WM, Stein JM. Clinical pharmacology of furosemide and ethacrynic acid. *Am J Cardiol* 22:162, 1968.

Kraus PE. Acute preload effects of furosemide. *Chest* 98:124, 1990.

Nelson GIC et al. Haemodynamic effects of furosemide and its influence of repetitive rapid volume loading in acute myocardial infarction. *Eur Heart J* 4:706, 1983.

Romano E et al. Chlorpromazine and furosemide in treatment of acute left ventricular failure. *Lancet* 1:1000, 1980.

Stason WB et al. Furosemide: A clinical evaluation of its diuretic action. *Circulation* 34:910, 1966.

HYDROCORTISONE AND OTHER CORTICOSTEROIDS

TRADE NAMES	Solu-Cortef (hydrocortisone) Solu-Medrol (methylprednisolone) Decadron (dexamethasone)
THERAPEUTIC EFFECTS	Not fully understood. May diminish the severity of allergic and inflammatory reactions.
INDICATIONS	• As an ancillary measure in the treatment of SEVERE ALLERGIC STATES, such as anaphylaxis or status asthmaticus. • To decrease CEREBRAL EDEMA (dexamethasone or methylprednisolone only). • For treatment and perhaps prevention of ACUTE MOUNTAIN SICKNESS. • May prove useful in minimizing damage from SPINAL CORD INJURY. • To treat certain PULMONARY INJURIES, such as near drowning, aspiration, and toxic inhalations. (This use of the drug is controversial.)
CONTRAINDICATIONS	No contraindications to a single IV dose in the field.
SIDE EFFECTS	If administered too rapidly, especially in large doses, may cause *hypotension* and *cardiovascular collapse*. Otherwise, there are no significant side effects to a *single* dose of corticosteroid.
HOW SUPPLIED	• Hydrocortisone: powder in vials of 100 mg, 250 mg, 500 mg, and 1,000 mg, for reconstitution in the diluent fluid supplied. • Methylprednisolone: powder in vials containing 40 mg, 125 mg, 500 mg, and 1,000 mg, for reconstitution in the diluent fluid supplied. • Dexamethasone: 1-ml, 5-ml, and 25-ml vials; in 1-ml prefilled syringes, each containing 4 mg/ml.
ADMINISTRATION AND DOSAGE	In the field, corticosteroids are given by **slow intravenous injection.** • For *severe allergic reactions*: Hydrocortisone: **100 mg** slowly IV. Methylprednisolone: **20 mg** slowly IV. Dexamethasone: **4 mg** slowly IV. • For *cerebral edema* or *pulmonary injury*: Methylprednisolone: **50 mg** slowly IV. Dexamethasone: **10 mg** slowly IV. • For *spinal cord injury*: Methylprednisolone: Bolus of 30 mg/kg slowly IV followed by 5.4 mg/kg/hr by infusion (still experimental as of this writing). *Note*: It is advisable for each rescue service to stock only *one* of the steroid preparations listed and to learn the doses appropriate for that drug.

Further Discussion

Chapters 16, 22, 26, and 30.

References

Bowler SD et al. Corticosteroids in acute severe asthma: Effectiveness of low doses. *Thorax* 47:548, 1992.

Braakman R et al. Megadose steroids in severe head injury: Results of a prospective double-blind clinical trial. *J Neurosurg* 58:326, 1983.

Bracken MB et al. A randomized, controlled trial of methylprednisolone or naloxone in the treatment of acute spinal-cord injury. *N Engl J Med* 322:1405, 1990.

Bracken MB et al. Methylprednisolone or naloxone treatment after acute spinal cord injury: 1-year follow-up data. *J Neurosurg* 76:23, 1992.

Braughler JM et al. Current application of "high-dose" steroid therapy for CNS injury: A pharmacologic perspective. *J Neurosurg* 62:806, 1985.

Engel T et al. Glucocorticoid therapy in acute severe asthma: A critical review. *Eur Resp J* 4:881, 1991.

Fanta CH et al. Glucocorticoids in acute asthma: A critical controlled trial. *Am J Med* 74:845, 1983.

Giannotta SL et al. High dose glucocorticoids in the management of severe head injury. *Neurosurgery* 15:497, 1984.

Glenn TM (ed.). *Steroids and Shock.* Baltimore: University Park Press, 1974.

Hackett PH et al. Dexamethasone for prevention and treatment of acute mountain sickness. *Aviat Space Environ Med* 59:950, 1988.

Haskell RJ. A double-blind, randomized clinical trial of methylprednisolone in status asthmaticus. *Arch Intern Med* 143:1324, 1983.

Lucas CE et al. The cardiopulmonary response to massive doses of steroids in patients with septic shock. *Arch Surg* 119:537, 1984.

Molofsky WJ. Steroids and head trauma. *Neurosurgery* 15:424, 1984.

Munt PW, Fleetham JA. Corticosteroids and near-drowning. *Lancet* 1:665, 1978.

O'Neil BJ. Steroids: Drugs of a new age? *Emergency* 23(9):60, 1991.

Paris PM, Stewart RD, Deggler F. Prehospital use of dexamethasone in pulseless idioventricular rhythm. *Ann Emerg Med* 13:1008, 1984.

Peulen JG. *Steroids and Brain Edema.* New York: Springer-Verlag, 1972.

Quinn S et al. Corticosteroid therapy for septic shock: Review and analysis. *Drug Intell Clin Pharm* 14:247, 1980.

Rowe BH et al. Effectiveness of steroid therapy in acute exacerbations of asthma: A meta-analysis. *Am J Emerg Med* 10:301, 1992.

Sheagren J. Septic shock and corticosteroids. *N Engl J Med* 305:456, 1981.

Sladen A, Zauder HL. Methylprednisolone therapy for pulmonary edema following near drowning. *JAMA* 215:1793, 1971.

Sprung CL et al. The effects of high-dose corticosteroids in patients with septic shock: A prospective controlled study. *N Engl J Med* 311:1137, 1984.

Stein LM et al. Early administration of corticosteroids in emergency room treatment of acute asthma. *Ann Intern Med* 112:822, 1990.

Todd JK et al. Corticosteroid therapy for patients with toxic shock syndrome. *JAMA* 252:3399, 1984.

Weinberger M. Corticosteroids for exacerbations of asthma: Current status of the controversy. *Pediatrics* 8:726, 1988.

White B et al. Incidence, etiology, and outcome of pulseless idioventricular rhythm treated with dexamethasone during advanced CPR. *JACEP* 8:188, 1979.

Wilson RF, Fisher RR. The hemodynamic effects of massive steroids in shock. *Surg Gynecol Obstet* 127:769, 1968.

ISOETHARINE

TRADE NAME	Bronkosol
THERAPEUTIC EFFECTS	Sympathomimetic drug with predominant beta-2 activity; therefore relaxes bronchial smooth muscle to produce bronchodilatation.
INDICATIONS	For the control of bronchospasm in ASTHMA and other conditions complicated by bronchospasm, such as chronic obstructive pulmonary disease.
CONTRAINDICATIONS	• **Allergy** to any components of the mixture, including the acetone sodium bisulfite, to which some asthmatics are sensitive. • Must be used with *caution* in patients with **angina, hypertension,** and **tachyarrhythmias.**
SIDE EFFECTS	• *Tachycardia, palpitations.* • *Headache, dizziness, weakness.* • *Anxiety, restlessness.* • May cause paradoxical *bronchospasm* after excessive use. • May make *sputum pink* (which can be mistaken for hemoptysis).
HOW SUPPLIED	• In metered-dose inhaler (MDI). • As a 1% solution in bottles of 10 ml and 30 ml.
ADMINISTRATION AND DOSAGE	Given by **metered-dose inhaler** OR by **nebulizer.** *Dosage for MDI:* **1 to 2 inhalations**, preferably with a spacer. *Dosage for nebulizer.* Dilute **0.5 ml in 3 ml of saline** and administer **over 15 to 20 minutes.**
INCOMPATIBILITY	**Do not administer with epinephrine** or other sympathomimetic agents, since together they may cause excessive tachycardia.

Further Discussion

Chapters 22 and 30.

References

Emmerman CL et al. A randomized, controlled comparison of isoetharine and albuterol in the treatment of acute asthma. *Ann Emerg Med* 20:1090, 1991.

Newman LJ et al. Isoetharine-isoproterenol: A comparison of effects on childhood status asthmaticus. *Ann Allergy* 48:230, 1982.

ISOPROTERENOL

TRADE NAME	Isuprel
THERAPEUTIC EFFECTS	Pure beta sympathomimetic agent, hence increases the rate, force, and automaticity of the heart and decreases peripheral resistance (through vasodilatation). In addition, relaxes bronchial smooth muscles to produce bronchodilation.
INDICATIONS	Isoproterenol is no longer a first-line drug for any indication. In the field, it is used as a last resort in SYMPTOMATIC BRADYCARDIA when atropine and epinephrine have not been effective. It is also used (rarely) to treat inadvertent overdose with beta blockers such as labetalol.
CONTRAINDICATIONS	• Since isoproterenol markedly increases myocardial oxygen demand, the drug should not be given in **acute myocardial infarction** or **cardiogenic shock.** • Should not be given when there are **tachyarrhythmias.** • Should not be given together with **epinephrine,** since the effects may be additive.
SIDE EFFECTS	• *Tachycardia, palpitations, angina,* and sometimes *premature ventricular contractions (PVCs).* • May *increase infarct size* in acute myocardial infarction. • *Flushing, sweating, hypotension.* • *Anxiety, dizziness, tremor.*
HOW SUPPLIED	Solution of 0.2 mg/ml in ampules of 1 ml and 5 ml.
ADMINISTRATION AND DOSAGE	Given by **titrated intravenous infusion** (microdrip administration set). To prepare the infusion, add 1 mg (5 ml) of isoproterenol to 500 ml of D5/W, to yield a solution containing 2 μg/ml. START the infusion at **2 μg/min** (1 ml/min of the above dilution), and slowly increase the rate up to a maximum of 10 μg/min, as needed to produce an increase in heart rate to 60 beats/min.
INCOMPATIBILITY	Do not mix with *sodium bicarbonate,* since isoproterenol may be inactivated by alkaline solutions.

Further Discussion

Chapter 23.

References

Emergency Cardiac Care Committee and Subcommittees, American Heart Association. Guidelines for cardiopulmonary resuscitation and emergency cardiac care. *JAMA* 268:2171, 1992.

Holmes HR et al. Influence of adrenergic drugs upon vital organ perfusion during CPR. *Crit Care Med* 8:137, 1980.

Stamler JS et al. Treatment of complete heart block with inhaled beta-agonists. *Am Heart J* 124:1093, 1992.

Stark MF et al. Cardiovascular hemodynamic function in complete heart block and the effect of isopropyl norepinephrine. *Circulation* 17:526, 1950.

LABETALOL

TRADE NAMES	Normodyne, Trandate
THERAPEUTIC EFFECTS	• Alpha sympathetic *blocker* that reverses vasoconstriction.
	• Also a beta blocker, opposing the effects of beta agents on the heart, blood vessels, and lungs.

Thus labetalol can lower blood pressure (vasodilator effect) without producing the reflex tachycardia that usually accompanies a fall in blood pressure. The net effect, then, is to *reduce heart rate, cardiac output, and peripheral resistance.*

INDICATIONS	Control of blood pressure in HYPERTENSIVE CRISIS.
CONTRAINDICATIONS	• **Asthma.**
	• **Cardiac failure.**
	• **Heart block.**
	• **Cardiogenic shock.**
	• **Severe bradycardia.**
SIDE EFFECTS	• *Postural hypotension* if the patient is allowed to assume an upright posture within 3 hours of receiving the drug.
	• Occasional *dizziness* and *nausea.*
HOW SUPPLIED	20-ml and 40-ml ampules and 20-ml and 60-ml multidose vials in a concentration of 5 mg/ml.
ADMINISTRATION AND DOSAGE	Best given by **continuous infusion.** Add the contents of two 20-ml ampules (200 mg) to 160 ml of D5/W to yield a concentration of 1 mg/ml. Administer at a rate of **2 mg/min** (2 ml/min).
	• THE PATIENT MUST REMAIN SUPINE THROUGHOUT ADMINISTRATION OF THE DRUG AND FOR AT LEAST THREE HOURS AFTERWARD.
	• Continue the infusion until blood pressure falls to target level, then *stop the infusion.*
	• MONITOR blood pressure, pulse, and electrocardiogram throughout.
	• Have atropine and isoproterenol at hand.

Further Discussion

Chapter 23.

References

Cressman MD et al. Intravenous labetalol in the management of severe hypertension and hypertensive emergencies. *Am Heart J* 107:980, 1984.

Ferguson RK, Vlasses PH. Hypertensive emergencies and urgencies. *JAMA* 255:1605, 1986.

Huey J et al. Clinical evaluation of intravenous labetalol for the treatment of hypertensive urgency. *Am J Hypertens* 1(3, Part 3): 2845, 1988.

Labetalol for hypertension. *Med Lett* 26:83, 1984.

Lebel M et al. Labetalol infusion in hypertensive emergencies. *Clin Pharmacol Ther* 37:615, 1985.

Smith WB et al. Antihypertensive effectiveness of intravenous labetalol in accelerated hypertension. *Hypertension* 5:579, 1983.

LIDOCAINE

TRADE NAME	Xylocaine
THERAPEUTIC EFFECTS	• Suppresses ventricular ectopic activity by decreasing the excitability of heart muscle and of the electric conduction system of the heart.
	• Local anesthetic.

INDICATIONS

Lidocaine is the drug of first choice:
• To SUPPRESS PREMATURE VENTRICULAR CONTRACTIONS (PVCs) when
   1. They occur in the context of *myocardial ischemia.*
   2. They are *frequent* (more than 6/min).
   3. They occur in *salvos* (two or more in a row).
   4. They fall on the T wave (*R-on-T* phenomenon).
   5. They are *multifocal* (of different shapes and sizes).
• To PREVENT RECURRENCE OF VENTRICULAR FIBRILLATION after electric defibrillation.
• To treat VENTRICULAR TACHYCARDIA.
• For WIDE-COMPLEX PAROXYSMAL SUPRAVENTRICULAR TACHYCARDIA of uncertain type.
(*Note*: No longer considered useful as a prophylactic measure against ventricular fibrillation in myocardial infarction.)

CONTRAINDICATIONS

• Known history of **allergy** to lidocaine or local anesthetics (e.g., Novocain).
• Second or third-degree **heart block.**
• PVCs occurring in the context of **sinus bradycardia** or sinus arrest.
• **Idioventricular rhythm.**

SIDE EFFECTS

• By decreasing the force of cardiac contractions as well as decreasing peripheral resistance, may cause a *fall in cardiac output and blood pressure.*
• May cause *numbness, drowsiness,* or *confusion.*
• *Anxiety, tremors, muscle twitching, slurred speech, paresthesias.*
• When given in high doses, especially to the elderly or to patients in heart failure, may cause *seizures.*

HOW SUPPLIED

• Ampules and prefilled syringes containing 100 mg in 5 ml (20 mg/ml) for bolus injection.
• Vials of 1 or 2 gm for making up an infusion solution.

ADMINISTRATION AND DOSAGE

Given by **intravenous bolus and infusion.** If an intravenous route cannot be established, lidocaine may be given via the **endotracheal tube.**
Dosage:
• *In cardiac arrest, for recurrent ventricular fibrillation:* **1.5 mg/kg IV bolus.** May be repeated in 5 to 10 minutes if needed. When spontaneous circulation returns, start an **infusion of 2 mg/min.** To prepare the infusion, add 0.5 gm (500 mg) of lidocaine to 250 ml of D5/W, yielding a solution of 2 mg/ml. Use a microdrip infusion set for administration.
• *For PVCs and ventricular tachycardia:* Give **1 mg/kg IV push,** followed by an **infusion of 2 mg/min.** Prepare the infusion as described above.

> **Reduce the dosage of lidocaine (both bolus and infusion) by half for patients in congestive heart failure or shock and for patients over 70 years old.**

INCOMPATIBILITY   Do not give together with *beta blockers* or *dopamine*.

Further Discussion

Chapter 23.

References

Baron DW et al. Protective effect of lidocaine during regional myocardial ischemia. *Mayo Clin Proc* 57:442, 1982.

Bernsten RF et al. Lidocaine to prevent ventricular fibrillation in the prehospital phase of suspected acute myocardial infarction: The north Norwegian lidocaine intervention trial. *Am Heart J* 124:1478, 1992.

Borak J et al. Prophylactic lidocaine: Uncertain benefits in emergency settings. *Ann Emerg Med* 11:493, 1982.

Boster SR et al. Translaryngeal absorption of lidocaine. *Ann Emerg Med* 11:461, 1982.

Brown DL, Skiendzielewski JJ. Lidocaine toxicity. *Ann Emerg Med* 9:627, 1980.

Carruth JE, Silverman ME. Ventricular fibrillation complicating acute myocardial infarction: Reasons against the routine use of lidocaine. *Am Heart J* 104:545, 1982.

Chow MSS et al. Antifibrillatory effects of lidocaine and bretylium immediately postcardiopulmonary resuscitation. *Am Heart J* 110:938, 1985.

Dunn HM et al. Prophylactic lidocaine in the early phase of suspected myocardial infarction. *Am Heart J* 110:353, 1985.

Emergency Cardiac Care Committee and Subcommittees, American Heart Association. Guidelines for cardiopulmonary resuscitation and emergency cardiac care. *JAMA* 268:2171, 1992.

Hargarten K et al. Prehospital prophylactic lidocaine does not favorably affect outcome in patients with chest pain. *Ann Emerg Med* 19:1274, 1990.

Harrison DC et al. Should prophylactic antiarrhythmic drug therapy be used in acute myocardial infarction? *JAMA* 247:2019, 1982.

Harrison EE. Lidocaine in prehospital countershock refractory ventricular fibrillation. *Ann Emerg Med* 10:420, 1981.

Koster RW, Dunning AJ. Intramuscular lidocaine for prevention of lethal arrhythmias in the prehospitalization phase of acute myocardial infarction. *N Engl J Med* 313:1105, 1985.

Levy DB. Update on lidocaine. *Emergency* 20(9):15, 1988.

Lie KI. Pre- and in-hospital antiarrhythmic prevention of ventricular fibrillation complicating acute myocardial infarction. *Eur Heart J* 5(Suppl B):95, 1984.

Lie KI et al. Lidocaine in the prevention of primary ventricular fibrillation. *N Engl J Med* 291:1324, 1974.

MacDonald JL. Serum lidocaine levels during cardiopulmonary resuscitation after intravenous and endotracheal administration. *Crit Care Med* 13:914, 1985.

Mace SE. Effect of technique of administration on plasma lidocaine levels. *Ann Emerg Med* 15:552, 1986.

Mace SE. Effect of dilution on plasma lidocaine levels with endotracheal administration. *Ann Emerg Med* 16:522, 1987.

MacMahon S et al. Effects of prophylactic lidocaine in suspected acute myocardial infarction: An overview of results from the randomized, controlled trials. *JAMA* 260:1910, 1988.

Teo KK et al. Effects of prophylactic antiarrhythmic drug therapy in acute myocardial infarction: An overview of results from randomized controlled trials. *JAMA* 270:1589, 1993.

Valentine PA et al. Lidocaine in the prevention of sudden death in the prehospital phase of acute infarction. *N Engl J Med* 291:1327, 1974.

Waller ES. Appropriate lidocaine doses: Science added to the art. *Tex Med* 77:55, 1981.

Wennerblom B et al. Antiarrhythmic efficacy and side-effects of lidocaine given in the prehospital phase of acute myocardial infarction. *Eur Heart J* 3:516, 1982.

White RD. Lidocaine. *EMT J* 4(3):64, 1980.

Wyse DG, Kellen J, Rademaker AW. Prophylactic versus selective lidocaine for early ventricular arrhythmias of myocardial infarction. *J Am Coll Cardiol* 12:507, 1988.

MAGNESIUM SULFATE

THERAPEUTIC EFFECTS	• Central nervous system depressant.
	• Stabilizes muscle cell membranes by interacting with the sodium/potassium exchange system.
	• Smooth muscle relaxation, hence vasodilation and bronchodilation.
INDICATIONS	• For the treatment of ECLAMPSIA.
	• For PROPHYLAXIS OF CARDIAC DYSRHYTHMIAS in acute myocardial infarction.
	• For treatment of selected TACHYARRHYTHMIAS.
	• In the management of ACUTE ASTHMATIC ATTACKS.
CONTRAINDICATIONS	• **Renal disease.**
	• **Heart block.**
SIDE EFFECTS	Excessive dose may cause *respiratory depression* or even *cardiac arrest*.
HOW SUPPLIED	Ampules of 10%, 25%, or 50% solution.
ADMINISTRATION AND DOSAGE	In the field, given by **slow intravenous injection.** The patient should be monitored by electrocardiogram and also watched closely for respiratory depression. Deep tendon reflexes (e.g., knee jerk) should be tested frequently; if deep tendon reflexes become absent, the patient may be overdosed with magnesium, and it may be necessary to administer calcium gluconate as an antidote.

Dosage:
* For *eclampsia*: **2 to 4 gm IV** (i.e., 20–40 ml of a 10% solution) given **over at least 3 minutes.**
* For *acute myocardial infarction*: Add **2.4 gm** to 50 ml of D5/W and infuse over 20 to 60 minutes.
* For *tachyarrhythmias*: **2 gm IV** over 1 minute.
* For *acute asthmatic attacks*: **1.2 gm in 50 ml saline IV over 20 minutes.**

Keep calcium gluconate (10 ml of a 10% solution) ready in the event of inadvertent overdose and respiratory depression.

Further Discussion

Chapters 22, 23, and 35.

References

Abraham AS et al. Magnesium in the prevention of lethal arrhythmias in acute myocardial infarction. *Arch Intern Med* 147:753, 1987.

Allen BJ et al. Magnesium sulfate therapy for sustained monomorphic ventricular tachycardia. *Am J Cardiol* 64:1202, 1989.

Cannon LA. Magnesium levels in cardiac arrest victims: Relationship between magnesium levels and successful resuscitation. *Ann Emerg Med* 16:1195, 1987.

Carnes CA et al. Magnesium in the treatment of bronchial constriction. *Drug Intell Clin Pharm* 22:721, 1988.

Ceremuzynski L et al. Threatening arrhythmias in acute myocardial infarction are prevented by intravenous magnesium sulfate. *Am Heart J* 118:1333, 1989.

Eisenberg MJ. Magnesium deficiency and sudden death. *Am Heart J* 124:544, 1992.

Finklestein JA, O'Keefe KP, Butzin CA. Magnesium in acute myocardial infarction. *Ann Emerg Med* 22:754, 1993.

Gottlieb SS et al. Effects of intravenous magnesium sulfate on arrhythmias in patients with congestive heart failure. *Am Heart J* 125:1645, 1993.

Gullestad L et al. The effect of magnesium versus verapamil on supraventricular arrhythmias. *Clin Cardiol* 16:429, 1993.

Higgins GL. Magnesium medicine comes of age. *Emerg Med* 23(4):83, 1991.

Kaplan PW et al. No, magnesium sulfate should not be used in treating eclamptic seizures. *Arch Neurol* 45:1361, 1988.

Kuitert LM, Kletchko SL. Intravenous magnesium sulfate in acute life-threatening asthma. *Ann Emerg Med* 20:1243, 1991.

Noppen M et al. Bronchodilating effect of intravenous magnesium sulfate. *Chest* 97:373, 1990.

Okayama H et al. Treatment of status asthmaticus with intravenous magnesium sulfate. *J Asthma* 28:11, 1991.

Pritchard JA. The use of magnesium sulfate in preeclampsia-eclampsia. *J Reprod Med* 23:107, 1979.

Rasmussen HS et al. Intravenous magnesium in acute myocardial infarction. *Lancet* 1:234, 1986.

Rasmussen HS et al. Magnesium and acute myocardial infarction. *Arch Intern Med* 146:872, 1986.

Rasmussen HS et al. Magnesium deficiency in patients with ischemic heart disease with and without acute myocardial infarction uncovered by an intravenous loading test. *Arch Intern Med* 148:329, 1988.

Roden DM. Magnesium treatment of ventricular arrhythmias. *Am J Cardiol* 63:436, 1989.

Rubeiz GJ et al. Association of hypomagnesemia and mortality in acutely ill medical patients. *Crit Care Med* 21:203, 1993.

Salem M et al. Hypomagnesemia is a frequent finding in the emergency department in patients with chest pain. *Arch Intern Med* 151:2185, 1991.

Schecter M. Magnesium for acute MI. *Emerg Med* 25(9):135, 1993.

Sibai BM et al. Eclampsia: Observations from 67 recent cases. *Obstet Gynecol* 58:609, 1981.

Skobeloff EM et al. Intravenous magnesium sulfate for the treatment of acute asthma in the emergency department. *JAMA* 262:1210, 1989.

Smith LF et al. Intravenous infusion of magnesium sulphate after acute myocardial infarction: Effects on arrhythmias and mortality. *Int Cardiol* 12:175, 1986.

Teo KK et al. Effects of intravenous magnesium in suspected acute myocardial infarction: An overview of randomised trials. *Br Med J* 303:1499, 1991.

White JD. Treatment for hypertension with eclampsia. *Ann Emerg Med* 10:166, 1981.

Woods KL et al. Intravenous magnesium sulphate in suspected acute myocardial infarction: Results of the second Leicester intravenous magnesium intervention trial (LIMIT 2). *Lancet* 339:1553, 1992.

Yusuf S et al. Intravenous magnesium in acute myocardial infarction: An effective, safe, simple, and inexpensive intervention. *Circulation* 87:2043, 1993.

MANNITOL

TRADE NAME	Osmitrol
THERAPEUTIC EFFECTS	Because it remains in the vascular space, mannitol acts as an *osmotic diuretic*, to draw fluid out of cells and promote excretion of fluid from the body.
INDICATIONS	• For the treatment of CEREBRAL EDEMA after closed head injury, cardiac arrest, and other conditions. • To promote diuresis and thereby minimize the damaging effects of myoglobinuria in CRUSH INJURY or ELECTRIC INJURY. • To promote diuresis in selected DRUG OVERDOSES.
CONTRAINDICATIONS	• **Anuria** (absence of urine flow) or severe renal impairment. • **Intracranial hemorrhage.** • **Pregnancy.** • **Dehydration** or sodium depletion.
SIDE EFFECTS	• *Headache* and *nausea* in conscious patients. • *Fall in serum sodium* concentration. • May precipitate *congestive heart failure* in susceptible patients. • Extravasation will cause local *tissue necrosis*.
HOW SUPPLIED	• As a 5% or 10% solution in 1,000 ml. • As a 15% or 20% solution in 500 ml. READ THE LABEL CAREFULLY!
ADMINISTRATION AND DOSAGE	Given by **intravenous infusion** using an administration set containing an *in-line filter.* • The solution should be inspected to be certain it does not contain crystals. • The patient should have a urinary catheter in place before receiving a mannitol infusion. *Dosage*: **500 mg/kg** by IV infusion **over 15 minutes.** (Example: For a 70-kg man, dosage is 35 gm. If you are using a 20% solution, containing 200 mg/ml, you would thus give 175 ml.)

Further Discussion

Chapters 15 and 16.

References

Better OS et al. Early management of shock and prophylaxis of acute renal failure in traumatic rhabdomyolysis. *N Engl J Med* 322:825, 1990.

Domaingue CM et al. Hypotensive effect of mannitol administered rapidly. *Anaesth Intens Care* 13:134, 1985.
McGraw CP, Howard G. Effect of mannitol on increased intracranial pressure. *Neurosurgery* 13:269, 1983.
Nissenson AR et al. Mannitol. *West J Med* 131:277, 1979.
Safar P, Bircher NG. *Cardiopulmonary Cerebral Resuscitation.* Philadelphia: Saunders, 1988. P.249.
Wise BL, Chater M. Use of hypertonic mannitol solution to lower CSF pressure and decrease brain bulk in man. *Surg Forum* 12:398, 1961.

METARAMINOL

TRADE NAME	Aramine
THERAPEUTIC EFFECTS	Effects are about midway between those of epinephrine and norepinephrine; that is, metaraminol has some of the *beta* properties of epinephrine (producing an increased rate and force of cardiac contractions) as well as some of the *alpha* properties of norepinephrine (producing vasoconstriction). It is usually used as an alternative to norepinephrine for raising the blood pressure.
INDICATIONS	To increase blood pressure in certain cases of NEUROGENIC SHOCK or CARDIOGENIC SHOCK.
CONTRAINDICATIONS	Should not be used as first-line therapy in hypotension due to **hypovolemia,** where fluid replacement should precede the use of vasopressors.
SIDE EFFECTS	• Essentially the same as for norepinephrine. • Extravasation can cause local *tissue necrosis.* • Excessive dosage leads to *sweating, headache,* and *dysrhythmias.*
HOW SUPPLIED	1-ml ampules and 10-ml vials, in a concentration of 10 mg/ml.
ADMINISTRATION AND DOSAGE	Given by **titrated intravenous infusion** (microdrip infusion set). *Dosage:* To prepare the infusion, add 100 mg (10 ml) of metaraminol to 250 ml of D5/W, to yield a concentration of 0.4 mg/ml. START the infusion at a rate of about **0.2 mg/min** (0.5 ml/min), and gradually increase the rate of the infusion until the systolic blood pressure reaches about 90 mm Hg.

Further Discussion

Chapter 23.

References

Emergency Cardiac Care Committee and Subcommittees, American Heart Association. Guidelines for cardiopulmonary resuscitation and emergency cardiac care. *JAMA* 268:2171, 1992.

Zaimis E. Vasopressor drugs and catecholamines. *Anesthesiology* 29:732, 1968.

MORPHINE SULFATE

THERAPEUTIC EFFECTS	• Vasodilator: Decreases pulmonary edema by pooling blood in the peripheral circulation ("internal phlebotomy") and thereby reducing venous return to the heart; helps as well to allay the anxiety associated with pulmonary edema.
	• Potent analgesic, providing relief of pain in myocardial infarction and other conditions.
	• Lowers myocardial oxygen consumption.
INDICATIONS	• To treat PULMONARY EDEMA associated with congestive heart failure.
	• To relieve PAIN in myocardial infarction, burns, and other, selected conditions.
CONTRAINDICATIONS	• Significant **hypotension.**
	• **Respiratory depression,** except that caused by pulmonary edema, where the drug may be used if ventilatory support is provided.
	• **Asthma** and **chronic obstructive pulmonary disease.**
	• In patients who have taken **other depressant drugs,** such as alcohol or barbiturates.
	• **Head injury.**
	• Possible *inferior*-wall AMI (relative contraindication).
	• Undiagnosed **abdominal pain.**
	• Patients taking **monoamine oxidase (MAO) inhibitor** antidepressant drugs.
SIDE EFFECTS	• *Hypotension* (most likely in volume-depleted patients).
	• Increased vagal tone, leading to *bradycardia* (this effect can be reversed with atropine).
	• *Respiratory depression* (this effect can be reversed with naloxone).
	• *Nausea* and *vomiting.*
	• *Urinary retention.*
HOW SUPPLIED	• Prefilled 10-ml syringes containing 1 mg/ml.
	• 1-ml Tubex syringe containing 10 mg/ml.
ADMINISTRATION AND DOSAGE	Given by **titrated intravenous injections.**
	Dosage: 0.1 mg/kg. In the field, we usually give **2 to 5 mg** by slow IV push every 5 to 30 minutes until the desired therapeutic effect is achieved. **Do not exceed 15 mg in the field.**
	• If hypotension occurs, keep the patient flat, and do not give more of the drug.
	• Have *atropine* and *naloxone* immediately at hand to treat possible bradycardia or respiratory depression.
INCOMPATIBILITY	Should not be given to patients taking *tricyclic antidepressants* or *MAO inhibitors.*

Further Discussion

Chapters 15 and 23.

References

Alderman EL. Analgesics in the acute phase of myocardial infarction. *JAMA* 229:1646, 1974.

Chambers JA, Guly HR. The need for better pre-hospital analgesia. *Arch Emerg Med* 10(3):187, 1993.

Hoffman JR, Reynolds S. Comparison of nitroglycerin, morphine and furosemide in treatment of presumed pre-hospital pulmonary edema. *Chest* 92:586, 1987.

Lowenstein EL et al. Cardiovascular response to large doses of intravenous morphine in man. *N Engl J Med* 281:1389, 1969.

Robin ED, Cross CE, Zelis R. Pulmonary edema. *N Engl J Med* 288:239, 1973.

Semenkovich CF, Jaffe AS. Adverse effects due to morphine sulfate. *Am J Med* 79:325, 1985.

Zelis R et al. The cardiovascular effects of morphine. *J Clin Invest* 54:1247, 1974.

NALOXONE

TRADE NAME	Narcan
THERAPEUTIC EFFECTS	Specific antidote for narcotic agents. Reverses the effects of all narcotic drugs, including heroin, morphine, methadone, codeine, meperidine (Demerol, Pethidine), hydromorphone (Dilaudid), paregoric, fentanyl, and Percodan. Also effective against pentazocine (Talwin), propoxyphene (Darvon), nalbuphine (Nubain), and butorphanol (Stadol). Naloxone will reverse stupor, coma, and respiratory depression *when they are due to narcotic overdose.* Naloxone is not usually effective in reversing coma from other causes.
INDICATIONS	• To treat known NARCOTIC OVERDOSE. • To treat COMA OF UNKNOWN CAUSE when patient has failed to respond to D50.
CONTRAINDICATIONS	None.
SIDE EFFECTS	• Too rapid administration may precipitate *vomiting* and *ventricular dysrhythmias.* • Administration to people who are physically dependent on narcotics may precipitate an *acute withdrawal syndrome.* For that reason, naloxone should be given very slowly, using improvement of respiratory status as an end point. • In general, the duration of action of naloxone is shorter than that of the narcotics it is used to counteract. Thus, the patient who has been successfully roused with naloxone may *fall back into stupor or coma* as the naloxone wears off. Patients treated with naloxone must therefore be watched closely, and the dose of naloxone should be repeated as necessary. • Has been reported to cause pulmonary edema and sudden death in very rare cases.
HOW SUPPLIED	• 1-ml ampules or prefilled syringes of 0.4 mg/ml. • 2-ml ampules of 1 mg/ml. • 10-ml vials of 0.4 mg/ml or 1 mg/ml. • 1-ml and 2-ml prefilled syringes of 1 mg/ml. READ THE LABEL CAREFULLY!
ADMINISTRATION AND DOSAGE	In the field, given by **slow intravenous injection,** but may be given via **endotracheal tube** (diluted) or by **intralingual injection** if intravenous access cannot be secured. *Dosage* (for intravenous administration): Draw up **0.8 mg** of naloxone in a 10-ml syringe. Fill the remainder of the syringe with D5/W. Administer this solution SLOWLY IV while monitoring the rate and depth of the patient's respirations. As soon as there is improvement in the respirations, stop giving the drug. It is preferable NOT to wake the patient up completely in the field, since many of these patients "come up fighting." If there is no response to the first dose, repeat the dose up to two more times (i.e., a total dose of 2.4 mg). If there is still no response, suspect another cause for the patient's coma. For *endotracheal administration*, dilute **0.8 mg in 5 to 10 ml normal saline.** For *intralingual injection*, give **2.0 mg** in a single injection into the vascular plexus beneath the tongue.

Further Discussion

Chapters 24 and 27.

References

Andress RA. Sudden death following naloxone administration. *Anesth Analg* 59:782, 1980.

Baskin DS, Hosobuchi Y. Naloxone reversal of ischaemic neurologic deficits in man. *Lancet* 2:272, 1981.

Bradberry JC et al. Continuous infusion of naloxone in the treatment of narcotic overdose. *Drug Intell Clin Pharm* 15:945, 1981.

Cuss FM et al. Cardiac arrest after reversal of effects of opiates with naloxone. *Br Med J* 288:363, 1984.

Fallis RJ et al. A double blind trial of naloxone in the treatment of acute stroke. *Stroke* 15:627, 1984.

Goldfrank LR. The several uses of naloxone. *Emerg Med* 16(10):105, 1984.

Handal KA, Schauben JL, Salamone FR. Naloxone. *Ann Emerg Med* 12:438, 1983.

Hoffman J et al. The empiric use of naloxone in patients with altered mental status: A reappraisal. *Ann Emerg Med* 20:246, 1991.

Kunkel DB. Narcotic antagonist update. *Emerg Med* 19(5):97, 1987.

Levy DB. Naloxone: Negating narcotics. *Emergency* 22(7):16, 1990.

Levy DB. Naloxone: Use in shock. *Emergency* 22(8):14, 1990.

Lewis JM et al. Continuous naloxone infusion in pediatric narcotic overdose. *Am J Dis Child* 138:944, 1984.

Martin WR. Naloxone. *Ann Intern Med* 85:765, 1976.

McFeely EJ. Naloxone: A narcotic antagonist. *Emerg Med Serv* 14(10):70, 1985.

Michiels TM et al. Naloxone reverses ethanol-induced depression of hypercapnic drive. *Am Rev Respir Dis* 128:823, 1983.

Milme B et al. Naloxone: New therapeutic roles. *Can Anaesth Soc J* 31:272, 1984.

Moore RA et al. Naloxone: Underdosage after narcotic poisoning. *Am J Dis Child* 134:156, 1980.

Neal JM. Complications of naloxone. *Ann Emerg Med* 17:765, 1988.

Pallasch TJ, Gill CJ. Naloxone-associated morbidity and mortality. *Oral Surg Oral Med Oral Pathol* 52:602, 1981.

Prough DS et al. Acute pulmonary edema in healthy teenagers following conservative doses of intravenous naloxone. *Anesthesiology* 60:485, 1984.

Tandberg D, Abercrombie D. Treatment of heroin overdose with endotracheal naloxone. *Ann Emerg Med* 11:443, 1982.

Yealy DM et al. The safety of prehospital naloxone administration by paramedics. *Ann Emerg Med* 19:902, 1990.

NIFEDIPINE

TRADE NAMES	Adalat, Procardia
THERAPEUTIC EFFECTS	Calcium channel blocker; acts by inhibiting the influx of calcium ions into cardiac and smooth muscle, thereby inhibiting the contractile process. Nifedipine thus *dilates coronary arteries, reduces afterload* (by dilating peripheral arteries), and thereby both increases myocardial blood supply *and* decreases myocardial work (thus myocardial oxygen demand).
INDICATIONS	• ANGINA, especially that caused by coronary artery spasm. (This is the only FDA-approved indication.) • HYPERTENSIVE CRISIS (not yet FDA-approved for this indication.)
CONTRAINDICATIONS	Known **allergy** to the drug.
SIDE EFFECTS	• May produce *excessive hypotension.* • *Dizziness.* • *Flushing* or sensations of heat. • *Weakness.* • *Nausea, heartburn.*
HOW SUPPLIED	Soft gelatin capsules of 10 mg and 20 mg.
ADMINISTRATION AND DOSAGE	In hypertensive crisis, use a hypodermic needle to puncture several holes in a **10-mg** capsule; then place the capsule **under the patient's tongue.** Alternatively, the patient may bite open the capsule and swallow the contents.
INCOMPATIBILITY	May potentiate the effects of *beta blocking agents*, leading to heart failure.

Further Discussion

Chapter 23.

References

Bertel O. Nifedipine in hypertensive emergencies. *Br Med J* 286:19, 1983.

Haft JI. Use of the calcium channel blocker nifedipine in the management of hypertensive emergency. *Am J Emerg Med* Suppl 3(6):25, 1985.

Haft JI, Litterer WE. Chewing nifedipine to rapidly treat hypertension. *Arch Intern Med* 144:2357, 1984.

Houston MC. Comparative effects of clonidine hydrochloride and nifedipine in the treatment of hypertensive crisis. *Am Heart J* 115:1, 1988.

Jaker M et al. Oral nifedipine vs. oral clonidine in the treatment of urgent hypertension. *Arch Intern Med* 149:260, 1989.

Olivari MT et al. Treatment of hypertension with nifedipine, a calcium antagonist agent. *Circulation* 59:1056, 1979.

Phillips RA. Nifedipine and hypertensive urgencies. *Emerg Med* 22(15):91, 1990.

Romaska EA et al. A one-year evaluation of calcium channel blocker overdoses: Toxicity and treatment. *Ann Emerg Med* 22:196, 1993.

Wright S. Use of nifedipine in hypertensive emergencies. *J Emerg Med* 6:548, 1988.

NITROGLYCERIN

THERAPEUTIC EFFECTS

The primary pharmacologic effect of nitroglycerin and related drugs is to *relax smooth muscle,* and the effects of nitroglycerin on the cardiovascular system are chiefly due to relaxation of *vascular* smooth muscle—hence, *vasodilation.*
- Nitroglycerin provides relief of pain in angina, probably by dilating coronary arteries and thereby increasing blood flow through them as well as by decreasing myocardial oxygen demand.
- Through its vasodilating action on peripheral vessels, nitroglycerin promotes pooling of the blood in the systemic circulation ("internal phlebotomy") and decreases the resistance against which the heart has to pump (the afterload); those effects are useful in treating congestive heart failure.

INDICATIONS

- To relieve the pain of ANGINA.
- To reduce infarct size in MYOCARDIAL INFARCTION.
- To treat selected cases of PULMONARY EDEMA due to CONGESTIVE HEART FAILURE.
- When applied topically, to DILATE VEINS FOR VENIPUNCTURE to facilitate starting an IV.

CONTRAINDICATIONS

- **Increased intracranial pressure.**
- **Glaucoma.**
- **Hypovolemia.**
- **Hypotension**, especially with brady- or tachycardia.
- **Epigastric distress** or **hiccups** accompanying symptoms of AMI (because they suggest *inferior*-wall AMI).

SIDE EFFECTS

- Transient, throbbing *headache.* (If the headache does *not* occur, suspect that the nitroglycerin is outdated and no longer potent.)
- *Hypotension, dizziness, weakness.*
- *Flushing,* feelings of warmth.

HOW SUPPLIED

Many forms, including tablets, sustained-release capsules, ointments, patches. For use in the field, tablets of 0.3 or 0.4 mg are preferred. (For topical application, use the ointment or paste form.)

ADMINISTRATION AND DOSAGE

Given **sublingually** (under the tongue).
Dosage: One **0.3- or 0.4-mg tablet** under the tongue for angina, AMI, or congestive heart failure. May repeat once after 3 minutes. If hypotension occurs, elevate the patient's legs and give IV fluids as per physician's order.
For dilating a vein to facilitate starting an IV in children, apply the nitroglycerin ointment to the skin over the vein and wait at least 5 minutes.

INCOMPATIBILITY

Do not give to a patient who has been drinking alcohol.

Further Discussion

Chapters 23 and 30.

References

Abrams J. Nitroglycerin and long-acting nitrates. *N Engl J Med* 302:1234, 1980.

Abrams J. Vasodilator therapy for chronic congestive heart failure. *JAMA* 254:3070, 1985.

Abrams J. A reappraisal of nitrate therapy. *JAMA* 259:396, 1988.

Armstrong PW et al. Pharmacokinetic-hemodynamic studies of nitroglycerin ointment in congestive heart failure. *Am J Cardiol* 4:670, 1980.

Brandes W et al. Nitroglycerin-induced hypotension,

bradycardia, and asystole: Report of a case and review of the literature. *Clin Cardiol* 13:741, 1990.

Chatterjee K et al. Combination vasodilator therapy for severe chronic congestive heart failure. *Ann Intern Med* 85:467, 1976.

Cohn JN, Franciosa JA. Vasodilator therapy of cardiac failure. *N Engl J Med* 297:27, 254, 1977.

Hecker JF et al. Nitroglycerin ointment as an aid to venepuncture. *Lancet* 1:332, 1983.

Herman LL et al. The prehospital use of nitroglycerin according to standing medical orders in an urban EMS system. *Prehosp Disaster Med* 8:29, 1993.

Hoffman JR, Reynolds S. Comparison of nitroglycerin, morphine and furosemide in treatment of presumed pre-hospital pulmonary edema. *Chest* 92:586, 1987.

Markiewicz W et al. Sublingual isosorbide dinitrate in severe congestive failure. *Cardiology* 67:172, 1981.

Nitroglycerin patches. *Med Lett* 26:59, 1984.

Pit WA et al. Effect of intravenous nitroglycerin on hemo-dynamics of congestive heart failure. *Angiology* 33:294, 1982.

Rajfer SI et al. Sustained beneficial hemodynamic responses to large doses of transdermal nitroglycerin in congestive heart failure and comparison with intravenous nitroglycerin. *Am J Cardiol* 54:120, 1984.

Roberge RJ. Facilitated intravenous access through local application of nitroglycerin ointment. *Ann Emerg Med* 16:546, 1987.

Rottman SJ, Larmon B. Nitroglycerin lingual aerosol in prehospital care. *Prehosp Disaster Med* 4(1):11, 1989.

Vaksmann G et al. Nitroglycerin ointment as an aid to venous cannulation in children. *J Pediatr* 111:89, 1987.

Wuerz R et al. Safety of prehospital nitroglycerin. *Ann Emerg Med* 23:31, 1994.

Wulf-Dirk B, Schupp D. Effect of sublingual nitroglycerin in emergency treatment of severe pulmonary edema. *Am J Cardiol* 41:931, 1978.

NITROUS OXIDE

TRADE NAMES	Nitronox, Entonox
THERAPEUTIC EFFECTS	Provides rapid, easily reversible relief of pain.
INDICATIONS	Relief of PAIN from

Relief of PAIN from
- Acute myocardial infarction.
- Musculoskeletal trauma.
- Burns.
- Other conditions (*e.g.,* ureteral colic, labor).

CONTRAINDICATIONS
- Any **altered state of consciousness,** such as **head injury** (masks neurologic signs one needs to monitor).
- **Chronic obstructive pulmonary disease.**
- Acute **pulmonary edema** (these patients need 100% oxygen).
- Known **pneumothorax** or **chest injury** where pneumothorax may be present (nitrous oxide collects in dead air spaces and may thus expand a pneumothorax).
- **Abdominal distention** or abdominal trauma where bowel sounds are absent.
- Major **facial injury.**
- **Shock.**
- **Decompression sickness.**
- **Air embolism** from any source.

SIDE EFFECTS
- *Light-headedness, drowsiness.*
- Occasional *nausea* and *vomiting.*
- Ambulance crew may experience *giddiness* if the vehicle is not properly vented.

HOW SUPPLIED

In the United States, nitrous oxide for field use is supplied as Nitronox, a set containing an oxygen cylinder and a nitrous oxide cylinder, joined by a valve that regulates flow to provide a fixed 50 : 50 mixture of the two gases. The gas mixture is piped to a demand valve apparatus. In Canada, D and E cylinders color-coded blue and white contain a premix of the two gases; such cylinders must be inverted several times before use to ensure thorough mixing.

ADMINISTRATION AND DOSAGE

Nitrous oxide is **self-administered by inhalation.** The patient is instructed to hold the mask to his or her face, to form a tight seal around the nose and mouth, and to breathe normally. As the patient becomes drowsy, the mask will drop away from his or her face. THE PATIENT MUST CONTROL THE DEMAND VALVE HIMSELF. The paramedic should not hold the face mask in place for the patient, for overdosage may result.

Further Discussion

Chapter 23.

References

Amey BD et al. Prehospital administration of nitrous oxide for control of pain. *Ann Emerg Med* 10:279, 1981.

Ancker K et al. Nitrous oxide analgesia during ambulance transportation: Airborne levels of nitrous oxide. *Acta Anaesthesiol Scand* 24:497, 1980.

Ballinger JA. Experience with prehospital administration of nitrous oxide. *Emerg Med Serv* 8(5):14, 1979.

Baskett PJ. Entonox. *Proc R Soc Med* 65:7, 1972.

Baskett PJ, Withnell A. Use of Entonox in the ambulance service. *Br Med J* 2:41, 1970.

Donen N et al. Pre-hospital analgesia with Entonox. *Can Anaesth Soc J* 29:275, 1982.

Gamis AS, Knapp JF, Glenski JA. Nitrous oxide analgesia in a pediatric emergency department. *Ann Emerg Med* 18:177, 1989.

James MFM et al. Nitrous oxide analgesia and altitude. *Anaesthesia* 37:285, 1982.

Johnson JL, Atherton GL. Effectiveness of nitrous oxide in a rural EMS system. *J Emerg Med* 9:45, 1991.

Kunkel DB. Nitrous oxide: Not a laughing matter anymore. *Emerg Med* 21(3):117, 1989.

McKinnon DDL. Prehospital analgesia with nitrous oxide/oxygen. *Can Med Assoc J* 125:836, 1981.

McKinnon DDL et al. Nitrous oxide analgesia in emergency care. *Can Fam Physician* 26:83, 1980.

Mitchell MM et al. Nitrous oxide does not induce myocardial ischemia in patients with ischemic heart disease and poor ventricular function. *Anesthesiology* 7:526, 1989.

Stewart RD. Nitrous oxide sedation/analgesia in emergency medicine. *Ann Emerg Med* 14:139, 1985.

Stewart RD et al. Patient-controlled inhalation analgesia in prehospital care: A study of side effects and feasibility. *Crit Care Med* 11:851, 1983.

Thal ER et al. Self-administered analgesia with nitrous oxide. *JAMA* 242:2418, 1979.

Thompson PL, Lown B. Nitrous oxide as an analgesic in acute myocardial infarction. *JAMA* 235:924, 1976.

Wright PM Jr. Nitrous oxide: An analgesic for field use. *Emerg Med Serv* 13(3):61, 1984.

NOREPINEPHRINE

TRADE NAME	Levophed
THERAPEUTIC EFFECTS	Chiefly an *alpha* sympathetic agent; therefore, it increases blood pressure by constricting arteries. It also has some beta activity, although less than epinephrine, and thus increases the force of cardiac contractions.

INDICATIONS
- To increase blood pressure in states of low total peripheral resistance, such as NEUROGENIC SHOCK or some cases of CARDIOGENIC SHOCK.
- For BLOOD PRESSURE SUPPORT AFTER cardiopulmonary resuscitation.

CONTRAINDICATIONS
- Should not be used as first-line therapy in **hypovolemic shock,** where fluid replacement should precede the use of vasopressors.
- Should not be used in patients with severe **hypoxia** or **hypercarbia.**
- Should be used with extreme caution in patients with **myocardial infarction,** since norepinephrine increases myocardial oxygen requirements.

SIDE EFFECTS
- *Necrosis* of tissue surrounding the IV catheter can occur if the IV infiltrates or if the norepinephrine solution leaks from the vein. For that reason, the IV should be established in a large vein and checked closely before a norepinephrine drip is hung. Do not use hand veins or leg veins for norepinephrine infusions. If extravasation occurs, phentolamine, 5 to 10 mg in 10 to 15 ml of saline, should be infiltrated as soon as possible into the area of extravasation to prevent sloughing of soft tissues.
- Within the therapeutic range, there are few other side effects. However, if the IV is inadvertently speeded up and the patient receives more than the therapeutic dose, he may experience severe *headache, sweating, nausea, vomiting, anxiety, ventricular dysrhythmias,* and severe *hypertension.*

> **WATCH A NOREPINEPRHINE DRIP LIKE A HAWK!**

HOW SUPPLIED	Ampules of 4 ml containing 4 mg (1 mg/ml).
ADMINISTRATION AND DOSAGE	Given by **titrated intravenous infusion** (microdrip infusion set). To make up the infusion, add 4 mg (4 ml) of norepinephrine to 500 ml of D5/W to yield a solution containing 8 µg/ml. START the infusion at **4 µg/min** (0.5 ml/min of the above dilution), and slowly increase the rate, rechecking the blood pressure after each increase, until the systolic blood pressure reaches about 90 mm Hg. Run the infusion at the rate necessary to maintain that level of blood pressure.
INCOMPATIBILITY	May cause severe, prolonged hypertension in patients taking *antidepressant medications.* Do not administer norepinephrine in the same IV line with *alkaline solutions* (e.g., sodium bicarbonate), which may inactivate the norepinephrine.

Further Discussion

Chapter 23.

References

Emergency Cardiac Care Committee and Subcommittees, American Heart Association. Guidelines for cardiopulmonary resuscitation and emergency cardiac care. *JAMA* 268:2171, 1992.

OXYGEN

THERAPEUTIC EFFECTS	Reverses the deleterious effects of hypoxemia on the brain, heart, and other vital organs.
INDICATIONS	Any condition in which systemic or local hypoxemia may be present:

- CARDIAC or RESPIRATORY ARREST (given with artificial ventilation).
- DYSPNEA or RESPIRATORY DISTRESS from any cause.
- CHEST PAIN.
- SHOCK.
- COMA from any cause.
- CHEST TRAUMA.
- NEAR DROWNING.
- PULMONARY EDEMA.
- TOXIC INHALATIONS (smoke, chemicals, carbon monoxide).
- Acute ASTHMATIC ATTACK.
- ACUTE DECOMPENSATION OF COPD.
- STROKE, HEAD INJURY.
- STATUS EPILEPTICUS.
- Any patient in CRITICAL CONDITION.

CONTRAINDICATIONS	**None.** May depress respirations in *rare* patients with chronic obstructive pulmonary disease. That is *not* a contraindication to its use, but simply means that such patients must be closely monitored and assisted to breathe if the respiratory rate declines.
SIDE EFFECTS	None when given for short periods (less than 24 hours) to adults.
HOW SUPPLIED	As a compressed gas in cylinders of various sizes.
ADMINISTRATION AND DOSAGE	Administered by **inhalation** from a mask, nasal cannula, endotracheal tube, etc. A patent airway and adequate ventilation must be ensured. Dosage depends on the condition being treated. For cardiac arrest and other conditions of large shunt, **100% oxygen** should be given as soon as possible.

Further Discussion

Chapter 8 and all chapters on clinical conditions.

References

Aberman A. On understanding oxygen transport. *Emerg Med* 14(7):116, 1982.

Aubier M et al. Central respiratory drive in acute respiratory failure of patients with chronic obstructive pulmonary disease. *Am Rev Respir Dis* 122:191, 1980.

Bourne S. Gearing for oxygen delivery. *JEMS* 13(8):58, 1988.

Campbell EJ et al. Subjective effects of humidification of oxygen for delivery by nasal cannula: A prospective study. *Chest* 93:289, 1988.

Campbell TP et al. Oxygen enrichment of bag-valve-mask units during positive-pressure ventilation: A comparison of various techniques. *Ann Emerg Med* 17:232, 1988.

Caroline NL. *Emergency Medical Treatment: A Text for EMT-As and EMT-Intermediates* (3rd ed.). Boston: Little, Brown, 1991. Chap. 9.

Christopher KL et al. Transtracheal oxygen therapy for refractory hypoxemia. *JAMA* 256:494, 1986.

Corley M et al. The myth of 100% oxygen delivery through manual resuscitation bags. *J Emerg Nursing* 19:45, 1993.

Doyle DJ. The rational use of medical oxygen. *Emerg Med* 24(12):215, 1992.

Feinsilver SH. Oxygen toxicity. *Emerg Med* 23(3):89, 1991.

Gaull ES. Are you overlooking O_2? *Emerg Med Serv* 22(6):31, 1993.

Peters WR, Jolly PC. Gastric rupture from nasal oxygen catheter. *Bull Mason Clin* 26:70, 1972.

Sassoon CSH, Hassell KT, Mahutte CK. Hyperoxic-induced hypercapnia in stable chronic obstructive pulmonary disease. *Am Rev Respir Dis* 135:907, 1987.

Selinger SR et al. Effects of removing oxygen from patients with chronic obstructive pulmonary disease. *Am Rev Respir Dis* 136:85, 1987.

Shannon T, Celli B. Oxygen therapy. *Emerg Med* 23(21):63, 1991.

Shelly RW. Oxygen administration. *JEMS* 7(7):37, 1983.

Skorodin MS. Current oxygen prescribing practices: Problems and prospects. *JAMA* 255:3283, 1986.

Tinits P. Oxygen therapy and oxygen toxicity. *Ann Emerg Med* 12:321, 1983.

Waxman K. Oxygen delivery and resuscitation. *Ann Emerg Med* 15:1420, 1986.

White RD. Essential drugs in emergency care. *EMT J* 1(4):51, 1977.

OXYTOCIN

TRADE NAMES	Pitocin, Syntocinon
THERAPEUTIC EFFECTS	Promotes contraction of the uterus toward its normal size after delivery; the contracting uterine muscle squeezes down on uterine blood vessels and thereby reduces postpartum bleeding.
INDICATIONS	To improve uterine contraction and thereby CONTROL POST-PARTUM BLEEDING *after delivery of the placenta.*
CONTRAINDICATIONS	• Previous **cesarean section.** • **Twin pregnancy,** before the birth of the second baby.
SIDE EFFECTS	Side effects are rare when oxytocin is given after the second stage of labor, but may include • *Nausea* and *vomiting.* • Cardiac *dysrhythmias.* • *Allergic reactions* to the drug.
HOW SUPPLIED	Ampules and prefilled syringes containing 10 units in 1 ml.
ADMINISTRATION AND DOSAGE	Given by **intravenous infusion.** Inject **10 units** (1 ml) of oxytocin into **1,000 ml of normal saline,** and infuse at the rate ordered.
INCOMPATIBILITY	Do not administer to patients receiving *vasopressor* drugs, as the combination may cause dangerous levels of hypertension.

Further Discussion

Chapter 35.

References

Doan-Wiggins L. Oxytocin use in prehospital care. *Emerg Med Serv* 21(8):27, 1992.

Levy DB et al. A last resort for postpartum hemorrhage. *Emergency* 22(5):16, 1990.

Schwartz RH. *Handbook of Obstetric Emergencies.* Flushing, N.Y.: Medical Examination Publishing, 1975.

PROPRANOLOL

TRADE NAME	Inderal
THERAPEUTIC EFFECTS	Nonselective beta-1 and beta-2 blocker; thus it opposes the effects of beta agents on the heart, lungs, and blood vessels. The most important effects are on the heart, where propranolol

- Decreases the sinus rate.
- Slows atrial conduction.
- Delays conduction through the atrioventricular (AV) node.
- Depresses spontaneous electric activity and muscular force.

INDICATIONS	

- Control of SUPRAVENTRICULAR TACHYCARDIAS.
- Prevention of recurrent VENTRICULAR TACHYCARDIA.
- To slow the ventricular rate in ATRIAL FLUTTER and ATRIAL FIBRILLATION when digitalis is contraindicated.
- To reduce the incidence of ventricular fibrillation AFTER ACUTE MYOCARDIAL INFARCTION in patients who did not receive thrombolytic therapy.

CONTRAINDICATIONS	

- **Asthma** or **chronic obstructive pulmonary disease.**
- Patients with **hay fever** during the pollen season.
- Sinus bradycardia; second- or third-degree **heart block.**
- Congestive **heart failure.**
- Any state in which **cardiac function** is **depressed** (e.g., immediately after resuscitation from cardiac arrest).

SIDE EFFECTS	

- *Hypotension* and/or *heart failure.*
- *Bronchospasm.*
- *Nausea* and *vomiting.*
- May *mask symptoms of hypoglycemia* in diabetics.

HOW SUPPLIED	Ampules of 1 ml containing 1 mg.
ADMINISTRATION AND DOSAGE	In the field, given by **slow intravenous injection.** *Dosage:* **1 mg** injected IV **over 5 minutes.** If there is no response, a second dose of 0.5 mg may be given slowly IV 5 to 10 minutes after the first dose.
INCOMPATIBILITY	Do not give together with *sympathomimetics* (such as epinephrine), *aminophylline,* or known cardiac depressants.

Further Discussion

Chapter 23.

References

Coodley EL, Snyder S. Propranolol and management of arrhythmias. *Am Fam Physician* 14(5):146, 1976.

Danahy DT, Aronow WS. Assessing antiarrhythmic actions: III. Propranolol. *Drug Ther Bull* 1:48, 1977.

Miller CD. Get up to speed on beta blockers. *JEMS* 19(1):78, 1994.

Morrelli HF. Propranolol. *Ann Intern Med* 78:913, 1973.

Norris RM et al. Prevention of ventricular fibrillation during acute myocardial infarction by intravenous propranolol. *Lancet* 2:833, 1984.

Shand DG. Propranolol. *N Engl J Med* 293:280, 1975.

Zharadwaja K, Promisloff R. Clinical pharmacology of propranolol. *Drug Ther Bull* 3:22, 1977.

SODIUM BICARBONATE

THERAPEUTIC EFFECTS	By neutralizing excess acid, helps return the blood and body fluids toward a physiologic pH, in which metabolic processes and sympathomimetic agents work more effectively.

INDICATIONS	• To treat METABOLIC ACIDOSIS as in
	  1. Certain POISONINGS (e.g., ethylene glycol).
	  2. SHOCK and other low-output states (e.g., after resuscitation from cardiac arrest).
	• To treat HYPERKALEMIA (high serum potassium).
	• To promote the excretion of some types of BARBITURATES taken in OVERDOSE.
	• To promote excretion of myoglobin in CRUSH INJURIES and ELECTROCUTION.
	• In some cases of STATUS ASTHMATICUS.
	• In PROLONGED CARDIOPULMONARY RESUSCITATION (CPR).

CONTRAINDICATIONS	• **Hypokalemia** (low serum potassium), sometimes detectable by large, prominent P waves, large U waves, and flattened T waves on the ECG. • Conditions in which the patient cannot tolerate a salt load, such as **congestive heart failure.**
SIDE EFFECTS	• Because each milliequivalent of bicarbonate comes along with a milliequivalent of sodium, sodium bicarbonate has the same effect as any other salt-containing solution; that is, it *increases the vascular volume.* Three 50-ml syringes of sodium bicarbonate (1 mEq/ml) contain approximately the same amount of salt as 1 liter of normal saline. Patients in borderline heart failure cannot tolerate salt loads of that magnitude and may be plunged into *pulmonary edema.* • Administration of sodium bicarbonate *lowers the serum potassium.* When bicarbonate is used to treat hyperkalemia, that is the desired effect. However, in cardiac patients, the heart becomes irritable if the potassium falls too low, and *dysrhythmias* may occur, especially in patients taking diuretics. • Sodium bicarbonate administration transiently *raises the arterial* PCO_2, so its administration must be accompanied by controlled hyperventilation (e.g., with a bag-valve-mask) to blow off the excess carbon dioxide.
HOW SUPPLIED	Vials and prefilled syringes of 50 ml containing 1 mEq/ml.
ADMINISTRATION AND DOSAGE	Given by **bolus injection.** *Dosage*: • For *cardiac arrest*: If used at all, **1 mEq/kg** after the first 10 minutes of CPR. Acidosis should thereafter be prevented by hyperventilation. • For *other conditions,* as ordered by physician.
INCOMPATIBILITY	• Do not give together with *calcium* salts, for the combination will produce a chalky precipitate of calcium carbonate. • Do not give together with *sympathomimetic* drugs (e.g., epinephrine), which will be inactivated in an alkaline solution.

Further Discussion

Chapters 9, 22, 23, 27, and 30.

References

Aufderheide TP et al. Prehospital bicarbonate use in cardiac arrest: A 3-year experience. *Am J Emerg Med* 10:4, 1992.

Bersin RM et al. Metabolic and hemodynamic consequences of sodium bicarbonate administration in patients with heart disease. *Am J Med* 87:7, 1989.

Better OS et al. Early management of shock and prophylaxis of acute renal failure in traumatic rhabdomyolysis. *N Engl J Med* 322:825, 1990.

Bishop RL, Weisfeldt ML. Sodium bicarbonate administration during cardiac arrest. *JAMA* 235:506, 1976.

Cooper DJ et al. Bicarbonate does not improve hemodynamics in critically ill patients who have lactic acidosis. *Ann Intern Med* 112:492, 1990.

Emergency Cardiac Care Committee and Subcommittees, American Heart Association. Guidelines for cardiopulmonary resuscitation and emergency cardiac care. *JAMA* 268:2171, 1992.

Frederick C et al. The effect of bicarbonate on resuscitation from cardiac arrest. *Ann Emerg Med* 20:1173, 1991.

Graf H et al. The use of sodium bicarbonate in the therapy of organic acidosis. *Intensive Care Med* 12:285, 1986.

Kettle F et al. Buffer solutions may compromise cardiac resuscitation by reducing coronary perfusion pressure. *JAMA* 266:2121, 1991.

Mansel JK et al. Face-mask CPAP and sodium bicarbonate infusion in acute, severe asthma and metabolic acidosis. *Chest* 96:943, 1989.

Sanders AB et al. The role of bicarbonate and fluid loading in improving resuscitation from prolonged cardiac arrest with rapid manual chest compression CPR. *Ann Emerg Med* 19:1, 1990.

Weil MH et al. Sodium bicarbonate during CPR: Does it help or hinder? *Chest* 88:487, 1985.

Weisfeldt M, Guerci A. Sodium bicarbonate in CPR (editorial). *JAMA* 266:2129, 1991.

STREPTOKINASE

TRADE NAME	Streptase
THERAPEUTIC EFFECTS	Lyses (dissolves) thrombi that have recently formed in the coronary arteries, thereby enabling renewed blood flow through blocked coronaries in the acute phase of myocardial infarction.
INDICATIONS	Evolving ACUTE MYOCARDIAL INFARCTION within the first 6 hours if inclusion criteria are met (see Chap. 23).
CONTRAINDICATIONS	• Active **internal bleeding** (e.g., peptic ulcer). • Recent **stroke** or **intracranial surgery.** • Severe, uncontrolled **hypertension.** • Recent **trauma, surgery.**
SIDE EFFECTS	• *Bleeding tendency;* fatal hemorrhage has occurred. • **Allergic reactions** to the drug, with itching, hives, flushing, nausea, headache, and myalgias. (Can be minimized by pretreatment with diphenhydramine.) • *Fever.* • *Hypotension.* • Reperfusion *dysrhythmias.*
HOW SUPPLIED	6.5-ml vials of powdered drug with a color-coded label corresponding to the amount of purified streptokinase in each vial: • Green: 250,000 IU. • Blue: 750,000 IU. • Red: 1,500,000 IU.
ADMINISTRATION AND DOSAGE	Given by **intravenous infusion.** Reconstitute the powdered drug with 5 ml of normal saline injected down the side of the vial. Then roll the vial gently (don't shake it) to dissolve the powder. Inspect for particulate matter. *Dosage:* 1,500,000 IU diluted in at least 45 ml of normal saline and infused **over 60 minutes.**

Further Discussion

Chapter 23.

References

Anderson HV, Willerson JR. Thrombolysis in acute myocardial infarction. *N Engl J Med* 329:703, 1993.

Applebaum D et al. Feasibility of pre-hospital fibrinolytic therapy in acute myocardial infarction. *Am J Emerg Med* 4:201, 1986.

Bresler MJ. Future role of thrombolytic therapy in emergency medicine. *Ann Emerg Med* 18:1331, 1989.

Buchalter MB et al. Streptokinase resistance: When might streptokinase administration be ineffective? *Br Heart J* 68:449, 1992.

Eisenberg MS et al. Thrombolytic therapy. *Ann Emerg Med* 22:417, 1993.

Grim PS, Feldman T, Childers RW. Evaluation of patients for the need of thrombolytic therapy in the prehospital setting. *Ann Emerg Med* 18:483, 1989.

Hartman JR et al. Intravenous streptokinase in acute myocardial infarction: Experience in community hospitals served by paramedics. *Am Heart J* 111:1030, 1986.

Hartman JR et al. A system approach to intravenous thrombolysis in acute myocardial infarction in community hospitals: The influence of paramedics. *Clin Cardiol* 11:812, 1988.

Peppers MP. Thrombolytics update. *Emergency* 25(2):24, 1993.

Rappaport E. Thrombolytic agents in acute myocardial infarction. *N Engl J Med* 320:861, 1989.

Sherrod M et al. A pilot study of paramedic-administered, prehospital thrombolysis for acute myocardial infarction. *Clin Cardiol* 13:421, 1990.

Tisdale JE et al. Streptokinase-induced anaphylaxis. *Ann Pharmacother* 23:984, 1989.

Weaver WD et al. Myocardial infarction triage and intervention project—Phase I: Patient characteristics and feasibility of prehospital initiation of thrombolytic therapy. *J Am Coll Cardiol* 15:925, 1990.

Weiss AT et al. Prehospital coronary thrombolysis: A new strategy in acute myocardial infarction. *Chest* 92:124, 1987.

SUCCINYLCHOLINE

TRADE NAME	Anectine
THERAPEUTIC EFFECTS	Short-acting skeletal muscle relaxant that works by depolarizing the receptors on skeletal muscle. By occupying those receptors, it prevents the normal transmitting chemical from reaching the receptors and thereby blocks neuromuscular transmission. The result is a transient paralysis of skeletal muscles.
INDICATIONS	To facilitate ENDOTRACHEAL INTUBATION.

CONTRAINDICATIONS

- Patients known to have had **problems during anesthesia** in the past.
- Penetrating **eye injury.**
- Severe **burns.**
- **Organophosphate poisoning.**
- Known **neuromuscular disease** (e.g., myasthenia gravis).
- Operator who is **not highly skilled in intubation.**
- Patients in whom you **cannot control the airway manually.**

SIDE EFFECTS

- Produces generalized *muscle fasciculations* immediately after administration (depolarizing effect).
- *Hypersalivation* (may be prevented by pretreating with atropine).
- *Bronchospasm.*
- *Bradycardia* (may be prevented by pretreating with atropine).
- *Prolonged respiratory depression.*
- In very rare cases, *malignant hyperpyrexia,* heralded by muscle rigidity, tachycardia, hypertension.

HOW SUPPLIED

- 20-ml vials containing 20 mg/ml (should be stored in a refrigerator).
- 2-ml and 5-ml ampules of 20 mg/ml.

ADMINISTRATION AND DOSAGE

Given by **intravenous bolus injection.**

- **Preoxygenate** the patient for at least 3 minutes with 100% oxygen.
- Have all **intubation equipment ready.**
- Have **atropine,** 0.01 mg/kg, drawn up in a syringe and ready to administer. Give for bradycardia or hypersecretion.
- **Premedicate:**
  1. Awake *adults*: 3–5 mg of DIAZEPAM slowly IV.
  2. Patients with *head injury*: LIDOCAINE, 1 mg/kg IV.
  3. *Children*: ATROPINE, 0.01 mg/kg IV.
- Give succinylcholine, **1 mg/kg IV.**
- Wait until fasciculations have stopped.
- Have an assistant apply **cricoid pressure** to block the esophagus.
- **Intubate** the trachea.
- Provide **controlled ventilation** with 100% oxygen until the patient resumes breathing spontaneously (usually within 4 to 6 minutes, but may take longer).

INCOMPATIBILITY

Drugs that may add to the paralytic effects of succinylcholine should not be given: oxytocin, procainamide, lidocaine, magnesium salts, beta blockers (e.g., propranolol).

Further Discussion

Chapter 7.

References

Berve MO. Easing intubation with succinylcholine. *JEMS* 15(11):60, 1990.

DeGarmo BH et al. Pharmacology and clinical use of neuromuscular blocking agents. *Ann Emerg Med* 12:48, 1983.

Hedges JR et al. Succinylcholine-assisted intubations in pre-hospital care. *Ann Emerg Med* 17:49, 1988.

Koenig KL. Rapid-sequence intubation of head trauma patients: Prevention of fasciculations with pancuronium versus minidose succinylcholine. *Ann Emerg Med* 21:929, 1992.

Ligier B et al. The role of anesthetic induction agents and neuromuscular blockade in the endotracheal intubation of trauma victims. *Surg Gynecol Obstet* 17:478, 1991.

Miller K. Paralysis for intubation. *Emergency* 21(5):19, 1989.

Murphy-Macabobby M et al. Neuromuscular blockade in aeromedical airway management. *Ann Emerg Med* 21:664, 1992.

Rhee KJ, O'Malley RJ. Neuromuscular blockade-assisted oral intubation versus nasotracheal intubation in the prehospital care of injured patients. *Ann Emerg Med* 23:37, 1993.

Roberts DJ, Clinton JE, Ruiz E. Neuromuscular blockade for critical patients in the emergency department. *Ann Emerg Med* 15:152, 1986.

Rotondo MF et al. Urgent paralysis and intubation of trauma patients: Is it safe? *J Trauma* 34:242, 1993.

Syverud SA et al. Pre-hospital use of neuromuscular blocking agents in a helicopter ambulance. *Ann Emerg Med* 17:236, 1988.

Thompson JD, Fish S, Ruiz E. Succinylcholine for endotracheal intubation. *Ann Emerg Med* 11:526, 1982.

Tressa J. Neuromuscular blocking agents. *Emergency* 24 (7):57, 1992.

Walls RM. Rapid-sequence intubation in head trauma. *Ann Emerg Med* 22:1008, 1993.

SYRUP OF IPECAC

THERAPEUTIC EFFECTS	Induces vomiting and thereby effectively empties the stomach of ingested poisons or drugs taken in excess.
INDICATIONS	To induce vomiting in POISONING or OVERDOSE by ingestion in a conscious patient.

CONTRAINDICATIONS	• **Stupor** or **coma.**
	• **Absent gag** reflex.
	• **Seizures.**
	• **Pregnancy.**
	• Acute **myocardial infarction.**
	• Children **under 6 months old.**
	• Ingestion of
	   1. **Corrosives** (strong acids or alkalis).
	   2. Volatile **hydrocarbons.**
	   3. **Strychnine** or **iodides.**

SIDE EFFECTS	None from the syrup of ipecac itself, BUT the patient induced to vomit—by whatever means—is at risk of aspiration.
HOW SUPPLIED	16-oz (480-ml) bottles containing 70 mg/ml.
ADMINISTRATION AND DOSAGE	Syrup of ipecac is given **by mouth.** *Dosage*: • Children: **3 to 5 teaspoons** (15–25 ml) followed by a glass of water. • Adults: **1 to 2 tablespoons** (15–30 ml) followed by a glass of water. The patient should be encouraged to walk around after taking the syrup of ipecac, until he feels the urge to vomit. He should then be positioned with his head lower than his waist and his face over a suitable receptacle. Save a sample of the emesis for laboratory analysis.

Further Discussion

Chapter 27.

References

Albertson T et al. Superiority of activated charcoal alone compared with ipecac and activated charcoal in the treatment of acute toxic ingestions. *Ann Emerg Med* 18:101, 1989.

Auerbach PS et al. Efficacy of gastric emptying: Gastric lavage versus emesis induced with ipecac. *Ann Emerg Med* 15:692, 1986.

Chafee-Bahamon C et al. Risk assessment of ipecac in the home. *Pediatrics* 75:1105, 1985.

Czajka, PA, Russell Sl. Nonemetic effects of ipecac. *Pediatrics* 75:1101, 1985.

Dean BS et al. Syrup of ipecac: 15 ml versus 30 ml in pediatric poisonings. *Clin Toxicol* 23(2–3):165, 1985.

Eason J et al. Efficacy and safety of gastrointestinal decontamination in the treatment of oral poisoning. *Pediatr Clin North Am* 26:827, 1979.

Flomenbaum NE, Hoffman R. GI evacuation: Is it still worthwhile? *Emerg Med* 22(2):80, 1990.

Grande GA et al. The effect of fluid volume on syrup of ipecac emesis time. *Clin Toxicol* 25:473, 1987.

Hoffman R. Choices in gastric decontamination. *Emerg Med* 24(10):212, 1992.

Ipecac syrup and activated charcoal for treatment of poisoning in children. *Med Lett* 21:70, 1979.

King WD. Syrup of ipecac: A drug review. *Clin Toxicol* 19:353, 1980.

Kornberg AE, Dolgin J. Pediatric ingestions: Charcoal alone versus ipecac and charcoal. *Ann Emerg Med* 20:648, 1991.

Krenzelok EP et al. Syrup of ipecac in children less than one year of age. *Clin Toxicol* 23(2–3):171, 1985.

Krenzelok EP et al. Effectiveness of 15-ml versus 30-ml doses of syrup of ipecac in children. *Clin Pharm* 6:715, 1987.

Kulig K et al. Management of acutely poisoned patients without gastric emptying. *Ann Emerg Med* 14:562, 1985.

Levy DB. Syrup of ipecac review. *Emergency* 21(12):20, 1989.

Manoguerra AS. Syrup of ipecac. *Emergency* 11(3):29, 1979.

McCray EA, Bonfiglio JF, Sigell LT. Home administration of syrup of ipecac to infants. *Drug Intell Clin Pharm* 18:792, 1984.

Mofenson HC. Benefits and risks of syrup of ipecac. *Pediatrics* 77:551, 1986.

Tenenbein M. Inefficacy of gastric emptying procedures. *J Emerg Med* 3:133, 1984.

Tenenbein M, Cohen S, Sitar D. Efficacy of ipecac-induced emesis, orogastric lavage, and activated charcoal for acute drug overdose. *Ann Emerg Med* 16:838, 1987.

Vasquez TE, Evans DG, Ashburn WL. Efficacy of syrup of ipecac–induced emesis for emptying gastric contents. *Clin Nucl Med* 13:638, 1988.

Wrenn K et al. Potential misuse of ipecac. *Ann Emerg Med* 22:1408, 1993.

Young WF, Bivins HG. Evaluation of gastric emptying using radionuclides: Gastric lavage versus ipecac-induced emesis. *Ann Emerg Med* 22:1423, 1993.

TERBUTALINE

TRADE NAMES	Bricanyl, Brethine, Brethaire
THERAPEUTIC EFFECTS	Beta sympathomimetic agent affecting primarily the bronchial musculature rather than the myocardium (i.e., a beta-2 agent). Terbutaline thus relaxes bronchial smooth muscle and thereby *relieves bronchospasm* in asthma.
INDICATIONS	• Moderate to severe ASTHMA. • Reversible bronchospasm in CHRONIC OBSTRUCTIVE PULMONARY DISEASE.
CONTRAINDICATIONS	• Should be used with *caution* in patients with **angina, hypertension,** or **cardiac dysrhythmias.** • Manufacturer does not recommend use in **children < 12 years old.**
SIDE EFFECTS	• *Tremor* and *nervousness.* • *Palpitations, dizziness.* • Sometimes transient *headache, sweating, drowsiness, nausea,* and *muscle cramps.*
HOW SUPPLIED	Several forms, but for field use, as an alternative to subcutaneous epinephrine, the solution for subcutaneous injection is preferred. That solution is supplied as 1-ml ampules containing 1 mg of terbutaline.
ADMINISTRATION AND DOSAGE	In the field, given primarily by **subcutaneous injection.** *Dosage*: • Children: **0.01 mg/kg SQ;** may repeat in 15 minutes. • Adults: **0.25 mg** (0.25 ml) **SQ** over the lateral deltoid. May also be given by **nebulizer** in a dose of **0.03 mg/kg** added to 3 ml of normal saline.
INCOMPATIBILITY	Do not give together with other *sympathomimetic drugs* (e.g., epinephrine).

Further Discussion

Chapters 22 and 30.

References

Amory DW, Burnham SC, Cheney Jr FW. Comparison of the cardiopulmonary effects of subcutaneously administered epinephrine and terbutaline in patients with reversible airway obstruction. *Chest* 67:279, 1975.

Baughman RP et al. A comparison study of aerosolized terbutaline and subcutaneously administered epinephrine in the treatment of acute bronchial asthma. *Ann Allergy* 53:131, 1984.

Pancorbo S et al. Subcutaneous epinephrine versus nebulized terbutaline in the emergency treatment of asthma. *Clin Pharm* 2:45, 1983.

Smith JA et al. Theophylline and aerosolized terbutaline in the treatment of bronchial asthma: Double-blind comparison of optimal doses. *Chest* 78:816, 1980.

Smith PR et al. A comparative study of subcutaneously administered terbutaline and epinephrine in the treatment of acute bronchial asthma. *Chest* 71:129, 1977.

Spiteri MA et al. Subcutaneous adrenaline versus terbutaline in the treatment of acute severe asthma. *Thorax* 43:19, 1988.

THIAMINE (Vitamin B₁)

THERAPEUTIC EFFECTS	Acts as a co-enzyme in carbohydrate metabolism and is therefore essential for the normal metabolism of glucose.
INDICATIONS	• Prior to administration of 50% DEXTROSE in patients with coma of unknown etiology, to prevent precipitation of Wernicke's encephalopathy. • Known THIAMINE DEFICIENCY (beriberi). • Chronic ALCOHOLISM and other states of generalized malnutrition.
CONTRAINDICATIONS	None.
SIDE EFFECTS	• Slight, transient *vasodilation* and *hypotension* after rapid IV administration. • Overdosage may produce toxicity (weakness, dyspnea, respiratory failure). • Rare *anaphylactic reactions.*
HOW SUPPLIED	• Vials of 50 mg/ml. • 1-ml, 5-ml, 10-ml, and 30-ml vials of 100 mg/ml. • Tubex syringes of 100 mg.
ADMINISTRATION AND DOSAGE	For coma, preceding the administration of D50, give **50 mg IV and 50 mg IM** (or, if there are signs of poor peripheral perfusion, give the entire 100 mg *slowly* IV).

Further Discussion

Chapters 24 and 27.

References

Goldfrank L, Flomenbaum N. Thiamine omitted from ACEP ALS medications document (letter). *Ann Emerg Med* 13:122, 1984.

Victor M, Adams RD, Collins GH. *The Wernicke-Korsakoff Syndrome*. Philadelphia: Davis, 1971.

Wrenn KD et al. A toxicity study of parenteral thiamine hydrochloride. *Ann Emerg Med* 18:867, 1989.

TISSUE PLASMINOGEN ACTIVATOR (rt-PA)

TRADE NAME	Activase
THERAPEUTIC EFFECTS	Enzyme that initiates the lysis of thrombi and thereby helps to re-open blocked coronary arteries in the acute phase of myocardial infarction.
INDICATIONS	Evolving ACUTE MYOCARDIAL INFARCTION within the first 6 hours if inclusion criteria are met (see Chap. 23).
CONTRAINDICATIONS	• Active **internal bleeding** (e.g., peptic ulcer).
	• Recent **stroke** or **intracranial surgery.**
	• Severe, uncontrolled **hypertension.**
	• Recent **trauma, surgery**
SIDE EFFECTS	• *Bleeding tendency;* fatal hemorrhage has occurred.
	• *Fever.*
	• *Hypotension.*
	• *Nausea* and *vomiting.*
	• Mild *allergic reactions*
HOW SUPPLIED	Powder in 20-mg and 50-mg vacuum-sealed vials packaged with diluent for reconstitution.
ADMINISTRATION AND DOSAGE	Given by **intravenous infusion** through a filter.
	Dosage: Recommended dosage is 100 mg, of which
	• **6 mg** is given as a **bolus over the first 1 to 2 minutes.**
	• **54 mg** is then infused over the **first hour.**
	• **20 mg** is infused over the second hour.
	• **20 mg** is infused over the third hour.

Further Discussion

Chapter 23.

References

Aufderheide TP et al. Feasibility of prehospital r-TPA therapy in chest pain patients. *Ann Emerg Med* 21:379, 1992

Califf RM et al. Experience with the use of tPA in the treatment of acute myocardial infarction. *Ann Emerg Med* 17:1176, 1988.

The GUSTO Investigators. An international randomized trial comparing four thrombolytic strategies for acute myocardial infarction. *N Engl J Med* 329:673, 1993.

Levy DB. Rt-PA . . . A new era. *Emergency* 21(1):19, 1989.

Linnik W, Tintinalli JE, Tamos R. Associated reactions during and immediately after rtPA infusion. *Ann Emerg Med* 18:234, 1989.

Loscalzo J et al. Tissue plasminogen activator. *N Engl J Med* 319:925, 1988.

Neuhaus KL et al. Improved thrombolysis with modified dose regimen of recombinant tissue-type plasminogen activator. *J Am Coll Cardiol* 14:1556, 1989.

Peppers MP. Thrombolytics update. *Emergency* 25(2):24, 1993.

Tebbe U et al. Single-bolus injection of recombinant tissue-type plasminogen activator in acute myocardial infarction. *Am J Cardiol* 64:448, 1989.

Thrombolysis Early in Acute Heart Attack Trial Study Group. Very early thrombolytic therapy in suspected acute myocardial infarction. *Am J Cardiol* 65:401, 1990.

Topol EJ et al. Comparison of two dose regimens of intravenous tissue plasminogen activator for acute myocardial infarction. *Am J Cardiol* 61:723, 1988.

Yon TC. Thrombolytic therapy in acute myocardial infarction. *J Prehosp Med* 2(2):24, 1988.

VERAPAMIL

TRADE NAME	Isoptin, Calan
THERAPEUTIC EFFECTS	Calcium channel blocker; antagonizes the effects of calcium ion, thereby slowing sinoatrial (SA) node discharge and delaying conduction through the atrioventricular (AV) junction.
INDICATIONS	• Second-line drug for the treatment of SUPRAVENTRICULAR TACHYCARDIAS that do not respond to vagal maneuvers or adenosine. • To decrease the ventricular rate in some cases of ATRIAL FLUTTER and ATRIAL FIBRILLATION.
CONTRAINDICATIONS	• **Cardiogenic shock** or **heart failure.** • Sinus node disease ("**sick sinus syndrome**"). • **Hypotension** not due to tachyarrhythmia. • Patient taking a **beta blocking drug** such as propranolol. • Acute **myocardial infarction.** • Wide-complex tachycardia • Use with *caution* in elderly patients and in patients taking digitalis.
SIDE EFFECTS	• *Hypotension.* • *Headache, dizziness, sweating.* • *AV block* or *bradycardia.* • May cause *cardiac arrest.* • May precipitate *heart failure* with *pulmonary edema.*
HOW SUPPLIED	2-ml ampules and 4-ml vials containing 2.5 mg/ml.
ADMINISTRATION AND DOSAGE	Given by **slow intravenous injection** (over 1–2 minutes). *Dosage:* **0.1 mg/kg** (usual adult dose, then, is 5–10 mg). May be repeated in 30 minutes.
INCOMPATIBILITY	Do not use together with *beta blockers*, which may potentiate the effects of verapamil and precipitate heart failure.

Further Discussion

Chapter 23.

References

Barbarash RA et al. Verapamil infusions in the treatment of atrial tachyarrhythmias. *Crit Care Med* 14:886, 1986.

Belhassen B et al. What is the drug of choice for the acute termination of paroxysmal supraventricular tachycardia: Verapamil, adenosine triphosphate, or adenosine? *Pace* 16:1735, 1993.

Coburn JP et al. Verapamil: An effective calcium blocking agent for pediatric patients. *Pediatrics* 71:748, 1983.

Deedwania PC. Calcium channel blockers. *West J Med* 137:24, 1982.

Garratt C et al. Misuse of verapamil in pre-excited atrial fibrillation. *Lancet* 1:367, 1989.

Haft JI et al. Treatment of atrial arrhythmias: Effectiveness of verapamil when preceded by calcium infusion. *Arch Intern Med* 146:1085, 1986.

Klein HO et al. Digitalis and verapamil in atrial fibrillation and flutter: Is verapamil now the preferred agent? *Drugs* 31:185, 1986.

Kuhn M. Verapamil in the treatment of PSVT. *Ann Emerg Med* 10:538, 1981.

Kuhn M et al. Low-dose calcium pretreatment to prevent verapamil-induced hypotension. *Am Heart J* 124:231, 1992.

O'Toole KS et al. Intravenous verapamil in the prehospital treatment of paroxysmal supraventricular tachycardia. *Ann Emerg Med* 19:291, 1990.

Peppers M. Verapamil and calcium use. *Emergency* 23(3):22, 1991.

Reedy DP et al. Effects of verapamil on acute focal cerebral ischemia. *Neurosurgery* 12:272, 1983.

Resnekov L. Calcium antagonist drugs: Myocardial preservation and reduced vulnerability to ventricular fibrillation during CPR. *Crit Care Med* 9:360, 1981.

Schamroth L. The clinical uses of intravenous verapamil. *Am Heart J* 100:1070, 1980.

Sung RJ et al. Intravenous verapamil for termination of reentrant supraventricular tachycardias. *Ann Intern Med* 93:682, 1980.

Waxman HL et al. Verapamil for control of ventricular rate in paroxysmal supraventricular tachycardia and atrial flutter. *Ann Intern Med* 94:1, 1981.

White BC et al. Calcium blockers in cerebral resuscitation. *J Trauma* 23:788, 1983.

Yee R et al. Combined verapamil and propranolol for supraventricular tachycardia. *Am J Cardiol* 53:757, 1984.

Zaloga GP et al. Verapamil reverses calcium cardiotoxicity. *Ann Emerg Med* 16:637, 1987.

B
Index to Commonly Prescribed Drugs

This listing of prescription drugs is intended to help you identify the medications a patient may be taking at home and to make an educated guess as to the conditions for which the patient is being treated. The drugs are listed alphabetically by *trade name*. For each drug, there is an indication of its generic name, its general class (e.g., antihypertensive, antidepressant), and the condition(s) for which it is most commonly prescribed. Various classes of prescription drugs are described in more detail elsewhere in the text. Bronchodilators, for example, are discussed in Chapter 22, Respiratory Emergencies; cardiac medications are discussed in Chapter 23, Cardiovascular Emergencies; psychotropic drugs are discussed in Chapter 38, Disturbances of Behavior.

TRADE NAME	GENERIC NAME	CLASS	COMMONLY PRESCRIBED FOR
Aarane	cromolyn	Mast cell inhibitor	Asthma
Actifed	pseudoephedrine	Beta sympathomimetic	Asthma
Adapin	doxepin	Tricyclic antidepressant	Depression
Aldactazide	hydrochlorothiazide plus spironolactone	Diuretic	Hyptertension
Aldactone	spironolactone	Diuretic	Hypertension
Aldoril	hydrochlorothiazide	Diuretic	Hypertension; CHF
Alupent	metaproterenol	Beta-2 sympathomimetic	Asthma
Amitril	amitriptyline	Tricyclic antidepressant	Depression
Amytal	amobarbital	Barbiturate	Sedation
Anaprox	naproxen	Nonsteroidal anti-inflammatory	Arthritis; pain; inflammation
Anhydron	cyclothiazide	Diuretic	Hypertension
Antabuse	disulfiram	Metabolic blocker	Alcoholism
Antivert	meclizine	Antihistamine	Vertigo
Apresoline	hydralazine	Vasodilator	Hypertension
Artane	trihexyphenidyl	Antispasmodic	Parkinson's disease
Asendin	amoxapine	Tricyclic antidepressant	Depression
Atarax	hydroxyzine	Antihistamine	Sleep
Ativan	lorazepam	Benzodiazepine tranquilizer	Anxiety; sleep
Atromid-S	clofibrate	Antilipidemic	To lower cholesterol
Atrovent	ipratropium	Bronchodilator	Asthma
Aventyl	nortriptyline	Tricyclic antidepressant	Depression
Azolid	phenylbutazone	Anti-inflammatory	Arthritis; other inflammations
Bactrim	trimethoprim	Antibiotic	COPD; urinary tract infections
Beclovent	beclomethasone	Corticosteroid	Asthma
Beconase	beclomethasone	Corticosteroid	Asthma

1009

TRADE NAME	GENERIC NAME	CLASS	COMMONLY PRESCRIBED FOR
Benadryl	diphenhydramine	Antihistamine	Allergies; hay fever
Benemid	probenecid	Uricosuric	Gout; hyperuricemia
Bentyl	dicyclomine	Anticholinergic	Nausea and vomiting
Blocadren	timolol maleate	Beta blocker	Angina; hypertension
Brethaire	terbutaline	Beta-2 sympathomimetic	Asthma
Brethine	terbutaline	Beta-2 sympathomimetic	Asthma
Bretylol	bretylium tosylate	Antiarrhythmic	Ventricular tachycardia
Bricanyl	terbutaline	Beta-2 sympathomimetic	Asthma
Bronkosol	isoetharine	Bronchodilator	Asthma
Butazolidin	phenylbutazone	Anti-inflammatory	Arthritis; other inflammations
Calan	verapamil	Calcium channel blocker	Coronary artery spasm; PSVT
Capastat	capreomycin	Antibiotic	Tuberculosis
Cardioquin	quinidine	Antiarrhythmic	Atrial/ventricular dysrhythmias
Cardizem	diltiazem	Calcium channel blocker	Angina
Catapres	clonidine	Vasodilator	Hypertension
Cibalith-S	lithium citrate	Anti-manic	Manic-depressive disorder
Clinoril	sulindac	Nonsteroidal anti-inflammatory	Arthritis
Cogentin	benztropine	Anticholinergic	Parkinson's disease
Compazine	prochlorperazine	Phenothiazine	Nausea; psychosis
Cordarone	amiodarone	Antiarrhythmic	Ventricular tachycardia
Corgard	nadolol	Beta blocker	Angina, hypertension
Corzide	nadolol	Beta blocker	Angina, hypertension
Cotrim	trimethoprim	Antibiotic	COPD; urinary tract infection
Coumadin	warfarin	Anticoagulant	Previous AMI; pulmonary embolism
Crystodigin	digitoxin	Cardiac glycoside	CHF; atrial dysrhythmias
Cyclospasmol	clyclandelate	Vasodilator	Nighttime leg cramps
Dalmane	flurazepam	Benzodiazepine tranquilizer	Sleep
Darvon	propoxyphene	Narcotic	Pain
Datril	acetaminophen	Analgesic	Pain, fever
Daxolin	loxapine	Antipsychotic	Psychosis
Depakene	valproic acid	Anticonvulsant	Seizures
Demerol	meperidine	Narcotic	Pain
Demulen	ethinyl estradiol	Estrogen	Contraception
Desyrel	trazodone	Antidepressant	Depression
DiaBeta	glyburide	Oral hypoglycemic	Diabetes
Diabinese	chlorpropamide	Oral hypoglycemic	Diabetes
Diamox	acetazolamide	Diuretic	Glaucoma
Dilantin	phenytoin	Anticonvulsant	Seizures
Dilaudid	hydromorphone	Narcotic	Pain
Diuril	chlorothiazide	Diuretic	Hypertension
Dolobid	diflunisal	Nonsteroidal anti-inflammatory	Arthritis; other inflammations
Donnatal	atropine/ scopolamine/ phenobarbital	Antispasmodic	Gastric or intestinal spasms
Doriden	glutethimide	Hypnotic	Sleep
Duraquin	quinidine	Antiarrhythmic	Atrial/ventricular dysrhythmias
Dyazide	hydrochlorothiazide	Diuretic	Hypertension; CHF

TRADE NAME	GENERIC NAME	CLASS	COMMONLY PRESCRIBED FOR
Dymelor	acetohexamide	Oral hypoglycemic	Diabetes
Dyrenium	triamterene	Diuretic	Hypertension
Edecrin	ethacrynic acid	Diuretic	Hypertension
Elavil	amitriptyline	Tricyclic antidepressant	Depression
Elixophyllin	theophylline	Xanthine bronchodilator	Asthma
Endep	amitriptyline	Tricyclic antidepressant	Depression
Enduron	methyclothiazide	Diuretic	Congestive heart failure
Equanil	meprobamate	Barbiturate-like tranquilizer	Anxiety
Ery-Tab	erythromycin	Antibiotic	COPD; many infections
Esidrix	hydrochlorothiazide	Diuretic	Hypertension; CHF
Eskalith	lithium carbonate	Anti-manic	Manic-depressive disorder
Feldene	piroxicam	Nonsteroidal anti-inflammatory	Arthritis; other inflammations
Feosol	ferrous sulfate	Iron	Iron deficiency anemia
Fiorinal	aspirin/butalbital/ caffeine	Analgesic	Pain
Flagyl	metronidazole	Antimicrobial	Amoebic infection; vaginal infection
Flexeril	cyclobenzaprine	Smooth muscle relaxant	Muscle spasms
Gantanol	sulfisoxazole	Antimicrobial sulfa drug	Urinary tract infection
Glucotrol	glipizide	Oral hypoglycemic	Diabetes
Halcion	triazolam	Benzodiazepine tranquilizer	Sleep
Haldol	haloperidol	Antipsychotic	Psychosis
Humulin	insulin	Hormone	Diabetes
HydroDIURIL	hydrochlorothiazide	Diuretic	Hypertension; CHF
Hydropres	hydrochlorothiazide	Diuretic	Hypertension; CHF
Hygroton	chlorthalidone	Diuretic	Hypertension; CHF
Iletin	insulin	Hormone	Diabetes
Imavate	imipramine	Tricyclic antidepressant	Depression
Inapsine	droperidol	Antipsychotic	Psychosis
Inderal	propranolol	Beta blocker	Angina, tachyarrhythmias, hypertension
Indocin	indomethacin	Nonsteroidal anti-inflammatory	Arthritis
Intal	cromolyn	Mast cell inhibitor	Asthma
Ismelin	guanethidine	Vasodilator	Hypertension
Isoptin	verapamil	Calcium channel blocker	Coronary artery spasm; PSVT
Isordil	isosorbide dinitrate	Nitroglycerin preparation	Angina
Isosorb	isosorbide dinitrate	Nitroglycerin preparation	Angina
Janimine	imipramine	Tricyclic antidepressant	Depression
Klonopin	clonazepam	CNS depressant	Seizures
K-Lyte	potassium chloride	Electrolyte	Potassium replacement
Lanoxin	digoxin	Cardiac glycoside	CHF; atrial dysrhythmias
Larodopa	levodopa	Dopamine precursor	Parkinson's disease
Lasix	furosemide	Diuretic	CHF; hypertension
Librium	chlordiazepoxide	Benzodiazepine tranquilizer	Anxiety
Lithane	lithium carbonate	Anti-manic	Manic-depressive disorder
Lithobid	lithium carbonate	Anti-manic	Manic-depressive disorder

TRADE NAME	GENERIC NAME	CLASS	COMMONLY PRESCRIBED FOR
Lithonate	lithium carbonate	Anti-manic	Manic-depressive disorder
Lomotil	diphenoxylate	Anticholinergic	Diarrhea
Lopressor	metoprolol	Beta blocker	Hypertension
Loxitane	loxapine	Antipsychotic	Psychosis
Ludiomil	maprotiline	Tricyclic antidepressant	Depression
Luminal	phenobarbital	Barbiturate	Seizures; sleep
Marax	ephedrine/ theophylline	Bronchodilator	Asthma
Marplan	isocarboxazid	MAO inhibitor	Depression
Mellaril	thioridazine	Antipsychotic	Psychosis
Mesantoin	mephenytoin	Anticonvulsant	Seizures
Methahydrin	trichlormethiazide	Diuretic	Hypertension
Mexitil	mexiletine	Antiarrhythmic	Ventricular dysrhythmias
Micronase	glyburide	Oral hypoglycemic	Diabetes
Miltown	meprobamate	Barbiturate-like tranquilizer	Anxiety
Minipress	prazosin	Beta blocker	Hypertension
Mixtard	insulin	Hormone	Diabetes
Moban	molindone	Antipsychotic	Psychosis
Motrin	ibuprofen	Nonsteroidal anti-inflammatory	Arthritis
Myambutol	ethambutol	Antibiotic	Tuberculosis
Mysoline	primidone	Anticonvulsant	Seizures
Nalfon	fenoprofen	Nonsteroidal anti-inflammatory	Arthritis
Naprosyn	naproxen	Nonsteroidal anti-inflammatory	Arthritis
Naqua	trichlormethiazide	Diuretic	Hypertension
Nardil	phenelzine	MAO inhibitor	Depression
Navane	thiothixene	Antipsychotic	Psychosis
Nembutal	pentobarbital	Barbiturate	Sleep
Nitro-Bid	nitroglycerin	Nitroglycerin	Angina
Nitro-Dur	nitroglycerin	Nitroglycerin	Angina
Nitrostat	nitroglycerin	Nitroglycerin	Angina
Noctec	chloral hydrate	Hypnotic	Sleep
Noludar	methyprylon	Barbiturate-like hypnotic	Sleep
Norinyl	ethinyl estradiol	Estrogen	Contraception
Normodyne	labetalol	Beta blocker	Angina; hypertension
Norpace	disopyramide	Antiarrhythmic	PVCs
Norpramin	desipramine	Tricyclic antidepressant	Depression
Novolin	insulin	Hormone	Diabetes
Omnipen	ampicillin	Antibiotic	COPD; other infections
Orap	pimozide	Antipsychotic	Psychosis
Oretic	hydrochlorothiazide	Diuretic	Hypertension; CHF
Orinase	tolbutamide	Oral hypoglycemic	Diabetes
Ortho-Novum	ethinyl estradiol	Estrogen	Contraception
Oxalid	oxyphenbutazone	Nonsteroidal anti-inflammatory	Arthritis
Pamelor	nortriptyline	Tricyclic antidepressant	Depression
Parnate	tranylcypromine	MAO inhibitor	Depression
Paxipam	halazepam	Benzodiazepine tranquilizer	Anxiety
Percodan	oxycodone	Narcotic	Pain
Periactin	cyproheptadine	Antihistamine	Colds; allergies
Permitil	fluphenazine	Antipsychotic	Psychosis
Persantine	disopyramide	Antiarrhythmic	Ventricular dysrhythmias
Pertofrane	desipramine	Tricyclic antidepressant	Depression
Phenergan	promethazine	Antihistamine	Sedation
Placidyl	ethchlorvynol	Tranquilizer	Anxiety

TRADE NAME	GENERIC NAME	CLASS	COMMONLY PRESCRIBED FOR
Premarin	conjugated estrogens	Hormone	Menopausal symptoms
Presamine	imipramine	Tricyclic antidepressant	Depression
Pro-Banthine	propantheline bromide	Anticholinergic	Spastic colon
Procan	procainamide	Antiarrhythmic	Ventricular dysrhythmias
Prolixin	fluphenazine	Antipsychotic	Psychosis
Procardia	nifedipine	Calcium channel blocker	Coronary artery spasm
Proloid	thyroglobulin	Thyroid hormone	Hypothyroidism
Pronestyl	procainamide	Antiarrhythmic	Ventricular dysrhythmias
Proventil	albuterol	Beta-2 sympathomimetic	Asthma; COPD
Prozac	fluoxetine	Antidepressant	Depression
Quadrinal	theophylline	Xanthine bronchodilator	Asthma
Quibron	theophylline	Xanthine bronchodilator	Asthma
Quinaglute	quinidine	Antiarrhythmic	Atrial/ventricular dysrhythmias
Quinidex	quinidine	Antiarrhythmic	Atrial/ventricular dysrhythmias
Quinora	quinidine	Antiarrhythmic	Atrial/ventricular dysrhythmias
Regroton	reserpine/ chlorthalidone	Vasodilator/diuretic	Hypertension
Restoril	triazolam	Benzodiazepine tranquilizer	Sleep
Retrovir	zidovudine	Antiviral	AIDS
Rifadin	rifampin	Antibiotic	Tuberculosis
Rifamate	rifampin	Antibiotic	Tuberculosis
Ritalin	methylphenidate	CNS stimulant	Hyperactivity in children
Sandril	reserpine	Vasodilator	Hypertension
Seconal	secobarbital	Barbiturate	Sleep
Sectral	acebutolol	Beta blocker	Hypertension
Ser-Ap-Es	reserpine	Vasodilator	Hypertension
Serax	oxazepam	Benzodiazepine tranquilizer	Anxiety
Serentil	mesoridazine	Antipsychotic	Psychosis
Serpasil	reserpine	Vasodilator	Hypertension
Sinemet	levodopa	Dopamine precursor	Parkinson's disease
Sinequan	doxepin	Tricyclic antidepressant	Depression
SK-Pramine	imipramine	Tricyclic antidepressant	Depression
SK-65	propoxyphene	Narcotic	Pain
Slo-Phyllin	theophylline	Xanthine bronchodilator	Asthma
Slow-K	potassium	Electrolyte	Potassium replacement
Sorbitrate	isosorbide dinitrate	Nitroglycerin	Angina
Stelazine	trifluoperazine	Antipsychotic	Psychosis
Sudafed	pseudoephedrine	Beta sympathomimetic	Asthma
Surmontil	trimipramine	Tricyclic antidepressant	Depression
Synthroid	levothyroxine	Thyroid hormone	Hypothyroidism
Tagamet	cimetidine	Antihistamine	Peptic ulcer disease
Talwin	pentazocine	Narcotic	Pain
Tambocor	flecainide	Antiarrhythmic	Ventricular dysrhythmias
Tapazole	methimazole	Thyroid inhibitor	Hyperthyroidism
Taractan	chlorprothixene	Antipsychotic	Psychosis
Tedral	theophylline	Xanthine bronchodilator	Asthma
Tegretol	carbamazepine	Anticonvulsant	Seizures; trigeminal neuralgia

TRADE NAME	GENERIC NAME	CLASS	COMMONLY PRESCRIBED FOR
Tenormin	atenolol	Beta blocker	Angina; hypertension; PSVT
Theo-Dur	theophylline	Xanthine bronchodilator	Asthma
Thorazine	chlorpromazine	Antipsychotic	Psychosis
Tigan	trimethobenzamide	Antiemetic	Nausea and vomiting
Tofranil	imipramine	Tricyclic antidepressant	Depression
Tolectin	tolmetin	Nonsteroidal anti-inflammatory	Arthritis; pain
Tolinase	tolazamide	Oral hypoglycemic	Diabetes
Tonocard	tocainide	Antiarrhythmic	Ventricular dysrhythmias
Trandate	labetalol	Beta blocker	Angina; hypertension
Tranxene	clorazepate	Benzodiazepine tranquilizer	Anxiety
Trental	pentoxifylline	Antiviscosity agent	Intermittent claudication
Triavil	amitriptyline	Tricyclic antidepressant	Depression
Trilafon	perphenazine	Antipsychotic	Psychosis
Tylenol	acetaminophen	Analgesic	Pain; fever
Valium	diazepam	Benzodiazepine tranquilizer	Anxiety
Vancenase	beclomethasone	Corticosteroid	Asthma
Vanceril	beclomethasone	Corticosteroid	Asthma
Vasotec	enalapril	Angiotensin inhibitor	Hypertension
Velosulin	insulin	Hormone	Diabetes
Vesprin	triflupromazine	Antipsychotic	Psychosis
Visken	pindolol	Beta blocker	Angina; hypertension
Vistaril	hydroxyzine	Antihistamine	Anxiety; nausea and vomiting; sleep
Wellbutrin	bupropion	Antidepressant	Depression
Xanax	alprazolam	Benzodiazepine tranquilizer	Anxiety
Zantac	ranitidine	Antihistamine	Peptic ulcer disease
Zaroxolyn	metolazone	Diuretic	Hypertension
Zyloprim	allopurinol	Uric acid blocker	Gout; hyperuricemia

AMI = acute myocardial infarction; CHF = congestive heart failure; CNS = central nervous system; COPD = chronic obstructive pulmonary disease; MAO = monoamine oxidase; PVCs = premature ventricular contractions; PSVT = paroxysmal supraventricular tachycardia.

GLOSSARIES

A
Glossary of Medical Root Words

a-, an- Without
ab- Away from
acro- An extremity
ad- Toward
adeno- Gland
aer(o)- Air
alb- White
-algia Pain
ambi- On both sides
andro- Male
angio- Blood vessel
ante- Before
anti- Against
arterio- Artery
arthro- Joint
-asthenia Weakness
auto- Self

bi- Twice, two
bio- Life
blepharo- Eyelid
brachio- Arm
brady- Slow
broncho- Bronchi

cardio- Heart
carpo- Wrist
-cele Cavity, swelling, protrusion
-centesis Puncturing
cephalo- Head
cerebro- Brain
chole- Bile, gall
chondro- Cartilage
-cide Killing of
circum- Around
co-, con- Together, with
contra- Against
costo- Rib
cranio- Skull
cyano- Blue

cyst- Bladder
-cyte, cyto- Cell

dento- Tooth
dermato- Skin
dia- Through
diplo- Double
-dipsia Thirst
dorso- Posterior, back
-dynia Pain
dys- Abnormal, painful, difficult

ec- Out
-ectasis Expansion, dilatation
ecto- Out from
-ectomy Surgical removal
-emia Blood
en- Into, within
endo- Within, innermost
entero- Intestines
epi- Upon, after, in addition to
equi- Equal
erythro- Red
-esthesia Feeling
eu- Normal, good
exo- Outward, outer
extra- Outside of, in addition to

gastro- Stomach
-genic Causing, caused by
glosso- Tongue
glyco- Sugar
-gram A written record
-graphy Visualization
gyn-, gyne-, gyneco- Woman

hem-, hema-, hemato- Blood
hemi- Half
hepato- Liver
hetero- Different

homeo-, homo- Same
hydro- Water
hyper- Above, excessive
hypo- Below, deficient
hystero- Uterus

-iasis State, condition
iatro- Physician
idio- Peculiar, self
ile- Ileum
ili- Ilium
in- Within, into, inside
infra- Beneath
inter- Between
intra- Within
ipsi- Same
irido- Iris
iso- Equal
-itis Inflammation

lacto- Milk
laryngo- Larynx
leuko- White
lingua- Tongue
lipo- Fat
litho- Stone
-lysis Dissolution

macro- Large
mal- Bad, poor
-malacia Softening
mammo- Breast, mammary gland
masto- Breast
mega-, megalo-, -megaly Enlargement
melano- Black
meningo- Meninges
meno- Month
metro- Uterus
micro- Small
mono- One, single
-morphic Shape, form
myelo- Spinal cord; also, bone marrow
myo- Muscle
myringo- Eardrum

narco- Stupor, numbness, sleep
naso- Nose
necro- Death
neo- New
nephro- Kidney
neuro- Nerve
noct- Night

oculo- Eye
-oid Like

oligo- Few, little, sparse
-ology Science of
-oma Tumor, swelling
onco- Tumor
onycho- Fingernail or toenail
oophor- Ovary
ophthalmo- Eye
-opia Vision
orchi- Testicle
ortho- Straight
-osis Disease, abnormal condition
osteo- Bone
-ostomy Surgical opening, outlet
oto- Ear
-otomy Cutting into

pan- All
para- Beside
-paresis Weakness
-pathy Disease
-penia Lack of, scarcity
per- Through
peri- Around
-phagia Swallowing, eating
pharyngo- Pharynx, throat
-phasia Speech
-philia Affinity for
phlebo- Vein
-phobia Fear
-phonia Sound, speech
photo- Light
phren- Diaphragm
pilo- Hair
-plasia Growth (of cells)
-plasty Surgical repair
-plegia Paralysis
pleuro- Pleura
-pnea Breathing
pneumo- Breath, air, lung
pod(o)- Foot
poly- Many
post- After
postero- Back
pre- Before, in front of
pro- In front of, before, forward
procto- Rectum
pseudo- False
psych- Mind
-ptosis Drooping, falling
pulmo- Lung
pyelo- Pelvis of the kidney
pyloro- Pylorus of the stomach
pyo- Pus

quad-, quadri- Four

reno-   Kidney
retro-   Behind, backward, back of
rhino-   Nose
-rrhage, -rrhagia   Excessive flow, bursting forth
-rrhaphy   Suture, repair
-rrhea   Profuse flow

salping-   Tube (usually fallopian or eustachian tube)
sclero-   Hardness
-scope   Instrument for looking at something
-scopy   Looking at
semi-   Half
sero-   Watery
-spasm   Involuntary contractions
spleno-   Spleen
spondylo-   Vertebra
-stasis   Stopping, stagnation of flow
sub-   Under

super-, supra-   Above, in addition
syn-, sym-   With, together

tachy-   Fast
thoraco-   Chest
thrombo-   Clot
trans-   Across, over
tri-   Three
-tripsy   Crushing

ultra-   Beyond, excessive
un-   Not, reversal
uni-   One
-uresis   Urination
-uria   Of the urine
uro-   Urine, urinary organs

vaso-   Vessel
ven-, veni-, veno-   Vein

B
Glossary of Common Medical Abbreviations

a   Before (from *a*nte)
AAL   Anterior axillary line
ABC   Airway, breathing, and circulation
ac   Before meals
AC   Alternating current
ad lib   As much as desired
AIDS   Acquired immunodeficiency syndrome
aq   Water
ALS   Advanced life support
AM   Amplitude modulation
AMI   Acute myocardial infarction
APC   Aspirin/phenacetin/caffeine
ASA   Acetylsalicylic acid (aspirin)
ASAP   As soon as possible
ASCVD   Arteriosclerotic cardiovascular disease
ATA   Atmospheres absolute
ATLS   Advanced trauma life support
AV   Atrioventricular

bid   Twice a day
BLS   Basic life support
BP   Blood pressure
BSA   Body surface area

c̄   With
CA   Cancer
CAD   Coronary artery disease
CAT   Computed axial tomography
CBC   Complete blood count
cc   Cubic centimeter (equivalent to a milliliter)
C.C.   Chief complaint
CCU   Coronary care unit
CHB   Complete heart block
CHF   Congestive heart failure
CHI   Closed head injury
CNS   Central nervous system
c/o   Complains of
CO   Carbon monoxide; also, cardiac output
CO$_2$ Carbon dioxide
COPD   Chronic obstructive pulmonary disease
CPR   Cardiopulmonary resuscitation

CSF   Cerebrospinal fluid
CSM   Carotid sinus massage
CVA   Cerebrovascular accident
CVP   Central venous pressure

D/C   Discontinue
DC   Direct current
DIP   Distal interpharyngeal joint (joint nearest fingertip)
DOA   Dead on arrival
DOB   Date of birth
DOE   Dyspnea on exertion
DP   Dorsalis pedis
DTs   Delirium tremens
DTR   Deep tendon reflex
D5/W   5% dextrose in water (IV solution)
Dx   Diagnosis

EBL   Estimated blood loss
ECF   Extracellular fluid
ECG, EKG   Electrocardiogram
ED   Emergency department
EDC   Estimated date of confinement (due date for delivery)
EEG   Electroencephalogram
EMS   Emergency medical services
EMT   Emergency medical technician
ENT   Ear, nose, and throat
EOA   Esophageal obturator airway
EOM   Extraocular movements
ER   Emergency room
ET   Endotracheal
ETA   Estimated time of arrival
EtOH   Alcohol

FB   Foreign body
FCC   Federal Communications Commission
FDA   Food and Drug Administration
FM   Frequency modulation
fsw   Feet of sea water
FUBAR   Fouled up beyond all recognition

FUO Fever of unknown origin
fx Fracture

G Gravida
GB Gall bladder
gc Gonorrhea
GI Gastrointestinal
gm Gram
GSW Gunshot wound
gtt Drop
GU Genitourinary

h, hr Hour
HAPE High-altitude pulmonary edema
Hb, Hgb Hemoglobin
Hct Hematocrit
HCVD Hypertensive cardiovascular disease
Hg Mercury
HIV Human immunodeficiency virus
H&P History and physical examination
HPI History of the present illness
HR Heart rate
hs At bedtime
Hx History

IC Intracardiac
ICF Intracellular fluid
ICS Intercostal space
ICU Intensive care unit
IM Intramuscular
I&O Intake and output
IPPB Intermittent positive pressure breathing
IUCD Intrauterine contraceptive device
IV Intravenous
IVC Inferior vena cava

JVD Jugular venous distention

kg Kilogram
KVO Keep vein open

L Liter
LCM Left costal margin
LLQ Left lower quadrant
LMP Last menstrual period
LOC Level of consciousness
LRS Lactated Ringer's solution
LSB Left sternal border
LUQ Left upper quadrant
LVH Left ventricular hypertrophy

MAP Mean arterial pressure
MAST Military anti-shock trousers
MCL Midclavicular line
mEq Milliequivalent
mg Milligram

μg Microgram
MI Myocardial infarction
MICU Mobile intensive care unit; medical intensive care unit
ml Milliliter
mm Millimeter
mm Hg Millimeters of mercury (units of pressure)
MS Morphine sulfate; multiple sclerosis; mitral stenosis; musculoskeletal
MSL Midsternal line
mV Millivolt

N/A Not applicable
NAD No apparent distress
NG Nasogastric
NKA No known allergies
NKDA No known drug allergies
N₂O Nitrous oxide
NPO Nihil per os (= nothing by mouth)
NS Normal saline
NSR Normal sinus rhythm
NTG Nitroglycerin
N&V Nausea and vomiting

O₂ Oxygen
OB Obstetrics
OD Overdose; right eye
OPC Outpatient clinic
OR Operating room
OS Left eye

p After (from *post*)
P Pulse
PAC Premature atrial contraction
PASG Pneumatic anti-shock garment
PAT Paroxysmal atrial tachycardia
pc After meals
PCO₂ Partial pressure of carbon dioxide
PE Physical examination
PEEP Positive end-expiratory pressure
PERRLA Pupils equal, round, and reactive to light and accommodation
pH Hydrogen ion concentration (acidity)
PH Past history
PID Pelvic inflammatory disease
PIP Proximal interphalangeal joint
PMH Past medical history
PMI Point of maximal impulse
PND Paroxysmal noctural dyspnea
po By mouth
PO₂ Partial pressure of oxygen
POPS Pulmonary overpressurization syndrome
prn As needed
PROM Premature rupture of the membranes (in pregnancy)
psi Pounds per square inch

PSVT Paroxysmal supraventricular tachycardia
pt Patient
PT Physical therapy
PTA Prior to admission
PUD Peptic ulcer disease
PVC Premature ventricular contraction
PVR Peripheral vascular resistance

q Every
qh Every hour
qid Four times a day

R Respirations
rad Radiation absorbed dose (unit of measure for x-rays)
RBC Red blood cell
RCM Right costal margin
Rh Rhesus factor, in blood grouping
RL Ringer's lactate
RLQ Right lower quadrant
RN Registered nurse
R/O Rule out
ROM Range of motion
RSB Right sternal border
RUQ Right upper quadrant
Rx Prescription, treatment

s̄ Without
SA Sinoatrial
SC Subcutaneous
SCUBA Self-contained underwater breathing apparatus
SIDS Sudden infant death syndrome
SL Sublingual
SNAFU Situation normal, all fouled up

SOB Shortness of breath
SQ Subcutaneous
stat Immediately
STD Sexually transmitted disease
SVC Superior vena cava
Sx Symptoms

T Temperature
TBW Total body water
TIA Transient ischemic attack
tid Three times a day
TKO To keep open
TMJ Temporomandibular joint
TNS Transcutaneous nerve stimulation
TPR Temperature, pulse, respirations

UGI Upper gastrointestinal
UHF Ultrahigh frequency
URI Upper respiratory infection
UTI Urinary tract infection
UV Ultraviolet

VD Venereal disease
VF Ventricular fibrillation
VHF Very high frequency
VS Vital signs
VT Ventricular tachycardia

WBC White blood cell
WDWN Well developed, well nourished
WNL Within normal limits
WPW Wolff-Parkinson-White syndrome

y/o Year old

C
Glossary of Medical Terms

This glossary is intended to provide brief definitions of terms used in the text. Words highlighted in *italic* type within the definitions are defined elsewhere in the glossary.

abandonment Abrupt termination of contact with the patient without giving the patient sufficient opportunity to find another health professional to take over his medical treatment.

ABCs *Airway, Breathing,* and *Circulation*—the first three items to evaluate and manage in the examination of any victim. These are the steps of *basic life support.*

abdomen The large cavity below the *diaphragm* and above the *pelvis.*

abdominal Pertaining to the abdomen.

abduct To draw away from the midline of the body or from a neighboring part or limb.

abduction Movement away from the midline of the body.

abnormality The quality of being abnormal or malformed.

abortion The premature expulsion from the *uterus* of the *embyro* or a nonviable *fetus.*

   criminal abortion Illegal attempt to produce an abortion, often under highly unsterile conditions hazardous to the mother's life.

   incomplete abortion Abortion in which some of the products of conception remain in the uterus.

   inevitable abortion Situation in which there is vaginal bleeding, uterine contractions, and cervical dilatation before term and no possibility that the pregnancy will go to term.

   missed abortion Prolonged retention in the uterus of a fetus who died during the first 20 weeks of gestation.

   spontaneous abortion An abortion occurring naturally.

   therapeutic abortion An abortion induced for justifiable medical reasons in an authorized medical setting.

   threatened abortion Situation in which there are bleeding and cramps during pregnancy, which may go on to incomplete abortion or may subside, allowing the pregnancy to go to term.

abrasion Portion of the body denuded of *epidermis* by scraping, rubbing, and so on.

abruptio placenta Premature separation of a normally implanted *placenta* from the uterine wall, usually with massive hemorrhage, occurring during the third trimester of pregnancy.

abscess Collection of pus in a sac, formed by necrotic tissues and an accumulation of *white blood cells.*

absolute refractory period Early phase of cardiac *repolarization,* wherein the heart muscle cannot be stimulated to depolarize.

absorption Passage of a substance through a membrane into the blood.

acceleration The rate of change in *velocity.*

accessory muscles Muscles other than the *diaphragm* and the *intercostal muscles* that are brought into play to assist breathing when a person is in respiratory distress, e.g., the *sternocleidomastoid muscle* of the neck.

acetabulum Cup-shaped cavity in which the rounded head of the *femur* rotates.

acetone breath Breath characterized by a sweet, fruity odor, found especially in *diabetic ketoacidosis.*

acetylcholine Chemical mediator of the *parasympathetic nervous system.*

acid Compound that dissociates with formation of hydrogen *ions* (H^+); solution with a *pH* less than 7.0.

acidosis Disturbance in the acid-base balance of the body caused by excessive amounts of *carbon dioxide* (respiratory acidosis) or of lactic and organic acids (metabolic acidosis). It is characterized by a pH less than 7.35.

acquired immunodeficiency syndrome (AIDS) Viral illness characterized by severe impairment of the body's immune defense system, which renders the patient vulnerable to many other infections.

acromion   Lateral extension of the *scapula* that forms the highest point of the shoulder.

activated charcoal   Substance used to adsorb ingested poisons.

acute   Having a rapid onset and severe symptoms and being of short duration.

acute abdomen   Condition caused by abdominal injury or by irritation or inflammation of the peritoneal lining, accompanied by severe pain.

acute myocardial infarction (AMI)   Condition present when a period of cardiac *ischemia* caused by sudden narrowing or complete occlusion of a coronary artery leads to death (*necrosis*) of myocardial tissue.

acute respiratory insufficiency   Any condition in which breathing is inadequate to suppply oxygen to or remove carbon dioxide from body tissues.

addiction   Overwhelming involvement in the use of drug, characterized by psychologic dependence, compulsive drug use, *tolerance*, and physical dependence.

adduction   Movement toward the midline of the body.

adipose   Referring to fat tissue.

ad lib   Abbreviation meaning "as desired."

Adrenalin   A trade name for *epinephrine*, the *hormone* produced by the *adrenal* gland with alpha and beta *sympathomimetic* properties.

adrenals   Paired glands, each situated on the superior pole of the kidney. The adrenals produce *corticosteroids*, *catecholamines*, and a variety of other *hormones*.

adrenergic   Referring to the *sympathetic nervous system* (deriving from the word Adrenalin).

adsorption   Adherence of a substance onto the surface of another substance.

advanced life support (ALS)   *Basic life support* (the *ABCs*) plus definitive therapy, including the use of invasive procedures, drugs, and *defibrillation*.

aerobic metabolism   Metabolism that can proceed only in the presence of *oxygen*.

afebrile   Without fever.

affect   The outward expression of a person's mood.

afterbirth   *Placenta*.

afterdrop   Continued fall in core temperature after a victim of *hypothermia* has been removed from a cold environment.

afterload   The resistance against which the *ventricle* contracts.

agglutination   Clumping together of *red blood cells*.

agitation   Extreme restlessness and anxiety.

agonal   Pertaining to the period of dying.

agonal rhythm   Cardiac *dysrhythmia* seen just before the heart stops altogether; essentially *aystole* with occasional *QRS complexes* that are not associated with any *cardiac output*.

agoraphobia   Literally, fear of the marketplace; fear of entering a place from which escape may be impeded.

air   Gas composed of approximately 20% oxygen and 80% nitrogen, with trace amounts of other gases.

air embolism   Air bubble introduced into the circulation.

air hunger   *Dyspnea*, or shortnesss of breath with rapid, labored breathing.

alarm reaction   First stage of the acute *stress* response.

alcoholic   Pertaining to or containing alcohol; one addicted to alcohol.

alerting response   Beginning of the *alarm reaction*, in which the animal suddenly stops all activity and orients toward the source of stimulation.

algorithm   Step-by-step procedure for solving a problem.

alimentary tract   The digestive tract as a whole.

alkaline   Having a *pH* greater than 7.0; in physiology, having a pH greater than 7.35.

alkalinizing agent   Substance, such as *sodium bicarbonate*, used to increase the *pH* or alkalinity of body fluids.

alkalosis   Abnormal condition of acid-base balance that results when the body loses too much carbon dioxide by *hyperventilation* (respiratory alkalosis) or too much acid (metabolic alkalosis), for example, from vomiting. Alkalosis may also be caused by excessive intake of alkaline substances, such as antacids or *sodium bicarbonate*.

allergen   Substance that produces allergic symptoms in a patient.

allergy   Abnormal susceptibility on reexposure to a substance that does not ordinarily cause adverse symptoms in the average person.

alopecia   Baldness.

alpha particle   Positively charged subatomic particle corresponding to the nucleus of a helium atom, with high ionizing ability but low penetration.

alpha receptor   Center located in the walls of small arteries and veins that, when simulated by alpha (*sympathomimetic*) drugs, causes the vessels to constrict.

alpha stimulator   Drug or hormone that activates *alpha receptors*, e.g., *norepinephrine*.

alternating current (AC)   Electric current whose direction reverses at regular intervals. Contact with alternating current can cause the victim to "freeze" to the current source.

alveolar air   That portion of the *tidal volume* that reaches the *alveoli* and participates in gas exchange there.

alveoli   Saccular units at the end of the *bronchioles* where gas exchange takes place (singular: alveolus).

amenorrhea   Absence of *menstruation*.

aminophylline   Xanthine drug used to relax smooth muscle in the air passages. It is sometimes used together with other agents in the treatment of *asthma, chronic obstructive pulmonary disease,* and *congestive heart failure*.

amnesia   Loss of memory.

amniotic fluid   Fluid that surrounds the *fetus* in the *uterus,* contained in the *amniotic sac*.

amniotic sac   Thin, transparent sac that holds the fetus suspended in *amniotic fluid*; popularly called the bag of waters.

amobarbital   A *barbiturate* sedative-hypnotic drug.

amplitude   Height, usually of an *ECG* wave or complex.

amputation   Severing of a part of the body.

anaerobic metabolism   Metabolism that takes place in the absence of *oxygen,* whose principal product is *lactic acid*.

analgesic   Agent that relieves pain.

analog signal   Continuous signal varying in amplitude and direction in proportion to the signal source, e.g., an *ECG* signal.

anaphylactic shock   An exaggerated allergic reaction with severe *bronchospasm* and vascular collapse, which may be rapidly fatal.

anasarca   Severe *edema* throughout the whole body.

anastomosis   Joining together of two tubelike structures, such as segments of intestine or blood vessels.

anatomic   Pertaining to anatomy or to the structure of an organism.

anatomy   The study of body structure.

anemia   State in which the volume of *red blood cells* or *hemoglobin* is deficient.

anesthesia   Absence of sensation to the point that pain is wholly abolished.

aneurysm   Sac or bulge resulting from the weakening of the wall of a blood vessel or *ventricle*.

angina   Condition marked by attacks of choking or suffocation.

    angina pectoris   Sudden pain from myocardial *ischemia,* caused by embarrassment of circulation to the cardiac muscle. The pain is usually *substernal* and often radiates to the arms, jaw, or abdomen. Usually it lasts 3 to 5 minutes and disappears with rest.

    stable angina   Angina pectoris characterized by periodic pain with a predictable pattern.

    unstable angina (preinfarction angina)   Angina pectoris characterized by a changing, unpredictable pattern of pain, which may signal an impending *acute myocardial infarction*.

Angiocath   A Teflon *catheter* inserted over a needle.

angiogram   A radiographic depiction of blood vessels, through the use of contrast medium.

angioneurotic edema   A condition of allergic origin characterized by hives and swelling of various tissues. It may involve laryngeal *edema,* facial swelling, and sometimes vascular collapse.

angle of Louis   Prominence on the *sternum* that lies opposite the second intercostal space.

anion   Negatively charged *ion,* e.g., Cl^- (chloride ion).

anisocoria   Inequality of the size of the pupils.

anomaly   Any feature that departs significantly from the normal.

anorexia   Lack of appetite.

anoxia   Absence of oxygen in a tissue.

antagonism   Opposition between the effects of medications.

antecubital   Situated in front of the forearm.

antenatal   Before birth.

antepartum   Before delivery.

anterior   Situated in front or in the forward part of. In anatomy, used in reference to the ventral or belly surface of the body.

anterior chamber   The portion of the eye between the *cornea* and the *lens*.

antiarrhythmic drug   Drug given to prevent or terminate cardiac *dysrhythmias*.

antibiotic   Agent derived from living sources that kills or inhibits the growth of bacteria.

antibody   Protein produced in the body in response to a specific *antigen* (foreign protein) that destroys or inactivates the antigen.

anticoagulant   Substance that prevents the *coagulation,* or clotting, of blood.

anticonvulsant   Substance used to stop seizures.

antidote   Substance used to counteract the effects of a drug or combat the effects of a poison.

antigen   Agent that, when taken into the body, stimulates the formation of specific protective proteins called *antibodies*.

antihypertensive agents   Drugs used to lower blood pressure, e.g., hydralazine, guanethidine.

antipyretic   Drug that reduces fever.

antiseptic   Preparation that prevents the growth or multiplication of bacteria.

antiserum   Serum that contains *antibodies* against a specific disease-producing agent, e.g., rabies antiserum.

antivenin   *Antiserum* against an animal or insect venom.

anus   The outlet of the *rectum*, lying in the fold between the buttocks.

anxiety   Feeling of apprehension, uncertainty, and fear.

aorta   Largest *artery* in the body, originating from the *left ventricle*.

aortic arch   Portion of the aorta that curves and begins to descend.

aortic valve   Valve between the left *ventricle* and the *aorta*.

apathy   Lack of feeling or interest.

apex of the heart   Caudal end of the *ventricles* located in the fifth left intercostal space in normal adults; also known as the *point of maximal impulse (PMI)*.

Apgar score   Method of assessing the newborn, developed by Virginia Apgar, that assigns scores between zero and two to the infant's color, heart rate, reflex irritability, muscle tone, and respiratory effort, as measured at 1 minute and 5 minutes after birth.

aphasia   Defect in speaking or understanding speech, caused by injury or disease affecting the brain centers that regulate speech.

　motor aphasia   Loss of speech or some component thereof (e.g., the ability to name things).

　sensory aphasia   Loss of the ability to comprehend speech.

aphonia   Loss of voice.

apical   Pertaining to the *apex of the heart*.

apical pulse   Pulse obtained by auscultating over the apical portion of the heart.

apnea   Absence of breathing.

apothecary system   System of weights and liquid measures utilizing pounds, pints, quarts, fluidounces, fluidrams, minims, ounces, drams, and grains. No longer in widespread use for medical purposes, having been replaced by the *metric system*.

appendicitis   Inflammation of the *appendix*.

appendicular skeleton   The part of the skeleton comprising the upper and lower extremities.

appendix   Wormlike structure attached to the *cecum*, in the right lower quadrant of the *abdomen*.

aqueous humor   Fluid in the anterior chamber of the eye.

arachnoid   Middle *meningeal* membrane.

arrest   Stoppage, usually referring to *pulse* or *respirations*.

arrhythmia   Disturbance in the normal rhythm of the heart. It is more correctly called a *dysrhythmia*.

arterial blood   Oxygenated blood. Blood is oxygenated in the *lungs* and then passes from the lungs to the left side of the heart, through the *pulmonary veins*. It is then pumped out of the left heart into the arteries supplying all parts of the body.

arteriole   Small blood vessel that carries oxygenated blood, branching into yet smaller vessels called *capillaries*.

arteriosclerosis   Pathologic condition in which the arterial walls become thickened and inelastic.

arteriovenous fistula (AV fistula)   Surgically created *anastomosis* between an artery and a vein, for purposes of facilitating *hemodialysis*.

artery   Muscular, thick-walled blood vessel that carries blood away from the heart.

arthralgia   Pain in one or more *joints*.

arthritis   Inflammation of the *joints*.

articulation   Place where two bones meet to form a *joint*.

artifact   Artificial product; used to refer to noise or interference in an *ECG* tracing.

arytenoid cartilage   One of the paired, pitcher-shaped *cartilages* at the back of the *larynx*, at the upper border of the *cricoid cartilage*.

ascending aorta   Portion of the aorta that rises out of the heart.

ascites   Accumulation of fluid in the abdominal cavity.

asepsis   Technique having the objective of preventing bacterial contamination of a wound or instrument.

asphyxia   Suffocation; a condition characterized by *hypercarbia* and *hypoxemia*.

aspirate   To inhale foreign material into the lungs; to remove by suction.

assault   To create in another person a fear of immediate bodily harm or invasion of bodily security.

assisted ventilation   Use of adjunctive equipment, such as a bag-valve-mask or demand valve, to boost the *tidal volume* of a spontaneously breathing patient.

asthma   Condition characterized by *dyspnea*, *bronchoconstriction*, *mucous* plugs, and *wheezing*.

asymptomatic   Not experiencing any symptoms.

asystole   Absent ventricular contractions; a "straight-line ECG."

ataxia   Inability to coordinate the muscles properly; often used to describe a staggering gait.

atelectasis   Collapse of the *alveolar air* spaces of the *lungs*.

atheroma   Mass of fatty tissue that develops in the *intima* of arteries.

atherosclerosis   Common type of *arteriosclerosis* affecting the *coronary* and *cerebral* arteries.

atlas   The first *cervical vertebra*.

atmospheres absolute (ATA)   Measurement of ambient pressure.

atrial arrhythmia   A *dysrhythmia* arising in the *SA node* or atrial tissue.

atrial depolarization   Electric process causing atrial

contraction. It is represented on the *ECG* by the *P wave*.

atrial fibrillation A *dysrhythmia* characterized by discharge of multiple atrial *ectopic foci* and an irregularly irregular ventricular rhythm.

atrial flutter A *dysrhythmia* characterized by rapid discharge of an atrial *ectopic focus*, with varying degrees of block through the *atrioventricular (AV) junction*.

atrial kick The addition to ventricular volume contributed by contraction of the atria.

atrial systole The period of atrial contraction that precedes ventricular contraction.

atrioventricular block (AV block) Condition in which the passage of impulses from the atrium through the *atrioventricular (AV) junction* is hindered or prevented altogether.

atrioventricular dissociation (AV dissociation) Condition in which the *atria* and *ventricles* contract independently of one another, associated with *complete heart block*.

atrioventricular junction (AV junction) Portion of the electric conduction system of the heart located in the upper part of the *interventricular septum* that conducts the *excitation impulse* from the *atria* to the *bundle of His*.

atrioventricular node (AV node) Specialized structure located in the *atrioventricular junction* that slows conduction through the AV junction.

atrioventricular valves (AV valves) The *mitral* and *tricuspid* valves.

atrium Thin-walled chamber of the heart. The right atrium receives venous blood from the *venae cavae*; the left atrium receives oxygenated blood from the *pulmonary veins*.

atrophy Wasting away of a tissue.

atropine *Parasympathetic* blocking agent, used to increase the heart rate in *bradycardia* or counteract the effects of poisoning with organophosphate insecticides.

auditory nerve The eighth cranial nerve, which mediates hearing and balance.

aura Premonitory sensation of impending illness; the term is usually used in connection with an epileptic attack.

auricle Atrium.

auscultation Technique of listening for and interpreting sounds that occur within the body, usually with a *stethoscope*.

automaticity Spontaneous initiation of depolarizing electric impulses by *pacemaker sites* within the *electric conduction system* of the heart.

autonomic nervous system Subdivision of the nervous system that controls primarily involuntary body functions. It comprises the *sympathetic* and *parasympathetic nervous systems*.

avulsion Injury that leaves a piece of skin or other tissue either partially or completely torn away from the body.

axial skeleton The part of the skeleton comprising the skull, spinal column, and rib cage.

axilla Armpit.

axis Second cervical *vertebra*.

Babinski reflex Reflex response of the big toe seen in patients with injury to the brain. When the sole of the foot is stroked with a sharp object, the big toe turns upward, instead of in the normal downward direction.

ball-and-socket joint Type of *joint* found in the hip and shoulder.

bandage Any material used to hold a *dressing* in place.

barbiturate Class of drugs that produces a calming, sedative effect, e.g., phenobarbital.

baroreceptor Special sensing device located in the *aortic arch* and *carotid sinus* that detects changes in pressure (volume) within the vascular system.

barotrauma Injury resulting from pressure disequilibrium across body surfaces.

base Compound that dissociates to form hydroxyl ions (OH⁻); solution having a *pH* greater than 7.0.

base station Assembly of radio equipment consisting of at least a transmitter, receiver, and antenna connection at a fixed location.

basic life support (BLS) The *ABCs*, without adjunctive equipment.

basophil White blood cell that contains chemical mediators of the immune/inflammatory reaction.

battery Any act of touching another person without that person's consent.

Battle's sign Bluish discoloration over the tip of the *mastoid* bone behind the ear, signifying basilar skull fracture.

Beck's triad Muffled heart sounds, *hypotension*, and neck vein distention, characteristic of *cardiac tamponade*.

Benadryl Trade name for diphenhydramine, an antihistamine drug.

bends Syndrome caused by bubbles of gas in the blood that evolve during too rapid ascent from deep water in diving.

benign Noncancerous; nonmalignant; not dangerous.

Benzedrine Trade name for one of the amphetamines.

beta particle Negatively charged subatomic particle, with slightly greater penetrating ability than an *alpha particle*.

beta receptor Structure located in the myocardium, blood vessels, and bronchi that, when stimulated, produces an increase in cardiac rate and contractile force, *vasodilation,* and *bronchodilation.*

beta stimulator   Any agent that activates the *beta receptors* of the body, e.g., isoproterenol.

bevel   The slanting edge of the point of a hollow needle.

bicarbonate   Any salt having two equivalents of carbonic acid to one of any basic substances; often used as an abbreviated name for *sodium bicarbonate.*

biceps   The large muscle of the front part of the upper arm, which bends the forearm at the elbow.

bifurcation   Division into two branches.

bigeminy   *Dysrhythmia* in which every other beat is a *premature contraction.*

bile   Fluid secreted by the liver, concentrated and stored in the *gallbladder,* and discharged into the intestine, where it aids in the digestion of fats.

biologic death   See *death, biologic.*

biopsy   Removal of a small piece of tissue from the body for microscopic examination.

biotelemetry   Transmission of physiolgic data, e.g., an *ECG,* from the patient to a distant point of reception.

biotransformation   Metabolic process by which a drug is inactivated.

bivalent   Having two charges, e.g., Ca^{++} (calcium ion).

bladder   An organ of the urinary system, located in the *pelvis* just behind the pubic bone, that stores *urine* produced by the *kidneys.*

blind panic   Type of reaction seen in situations of mass casualties in which an individual's judgment is severely impaired.

blocker   Drug that counteracts or inhibits the action of another drug or agent. For example, *atropine* is a parasympathetic blocker.

blood pressure (BP)   The pressure exerted by the pulsatile flow of blood against the arterial walls.

   diastolic blood pressure   Blood pressure measured during ventricular relaxation (diastole).

   systolic blood pressure   Blood pressure measured during ventricular contraction (systole).

blood type   One of several groups into which human blood is divided according to its *antigens.*

blood volume   Total amount of blood in the heart and blood vessels, representing about 8 to 9 percent of body weight.

bloody show   Mucus and blood passed from the *vagina* when *labor* begins.

bradycardia   Slow heart rate, less than 60 per minute.

brain   Organ located in the skull that controls all body functions and is the seat of consciousness.

brainstem   Portion of the brain inferior to the *cerebrum* and continuous with the *spinal cord.*

Braxton Hicks contractions   Intermittent contractions of the *uterus* after the third month of pregnancy.

breech birth   Delivery in which the *presenting part* is the buttocks or foot.

bronchiole   Small subdivision of a *bronchus,* or airway.

bronchiolitis   Condition seen in children under 2 years old, characterized by *dyspnea* and *wheezing.*

bronchitis   Inflammation of the bronchi.

bronchoconstriction   Narrowing of the bronchial tubes.

bronchodilation   Widening of the bronchial tubes.

bronchodilator   Agent that causes dilation of the bonchi.

bronchospasm   Severe constriction of the bronchial tree.

bronchus   One of the main branches of the *trachea* carrying air into various parts of the lung.

bruise   Injury that does not break the skin but causes rupture of small, underlying blood vessels with resulting tissue discoloration; a *contusion.*

buccal   Pertaining to the cheek.

buffer   Substance in a fluid that tends to minimize changes in *pH* that would otherwise result from addition of *acid* or *base* to the fluid.

bundle branch block   Disturbance in *electric conduction* through the right or left *bundle branch* from the *bundle of His.*

bundle branches   The portion of the *electric conduction system* in the ventricles that conducts the *depolarizing* impulse from the *bundle of His* to the *Purkinje network* in the myocardium. They are subdivided into a right bundle branch and a left bundle branch.

bundle of His   Portion of the *electric conduction system* in the *interventricular septum* that conducts the *depolarizing* impulse from the *atrioventricular junction* to the right and left *bundle branches.*

burn   Injury caused by extremes of temperature, electric current, or certain chemicals.

   first-degree burn   Burn affecting only the outer skin layers (*epidermis*).

   second-degree burn   Burn penetrating beneath the superficial skin layers, producing *edema* and blistering.

   third-degree burn   Full-thickness burn, involving all layers of the skin and underlying tissue as well, having a charred or white, leathery appearance.

burnout   Exhaustion of physical or emotional strength as a result of chronic *stress.*

cachexia   Severe malnutrition and poor health as a result of disease or lack of nourishment.

café coronary   Choking incident, so named because

its suddenness may lead observers to mistake it for a heart attack.

calcium   Bivalent *cation* required for proper functioning of heart muscle and normal bone metabolism.

cancer   Growth in any tissue that has the power to invade other tissues and spread to other parts of the body.

cannula   Tube for insertion into a blood vessel.

capillary   Extremely narrow blood vessel, composed of a single layer of cells through which oxygen and nutrients pass to the tissues. Capillaries form a network between *arterioles* and *venules*.

capsule   Cylindrical gelatin container enclosing a dose of medication, usually in powdered form; ligamentous structure surrounding a *joint*.

carbohydrate   Element of food containing carbon, hydrogen, and oxygen, e.g., sugar or starch.

carbon dioxide (CO_2)   End product of *carbohydrate metabolism*, eliminated from the body by respiration.

carbon monoxide (CO)   Colorless, odorless, tasteless gas produced by incomplete combustion of organic materials.

carboxyhemoglobin   *Hemoglobin* that is combined with *carbon monoxide* instead of *oxygen*.

cardiac   Pertaining to the heart; sometimes used to refer to a person who has heart disease.

cardiac arrest   Sudden and unexpected cessation of adequate cardiac output.

cardiac asthma   *Left heart failure* and *pulmonary edema* with *wheezing* respirations.

cardiac axis   The average direction of current flow across the myocardium.

cardiac cycle   The period from one cardiac contraction to the next. Each cardiac cycle consists of ventricular contraction (*systole*) and relaxation (*diastole*).

cardiac output   Amount of blood pumped by the heart per minute, calculated by multiplying the *stroke volume* times the heart rate per minute.

cardiac rupture   Life-threatening complication of *acute myocardial infarction* that can involve the *papillary muscle, interventricular septum,* or *myocardium.*

cardiac standstill   *Asystole;* absence of cardiac contractions.

cardiac tamponade   Restriction of cardiac contraction, failing *cardiac output,* and *shock,* caused by the accumulation of fluid or blood in the *pericardium.*

cardiac work   The energy consumed by the heart in maintaining *cardiac output.* Cardiac work is increased by increases in heart rate or *peripheral vascular resistance.*

cardiogenic   Of cardiac origin.

cardiogenic shock   Serious complication of *acute myocardial infarction* in which ventricular damage is so extensive that the heart is unable to maintain adequate output to vital organs.

cardiopulmonary arrest   Cessation of cardiac and respiratory activity.

cardiopulmonary resuscitation (CPR)   Artificial ventilation and *external chest compressions.*

cardiotonic drugs   Drugs that increase the rate and force of myocardial contractions.

cardiovascular   Pertaining to the heart and blood vessels.

cardiovascular collapse   Failure of the heart and blood vessels; *shock.*

cardioversion   Use of synchronized *direct current* (DC) electric shock to convert *tachyarrhythmias* (e.g., atrial flutter) to *normal sinus rhythm.*

carina   Point at which the *trachea* bifurcates into the right and left main *bronchi.*

carotid   One of the main arteries of the neck supplying blood to the head.

carotid sinus   A dilated area in the internal *carotid artery,* usually found just above the *bifurcation* of the common carotid artery, containing very sensitive nerve endings that participate in regulation of heart rate and *blood pressure.* Massage of the carotid sinus can produce marked slowing of the heart through *vagal* stimulation.

carotid sinus massage (CSM)   Use of pressure on the *carotid sinus* to convert certain supraventricular *tachyarrhythmias,* especially *paroxysmal atrial tachycardia,* to *normal sinus rhythm.*

carpals   The eight small bones of the wrist.

carpopedal spasm   Contorted position of the hand in which the fingers flex in a clawlike attitude and the thumb curls toward the palm; may be caused by *hyperventilation.*

carrier   Person who harbors an infectious agent and, although not himself ill, can transmit the infection to another person.

cartilage   Tough, elastic substance that covers opposable surfaces of moveable *joints* and also forms parts of the *skeleton.*

cataract   Opacity of the crystalline *lens* of the eye or its capsule, causing impaired vision and eventually blindness.

catecholamine   Substance, such as *epinephrine* or *norepinephrine,* that acts on receptors of the *sympathetic nervous system* in the heart and small peripheral blood vessels to increase *cardiac output* and *blood pressure.*

catheter   Tube used for withdrawing fluid from various structures of the body or for irrigating hollow organs, such as the bladder.

catheter embolism   Accidental loss of a *catheter* fragment in a vein from shearing of an indwelling intravenous catheter.

cation   Positively charged *ion,* e.g., Na^+ (sodium ion).

caudad   Toward the foot end of the body.

cecum   First portion of the *large intestine* into which the *small intestine* empties. The vermiform *appendix* is attached to the cecum.

central nervous system (CNS)   The *brain* and *spinal cord*.

central neurogenic hyperventilation   Abnormal pattern of breathing seen in severe illness and injury involving the brain, characterized by marked *tachypnea* and *hyperpnea*.

cephalhematoma   Collection of blood beneath the periosteum of a baby's skull, presenting as a boggy mass in the scalp.

cephalic   Pertaining to the head.

cerebellum   Portion of the brain, located behind and below the *cerebrum*, whose general function is coordination of movement.

cerebral   Relating to the *brain*.

cerebral hemorrhage   Bleeding into the *cerebrum*; one of the forms of *stroke* or *cerebrovascular accident*.

cerebrospinal fluid (CSF)   The fluid that bathes the *brain* and *spinal cord*.

cerebrovascular accident (CVA)   Sudden cessation of circulation to a region of the brain, caused by *thrombus*, *embolism*, or *hemorrhage*; also called *stroke*.

cerebrum   Portion of the *brain* that controls higher functions, such as memory, perception, thought, and judgment.

certification   Process by which a professional association grants recognition to an individual who has met predetermined qualifications specified by that association.

cervical   Pertaining to the neck.

cervix   The lower portion, or neck, of the *uterus*.

cesarean section   The *delivery* of a baby by an operation in which an opening is made directly into the *uterus* through an abdominal incision.

chancre   Ulcerated lesion characteristic of primary syphilis.

channel   In EMS radio systems, a pair of radio frequencies (one for transmitting, the other for receiving).

chemotherapy   Treatment of a disease with drugs.

Cheyne-Stokes respirations   An abnormal breathing pattern characterized by rhythmic waxing and waning of the depth of respiration, with regularly occurring periods of *apnea*; seen in association with *central nervous system* dysfunction.

chief complaint   The problem for which a patient seeks help, stated in a word or short phrase.

chin lift   Technique of opening the airway by supporting the chin in a forward position.

chloride   *Monovalent anion* important in cellular function.

chock   A block of wood or similar object placed in front of or behind a wheel of a vehicle to prevent the vehicle from moving.

cholecystitis   Inflammation of the gallbladder.

cholesterol   Chemical found in various foods (e.g., animal tissue, egg yolks, certain oils and fats) that, when ingested in excess, is believed to contribute to the development of *atherosclerosis*.

cholinergic   Referring to the *parasympathetic nervous system*; derived from the word *acetylcholine*.

cholinesterase   Enzyme that inactivates *acetylcholine* released at the nerve cell junction.

chordae tendinae   Fibrous strands shaped like umbrella stays that attach the free edges of the leaflets, or cusps, of the *atrioventricular valves* to the *papillary muscles*.

chronic   Of long duration.

chronic obstructive pulmonary disease (COPD)   Term comprising chronic bronchitis, *emphysema*, and sometimes *asthma*—illnesses that cause obstructive problems in the lower airways.

chronotropic   Affecting the time or rate, applied especially to nerves whose stimulation or to agents whose administration affects the rate of contraction of the heart.

circulatory   Pertaining to the heart and blood vessels.

cirrhosis   Chronic, progressive fibrosis of the *liver*, often associated with chronic and excessive alcohol ingestion.

CISD   Critical incident stress debriefing.

civil suit   Action instituted by a private individual against another private individual.

clavicle   Collar bone, attached at right angles to the uppermost part of the *sternum*.

clonic   Characterized by rapid contraction and relaxation of a muscle or group of muscles.

clot   Lump or solid coagulum.

coagulation   Process of changing from a liquid to a thickened or solid state; the formation of a *clot*.

coccyx   Lowermost part of the spine, composed of four small, fused bones. Also called the tail bone.

cold diuresis   Secretion of large amounts of urine in response to cold exposure and the consequent shunting of blood volume to the body *core*.

colic   Crampy pain associated with obstruction of a hollow organ.

colitis   Inflammation of the *colon*.

collagen   Protein that gives tensile strength to the connective tissues of the body.

collateral circulation   Mesh of arteries and capillaries that furnishes blood to a segment of tissue whose original arterial supply has been obstructed.

colloid An intravenous solution containing proteins or other large molecules, e.g., albumin.

colon The large intestine.

colostomy Establishment of an opening between the *colon* and the surface of the body for the purpose of providing drainage of the bowel.

coma State of unconsciousness from which a person cannot be roused, even by noxious stimulation.

comatose Affected with *coma*.

comminuted fracture Fracture in which the bone is shattered or crushed into several small pieces.

communicable disease Disease that is transmissible from one person to another.

communicable period Period during which an infected person is capable of transmitting his illness to someone else.

compensatory pause The *R–R interval* between a premature beat and the following normal beat when that interval is longer than the R–R interval between the premature beat and the preceding normal beat. If the pause is fully compensatory, the R–R interval from the premature beat to the next beat, together with the preceding, shortened R–R interval, should equal two normal R–R intervals.

complete heart block *Third-degree heart block*; complete absence of electric conduction from the atria to the ventricles. The block can occur anywhere in the conduction system, from the *atrioventricular junction, atrioventricular node,* or *bundle of His* to the *bundle branches*. The *ventricles* are driven by an ectopic *pacemaker* below the block, and atrial and ventricular contractions become dissociated.

compress Folded cloth or pad used for applying pressure to stop *hemorrhage* or as a wet *dressing*.

compulsion Repetitive action carried out to relieve the anxiety of *obsessive* thoughts.

concussion Violent jar or shock; the injury that results from a violent jar or shock.

conduction Transfer of heat to a liquid or solid object.

conductivity Potential of the *electric conduction system* of the heart to transmit electric impulses.

confabulation Invention of experiences to cover over gaps in memory, seen in patients with certain organic brain syndromes.

confrontation Interviewing technique in which the interviewer points out to the patient something of interest in his conversation or behavior.

congenital Any condition that exists at or was acquired before birth.

congestive heart failure (CHF) Failure of adequate ventricular function with resulting backup of blood or fluid into the lungs or body tissues.

conjunctiva Delicate membrane that lines the eyelids and covers exposed surfaces of the eyeball. Normally pink, it may be pale in anemia or red in infection (conjunctivitis).

conscious Capable of responding to sensory stimuli and having subjective experiences.

consensual reaction Similar reaction of both *pupils* (e.g., constriction) to a stimulus applied to only one of them (e.g., bright light).

consent Agreement by a patient to accept medical intervention.

constrict To make smaller or narrower, e.g., constricted pupils.

constricting band Tourniquet-like device formerly used in treating snakebites of the extremities, to restrict venous flow of blood back to the heart; no longer recommended.

constriction Narrowing, as in the term *vasoconstriction*, which is a narrowing of the internal diameter of the blood vessels.

contact burn Burn produced by touching a hot object.

contagious Describing a disease that is readily transmissible from one person to another.

contaminated Infected with bacteria, such as a wound or other surface; may also refer to polluted water, foods, or drugs.

contractility Ability of a muscle to contract when depolarized by an electric impulse.

contraction Shortening of a part, such as a muscle.

contraindication Situation that prohibits use of a drug.

contralateral On the opposite side.

contrecoup Head injury resulting from a blow at another site.

controlled ventilation Artificial ventilation of a patient who is not breathing spontaneously.

contusion A *bruise*; an injury that causes *hemorrhage* into or beneath the skin but does not break the skin.

convection Mechanism by which body heat is picked up and carried away by moving air currents.

conversion hysteria Condition in which a person unconsciously translates an emotional conflict into a physical symptom, such as *paralysis*.

convulsion Violent, involuntary *contraction* or series of contractions of the *voluntary muscles*; a "fit" or *seizure*.

core The part of the body comprising the heart, lungs, brain, and abdominal viscera.

cornea The transparent structure covering the *pupil*.

coronary Term applied to the blood vessels of the heart that supply blood to its walls; also used by lay persons to refer to an *acute myocardial infarction*.

coronary artery disease (CAD) Pathologic process caused by *atherosclerosis* that leads to progressive narrowing and eventual obstruction of the coronary arteries.

coronary occlusion Obstruction in a coronary artery that hinders or prevents the flow of blood to some portion of the heart muscle. The term is used synonymously with *heart attack.*

coronary sinus Large vessel in the posterior part of the *coronary sulcus* into which the coronary veins empty.

coronary sulcus Groove along the exterior surface of the heart that separates the *atria* from the *ventricles.*

cor pulmonale Heart disease that develops secondary to a chronic lung disease, usually affecting primarily the right side of the heart.

corpus luteum Part of the *ovarian follicle* that remains and produces *progesterone* after the *ovum* has been released.

corticosteroid One of several drugs used to counteract inflammation whose structure is similar to that of naturally occurring steroid *hormones.*

costal Pertaining to the *ribs.*

costochondral Pertaining to a *rib* and the *cartilage* by which it is attached to the *sternum.*

coup A head injury occurring at the site of a blow.

crackles Any discontinuous adventitious sounds in the lungs, caused by the popping open of air spaces.

craniad Toward the head end of the body.

cranial Pertaining to the skull.

cravat Type of bandage made from a large, triangular piece of cloth that has been folded into a wide strip.

crepitus Grating sound heard and a sensation felt when the fractured ends of a bone rub together.

cribbing Timber used to provide a support or framework.

crib death *Sudden infant death syndrome,* of unknown cause.

cricoid cartilage Ringlike cartilage forming the lower and back part of the *larynx.*

cricothyroid membrane Membrane between the cricoid and thyroid cartilages of the *larynx.*

cricothyrotomy Puncture of the *cricothyroid membrane* for the purpose of establishing an emergency airway in cases of upper airway obstruction.

criminal suit Action instituted by the government against a private individual for violation of criminal law.

critical incident Incident that overwhelms a person's ability to adjust emotionally.

croup Common disease of childhood characterized by spasm of the *larynx* and resulting upper airway obstruction.

crowning Stage of birth when the *presenting part* of the baby is visible at the vaginal orifice.

crystalloid Intravenous solution that does not contain protein or other large molecules, e.g., 5% dextrose in water (D5/W), normal saline, *Ringer's solution.*

cumulative action Action of increased intensity evidenced after several doses of a drug.

cutaneous Pertaining to the skin.

cutdown Surgical exposure of a *vein* to insert a *cannula* for administration of *intravenous* fluids.

cyanosis Bluish discoloration of the skin caused by large quantities of reduced *hemoglobin* in the blood; a sign of *hypoxemia.*

damages Compensation for injury awarded by a court.

dead space Portion of the *tidal volume* that does not reach the alveoli and thus does not participate in gas exchange.

death, biologic Irreversible brain damage, usually occurring after 3 to 10 minutes of *cardiac arrest.*

death, clinical The moment the pulse and blood pressure are absent. Clinical death occurs immediately after the onset of *cardiac arrest.*

debriefing Formal session usually conducted 24 to 72 hours after a *critical incident* to deal with the feelings and reactions of the personnel involved.

deceleration Negative acceleration, i.e., a slowing down.

decerebrate posture Posture assumed by patients with severe brain dysfunction, characterized by extension and internal rotation of the arms and extension of the legs.

decimal A unit of 10; a system based on 10s.

decompensation Failure of an organ system; most often used to indicate the failure of the heart, as a result of disease, to maintain sufficient circulation of blood to meet the demands of the body.

decorticate posture Posture assumed by patients with severe brain dysfunction, characterized by extension of the legs and flexion of the arms.

decubitus ulcer A bedsore; an eroded wound acquired by sustained pressure on a single area of skin.

defibrillation Use of unsynchronized *direct current (DC) electric shock* to terminate *ventricular fibrillation.*

defibrillator Device that delivers *direct current (DC) electric shock* for the purpose of terminating *ventricular fibrillation.*

definitive care The D of the ABC-D sequence in *advanced life support.* Definitive care includes ECG monitoring, diagnosis and treatment of cardiac dysrhythmias, *defibrillation,* and administration of *intravenous* fluids and drugs.

deformity Unusual alteration in the shape of a part or organ.

defusing Brief meeting shortly after a potentially *critical incident* to ventilate feelings and prevent psychologic sequelae.

dehydration Condition that results from excessive loss of body water.

delirium Acutely disturbed mental condition, usually resulting from fever, injury, or intoxication; an acute confusional state.

delirium tremens (DTs) Potential complication of alcohol withdrawal, characterized by agitation, frightening hallucinations, and sometimes *cardiovascular collapse.*

delivery Expulsion or extraction of the child at birth.

delusion Belief or feeling that has no basis in fact, seen in *psychosis.*

dementia Chronic deterioration of mental functions.

denial Psychologic defense mechanism for dealing with unwanted feelings or data by ignoring them; seen, for example, in the patient who dismisses his chest pain as "just a little indigestion."

dependency Condition of leaning on or requiring support from another.

depolarization Process of discharging resting cardiac muscle fibers by an electric impulse that causes them to contract.

depolarization wave The electric movement produced by the progressive depolarization from the atria through the *ventricles* and recorded on the *ECG* as the *P wave* (atrial depolarization) and the *QRS complex* (ventricular depolarization).

depressant Drug that lessens the activity of the body or any of its organs.

depression Sadness, dejection; a decrease of functional activity.

dermis Inner layer of skin, containing hair follicle roots, glands, blood vessels, and nerves.

dextrose Preparation obtained by hydrolysis of starch, used as an *intravenous* nutrient.

diabetes mellitus Systemic disease affecting many organs, including the *pancreas,* whose failure to secrete *insulin* causes an inability to metabolize carbohydrate and consequent elevations in blood sugar.

diabetic ketoacidosis Condition resulting from uncontrolled diabetes, characterized by excessive thirst, hunger, urination, vomiting, and sometimes coma, with the production of ketones in *metabolism* as well as an excess of organic acids.

diagnosis Distinguishing one disease from another; the determination of the nature of a disease.

diaphoresis Profuse perspiration.

diaphragm Large skeletal muscle that plays a major role in breathing and that separates the chest cavity from the *abdominal* cavity.

diaphysis The shaft of a long bone.

diarrhea Increased frequency of defecation with discharge of watery or loose stools.

diastole Period of ventricular relaxation during which the *ventricles* passively fill with blood.

diastolic blood pressure The *blood pressure* obtained during ventricular *diastole;* the lowest arterial pressure between two *systolic* peaks.

diffusion Passage of fluid and chemicals through a membrane.

digitalis Drug used in the treatment of *congestive heart failure* and certain atrial *dysrhythmias.*

digitalization Process of giving *digitalis* to the point where maximum therapeutic effects are achieved without untoward side effects.

digitoxicity Toxicity from *digitalis,* which may be manifested by *anorexia, nausea,* vomiting, yellow vision, or cardiac *dysrhythmias.*

dilatation The condition of being dilated or stretched beyond normal dimensions.

diplopia Double vision.

direct current (DC) Electric current that flows at a steady rate in a single direction.

direct current (DC) electric shock Electric shock delivered with a *defibrillator* to the heart directly or through the chest wall to terminate certain *dysrhythmias,* such as *ventricular fibrillation,* or to convert various *tachyarrhythmias.*

disc Cartilaginous material that separates each of the *vertebrae.*

dislocation Disruption of the normal anatomy of a *joint.*

disorganization Disturbed mental state characterized by incoherence.

disorientation Disturbed mental state characterized by confusion regarding one's relationship to physical surroundings, time, or person.

displacement Redirection of an emotion from the original object to a substitute object more acceptable to the patient.

dissecting aneurysm *Aneurysm,* or bulge, formed by the separation of the layers of an arterial wall.

distal Farther from a point of reference; generally the point of reference is the heart.

distention State of being inflated or enlarged, particularly of the abdomen.

diuresis Secretion of large amounts of *urine* by the kidney.

diuretic Drug used to promote elimination of excess *extracellular fluid* by increasing the renal secretion of *urine.* Diuretics are often used in the treatment of *congestive heart failure.*

diverticulitis Inflammation of *diverticula,* which may produce an acute abdomen.

diverticulum   Pocket formed by a weakened area in the wall of the colon (plural: diverticula).

doll's eyes   Normal phenomenon in which the eyes move in the direction opposite to that in which the head is turned.

dominant pacemaker   The *sinoatrial (SA) node*. Other pacemakers are normally secondary.

dorsal   Referring to the back or posterior side of the body or an organ.

dorsiflexion   Backward bending of the hand or foot.

dressing   Protective covering for a wound, used to stop bleeding and to prevent contamination of the wound.

drowning   Death by submersion in water.

drowsiness   State in which a person appears to be asleep but can be roused by vocal stimuli.

ductus arteriosus   Direct communication between the *pulmonary artery* and the *aorta* in the fetal circulation.

ductus venosus   Muscular tube through which the umbilical vein enters the fetal abdomen.

duodenum   Name given to the first 11 inches of the *small intestine*.

duplex   Radio system employing more than one frequency.

dura mater   Tough *meningeal* membrane that covers the brain.

duty to act   Legal obligation of public and certain other ambulance services to respond to a call for help in their jurisdiction.

dying heart   Heart that contracts weakly and ineffectually and produces an *ECG* showing marked broadening of the *QRS complexes*.

dysarthria   Interference with proper articulation in speech; slurring of speech.

dysconjugate gaze   Gaze in which the two eyes are not aligned but instead stare in different directions.

dysfunction   Lack of function; abnormal function.

dysmenorrhea   Pain or cramps during *menstruation*.

dysphagia   Interference with the act of swallowing; pain or difficulty in swallowing.

dyspnea   Sensation of difficulty in breathing, with resultant rapid, shallow respirations.

dysrhythmia   Disturbance in cardiac rhythm.

dysuria   Painful or difficult urination.

eardrum   Flexible structure stretched across the far end of the ear canal, whose vibrations conduct sound to the middle ear.

ecchymosis   *Extravasation* of blood under the skin causing a "black-and-blue mark."

ECG   Abbreviation for *electrocardiogram*.

echolalia   Meaningless echoing of the interviewer's words by the patient.

eclampsia   Toxic condition that may occur during pregnancy, characterized by *hypertension*, *edema*, proteinuria, and *seizures*; also called *toxemia of pregnancy*.

ectopic   Located away from normal position, as in *ectopic pregnancy* or *ectopic focus*.

ectopic focus   A *pacemaker site* located in some part of the *electric conduction system* other than the *sinoatrial node*.

ectopic pregnancy   Pregnancy in which the *fetus* is implanted elsewhere than in the *uterus*, e.g., in the *fallopian tube* or in the abdominal cavity.

edema   Condition in which excess fluid accumulates in tissues, manifested by swelling.

effacement   Thinning of the *cervix* as the lower segment of the *uterus* retracts during the first stage of *labor*.

effusion   Leakage of fluid from tissues into a cavity, such as into the *pleural cavity*.

elastin   Protein that gives the skin its elasticity.

electric conduction system   Specialized cardiac tissue that initiates and conducts electric impulses. The system includes the *SA node*, internodal atrial conduction pathways, *atrioventricular junction*, *atrioventricular node*, *bundle of His*, and the *Purkinje network*.

electric instability   Condition in which there are *ectopic foci* in the *ventricles* capable of producing *life-threatening dysrhythmias*.

electrocardiogram (ECG)   Graphic display of the electric activity produced by *depolarization* and *repolarization* of the *atria* and *ventricles*.

electrocardiograph   Instrument that records electric currents produced by the heart.

electrode   Probe used to sense electric activity.

electroencephalogram (EEG)   Graph of brain waves.

electrolyte   Substance whose molecules dissociate into charged components (*ions*) when placed in water.

electrolyte imbalance   Abnormal concentrations of serum electrolytes caused by excessive intake or loss.

electromechanical dissociation   Condition in which *ECG* complexes are present without effective cardiac contractions.

elixir   Syrup with alcohol and flavoring added, e.g., terpin hydrate elixir, a cough medication.

emaciation   Excessive leanness; a wasted condition of the body.

embolism   A mass (embolus, sing.; emboli, pl.) of solid, liquid, or gaseous material that is carried in the circulation and may lead to occlusion of blood vessels, with resultant *infarction* and *necrosis* of tissue supplied by those vessels.

embryo   The human *fetus* during the first 8 weeks after conception.

emergency doctrine   Form of implied *consent* to medical treatment when a person's life or limb is in imminent danger.

emesis Vomiting.

emetic Medication that produces vomiting, e.g., syrup of ipecac.

emphysema Infiltration of any tissue by air or gas; a *chronic obstructive pulmonary disease* characterized by *distention* of the *alveoli* and destructive changes in the lung parenchyma.

emulsion Preparation of one liquid (usually an oil) distributed in small globules in another liquid (usually water) used as a lubricant.

encephalitis Inflammation of the *brain*.

endocardium Thin membrane lining the inside of the heart.

endometrium Lining cells of the *uterus* on which the fertilized *ovum* implants.

endothelium Thin, inner lining of blood vessels.

endotracheal (ET) Within or through the *trachea*.

endotracheal intubation Insertion of a tube into the *trachea* through the mouth or nose to establish a patent airway.

enteritis Inflammation of the *small intestine*.

entrance wound Point at which a penetrating object enters the body.

envenomation Process by which a venom is injected into a wound.

enzyme Protein that acts as an organic catalyst. When *myocardial* tissue is damaged, enzymes from that tissue are released into the circulation, and measurement of the blood levels of those enzymes provides evidence for *acute myocardial infarction*.

epicardium Thin membrane lining the outside of the heart.

epidemic Occurrence of a disease in many people, over a large area.

epidermis Outermost layer of the skin.

epidural Outside or above the *dura mater*, the heavy sheath that covers the brain.

epigastrium Upper middle region of the abdomen, within the sternal angle.

epiglottis Thin structure, located behind the root of the tongue, that shields the entrance of the *larynx* during swallowing, thus preventing the *aspiration* of food into the *trachea*.

epiglottitis Common illness of childhood, characterized by swelling of the *epiglottis*, high fever, and pain on swallowing. Complete airway obstruction may result with alarming rapidity.

epilepsy Disease characterized by *seizures*.

epinephrine Hormone and drug that has powerful *beta stimulating* properties, used in the treatment of *asthma, anaphylactic shock, asystole,* and fine *ventricular fibrillation* (trade name: Adrenalin).

epiphysis End of a long bone.

epistaxis Nosebleed.

epithelium The layer of cells covering the surface of body cavities.

erythrocyte A *red blood cell*; the cellular element of blood that carries *oxygen*.

esophageal obturator airway (EOA) Device used to prevent *regurgitation* and provide an adequate airway by blocking off the esophageal opening with a cuffed obturator and providing *ventilation* through a series of sideholes in the obturator tube.

esophageal varices Widened, tortuous blood vessels in the *esophagus* that develop as a result of elevated pressure in the vasculature of the liver.

esophagus Portion of the digestive tract that lies between the *pharynx* and the *stomach*.

estrogen One of the classes of female sex *hormones*.

ethanol Ethyl alcohol; the type of alcohol consumed in alcoholic beverages.

etiology The causative agent of a disease.

eustachian tube Tube leading from the back of the throat to the middle ear, whose purpose is to equalize pressure in the middle ear.

evert To turn a part, such as the foot, outward.

eviscerate To remove the intestines; to disembowel.

exacerbation A flare-up or worsening of a disease condition.

excitability Ability of the heart to initiate, conduct, and be stimulated by electric impulses.

excitation impulse Electric impulse that arises automatically in the *electric conduction system* of the heart and causes *depolarization* of the heart muscles.

exhalation The act of breathing out; *expiration*.

exit wound Point at which a penetrating object leaves the body.

expectorant Drug that loosens the mucus secretions of the bronchial tree and facilitates their removal.

expiration The act of breathing out; *exhalation*.

exsanguinate Bleed to death.

extension Movement that brings two members of a limb into or toward a straight condition.

external chest compressions Mechanical depression of the lower half of the sternum with the aim of compressing the *ventricles* and increasing intrathoracic pressure, thereby squeezing blood into the *systemic circulation* and the *pulmonary circulation*.

external rotation Rotation of an extremity in a lateral direction.

extracellular fluid (ECF) The portion of the *total body water* outside the cells, comprising the *interstitial fluid* and the *plasma*.

extract Concentrated form of a drug prepared by putting the drug into *solution* in alcohol or water and evaporating off the excess solvent to a prescribed standard.

extraocular motions Movements of the eyes.

extrasystole Extra heart beat, often a premature contraction.

extravasation   Leakage of *intravenous* fluid into surrounding tissues, often caused by penetration of the opposite wall of the vein used for *venipuncture*.

extremity   A limb; an arm or a leg.

extrication   Freeing an entrapped victim.

extruded   Being pushed out of normal position.

exudate   Accumulation of fluid in body tissue or cavities.

facies   The expression or appearance of the face, which may be characteristic of various disease conditions.

facilitation   Interviewing technique in which the interviewer uses noncommital words and gestures to encourage the patient to proceed.

fainting   A momentary loss of consciousness caused by insufficient blood supply to the brain; *syncope*.

fallopian tube   Tube extending from an *ovary* to the *uterus*.

false imprisonment   Intentional and unjustified detention of a person against his will.

fasciculations   Rippling movements in individual muscle bundles.

febrile   Characterized by fever.

feces   Bowel movement; the stool.

femoral   Pertaining to the *femur* or the thigh.

femoral artery   The main *artery* supplying the thigh and leg.

femur   The bone that extends from the *pelvis* to the knee. It is the longest and largest bone of the body.

fetus   The unborn human after the second month of pregnancy.

fibrillation   Disorganized, uncoordinated movements of the heart muscle, resulting in quivering and ineffectual contractions of the atria or *ventricles*.

fibrillatory waves (f waves)   On the *ECG*, these waves appear as frequent, irregular waves caused by rapid, disorganized firing of multiple *ectopic foci* in the atria or *ventricles*.

fibrosis   The formation of fibrous tissue in the place of *necrotic* muscle.

fibula   The smaller of the two bones of the lower leg.

fight-or-flight reaction   Instinctive response to acute *stress*, mediated by the *sympathetic nervous system*.

flaccid   Soft; limp.

flail chest   Condition in which several *ribs* are broken, each in at least two places, or in which there is sternal fracture or separation of the ribs from the *sternum*, producing a free or floating segment of the chest wall that moves paradoxically with respiration.

flash burn   Electrothermal injury caused by arcing of electric current.

flexion   The act of bending.

flight of ideas   Accelerated thinking in which the mind skips very rapidly from one thought to the next.

fluidextract   Concentrated form of a drug prepared by dissolving the crude drug in the fluid in which it is most readily soluble. Fluidextracts are standardized so that 1 ml contains 1 gm of the drug.

flutter   Repetitive, regular, and rapid beating of the atrial muscle.

flutter waves (F waves)   Coarse, sawtooth waves on the *ECG* characteristic of *atrial flutter*.

follicle (graafian follicle)   Immature *ovum* and the epithelial cells that surround it.

fomite   Inanimate object contaminated with microorganisms that serves as a means of transmitting an illness.

fontanelles   Openings between the bones of the *skull* in very young children. As the child grows older, the bones of the skull fuse, and the fontanelles close.

foramen   Any natural opening through a bone or other structure of the body.

foramen magnum   Large opening in the inferoanterior part of the *occipital* bone, through which the *brainstem* passes.

foramen ovale   Opening between the right and left atria of the fetal heart.

forearm   The part of the upper extremity between the elbow and the wrist.

Fowler's position   Semisitting position.

fracture   Break or rupture in a bone.

  closed fracture   Fracture that does not produce an open wound in the skin; a *simple fracture*.

  comminuted fracture   Fracture in which the bone is shattered or crushed into several small pieces.

  compound fracture   Fracture in which bone ends pierce the skin; an *open fracture*.

  greenstick fracture   Type of fracture occurring most frequently in children in which there is an incomplete breakage of bone.

  impacted fracture   Fracture in which the broken ends of the bone are jammed into each other.

  oblique fracture   Injury in which the fracture line crosses the bone at an oblique angle.

  open fracture   Fracture involving disruption of the skin over the fracture site; a *compound fracture*.

  simple fracture   Fracture that does not cause disruption of the skin; a *closed fracture*.

  spiral fracture   Injury in which the fracture line twists around and through the bone.

  transverse fracture   Injury in which the fracture line is straight across the bone at right angles to its long axis.

frequency   The number of cycles per second of a radio signal, inversely related to wavelength.

frequency modulation (FM) Method of converting an *analog signal* (e.g., an *ECG*) into a tone of varying pitch, which can then be transmitted over radio frequencies.

frequency spectrum The range of radio frequencies.

frontal Pertaining to the forehead region.

frontal bone Large, flat bone that forms the front of the *skull*.

frontal lobe The front portion of the *brain*.

frostbite Localized damage to tissues resulting from prolonged exposure to freezing temperatures.

frost nip First-degree *frostbite*, characterized by numbness and pallor without significant tissue damage.

fundus (uterine) Part of the uterus above the entrance of the fallopian tubes.

fused joint Joining of bones to form a rigid structure, such as in the *skull*.

F waves *Flutter waves.*

f waves *Fibrillatory waves.*

gag reflex Automatic spasm of the airway in response to irritation of the throat.

gait The way a person walks.

galea aponeurotica Tendinous structure of the scalp that connects various facial muscles.

gallbladder Sac located just beneath the *liver* that concentrates and stores *bile*.

gamma ray Radioactive emission from the nucleus of an atom, with high penetrating ability.

gastric Pertaining to the *stomach*.

gastrointestinal Pertaining to the *stomach* and intestines.

gauge Measurement referring to the diameter of a needle *cannula*. Sizes range from 12-gauge (very large) to 25-gauge (very small) needles. The larger the gauge number, the smaller the *lumen* of the needle.

generic name Name given to a drug by the company that first manufactures it. It is usually a simplified version of the chemical name.

genitalia Male and female external sex organs.

geriatric Referring to the elderly.

gestation Pregnancy.

gingiva Gums.

gland Any organ or group of cells that produces any type of secretion.

glaucoma Disease that produces increased pressure within the eyeball and may lead to blindness.

glenoid Socket in the *scapula* in which the head of the *humerus* rotates.

globe Eyeball.

glottis Opening between the vocal cords.

glucose Simple sugar. Its dextro- form (*dextrose*) is commonly used in intravenous solutions.

Good Samaritan Act Statute providing limited immunity from liability to persons responding voluntarily and in good faith to the aid of an injured person outside the hospital.

graafian follicle Immature *ovum* and the epithelial cells that surround it.

gram (gm) Unit of weight in the metric system, equivalent to about 0.035 ounces.

grand mal seizure Generalized motor seizure.

gravid Pregnant.

gravidity The number of times a woman has been pregnant, regardless of the outcome of the pregnancies.

gravity The acceleration of a body by the attraction of the earth's gravitational force, normally 32.2 feet/second^2.

groin Inguinal region; the junction of the abdomen with the thigh.

habituation Situation in which the effects produced by a drug are necessary to maintain a person's feeling of well-being.

hallucination Sense perception not founded on objective reality.

hallucinogen Agent or drug that has the capacity to induce *hallucinations*.

head tilt Maneuver to open the airway by hyperextending the head.

heart attack Layman's term for a condition resulting from blockage of a coronary artery with subsequent death of part of the heart muscle; an *acute myocardial infarction*; a "coronary."

heart block Condition in which the passage of electric impulses from the *atrium* through the *atrioventricular junction* is hindered or prevented altogether.

first-degree heart block Partial disruption of the conduction of the depolarizing impulse from the atria to the *ventricles*, causing prolongation of the *P–R interval*.

second-degree heart block Type of incomplete heart block in which a variable percentage of the *P waves* are not followed by a *QRS complex*.

third-degree heart block *Complete heart block*; complete absence of conduction of the depolarizing impulse from the atria to the *ventricles*. An *ectopic focus* below the block becomes the *pacemaker* for the ventricles, and atrial and ventricular contractions become dissociated.

heat cramps Painful muscle cramps resulting from excessive loss of salt and water through sweating.

heat exhaustion *Prostration* caused by excessive loss of water and salt through sweating. It is characterized by cold, clammy skin and a weak, rapid pulse.

heat stroke Life-threatening condition caused by a

disturbance in the temperature-regulating mechanism. It is characterized by extreme fever, hot and usually dry skin, bounding *pulse,* and *delirium* or *coma.*

hematemesis   Vomiting blood.

hematocrit (hct)   The percentage of a sample of whole blood occupied by *red blood cells.*

hematoma   Localized collection of blood in the tissues as a result of injury or a broken blood vessel.

hematuria   Discharge of blood in the urine.

hemiparesis   Weakness on one side of the body.

hemiplegia   *Paralysis* of the lower half of the body.

hemodialysis   Process of removing certain noxious agents from the blood by diffusion through a semipermeable membrane.

hemoglobin (hb, hgb)   Oxygen-carrying pigment of the *red blood cells.* When it has absorbed oxygen in the lungs, hemoglobin is bright red and is called oxyhemoglobin. After it has given up its oxygen in the tissues, it is purple and is called reduced hemoglobin.

hemolysis   Disintegration of red blood cells resulting from some adverse factor, such as a *transfusion reaction.*

hemoperitoneum   Blood in the *peritoneal cavity.*

hemophilia   Inherited blood disease of males, characterized by inability of the blood to clot normally.

hemoptysis   Coughing up blood.

hemorrhage   Bleeding, especially profuse bleeding.

hemorrhagic shock   State of inadequate tissue *perfusion* caused by blood loss.

hemostasis   Stopping *hemorrhage.*

hemostat   Instrument that stops *hemorrhage* by compressing the bleeding vessel; type of clamp.

hemothorax   Bleeding into the *pleural cavity.*

heparin   *Anticoagulant* medication given *intravenously.*

hepatitis   *Inflammation* of the *liver.*

hepatomegaly   Enlargement of the *liver.*

hernia   Protrusion of any organ through an opening into a body cavity where it does not belong. The most common is an inguinal hernia in which a loop of intestine descends into the inguinal canal in the *groin.*

herniation, cerebral   Extrusion of part of the brain through the *tentorium* or *foramen magnum* in the context of increased intracranial pressure.

hertz   Cycles per second.

hiatus hernia   Protrusion of the *stomach* into the *mediastinum* through an opening in the *diaphragm;* can mimic the chest pain of *angina pectoris* or *acute myocardial infarction.*

hinge joint   Specialized joint found in the elbow, knee, and fingers.

His-Purkinje system   Portion of the *electric conduction system,* located in the lower part of the *interventricular septum* and in the ventricular walls, that conducts the electric impulse from the *atrioventricular junction* to the *Purkinje network* in the ventricles.

history   Information about the patient's chief complaint, present symptoms, and previous illnesses.

history of the present illness   Elaboration of the patient's *chief complaint.*

homeostasis   Tendency to constancy or stability in the body's internal environment.

homicide   Taking of another's life.

hormone   Substance secreted by an endocrine gland that has effects on other glands or organs of the body.

humerus   The bone of the upper arm.

hydration   State of water balance of the body.

hydrothorax   Fluid in the *pleural cavity.*

hygroscopic   Tending to absorb water.

hyoid bone   U-shaped bone in the throat just above the *larynx* at the base of the tongue.

hypercarbia   Excessive partial pressure of *carbon dioxide* in the blood; an arterial PCO_2 greater than 40–50 torr.

hyperemia   Increased blood flow to a region or tissue.

hyperextension   Extension of a limb or other body part beyond its usual range of motion.

hyperglycemia   Abnormally high concentration of sugar in the blood.

hyperkalemia   Excessive amount of *potassium* in the blood.

hyperpnea   Abnormally deep breaths.

hyperpyrexia   Abnormally high fever; *hyperthermia.*

hyperreflexia   Overactive *reflexes.*

hyperresonance   Abnormally increased resonance to *percussion,* as in the chest of an asthmatic during a severe attack.

hypersensitivity   Having the ability to react with characteristic symptoms to contact with certain substances; *allergy.*

hypertension   High blood pressure, usually referring to a diastolic pressure greater than 90 to 95 mm Hg.

hyperthermia   Abnormally increased body temperature; *hyperpyrexia.*

hypertonic   Having an *osmotic pressure* greater than a *solution* to which it is being compared, usually the *intracellular fluid.*

hypertrophy   Enlargement of an organ caused by an increase in size of its constituent cells rather than an increase in the number of cells.

hyperventilation   Increased rate and/or depth of respiration that results in abnormal lowering of the arterial *carbon dioxide* tension (PCO$_2$).

hyphema *Hemorrhage* into the anterior chamber of the eye.

hypocarbia Abnormally low *carbon dioxide* tension in the blood; an arterial PCO$_2$ less than 35 torr.

hypoglycemia Abnormally low concentration of sugar in the blood.

hypokalemia Abnormally low concentration of *potasssium* in the blood.

hyponatremia Abnormally low concentration of *sodium* in the blood.

hypopharynx The most *distal* portion of the *pharynx*, which leads to the *larynx* and *esophagus*.

hypotension Low *blood pressure*.

hypothalamus Portion of the brain that regulates a multitude of bodily functions, including core temperature.

hypothermia A body temperature significantly below normal.

hypotonic Having an *osmotic pressure* less than a solution to which it is being compared, usually the *intracellular fluid*.

hypoventilation *Ventilation* that is inadequate to maintain the arterial PCO$_2$ at levels less than 45 torr.

hypovolemia Abnormally decreased amount of blood and fluids in the body.

hypoxemia Inadequate oxygen in the blood; an arterial PO$_2$ less than 60 torr.

hypoxic drive Situation when a person's stimulus to breathe comes from a fall in arterial PO$_2$ rather than the normal stimulus, a rise in arterial PCO$_2$.

icterus *Jaundice*, the yellow appearance of the skin and other tissues caused by an accumulation of bile pigments; often seen in liver disease.

idiopathic Of unknown cause.

idiosyncrasy Abnormal sensitivity to a drug, peculiar to an individual.

idioventricular Relating to or affecting the *ventricle* only. An idioventricular rhythm is one that arises in the *ventricles*.

ileum Third portion of the *small intestine*.

ilium Broad, uppermost bone of the pelvis.

illusion A misinterpretation of sensory stimuli.

immobilization Holding of a part firmly in place, as with a *splint*.

impaled object Object that has caused a puncture wound and that remains embedded in the wound.

implantation Process by which the fertilized egg attaches to the *endometrium*.

incision Wound usually made deliberately in connection with surgery; a clean cut, as opposed to a *laceration*.

incompatibility In blood typing, the situation in which the donor and recipient blood cannot be mixed without clumping or other adverse reactions.

incomplete AV block First- or second-degree *atrioventricular block*.

incontinence Inability to control the elimination of urine or feces.

incubation period Period from infection until the appearance of the first symptoms of a communicable disease.

indication Circumstances under which a drug is suited for use.

infant Child less than a year of age.

infarction Death (*necrosis*) of a localized area of tissue caused by the cutting off of its blood supply.

infection Invasion of the body by *pathogenic* microorganisms.

inferior In anatomy, situated below, or directed downward; the lower surface of an organ or structure.

inferior vena cava Major *vein* that empties blood from the lower extremities and abdominal organs into the *right atrium*.

infiltration Deposit of fluid into the tissues, often occurring as the result of administering fluid through an *intravenous cannula* that has penetrated the opposite wall of the *vein*.

inflammation Tissue reaction to chemical or physical injury or infection, manifested by pain, heat, redness, and swelling.

infusion Administration of fluid into a *vein*.

ingestion The taking of food or other substances through the mouth.

inhalation Active phase of respiration in which air is drawn into the lungs; *inspiration*.

innocuous Not harmful or poisonous.

inoculation Injection of any biologic substance intended to confer protection against disease.

inotropic Tending to increase the force of *cardiac* contractions.

inspection First part of the physical examination, involving a careful visual examination of the patient.

inspiration Breathing of air into the lungs; *inhalation*.

insufficiency Condition of being inadequate to normal performance.

insulin *Hormone* secreted by the pancreatic islets that promotes utilization of sugar by the body.

insulin shock Severe *hypoglycemia* caused by excessive *insulin* dosage with respect to sugar intake;

may be characterized by bizarre behavior, sweating, *tachycardia,* or coma.

integument Skin.

intercostal Between the *ribs.*

intercostal muscles The muscles between the *ribs.*

intercostal space The area between two adjacent *ribs,* containing intercostal muscles, arteries, veins, and nerves.

intermammary line Imaginary line between the nipples.

intermittent positive pressure breathing (IPPB) Assisted *ventilation* under positive pressure to the spontaneously breathing patient.

intermittent positive pressure ventilation (IPPV) Controlled *ventilation* under positive pressure to the patient who is not breathing spontaneously.

interstitial fluid Fluid bathing the cells; one component of the *extracellular fluid.*

interventricular septum Thin, muscular wall dividing the right and left *ventricles.*

intima Innermost layer of a blood vessel.

intoxication State of being poisoned; condition caused by excessive use of drugs, including alcohol.

intracardiac injection Injection of medication, such as *epinephrine,* directly into a heart chamber through the chest wall.

intracellular fluid (ICF) The portion of *total body water* contained within the cells, usually about 45 percent of body weight.

intracranial Within the *skull.*

intracranial pressure (ICP) Pressure within the skull.

intramuscular (IM) injection Injection of medication directly into a muscle of the patient.

intraosseous Within or into a bone.

intravascular fluid Portion of the *total body water* contained within the blood vessels; *plasma.*

intravenous (IV) Within or into a *vein.*

intravenous solution Sterile water mixed with various concentrations of *electrolytes* and/or dextrose and prepared in sterile plastic or glass containers.

intubation The placement of a tube through the *glottis* into the *trachea* (*endotracheal intubation*) or into the *esophagus* (*esophageal obturator airway* intubation); may also refer to intubation of the stomach with a nasogastric tube.

involuntary muscles Muscles that function without voluntary control; smooth muscles (as opposed to skeletal muscles).

ion Electrically charged molecule, e.g., Na^+ or Cl^-.

ionizing radiation Transmission of energy in the form of waves or particles that has the ability to disrupt atoms in its path into their component *ions.*

ipecac, syrup of Medication used to induce vomiting.

iris Colored portion of the eye surrounding the *pupil.*

irritation Drug action that produces slight or temporary damage to tissues.

ischemia Tissue *anoxia* from diminished blood flow, usually caused by narrowing or *occlusion* of the artery to the tissue.

ischial tuberosity Protuberance on the inferior portion of the *ischium* (the part of the ischium we sit on).

ischium Lowermost portion of pelvic bone.

islets of Langerhans Clusters of cells in the *pancreas* that produce *insulin.*

isoelectric line Baseline of the *ECG.*

isotonic Having the same *osmotic pressure* as that of a reference *solution,* usually the *intracellular fluid.*

jaundice Presence of excessive *bile* pigments in the bloodstream, which give the skin, mucous membranes, and eyes a distinct yellow color; often associated with liver disease.

jaw thrust Maneuver to open the airway by pushing forward on the *mandible.*

jejunum Second portion of the *small intestine.*

joint Point at which two or more bones articulate or come together.

joint capsule Saclike envelope that encloses the cavity of a *synovial joint.*

jugular notch Top border of the *sternum.*

jugular veins *Veins* that return blood from the head, neck, and face to the *superior vena cava.*

junctional rhythm *Dysrhythmia* arising from *ectopic foci* in the area of the *atrioventricular junction;* often shows an absence of the *P wave,* a short *P–R interval,* or a P wave appearing after the *QRS complex.*

K^+ Chemical symbol for *potassium ion.*

Kehr's sign Pain in the left shoulder after rupture of the spleen.

keratin Horny, proteinlike substance in the upper layers of the skin that is also the principal constituent of the hair and fingernails.

ketoacidosis Condition arising in diabetics whose *insulin* dose is insufficient to meet their needs, wherein blood sugar reaches high levels and fat is metabolized to ketones and *acids;* characterized by excessive thirst, urination, *nausea,* and vomiting, sometimes *coma.* Ketoacidosis may also occur in conditions other than diabetes.

kidneys Paired organs located in the *retroperitoneum* that filter the blood and produce *urine.*

kilogram (kg) Unit of measurement in the *metric system,* equal to 1,000 gm or 2.2 pounds.

kinetic energy The energy associated with bodies in motion, expressed mathematically as half the mass times the square of the *velocity.*

Kussmaul's breathing Respiratory pattern characteristic of the diabetic in *ketoacidosis,* with marked *hyperpnea* and *tachypnea.*

labia The folds of skin and mucous membrane that make up the *vulva.*

labor Muscular contractions of the *uterus* designed to expel the *fetus* from the mother.

laceration Wound made by a tearing or cutting action on the tissues.

lactate Salt of lactic acid.

lactated Ringer's solution A sterile *intravenous solution* containing *sodium, potassium, calcium,* and *chloride ions* in concentrations similar to those present in the blood, as well as *lactate* added as a *buffer.*

lactation Secretion of milk.

lactic acid Metabolic end product of the breakdown of *glucose;* lactic acid accumulates when *metabolism* proceeds in the absence of oxygen (*anaerobically*).

lactic acidosis Excess of *lactic acid* in the blood, causing the blood *pH* to fall below 7.35.

landline Communications link by wires, usually in reference to conventional telephone.

large intestine Portion of the intestine between the *small intestine* and the *rectum;* the *colon.*

laryngectomee Person who has had total or partial surgical removal of the *larynx;* a "neck breather."

laryngectomy Removal of the *larynx.*

laryngoscope Instrument for directly visualizing the *larynx* and its related structures.

larnygospasm Severe *constriction* of the *larynx,* often in response to *allergy* or noxious stimuli.

larynx The organ of voice production.

lassitude Condition of listlessness and fatigue.

lateral Of or toward the side; away from the midline of the body.

lavage Washing out of a hollow organ, such as the stomach.

lead Any one of the records made by the *ECG,* depending on the direction of current flow.

left atrium Upper left chamber of the heart, which receives blood from the *pulmonary veins.*

left heart The *left atrium* plus the *left ventricle.*

left heart failure Failure of the *left ventricle* to pump blood forward effectively, causing backup of blood into the *pulmonary circulation, extravasation* of fluid into the *lungs,* and consequent *pulmonary edema.*

left ventricle Thick-walled, muscular, lower left chamber of the heart, which receives blood from the *left atrium* and pumps it out through the *aorta* into the systemic arteries.

lens Portion of the eye that focusses light rays on the *retina.*

lesion *Pathologic* or traumatic discontinuity of tissue or loss of function of a part.

lethargy Lack of ambition to do anything, coupled with a feeling of sleepiness.

leukemia Disease of the blood-forming organs characterized by proliferation of *white blood cells* and pathologic changes in the bone marrow and other lymphoid tissue.

leukocyte *White blood cell.*

liability Finding in civil cases that the preponderance of evidence shows the defendant was responsible for the plaintiff's injuries.

licensure Process by which a governmental agency grants permission to an individual to engage in a given occupation.

life-threatening dysrhythmias *Dysrhythmias* characterized by extreme *bradycardia* (less than 40 beats/min), extreme *tachycardia* (more than about 140 beats/min), where electric instability is present or the *cardiac output* is markedly decreased, especially in the context of *acute myocardial infarction.*

ligament Tough band of fibrous tissues that connects bone to bone around a joint or supports an organ.

ligate To tie off, as a bleeding artery.

liniment Preparation of a drug for external use, usually to relieve some discomfort or protect the skin.

liter (L) Metric volume measurement, equal to 1,000 ml or 1.1 quarts.

litigation Lawsuit.

liver Large solid organ in the right upper quadrant of the *abdomen* that secretes *bile,* produces many essential proteins, detoxifies drugs, and performs many other vital functions.

loading dose An initial, large dose of a drug that provides the blood level of the drug necessary to achieve its therapeutic effects.

lotion Preparation of a drug for external use, usually to relieve some discomfort or protect the skin.

lumbar Region of the spine and surrounding trunk between the *thorax* and the brim of the *pelvis.*

lumen Cavity or channel within a tube, such as within an IV *cannula.*

lungs Paired organs in the *thorax* responsible for *ventilation* and oxygenation.

lung squeeze Injury to the lung caused by breath-holding during descent through water.

lymph Nearly colorless nutrient fluid that circulates in the lymphatic vessels.

malaise Generalized feeling of vague bodily discomfort.

malignant Cancerous; tending to become progressively worse and to result in death.

malleolus Large, rounded, bony protuberance on either side of the ankle joint.

malocclusion Failure of proper alignment of the upper and lower teeth.

mandible Lower jaw bone.

mania Mental disorder characterized by hyperactivity, insomnia, and grandiose ideas.

manubrium Upper portion of the *sternum* to which the *clavicles* are attached.

marrow cavity Central cavity in the shaft of a long bone where the yellow marrow is contained.

mast cell Mobile chemical-mediator factory that releases histamine and related substances in response to an *antigen/antibody* reaction.

mastoid Large, spongy bone behind the ear.

maxilla Upper jaw bone.

mean arterial pressure (MAP) Pressure approximately midway between the *systolic* and *diastolic* *blood pressures.*

mechanism of injury Way in which an injury occurred and the forces involved in producing the injury.

meconium Fetal stool.

medial Toward the midline of the body.

mediastinum Space within the chest that contains the heart, major blood vessels, *vagus nerve, trachea,* and *esophagus;* located between the two *lungs.*

medical control The supervision of paramedics by physicians that provides the legal framework for paramedics to function.

medulla oblongata Lower portion of the *brainstem* continuous with the *spinal cord* that contains the centers for control of *respiration* and heart beat, together with other major control centers.

melanin Pigment that gives the skin its color.

melena The passage of dark, tarry stools, signifying blood in the gastrointestinal tract.

menarche The onset of menstrual periods.

meninges The three membranes covering the *spinal cord* and *brain;* the *dura mater* (external), *arachnoid* (middle), and *pia mater* (internal).

meningitis Inflammation of the *meninges;* may present with fever, stiff neck, and *delirium.*

menopause The time in a woman's life when her menstrual periods have ceased altogether.

menorrhagia Excessive flow during a menstrual period.

menses Discharge of blood that occurs with the menstrual period.

menstruation Process by which the uterine lining is shed each month by women between the ages of puberty and *menopause.*

mesentery Tissues by which the intestines are connected to the back surface of the abdominal cavity and that contain the blood vessels, lymphatics, and nerves supplying the intestines.

metabolism The conversion of food into energy and waste products.

metacarpal bones The five bones that form the palm and back of the hand.

metatarsal bones The five long bones extending from the tarsus to the *phalanges* of the foot.

meter Metric linear measurement, equal to 1,000 millimeters or 39.37 inches.

methanol Methyl alcohol; wood alcohol; poisonous if ingested, causing extreme metabolic *acidosis* and sometimes blindness.

metric system System of weights and measures based on *decimal* units.

metrorrhagia Vaginal bleeding between menstrual periods.

microdrip fluid administration set Set used to deliver *intravenous solutions* or medication at a very slow rate, thus permitting accurate *titration* of dosage.

microgram (μg) Metric unit of weight, equal to 0.001 mg.

micturition syncope Fainting during urination.

midclavicular line Imaginary vertical line beginning in the middle of the *clavicle* and running parallel to the *sternum* slightly inside the nipple.

military anti-shock trousers (MAST) Inflatable garment applied around the legs and *abdomen,* used in the treatment of *shock;* also known as pneumatic anti-shock garment (PASG).

milk In pharmacology, an aqueous suspension of insoluble drugs, e.g., milk of magnesia.

milliampere Unit of current, equal to 0.001 ampere.

milliequivalent (mEq) Unit of measurement for *electrolytes* based on chemical combining power; defined as the weight of a substance present in 1 ml of normal *solution.*

milligram (mg) Metric weight measurement, equal to 0.001 gm.

milliliter (ml) Metric volume measure, equal to 0.001 liter.

millimeter (mm) Metric linear measurement, equal to 0.001 meter.

millimeter of mercury (mm Hg) Metric measurement used in determination of *blood pressure;* commonly referred to as torr (Torricelli unit) when used to designate gas tensions in blood.

millivolt (mV) Unit of electric energy, equal to 0.001 volt.

minute volume Volume of air inhaled or exhaled during 1 minute, calculated by multiplying the *tidal volume* times the respiratory rate.

miosis Pupillary *constriction*.

miscarriage Layman's term for an *abortion*, or the premature expulsion of a *fetus* from the *uterus*.

mitral valve Valve located between the *left atrium* and the *left ventricle* of the heart.

mobile intensive care unit (MICU) Ambulance staffed and equipped to give *advanced life support*.

monovalent Having a single charge, e.g., the *sodium ion* (Na$^+$).

mood A person's sustained and pervasive emotional state.

morbidity Synonym for illness; generally used to refer to an untoward effect of an illness or injury.

mortality Death from a given disease or injury.

motor nerves Nerves that send messages from the brain to various organs and muscles to stimulate voluntary and involuntary actions.

mouth-to-mouth ventilation Preferred emergency method of artificial *ventilation* without adjuncts in which the rescuer exhales through his mouth into the mouth of the victim.

mouth-to-nose ventilation Emergency method of artificial *ventilation*, used when the mouth-to-mouth technique cannot be performed. In this method, the rescuer exhales through his mouth into the nose of the victim.

mucosa Any mucous membrane.

mucous membrane Membrane that lines many organs of the body and contains small, mucus-secreting glands.

mucus Viscid, slippery secretion that serves as a lubricant and protects various surfaces.

multifocal Arising from or pertaining to many foci or locations.

multigravida Woman who has had two or more pregnancies.

multipara Woman who has had more than two deliveries; also called "multip."

multiplex Method by which simultaneous transmission and reception of voice and *ECG* signals can be achieved over a single radio frequency.

murmur Sound that may be detected by *auscultation* of the heart when one of its valves is leaking or partially shut.

muscle Tissue comprising fibers that have the ability to shorten, thus causing bones and *joints* to move.

muscle tremor artifact Numerous extraneous deflections in the *ECG* caused by muscle movement or shivering.

mutism The absence of speech.

myalgia Pain in muscles.

myasthenia gravis Progressive disease of the *muscles* characterized by slow *paralysis* of various muscle groups.

mydriasis Pupillary *dilatation*.

myocardial Pertaining to the musculature of the heart.

myocardial infarction Damage or death of an area of heart *muscle* resulting from a reduction in the blood supply to that area.

myocardial rupture The bursting of a *necrotic* area of cardiac *muscle*, which may occur several days after the onset of an *acute myocardial infarction*; results in *cardiac tamponade* and is rapidly fatal if untreated.

myocardium *Cardiac muscle*.

myoglobin Protein found in *muscle* that is released into the circulation after crush injury or other muscle damage and whose presence in the circulation can result in damage to the kidneys.

Na$^+$ Chemical symbol for *sodium ion*.

NaHCO$_3$ Chemical symbol for *sodium bicarbonate*.

narcosis Unconscious state caused by *narcotics* or the accumulation of *carbon dioxide* or other toxic substances in the blood; the term usually implies respiratory depression leading to *apnea*.

narcotic Drug that relieves pain and produces sleep by its *depressant* effect on the *central nervous system*.

naris Nostril (plural: nares).

nasal flaring Marked widening of the nostrils on inhalation—a sign of respiratory distress.

nasal septum Partition separating the two nasal cavities in the midline, composed of *cartilage*, membrane, and bone.

nasopharynx The part of the *pharynx* that is continuous with the nasal passages.

nausea Unpleasant sensation in the *epigastrium* and *abdomen*, often preceding vomiting.

near drowning Submersion in water with temporary or long-term survival thereafter.

nebulizer Device that delivers water or liquid medication in the form of very fine spray.

neck lift Maneuver to open the airway by lifting upward on the patient's neck.

necrosis Death of tissue, usually caused by a cessation of its blood supply.

necrotic Pertaining to dead tissue.

negligence Failure to exercise the care that circumstances demand; an act of omission or commission that results in injury.

neologism A made-up word.

neonate A newborn.

nervous system The *brain*, the *spinal cord*, and the nerves branching from both.

neurogenic Originating in the *nervous system*.

neurogenic shock *Shock* caused by massive *vasodilation* and pooling of blood in the *peripheral* vessels to the degree that adequate *perfusion* cannot be maintained.

nitrogen　An element making up about 80 percent of the air we breathe, present in all plant and animal tissues.

nitrogen narcosis　State resembling alcohol intoxication produced by nitrogen gas dissolved in the blood at high ambient pressure; "rapture of the deep."

nodal　Usually, pertaining to the *atrioventricular node*.

noise　Extraneous deflections in the *ECG* signal; may be caused by muscle tremor, 60-cycle interference, loose electrodes, or (in biotelemetry) weak radio transmission.

norepinephrine　A neurotransmitter and drug sometimes used in the treatment of shock. It produces *vasoconstriction* through its *alpha stimulator* properties.

normal saline　*Intravenous solution* containing 0.9% sodium chloride, used when volume replacement is desired.

normal sinus rhythm (NSR)　Normal rhythm of the heart, wherein the *excitation impulse* arises in the *SA node*, travels through the internodal pathways to the *atrioventricular junction,* thence down the *bundle of His*, through the *bundle branches,* and into the *Purkinje network* without interference.

nosocomial　Pertaining to a hospital or health care setting.

nullipara　A woman who has never been delivered of a baby.

O₂　Chemical symbol for oxygen.

obsession　Persistent idea that a person cannot dismiss from his thoughts.

occipital　Region of the back part of the head.

occlusion　Stoppage, as of a blood vessel by a *clot* or *thrombus.*

occlusive dressing　Watertight or airtight covering for a wound.

ocular　Pertaining to the eyes.

odontoid process　Toothlike structure projecting from the second cervical *vertebra.*

ointment　Semisolid substance used externally, usually containing a medication.

olecranon　Proximal bony projection of the *ulna* at the elbow; the part of the ulna that constitutes the "funny bone."

oliguria　Very small *urine* output.

open pneumothorax　*Pneumothorax* caused by an opening in the chest wall; a *sucking chest wound.*

opiate　Technically, various alkaloids derived from the opium or poppy plant; often used in a general sense to refer to any drug that produces sleep.

opisthotonos　Convulsive, rigid arching of the back that is seen in *tetanus* and severe *meningitis.*

optic nerve　Nerve of the eye that transmits visual impulses from the eye to the *brain.*

orbit　Eye socket.

orchitis　Inflammation of the testes.

orifice　Entrance or outlet of any body cavity.

oropharyngeal airway　Ventilatory adjunct placed in the patient's mouth in such a way that the curved, *distal* part slides behind the base of the tongue, thereby holding the tongue forward, away from the *posterior* wall of the *pharynx.*

oropharynx　Area behind the base of the tongue between the soft palate and the upper portion of the *epiglottis.*

orthopnea　Severe *dyspnea* experienced when lying down, relieved by sitting up.

orthostatic hypotension　Fall in *blood pressure* in assuming an erect position.

oscilloscope　Display device with a screen for viewing an *ECG* or other physiologic data.

osmosis　The passage across a semipermeable membrane of pure solvent from a *solution* of lower solute concentration to one of higher concentration.

osmotic diuresis　Passage of large volumes of urine as a consequence of a high solute concentration in the blood.

osmotic pressure　Pressure exerted by a *solution* of greater solute concentration on water in a *solution* of lower solute concentration.

osteoporosis　Pathologic reduction in bone mass to the degree that the skeleton can no longer perform its supportive function.

ovary　The female sex organ in which eggs and female *hormones* are produced.

overhydration　Condition that results from excessive retention of fluids.

ovulation　Process by which an *ovum* is released from a *graafian follicle,* usually occurring once a month in nonpregnant women of childbearing age.

ovum　Egg (plural: ova).

oxygen (O₂)　Colorless, odorless, tasteless gas essential to life, composing 21 percent of the air we breathe.

pacemaker　Specialized tissue within the heart that initiates *excitation impulses*; an electronic device used to stimulate cardiac contraction when the *electric conduction system* of the heart is malfunctioning, especially in *complete heart block*. An electronic pacemaker consists of a battery-powered pulse generator and a wire that transmits the electric impulse to the *ventricles.*

pacemaker site　Site in any part of the *electric conduction system* of the heart where *excitation impulses* arise.

palate　The roof of the mouth.

pallor   Paleness of the skin.

palpation   Feeling a part of the patient's body with the hand to assess the consistency of the parts beneath.

palpitation   Sensation, felt under the left breast, of the heart "skipping a beat," usually caused by a *premature ventricular contraction.*

palsy   *Paralysis.*

pancreas   Intra-abdominal *gland* that secretes *insulin* and important digestive enzymes.

papillary muscle   Protrusions of the *myocardium* into the ventricular cavities to which the *chordae tendinae* are attached.

paracentesis   Draining of fluid from the *peritoneal cavity* by means of a needle or *catheter* inserted through the *abdominal* wall.

paradoxical respiration   Situation in which attempts to inhale cause collapse of a portion of the chest wall instead of expansion; seen in *flail chest.*

paralysis   Loss of motor function.

paranoia   Mental disorder characterized by abnormal suspicions or other *delusions* (often of persecution or grandeur).

paraplegia   Loss of both motion and sensation in the legs and lower part of the body, most commonly caused by damage to the *spinal cord.*

parasympathetic nervous system   Subdivision of the *autonomic nervous system,* involved in control of involuntary, vegetative functions, mediated largely by the *vagus nerve* through the chemical *acetylcholine.*

parenchyma   The substance of a gland or solid organ.

parenteral   Administration of a medication or fluid by means other than through the digestive tract, e.g., *intravenous, intramuscular.*

paresis   Weakness.

paresthesia   Abnormal sensation, often of the pins-and-needles variety, indicating disturbance in nerve function.

parietal lobe   Portion of the *brain* containing sensory areas and areas of muscle control.

parietal pleura   Membrane lining the inside of the chest wall and the *pericardium.*

parity   The number of times a woman has carried a fetus to at least 28 weeks' gestation.

paroxysm   Sudden and intense occurrence of symptoms.

paroxysmal nocturnal dyspnea (PND)   Severe shortness of breath occurring at night after several hours of recumbency, during which fluid pools in the *lungs.* The patient is forced to sit up to breathe. PND is caused by *left heart failure* or decompensation of *chronic obstructive pulmonary disease.*

partial pressure   The fractional concentration of a gas in a gas mixture.

parturition   The act of giving birth.

patch   Connection between a telephone line and a radio communications system, enabling a caller to get "on the air" by dialing in to a special phone.

patella   Small, flat bone that protects the knee *joint;* the knee cap.

patent   Open; unobstructed.

pathogenic   Capable of causing a disease process.

pathognomonic   Symptom or sign that is sufficiently characteristic of a disease process to make *diagnosis* possible on the basis of that finding alone.

pathologic   Indicative of or caused by a morbid condition.

PCO$_2$ Chemical symbol for the *partial pressure* of carbon dioxide in a gas.

pedal   Pertaining to the foot.

pediatrics   Medical specialty devoted to the *diagnosis* and treatment of diseases of children.

pedicle   Narrow strip of tissue by which an *avulsed* piece of tissue remains connected to the body.

pelvic girdle   The large bone that arises in the area of the last nine vertebrae and sweeps around to form a complete ring.

pelvis   The lower bony structure of the trunk.

peptic ulcer   An *ulcer* produced by acidic gastric juice acting on the wall of the *stomach* and *duodenum.*

percussion   Striking a part of the patient's body with short, sharp blows to produce a sound that will indicate the condition of the structures within.

percutaneous   Through the skin.

perfusion   The flow of blood through tissues.

pericardial cavity   Potential space between the two layers of the *pericardium,* the outer (parietal) pericardium and the inner (visceral) *epicardium.* Normally that space contains only a small amount of lubricating fluid.

pericardial effusion   Excess fluid within the pericardial sac.

pericardial tamponade   Accumulation of excess fluid or blood in the pericardial sac to the point that it interferes with cardiac function.

pericardiocentesis   Aspiration of blood or fluid from the *pericardium.*

pericardium   Double-layered sac containing the heart and the origins of the *superior vena cava, inferior vena cava,* and *pulmonary artery.*

perineum   Region between the *genitalia* and the *anus.*

periodic breathing   *Cheyne-Stokes respirations.*

periorbital   The region around the eyes.

periosteum   Dense, fibrous tissue covering bone.

peripheral   Pertaining to an outside surface or distant area.

peripheral vascular resistance (PVR)   Resistance to

blood flow in the *systemic circulation* depending on the degree of *constriction* within the network of blood vessels making up the peripheral vascular system.

peripheral vasoconstriction *Constriction* of peripheral blood vessels, causing the skin to grow pale and cool.

peripheral vasodilatation *Dilatation* of peripheral blood vessels, causing a decrease in *blood pressure* and warm, flushed skin.

peristalsis Successive waves of muscular *contraction* and relaxation proceeding uniformly along a hollow tube, such as the *esophagus* or intestines, which propel the contents of the tube forward.

peritoneal cavity *Abdominal* cavity.

peritoneal dialysis Process of removing noxious agents from the body by infusing balanced *electrolyte* solutions into the abdominal cavity and then withdrawing the solutions after they have equilibrated with the blood.

peritoneum Membrane that lines the *abdominal* cavity.

peritonitis *Inflammation* of the *peritoneum*.

permanent cavity The path of crushed tissue produced by a missile traversing part of the body.

perseveration Repeating the same idea over and over again.

pertinent negative *Symptom* or *sign* that the patient does NOT have but might be expected to have, given the chief complaint.

petit mal seizure Type of epileptic attack seen in children, characterized by momentary loss of awareness without loss of motor tone.

pH Measure of the hydrogen ion (H^+) concentration, hence the acidity or alkalinity of a fluid.

phalanx Any bone of a finger or toe.

pharmacology The science that deals with the study of drugs in all their aspects.

pharyngeal Pertaining to or situated near the *pharynx*.

pharynx Portion of the airway between the nasal cavity and the larynx, consisting of the nasopharynx, oropharynx, and laryngopharynx.

phlebitis Inflammation of the wall of a *vein*, sometimes caused by an IV line, manifested by tenderness, redness, and slight *edema* along part of the length of the *vein*.

phlebotomy The withdrawal of blood from a vein.

phobia Abnormal and persistent dread of some specific thing.

physiologic action Action caused by a drug when given in the concentrations normally present in the body (applies only to drugs that are derived from normal body chemicals, e.g., *epinephrine*).

physiology The study of body functions.

pia mater Innermost layer of the *meninges*.

piggyback Adding *solution* to an *infusion* by inserting a needle connected to another infusion set.

pill Drug shaped into a ball or oval to be swallowed, often coated to disguise an unpleasant taste.

pinna Outer portion of the ear, leading to the ear canal.

pitting edema Severe *edema* that renders the tissue boggy and capable of being indented by moderate pressure.

pituitary Master *gland* of the body, located in the *brain* behind the eyes; influences the secretions of all other glands.

placenta Vascular organ attached to the uterine wall, supplying *oxygen* and nutrients to the *fetus*; also called the afterbirth.

placenta previa Delivery in which the *placenta* is the *presenting part*; may result in *exsanguinating hemorrhage*.

plantar Relating to the sole of the foot.

plaque Calcified *atheroma*.

plasma Fluid portion of the blood from which the cells have been removed.

plasmin Naturally occurring clot-dissolving enzyme, usually present in the body in its inactive form, plasminogen.

platelet Small, cellular element in the blood that plays an important role in blood clotting.

pleura Membrane lining the outer surface of the *lungs* (*visceral pleura*), the inner surface of the chest wall, and the *thoracic* surface of the *diaphragm* (*parietal pleura*).

pleural cavity Thoracic cavity.

pleural effusion Excessive accumulation of fluid in the *pleural space*.

pleural space Potential space between the two layers of the *pleura*.

pleuritic pain Chest pain that is sharp and made worse by deep *inhalation*, coughing, or laughing; characteristic of pleural inflammation.

pneumonia Acute infectious disease of the *lungs*.

pneumothorax Air in the *pleural space*.

PO₂ Symbol for the *partial pressure* of *oxygen* in a gas.

point of maximal impulse (PMI) Palpable beat of the *apex of the heart* against the chest wall during ventricular contraction; normally palpated in the fifth left *intercostal space* in the *midclavicular line*.

polydipsia Excessive thirst and/or excessive intake of fluids.

polyphagia Excessive hunger and eating.

polyuria Excessive urination.

popliteal Area or space behind the knee *joint*.

positive end-expiratory pressure (PEEP) Application of slight positive pressure at the end of *exhalation* for the purpose of preventing small airways from collapsing.

posterior   Situated in the back of or on the *dorsal* surface.

postictal   Referring to the period after the convulsive state of a *seizure*.

postmortem   After death.

potassium (K⁺)   *Monovalent cation* required for the proper functioning of muscle, particularly the *electric conduction system* of the heart.

potentiation   Enhancement of the effect of one drug by another.

powder   Drug that has been ground into very fine particles.

P-QRS-T   The *ECG* representation of one cycle of *depolarization* and *repolarization* of the *atria* and *ventricles*.

precordial   Referring to the general area over the heart and left lower *thorax*.

precordial thump   Sharp blow to the midsternum delivered in an attempt to terminate *ventricular tachycardia* or stimulate the heart to beat in *asystole*.

preeclampsia   Condition that precedes *eclampsia*, or *toxemia of pregnancy*, characterized by *hypertension* and *edema*.

preinfarction angina   Unstable *angina pectoris*.

preload   Pressure under which the ventricle fills.

premature atrial contractions (PACs)   Extra atrial *contractions* followed by ventricular *contractions* with normal or abnormal *QRS complexes*, caused by *ectopic foci* in the interatrial conduction pathways.

premature infant ("preemie")   Infant born before 37 weeks' gestation.

premature junctional contractions (PJCs)   Also called *premature nodal contractions*; extra ventricular *contractions* with normal or abnormal *QRS complexes* caused by *ectopic foci* in the *atrioventricular junction*.

premature nodal contractions (PNCs)   *Premature junctional contractions*.

premature ventricular contractions (PVCs)   Extra ventricular *contractions* caused by *ectopic foci* in the *His-Purkinje system* of the *ventricles* and characterized on the *ECG* by bizarre, widened *QRS complexes* and usually a *T wave* oppositely directed to the normal T wave.

prenatal   Before birth.

presenting part   The part of the baby that comes out first during *delivery*.

pressure of speech   Speech in which words seem to tumble out under immense emotional pressure.

priapism   Sustained erection of the penis, sometimes seen in *spinal cord* injury.

primigravida   Woman who is pregnant for the first time.

primipara   Woman who has had one previous delivery.

P–R interval   Period of time between the beginning of the *P wave* (atrial *depolarization*) and the onset of the *QRS complex* (ventricular *depolarization*), signifying the time required for atrial depolarization and passage of the *excitation impulse* through the *atrioventricular junction*.

progesterone   Female *hormone* produced by the *corpus luteum* that governs the secretory phase of the menstrual cycle.

prognosis   Probable outlook for recovery from disease.

projection   Attributing to others one's own unacknowledged feelings.

prolapsed cord   *Delivery* in which the *umbilical cord* emerges from the uterus ahead of the presenting part.

pronation   The act of turning the palm of the hand backward or downward, performed by internal rotation of the forearm.

prone   Lying flat with the face downward.

prophylaxis   Measures to prevent the occurrence of a given disease or abnormal state.

proprioception   The ability to perceive the position and movement of one's body or one's limbs.

prostate   *Gland* at the base of the male *bladder* that often becomes enlarged later in life, causing obstruction to *urine* flow.

prosthesis   Artificial part made to replace a natural one.

prostration   Collapse.

protocol   Written procedure, usually established by the medical director of an EMS system and forming part of the official policy of the system, for diagnosis, *triage*, treatment, or transport of specified emergency medical cases.

proximal   Closer to a point of reference, usually the heart.

pruritus   Itching.

psi   Pounds per square inch, a measurement of pressure.

psychosis   Mental disorder causing disintegration of personality and loss of contact with reality.

psychosomatic   Pertaining to bodily manifestations of any disorder of the mind.

pubis   One of the two bones that form the anterior portion of the *pelvic ring*.

puerperium   Convalescent period after giving birth to a baby.

pulmonary   Referring to the *lungs* or related structures.

pulmonary arteries   *Arteries* that carry blood poor in *oxygen* from the *right ventricle* to the *lungs*.

pulmonary circulation   Flow of blood from the *right ventricle* through the *pulmonary arteries* and all of their branches and *capillaries* in the *lungs* and thence back to the *left atrium* through the *venules* and *pulmonary veins*; also called the lesser circulation.

pulmonary edema   Congestion of the *pulmonary* air spaces with *exudate* and foam, often secondary to *left heart failure*.

pulmonary embolism   Obstruction of a *pulmonary artery* or arteries by solid, liquid, or gaseous material swept through the *right heart* into the *lungs*.

pulmonary veins   Vessels that carry oxygenated blood from the *lungs* to the *left atrium*.

pulmonic valve   Valve between the *right ventricle* and the *pulmonary artery*.

pulsatile   Characterized by rhythmic beating.

pulse   Expansion and *contraction* of an arterial wall caused by ventricular *systole* and *diastole*.

pulse pressure   Difference between the *systolic* and *diastolic blood pressures*, indicative of the *stroke volume*.

pulse rate   Heart rate determined by counting the number of pulsations per minute palpated in any superficial artery.

pulsus paradoxus   Weakening or loss of a palpable pulse during inhalation, characteristic of cardiac tamponade and severe asthma.

pump failure   Inability of the heart to maintain *cardiac output*, resulting in *congestive heart failure* and *cardiogenic shock*.

pupil   Small opening in the center of the *iris*.

Purkinje network   System of fibers in the *ventricles* that conducts the *excitation impulse* from the *bundle branches* to the *myocardium*.

purulent   Full of pus.

P wave   First wave of the *ECG* complex, representing *depolarization* of the ventricles.

pyrogen   Foreign protein capable of causing fever.

QRS complex   Deflections of the *ECG* produced by ventricular *depolarization*.

Q–T interval   Period between the onset of the *QRS complex* and the end of the *T wave*, representing ventricular *depolarization* and *repolarization*.

quadrant   Term used to designate one quarter of the abdomen.

quadriplegia   *Paralysis* of both arms and legs.

quickening   The first recognizable movements of the *fetus* in the *uterus*, usually occurring around the sixteenth to twentieth week of *gestation*.

Q wave   First negative deflection of the *QRS complex* not preceded by an *R wave*.

raccoon sign   Also called "coon's eyes"; bilateral symmetric *periorbital ecchymoses* seen with some skull fractures.

rad   Abbreviation for "radiation absorbed dose," a measure of radiation received at a given target.

radial   Pertaining to the wrist.

radiation   Emission of heat from an object into surrounding, colder air.

radioactive   Having the property of emitting ionizing radiation.

radius   Bone on the thumb side of the forearm.

rales   Old terminology for abnormal breath sounds that have a fine, crackling quality; now called *crackles*.

rape   Sexual intercourse inflicted forcibly on another person, against that person's will.

recanalization   Opening up of new channels through a blocked artery.

receptor   Specialized area in a tissue that initiates certain actions upon specific stimulation.

rectum   Distal portion of the *small intestine*.

recumbent   Lying down.

red blood cell (RBC)   *Erythrocyte*; cell that carries *oxygen*.

reduce   To restore a part to its normal position, as a fractured bone.

reducing valve   The pressure regulator on an oxygen cylinder that decreases the high pressures inside the cylinder to much lower pressures that can be delivered safely to the patient.

reflex   Involuntary muscular action in response to some stimulation.

regression   In psychiatry, a return to an earlier behavior pattern.

regurgitation   Passive, retrograde flow of gastric contents from the stomach into the *pharynx* and mouth (to be distinguished from the active process of *vomiting*).

relative refractory period   Stage of ventricular *diastole* during which the *cardiac muscle* is recharging (*repolarizing*) to a resting state following *depolarization*. During this phase of the refractory period, the heart can be stimulated to contract prematurely.

rem   Abbreviation for "roentgen equivalent man," a measure of radiation dose that takes into account the potential destructiveness of the type of radiation emitted.

renal   Pertaining to the *kidney*.

repeater   Miniature transmitter that picks up a radio signal and rebroadcasts it, thus extending the range of a radio communications system.

reperfusion   Resumption of blood flow through an *artery*.

repolarization   Electric process of recharging depolarized *muscle* fibers back to their resting state.

reservoir   Place where germs live and multiply.

residual volume   Volume of air remaining in the *lungs* after a maximal *exhalation*.

respiration   Broadly, the exchange of gases between a living organism and its environment; the act of breathing; the exchange of *oxygen* and *car-*

bon dioxide among the tissues, *lungs*, and atmosphere.

respiratory arrest   Cessation of breathing.

respiratory failure   Failure of the respiratory system to maintain an arterial PO_2 greater than 60 torr and an arterial PCO_2 less than 50 torr.

resting potential   Electric charge of the *muscle* fibers during the resting, polarized state.

resuscitation   The act of reviving an unconscious person by any means.

retention   Inability to pass urine.

reticular activating system   Center in the brainstem that controls the state of wakefulness.

retina   Lining of the back of the eye that receives visual images and transmits them through the *optic nerve* to the *brain.*

retractions   Drawing in of the *intercostal muscles* and the *muscles* above the *clavicles* in respiratory distress.

retroperitoneum   Area behind the *peritoneum,* containing the *kidneys* and other important structures.

retrosternal   Situated or occurring behind the *sternum.*

rewarming shock   Shock caused by sudden expansion of the circulation that follows dilatation of peripheral vessels as the body surface is warmed.

Rh factor   *Antigen* present on the *red blood cells* of some individuals; when Rh factor is present, the individual is said to be Rh-positive; when Rh factor is absent, the individual is Rh-negative.

rhonchi   Old terminology for coarse, rattling respiratory sounds; now called *crackles.*

rib   One of the 12 bones forming the *thoracic* cavity wall.

rib cage   The supporting structure of the chest.

right atrium   Upper right chamber of the heart, which receives blood from the *venae cavae* and supplies blood to the *right ventricle.*

right heart   The *right atrium* plus the *right ventricle.*

right heart failure   Inability of the *right ventricle* to pump blood forward effectively, causing backup of blood into the systemic veins, with consequent *edema* of body tissues.

right ventricle   Lower right chamber of the heart, which receives blood from the *right atrium* and pumps blood out through the *pulmonic valve* into the *pulmonary artery.*

rigor   A shaking chill, often heralding *pneumonia.*

Ringer's solution   Sterile *intravenous solution* containing *sodium, potassium, calcium,* and *chloride ions* in concentrations similar to those present in blood; useful for replacing fluid losses, as in *dehydration.*

risk factor   Factor that leads to and perpetuates a disease process.

roentgen (R)   Unit of measurement for radioactive emissions, named for the discoverer of x-rays.

R-on-T pattern   Dangerous kind of *premature ventricular contraction* that is seen on the *ECG* to fall on the *T wave* of the preceding *QRS–T complex,* representing the occurrence of an *extrasystole* during the vulnerable period of ventricular *repolarization* and often triggering *ventricular tachycardia* or *fibrillation.*

R–R interval   Period of time between the onset of one *QRS complex* and the onset of the succeeding *QRS complex.*

R wave   The positive wave or deflection in the *QRS complex.*

sacral   Pertaining to the *sacrum,* part of the lower spine.

sacroiliac joint   Point of attachment of the *ilium* to the *sacrum.*

sacrum   Part of the lower spine formed by five fused *vertebrae.*

saddle joint   *Joint* formed where a portion of one bone hangs over another, as in the thumb.

safe residual   Minimum permissible pressure in an oxygen cylinder, defined as 200 *psi.*

salicylate   Class of drugs that includes aspirin.

saline   *Solution* containing salt.

salivary glands   *Glands* that produce and secrete saliva, connected to the mouth through ducts.

SA node   Abbreviation for *sinoatrial node,* the principal *pacemaker* of the heart.

scalp vein set   *Intravenous* needle with butterfly "wings."

scapula   Shoulder blade.

sclera   Tough, white covering of the eyeball.

sebaceous gland   *Gland* in the *dermis* that secretes an oily substance known as sebum.

secondary pacemaker   *Pacemaker site* or *ectopic focus* in the *electric conduction system* of the heart other than the *SA node.*

sedative   Drug that depresses the activity of the *central nervous system,* thus having a calming effect, e.g., *barbiturates,* chloral hydrate.

seizure   An attack of *epilepsy;* a *convulsion.*

Sellick maneuver   Pressure applied over the cricoid to seal off the esophagus and prevent reflux of gastric contents.

semicircular canals   Small structures in the inner ear that maintain one's equilibrium.

semilunar valves   The *aortic* and *pulmonic valves* of the heart.

seminal duct   Duct through which sperm pass into the seminal vesicles.

sensory nerves   Nerves that send messages of various sense modalities (e.g., temperature, pain, touch, taste) through the *spinal cord* to the *brain.*

sepsis Generalized body poisoning by the products of bacteria.

septic shock *Shock* resulting from severe bacterial *infection*.

septum Dividing wall or partition, usually separating two cavities.

sequelae Aftereffects of disease or injury.

seropositive Having a positive blood test for an infectious agent, such as HIV or hepatitis B virus.

serum The liquid portion of clotted blood.

shell The skin, subcutaneous tissues, skeletal muscles, and extremities, which enclose the body *core*.

shock State of inadequate *tissue perfusion*, which may be caused by pump failure (*cardiogenic shock*), volume loss (*hypovolemic shock*), vasodilatation (*neurogenic shock*), or any combination thereof.

shunt (1) Situation in which a portion of the output of the *right heart* reaches the *left heart* without being oxygenated in the *lungs*; may be caused by *atelectasis*, *pulmonary edema*, or a variety of other conditions. (2) In *hemodialysis*, an *anastomosis* between a peripheral *artery* and *vein*.

sickle cell anemia Hereditary, genetically determined hemolytic *anemia* occurring in the Black population, characterized by *arthralgias*, acute attacks of *abdominal* pain, and recurrent embolic episodes.

side effect An expected and predictable effect of a drug that is not part of its therapeutic effect.

sigmoid S-shaped, terminal portion of the descending *colon*.

sign Bodily evidence of disease found on physical examination; an indication of illness or injury that the examiner OBSERVES.

silent acute myocardial infarction Painless *acute myocardial infarction*, occurring in 10 to 20 percent of patients with AMI, especially the elderly.

simplex Method of radio communication utilizing a single frequency that enables either transmission or reception of either voice or an *ECG* signal but is incapable of simultaneous transmission and reception.

singultus Hiccups.

sinoatrial node (SA node) The *dominant pacemaker* of the heart, located at the junction of the *superior vena cava* and the *right atrium*.

sinus arrhythmia Slight irregularity of the heart rate caused by changes in *parasympathetic* tone during breathing.

sinus bradycardia Sinus rhythm with a rate less than 60 per minute

sinus tachycardia Sinus rhythm with a rate greater than 100 per minute.

skeleton The hard, bony structure that forms the main scaffolding of the body.

skull Bony structure surrounding the *brain*; *cranium*.

sling Triangular bandage applied around the neck to immobilize an arm.

small intestine Portion of the intestine between the *stomach* and the *colon*.

sniffing position Position of a patient for *endotracheal intubation*, with the neck flexed and the head extended.

snoring Noise made on inhalation when the upper airway is partially obstructed by the tongue.

socket Hollow in a bone into which a rounded part fits.

sodium The major *cation* of the *extracellular fluid*.

sodium bicarbonate (NaHCO₃) Chemical *buffer* used to raise *pH* when *acidosis* is present.

solution Liquid consisting of a mixture of two or more substances that are molecularly dispersed through one another in a homogenous manner.

somnolence Sleepiness.

soporific Drug that induces deep sleep.

spasm Sudden, involuntary contraction of a *muscle* or group of muscles; sudden but transitory *constriction* of a passage, canal, or *orifice*, as in *laryngospasm*.

sphincter Circularly arranged *muscle* that acts as a valve to control the retention or release of fluids or semisolid materials in the body.

sphygmomanometer Device for measuring *blood pressure*.

spinal canal Area filled with spinal fluid immediately surrounding the *spinal cord*.

spinal cord Collection of nerve tracts extending from the *brain* down the *foramen* of the *vertebral* column.

spirits Preparations of volatile substances dissolved in alcohol, e.g., spirits of ammonia.

spleen Organ located in the left upper *quadrant* of the *abdomen* that destroys old *red blood cells*.

splenomegaly Enlargement of the spleen.

splint Any device used to immobilize a part of the body.

spondylosis Abnormal immobility and consolidation of a vertebral joint.

spontaneous pneumothorax Rupture of the *lung parenchyma* without *trauma*, leading to the accumulation of air in the *pleural space*.

sprain *Trauma* to a *joint* that causes injury to the *ligaments*.

squelch To eliminate unwanted *noise* on a radio frequency.

stable side position Position in which the patient is lying on his left side with his left thigh and leg flexed and his head resting on his extended left arm.

staging area At a mass casualty incident, area in which the ambulances are stationed until they are needed to evacuate patients.

stasis The slowing down or cessation of blood flow to an area.

status asthmaticus Severe, prolonged asthmatic attack that cannot be broken with *epinephrine*.

status epilepticus The occurrence of two or more *seizures* without a period of complete consciousness between them.

stenosis Narrowing or *stricture* of a hollow tube.

stereotyped activity Repetitive movements that do not seem to serve any useful purpose.

sterile Free from living organisms such as bacteria.

sternocleidomastoid muscle Large *muscle* that is easily felt at the side of the neck.

sternum Long, flat bone located in the midline in the anterior part of the *thoracic* cage; breast bone.

stethoscope Instrument for performing *auscultation*.

stimulant Agent that increases the level of bodily activity.

stoma Small opening, especially an artificially created opening, such as that made by *tracheostomy*.

stomach Hollow digestive organ in the *epigastrium* that receives food material from the *esophagus*.

strain Overstretching of a *muscle*; soft tissue injury involving a *muscle*.

stress The nonspecific response of the body to any demand made upon it.

stricture Narrowing of a duct or any natural passage by an inflammatory process.

stridor Harsh, high-pitched sound associated with severe upper airway obstruction, such as that caused by laryngeal *edema*.

stroke Relatively sudden onset of a neurologic deficit that corresponds to the distribution of a cerebral artery and lasts more than 24 hours.

stroke volume Volume of blood pumped forward with each ventricular *contraction*.

S–T segment Interval between the end of the *QRS complex* and the beginning of the *T wave*; often elevated or depressed with respect to the *isoelectric line* when there is significant *myocardial ischemia*.

stupor State of reduced sensibilities; mental confusion.

subarachnoid hemorrhage Bleeding into the space around the *brain*, usually caused by rupture of an *aneurysm*.

subclavian vein Large *vein* located beneath the *clavicle*, joining the internal *jugular vein*.

subcutaneous (SQ) Beneath the skin.

subcutaneous emphysema Condition in which *trauma* to the *lung* or airway results in the escape of air into tissues of the body, especially the chest wall, neck, and face, causing a crackling sensation on palpation of the skin.

subdural Occurring beneath the dura, i.e., beneath the heavy, sheathlike covering of the *brain*. The term is often used in connection with the subdural *hematoma* following *trauma* to the head.

sublingual (SL) Under the tongue.

substernal Under the *sternum*; *retrosternal*.

sucking chest wound *Open pneumothorax*.

sudden infant death syndrome (SIDS) *Crib death*; death of an infant after the first few weeks of life, the cause of which cannot be established by careful autopsy.

suicide The taking of one's own life.

sunstroke Form of *heat stroke* caused by prolonged sun exposure.

superficial On the surface; the opposite of deep.

superior *Anatomic* term referring to an organ or part that is located above another organ or part of the body.

superior vena cava Major *vein* that empties *venous blood* from the upper extremities, head, and neck into the *right atrium*.

supinate To turn the forearm so that the palm faces upward.

supine Lying flat with the face upward.

suppository Drug mixed in a firm base that melts at body temperature, shaped to fit various body *orifices*.

supraventricular dysrhythmia *Dysrhythmia* arising from any portion of the *electric conduction system* above the *ventricles*.

supraventricular tachycardia *Tachyarrhythmia* arising from above the *ventricles*.

suspension Preparation of a pulverized drug in liquid; requires thorough shaking before use.

suture (1) Type of *joint* in which the articulating surfaces are united, as in the *skull*. (2) Special type of thread used in closing a wound.

swath *Cravat* tied around the body to enhance immobilization of a part.

S wave The first downward deflection of the *QRS complex* that is preceded by an *R wave*.

sweat gland *Gland* that secretes water and *electrolytes* through the skin.

sympathetic nervous system Subdivision of the *autonomic nervous system* that governs the body's "fight-flight" reactions, stimulating *cardiac* activity.

sympathomimetic Producing effects similar to those engendered by stimulation of the *sympathetic nervous system*, hence an alpha or beta sympathetic drug.

symphysis pubis Midline *articulation* of the pubic bones.

symptom Abnormal feeling of distress and/or awareness of disturbances of bodily function experienced by a patient; symptoms are elicited in the *history*.

synapse The junction between two nerve cells.

syncope Fainting; brief loss of consciousness caused by transiently inadequate blood flow to the *brain*.

syndrome Complex of *symptoms* and *signs* characteristic of a specific condition.

synergism   Combined effect of two or more drugs such that their action in combination is greater than the sum of their individual actions.

synovial joint   *Joint* that permits movement of its component bones.

syrup   Drug suspended in sugar and water to improve its taste.

syrup of ipecac   Drug commonly used to induce vomiting.

systemic   Referring to anything that affects the body as a whole.

systemic circulation   The flow of blood from the *left ventricle* through the *aorta,* to all of its branches and *capillaries* in the tissues, and thence back to the *right atrium* through the *venules, veins,* and *venae cavae;* also called the greater circulation.

systole   Period during which the *ventricles* contract.

systolic blood pressure   Peak pressure exerted by the blood on the arterial walls during ventricular *contraction.*

tablet   Powdered drug that has been molded or compressed into a small disc.

tachyarrhythmia   Rapid *dysrhythmia* (heart rate over 120–140/min).

tachycardia   Rapid heart rate, over 100 per minute.

tachypnea   Excessively rapid rate of breathing (over 25/min in adults).

tamponade (cardiac)   Acute compression of the heart caused by accumulation of fluid or blood in the *pericardium.*

tarsal   Pertaining to the ankle.

telemetry   Process of communicating *physiologic* data, such as the *ECG,* over long distances by radio or telephone.

tempered glass   Glass that breaks into small pieces when struck with a sharp-pointed object; safety glass.

temple   Region on each side of the head above and *anterior* to the ears.

temporal   Region of the *temples.*

temporal lobe   Lobe of the *brain* containing the control centers for speech.

temporary cavity   Transient hollow produced by a missile traversing part of the body.

temporomandibular joint   *Articulation* of the *mandible* with the *skull.*

ten-code   Radio code system using the number 10 plus another number.

tendon   Fibrous portion of *muscle* that attaches to bone.

tension pneumothorax   Situation in which air enters the *pleural space* through a one-way valve defect in the *lung,* causing progressive increase in intrapleural pressure, with collapse of the lung and impairment of circulation.

tentorium   The extension of *dura mater* that forms a partition between the *cerebrum* and *cerebellum.*

term   Forty weeks' *gestation;* the time when the *fetus* is fully mature and ready to be born.

testes   Male gonads, which are normally situated in the scrota and which produce sperm.

tetanus   Acute infectious disease caused by a bacterial toxin, with spasm of the jaw muscles causing *trismus* ("lockjaw") and of the back muscles causing *opisthotonos.*

tetany   Sustained *contraction* of a *muscle* group.

therapeutic action   A beneficial action of a drug to correct a bodily dysfunction.

thermal   Pertaining to heat.

thoracic   Pertaining to the chest.

thorax   The part of the body between the neck and the *diaphragm,* encased by the *ribs.*

thready   Describing a *pulse* that is weak or feeble.

thrombocyte   *Platelet;* a cellular element of the blood involved in clotting.

thrombolysis   The process of dissolving blood clots.

thrombophlebitis   Condition in which *inflammation* of a *vein* leads to the formation of a plug (*thrombus*) in the vein.

thrombosis   Formation of a blood *clot* or *thrombus* within a blood vessel.

thrombus   Fixed blood *clot* that forms inside a blood vessel.

thyroid   *Gland* located in the neck that produces *hormones* involved in the regulation of *metabolism.*

thyroid cartilage   The largest *cartilage* of the *larynx* whose two plates join anteriorly in a V shape to form the Adam's apple.

tibia   Shin bone, located in the front part of the lower leg.

tic   Spasmodic twitching of a facial *muscle.*

tidal volume   Amount of air inhaled or exhaled during normal, quiet breathing; the volume of one breath.

tincture   Dilute alcoholic *extract* of a drug, e.g., tincture of iodine.

tinnitus   Ringing, buzzing, or roaring noise in the ears.

tissue   Collection of cells of similar type that are specialized for performance of a particular function.

titration   In pharmacologic treatment, the method of administering a drug dose in very small increments at a time while carefully gauging the effect of each increment.

tolerance   Progressive diminution of susceptibility to the effects of a drug after repeated doses.

tonic-clonic   Referring to the repetitive contraction and relaxation of *muscle* groups in a *seizure.*

torr   Torricelli unit, equivalent to 1 mm Hg.

tort   Wrongful conduct that gives rise to a civil suit.

total body water (TBW) Total fluid content of the body, equivalent to about 60 percent of body weight in the adult male.

total lung capacity The volume of gas contained in the *lung* at the end of maximal *inhalation*.

tourniquet Constricting device applied circumferentially around an extremity to impede venous outflow or obstruct arterial inflow.

toxemia Generalized poisoning of the system caused by absorption of bacterial products.

toxemia of pregnancy *Eclampsia.*

toxic Pertaining to a poison; harmful.

toxin Poison manufactured by bacteria or other forms of animal or vegetable life.

toxoid Chemically modified *toxin* that, when injected, stimulates the development of immunity against a specific disease but that is not itself harmful, e.g., *tetanus* toxoid.

trachea Cartilaginous tube extending from the *larynx* to its division into the main bronchi; the windpipe.

tracheostomy Surgical opening of the *trachea* to create an airway.

traction Pulling or exerting force to straighten the alignment of a part of the body.

trade name Name under which a drug is marketed by a given manufacturer.

transceiver A radio with which one can both transmit and receive; a two-way radio.

transfusion Infusion of blood into a *vein.*

transfusion reaction Adverse response to receiving blood or blood products.

transient ischemic attack (TIA) "Little stroke"; temporary loss of function resulting from a transitory decrease in circulation to a part of the *brain*; may warn of an impending *stroke.*

transverse lie Abnormal presentation in which the *fetus* lies crosswise in the *uterus.*

trauma Injury.

traumatic asphyxia *Syndrome* resulting from a very severe compression injury of the chest, with *cyanosis* of the face and neck, bulging of the eyes, and caved-in chest.

tremor Involuntary twitching of an extremity.

Trendelenburg position Position in which a patient is placed on his back with legs raised and head lowered; also called shock position.

triage System used for categorizing and sorting patients according to the severity of their injuries.

tricuspid valve Valve between the *right atrium* and *right ventricle* of the heart.

trimester Period of 3 months.

trismus Spasm of the jaw muscles causing the teeth to be clenched shut, characteristic of *tetanus.*

trochanter Either of the two processes below the neck of the *femur.*

tuberculin test Skin test to determine if a person has ever been infected with tuberculosis.

T wave Upright, flat, or inverted wave following the *QRS complex* of the *ECG*, representing ventricular *repolarization.*

UHF Ultrahigh frequency; the portion of the radio frequency spectrum between 300 and 3,000 mHz.

ulcer Open lesion of the skin or *mucous membrane.*

ulna The larger bone of the forearm, on the side opposite that of the thumb.

umbilical cord Flexible structure connecting the *fetus* to the *placenta.*

umbilicus The navel; the "belly button."

unconscious State of being insensible or *comatose.*

unifocal Arising from a single site.

urea An end product of protein metabolism that may accumulate in the blood of patient with impaired *renal* function.

uremia *Toxic* condition caused by the inability of the *kidneys* to remove waste products of *metabolism* from the blood.

ureter Tube leading from the *kidney* to the *bladder.*

urethra Tube leading from the *bladder* to the outside of the body.

urine Fluid secreted by the *kidneys*, stored in the *bladder*, and discharged through the *urethra.*

urticaria Hives.

uterus Muscular organ lying in the female *pelvis* that houses the developing *fetus*; the womb.

uvula Small dangling protrusion attached to the soft *palate* in the midline.

vagal activity *Parasympathetic* activity.

vagina Genital canal in the female extending from the *uterus* to the *vulva*; the birth canal.

vagotonic Mimicking the action of the *vagus* nerve, hence stimulating *parasympathetic* effects like *bradycardia.*

vagus Tenth *cranial* nerve, chief mediator of the *parasympathetic nervous system.*

vallecula Groove between the base of the tongue and the *epiglottis.*

Valsalva maneuver Forced *exhalation* against a closed *glottis*, the effect of which is to stimulate the *vagus* nerve and thereby slow the heart rate.

vasoconstriction Narrowing of the diameter of a blood vessel.

vasoconstrictor Substance that causes narrowing of the diameter of a blood vessel; an alpha *sympathomimetic* agent.

vasodilation Widening of the diameter of a blood vessel.

vasodilator Substance that causes widening of the diameter of blood vessels.

vasopressor Agent that raises the *blood pressure* by causing *vasoconstriction*.

vasovagal Having vascular and vagal components; often used to refer to a *syndrome* consisting of *precordial* distress, *anxiety, nausea*, and sometimes *syncope*.

vein Blood vessel that carries blood to the heart.

velocity The speed of an object in a given direction.

venae cavae The largest *veins* of the body, which return blood to the *right atrium*.

venipuncture Puncture of a *vein* to obtain a blood sample or to introduce a *catheter*.

venom Poison, usually the poisonous substances derived from snakes, spiders, bees, wasps, and other such creatures.

venous blood Blood poor in *oxygen*, containing *hemoglobin* in the reduced state.

ventilation Breathing; moving air in and out of the *lungs*.

ventral Referring to the front of the body; *anterior*.

ventricle Thick-walled, muscular chamber that receives blood from the *atrium* and pumps it into the *pulmonary* or *systemic circulation*.

ventricular aneurysm Localized bulge in the wall of the *ventricle*, often the late result of *myocardial infarction*.

ventricular arrhythmia *Dysrhythmia* arising in the *His-Purkinje system*.

ventricular ectopic activity Initiation of electric impulses by a *secondary pacemaker* in the *ventricles*.

ventricular fibrillation Rapid, tremulous, and ineffectual *contractions* of the *cardiac ventricles*; a form of *cardiac arrest*.

ventricular standstill *Asystole*.

ventricular tachycardia Rapid, repetitive firing of a ventricular *ectopic focus*; a *life-threatening dysrhythmia*.

venule Very small *vein*.

vernix White, cheesy substance covering the skin of the newborn.

vertebra One of the 33 bones of the spinal column.

vertebral Pertaining to the spinal column.

vertex The top of the head.

vertigo Dizziness; a hallucination of movement; a sensation that the external world is spinning around.

vesicle Tiny, fluid-filled sac; a small blister.

VHF Very high frequency; the portion of the radio frequency spectrum between 30 and 150 mHz.

viable Capable of living.

vial Glass container storing a sterile powdered or liquid drug for *parenteral* use, sealed with a rubber stopper, and often containing multiple doses.

visceral Pertaining to organs of the chest or abdomen.

visceral pleura Outer, membranous covering of the *lungs*.

viscus Any large internal organ of the *abdomen, pelvis*, or *thorax* (plural: viscera).

vital capacity Volume of air that can be forcefully exhaled from the *lungs* following a full inhalation.

vital signs Measurements of body functions, including *pulse, respirations*, temperature, and *blood pressure*.

vitreous fluid Jellylike, transparent substance filling the inside of the eye.

vocal cords Paired structures in the *larynx* whose vibrations produce sound.

vocal fremitus The vibrations palpable on the chest wall when someone speaks.

volar Pertaining to the palm side of the arm.

Volkmann's ischemic contracture Contraction of the fingers and sometimes also the wrist, with loss of muscular power, that sets in rapidly after severe injury around the elbow joint.

volume expander *Intravenous solution* that stays in the vascular space, usually a *colloid*.

voluntary commitment Situation in which a patient signs himself into a psychiatric facility of his own free will.

voluntary muscles *Muscles* that function under the conscious control of the *brain*.

vomiting Forceful, active expulsion of stomach contents through the mouth (as opposed to *regurgitation*, which is a passive process).

vulnerable period Interval during the *relative refractory period* of ventricular *repolarization*, corresponding to the upstroke of the *T wave*, in which an *ectopic* impulse or an unsynchronized current can produce *ventricular tachycardia* or *fibrillation*.

vulva External parts of the female *genitalia*.

watt Unit of electric energy obtained by multiplying amperes times volts.

watt-seconds Units of electric energy expressed as *watts* delivered for 1 second; joules.

wavelength The distance in a propagating wave from one point to the corresponding point on the next wave.

Wernicke's encephalopathy Nutritional deficiency syndrome involving mental disturbance, paralysis of eye movements, and *ataxia* of gait that can be precipitated by administering 50% *glucose* to susceptible individuals, such as chronic *alcoholics*.

wheeze High-pitched, whistling sound characterizing obstruction or spasm of the lower airways.

white blood cell *Leukocyte*; the cellular element of the blood that produces *antibodies* and participates in the inflammatory response.

windchill factor   Factor that takes into account both the temperature and wind velocity in calculating the effect of a given ambient temperature on living organisms.

withdrawal   *Symptoms* produced by abstinence from a drug to which one is addicted.

xiphoid   Small cartilaginous and bony portion of the *sternum* attached to the lower end of the body of the sternum.

yaw   Oscillation around the vertical axis.

zygoma   Cheek bone.

Additional Reading

The following general references may be of interest to those who wish to read further about some of the topics covered in this text. The list is not intended to be comprehensive but merely to suggest some additional resource material. A list of references for specific topics is appended to each chapter as well.

Baldwin GA (ed.). *Handbook of Pediatric Emergencies*. Boston: Little, Brown, 1989.

Bassuk EL, Fox SS, Prendergast KJ. *Behavioral Emergencies: A Field Guide for EMTs and Paramedics*. Boston: Little, Brown, 1983.

Caroline NL. *Ambulance Calls: Review Problems in Emergency Care* (3rd ed.). Boston: Little, Brown, 1991.

Caroline NL. *Emergency Medical Treatment: A Text for EMT-As and EMT-Intermediates* (3rd ed). Boston: Little, Brown, 1991.

Caroline NL. *Study Guide for Emergency Care in the Streets, Fifth Edition*. Boston: Little, Brown, 1995.

Caroline NL. *Workbook for Emergency Medical Treatment: Review Problems for EMTs* (3rd ed.). Boston: Little, Brown, 1991.

Cassell EJ. *The Healer's Art*. Cambridge, MA: MIT Press, 1985.

Cooper RK. *Health & Fitness Excellence*. Boston: Houghton Mifflin, 1989.

Copass MK, Soper RG, Eisenberg MS. *EMT Manual* (2nd ed.). Philadelphia: Saunders, 1991.

Copass MK, Eisenberg MS, MacDonald SC. *Paramedic Manual* (2nd ed.). Philadelphia: Saunders, 1987.

Cousins N. *Head First: The Biology of Hope*. New York: Dutton, 1989.

Eisenberg MS, Copass MK. *Manual of Emergency Medical Therapeutics* (2nd ed.). Philadelphia: Saunders, 1982.

Eisenberg MS, Cummins RO, Ho MT. *Code Blue: Cardiac Arrest and Resuscitation*. Philadelphia: Saunders, 1987.

Frey R, Nagel E, Safar P (eds.). *Mobile Intensive Care Units*. New York: Springer-Verlag, 1976.

Jenkins JL, Loscalzo J. *Manual of Emergency Medicine*. Boston: Little, Brown, 1990.

MacDonald MG, Miller MK (eds.). *Emergency Transport of the Perinatal Patient*. Boston: Little, Brown, 1989.

McNeil EL. *Airborne Care of the Ill and Injured*. New York: Springer-Verlag, 1983.

Mills K, Morton R, Page G. *A Color Atlas of Accidents and Emergencies*. London: Wolfe Medical, 1984.

Safar P, Bircher NG. *Cardiopulmonary Cerebral Resuscitation* (3rd ed.). Philadelphia: Saunders, 1988.

Stine RJ, Marcus RH (eds.). *A Practical Approach to Emergency Medicine*. Boston: Little, Brown, 1987.

Yeshua I, Caroline NL. *CPR for All: Cardiopulmonary Resuscitation in Adults, Children and Infants*. Singapore: Longman, 1991.

The following medical journals are also likely to be of interest to the paramedic:

American Journal of Emergency Medicine
Annals of Emergency Medicine
Emergency
Emergency Medical Services
Emergency Medicine
Journal of Emergency Medical Services (JEMS)
Journal of Prehospital and Disaster Medicine
Journal of Trauma
Rescue

Index

Page numbers in **boldface** indicate an illustration. Page numbers in *italics* indicate a table.

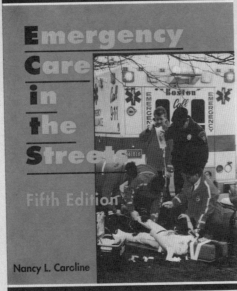

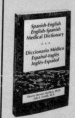
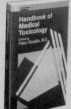